DENTAL MANAGEMENT
of the Medically
Compromised Patient

DENTAL MANAGEMENT
of the Medically
Compromised Patient

SIXTH EDITION

James W. Little, DMD, MS

Professor Emeritus
University of Minnesota
School of Dentistry
Minneapolis, Minnesota; Naples, Florida

Donald A. Falace, DMD

Professor and Section Leader, Oral Diagnosis
Department of Oral Health Science
The University of Kentucky
College of Dentistry
Lexington, Kentucky

Craig S. Miller, DMD, MS

Professor
Department of Oral Health Science
Department of Microbiology, Immunology, and Genetics
The University of Kentucky
College of Dentistry and College of Medicine
Lexington, Kentucky

Nelson L. Rhodus, DMD, MPH

Morse Distinguished Professor and Director
Division of Oral Medicine, Oral Diagnosis and Oral Radiology
University of Minnesota
School of Dentistry and College of Medicine
Minneapolis, Minnesota

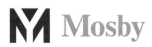

An Affiliate of Elsevier Science

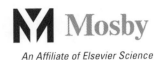

An Affiliate of Elsevier Science

Publishing Director: Linda Duncan
Senior Acquisition Editor: Penny Rudolph
Developmental Editor: Jaime Pendill
Project Manager: Linda McKinley
Production Editor: Jim Rygelski
Designer: Julia Dummitt
Cover Art: Jen Brockett

Sixth Edition

A NOTE TO THE READER

The authors and publisher have made every attempt to check dosages and nursing content for accuracy. Because the science of pharmacology is continually advancing, our knowledge base continues to expand. Therefore we recommend that the reader always check product information for changes in dosage or administration before administering any medication. This is particularly important with new or rarely used drugs.

Mosby, Inc.
An Affiliate of Elsevier Science
11830 Westline Industrial Drive
St. Louis, Missouri 63146

Printed in the United States of America

International Standard Book Number: 0-323-01171-3

03 04 05 06 TG/FF 9 8 7 6 5 4 3 2

The sixth edition of this textbook is dedicated to
those who have faithfully stood by all of us, our wives
and significant others, namely: Anne, Peggy, Sherry and Patti.
We are grateful to them for their love, support,
and undying patience with us.

Foreword

*D*ental management of medically compromised patients has assumed great importance in oral healthcare delivery. An important reason for that is the relationship between disease and aging; almost 14% of Americans are over age 65, a percentage expected to grow to 20% by the year 2020. With extended longevity, an increase in diseases and disabilities will demand larger responsibilities and challenges from healthcare providers. Ever increasing identification of abnormalities is occurring through a greater use of diagnostic techniques, recognition and popularity for prevention, and the widespread use of drugs. As a consequence, a growing number of individuals will be seeking oral healthcare, leading to a concomitant expansion of patients with health risks that may complicate dental-oral diseases and treatments.

A multitude of diseases have an impact on oral healthcare services. Cancer is an age-related disease that serves as an example. More than 1.3 million new cancers are diagnosed each year in the United States that in turn account for almost 25% of all deaths. Because of the ever-increasing number of new malignancies and the complications caused by aggressive therapy, dental services and knowledge in this area take on significant importance. Other examples that commonly affect dental-oral care are cardiovascular disease, the number-one killer of Americans, and diabetes, which affects 16 million Americans. The list could go on endlessly. This underscores the need for current, reliable, and practical information to minimize or prevent potential problems related to general health and ongoing oral health-dental care.

Interrelationships between oral and general health involve most organ systems. A most dramatic example of medical-dental interaction relates to infectious diseases that strike both the young and the elderly. This includes HIV infection, hepatitis, tuberculosis, sexually transmitted diseases, and many other bacterial, viral, and fungal infections. The problem involves recognition and management of oral manifestations, control of blood-borne pathogens, and avoidance of complications when providing dental treatment. Again, to meet this challenge, updated information in a concise and understandable format is required.

Because the majority of medically compromised patients need or want oral healthcare, a working knowledge of the multitude of compromised conditions is essential for dental professionals. This knowledge will support high standards for dental-oral healthcare delivery, which include understanding medical conditions and compromised states, preventing adverse side effects from procedures and drugs used in dentistry, and formulating treatment plans that are compatible with a patient's medical status.

Treating the compromised patient is a complex part of dentistry, requiring competent practitioners with many attributes: sound technical skills, insight into medicine, familiarity with pharmacotherapeutics, and the capability of analyzing findings from patient histories and signs and symptoms. Therefore the usefulness of this text as a reference at all levels of dentistry, for the student and the practitioner, is evident.

Care of the medically compromised patient often is complicated, requiring specialists. However, occurrence of compromised patients is so common that practitioners and students must know how to recognize and prevent problems associated with dental management, and to use consultations and referrals appropriately. This updated, revised, and expanded text recognizes and supplies this type of information with practical and organized overviews of diagnosis and management. This is accomplished by comprehensively covering, in 26 well-organized and revised chapters, conditions that lead to compromised states that affect a person's well-being. The material is supported by summary tables for easy access to information, some figures to supplement text, and appendices that allow the reader to recognize disease states, be aware of potential complications, and select an approach to drug management. Although the main focus is on the management of compromised patients during dental procedures, the text effectively includes causation, medical treatment, pathophysiology, and prognosis. In its present format, it serves as both a quick reference and a somewhat in-depth resource for this critical interface of medicine and dentistry. It will help ensure high standards of care and reduce the occurrence of adverse reactions by improving knowledge and encouraging judgment in the management of at-risk patients.

Sol Silverman, Jr.
Professor of Oral Medicine
University of California, San Francisco

Preface

The need for a sixth edition of *Dental Management of the Medically Compromised Patient* became apparent because of the continued, ever-increasing flow of new knowledge and changing concepts in medicine and dentistry.

The purpose of the book remains to give the dental provider an up-to-date, concise, factual reference work describing the dental management of patients with selected medical problems. The more common medical disorders that may be encountered in a dental practice continue to be the focus. This book is not a comprehensive medical reference but rather a book containing enough core information about each of the medical conditions covered to enable the reader to recognize the basis for various dental management recommendations. Medical problems are organized to provide a brief overview of the basic disease process, epidemiology, pathophysiology, signs and symptoms, laboratory findings, and currently accepted medical therapy of each disorder. This is followed by a detailed explanation and recommendations for specific dental management. The accumulation of evidence-based research over the years has allowed us to make more specific dental management guidelines that should benefit those who read this text. This includes practicing dentists, practicing dental hygienists, dental graduate students in specialty or general practice programs, and dental and dental hygiene students. In particular, the text is intended to give the dental provider an understanding of how to ascertain the severity and stability of common medical disorders and make dental management decisions that afford the patient the utmost health and safety.

Several major changes have been made in this sixth edition. A new chapter on the special problems presented in the dental management of older adults has been added. The chapters on rheumatic fever, rheumatic heart disease, and murmurs (old Chapter 3); congenital heart disease (old Chapter 4); surgically corrected cardiac and vascular disease (old Chapter 5) have been combined into a new Chapter 3, Cardiac Conditions Associated with Endocarditis. The material from old Chapter 28 on prosthetic implants has been moved to appropriate chapters in this edition. A new summary table on the management of medical emergencies in the dental office has been added to the front of the book for quick and easy access. A third appendix (Appendix C) has been added, covering important drug interactions that may occur among medications used to treat the medical conditions discussed in the book and agents used by the dentist.

All chapters have been updated where necessary, and many have been provided with new figures and tables. In keeping with the nature of the book, the chapter on oral cancer has been expanded to discuss cancer in general. Several new topics have been added. These include multiple sclerosis, antithrombotic agents, Lymes disease, Sjögren's syndrome, and others. Appendix B has been updated by including the most recent (fifth) edition of the American Academy of Oral Medicine's *Clinician's Guide to Treatment of Common Oral Conditions*.

Even more emphasis has been placed on the medications used to treat the medical conditions covered in this sixth edition. Dosages, side effects, and drug interactions with agents used in dentistry—including those used during pregnancy—are discussed in greater detail. Emphasis also has been placed on having contemporary equipment and diagnostic information to assess and monitor patients with moderate to severe medical disease. Tables have been added, and all tables have been made to stand out and be easier to read. More than 60 figures have been added to better illustrate certain concepts and clinical findings. A great deal of gratitude goes to Dr. Richard Estensen, emeritus professor of pathology at the University of Minnesota, for his generous contribution of many clinical photographs.

Our sincere thanks and appreciation are extended to those many individuals who have contributed their time and expertise to the writing and revision of this text. Particular thanks is extended to Rebecca Turpin and Joyce Wallace for their typing and editing of the drafts of new chapters and revisions of the old.

James W. Little
Donald A. Falace
Craig S. Miller
Nelson L. Rhodus

Contents

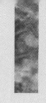

DENTAL MANAGEMENT
of the Medically
Compromised Patient

Dental Management

A Summary

*T*his table presents the more important factors to be considered in the dental management of medically compromised patients. Each medical problem is outlined according to the potential problems related to dental treatment, oral manifestations, the prevention of these problems, and the effect of the complications on dental treatment planning.

The table has been designed for use by dentists, dental students, graduate students, dental hygienists, and dental assistants as a convenient reference work for the dental management of patients who have medical diseases covered in this book.

Dental Management: A Summary—cont'd

Potential Problems Related to Dental Care	Oral Manifestations

High-Risk Conditions: Prosthetic valves, previous bacterial endocarditis, single ventricle states, transposition of the great arteries, tetralogy of Fallot
Chapters 2-3

1. Patients with these conditions are at high risk for bacterial endocarditis secondary to dental treatment resulting in significant bleeding, even if they have had surgical repair 2. Patients with mechanical prosthetic valves may be at risk for excessive bleeding because of long-term anticoagulant therapy 3. Patients with cyanosis (right to left shunt) may have excessive bleeding and be prone to infection	Usually none with prosthetic valves or history of previous bacterial endocarditis; possible cyanotic appearance of oral mucous membranes with complex cyanotic congenital heart disease and petechiae or ecchymosis because of hematologic abnormalities

Moderate-Risk Conditions: Other uncorrected congenital cardiac malformations, acquired valvular dysfunction, hypertrophic cardiomyopathy, mitral valve prolapse with regurgitation
Chapters 2-3

1. Patients with these conditions are at moderate risk for bacterial endocarditis, secondary to dental treatment resulting in significant bleeding 2. Patients with surgically repaired congenital defects *without residual dysfunction* do not require antibiotic prophylaxis 3. Patients with a history of rheumatic fever but *without evidence of rheumatic heart disease* do not require antibiotic prophylaxis 4. Patients with mitral valve prolapse *without regurgitation* do not require antibiotic prophylaxis	Usually none

Heart Murmurs
Chapter 2-3

1. None exist if murmur is functional or innocent, murmurs that appear only during childhood or pregnancy do not require prophylactic coverage unless history is unclear	Usually none

Prevention of Problems	Treatment Planning Modifications

1. Patients with prosthetic valves, a history of previous bacterial endocarditis or any form of repaired or unrepaired complex cyanotic congenital heart disease should receive prophylactic antibiotics for dental procedures likely to result in significant bleeding (See Chapter 19 for management of potential bleeding problems caused by anticoagulant therapy or cyanosis with right to left shunt.)
2. Based on 1997 American Heart Association recommendations (See Boxes 2-5, 2-6, 2-7) the antibiotic regimens are:
  a. Standard—oral amoxicillin
  b. Unable to take oral medications—IV or IM ampicillin
  c. Allergic to penicillin—oral clindamycin
  d. Allergic to penicillin and unable to take oral medications—IV clindamycin
	1. Patients with these conditions may receive any indicated dental care provided prophylactic antibiotics are administered before procedures likely to result in significant bleeding.
	2. As much treatment as possible should be performed in each treatment session during the 1-3 hours after administration of the antibiotic
	3. A second antibiotic dose may be indicated if the appointment lasts more than 4-6 hours or if multiple appointments occur on the same day
	4. The dose of anticoagulant may need to be altered depending on the level of anticoagulation and the extent of the planned procedure (see Chapter 19)
	5. Allow at least 9 days between treatment sessions so that penicillin-resistant organisms disappear from the oral flora If treatment becomes necessary sooner than 9 days, select one of the alternative antibiotics for prophylaxis

Patients with any of these conditions should receive prophylactic antibiotics before dental procedures likely to result in significant bleeding (See recommended American Heart Association regimes listed above.)	1. Patients with any of these conditions can receive any indicated dental care provided that prophylactic antibiotics are administered before those procedures likely to result in significant bleeding 2. As much treatment as possible should be performed in each treatment session during the 1-3 hours after administration of the antibiotic 3. A second antibiotic dose may be indicated if the appointment lasts more than 4-6 hours or if multiple appointments occur on the same day 4. Allow at least 9 days between treatment sessions so that penicillin-resistant organisms disappear from the oral flora If treatment becomes necessary sooner than 9 days, select one of the alternative antibiotics for prophylaxis
1. If a history of a murmur exists and its current status or origin is unknown, obtain medical consultation to determine its presence and type; if murmur is pathologic, provide antibiotic prophylaxis for dental treatment likely to result in significant bleeding	1. Patients with functional or innocent murmurs may receive any dental care without restriction

Dental Management: A Summary—cont'd

Potential Problems Related to Dental Care	Oral Manifestations

Heart Murmurs—cont'd
Chapters 2-3
2. If murmur is pathologic, antibiotic prophylaxis is indicated for dental procedures likely to result in significant bleeding

Synthetic Vascular Grafts or Patches
Chapter 3
Endothelial tissue may not completely line inside of graft material; potential for infection during transient bacteremia

None

Cardiac Pacemakers and Defibrillators
Chapter 3
1. Infection of cardiac lead(s)
2. Electrical interface with cardiac defects

None

Hypertension
Chapter 4
1. Stress and anxiety related to dental visit may cause increase in blood pressure, angina, myocardial infarction, or cerebrovascular accident
2. Patients being treated with antihypertensive agents may become nauseated or hypotensive, or may develop postural hypotension
3. Excessive use of vasopressors may cause significant elevation of blood pressure
4. Sedative medication used in patients taking certain antihypertensive agents may bring about hypotensive episodes

1. Xerostomia secondary to diuretics and other antihypertensive medications
2. Ulceration or stomatitis caused by mercurial diuretics
3. Lichenoid reactions seen with thiazides, methyldopa, propranolol, and labetalol
4. Lupus-like reaction rarely seen with hydralazine

Prevention of Problems

Treatment Planning Modifications

2. If medical consultation is not available and dental treatment is necessary, assume the murmur may be pathologic and provide antibiotic prophylaxis for dental treatment likely to result in significant bleeding (See recommended American Heart Association regimes listed above.)

2. Patients with a pathologic murmur may receive any indicated dental care when prophylactic antibiotics are administered for procedures likely to result in significant bleeding
3. As much treatment as possible may be performed in each session during the 1-3 hours after administration of the antibiotic
4. A second antibiotic dose may be indicated if the appointment lasted 4-6 hours or if multiple appointments occur on the same day
5. Allow at least 9 days between treatment sessions so that penicillin-resistant organisms disappear from the oral flora If treatment becomes necessary sooner than 9 days, select one of the alternative antibiotics for prophylaxis

1. Prophylactic antibiotics for invasive dental procedures?
2. American Heart Association suggests considering prophylaxis for first 6 months; after that no prophylaxis is recommended

American Heart Association has stated that evidence is inconclusive regarding need for antibiotic prophylaxis for prevention of endarteritis in patients with synthetic arterial grafts; it recommends that the need for prophylaxis be determined on an individual patient basis following consultation with physician; if prophylaxis is decided on, standard amoxicillin regimen of the AHA would be appropriate

1. Antibiotic prophylaxis is not recommended for patients with cardiac pacemakers or defibrillators
2. Avoid use of ultrasonic scanners or electrosurgery antibiotic prophylaxis for patients with cardiac pacemakers or debrillators

None

1. Detection and referral of patients with significant elevation of blood pressure for medical evaluation and treatment; for blood pressure ≥180/110, delay dental care and refer to physician
2. With patients being treated with antihypertensive agents the following procedures may be used:
   a. Reduce stress and anxiety of dental visit by premedication, short appointments, and open concerned atmosphere by dentist and staff; let patient talk about fears and concerns related to dental visit; use nitrous oxide but avoid hypoxia

1. For patients under good medical management with no complications, such as renal failure, any indicated treatment may be provided
2. For patients with complications, refer to appropriate section

Dental Management: A Summary—cont'd	
Potential Problems Related to Dental Care	**Oral Manifestations**

Hypertension—cont'd
Chapter 4

Angina Pectoris
Chapter 5

1. Stress and anxiety related to dental visit could precipitate an anginal attack, myocardial infarction, or sudden death in the office	Usually none as a direct result of angina; however, may see drug-related changes such as dry mouth, taste changes, or stomatitis; also may have excessive postsurgical bleeding due to platelet aggregation inhibition
2. For patient taking a non-selective beta blocker, the use of excessive amount of epinephrine could precipitate a dangerous elevation of blood pressure	
3. Patient taking aspirin or other platelet aggregation inhibitor could experience excessive bleeding	
4. Potential to cause endarteritis of coronary artery stent in the immediate post-placement period exists as a result of dentally induced bacteremia	

Prevention of Problems	Treatment Planning Modifications

b. If patient becomes overly stressed, terminate appointment
c. Avoid orthostatic hypotension by changing chair position slowly and supporting patient when getting out of chair
d. Avoid stimulating gag reflex
e. Select sedative medication that dosage cautiously
3. Drug considerations include the following:
a. Use local anesthetics judiciously with minimal concentration of vasopressor (epinephrine 0.036 mg; levonordefrin 0.20 mg); aspirate before injection and inject slowly
b. Use caution when using vasoconstrictors in patients taking a nonselective beta-blocker
c. Do not use gingival packing material that contains epinephrine
d. Reduce dosage of barbiturates and other sedatives whose actions may be enhanced by antihypertensive agents
e. Avoid use of general anesthesia in the office
f. Use epinephrine and levonordefrin judiciously in patients being treated with monoamine oxidase inhibitor

---

Unstable angina (major risk): Elective dental care should be postponed if possible; if care is necessary, it should be provided in consultation with physician. Management may include establishment of IV line, sedation, electrocardiogram, pulse oximeter, cautious use of vasoconstrictor, and prophylactic nitroglycerin

Stable angina (low-intermediate risk): Elective dental care may be provided with the following management considerations:
(1) Short, morning appointments, comfortable chair position, pretreatment vital signs, nitroglycerin available, stress reduction measures, limit quantity of vasoconstrictor, avoid epinephrine in retraction cords, avoid anticholinergics, ensure excellent intraoperative and postoperative pain control
(2) If patient taking aspirin, excess bleeding is usually controllable by local measures only
(3) If coronary artery stent in place, prophylactic antibiotics may be provided for dental procedures likely to result in significant bleeding for first 2-4 weeks only

Unstable angina: Dental treatment should be limited to that which is absolutely necessary, such as for infection or pain

Stable angina: Any desired dental treatment may be provided taking into consideration appropriate management considerations

Dental Management: A Summary—cont'd

Potential Problems Related to Dental Care	Oral Manifestations
Myocardial Infarction **Chapter 5** 1. Stress and anxiety related to dental visit could precipitate an anginal attack, myocardial infarction, or sudden death in the office 2. Patient may have some degree of congestive heart failure 3. Electrical interference could occur with the use of certain dental equipment if pacemaker in place 4. Use of excessive amount of epinephrine could precipitate a dangerous elevation of blood pressure if patient taking a nonselective beta-blocker 5. Patient taking aspirin, other platelet aggregation inhibitor, or Coumadin could experience excessive bleeding with invasive dental procedures 6. Potential exists for endarteritis of coronary artery stent in the immediate post-placement period as a result of dentally induced bacteremia	Usually none as a direct result of myocardial infarction; however, may see drug-related changes such as dry mouth, taste changes, or stomatitis; also may have excessive postsurgical bleeding due to platelet aggregation inhibition or anticoagulation
Cardiac Arrhythmias **Chapter 6** 1. Stress associated with dental treatment or excessive amounts of epinephrine can produce life-threatening arrhythmia in susceptible patient 2. Patients with existing arrhythmia are at increased risk for serious complications—cardiac arrest, etc. 3. Patients with cardiac pacemaker are at risk for possible malfunction of pacemaker because of electromagnetic interference from Cavitrons, electrocautery etc (see section on prosthetic devices)	Agents used to control arrhythmias may have side effects that can cause oral manifestations includes the following: a. Ulceration b. Lupus-like syndrome c. Xerostomia d. Petechiae

Prevention of Problems	Treatment Planning Modifications

Recent myocardial infarction (<1 month) (major risk): Elective dental care should be postponed if possible; if necessary, should be provided in consultation with physician. Management may include establishment of IV line, sedation, electrocardiogram, pulse oximeter, cautious use of vasoconstrictors, and prophylactic nitroglycerine

Recent myocardial infarction: Dental treatment should be limited to that which is absolutely necessary such as for infection or pain

Past myocardial infarction (more than 1 month) (minor-intermediate risk): Elective dental care may be provided with these considerations:

(1) Short, morning appointments, comfortable chair position, pretreatment of vital signs, nitroglycerine available, stress reduction measures, limit quantity of vasoconstrictor, avoid epinephrine in retraction cords, avoid anticholinergics, ensure pain control

(2) If patient taking aspirin, excess bleeding usually controllable by local measures only

(3) If patient taking coumadin, international normalized ratio should be 3.5 or less for invasive procedures.

(4) If coronary artery stent in place, prophylactic antibiotics should be provided for dental procedures likely to result in significant bleeding for first 2-4 weeks only

Past myocardial infarction: Any desired dental treatment may be provided, taking into consideration appropriate management considerations

1. Identify patients susceptible to developing cardiac arrhythmia by medical consultation on the following conditions:
   a. History of significant heart disease
   b. Thyroid disease
   c. Chronic pulmonary disease
   d. Open heart surgery
2. Identify patients with significant arrhythmia by history and clinical findings:
   a. Those taking medications to control arrhythmia—procainamide, quinidine, disopyramide, or propranolol
   b. Those with cardiac pacemaker to control arrhythmias
   c. Those with history of palpitation, dizziness, angina, dyspnea, and/or syncope (refer for medical evaluation)
   d. Those with abnormal physical findings—irregular pulse, very fast pulse, very slow pulse, high blood pressure (refer for medical evaluation)

1. Reduce anxiety through the following procedures:
   a. Prescribe premedication
   b. Provide open and honest communication
   c. Schedule morning or early afternoon appointments
   d. Schedule short appointments
   e. Nitrous oxide–oxygen inhalation
2. Avoid excessive amounts of epinephrine
   a. Use 1:100,000 epinephrine in local anesthetic except for patient with severe arrhythmia
   b. Use anesthetic without epinephrine in patients with severe arrhythmia (confirm by medical consultation)
   c. Use no more than two cartridges of anesthetic; aspirate before injection
   d. Do not use epinephrine in gingival packing
   e. Do not use epinephrine for control of local bleeding
3. Avoid use of general anesthesia
   (If above precautions are taken, any dental procedure can be performed)

Dental Management: A Summary—cont'd

Potential Problems Related to Dental Care	Oral Manifestations

Cardiac Arrhythmias—cont'd
Chapter 6

Congestive Heart Failure
Chapter 7

Potential Problems Related to Dental Care	Oral Manifestations
1. Sudden death resulting from cardiac arrest or arrhythmia	1. Infection
2. Myocardial infarction	2. Bleeding
3. Cerebrovascular accident	3. Petechiae
4. Infection	4. Ecchymoses
5. Infective endocarditis if heart failure is caused by rheumatic heart disease, congenital heart disease, etc	5. Drug related
6. Breathing difficulty	a. Xerostomia
7. Drug side effects include:	b. Lichenoid mucosal lesions
a. Orthostatic hypotension (diuretics, vasodilators)	
b. Arrhythmias (digoxin, overdosage)	
c. Nausea, vomiting (digoxin, vasodilators)	
d. Palpitations (vasodilators)	

Prevention of Problems	**Treatment Planning Modifications**

3. Medical consultation should occur before starting dental treatment to:
   a. Establish current status
   b. Determine presence of underlying cardiac problem and need for antibiotic prophylaxis
   c. Confirm medications patient is taking
   d. Review dental management plan
   e. Determine need for antibiotic prophylaxis because of presence of cardiac pacemaker (not recommended by American Heart Association, but some physicians may suggest it)
   f. Adjust dosage of coumarin (Coumadin) for patients with atrial fibrillation before surgery to less than 2.5 or less times normal prothrombin time or 3.5 or less of INR.
4. Be prepared to deal with life-threatening arrhythmias
5. Avoid use of instruments such as Cavitron or electrocautery in patients with pacemaker

---

1. Detection and referral to physician
2. No routine dental care until patient under good medical management (class I or II and possibly III)
3. Patients under good medical management—cause of heart failure and any other complications—must be controlled including:
   a. Hypertension
   b. Valvular disease (rheumatic heart disease)
   c. Congenital heart disease
   d. Myocardial infarction
   e. Renal failure
   f. Thyrotoxicosis
   g. Chronic obstructive lung disease
4. For class I or II patients, maximum 0.036 mg epinephrine or 0.20 mg levonordefrin to be used; vasoconstrictors avoided in class III or IV patients
5. Patients in semisupine or upright position during treatment to decrease collection of fluid in lung
6. Appointment terminated if patient becomes fatigued, etc
7. Drug considerations:
   a. Digitalis—patient more prone to nausea and vomiting
   b. Anticoagulants—dosage should be reduced so that prothrombin time is 2.5 times normal value or less (INR of 3.5 or less) (takes 3 or 4 days)
   c. Antidysrhythmic agents (see cardiac arrhythmias)
   d. Antihypertensive agents (see hypertension)
   e. Avoidance of outpatient general anesthesia

In patients under good medical management with no complications, any indicated dental care can be performed

Dental Management: A Summary—cont'd

Potential Problems Related to Dental Care	Oral Manifestations
Chronic Obstructive Pulmonary Disease **Chapter 8** Aggravation or worsening of compromised respiratory function	Leukoplakia, erythroplakia or frank carcinoma in chronic smokers
Asthma **Chapter 8** Precipitation of acute asthma attack	Oral candidiasis reported with use of inhaler without "spacer" but is rare Altered maxillofacial growth when asthma is severe during childhood

Prevention of Problems	Treatment Planning Modifications

1. Use of upright chair position
2. Minimize use of bilateral mandibular or palatal blocks
3. Do not use rubber dam in severe disease
4. Use of low-flow oxygen helpful
5. Do not use nitrous oxide–oxygen sedation in severe emphysema
6. Low-dose oral diazepam is acceptable
7. Avoid barbiturates, narcotics, antihistamines, and anticholinergics
8. May need additional steroid dose in patients taking systemic steroids for surgical procedures
9. Avoid macrolide antibiotics (erythromycin, clarithromycin) for patient taking theophylline
10. Outpatient general anesthesia contraindicated

None

---

1. Identification of asthmatic patient by history
2. Determination of character of asthma
   a. Type (allergic or nonallergic)
   b. Precipitating factors
   c. Age at onset
   d. Frequency, severity of attacks (mild, moderate, severe)
   e. Disease stability; and how usually managed
   f. Medications being taken
   g. Necessity for past emergency care
3. Avoidance of known precipitating factors
4. Consultation with physician for severe, active asthma
5. Reduce risk of an attack: have patient bring medication inhaler to each appointment and prophylax with inhaler prior to appointment
6. Drugs to avoid
   a. Aspirin containing medications
   b. Nonsteroidal anti-inflammatory drugs
   c. Narcotics and barbiturates
   d. Macrolide antibiotics (i.e., erythromycin) if patient taking theophylline
7. Avoidance of sulfite-containing local anesthetic solution
8. May need additional steroid dose in patients taking systemic steroids for surgical procedures
9. Premedication of anxious patient (nitrous oxide or diazepam)
10. Provide stress-free environment
11. Use of pulse oximeter

None required

Dental Management: A Summary—cont'd

Potential Problems Related to Dental Care	Oral Manifestations
Tuberculosis **Chapter 8** 1. Tuberculosis may be contracted by dentist from actively infectious patient 2. Patients and staff can be infected by dentist who is actively infectious	1. Oral ulceration (rare); tongue most common 2. Tuberculous involvement of cervical and submandibular lymph nodes (scrofula)

Prevention of Problems	Treatment Planning Modifications

Caveat: Many patients with infectious disease cannot be identified by history or examination; therefore all patients should be approached using universal precautions (Appendix A)

None required

1. Patient with active sputum-positive tuberculosis:
   a. Consultation with physician before treatment
   b. Treatment limited to emergency care (over age 6 years)
   c. Treatment in hospital setting with proper isolation, sterilization, mask, gloves, gown, ventilation
   d. Patient under age 6 years—treatment as normal patient (noninfectious) after consultation with physician
   e. Patient producing consistently negative sputum while undergoing chemotherapy—treatment as normal patient
2. Patient with past history of tuberculosis:
   a. Should be approached with caution; obtain good history of disease and its treatment, appropriate review of systems
   b. Should give history of adequate treatment, periodic chest radiographs, and examination to rule out reactivation
   c. Should have dental treatment postponed if:
      (1) Questionable history of adequate treatment
      (2) Lack of appropriate medical supervision since recovery
      (3) Signs or symptoms of relapse
   d. If present status free of clinical disease, should be treated as normal patient
3. Patients with recent conversion to positive tuberculin skin test (purified protein derivative [PPD])
   a. Should have been evaluated by physician to rule out clinical disease
   b. May be receiving isoniazid (INH) for 6 months to 1 year prophylactically
   c. Should be treated as normal patient when physician approves health status
4. Patients with signs or symptoms of tuberculosis
   a. Should be referred to physician and have treatment postponed
   b. If treatment necessary, treat as in 1 above

Dental Management: A Summary—cont'd

Potential Problems Related to Dental Care	Oral Manifestations

End-Stage Renal Disease
Chapter 9

1. Bleeding tendency	1. Mucosal pallor
2. Hypertension	2. Xerostomia
3. Anemia	3. Metallic taste
4. Intolerance to nephrotoxic drugs metabolized by kidney	4. Ammonia breath odor
5. Enhanced susceptibility to infection	5. Stomatitis
	6. Loss of lamina dura
	7. Bone radiolucencies
	8. Bleeding tendency

Hemodialysis
Chapter 9

1. Bleeding tendency	Oral ulcerations and candidiasis
2. Hypertension	
3. Anemia	
4. Intolerance to nephrotoxic drugs metabolized by kidney	
5. Bacterial endarteritis of arteriovenous fistula secondary to bacteremia	
6. Hepatitis (active or carrier)	
7. Bacterial endocarditis	
8. Collapse of shunt	

Viral Hepatitis, Types B, C, D, E
Chapter 10

1. Hepatitis may be contracted by dentist from infectious patient	Bleeding
2. Patients or staff can be infected by dentist with active hepatitis or who is a carrier	Lichenoid eruptions
3. With chronic active hepatitis patient may have bleeding tendency or altered drug metabolism	

Prevention of Problems	Treatment Planning Modifications
1. Consultation with physician 2. Pretreatment screening for hematologic disorder (bleeding time, prothrombin time, partial thromboplastin time, hematocrit, hemoglobin) 3. Close monitoring of blood pressure before and during treatment 4. Avoidance of drugs excreted by kidney or nephrotoxic drugs 5. Meticulous attention to good surgical technique to minimize risk of abnormal bleeding or infection 6. Aggressive management of infection	1. Major emphasis on oral hygiene and optimum maintenance care to eliminate possible sources of infection 2. No contraindications for routine dental care but extensive reconstructive crown and bridge procedures not recommended
Hemodialysis **Chapter 9** 1. Consultation with physician 2. Delay of dental treatment until off dialysis machine for at least 4 hours (because of heparin); best on day following 3. Pretreatment screening for bleeding disorder (bleeding time, prothrombin time, partial thromboplastin time) 4. Avoidance of drugs metabolized by kidney or nephrotoxic drugs 5. Consideration of antibiotic prophylaxis for dental work to minimize effects of bacteremia 6. Pretreatment screening for hepatitis viruses and HIV 7. Avoidance of blood pressure cuff on arm containing shunt	1. Major emphasis on oral hygiene and optimum maintenance care to eliminate possible sources of infection 2. No contraindications for routine dental care

Caveat: Because most carriers are undetectable by history, all patients should be treated using universal precautions (Appendix A); risk can be decreased by use of hepatitis B vaccine
1. For patient with active hepatitis, use following procedures:
  a. Consultation with physician
  b. Treatment on emergency basis only
2. For patients with history of hepatitis, use the following procedures:
  a. Consultation with physician
  b. Probable type determination:
    (1) Age at time of infection (type B uncommon under age 15 years)
    (2) Source of infection (if food or water, usually type A or E)
    (3) If blood transfusion—related, probably type C
    (4) If type indeterminate, assay for hepatitis B surface antigen (HBsAg) may be considered
	None required

Potential Problems Related to Dental Care	Oral Manifestations

Viral Hepatitis, Types B, C, D, E—cont'd
Chapter 10

Alcoholic Liver Disease (Cirrhosis)
Chapter 10

Bleeding tendencies; unpredictable drug metabolism	1. Neglect
	2. Bleeding
	3. Ecchymoses
	4. Petechiae
	5. Glossitis
	6. Angular cheilosis
	7. Impaired healing
	8. Parotid enlargement
	9. Candidiasis
	10. Oral cancer
	11. Alcohol breath odor
	12. Bruxism
	13. Dental attrition
	14. Xerostomia

Peptic Ulcer Disease
Chapter 11

1. Further injury to intestinal mucosa by aspirin and nonsteroidal antiinflammatory drugs	1. Rare—enamel dissolution associated with persistent regurgitation
2. Fungal overgrowth during or after systemic antibiotic use	2. Fungal overgrowth
	3. Rare vitamin B deficiency (glossopyrosis) with omeprazole use

Prevention of Problems	Treatment Planning Modifications

3. With patients in high-risk categories—consider screening for hepatitis B surface antigen or anti–hepatitis C virus
4. If hepatitis B surface antigen or hepatitis C virus positive (carrier):
   a. Consultation with physician, recommendation of early treatment
   b. Minimize use of drugs metabolized by liver
   c. Preoperative prothrombin time and bleeding time in chronic active hepatitis
5. Needle stick:
   a. Consult physician
   b. Consider hepatitis B immunoglobin

---

1. Identification of alcoholic patients through the following methods:
   a. History
   b. Clinical examination
   c. Detection of odor on breath
   d. Information from friends or relatives
2. Consultation with physician to verify current status
3. Clinical screening with CAGE questionnaire and attempt to direct patient into treatment
4. Laboratory screening to include the following:
   a. Complete blood count with differential
   b. Aspartate aminotransferase, alanine aminotransferase
   c. Bleeding time
   d. Thrombin time
   e. Prothrombin time
5. Minimize use of drugs metabolized by liver
6. If screening tests abnormal for surgery, consideration antifibrinolytic agents, fresh frozen plasma, vitamin K, platelets
7. Defer routine care if ascites (encephalopathy) present

Since oral neglect is commonly seen in alcoholics, patients should be required to demonstrate interest in and ability to care for dentition before any significant treatment is rendered

---

1. Avoid aspirin and nonsteroidal anti-inflammatory drugs
2. Avoid corticosteroids
3. Examine oral cavity for signs of fungal overgrowth

Reduce stressful environment

Dental Management: A Summary—cont'd

Potential Problems Related to Dental Care	Oral Manifestations
Inflammatory Bowel Disease **Chapter 11** In patients being treated with steroids, stress may lead to serious medical problems	1. Cobblestoned—aphthous lesions 2. Pyostomatitis vegetans
Pseudomembranous Colitis **Chapter 11** Fungal overgrowth during course of antibiotics	Rare—fungal overgrowth
Gonorrhea **Chapter 12** Remote possibility of transmission from oral or pharyngeal lesions of an infected patient	Rare but varied expression including generalized stomatitis, ulceration, and formation of pseudomembranous coating of oropharynx
Syphilis **Chapter 12** 1. Syphilis may be contracted by dentist from actively infectious patient 2. Patients or staff may be infected by dentist who has syphilis	1. Chancre 2. Mucous patch 3. Gumma 4. Interstitial glossitis 5. Congenital syphilis (associated with Hutchinson's incisors and mulberry molars)

Prevention of Problems	Treatment Planning Modifications
1. Additional steroids may be needed for surgical procedures 2. Complete blood count needed to monitor toxic hematologic effects of drugs	Schedule appointments during remissions
1. Select appropriate antibiotic and dosage 2. Precaution with prolonged antibiotic use in elderly and those previously affected	Schedule appointments when patient is free of disease

Caveat: Many patients with sexually transmitted disease cannot be identified by history or examination; therefore all patients must be approached using universal precautions (see Appendix A)
1. Patients currently receiving treatment for gonorrhea—provide necessary care
2. Patients with past history of gonorrhea, perform the following:
  a. Obtain good history of disease and its treatment
  b. Provide necessary care
3. Patients with signs or symptoms suggestive of gonorrhea, perform the following:
  a. Refer to physician for evaluation
  b. Provide necessary care after disease treatment initiated
	None required

Caveat: Many patients with sexually transmitted disease cannot be identified by history or examination; therefore all patients must be approached using universal precautions (see Appendix A)
1. Patients receiving treatment for syphilis:
  a. Consult with physician before treatment
  b. Provide necessary care
  c. Be aware that oral lesions of primary and secondary syphilis are infectious prior to initiation of antibiotic therapy
2. Patients with past history of syphilis:
  a. Approach with caution; obtain good history of disease, its treatment, and negative serologic tests for syphilis test following therapy
  b. Treat as normal patient if free of disease
3. Patients showing signs or symptoms suggestive of syphilis:
  a. Refer to physician and postpone treatment
  b. May elect to order serologic test for syphilis before referral
  c. Treat as in Category 1 if treatment necessary
	None required

Dental Management: A Summary—cont'd

Potential Problems Related to Dental Care	Oral Manifestations

Genital Herpes
Chapter 12
Inoculation of oral cavity and potential transmission to dentist's fingers

Autoinoculation of type 2 herpes to oral cavity

Antibody Positive for HIV (AIDS) But Asymptomatic
Chapter 13
1. Transmission of infectious agents to dental personnel and patients includes:
   a. AIDS virus (HIV)
   b. Hepatitis B virus (HBV)
   c. Hepatitis C virus (HCV)
   d. Epstein-Barr virus (EBV)
   e. Cytomegalovirus (CMV)
2. To date no dental health care workers have been HIV infected through occupational exposure; 6 patients may have been infected by an HIV-infected dentist; thus risk of HIV transmission in dental setting is very low, but potential exists
3. Individuals who are hepatitis carriers can transmit hepatitis B virus or hepatitis C virus infection

None in early stage; however, increased incidence of certain oral lesions associated with AIDS is found when compared to noninfected individuals (i.e., candidiasis)

HIV-infected, Asymptomatic Patient (CD4 lymphocyte count less than 500, more than 200)
Chapter 13
1. Transmission of infectious agents to dental personnel and patients includes the following:
   a. HIV
   b. Hepatitis B virus
   c. Hepatitis C virus
   d. Epstein-Barr virus
   e. Cytomegalovirus
2. To date, with the exception of possible transmission by a Florida dentist, HIV has not been found to be transmitted to patients in the dental setting; no dental health care workers have been HIV infected by occupational exposure; however, HBV and HCV transmission has been well documented on numerous occasions

1. Oral candidiasis
2. Hairy leukoplakia
3. Persistent lymphadenopathy
4. With the exception of Kaposi's sarcoma and non-Hodgkin's lymphoma, other lesions listed under AIDS can be found with increased frequency

Prevention of Problems	Treatment Planning Modifications
Caveat: Many patients with sexually transmitted disease cannot be identified by history or examination; therefore all patients must be approached using universal precautions (see Appendix A) 1. Localized genital infection poses no problem; however, be aware of possibility of autoinoculation to oral cavity by patient 2. Oral infection of type 1 or type 2—postpone elective dental care until lesion in scab phase	None usually required; patients prone to recurrences after dental treatment should be provided systemic antiviral drug for prophylactic use
1. Identification of HIV-infected patient is difficult; interview questions should address promiscuous sexual behavior; infectious disease control procedures must be used for *all* patients 2. Extreme care must be taken to avoid needle stick and instrument wounding 3. All dental personnel should be vaccinated to be protected from hepatitis B virus infection 4. All asymptomatic antibody-positive (HIV) individuals may go on to develop AIDS; however, can take as long as 15 years before diagnosis of AIDS is made 5. HIV-infected patient's CD4 count must be monitored	None indicated
1. Use infectious disease control procedure for *all* patients 2. Vaccinate dental personnel for protection from hepatitis B virus infection 3. Identify patients by presence of signs and symptoms associated with decreasing CD4 lymphocytes; refer for medical evaluation, counseling, and management 4. Establish platelet status and immune status of patients with decreasing CD4 lymphocytes before performing invasive dental procedures (see AIDS, next page) 5. Inform patients of various support groups available to help in terms of education and emotional, financial, legal, and other issues	None indicated

Dental Management: A Summary—cont'd

Potential Problems Related to Dental Care	Oral Manifestations

HIV-infected, Asymptomatic Patient (CD4 lymphocyte count less than 500, more than 200)—cont'd
Chapter 13

3. Patients with decreasing CD4 lymphocytes may have significant immune suppression and be at increased risk for infection
4. Patients with decreasing CD4 lymphocytes may be thrombocytopenic and hence potential bleeders

AIDS (CD4 lymphocyte count less than 200)
Chapter 13

1. Transmission of infectious agents to dental personnel and patients: a. HIV b. Hepatitis B virus c. Hepatitis C virus d. Epstein-Barr virus e. Cytomegalovirus 2. To date, HIV has not been found to be transmitted to patient in the dental setting (possible exception of 6 patients who may have been infected by a Florida dentist); no dental health care workers have been HIV infected through occupational exposure; however, HBV and HCV have been transmitted to patients or dental health care workers on a number of occasions in dental setting 3. Patients with advanced disease have significant suppression of their immune system and can be at risk for infection resulting from invasive dental procedures 4. Patients may be bleeders because of thrombocytopenia	1. Kaposi's sarcoma 2. Non-Hodgkin's lymphoma 3. Oral candidiasis 4. Lymphadenopathy 5. Hairy leukoplakia 6. Xerostomia 7. Salivary gland enlargement 8. Venereal warts 9. Linear gingivitis erythemia 10. Necrotizing ulcerative periodontitis 11. Necrotizing stomatitis 12. Herpes zoster 13. Primary or recurrent herpes simplex lesions 14. Major aphthous lesions 15. Herpetiform aphthous lesions 16. Petechiae, ecchymoses 17. Others (see Box 13-6)

Diabetes Mellitus
Chapter 14

1. In uncontrolled diabetic patients: a. Infection b. Poor wound healing 2. Insulin reaction in patients treated with insulin 3. In diabetic patients, early onset of complications relating to cardiovascular system, eyes, kidneys, and nervous system (angina, myocardial infarction, cerebrovascular accident, renal failure, peripheral neuropathy blindness, hypertension, congestive heart failure)	1. Accelerated periodontal disease 2. Gingival proliferations 3. Periodontal abscesses 4. Xerostomia 5. Poor healing 6. Infection 7. Oral ulcerations 8. Candidiasis 9. Mucormycosis 10. Numbness, burning, or pain in oral tissues

Prevention of Problems	Treatment Planning Modifications

1. Use infectious disease control procedures for *all* patients
2. Vaccinate dental personnel for protection from hepatitis B virus
3. By medical history and examination findings, identify undiagnosed cases and refer for medical evaluation, counseling, and management
4. Give patients with significant immune suppression antibiotic prophylaxis for surgical or invasive dental procedures if neutrophil count is less than 500 cu/m
5. Platelet count or bleeding time should be ordered before any surgical procedure; if significant thrombocytopenia present, platelet replacement may be needed

1. None for cases in "remission"; however, complex restorative procedures usually are not indicated because of poor prognosis (death occurs most often within 2 years after diagnosis)
2. Patients in advanced stages of disease should receive emergency and preventive dental care; elective dental treatment usually is not indicated at this stage

1. Detection by the following methods:
   a. History
   b. Clinical findings
   c. Screening blood glucose level
2. Referral for diagnosis and treatment
3. Monitoring and control of hyperglycemia
4. Patients receiving insulin—insulin reaction prevented by the following:
   a. Eating of normal meals before appointments
   b. Scheduling of appointments in morning or midmorning
   c. Informing the dentist of any symptoms of insulin reaction when they first occur
   d. Having sugar available in some form in case of insulin reaction

1. In well-controlled diabetic patients, no alteration of treatment plan is indicated unless complication of diabetes present such as:
   a. Hypertension
   b. Congestive heart failure
   c. Myocardial infarction
   d. Angina
   e. Renal failure
2. Defer prosthodontic care until periodontal disease well controlled

Potential Problems Related to Dental Care	Oral Manifestations

Diabetes mellitus—cont'd
Chapter 14

Intraocular Lenses
Chapter 14

No risks	None

Adrenal Insufficiency
Chapter 15

1. Inability to tolerate stress	1. Primary—pigmentation of oral mucous membranes
2. Delayed healing	2. Delayed healing
3. Susceptibility to infection	3. Susceptibility to infection
4. Hypertension (with steriod use)	

Hyperthyroidism (Thyrotoxicosis)
Chapter 16

1. Thyrotoxic crisis (thyroid storm) may be precipitated in untreated or incompletely treated patients with thyrotoxicosis by	1. Osteoporosis may occur
a. Infection	2. Periodontal disease may be more progressive
b. Trauma	3. Dental caries may be more extensive
c. Surgical procedures	4. Premature loss of deciduous teeth and early eruption of permanent teeth
d. Stress	5. Early jaw development
2. Patients with untreated or incompletely treated thyrotoxicosis may be very sensitive to actions of epinephrine and other pressor amines; thus these agents must not be used; once patient is well managed from medical standpoint, these agents can be resumed	6. Tumors found in midline of posterior dorsum of tongue must not be surgically removed until possibility of functional thyroid tissue has been ruled out by 1311 uptake tests

Prevention of Problems	Treatment Planning Modifications
5. Diabetic patients being treated with insulin who develop oral infection may require increase in insulin dosage; consult with physician in addition to aggressive local and systemic management of infection (including antibiotic sensitivity testing)	
6. Drug considerations include the following:	
a. Insulin—insulin reaction	
b. Hypoglycemic agents—on rare occasions aplastic anemia, etc.	
c. Avoidance of general anesthesia in severe diabetics	
No special precautions	None
1. For routine dental procedures (excluding extractions):	None required
a. Patients currently taking corticosteroids—no additional supplementation generally required; be sure to obtain good local anesthesia and good postoperative pain control	
b. Patients with past history of regular corticosteroid usage; none generally required	
c. Patients using topical or inhalational steroids— generally no supplementation required	
2. For extractions or other surgery, extensive procedures, or extreme patient anxiety, with local anesthetic include the following:	
a. Target dose of 25 mg hydrocortisone per day for minor oral and periodontal surgery	
b. Target dose of 50 to 100 mg hydrocortisone per day for major oral surgery or involving general anesthesia	
1. Detection of patients with thyrotoxicosis by history and examination findings	1. Once under good medical management, patient may receive any indicated dental treatment
2. Referral for medical evaluation and treatment	2. If acute infection occurs, physician should be consulted concerning management
3. Avoidance of any dental treatment for patient with thyrotoxicosis until under good medical control; however, any acute oral infection will have to be dealt with by antibiotic therapy and other conservative measures to prevent development of thyrotoxic crisis; suggest consultation with patient's physician during management of acute oral infection	
4. Avoidance of epinephrine and other pressor amines in untreated or incompletely treated patient	

Dental Management: A Summary—cont'd

Potential Problems Related to Dental Care	Oral Manifestations

Hyperthyroidism (Thyrotoxicosis)—cont'd
Chapter 16
3. Thyrotoxicosis increases risk for hypertension, angina, MI, congestive heart failure, and severe arrhythmias

Hypothyroidism
Chapter 16
1. Untreated patients with severe hypothyroidism exposed to stressful situations such as trauma, surgical procedures, or infection may develop hypothyroid (myxedema) coma
2. Untreated hypothyroid patients may be very sensitive to actions of narcotics, barbiturates, and tranquilizers
3. Type 1 diabetes and Sjögren's syndrome may coexist in some cases of Hashimoto's thyroiditis (see those sections)

1. Increase in tongue size
2. Delayed eruption of teeth
3. Malocclusion
4. Gingival edema

Pregnancy and Lactation
Chapter 17
1. Dental procedures could harm developing fetus via:
   a. Radiation
   b. Drugs
   c. Stress
2. Supine hypotension in late pregnancy
3. Poor nutrition and diet can affect oral health
4. Transmission of drugs to infant via breast milk

1. Exaggeration of periodontal disease, "pregnancy gingivitis"
2. "Pregnancy tumor"
3. Tooth mobility

Prevention of Problems	Treatment Planning Modifications

5. Recognition of early stages of thyrotoxic crisis:
   a. Severe symptoms of thyrotoxicosis
   b. Fever
   c. Abdominal pain
   d. Delirious, obtunded, or psychotic
6. Initiation of immediate emergency treatment procedures:
   a. Seek immediate medical aid
   b. Cool with cold towels, ice packs
   c. Hydrocortisone (100 to 300 mg)
   d. Monitor vital signs
   e. Start CPR if needed

---

1. Detection and referral of patients suspected of being hypothyroid for medical evaluation and treatment
2. Avoidance of narcotics, barbiturates, and tranquilizers in untreated hypothyroid patients
3. Recognition of initial stage of hypothyroid (myxedema) coma
  a. Hypothermia
  b. Bradycardia
  c. Hypotension
  d. Epileptic seizures
4. Start immediate treatment of myxedema coma
  a. Seek immediate medical aid
  b. Hydrocortisone (100 to 300 mg)
  c. CPR as indicated
	1. In hypothyroid patients under good medical management, indicated dental treatment may be performed
	2. In patients with congenital form of disease and severe mental retardation, assistance with hygiene procedures may be needed

---

1. Women of childbearing age:
  a. Always use contemporary radiographic techniques including lead apron when performing radiographic examination
  b. Do not prescribe drugs that are known to be harmful to fetus or whose effects are as yet unknown (Table 17-3)
  c. Encourage patients to maintain balanced, nutritious diet
2. Pregnant women
  a. Contact patient's physician to verify physical status, present management plan; ask for suggestions regarding patient's treatment especially relating to drug administration
  b. Maintain optimum oral hygiene, including prophylaxis, throughout pregnancy
  c. Minimize oral microbial load (consider chlorhexidine or fluoride).
	None, except that major reconstructive procedures, crown and bridge fabrication, or significant operations are best delayed until after delivery

Dental Management: A Summary—cont'd

Potential Problems Related to Dental Care	Oral Manifestations

Pregnancy and Lactation—cont'd
Chapter 17

Anaphylaxis
Chapter 18

Severe reaction following administration of agent patient is allergic to, such as:
  a. Drugs
  b. Local anesthetic
  c. Latex gloves or other rubber products (rubber dam, gutta percha)
	Usually none

Prevention of Problems	Treatment Planning Modifications

d. Avoid elective dental care during first trimester. Second trimester and most of third trimester are best times for elective treatment
e. Do not schedule radiographs during first trimester; thereafter take only those necessary for treatment, always using lead apron
f. Avoid drugs known to be harmful to fetus or whose effects are unknown (Table 20-3)
g. In advanced stages of pregnancy (late third trimester), do not place patient in supine position for prolonged periods; avoid aspirin, NSAIDs
3. Lactating mothers
   a. Most drugs are of little pharmacologic significance to lactation
   b. Do not prescribe drugs known to be harmful (Table 17-3)
   c. Administer drugs just after breast-feeding

	Usually none

1. Take careful history and identify patients who are allergic to agents used in dentistry and who have history of atopic reactions (asthma, hayfever, urticaria, angioneurotic edema).
2. Do not use agents that patient is allergic to as identified in medical history
3. Patients with history of atopic reactions—use care when giving drugs and materials with high incidence of allergy such as penicillin; be prepared to deal with severe allergic reaction in the following ways:
   a. Identify anaphylactic reaction
   b. Call for medical help
   c. Place patient in supine position
   d. Check for open airway
   e. Administer oxygen
   f. Check vital signs—respiration, blood pressure, pulse rate and rhythm
   g. If vital signs depressed or absent, inject 0.3-0.5 ml of epinephrine 1:1000 IM into tongue
   h. Provide CPR as indicated
   i. Repeat injection of epinephrine if no response
4. When prescribing drugs, inform patient regarding signs and symptoms of allergic reactions; advise patient to call dentist if such reaction occurs, or to report to nearest hospital emergency room

Dental Management: A Summary—cont'd

Potential Problems Related to Dental Care	Oral Manifestations
Urticaria (angioneurotic edema) **Chapter 18** 1. Nonemergency, edematous swelling of lips, cheek, etc, after contact with antigen 2. Emergency, edematous swelling of tongue, pharynx, and larynx with obstruction of airway	Soft tissue swelling

Bleeding Problem Suggested by Examination and History Findings But No Clues as to Underlying Cause
Chapter 19

Excessive blood loss following surgical procedures, scaling, etc.	Excessive bleeding after dental procedures

Prevention of Problems	Treatment Planning Modifications

1. Identify patients who have had allergic reactions by history and what drug or materials caused reaction
2. Avoid use of antigen in allergic persons
3. If patients develop allergic reaction to drug or material to which they gave no indication of being allergic consider the following:
  a. Nonemergency reaction, no further contact with agent—administer diphenhydramine, 50 mg up to qid, orally or IM
  b. Emergency reaction, put patient in supine position, patent airway, oxygen, inject 0.3-0.5 ml epinephrine 1:1000 IM, support respiration if necessary, check pulse, obtain medical assistance
4. Before administering local anesthetics, consider the following:
  a. Obtain from patient information about being allergic to a local anesthetic (Most patients who say they are allergic will describe, a fainting episode or toxic reaction)
  b. If allergic reaction occurred, identify kind of anesthetic used and select one from different chemical group
    (1) Inject 1 drop (aspirate first) of alternate anesthetic; wait 5 minutes, if no reaction, proceed with injection of remaining anesthetic
    (2) If anesthetic that patient reacted to cannot be identified, consider the following procedures:
      A. Refer to allergist for provocative dose testing, or
      B. Use diphenhydramine (Benadryl) with epinephrine 1:100,000 as local anesthetics (1% solution, 1 to 4 ml)
5. Allergy to penicillin
  a. Administer erythromycin or other macrolide antibiotic
  b. In nonallergic person, administer by oral route whenever possible—lowest incidence of sensitization
  c. Do not use in topical form
	1. Avoidance of drug or material to which patient is allergic
	2. In rare patient who is allergic to many local anesthetics, diphenhydramine (Benadryl) can be used as local anesthetic or refer to allergist for provocative dose testing

1. Screen patients with following (if one or more are abnormal, refer for diagnosis and medical treatment):
  a. Prothrombin time
  b. Activated partial thromboplastin time
  c. Thrombin time
  d. Platelet count
  e. Bleeding time
2. Avoid use of aspirin and related drugs
	None unless test(s) abnormal, then manage based on nature of underlying problem once diagnosis established by physician

Dental Management: A Summary—cont'd

Potential Problems Related to Dental Care	Oral Manifestations

Thrombocytopenia (primary or secondary) Caused by Chemicals, Radiation, or Leukemia
Chapter 19

1. Prolonged bleeding	1. Spontaneous bleeding
2. Infection in patients with bone marrow replacement or destruction	2. Prolonged bleeding following certain dental procedures
3. In patients being treated with steroids, serious medical emergency resulting from stress	3. Petechiae
	4. Ecchymoses
	5. Hematomas

Vascular Wall Alterations (scurvy, infection, chemical, allergic, autoimmune, other)
Chapter 19

Prolonged bleeding after surgical procedures or any insult to integrity of oral mucosa	1. Excessive bleeding after scaling and surgical procedures
	2. Petechiae
	3. Ecchymoses
	4. Hematomas

Congenital Disorders of Coagulation (hemophilia)
Chapter 19

Excessive bleeding following dental procedures	1. Spontaneous bleeding
	2. Prolonged bleeding after dental procedures that injure soft tissue or bone
	3. Hematomas
	4. Oral lesions associated with HIV infection in patients who receive infected replacement products (most occurred before 1986)

Prevention of Problems	Treatment Planning Modifications

1. Identification of patients to include the following:
  a. History
  b. Examination findings
  c. Screening tests—bleeding time, platelet count
2. Referral and consultation with hematologist
3. Correction of underlying problem or replacement therapy before surgery
4. Local measures to control blood loss—splint, gelfoam, thrombin, etc
5. Prophylactic antibiotics in surgical cases to prevent postoperative infection can be considered
6. Additional steroids for patients being treated with steroids if indicated (see section on adrenal insufficiency)
7. Asprin, aspirin-containing compounds, and nonsteroidal antiinflammatory drugs not to be used, acetaminophen (Tylenol) with or without codeine can be used
	No dental procedures unless replacement of platelets is done before procedure or unless underlying problem has been corrected
	In children with primary thrombocytopenia, many will respond to steroids, allowing surgical procedures to be performed

1. Identification of patients to include the following:
  a. History
  b. Clinical findings
  c. Screening test, bleeding time
2. Consultation with hematologist
3. Local measures to control blood loss
4. Prevention of allergy involved in etiology, and identification of antigen
5. Splints, gelfoam, Oxycel, surgical thrombin
	Surgical procedures must be avoided in these patients unless underlying problem has been corrected or patient has been prepared for surgery by hematologist, and dentist is prepared to control excessive loss of blood by local measures (see section on hemophilia)

1. Identification of patients includes the following:
  a. History—bleeding problems in relatives, excessive bleeding following trauma or surgery
  b. Examination findings:
    (1) Ecchymoses
    (2) Hemarthrosis
    (3) Dissecting hematomas
  c. Screening tests—prothrombin time (normal), activated partial thromboplastin time (prolonged), bleeding time (normal) and thrombin time (normal)
2. Consultation and referral for diagnosis and treatment and for preparation before dental procedures
3. Replacement options include the following:
  a. Cryoprecipitate
  b. Fresh frozen plasma
	No dental procedures unless patient has been prepared based on consultation with hematologist
	Avoid aspirin, aspirin-containing compounds, and NSAIDs—use acetaminophen (Tylenol) with or without codeine

Dental Management: A Summary—cont'd	
Potential Problems Related to Dental Care	**Oral Manifestations**

Congenital Disorders of Coagulation (hemophilia)—cont'd
Chapter 19

---

von Willebrand's Disease
Chapter 19

Excessive bleeding after invasive dental procedures	1. Spontaneous bleeding
	2. Prolonged bleeding following dental procedures that injure soft tissue or bone
	3. Petechiae
	4. Hematomas

Prevention of Problems	Treatment Planning Modifications

   c. Factor VIII concentrates, including:
     (1) Heat-treated concentrate
     (2) Purified factor VIII
     (3) Recombinant factor VIII
4. Mild and moderate factor VIII deficiency consider using
   a. 1-desamino-8-D-arginine vasopressin
   b. Epsilon-aminocaproic acid
   c. Tranexamic acid (Cyklokapron)
   d. Factor VIII replacement for some cases
5. Severe factor VIII deficiency alleviated by such measures as:
   a. Agents used in No. 4 above
   b. Higher dose(s) factor VIII
6. Stable level of inhibitors include:
   a. Agents used in No. 4 above
   b. Very high dose(s) factor VIII
7. Inducible inhibitors include:
   a. No elective surgery
   b. Agents used in No. 4 above
   c. High doses of porcine factor VIII concentrate
   d. Nonactivated prothrombin-complex concentrate
   e. Activated prothrombin-complex concentrate
   f. Plasmapheresis
   g. Factor VIIA
   h. Steroids
8. Treatment on outpatient basis allowed depending on results of consultation (mild to moderate deficiency, no inhibitors)
9. Local measures for control of bleeding—splints, thrombin, microfibrillar collagen, etc.
10. Avoidance of aspirin, aspirin-containing compounds, and nonsteroidal antiinflammatory drugs

---

1. Identification of patients to include:
   a. History of bleeding problems in relatives and of excessive bleeding after surgery or trauma, etc.
   b. Examination findings to include:
     (1) Petechiae
     (2) Hematomas
   c. Screening laboratory tests—prolonged bleeding time, or PFA-100, possible prolonged partial thromboplastin time
2. Consultation and referral for diagnosis and treatment and preparation before dental procedures

No invasive dental procedures unless patient has been prepared based on consultation with hematologist

Dental Management: A Summary—cont'd

Potential Problems Related to Dental Care	Oral Manifestations

von Willebrand's Disease—cont'd
Chapter 19

Acquired Disorders of Coagulation (liver disease, broad spectrum antibiotics, malabsorption syndrome, biliary tract obstruction, heparin, and others)
Chapter 19

Excessive bleeding following dental procedures that result in soft tissue or osseous injury	1. Excessive bleeding 2. Spontaneous bleeding 3. Petechiae 4. Hematomas

---

Anticoagulation with Coumarin Drugs
Chapter 19

Excessive bleeding after dental procedures that result in soft tissue or osseous injury	1. Excessive bleeding 2. Hematomas 3. Petechiae 4. In rare cases spontaneous bleeding

Prevention of Problems	Treatment Planning Modifications

3. Type I and many type II cases require the following:
   a. 1-desamino-8-D-arginine vasopressin
   b. Local measures (see No. 6 below)
4. Type III and some type II patients require the following:
   a. Fresh frozen plasma
   b. Cryoprecipitate
   c. Special factor VIII concentrates:
      (1) Humate-P
      (2) Koate HS
   d. Local measures (see No. 6 below)
5. Outpatient treatment possible based on results of consultation
6. Local measures for control of bleeding include:
   a. Splints
   b. Gelfoam with thrombin
   c. Oxycel, Surgicel
7. Avoid aspirin, aspirin-containing compounds, and nonsteroidal anti-inflammatory drugs
8. Acetaminophen with or without codeine, or Cox-2 specific inhibitors—Celecoxib, Rofecoxib can be used.

---

1. Identification of patients with disorder to include:
   a. History
   b. Examination findings
   c. Screening laboratory tests—prothrombin time (prolonged), bleeding time (in liver disease prolonged if hypersplenism present)
2. Consultation and referral
3. Preparation before dental procedure; may include vitamin K injection by physician
4. Local measurements to control blood loss
5. In patients with liver disease; drugs metabolized by the liver avoid or reduce dosage
6. No use of aspirin, aspirin-containing compounds, and nonsteroidal anti-inflammatory drugs

No dental procedures unless patient prepared based on consultation with hematologist

---

1. Identification of patients taking anticoagulants— coumarin drugs to include:
   a. History
   b. Screening lab test—prothrombin time (PT)

No dental procedures unless medical consult has been obtained and the level of anticoagulation is at an acceptable range; procedure may have to be delayed by 2 to 3 days if the dosage of anticoagulant has to be reduced

Dental Management: A Summary—cont'd

Potential Problems Related to Dental Care	Oral Manifestations
Anticoagulation with Coumarin Drugs—cont'd **Chapter 19**	
Disseminated Intravascular Coagulation (DIC) **Chapter 19** Excessive bleeding after invasive dental procedures; in chronic form of disease widespread thrombosis may occur	1. Spontaneous gingival bleeding 2. Petechiae 3. Ecchymoses 4. Prolonged bleeding following invasive dental procedures

Prevention of Problems	Treatment Planning Modifications

2. Consultation regarding level of anticoagulation:
  a. If PT ratio is 2.5 or less, most surgical procedures can be performed
  b. If international normalized ratio (INR) is 3.5 or less, most surgical procedures can be performed
  c. Reduction of the dosage of the anticoagulant if PT ratio is greater than 2.5 or if the INR is greater than 3.5 (it takes several days for the PT or INR to fall to the desired level; confirmation by new tests before surgery is done)
3. Local measures instituted to control blood loss after surgery	

1. Identification of patients includes the following:
  a. History—excessive bleeding after minor trauma; spontaneous bleeding from nose, gingiva, gastrointestinal tract, or urinary tract; recent infection, burns, shock and acidosis, or autoimmune disease; history of cancer most often associated with chronic form of DIC, in which thrombosis is usually the major clinical problem rather than bleeding
  b. Examination findings include the following:
    (1) Petechiae
    (2) Ecchymoses
    (3) Spontaneous gingival bleeding, bleeding from nose, ears, etc
  c. Screening laboratory findings include the following:
    (1) Acute DIC—prothrombin time (prolonged), partial thromboplastin time (prolonged), thrombin time (prolonged), bleeding time (prolonged), platelet count (decreased)
    (2) Chronic DIC—most tests may be normal but fibrin split products present
2. Referral and consultation with physician if invasive dental procedures must be performed and include information on:
  a. Acute DIC—cryoprecipitate, fresh frozen plasma, and platelets
  b. Chronic DIC—anticoagulants such as heparin or vitamin K antagonists
3. Aspirin or aspirin-containing products prohibited
4. Use of local measures to control bleeding
5. Consideration of antibiotic therapy to prevent postoperative infection
	Depending on cause of DIC treatment plan should be altered in following ways:
	1. Cases of acute DIC, no routine dental care until medical evaluation and correction of cause
	2. Cases of chronic DIC, no routine dental care until medical evaluation and correction of cause when possible; if prognosis is poor based on underlying cause (advanced cancer), limited dental care would be indicated

Dental Management: A Summary—cont'd

Potential Problems Related to Dental Care	Oral Manifestations

Disorders of Platelet Release
Chapter 19

Excessive bleeding after invasive dental procedures

1. Excessive bleeding may occur following surgery
2. Petechiae, ecchymoses, and hematomas may be found when other platelet or coagulation disorders are present

Primary Fibrinogenolysis
Chapter 19

Excessive bleeding after invasive dental procedures

1. Prolonged bleeding following invasive dental procedures
2. Jaundice of mucosa
3. Ecchymoses

Low-Molecular Weight Heparin Therapy: Enoxaparin (*Lovenox*), ardeparin (*Normiflo*), dalteparin (*Fragmin*), nadroparin (*Fraxiparine*), reviparin (*Clivarin*), tinzaparin (*Innohep*)
Chapter 19

1. Used in patients who have received prosthetic knee or hip replacement; patient takes medication for approximately 2 weeks after getting out of hospital
2. Complications include the following:
   a. Excessive bleeding
   b. Anemia
   c. Fever
   d. Thrombocytopenia
   e. Peripheral edema

1. Gingival bleeding
2. Petechiae
3. Ecchymoses
4. In rare cases excessive bleeding after dental procedures

Prevention of Problems	Treatment Planning Modifications

1. Identification of patient to include the following:
  a. History—recent use of aspirin, indomethacin, phenylbutazone, ibuprofen, or sulfinpyrazone; presence of other platelet or coagulation disorders
  b. Examination—often negative unless signs present relating to other platelet or coagulation disorder
  c. Screening laboratory tests—bleeding time (prolonged), PFA-100 (prolonged), partial thromboplastin time (prolonged)
2. Most patients on drugs noted above in 1a without an additional platelet or coagulation problem will not bleed excessively following surgery
3. Patients with prolonged bleeding time and/or partial thromboplastin time should be referred for evaluation prior to any surgical procedures being performed
4. Elective surgery can be performed following withdrawal of drug and management of other platelet or coagulation disorder by appropriate means
	Usually no modifications indicated for patients who have no other platelet or coagulation disorder

1. Identification of patients to include the following:
  a. History—liver disease, cancer of lung, cancer of prostate, and heat stroke may develop this condition
  b. Examination findings to consider:
    (1) Jaundice
    (2) Spider angiomas
    (3) Ecchymoses
    (4) Hematomas
  c. Screening laboratory tests—platelet count (often normal), prothrombin time (prolonged), bleeding time (usually normal), partial thromboplastin time (prolonged), thrombin time (prolonged)
2. Consultation and referral prior to any invasive dental procedure; epsilon-aminocaproic acid therapy will inhibit both plasmin and plasmin activators
	Patients with advanced cancer should have treatment limited to emergency dental procedures and preventive measures; complex dental restorations in general are not indicated; in other patients, once preparation to avoid excessive bleeding has occurred (epsilon-aminocaproic acid), most dental treatment can be rendered

1. Delay procedure until patient is off the medication 2. Have physician stop medication and perform the surgery the next day and once hemostasis obtained have physician resume medication 3. Perform the surgery and manage any excessive bleeding using local means (preferred if excessive bleeding is not anticipated)	Usually none needed

Dental Management: A Summary—cont'd

Potential Problems Related to Dental Care	Oral Manifestations

Antiplatelet Drug Therapy: Aspirin, aspirin plus dipyridamole (*Aggrenox*), ibuprofen (*Advil, Motrin*)
Chapter 19

1. Used for prevention of initial or recurrent myocardial infarction and stroke prevention
2. Complications include:
   a. Excessive bleeding
   b. GI bleeding
   c. Tinnitus
   d. Bronchospasm

1. Gingival bleeding
2. Petechiae
3. Ecchymoses
4. In rare cases excessive bleeding following dental procedures

Fibrinogen Receptor Therapy (GP IIb-IIIa inhibitors: Clopidogrel (*Plavix*), ticlopidine (*Ticlid*)
Chapter 19

1. Used for prevention of recurrent myocardial infarction and stroke
2. Complications include:
   a. Excessive bleeding
   b. GI bleeding
   c. Neutropenia
   d. Thrombocytopenia

1. Gingival bleeding
2. Petechiae
3. Ecchymoses
4. In rare cases excessive bleeding following dental procedures

Iron Deficiency Anemia
Chapter 20

1. Usually none
2. In rare cases severe leukopenia and thrombocytopenia may result in problems with infection and excessive loss of blood

1. Paresthesias
2. Loss of papillae from tongue
3. In rare cases infection and bleeding complications
4. In patients with dysphagia, increased incidence of carcinoma of oral and pharyngeal area (Plummer-Vinson syndrome)

G-6-PD Deficiency
Chapter 20

Accelerated hemolysis of red blood cells

Usually none

Pernicious Anemia
Chapter 20

1. Infection
2. Bleeding
3. Delayed healing

1. Paresthesias of oral tissues (burning, tingling, numbness)
2. Delayed healing (severe cases), infection, red tongue, angular cheilosis
3. Petechial hemorrhages

Prevention of Problems	Treatment Planning Modifications
If no other complications exist, dental procedures and surgery can usually be performed. Can screen with BT and if under 20 minutes most surgeries can be performed.	Usually none needed
If no other complications exist, dental procedure and surgery can be performed.	Usually none needed
1. Detection and referral for diagnosis and treatment 2. Recognition that in women most cases caused by physiologic process—menstruation or pregnancy 3. Recognition that in men most cases secondary to underlying disease—peptic ulcer, carcinoma of colon, etc.	Usually none
1. Control infection 2. Avoid drugs containing certain antibiotics, aspirin, acetaminophen 3. Be aware that these patients often have increased sensitivity to sulfa drugs, aspirin, chloramphenicol	Usually none unless anemia severe, then only urgent dental needs
Detection and medical treatment (early detection and treatment can prevent permanent neurologic damage)	None once patient under medical care

Dental Management: A Summary—cont'd

Potential Problems Related to Dental Care	Oral Manifestations

Sickle Cell Anemia
Chapter 20
Sickle cell crisis

1. Osteoporosis
2. Loss of trabecular pattern
3. Delayed eruption of teeth
4. Hypoplasia of teeth
5. Pallor of oral mucosa
6. Jaundice of oral mucosa
7. Bone pain

Agranulocytosis
Chapter 20
Infection

1. Oral ulcerations
2. Periodontitis
3. Necrotic tissue

Cyclic Neutropenia
Chapter 20
Infection

1. Periodontal disease
2. Oral infection
3. Oral ulceration similar to aphthous stomatitis

Prevention of Problems	Treatment Planning Modifications

1. Avoid any procedure that would produce acidosis or hypoxia
2. Consideration of the following drug situations:
  a. Avoid excessive use of barbiturates and narcotics, as suppression of respiratory center can occur, leading to acidosis, which can precipitate acute crisis
  b. Avoid excessive use of salicylates, as "acidosis" may result, again leading to possible acute crisis; codeine and acetaminophen in moderate dosage can be used for pain control
  c. Avoid use of general anesthesia, as hypoxia can lead to precipitation of acute crisis
  d. Nitrous oxide may be used, provided 50% oxygen is supplied at all times; critical to avoid diffusion hypoxia at termination of nitrous oxide administration
  For nonsurgical procedures use local without vasoconstrictor; for surgical procedures, use 1:100,000 epinephrine in anesthetic solution
    (1) Aspirate before injecting
    (2) Slow injection
    (3) Use no more than two cartridges
3. Need to prevent infection; if infection occurs manage aggressively
  a. Heat
  b. I & D
  c. Antibiotics
  d. Corrective treatment—extraction, pulpectomy, etc
4. Avoid dehydration in patients with infection or patients receiving surgical treatment
	Usually none unless symptoms of severe anemia present, and then only urgent dental needs should be met

1. Referral for medical diagnosis and treatment 2. Drug considerations—chloramphenicol not used for oral infection because of high incidence of agranulocytosis	Emergency care only during periods of low blood counts with use of antibiotics, supportive therapy for oral lesions (see Appendix B for specific treatment regimens)
1. Antibiotics to prevent infection 2. Serial white blood cell counts, to pick time in cycle when count is closest to normal level	As indicated; if white cell count depressed severely, antibiotics to avoid postoperative infection

Dental Management: A Summary—cont'd

Potential Problems Related to Dental Care	Oral Manifestations

Multiple Myeloma
Chapter 20

1. Excessive bleeding after invasive dental procedures
2. Risk of infection because of decrease in normal immunoglobulins
3. Risk of infection and bleeding in patients being treated by radiation or chemotherapy

1. Soft tissue tumors
2. Osseolytic lesions
3. Amyloid deposits in soft tissues
4. Unexplained mobility of teeth

Lymphomas: Hodgkin's disease, non-Hodgkin's lymphoma, Burkitt's lymphoma
Chapter 20

1. Increased risk for infection
2. Risk of infection and excessive bleeding in patients receiving chemotherapy
3. Minor risk of osteonecrosis in patients treated by radiation to head and neck region (this usually does not occur because radiation dosage seldom exceeds 6000 cGy)
4. Xerostomia may occur in patients treated by radiation to head and neck region
5. Non-Hodgkin's lymphoma can be found in patients with AIDS; hence transmission of infectious agents may be a potential problem

1. Extranodal oral tumors in Waldeyer's ring or osseous soft tissues
2. Xerostomia in patients treated by radiation; some of these patients prone to osteonecrosis
3. Burning mouth or tongue symptoms
4. Petechiae or ecchymoses if thrombocytopenia present because of tumor invasion of bone marrow
5. Cervical lymphadenopathy
6. Mucositis in patients treated by radiation therapy or chemotherapy

Radiation-Treated Patients (radiation to head and neck)
Chapter 21

1. Patients treated by radiation tend to develop the following problems during and just after completion of therapy
   a. Mucositis
   b. Xerostomia
   c. Loss of taste
   d. Constricture of muscles (trismus)
   e. Secondary infections—viral, bacterial, fungal (candidiasis)
   f. Tooth sensitivity
2. Chronic problems caused by radiation therapy include:
   a. Xerostomia
   b. Cervical caries
   c. Osteonecrosis
   d. Muscle trismus
   e. Tooth sensitivity
   f. Loss of taste

1. Mucositis
2. Candidiasis
3. Xerostomia
4. Loss of taste
5. Trismus
6. Sensitivity of teeth
7. Cervical caries
8. Osteonecrosis

Prevention of Problems	Treatment Planning Modifications
1. Patients with oral soft tissue lesions and/or osseous lesions should have them biopsied by dentist or referred for diagnosis and treatment as indicated 2. Medical history should identify patients with diagnosed disease; medical consultation is needed to establish current status (See sections on chemotherapy and radiation therapy concerning prevention and management of medical complications)	1. Supportive dental care only for patients in terminal stage 2. General prognosis is poor, so complex dental procedures are usually not indicated 3. If thrombocytopenia or leukopenia is present, special precautions needed to prevent bleeding and infection (platelet replacement, antibiotic therapy) when invasive dental procedures are performed 4. Patients may be bleeders due to presence of abnormal immunoglobulin M macroglobulins, which form complexes with clotting factors, thus inactivating the clotting factors (See sections on chemotherapy and radiation therapy for treatment plan modifications)
1. Patients with generalized lymphadenopathy, extranodal tumors, and osseous lesions need to be identified and referred for medical evaluation and treatment 2. Dentist can biopsy extranodal or osseous lesions to establish a diagnosis; patients with lesions involving lymph nodes should be referred for needle biopsy 3. Medical history should identify patients with diagnosed disease; medical consultation will be needed to establish current status (See sections on chemotherapy and radiation therapy concerning management and prevention of medical complications)	1. Patients in terminal phase should receive only supportive dental treatment 2. Patient under "control" can receive any indicated treatment; however, complex restorative treatment may not be indicated in cases with poor prognosis 3. Platelet replacement may be needed for patients with thrombocytopenia (See sections on radiation therapy and chemotherapy for treatment plan modifications)

1. Before radiation therapy is started, dentist should be involved; and after a complete examination the following procedures should be done:
  a. Extract teeth that cannot be repaired
  b. Extract teeth with advanced periodontal disease
  c. Perform preprosthetic surgery
  d. Restore large carious lesions
  e. Perform surgeries with adequate time for healing or consider hyperbaric oxygen therapy
  f. Establish good oral hygiene
  g. Start daily fluoride treatment using flexible tray and gel
  h. Treat endodontically or extract nonvital teeth
  i. Treat chronic infection in jaw bones
2. During radiation treatment, dentist can be involved with the following:
  a. Symptomatic treatment of mucositis (see Appendix B)
  b. Management of xerostomia (see Appendix B)
	1. One radiation treatment has been completed and more than 6000 cGy used, every effort must be made to avoid osteonecrosis:
	  a. Teeth should not be extracted
	  b. Diseased teeth should be endodontically treated if indicated
	2. Aggressive preventive measures are needed to prevent periodontal disease and cervical caries
	3. Most dental procedures other than extractions and surgical procedures can be done if performed atraumatically and without vascular compromise

| Dental Management: A Summary—cont'd |

Potential Problems Related to Dental Care	Oral Manifestations

Radiation-Treated Patients (radiation to head and neck)—cont'd
Chapter 21

Patients Receiving Chemotherapy for Cancer
Chapter 21

1. Excessive bleeding because of bone marrow suppression (thrombocytopenia)	1. Mucositis
2. Prone to infection because of bone marrow suppression (leukopenia)	2. Excessive bleeding following minor trauma
3. Severe anemia from bone marrow suppression	3. Spontaneous gingival bleeding
4. Thrombocytopenia, leukopenia, and anemia possible complications of underlying cancer	4. Xerostomia
	5. Infection
	6. Poor healing

Prevention of Problems	**Treatment Planning Modifications**

    c. Prevention of trismus by having patient (use several) tongue blades in mouth as daily exercise

    d. Chlorhexidine rinses for plaque and candidiasis control (see Appendix B)

    e. Diagnosis and treatment of secondary infection—candidiasis, etc (see Appendix B)

    f. Continue daily fluoride treatment

3. Following radiation treatment, dentist should ensure the following:

    a. Have patient back for frequent recall appointments (every 3 to 4 months)

    b. Continue emphasis on good oral hygiene

    c. Treat carious lesions when first detected

    d. Make every effort to avoid oral infection

    e. Manage xerostomia (see Appendix B)

    f. Manage chronic loss of taste (see Appendix B)

Patients Receiving Chemotherapy for Cancer
Chapter 21

1. Before starting chemotherapy, the dentist should:

    a. Eliminate gross infection in the following areas:

        (1) Periapical

        (2) Periodontal

        (3) Soft tissue

    b. Treat advanced carious lesions

    c. Smooth sharp tooth edges

    d. Remove appliances

    e. Provide oral hygiene instructions

    f. Ensure that in children and young adults the following occur:

        (1) Mobile primary teeth removed

        (2) Gingival operculum removed

        (3) Adequate time allowed for healing before induction

2. During chemotherapy the dentist should:

    a. Consult with oncologist prior to any invasive dental procedures

    b. Perform the following if invasive procedures are required:

        (1) Consider antibiotic prophylaxis if granulocyte count less than $2000/mm^3$ or absolute neutrophil count less than $500/mm^3$

        (2) Consider platelet replacement if platelet count less than $50,000/mm^3$

    c. Perform culture and antibiotic sensitivity testing of exudate from areas of infection:

    d. Control spontaneous bleeding by gauze, periodontal packing, soft mouth guard

1. Perform only emergency dental treatment during chemotherapy

2. Based on prognosis of underlying disease, consider limiting dental treatment to only immediate care needs for patients being treated in palliative sense; however, children and adults being treated for leukemia may have very good prognosis, and any indicated dental treatment can be performed; also many patients with lymphoma can have good prognosis

Dental Management: A Summary—cont'd

Potential Problems Related to Dental Care	Oral Manifestations

Patients Receiving Chemotherapy for Cancer—cont'd
Chapter 21

Penile Implants
Chapter 21

No evidence suggests that these implants are at risk for infection from transient dental bacteremias	None

Breast Implants
Chapter 21

No risks	None

Intravascular Access Devices (Uldall catheter, central IV line, Broviac-Hickman device)
Chapter 21

High rate of infection but role of transient dental bacteremias causing these infections has not been established	None

Stroke
Chapter 22

1. Dental treatment could precipitate stroke 2. Bleeding is secondary to drug therapy	May have unilateral atrophy and one-sided neglect

Prevention of Problems	Treatment Planning Modifications

e. Use topical fluoride for caries control
f. Apply chlorhexidine rinses for plaque and candidiasis control (see Appendix B)
g. Provide symptomatic relief of mucositis and xerostomia (see Appendix B)
h. If severe anemia is present, avoid general anesthesia
i. Consider modifying home care instructions based on oral status, reduce or stop flossing and brushing if excessive bleeding or tissue irritation result; can use damp gauze to wipe gingiva and teeth; use solution of water and baking soda to rinse mouth to clean ulcerated tissues
j. Minimize food aversion during chemotherapy—fast before treatment (4 hours), eat novel nonimportant food just before treatment, avoid nutritionally important foods during posttreatment nausea
3. Following completion of chemotherapy:
  a. Monitor patient until all side effects of therapy have cleared
  b. Place patient on dental recall program	

Antibiotic prophylaxis not indicated for these patients based on available evidence; however need should be decided on individual patient basis following medical consultation	None
No special precautions	None
Determine need for antibiotic prophylaxis on an individual patient basis following medical consultation	Depends on reason for intravascular device

1. Identification of stroke-prone patient from history (hypertension, smoking, transient ischemic attacks, etc.)
2. Reduction of patient's risk factors for stroke
3. For past history of stroke:
  a. For current transient ischemic attacks—no elective care
  b. Delay elective care for 6 months
	1. Consideration of periodic panoramic film to assess carotid patency
	2. Dependent on physical impairment
	3. All restorations made easily cleansable—porcelain occlusals to be prevented
	4. Modified oral hygiene aids may be needed

Dental Management: A Summary—cont'd

Potential Problems Related to Dental Care	Oral Manifestations
Stroke—cont'd **Chapter 22**	
Seizure Disorder (epilepsy) **Chapter 22** 1. Occurrence of generalized tonic-clonic seizure in dental office 2. Drug-induced leukopenia and thrombocytopenia (phenytoin, carbamazepine, valproic acid)	1. Gingival overgrowth secondary to phenytoin (Dilantin) 2. Traumatic oral injuries 3. Drug-induced erythema multiform
Cerebrospinal Fluid Shunts **Chapter 22** Infection following transient dental bacteremias caused by invasive dental procedures	None

Prevention of Problems	**Treatment Planning Modifications**

c. Drug considerations include:
   (1) Aspirin and dipyridamole—obtain pretreatment bleeding time (less than 20 minutes)
   (2) Warfarin (Coumadin)—obtain prothrombin time ratio of 2.5 or less or INR of 3.5 or less
d. Short, morning appointments
e. Monitor blood pressure
f. Use minimum amount of vasoconstrictor in local anesthetic
g. No epinephrine in retraction cord

---

1. Identification of epileptic patient by history, including:
  a. Type of seizure
  b. Age at time of onset
  c. Cause of seizures
  d. Medications
  e. Regularity of physician visits
  f. Degree of control
  g. Frequency of seizures, last seizure
  h. Precipitating factors
  i. History of seizure-related injuries
2. Well controlled—normal care provided
3. Poorly controlled—consultation with physician; medication change may be required
4. Awareness of adverse effects of anticonvulsants
5. Patients taking valproic acid—bleeding time obtained, aspirin and nonsteroidal anti-inflammatory drug avoided
6. Propoxyphene and erythromycin not given to patients taking carbamazepine
7. Seizure managed by using a ligated mouth prop at beginning of appointment
	1. Maintenance of optimum oral hygiene
	2. Surgical reduction of gingival hyperplasia if indicated
	3. Replacement of missing teeth with fixed prosthesis as opposed to removable
	4. Metal used instead of porcelain when possible

---

1. Antibiotic prophylaxis indicated for ventriculoatrial shunts but not for ventriculoperitoneal shunts; confirm by medical consultation 2. Standard American Heart Association regimens recommended for patients with ventriculoatrial shunt when receiving invasive dental procedures	Usually none

Dental Management: A Summary—cont'd

Potential Problems Related to Dental Care	Oral Manifestations

Anxiety
Chapter 23

1. Extreme apprehension
2. Avoidance of dentistry
3. Elevation of blood pressure
4. Precipitation of arrhythmias
5. Side effects and drug interactions with agents used in dentistry (see section below on medications)

1. Usually none
2. Oral lesions associated with side effects of medications (see section below on medications)

Depression and Bipolar Disorders
Chapter 23

1. Little or no interest in oral health
2. Factors increasing risk of suicide:
   a. Age, adolescent, and elderly male
   b. Chronic illness, alcoholism, drug abuse, and depression
   c. Recent diagnosis of serious condition such as AIDS or cancer
   d. Previous suicide attempts
   e. Recent psychiatric hospitalization
   f. Loss of a loved one
   g. Living alone or little social contact
3. Taking medications that have significant side effects and that may interact with agents used by dentist (see section on medications below)

1. Depression—Poor oral hygiene and xerostomia associated with agents used to treat depression increase risk for periodontal disease and caries; facial pain syndromes, glossodynia
2. Manic disorder—injury to soft tissue and abrasion of teeth from over flossing and over brushing
3. Oral lesions associated with side effects of medications (see section below on medications)

Cocaine Abuse
Chapter 23

1. Dilated pupils, elevated blood pressure, and cardiac arrhythmia may indicate recent use
2. Myocardial ischemia
3. Cardiac arrhythmias
4. Vasopressors such as epinephrine and levonordefrin can precipitate hypertensive crisis, myocardial infarction, arrhythmia, or stroke
5. Patients with rash secondary to cocaine use may react to ester-type local anesthetics
6. Injecting drug abuse increases risk of infection by hepatitis B virus, hepatitis C virus and HIV (needle tracks)

Rare gingival recession and tooth abrasion when chronically rubbed on facial gingiva

Prevention of Problems	Treatment Planning Modifications

1. For behavioral, the dentist should provide the following:
  a. Provide good communication (open, honest)
  b. Explain what is to happen
  c. Make procedures as "pain free" as possible
  d. Encourage patient to ask questions at any time
  e. Hypnosis, relaxation techniques
2. For pharmacologic, the dentist should provide the following as indicated:
  a. Oral sedation
  b. Inhalation sedation
  c. Intramuscular sedation
  d. Intravenous sedation
  e. Analgesics for pain control
	1. Postpone complex dental procedures until patient is more comfortable in dental environment
	2. Posttraumatic stress disorder—very important to attempt to develop trust and to establish communication with these patients
	3. May need to refer patients with panic attack or phobic symptoms related to dentistry for diagnosis and treatment

1. If patients appear very depressed:
  a. Ask if they have thought of suicide
    (1) Do they state a plan?
    (2) Do they have the means to carry out the plan?
  b. Immediately refer patients who are suicide candidates for medical intervention
  c. Involve a family member
2. Obtain good history including medications patient is taking and avoid using agents that have significant interactions (see Tables 23-10, 23-12)
3. If history and examination findings suggest presence of significant drug side effects refer patient to the patient's physician
	1. Patients often have little interest in dental health or home care procedures and poor dental repair is common
	2. Emphasis should be on maintaining best possible oral health during the depressive episode
	3. Dental treatment should be directed toward immediate needs with elective and complex procedures put off until effective medical treatment is obtained

1. Do not treat patients who are "high" on cocaine or show signs of recent use 2. Wait at least 6 hours after cocaine administration before performing any dental treatment (Cocaine effects take several hours to wear off) 3. Avoid ester-type local anesthetics in patients who have skin rash associated with cocaine use 4. Use infectious disease control procedures for all patients 5. Avoid narcotic analgesics for recovering addict	1. Care must be taken in selection of medications used for sedation and pain control 2. Tolerance may be present for sedative drugs and local anesthetics requiring increased dosage which increases risk for toxic side effects 3. Cocaine abusers may be using other drugs and may try to get prescriptions for strong pain medications, steal prescription pads or drugs 4. The dentist should not prescribe addictive substances 5. Anxiety control should be provided with propranolol if needed 6. Pain control using nonsteroidal anti-inflammatory drugs should be provided

Dental Management: A Summary—cont'd

Potential Problems Related to Dental Care	Oral Manifestations

Alzheimer's Disease
Chapter 23

1. Patient may be difficult to communicate with
2. Patient may be unable to perform home care procedures such as flossing and brushing
3. Patient may be unable to cooperate during dental treatment
4. Significant drug side effects and interactions with agents used by the dentist may occur (see section below on medications)

1. Oral injuries
2. Poor oral hygiene
3. Incrased risk for periodontal disease and caries
4. Oral lesions may develop due to side effects of medications used to control symptoms associated with the disease (see medications section below)

Schizophrenia
Chapter 23

1. Patient may be difficult to communicate with and uncooperative during dental care
2. Significant drug side effects are common and agents used by the dentist may interact with medications the patient is taking (see section below on medications)

1. Usually none
2. Oral lesions may be self-inflicted or develop as side effects of medications used to treat the patient (see section below on medications)

Eating Disorders: Anorexia nervosa, bulimia nervosa
Chapter 23

1. Patients with anorexia are in a state of self starvation (severe weight loss) and may be subject to hypotension, bradycardia, severe arrhythmias and death
2. Bulimic patients are at risk for serum electrolyte disturbances, esophageal or gastric rupture, cardiac arrhythmias and death
3. Patients with bulimia may induce vomiting by use of physical means (finger in throat) or use of ipecac (may cause myopathy or cardiomyopathy), laxatives and diuretics also are used by bulimics to purge
4. Some patients may show signs and symptoms of both anorexia and bulimia

1. In bulimia the following are noticed:
   a. Dental erosion of the lingual surfaces of teeth (usually maxillary teeth)
   b. Patients with poor oral hygiene may have increased risk for caries and periodontal disease
   c. Extensive dental caries (associated with the diet— lots of carbohydrates)
   d. Parotid gland swelling
   e. Tooth sensitivity to thermal changes
2. In anorexia, the following are noticed:
   a. Usually none
   b. Patients with poor oral hygiene may have increased risk for periodontal disease and caries

Prevention of Problems	Treatment Planning Modifications
1. Identify by history, medications and signs and symptoms 2. Refer patients with signs and symptoms of Alzheimer's disease 3. Consult with patient's physician concerning patient's current status, medications and review dental management plan 4. Work with relatives or health care providers who will need to provide dental home care for patients with advanced disease	1. Establish good oral hygiene and dental repair early in the course of the disease; initiate an aggressive preventive program with 3-month recall 2. Use an empathetic approach and provide positive nonverbal communication 3. Try to keep the patient's attention by using short words and sentences; repeat important ideas, concepts or directions; and look directly into the patient's eyes 4. Early in the disease plan fixed prostheses; this will eliminate the problem with misplacing or losing removable ones as the disease progresses 5. If sedation is needed use choral hydrate or oxazepam 6. With advancing disease shorten appointments 7. Use treatment plan that is realistic, flexible and dynamic with the emphasis on maintaining oral health and comfort
1. Have family member or attendant accompany patient 2. Schedule morning appointments 3. Avoid confrontational and authoritative attitude 4. Perform elective dental care only if patient is under good medical management 5. Consider sedation with chloral hydrate, diazepam, or oxazepam	1. Emphasis on maintaining oral health and comfort by preventing and controlling dental disease 2. Family member or attendant may have to assist patient with home care procedures 3. Complex dental procedures are usually not indicated
1. Patients with severe weight loss and no history of cancer or other illnesses and who are hypotensive should be referred for medical evaluation 2. Attempts should be made to ascertain the cause of dental erosion involving the lingual surfaces of the teeth. Consider referral for medical evaluation. 3. For the patient to act on these recommendations the dentist needs to point out to the patient the serious complications of anorexia (hypotension, severe arrhythmias and death) and bulimia (gastric and esophageal tears, cardiac arrhythmias and death	1. Avoid elective dental procedures until patient is stable from a cardiac standpoint 2. In general, for both anorexic and bulimic patients the emphasis should be on oral hygiene maintenance and noncomplex repair until significant improvement of their condition has occurred from a medical standpoint 3. Complex restorative procedures should be avoided in bulimic patients until the purging has been corrected. However, crowns may have to be placed to stabilize a tooth or protect it from thermal symptoms in patients who are actively purging

Dental Management: A Summary—cont'd

Potential Problems Related to Dental Care	Oral Manifestations

Antipsychotic (neuroleptic) Drugs
   chlorpromazine (Thorazine)
   fluphenazine (Prolixin)
   trifluoperazine (Stelazine)
   thiothixene (Navane)
   haloperidol (Haldol)
   risperidone (Risperdal)
   molindone (Moran)

Chapter 23

1. Drug side effects include the following:
   a. Hypotension
   b. Tardive dyskinesia
   c. Dystonia
   d. Xerostomia
   e. Neuroleptic malignant syndrome
   f. Agranulocytosis
2. Drug interactions include the following:
   a. Prolong/intensify effects of:
      (1) Sedatives, hypnotics
      (2) Opioids, antihistamines
   b. Epinephrine (hypotensive crisis)

No significant oral findings associated with medications unless following drug side effects are present:
   a. Agranulocytosis—ulceration, infection
   b. Xerostomia—mucositis, periodontal disease, dental caries
   c. Thrombocytopenia—bleeding
   d. Leukopenia—infection
   e. Uncontrollable movement of tongue and lips (tardive dyskinesia)

Antidepressant Drugs
   Heterocyclics—
      amitriptyline (Elavil)
      imipramine (Tofranil)
      amoxapine (Asendin)
   SSRIs—
      Fluoxetine (Prozac)
      Sertraline (Zoloft)
      Paroxetine (Paxil)
   SNRIs—
      Nefazodone (Serzone)
      Venlafaxine (Effexor)
   Monoamine oxidase inhibitors
      Phenelzine (Mardil)
      Isocarboxazid (Marplan)
      Tranylcypromine (Parnate)
   Others—
      Bupropion (Wellbutrin)
      Trazodone (Desyrel)

Chapter 23

1. Drug side effects include the following:
   a. Xerostomia
   b. Hypotension

1. No significant oral findings associated with medications unless following drug side effects are present:
   a. Xerostomia—periodontal disease, mucositis, dental caries

Prevention of Problems	**Treatment Planning Modifications**

1. Identification of patients:
  a. Obtain history of mental disorder (patient may be taking antipsychotic medication)
  b. Ask patient to list all drugs
  c. Identify patients with recent onset of side effects
2. Referral of patients with significant side effects
3. Consultation with physician to confirm current status and medications
4. Reduction of dosage or avoidance of:
  a. Epinephrine
  b. Sedatives, hypnotics, opioids, antihistamines
	1. Local anesthetic guidelines include:
	  a. Use without vasoconstrictor for most dental procedures if possible
	  b. For surgical or complex restorative procedures, epinephrine is vasoconstrictor of choice
	    (1) Use 1:100,000 concentration
	    (2) Aspirate before injecting
	    (3) Use no more than 2 cartridges
	2. Don't use topical epinephrine to control bleeding or in retraction cord
	3. Based on patient's needs and wants any dental procedure can be provided
	4. Provide treatment to deal with xerostomia (see Appendix B)
	5. Patients with tardive dyskinesia may be difficult to manage, if this side effect has just started refer the patient to the patient's physician for evaluation and possible change in medication

1. Identify patients by medical and drug history 2. Identify patients with significant drug side effects: a. History	1. Avoid elective dental procedures until depression has been managed by medication or behavioral means

Dental Management: A Summary—cont'd

Potential Problems Related to Dental Care	Oral Manifestations
Antidepressant Drugs—cont'd **Chapter 23** c. Orthostatic hypotension d. Arrhythmias e. Nausea and vomiting f. Leukopenia, anemia g. Thrombocytopenia h. Mania, seizures i. Myocardial infarction, stroke j. Hypertension (venlafaxine) k. Loss of libido 2. Drug interactions (Caveat: Don't mix the different classes of antidepressant drugs) include the following: a. Epinephrine (1) Hypertensive crisis (2) Myocardial infarction b. Sedatives, hypnotics, narcotics, barbiturates respiratory depression c. Atropine; increase intraocular pressure d. Warfarin metabolism may be inhibited—overdosage	b. Thrombocytopenia—bleeding c. Leukopenia—infection
Anxiolytic Drugs (anxiety control) Benzodiazepines— **chlordiazepoxide (Librium)** **diazepam (Valium)** **lorazepam (Ativan)** **oxazepam (Serax)** **alprazolam (Xanax)** **Chapter 23** 1. Drugs side effects include the following: a. Daytime sedation b. Aggressive behavior c. Amnesia (older adults) 2. Drug interactions (CNS depression): a. Antipsychotic agents b. Antidepressants c. Narcotics d. Sedative agents e. Antihistamines f. H_2 histamine receptor blockers	1. Usually no significant oral findings
Antimanic Drugs **lithium (Lithobid)** **valproic acid (Depacon)** **carbamazepine (Tegretol)** **Chapter 23** 1. Lithium a. Side effects include the following: (1) Nausea, vomiting, diarrhea (2) Metallic taste (3) Hypothyroidism	1. Lithium (metallic taste) 2. Carbamazepine and valproic acid show the following: a. Oral ulcerations b. Bleeding

Prevention of Problems	Treatment Planning Modifications

b. Examination—blood pressure, pulse, bleeding, soft tissue lesions infection
3. Refer patients with significant drug side effects
4. Consult with physician to confirm current status and medications
5. Minimize effects of orthostatic hypotension
  a. Change chair position slowly
  b. Support patient, as they get out of dental chair
6. Avoid atropine in patients with glaucoma
7. Use epinephrine with caution and only in small concentration
8. Look up specific medication patient is taking for significant side effects associated with the drug and possible drug interactions with agents used in dentistry
	2. Local anesthetic:
	  a. Use without vasoconstrictor for most dental procedures if possible
	  b. For surgical or complex restorative procedures, epinephrine is vasoconstrictor of choice
	    (1) Use 1:100,000 concentration
	    (2) Aspirate before injecting
	    (3) Use no more than 2 cartridges
	3. Do not use topical epinephrine to control bleeding or in retraction cord
	4. Provide treatment to deal with xerostomia (see Appendix B)

1. Advise patient not to drive when using these medications 2. Use reduced dosage in older adults 3. Do not dispense or reduce dosage for patients on other central nervous system depressant drugs 4. Use in reduced dosage in patients taking: cimetidine, ranitidine, or erythromycin 5. Do not dispense to patients with narrow-angle glaucoma	1. Do not give over-sedation when using sedative agents, narcotics, or antihistamines: reduce dosage or do not use these agents 2. All dental procedures can be provided to patients on these medications 3. Use the anxiolytic drugs in dentistry for short durations to avoid tolerance and dependency
1. Identify patients by medical and drug history who are taking these medications 2. Refer to physician when significant drug side effects occur	1. No special modifications in the treatment plan of patients well controlled with lithium or anticonvulsant drugs 2. Patients with signs or symptoms of lithium toxicity should be referred to their physician for evaluation

Dental Management: A Summary—cont'd	
Potential Problems Related to Dental Care	**Oral Manifestations**

Antimanic Drugs—cont'd

Chapter 23

    (4) Diabetes insipidus

    (5) Arrhythmias

    (6) Sedation

    (7) Seizures

  b. Drug interactions (toxicity) include the following:

    (1) Nonsteroidal anti-inflammatory drugs

    (2) Diuretics

    (3) Erythromycin

2. Valproic acid and carbamazepine

  a. Side effects include the following:

    (1) Nausea, ataxia, blurred vision

    (2) Tremor

    (3) Agranulocytosis (infection)

    (4) Platelet dysfunction (bleeding)

    (5) Seizures if abruptly stopped

  b. Drug interactions (toxicity) include the following:

    (1) Erythromycin

    (2) Isoniazid

    (3) Cimetidine

Oral Manifestations:

  c. Oral infections

  d. Tremor of the tongue

Osteoarthritis

Chapter 24

1. Joint pain, stiffness, and loss of mobility
2. Difficulty maintaining oral hygiene
3. Increased bleeding from aspirin or nonsteroidal anti-inflammatory drugs

Oral Manifestations:

1. Potential for plaque accumulation
2. Temporomandibular joint involvement

Rheumatoid Arthritis

Chapter 24

1. Joint pain and immobility
2. Difficulty maintaining oral hygiene
3. Increased bleeding secondary to aspirin and non-steroidal anti-inflammatory drugs
4. Bone marrow suppression from gold salts, penicillamine, sulfasalazine, or immunosuppressives—resulting in anemia, agranulocytosis, or thrombocytopenia

Oral Manifestations:

1. Potential for plaque accumulation
2. Temporomandibular joint involvement—anterior open-bite possible
3. Stomatitis secondary to gold salts, penicillamine, and immunosuppressives

Prevention of Problems	Treatment Planning Modifications
3. Avoid the use of nonsteroidal anti-inflammatory drugs and erythromycin or use in reduced dosage in patients on lithium 4. Avoid the use of erythromycin or use in reduced dosage in patients taking valproic acid or carbamazepine	3. Nonsteroidal anti-inflammatory drugs should be avoided or used in reduced dosage for pain control in patients taking lithium to prevent lithium toxicity 4. Erythromycin should not be used for infections as lithium toxicity could result 5. Patients on the anticonvulsant drugs (valproic acid or carbamazepine) who develop oral ulcerations, infection or bleeding should be referred for medical evaluation 6. Erythromycin should be avoided in patients taking valproic acid or carbamazepine

1. Short appointments
2. Physical comfort ensured by the following:
  a. Position changes
  b. Comfortable chair position
  c. Physical supports
3. Aspirin or nonsteroidal anti-inflammatory drugs may result in increased bleeding but usually not clinically significant
4. If joint prosthesis, antibiotic prophylaxis not necessary unless "high risk" (rheumatoid arthritis, diabetic, immunosuppressed, or previous infection) condition
	Dictated by severity of disability; if severe, extensive treatment not indicated; oral hygiene encouraged

1. Short appointments
2. Physical comfort
  a. Position changes
  b. Comfortable chair position
  c. Physical supports
3. Management of drug complications
  a. Aspirin or nonsteroidal antiinflammatory drugs (nonsteroidal anti-inflammatory drugs)—may result in increased bleeding but not usually clinically significant
	Dictated by severity of disability and temporomandibular joint involvement; if severe, extensive treatment not needed; temporomandibular joint surgery may be indicated; oral hygiene encouraged

Dental Management: A Summary—cont'd

Potential Problems Related to Dental Care	Oral Manifestations

Rheumatoid Arthritis—cont'd
Chapter 24

Systemic Lupus Erythematosus
Chapter 24

1. Systemic manifestations
2. Possible bleeding tendency
3. Infection susceptibility
4. Adrenal suppression (taking corticosteroids)
5. Infective endocarditis (rare)

Drug-induced stomatitis

Leukemia
Chapter 24

1. Prolonged bleeding
2. Infection
3. Delayed healing

1. Infection
2. Ulceration
3. Gingival bleeding
4. Ecchymoses
5. Petechiae
6. Gingival hyperplasia
7. Soft tissue and osseous lesions
8. Paresthesias—numbness, burning, tingling
9. Candidiasis
10. Lymphadenopathy

Prevention of Problems	Treatment Planning Modifications
b. Gold salts, penicillamine, sulfasalazine, or immunosuppressives—obtain complete blood count with differential and bleeding time c. Corticosteroids—possible need for supplements 4. If joint prosthesis, prophylactic antibiotics recommended	

1. Consultation physician re: systemic manifestations—manage appropriately (e.g., kidney failure)
 2. Drug considerations
   a. Aspirin and nonsteroidal anti-inflammatory drug can cause increased bleeding but not usually clinically significant
   b. Gold salts, penicillamine, sulfasalazine, or immunosuppressives—obtain CBC with differential; bleeding time
   c. Corticosteroids—possible need for supplements
 3. Leukopenia with corticosteroids—postsurgical antibiotics recommended
 4. Platelets $<50,000/mm^3$—consult physician
 5. Elevated PTT *not* associated with bleeding problems
 6. If susceptible to infective endocarditis—prophylactic antibiotics advised
	None

1. Detection and referral for diagnosis and treatment
 2. Determination of platelet status on day of any surgical procedure, including scaling of teeth; bleeding time is within normal range, proceed; if not, postpone procedure (platelet count less than $50,000/mm^3$)
 3. Prevention of postoperative infection when absolute neutrophil count less than $500/mm^3$ by prophylactic use of antibiotics (see below recommendations)
   a. Most situations covered by the following:
     (1) 2 g penicillin V orally at least 30 minutes before procedure
     (2) Give 500 mg penicillin V orally every 6 hours for remaining part of appointment day
   b. Alternative: give 1 g of cephalexin 1 hour before procedure, followed by 250 mg cephalexin every 6 hours for 1 week
   c. For patients allergic to penicillin give 300 mg of clindamycin orally 1 hour before procedure, 150 mg every 6 hours for the next 3 to 7 days
	1. During acute stages of disease, avoidance of dental care of any kind if at all possible
	 2. When patient is in state of remission, all active dental disease should be treated and patient placed on good hygiene maintenance program
	 3. Avoidance of long, drawn-out dental procedures
	 4. Complex restorative procedures usually not indicated for patients with poor prognosis
	 (See Appendix B for treatment regimens for oral complications of leukemia)

Dental Management: A Summary—cont'd

Potential Problems Related to Dental Care	Oral Manifestations

Leukemia—cont'd
Chapter 24

Joint Prostheses
Chapter 24

Deep infection is possible secondary to bacteremia caused by acute infection elsewhere in body; no evidence exists that transient bacteremias caused by invasive dental procedures can infect these prostheses

Several authors have suggested that patients with active rheumatoid arthritis, severe type I diabetes mellitus, congenital or acquired immune deficiency, hemophilia, patients with a loose prosthesis or history of infection of the prosthesis may be at risk, but little data exist to support this concept

None

Solid Organ Transplantation
Chapter 25

Common problems found in all patients

1. Infection from suppression of immune response by the following:
   a. Cyclosporine
   b. Azathioprine
   c. Prednisone
   d. Antithymocyte globulin
   e. Antilymphocyte globulin
   f. Orthoclone (monoclonal antibody)
2. Acute rejection, reversible
3. Chronic rejection, nonreversible, includes the following:
   a. Graft failure—endstage organ failure
   b. Bleeding—liver, kidney
   c. Drug overdosage—liver, kidney
   d. Death or need for transplantation—heart, liver
   e. Need for transplantation or hemodialysis—kidney
   f. Need for transplantation or insulin—pancreas

1. Usually none
2. Excessive immune suppression includes the following:
   a. Candidiasis
   b. Herpes simplex
   c. Herpes zoster
   d. Hairy leukoplakia
   e. Lymphoma
   f. Kaposi's sarcoma
   g. Aphthous stomatitis
   h. Squamous cell carcinoma of lip
3. Side effects of immunosuppressant drugs include:
   a. Bleeding (spontaneous)
   b. Infection
   c. Ulceration
   d. Petechiae
   e. Ecchymoses
   f. Gingival hyperplasia
   g. Salivary gland dysfunction

Prevention of Problems	Treatment Planning Modifications
d. Based on special conditions and medical consultation, other agents, dosage, and duration of treatment may be indicated	

1. Obtain good history from patient
2. Obtain medical consultation regarding need for prophylaxis (little data exist to support the use of antibiotic prophylaxis; in contrast, most orthopaedic surgeons still recommend prophylaxis)
3. If orthopedic consultant does not recommend prophylaxis, proceed without it
4. If orthopedic consultant recommends prophylaxis (most orthopedic surgeons recommend a cephalosporin), consider the following:
  a. Review current state of clinical and research data with consultant in an attempt to modify recommendation
  b. Inform patient of known data and lack of proven risk with dental procedures and infection of their prosthesis, based on informed consent proceed with or without prophylaxis
  c. Let orthopedic surgeon prescribe antibiotic prophylaxis
  d. Follow recommendation knowing there is little to no benefit with some risk for adverse reaction to antibiotic
	None

1. Dental evaluation and treatment before transplantation includes the following:
  a. Establish stable oral and dental status free of active dental disease
  b. Initiate aggressive oral hygiene program to maintain oral health
  c. Arrange medical consultation for patients with organ failure before performing needed dental treatment to establish the following:
    (1) Degree of failure
    (2) Current status of patient
    (3) Need for antibiotic prophylaxis
    (4) Need to modify drug selection or dosage
    (5) Need to take special precautions to avoid bleeding
    (6) If surgery is indicated, access to recent prothrombin time, partial thromboplastin time, bleeding time, and white cell count or differential may be needed
	1. Before transplantation consider the following:
	  a. For patients with poor dental status, consider extractions and full dentures
	  b. With patients with good dental status perform the following:
	    (1) Maintain dentition
	    (2) Establish aggressive oral hygiene program in the following areas:
	      (a) Toothbrushing, flossing
	      (b) Diet modification if indicated
	      (c) Topical fluorides
	      (d) Plaque control, calculus removal
	      (e) Chlorhexidine or Listerine mouth rinse
	    (3) Treat all active dental disease in the following areas:
	      (a) Extraction—nonrestorable teeth
	      (b) Endodontics—nonvital teeth

Dental Management: A Summary—cont'd

Potential Problems Related to Dental Care	Oral Manifestations

Solid Organ Transplantation—cont'd
Chapter 25
Common problems found in all patients—cont'd

4. Cancer associated with use of immunosuppressants:
   a. Squamous cell carcinoma of skin
   b. Squamous cell carcinoma of lip
   c. Lymphoma
   d. Kaposi's sarcoma
5. Side effects of drugs used to suppress the immune response include the following:
   a. Hypertension
   b. Diabetes mellitus
   c. Osteoporosis
   d. Psychoses
   e. Anemia
   f. Leukopenia
   g. Thrombocytopenia
   h. Gingival hyperplasia
   i. Adrenocortical suppression
   j. Tumors (listed above)
   k. Poor healing
   l. Bleeding
   m. Infection

4. Graft failure includes:
   a. Uremic stomatitis (kidney)
   b. Bleeding (liver)
   c. Petechiae (liver, kidney)
   d. Ecchymoses (liver)

Heart Transplantation Special Considerations
Chapter 25

1. Patient may be on long-term anticoagulation therapy; excessive bleeding may occur with surgical procedures
2. Graft atherosclerosis may occur, increasing risk for myocardial infarction
3. No nerve supply exists to the transplanted heart; thus pain will not be symptom of an MI
4. Some patients require cardiac pacing; electrical equipment may interfere with pacemaker

Usually none
See above

Prevention of Problems	**Treatment Planning Modifications**

2. Dental treatment after transplantation includes the following:
   a. Immediate posttransplant period (6 months):
      (1) Provide emergency dental care only
      (2) Continue oral hygiene procedures
   b. Stable graft period.
      (1) Maintain oral hygiene
      (2) Recall every 3 months
      (3) Use universal precautions
      (4) Vaccinate dental staff against HBV infection
      (5) Schedule medical consultation on the following topics:
         (a) Need for antibiotic prophylaxis
         (b) Need for precautions to avoid excessive bleeding
         (c) Need for supplemental steroids
         (d) Selection of drugs and dosage
      (6) Examine for clinical evidence of the following:
         (a) Organ failure or rejection
         (b) Overimmunosuppression (tumors, infection, etc)
      (7) Monitor blood pressure at every appointment
      (8) If evidence of drug side effects, graft rejection, or overimmunosuppression is found, refer patient to physician
   c. Chronic rejection period
      (1) Perform immediate or emergency dental care only
      (2) Follow guidelines for stable graft when treatment is performed

   (c) Carious teeth restoration
   (d) Complex dental prostheses, etc. deferred until after transplantation
   c. Patients with dental status between above extremes:
      (1) Decision to maintain natural dentition must be made on individual patient basis
      (2) Factors to be considered:
         (a) Extent and severity of dental disease
         (b) Importance of teeth to patient
         (c) Cost of maintaining natural dentition
         (d) Systemic status of patient and prognosis
      (3) Physical ability to maintain good oral hygiene
2. Following transplantation:
   a. Immediate posttransplantation period—limit dental care to emergency needs
   b. Stable graft period—base treatment plan on needs and desires of patient; recall every 3 to 6 months
   c. Chronic rejection period—limit dental care to immediate or emergency needs
   d. Maintain aggressive oral hygiene program throughout all periods
   e. Consult with physician to confirm patient's current status and need for special precautions

---

1. Have physician modify degree of anticoagulation to 2.5 normal prothrombin time or less (INR 3.5 or less) if surgical procedures are planned
2. Consult with physician to establish status of coronary vessels of transplanted heart; if advanced graft atherosclerosis is present, manage as described under section on coronary atherosclerotic heart disease
3. Be aware of signs and symptoms of MI other than pain; if these occur, obtain immediate medical assistance for patient
4. Do not use Cavitron or electrosurgery in patients with pacemaker

1. American Heart Association has stated that there is inconclusive evidence regarding need for antibiotic prophylaxis for prevention of endocarditis in patients with heart transplantation
2. American Heart Association recommends that the need for prophylaxis be determined on an individual patient basis following consultation with physician
3. If prophylaxis is decided on, standard amoxicillin regimen of American Heart Association would be appropriate

Dental Management: A Summary—cont'd

Potential Problems Related to Dental Care	Oral Manifestations
Liver Transplantation Special Considerations **Chapter 25** 1. Drugs that may be toxic to liver must not be prescribed 2. Some patients may be on anticoagulation medication 3. Excessive bleeding could occur with surgical procedures	See Solid Organ Transplantation, previous pages
Kidney Transplantation Special Considerations **Chapter 25** Drugs that may be toxic to kidney must not prescribed	See Solid Organ Transplantation, previous pages
Pancreas Transplantation **Chapter 25** No special considerations	See Solid Organ Transplantation, previous pages

Bone Marrow Transplantation
Chapter 25
1. Immune suppression and pancytopenia resulting from conditioning therapy includes:
  a. Total body irradiation
  b. Cyclophosphamide
  c. Busulfan
2. Problems during conditioning phase and critical phase (until transplanted marrow become functional) includes:
  a. Infection
  b. Bleeding
  c. Poor healing
3. Immune suppression resulting from maintenance medications used to prevent graft-versus-host disease and chronic rejection
  a. Cyclosporine
  b. Prednisone
  c. Methotrexate
4. Problems during maintenance phase include:
  a. Infection
  b. Others listed above under solid organ transplantation relating to medication(s) being used
5. Graft-vs.-host disease and chronic rejection:
  a. Infection
  b. Bleeding
	1. Mucositis
	2. Gingivitis
	3. Xerostomia
	4. Candidiasis
	5. Herpes simplex infections
	6. Osteoradionecrosis
	7. Gingival hyperplasia (with cyclosporine)

Older Adults: falls **Chapter 26** 1. Falling in dental reception area or in operatory. 2. Patient who is taking multiple medications may be at increased risk for falls	1. Tooth fracture 2. Jaw fracture

Prevention of Problems	Treatment Planning Modifications
1. Avoid drugs that are toxic to liver 2. Have physician modify degree of anticoagulant to $2\frac{1}{2}$ times normal prothrombin time or less	Need for prophylactic antibiotics for invasive dental procedures in patients with stable liver transplants should be determined on individual patient basis by medical consultation
Avoid drugs that are toxic to kidney	Need for prophylactic antibiotics for invasive dental procedures in patients with stable kidney transplants should be determined on individual patient basis by medical consultation
	Need for prophylactic antibiotics for invasive dental procedures in patients with stable pancreas transplants should be determined on individual patient basis by medical consultation

1. Avoid dental treatment during conditioning and critical phases of bone marrow transplantation
2. Treat all active dental disease prior to bone marrow transplantation
3. Observe requirements for antibiotic prophylaxis for invasive dental procedures:
   a. Indicated if procedures must be performed on emergency basis during conditioning or critical phases of bone marrow transplantation
   b. Need should be determined by medical consultation
   (See Solid Organ Transplantation [previous pages] for details of hygiene program and dental management)
	1. If possible, treat active dental disease before transplantation
	2. Prognosis varies based on reason for transplantation, source of marrow to be transplanted, and techniques used to condition and maintain patient; other factors affecting prognosis include age and general health status; complex dental prostheses may not be indicated for many patients
	(See Solid Organ Transplantation, previous pages, for other suggested treatment planning considerations)
	(For management of soft tissue complications, see Appendix B)

1. Move chair position slowly, help patient out of chair and support for first few steps	Usually none

Dental Management: A Summary—cont'd

Potential Problems Related to Dental Care	Oral Manifestations

Older Adults: falls—cont'd
Chapter 26

3. Patient with dementia, musculoskeletal disorders, proprioceptive dysfunction or peripheral neuropathy also may be at increased risk for falls

3. Soft tissue lacerations
4. Bleeding

Older Adults: poor eyesight, loss of hearing, dementia, advanced illness
Chapter 26

1. Difficult to fill out health and dental history questionnaire
2. Unable to hear questions or directions
3. Difficult to follow directions
4. Unable to sit still during appointment
5. Difficult or impossible to render effective home dental care

1. Usually none
2. Periodontal disease, recurrent caries, mucositis, xerostomia, fractured restorations, infections, and others depending on the medical illness and medications used to treat it

Older Adults: organ system, changes associated with advanced age
Chapter 26

1. General—increase in fat, decrease in body water
   a. Less effect of fat soluble drugs
   b. Increased effect of water soluble drugs
2. Immune system—decrease in numbers of lymphocytes and their response to antigens with increased risk for infection and cancer
3. Musculoskeletal—decrease in muscle mass and bone density with increased risk for fracture of bones and functional impairment
4. Cardiovascular—increased risk for syncope, heart failure and heart block
5. Respiratory system—decreased lung elasticity and increased chest wall stiffness decreasing ventilation and perfusion causing decrease in Po_2. Can lead to breathing difficulty during some dental procedures
6. Endocrine—blood glucose increase in response to illness, decreased vitamin D absorption and activation, and decreased T_4 clearance. These changes can complicate diabetes, increase risk for osteomalacia and fracture or cause thyroid dysfunction
7. Nervous system—decrease in catechol synthesis, dopaminergic synthesis and righting reflexes. These changes can result in benign forgetfulness, stiffer gait and increased body sway (increasing risk for falls)

1-3. Usually none, but in severe cases increased risk of fracture of mandible and loss of masculatory muscle function. Increased incidence of periodontal disease.
4. Usually none
Oral complications based on those associated with diabetes, hypothyroidism, renal failure, dementia, and major depression—see respective topics in summary table

Prevention of Problems	Treatment Planning Modifications
2. Consult with physician to see if number of medications can be reduced or dosage of any medications could be reduced 3. Plan short appointments, may have to transfer patient from wheelchair to dental chair 4. Have spouse or relative accompany patient to dental office	
1. Have spouse or relative help fill out questionnaire or take history orally 2. Speak slowly and directly to the patient increasing the volume of your voice 3. Use non-verbal communication to show what you want the patient to do 4. Schedule short appointments 5. Train spouse or relative to provide basic oral home care needs	1. None for patients with loss of hearing and poor eyesight who are in good general health 2. Patients with significant dementia or advanced illness are not candidates for complex dental procedures, the emphasis should be on maintaining as good of oral and dental health as possible
1. Increase dosage for fat soluble drugs and decrease dosage for water soluble drugs 2. Avoid oral infection and when it does occur treat with local and systemic means, search for oral cancer 3. Avoid accidents in the dental office, may impact on oral surgery and periodontal surgical procedures 4. Don't treat patients in active congestive heart failure (refer patients for medical treatment), avoid epinephrine in patients with severe arrhythmias 5. Do not use rubber dam and bilateral mandibular blocks if severe and drugs that will suppress the respiratory center such as barbiturates and narcotics. Treat in upright chair position if severe 6. Refer patients with signs or symptoms of diabetes mellitus, hypothyroidism, or history of fracture, consider vitamin D and calcium supplementation 7. Refer to rule out dementia, depression, and Parkinson's disease, take actions listed above to avoid falls in the dental office	1-3. The change in body composition seen with advancing age does not impact on the selection of treatment options for the older adult except for cases with extreme loss of muscle mass and bone density. In these cases certain complex oral surgery or periodontal surgery procedures may not be indicated 4. Complex or elective dental procedures are not indicated for patients with heart failure that is non-responsive to medical treatment 5. Avoid complex dental procedures for patients with severe pulmonary dysfunction 6. The changes seen in the endocrine system in general will not affect the selection of dental procedures unless complicated by diabetes, hypothyroidism, or renal failure 7. The changes seen in the nervous system in general will not affect the selection of dental procedures unless complicated by dementia, major depression, or severe peripheral neuropathy

A Guide to Management of Common Medical Emergencies in the Dental Office

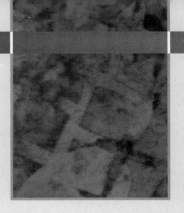

GENERAL CONSIDERATIONS

The best management of a dental office medical emergency is prevention. Dental practitioners must be prepared to treat the seemingly well but chronically ill patient whose condition is managed by a variety of drugs. Dentists and their office staffs must be aware of the pathophysiologic factors regulating disease processes and the pharmacodynamics of drug action and interaction. Patients frequently experience physical reactions and this places considerable responsibility on the dentist to meet any emergencies quickly, efficiently, and competently with adequate resuscitative procedures. The health professional is responsible and required to use those techniques that are known, practiced, safe, and efficient. An unfamiliar or unreliable maneuver should never be attempted. The dentist must be trained in providing basic cardiac life support (BCLS) and in many cases advanced cardiac life support (ACLS).

The dentist should be prepared to provide resuscitative procedures in emergency situations but should give even more consideration to preventing them. This can be accomplished by obtaining an adequate history of the patient, making an appropriate physical evaluation, and ensuring that the patient and environment are prepared before treatment. Sometimes emergencies may be prevented through the recognition of physical limitations before treatment begins.

The management of emergencies must begin long before a misadventure occurs. The dentist must be prepared

Much of the material contained herein is adapted, with permission, from: Malamed SF: *Medical Emergencies in the Dental Office*, ed 3, St Louis, 2000, Mosby; and American Heart Association Guidelines for Basic Cardiac Life Support and Advanced Cardiac Life Support (Current Emergency Cardiovascular Care, *Circulation* 102|Suppl I|1-384, 2000.)

with a plan of action and an adequate armamentarium to meet emergencies. Presenting a plan for every situation that may arise in the dental office is impossible. No cookbook solutions exist, and hurried emotional responses are hazardous. The actions of the dental team must be based on a thorough background, continued study, and carefully prepared and rehearsed emergency procedures in which each individual has specific duties and responsibilities. This necessitates the presence of appropriate resuscitative equipment and drugs to permit the team to work calmly and precisely. This teamwork must be based on knowledge, practice, sound judgment, and confidence. Every dental office should have a written plan including specific duties for all office staff, covering areas such as who will call the emergency medical support system (911), start CPR, begin an IV line, and administer drugs. A designated staff member should record every event and the time of each action.

A good medical history, appropriate physical evaluation, and proper consultation frequently may prevent the onset of a life-threatening situation. However, unforeseen circumstances do occur and the dentist should make every effort to prevent irreversible physiologic damage.

Physical evaluation of patients has become more important because of the introduction of more complicated and lengthy dental procedures, the increasing number of medical risk patients, the growing number of geriatric patients, and the use of conscious sedation techniques. The goal of evaluation is to determine the ability of a patient to tolerate a specific procedure safely at a given time. The goal is not to diagnose and treat medical conditions; rather, it is to gather reliable information so that intelligent decisions can be made in treatment. This approach eliminates the element of surprise, heightens the awareness of potential risk, produces confidence, establishes rapport with the patient, and provides a basis for communication with a physician when indicated.

Consultation with the physician should be made on the basis of adequate knowledge of the patient's particular problem and the proposed dental treatment plan. Generally, consultation with the physician does not alter the treatment plan, though occasionally it will do so significantly. Rarely, however, will consultation delay treatment. These consultations serve only as guidelines to patient management. The dentist must make final decisions regarding dental treatment.

In most emergencies the dentist should employ BCLS and call the 911 emergency medical system phone number. Dentists with ACLS training may start an IV line and administer drugs through it as indicated. The pulse oximeter/ECG can be an important adjunct for the monitoring of a patient's vital signs.

GENERAL PRINCIPLES OF EMERGENCY CARE

Most life-threatening office emergencies are caused by the patient's inability to withstand physical or emotional stress or the patient's reaction to drugs. Emergencies also can be caused by a complication of a preexisting systemic disease. Cardiopulmonary systems can be involved, thus requiring some emergency supportive therapy.

In all emergencies, the following must be performed:
1. Place the patient in the supine position if possible; if still conscious, the patient may prefer a more upright position
2. Give the patient the basics of life support (cardiopulmonary rescuscitation [CPR]):
   a. Air passage opened and cleared if necessary
   b. Breathing ensured (by artificial respiration if necessary)
   c. Carotid pulse checked as a way of ensuring circulation, CPR administered if no carotid pulse, and blood pressure checked if carotid pulse present

Once the emergency has been diagnosed, proper treatment in most cases includes the following:
1. Emergency medical system activated by 911 phone call.
2. Administering of oxygen (10 L/min. flow)
3. Use of IV line for rapid drug administration (with ACLS training)
4. Administering of CPR
5. Treating with drugs (ACLS training for IV line)
   Key points:
1. Quick recognition and diagnosis of signs and symptoms
2. Early response time (4 to 6 minutes without oxygen leading to irreversible brain damage)
3. Airway clearance (circulation meaningless without oxygen)

4. Proper monitoring of vital signs (e.g., carotid pulse)
5. Continued monitoring of patient status (e.g., color, ventilation, pulse, blood pressure, pupils)
6. Assurance that patient receives proper medical care

TYPES OF EMERGENCIES AND THEIR TREATMENT

UNCONSCIOUSNESS

Syncope and Psychogenic Shock
Cause
Cerebral hypoxia (reduced blood flow to brain)
Symptoms:
1. Early
   a. Pallor
   b. Sweating
   c. Nausea
   d. Anxiety
2. Late
   a. Pupillary dilation
   b. Yawning
   c. Decreased blood pressure
   d. Bradycardia (slow pulse)
   e. Convulsive movements
   f. Unconsciousness
Treatment
1. Lower head slightly and elevate legs and arms (for pregnant women, roll on left side)
2. Administer oxygen at 10 L flow/min
3. Administer spirits of ammonia
4. Apply cold compresses to forehead
5. Monitor and record vital signs
6. Reassure patient
   Low blood pressure or pulse (systolic is less than previous diastolic)
1. Low blood pressure
   a. Lower head and raise arms and legs
   b. Start 5% dextrose and lactated Ringer's IV
   c. Administer a vasopressor drug (epinephrine 0.3-0.5 mg SC or IM, IV with ACLS training)
2. Slow pulse (less than 60 beats per minute)
   A. Administer 0.4 mg atropine IV to increase heart rate
   B. Repeat up to 1.2 mg, then consider use of additional vasopressors

Cardiac Arrest
Signs and Symptoms
1. No pulse or blood pressure
2. Sudden cessation of respiration (apnea)
3. Cyanosis
4. Dilated pupils

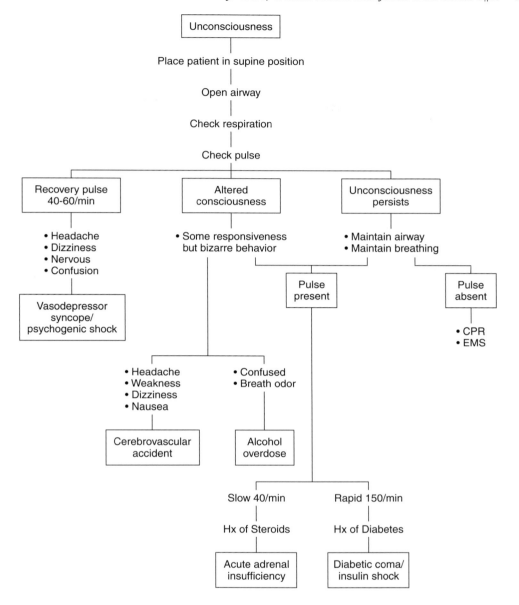

Treatment

1. Airway—lift chin, clear airway if necessary, and observe for breathing
2. Breathing—inflate lungs with mouth-to-mouth resuscitation, give 2 initial quick breaths, and perform endotracheal intubation and positive pressure oxygen
3. Circulation—check carotid pulse; if pulse is absent, compress sternum 1 to 2 inches (2 to 3) fingerwidths above xiphoid process
   a. One operator: 15 compressions, 2 inflations-rate of 80 compressions/min
   b. Two operators: 15 compressions, 2 inflation-rate of 80 compressions/min
   Continue resuscitation until spontaneous pulse returns
4. Drugs IV—start 5% dextrose lactated ringers (with ACLS training)
   a. Epinephrine 0.5-1.0 ml 1:1,000, repeat every 5 minutes prn
   b. Sodium bicarbonate 1 m Eq/kg initially and initial dose every 10 minutes until circulation is restored (or as governed by arterial blood gas measurement)

c. Atropine sulfate indicated if pulse is less than 60/min and systolic blood pressure below 90- initial dose of 0.5 mg; repeat every 5 minutes, not to exceed 2.0 mg total dose
5. Other drugs used for cardiac arrest (with ACLS training)
   a. Lidocaine (anti-arrhythmic agent)
   b. Calcium chloride (increase in myocardial contractility)
   c. Morphine sulphate (for pain relief)

Monitor and record all vital signs, drug administrations, and patient responses. Ambulance, emergency room, and medical assistance should be called.

Diabetic Coma Versus Insulin Shock

Diagnostic Factors	Diabetic Coma (no insulin)	Insulin Shock
History		
Food intake	Normal or excessive	May be insufficient
Insulin	Insufficient	Excessive
Onset	Gradual (days)	Sudden (hours)
Physical exam		
Appearance	Extremely ill	Very weak
Skin	Dry and flushed	Moist and pale
Infection	Frequent	Absent
Fever	Frequent	Absent
GI symptoms		
Mouth	Dry	Drooling
Thirst	Intense	Absent
Hunger	Absent	Occasional
Vomiting	Common	Rare
Abdominal pain	Frequent	Absent
Breath	Acetone odor	Normal
Blood pressure	Low	Normal
Pulse	Weak and rapid	Full and bounding
Tremor	Absent	Frequent
Convulsions	None	In late stages

Treatment

1. Place patient in supine position
2. Administer oxygen
3. If patient is conscious, give patient a high sugar-containing drink such as Glucola or orange juice
4. If patient is unconscious, a glucose paste can be applied to the buccal mucosa. A dentist with ACLS training can start an IV 5% dextrose (D5LR) and run IV as fast as possible
5. Monitor and record vital signs
6. Activate EMS system by calling 911
7. Transport patient to emergency room if some improvement is not fairly rapid
   NOTE: If in doubt, treat as insulin shock.

Response to Treatment

1. Insulin shock-rapid improvement following carbohydrate administration
2. Diabetic coma
   a. No improvement after carbohydrate administration
   b. Slow improvement (6-12 hours) after insulin administration

Acute Adrenal Insufficiency

Cause

Adrenal suppression (low adrenocorticotropic hormone) because exogenous steroids suppress adrenal production. The patient may be medicated with steroids for dozens of medical problem; or the cause may be primary or secondary malfunction of the adrenal cortex.

Signs and Symptoms

1. Altered consciousness
2. Confusion, weakness, fatigue
3. Headache
4. Pain in abdomen, legs
5. Nausea, vomiting
6. Hypotension and syncope
7. Coma

Treatment

Conscious

1. Position patient semireclining
2. Monitor and record vital signs
3. Administer oxygen
4. Administer steroids, hydrocortisone 100 mg, or dexamethasone 4 mg (IV with ACLS training)
5. May have to transfer to hospital for lack of fluids

Unconscious

1. Position patient supine
2. BCLS
3. Administer oxygen
4. Summon EMS (911 call)
5. Review patient's medical history
6. Administer steroids hydrocortisone 100 mg, or dexamethasone 4 mg
7. Administer vasopressor (epinephrine 0.5 ml)
8. Rapid transfer of patient to hospital

Cerebrovascular Accident
Signs and Symptoms
1. Early warning signs
   a. Dizziness (patient may fall)
   b. Vertigo and vision changes
   c. Nausea and vomiting
   d. Transient paresthesia
   e. Unilateral weakness or paralysis
2. General symptoms
   a. Headache
   b. Nausea
   c. Vomiting
   d. Convulsions, coma
   Note: Blood pressure and pulse are generally normal. Raised blood pressure and body temperature and lowered pulse and respiration indicate increased intracranial pressure.
Treatment
1. Call EMS (911)
2. Position patient in reclining, semisitting position with the head elevated
3. Provide the following support:
   a. Oxygen at 10 L/min. flow
   b. No sedative use
   c. Airway and breathing maintenance
4. Monitor and record vital signs
5. Keep patient quiet and still
6. Rapid transfer to hospital

Convulsions
Causes
1. Syncope
2. Drug reactions
3. Insulin shock
4. Cerebrovascular accident
5. Convulsive seizure disorder
Signs and Symptoms
1. Aura-flash of light or sound
2. Mental confusion
3. Excessive salivation
4. Tonic contractions and tremors
5. Convulsive movements of extremities
6. Rolling back of eyes
7. Loss of consciousness
Treatment
1. Protect patient from personal damage
2. After convulsion, make sure airway is open
3. Dispense oxygen at 10 L/min. flow
4. For status epilepticus, administer diazepam (Valium) 5-20 mg IV
5. Monitor and record vital signs
6. Support respiration (patient may have respiratory arrest)

Local Anesthesia Drug Toxicity
Causes
1. Too large a dose of local anesthetic per body weight
2. Rapid absorption of drug or inadvertent IV injection
3. Slow detoxification or elimination of drug
Signs and Symptoms
1. Early
   a. Talkative, restless, apprehensive, excited manner
   b. Convulsions
   c. Increase in blood pressure and pulse rate
   Note: The stimulation is followed by depression of the central nervous system.
2. Late signs and symptoms
   a. Convulsions followed by depression
   b. Drop in blood pressure
   c. Weak, rapid pulse or bradycardia
   d. Apnea
   e. Unconsciousness, death
   Note: Lidocaine is documented to have occasionally exhibited only the depression without the usual prodromal of the excitatory phase.
Treatment
1. Protect patient during the convulsive period (consider administration of 5-15 mg Valium IV if convulsive period is prolonged)
2. Monitor and record vital signs
3. Provide supportive therapy
   a. Keep patient in supine position
   b. Maintain oxygen at 10 L flow/min
   c. Maintain blood pressure
   d. Treat bradycardia (0.4 mg atropine IV, with ACLS training)
   e. Transport to hospital
   Note: If patient becomes unconscious, maintain the airway, administer CPR, and call for emergency medical service.

RESPIRATORY DIFFICULTY

Hyperventilation
Cause
1. Excess loss of CO_2
2. Respiratory alkalosis
Symptoms
1. Rapid, shallow breathing
2. Confusion
3. Dizziness
4. Paresthesia
5. Carpal-pedal spasms
Treatment
1. Explain the problem to the patient and reassure patient
2. Instruct the patient to be calm and breathe slowly

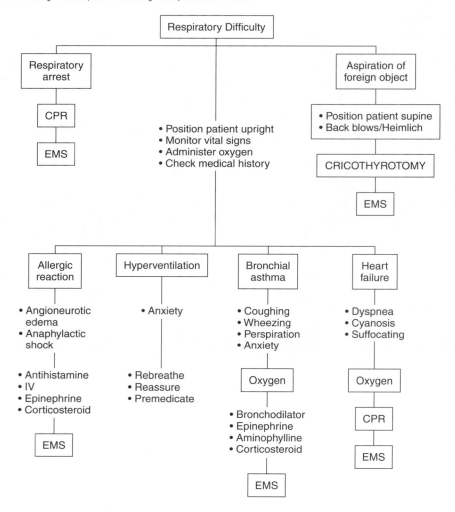

3. Have patient breathe slowly into a paper bag
4. Reappoint for presedation

Aspiration or Swallowing a Foreign Object
Cause
Foreign body in larynx or pharynx
Signs and Symptoms
1. Coughing or gagging associated with the loss of a foreign object; inability to speak
2. Possible cyanosis from airway obstruction
3. Violent respiratory effort
4. Suprasternal retraction
5. Rapid pulse
Treatment
1. Keep patient supine if unconscious; keep standing or sitting leaning forward if conscious

2. Establish airway (open and evaluate breathing)
3. Apply Heimlich maneuver
   Note: If cricothyrotomy necessary, refer to "Cricothyroid Membrane Puncture" that follows.
4. Administer oxygen
5. Maintain the supine position and transport patient to hospital for radiographs

   A. Posterior-anterior chest view
   B. Lateral chest view
   C. Flat plane abdominal view to establish location

   Note: If foreign object is in GI tract, follow with x-ray examination; if in trachea or lung, requires a bronchoscopy or thoracotomy. If foreign object has occluded the airway, the Heimlich maneuver may be of benefit before initiation of a cricothyrotomy.

Cricothyroid Membrane Puncture

The approach to a patient with acute airway obstruction should be:

1. Recognition of obstruction
2. Use of nonsurgical maneuvers to relieve obstruction (i.e., back blows, Heimlich maneuver)
3. Administration of mouth-to-mouth breathing to bypass obstruction or to diagnose obstruction
4. Activation of EMS (with 911 call)
5. Establishment of an emergency surgical airway (cricothyrotomy) if Heimlich maneuver unsuccessful

Cricothyrotomy

1. Place patient in head-down position with neck hyperextended
2. Ensure that chin and sternal notch are held in median plane
3. Perform 2-cm vertical incision through skin over cricothyroid cartilage
4. Perform 2-cm transverse incision over cricothyroid membrane
5. Insert small scissors or hemostats through cricothyroid membrane and into the tracheal space, or use large (8-gauge) needle
6. Expand instrument and dilate transversely
7. Insert tube into trachea between beaks of dilating instrument
8. Remove scissors or hemostats
9. Tape tube into place
10. Use positive pressure or enriched oxygen flow if patient is breathing independently
11. Rapid transfer patient to hospital

Bronchial Asthma

Signs and Symptoms

1. Sense of suffocation
2. Pressure in chest
3. Nonproductive cough
4. Expiratory wheezes
5. Prolonged expiratory phase
6. Increased respiratory effort
7. Chest distension
8. Thick, stringy mucous sputum
9. Cyanosis (in severe cases)

Treatment

1. Use Beta2-agonist inhaler (e.g., Isuprel mistometer) 1 to 2 deep inhalations
2. Activate EMS (911 call)
3. Dispense oxygen at 10L/min. flow
4. If unresponsive, administer epinephrine (0.3-0.5 ml, 1:1000 SC; repeat every 20 minutes prn)
5. Dispense theophylline ethylenediamine (aminophylline) 250-500 mg slowly by IV over a 10-minute period

6. Administer hydrocortisone sodium succinate (Solu-Cortef), 100 mg IV
7. Monitor and record vital signs
8. Rapid transport patient to hospital

Note: Because aminophylline may cause hypotension, it should be given with extreme caution to patients with asthma who are hypotensive.

Mild Allergic Reaction

Symptoms

1. Mild pruritus (itching)—slow appearance
2. Mild urticaria (rash)—slow appearance

Treatment

1. Administer diphenhydramine (Benadryl) 25-50 mg orally, IV, or IM (if dentist has ACLS training)
2. Repeat dose up to 50 mg every 6 hours orally for 2 days
3. If suspected allergy to medication, withdraw drug administration

Severe Allergic Reaction

Symptoms

1. Skin reactions—rapid appearance
   a. Severe pruritus (itching)
   b. Severe urticaria (rash)
2. Swelling of lips, eyelids, cheeks, pharynx and larynx (angioneurotic edema)
3. Anaphylactic shock
   a. Cardiovascular-fall in blood pressure
   b. Respiratory-wheezing, choking, cyanosis, hoarseness
   c. Central nervous system-loss of consciousness, dilation of pupils

Treatment

1. Call EMS (through 911)
2. Administer epinephrine 0.3-0.5 mg 1:1000 SC or IM (contraindication:severe hypertension) or IV if dentist has ACLS training; repeat every 5-10 minutes as needed
3. Administer theophylline ethylenediamine (aminophylline) 250-500 mg IV over 10 minutes (contraindication: hypotension) if dentist has ACLS training
4. Dispense steroids-hydrocortisone sodium succinate (Solu-Cortef), 100 mg SC or IM or IV if dentist has ACLS training
5. Administer oxygen
6. Monitor and record vital signs
7. Perform CPR if needed
8. Use cricothyrotomy if needed
9. Ensure rapid transfer of patient to hospital

Note: Aminophylline may cause hypotension and should be given with extreme caution to patients with asthma who also are hypotensive.

Respiratory Arrest
Cause
1. Physical obstruction of airway (tongue or foreign object)
2. Drug-induced apnea
Signs and Symptoms
1. Cessation of breathing
2. Cyanosis
Treatment
1. Place patient in supine position
2. Keep airway open by tilting head back and removing obstruction if possible; if not possible perform Heimlich manuever
3. Activate EMS (911 call)
4. Ventilate patient 12 to 15 times per minute
   a. If apnea is secondary to narcotic, give 0.4 mg naloxone hydrochloride (Narcan) IV, IM, or SC and administer oxygen
   b. If apnea is secondary to sedative barbiturate or diazepam overdose, the following should be performed:
      (1) Administer oxygen or artificial respiration
      (2) Keep patient awake

(3) Support blood pressure through position of patient, parenteral fluids, and vasopressors
(4) Take patient to hospital if necessary
Note: Monitor patient carefully for the duration of action of Narcan, which may be less than that of the narcotic. No reversal agent exists for sedative and barbiturate overdose. Flumazenil is an agent that can reverse the effects of diazepam. Dentists with ACLS training may select to have this drug available.

CHEST PAIN

Angina Pectoris
Cause
Blood supply to the cardiac muscle is insufficient (atherosclerosis or coronary artery spasm) and precipitated by stress, anxiety, and physical activity.
Signs and Symptoms
1. Substernal pain or pain referred to arms, neck, or abdomen
2. Pain lasting less than 15 minutes and possibly radiating to the left shoulder

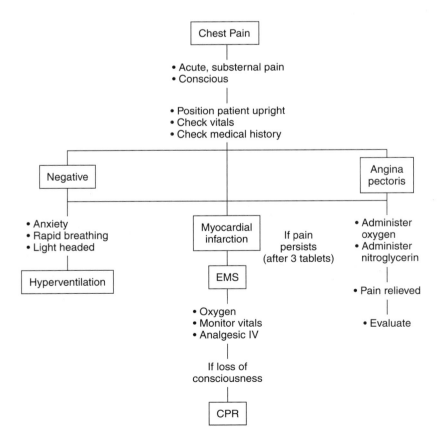

3. Positive response to nitroglycerine
4. Patient usually has a history of the condition
   Note: Vital signs are normal; no hypotension, sweating, or nausea occurs.
   ### Treatment
1. Place patient in semireclining or sitting-up position with head elevated
2. Administer nitroglycerin 0.3 mg tablet sublingual or spray amyl nitrate bud (3 tablets, 1 tablet every 5 minutes up to a total of 3 tablets)
3. Administer oxygen at 10 L/min. flow
4. Put patient at rest and give reassurance
5. Monitor and record vital signs
   Note: If any doubt exists about whether angina or myocardial infarction exists, call EMS (through 911) or transport patient to hospital emergency room. Once the nitroglycerin tablet container has been opened, the remaining tablets have a poor shelf life (30 days); a new supply should be stocked.

MYOCARDIAL INFARCTION

Cause
Most commonly occlusion of coronary vessels occurs. Anoxia, ischemia, and infarct are present.
Signs and Symptoms
1. Crushing chest pain
   a. More severe than angina, possibly radiating to neck, shoulder, jaw
   b. Longer than 15 minutes
   c. Not relieved by nitroglycerin tablets
   d. Squeezing or heavy feeling
2. Cyanosis, pale, or ashen appearance
3. Weakness
4. Cold sweat
5. Nausea, vomiting
6. Air hunger and fear of impending death
7. Increased, irregular pulse beat of poor quality and containing palpitations
8. Feeling of impending doom
   ### Treatment
1. Place patient in most comfortable position
2. Administer oxygen at 10 L/min. flow
3. Activate EMS (911 call)
4. Monitor and record vital signs
5. Reassure patient
   Note: Maintain patient in most comfortable position; this may not be the supine position since the air hunger may be associated with orthopnea. Nitrous oxide-oxygen (N_2O-30%, O_2 70%) Demerol (50 mg IV), or morphine (10 mg IV) may be administered if the dentist has ACLS training. The condition may progress to cardiac arrest.
6. CPR

OTHER REACTIONS

Intraarterial Injection of Drug Into the Arm
Symptoms
1. Pain and burning sensation distal to the injection site
2. Cold and blotching hand or fingers distal to the injection site

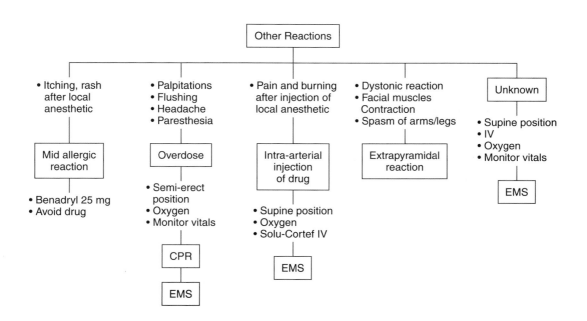

Treatment

1. Place patient in supine position
2. Administer oxygen
3. Leave needle in place and inject 40 to 60 mg 2% lidocaine (2-3ml) b 100 mg hydrocortisone sodium succinate (Solu-Cortef) IM
4. Later, transport patient to hospital where treatment may include heparinization and brachial plexus block

Extrapyramidal Reactions
Antipsychotic Drugs Producing Side Reactions

1. Phenothiazines (Compazine, Thorazine, Phenergan, Sparine, Stelazine, Trilafon, and Mellaril)
2. Butyrophenones (Haldol and Innovar [general anesthetic])
3. Thioxanthenes (Navane and Taractan)

Signs and Symptoms

1. Acute dystonic reaction (more frequent in young people, women)
   a. Rapid onset
   b. Involuntary movement of tongue, muscles of mastication, and muscles of facial expression
   c. Neck muscles affected frequently (torticollis), arms and legs less so frequently arms
2. Akathisia (constant motion)
3. Parkinsonism
4. Tardive dyskinesia ([buccolingomasticatory triad] sucking, smacking, chewing, fly-catching movement of tongue)

Treatment

1. Position patient in semierect position
2. Administer diphenhydramine HCI (Benadryl) 25-50 mg orally, IV if dentist has ACLS training
3. Administer oxygen
4. Monitor and record patient's vital signs
5. Transfer to hospital if necessary

Response to Unknown Cause

When a cause for the patient's response can not be rationally identified, a period of observation is justified.

1. Place patient in supine position
2. Activate EMS (911 call)
3. Support airway respiration and administer oxygen
4. Monitor and record vital signs
5. Start IV 5% dextrose with lactated ringers
6. Keep patient off all medication
7. Transfer to hospital if serious

EMERGENCY KIT

Review contents, expiration date, and clarity of all drugs periodically (at least monthly)

1. Oxygen setup
2. Blood pressure cuff
3. Stethoscope
4. Syringes (1, 5, 10, and 20 ml)
5. Lacrimal pocket mask
6. Disposable airway No. 2, 3, and 4
7. Butterflies No. 3, 21 gauge
8. 22 gauge needles
9. IV tubing set, Long No. 880-35
10. 250 cc dextrose, lactated ringers solution
11. Paper tape roll
12. Alcohol sponges
13. Drugs

   a. Atropine 0.4 mg ampule, 1 cc
   b. Benadryl (Diphenhydramine) 50 mg tablets or 50 mg/1 ml syringe/22 gauge, 1-inch needle
   c. Aminophylline (Theophylline Ethylenediamine) 250 mg/IO ml syringe/22 gauge, 1-inch needle
   d. Hydrocortisone sodium succinate (Solu-Cortef) 100 mg/2 cc syringe/22 gauge, 1 needle
   e. Epinephrine 1:1000 1.0 ml ampule
   f. Narcan (Naloxone hydrochloride) 0.4 mg/1 cc ampule/TB syringe
   g. Amyl nitrate 0.18 ml bud
   h. Nitroglycerine 0.3 mg tabs (packed as 30/bottle)
   i. Two ammonia inhalant buds
   j. Orange juice, Glucola, glucose paste or dextrose 50% 100 ml
   k. Sodium bicarbonate: 50 ml of 7.5% solution (44.6 mEq)-two bottles
   l. Isuprel mistometer (Isoproterenol hydrochloride)
   m. Diazepam (Valium) 5 mg/ml
   n. Lidocaine 2%, 2 ml ampules

14. Curved cricothyrotomy cannula
15. Padded tongue blade
16. Pulse oximeter/ECG (medical resources)
17. Automated external defibrillator (e.g., Heartstream FR-2, Medtronic Physio-control, Survivalink)
   Note: Commercial medical emergency kits for dentistry are available from companies such as Banyon International and Health First.

PEDIATRIC DRUG DOSES

These doses are presented on a weight basis, which can be simply multiplied. Though nomograms using weight, surface area, and other factors may be more accurate, the proposed method is suggested in an emergency situation.

1. Diphenhydramine HCL (Benadryl)
   Dose: 1-1.25 mg/kg up to SO mg maximum IV, then 1-1.25 mg/kg q 6 h orally or parenteral
2. Atropine sulfate
   Dose: 0.01 mg/kg up to 0.4 mg maximum IV or SC

3. Theophylline ethylenediamine (aminophylline)
   Dose: 3-5 mg/kg IV slowly—20 mg/minute maximum
4. Epinephrine (adrenaline) 1:1,000
   Dose: 0.05 mg-0.3 mg maximum SC or IM; diluted to 1:10,000 for IV administration
5. Isoproterenol sulfate 70 mEq /spray aerosol (MedVislet-Iso)
   Dose: 1 inhalation (70 mEq maximum
6. Amyl nitrate bud 0.3 mL
   Dose: Unlikely in children—same as adult
7. Ammonia inhalants
   Dose: same as adults
8. Hydrocortisone sodium succinate
   Dose: adult dose IV—50 mg, 100 mg and above
9. Sodium bicarbonate 44.6 mEq/50 ml
   Dose: 1 mEq/kg IV; 0.5-1 mEq/kg q 10 mm
10. Naloxone HCl (Narcan)
    Dose: No pediatric doses clearly established; 0.01 mg/kg IV (preferably) q 2-3 min x 2-3 doses maximum

11. 50% dextrose injection
    Dose: 0.5 mg/kg or 1 ml/kg
12. Diazepam (Valium)
    Dose: Not clearly established under age 12, but in range of 0.1-0.5 mg/kg for intractable seizures

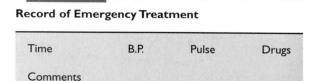

Record of Emergency Treatment

Time	B.P.	Pulse	Drugs
Comments			

Physical Evaluation and Risk Assessment

entistry today is far different from what was practiced only a decade or two ago, in not only techniques and procedures but also types of patients seen. As a result of advances in medical science, people are living longer and receiving medical treatment for disorders that were fatal only a few years ago. For example, damaged heart valves are surgically replaced, occluded coronary arteries are surgically bypassed or opened by balloons, organs are transplanted, severe hypertension is medically controlled, and many types of malignancies and immune deficiencies are being managed or controlled.

Because of the increasing numbers of dental patients, especially the elderly, with chronic medical problems, the dentist must remain knowledgeable about patients' medical conditions. Many chronic disorders or their treatments necessitate alterations in the provision of dental treatment. Failure to make appropriate treatment modifications can result in serious consequences.

The key to the successful dental management of a medically compromised patient requires a thorough evaluation and assessment of risk to determine whether a patient can safely tolerate a planned procedure. Risk assessment involves the determination of at least three components: (1) the nature, severity, and stability of the patient's medical condition; (2) the emotional state of the patient; and (3) the type and magnitude of the planned procedure (invasive or noninvasive). All factors must be carefully weighed for each patient (Fig. 1-1).

For example, a patient may have severe congestive heart failure, but the risk is minimal if the planned procedure is limited to taking radiographs (noninvasive) and the patient is not anxious or fearful. Conversely, the risk may be significant if the congestive failure is only moderate but the procedure planned is a full mouth extraction (invasive) and the patient is very anxious. Therefore the dentist much carefully weigh the physical and emotional state of the patient against the invasiveness and

trauma of the planned procedure. The cornerstone of patient evaluation and risk assessment is the medical history, supplemented by physical examination, laboratory tests, and medical consultation as appropriate.

MEDICAL HISTORY

A medical history must be taken on every patient who is to receive dental treatment. A number of techniques and forms may be used to obtain a medical history, ranging from an interview format, in which the questioner records the patient's responses on a blank sheet, to the use of a printed questionnaire that the patient fills out independently. The latter is most commonly used in dental practice and prevents omissions that may occur in an interview format. Many types of questionnaires are commercially available today, including one from the American Dental Association. Dentists often develop questionnaires that meet the specific needs of individual practice. Fig. 1-2 is the medical history questionnaire used at the University of Kentucky College of Dentistry. It provides a comprehensive review of a patient's medical history and a limited review of systems. It also serves as a basis for teaching and discussion. The medical history is designed to allow the dentist to conduct a follow-up interview to review selected questions or positive responses.

Although medical history questionnaires differ in organization and content detail, most attempt to elicit information about the same basic medical problems. The form in Fig. 1-2 is organized into two sections. The first comprises 23 questions followed by the signatures of patient and dentist (student and faculty). The second provides for the recording of vital signs, health comments and summary, and the American Society of Anesthesiologists classification of physical status. The comments section is intended for explanation and treatment of

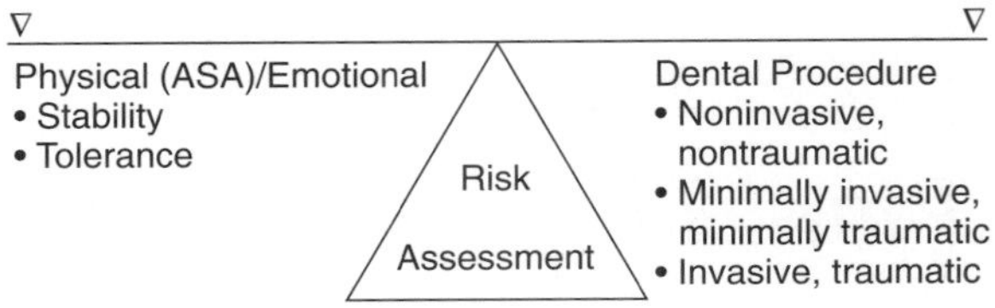

Fig. 1-1 Risk assessment by weighing key determining factors.

Physical (ASA)/Emotional
• Stability
• Tolerance

Risk

Assessment

Dental Procedure
• Noninvasive, nontraumatic
• Minimally invasive, minimally traumatic
• Invasive, traumatic

University of Kentucky
College of Dentistry

PATIENT'S NAME_____   DATE_____

Please check the box for any condition that you have had in the past or have now. Parents or Guardian, if you are completing this form for your child, please indicate your child's health status by checking the appropriate box.

(1) CARDIOVASCULAR

Congestive Heart Failure ☐
Heart Attack ☐
Angina Pectoris or
    Chest Pain ☐
High Blood Pressure ☐
Heart Murmer ☐
Mitral Valve Prolapse ☐
Rheumatic Fever ☐
Congenital Heart Defect ☐
Artificial (Prosthetic)
    Heart Valve ☐
Arrhythmias ☐
Heart Pacemaker or
    Difibrillator ☐
Coronary Bypass ☐
Coronary Angioplasty ☐
Heart Transplant ☐
Aneurysm ☐
Other Heart Problem ☐

(2) HEMATOLOGIC

Blood Transfusion ☐
Anemia ☐
Hemophilia ☐
Leukemia ☐
Sickle Cell Anemia ☐
Tendency to Bleed
    Longer than Normal ☐

(3) NEUROLOGIC

Vision Problems ☐
Glaucoma ☐
Earaches, Ringing in Ears ☐
Hearing Loss ☐
Severe Headaches ☐
Fainting or Dizzy Spells ☐
Stroke ☐
Epilepsy, Seizures, or
    Convulsions ☐
Psychiatric Treatment ☐
Panic Attacks ☐
Phobias ☐

(4) GASTROINTESTINAL

Stomach/Intestinal
    Ulcers ☐
Colitis ☐
Persistent Diarrhea ☐
Hepatitis ☐
Liver Disease ☐
Yellow Jaundice ☐
Cirrhosis ☐
Eating Disorder ☐

(5) PULMONARY

Hay Fever ☐
Sinus Trouble ☐
Allergies or Hives ☐
Asthma ☐
Chronic Cough ☐
Emphysema ☐
Chronic Bronchitis ☐
Tuberculosis (TB) ☐
Breathing Difficulties ☐

(6) DERMAL/
MUSCULOSKELETAL

Allergy to Latex (Rubber) ☐
Skin Rash ☐
Dark Mole(s) (Recent
    changes in appearance) ☐
Night Sweats ☐
Osteoarthritis ☐
Rheumatoid Arthritis ☐
Systemic Lupus ☐
Artificial (Prosthetic) Joint ☐

(7) ENDOCRINE

Diabetes ☐
Thyroid Disease ☐
Taking Cortisone or
    Other Steroid ☐

(8) GENITOURINARY

Urinate Frequently ☐
Kidney, Bladder Problem ☐
Dialysis ☐
Kidney Transplant ☐
Sexually Transmitted
    Disease (Syphilis,
    Gonorrhea, Chlamydia or
    Genital Herpes) ☐
HIV Positive ☐
Multiple Sexual Partners ☐

(9) OTHER CONDITIONS

Frequent Sore Throats ☐
Enlarged Lymph Node or
    "Gland" ☐
Use Tobacco ☐
Use Alcohol ☐
Use Injectable Drugs ☐
Drug or Alcohol Addiction
    (Recovering or Current) ☐
Tumor or Cancer ☐
Radiation Therapy ☐
Chemotherapy ☐
Disease, Problem or
    Condition not Listed ☐
If yes, list

_____

_____

_____

_____

_____

_____

Fig. 1-2 Health questionnaire in use at the University of Kentucky College of Dentistry. (Courtesy, University of Kentucky College of Dentistry.)

10. Who is your physician?
    Physician's Name_____ Address_____
    Phone #_____ Last Appointment Date_____
    For What?_____

11. Are you taking (or supposed to be taking) any medicine, drugs or pills of any kind?   **Yes No**
    If yes, what kind and dose   ☐   ☐
    _____
    _____

12. Do you have reactions or allergies to drugs or medicines?   ☐   ☐
    What kind?_____

13. Have you had an adverse reaction to dental or general anesthetic?   ☐   ☐

14. Have you ever had any operations or surgery?   ☐   ☐
    Describe the problem and any complications
    _____
    _____
    _____

15. When you walk up stairs or take a walk, do you ever have to stop because of pain in your chest,   ☐   ☐
    shortness of breath, or because you are very tired?

16. Do your ankles swell during the day?   ☐   ☐

17. Have you unintentionally lost or gained more than 10 pounds in the past year?   ☐   ☐

18. Are you on a special diet?   ☐   ☐

19. (WOMEN) Are you pregnant, or possibly pregnant?   ☐   ☐

To the best of my knowledge, all of the preceding answers are true and correct. If I ever have any change in my health, abnormal laboratory test, or if my medicines change, I will inform the dentist at the next appointment without fail.

_____   _____   _____
Date   Patient, Parent, or Guardian Signature   Student Dentist Signature

                                                               _____
                                                               Faculty Signature

Initial Blood Pressure_____ Pulse_____
Review and Update (a new medical history 3A should be completed every 2 years)

_____ _____ _____ _____ _____
_____ _____ _____ _____ _____

_____ _____ _____ _____ _____
Date   BP   Change in Health Status   Student Signature   Faculty Signature

****

HEALTH COMMENTS & SUMMARY: ASA   I   II   III
_____
_____

Fig. 1-2, cont'd

modifications for significant positive responses that the patient makes on the medical history form, and serves as a capsular summary of the patient's health status. The following information provides the rationale for asking certain questions and the significance of positive responses. Detailed information concerning most of these medical problems is found in the following chapters.

CARDIOVASCULAR DISEASES

Patients with various forms of cardiovascular disease are especially vulnerable to physical or emotional challenges that may be encountered during dental treatment.

Heart Failure

Heart failure is not a disease per se but rather a clinical syndrome complex that is the result of an underlying cardiovascular problem such as valvular disease or an arrhythmia. The underlying problem should be identified and its potential significance assessed. Patients with untreated or poorly controlled congestive heart failure generally should not receive elective dental treatment. Chair position may influence a patient's ability to breathe, with some patients being unable to tolerate a supine or semisupine position. Vasoconstrictors should be used cautiously in patients taking digitalis glycosides (digoxin) because the combination can precipitate arrhythmias (see Chapter 7). Stress reduction measures also may be necessary (Box 1-1).

Heart Disease or Heart Attack

A history of a heart attack (myocardial infarction) within the recent past may preclude elective dental care because during the immediate postinfarction period, patients have increased susceptibility to repeat infarctions, arrhythmias, and heart failure. Many patients may be taking medications such as antianginals, anticoagulants, adrenergic-blocking agents, calcium channel blockers, antiarrhythmic agents, and digitalis. Some of these drugs may alter the dental management of these patients because of the potential interaction with vasoconstrictor in the local anesthetic, drug side effects, or other considerations (see Chapter 5). Stress reduction measures may be appropriate (see Box 1-1).

Angina Pectoris

Brief substernal pain resulting from myocardial ischemia, commonly provoked by physical activity or emotional stress, is a common and significant symptom of coronary heart disease. Patients with angina, especially unstable angina, are candidates for arrhythmias, myocardial

infarction, and sudden death. A variety of vasoactive medications are used to treat angina, such as nitroglycerin, beta-blocking agents, and calcium channel blockers. Vasoconstrictors should be used cautiously. Patients with unstable or progressive angina are not candidates for elective dental care (see Chapter 5). Stress-reduction measures may be appropriate (see Box 1-1).

High Blood Pressure

Patients with hypertension (more than 140/90 mm Hg) should be identified. This includes the questioner or medical history determining whether the patient has been diagnosed with high blood pressure or is supposed to be taking antihypertensive medication; patients often stop taking their medications without their doctor's knowledge. Current blood pressure readings and any symptoms that may be associated with hypertension such as visual changes, dizziness, and headaches should be noted. Some antihypertensive medications such as some beta-blocking agents may require special consideration during dental treatment. Vasoconstrictors should be used cautiously (see Chapter 4). Stress-reduction measures also may be appropriate (see Box 1-1).

Heart Murmur

The presence of a heart murmur may be of special significance in the dental patient. A heart murmur is caused by turbulence of blood flow producing vibratory sounds during the beating of the heart. This turbulence

---

BOX 1-1

General Stress Management Protocol

- Open communication about fears/concerns
- Short appointments
- Morning appointments
- Preoperative vital signs
- Preoperative sedation
  - Short-acting benzodiazepine (e.g., triazolam 0.125-0.25 mg)
    - night before appointment
    - 1 hr before appointment
- Intraoperative sedation (N_2O/O_2)
- Profound local anesthesia; topical used prior to injection
- Adequate postoperative pain control
- Patient contacted evening of the procedure

may result from either physiologic (normal) factors or pathologic abnormalities of the heart valves, vessels or both. The primary goal in the medical history is to determine the nature of the heart murmur. If a murmur is caused by a pathologic condition, patients may be susceptible to an infection inside the heart (on or near the heart valves) as a result of microorganisms entering the bloodstream from dental treatment that caused significant bleeding. This infection is called *infective* or *bacterial endocarditis* and is a serious problem that can be fatal. A patient identified as having a heart murmur of pathologic or unknown origin may need to be placed on antibiotics prophylactically (preventively) for certain dental procedures in an attempt to prevent bacterial endocarditis. Currently, oral amoxicillin is the drug of choice for this purpose (see Chapters 2 and 3).

Mitral Valve Prolapse

In mitral valve prolapse (MVP) leaflets of the mitral valve are thickened and redundant and prolapse into the left atrium during systole. As a result, the tight closure of the leaflets may not occur, which can result in backflow of blood (regurgitation) from the ventricle to the atrium. Patients with MVP and regurgitation may require antibiotic prophylaxis for certain dental procedures likely to result in significant bleeding. Currently, oral amoxicillin is the drug of choice for antibiotic prophylaxis. Patients with MVP without regurgitation are not considered to be at risk for bacterial endocarditis (see Chapter 3).

Rheumatic Fever

Rheumatic fever is an autoimmune condition that can follow an upper respiratory beta-hemolytic streptococcal infection and can lead to permanent damage to the heart valves. When the heart valves are damaged, the condition is called *rheumatic heart disease*. Patients with rheumatic heart disease are susceptible to bacterial endocarditis as a result of bacteria entering the bloodstream during the course of certain dental procedures that cause significant bleeding. Patients with rheumatic heart disease are given prophylactic antibiotics for certain dental procedures likely to result in significant bleeding in an attempt to prevent bacterial endocarditis. Currently, oral amoxicillin is the drug of choice for this purpose (see Chapter 3).

Congenital Heart Defect or Lesion

Patients with many forms of persistent or unrepaired congenital heart defects are considered susceptible to bacterial endocarditis and given prophylactic antibiotics for certain dental procedures likely to result in significant bleeding. Currently, oral amoxicillin is the drug of choice for this purpose (see Chapter 3).

Many patients with surgically repaired congenital defects are not considered at risk for bacterial endocarditis and do not require antibiotic prophylaxis. One exception is the patient who has an artificial heart valve. These patients have an *increased* risk of bacterial endocarditis.

Artificial Heart Valve

Patients with artificial heart valves are considered highly susceptible to bacterial endocarditis from bacterial seeding that results from significant bleeding during certain dental procedures. This is significant in view of the high mortality rate for patients with artificial heart valves who contract bacterial endocarditis (prosthetic valve endocarditis). These patients are given prophylactic antibiotics for dental procedures likely to result in significant bleeding. Currently, oral amoxicillin is the drug of choice. However, parenteral drugs may be administered in place of or in addition to the oral regimen (see Chapter 3).

Arrhythmias

Arrhythmias are frequently related to heart failure or ischemic heart disease. Stress, anxiety, physical activity, drugs, and hypoxia are some elements that can precipitate arrhythmias. Vasoconstrictors in local anesthetic should be used cautiously in patients prone to arrhythmias because they can be precipitated by excessive quantities or inadvertant intravascular injections. The use of vasoconstrictors in patients with serious arrhythmias refractory to treatment is not recommended. Stress-reduction measures may be necessary (see Box 1-1).

Some of these patients take antiarrhythmic drugs; certain agents may cause oral manifestations or other effects. Patients with arrhythmias may require a pacemaker or defibrillator to artificially regulate or pace heart rhythm. These patients do not require antibiotic prophylaxis. Caution is advised with the use of certain electrical equipment (e.g., electrosurgery, ultrasonic scalers) in these patients because of the possibility of interference with the function of the pacemaker (see Chapter 6).

Heart Surgery or Transplant

One of the most common forms of cardiac surgery performed today is the coronary artery bypass graft. Vasoconstrictors should be used cautiously during the immediate postoperative period because of the possibility of precipitating arrhythmias. These patients do not require antibiotic prophylaxis. Likewise, most patients with surgically repaired congenital defects do not require antibiotic prophylaxis. Heart transplant patients are not seen frequently. As with any organ transplant, however, the administration of powerful immunosuppressive drugs renders a patient susceptible to infection and gingival bleeding. In addition, some physicians may

recommend antibiotic prophylaxis for dental treatment (see Chapter 3).

Stroke

Efforts should be made to minimize stress and hypoxia in patients with a history of stroke (see Box 1-1). Problems that may predispose to stroke such as hypertension and diabetes must be identified so appropriate management alterations are determined. Elective dental care should be avoided for the first 6 months after a stroke because of the patient's increased susceptibility for subsequent strokes. Vasoconstrictors should be used cautiously. Anticoagulant medications and antiplatelet medications can result in prolonged bleeding. Stress-reduction measures may be necessary. Some stroke victims may have hemiplegia, speech impairment and other physical handicaps. Occasionally, calcified atheromatous plaques may be seen in the carotid arteries on panoramic films; thus identifying patients susceptible to a stroke (see Chapter 22).

Aneurysm

A patient with a known, unrepaired aneurysm is not a candidate for elective dental care. If care is necessary, stress, hypoxia, hypertension, and excessive physical exertion should be avoided. Patients with a surgically repaired aneurysm do not require antibiotic prophylaxis for dental procedures if more than 6 months has elapsed since the repair.

HEMATOLOGIC DISORDERS

Blood Transfusion

Patients with a history of blood transfusions are of concern from at least two aspects. The underlying problem that necessitated a blood transfusion such as a bleeding disorder needs to be determined. Patients at risk to be carriers of hepatitis B or C or infected with the AIDS virus need to be identified. Laboratory screening or medical consultation may be appropriate, and as always, universal infection control procedures are mandatory (see Chapters 10 and 19).

Anemia

A significant reduction in the oxygen-carrying capacity of the red blood cells can be the result of an underlying pathologic process such as blood loss, decreased production of red blood cells, or hemolysis. Some anemias, such as glucose-6-phosphate dehydrogenase deficiency and sickle cell disease, require dental management considerations. Oral lesions, infections, delayed wound healing, and adverse response to hypoxia are all potential concerns (see Chapter 20).

Leukemia

Depending on the type of leukemia, status of the disease, and type of treatment, some patients may have bleeding problems, or delayed healing, or be prone to infection and gingival enlargement. Some adverse effects can result from their use of powerful chemotherapeutic agents and require management considerations (see Chapters 20 and 21).

Tendency to Bleed Longer Than Normal

A potentially significant problem is that of a patient with a history of abnormal bleeding. This is of obvious concern, especially if any surgical treatment is planned. Bleeding disorders may be genetic or acquired. An example of a common genetic bleeding disorder is hemophilia A (factor VIII deficiency). Examples of acquired bleeding disorders include some forms of leukemia and conditions caused by various medications such as warfarin (Coumadin) or aspirin. However, many complaints of abnormal bleeding are more apparent than real; further questioning or screening laboratory tests may allow the dentist to make this distinction (see Chapter 19).

NEURAL AND SENSORY DISEASES

Headache, Dizziness, and Fainting

Positive responses to this section of the medical history such as to the presence of headache, dizziness, or fainting spells, may signify that a patient has signs or symptoms related to a central nervous system disorder or other systemic disease. Some of these underlying conditions may be undiagnosed and that these responses may be the first indication of the problem (see Chapter 22).

Glaucoma

Patients with closed-angle glaucoma can experience an acute increase in intraocular pressure if anticholinergic drugs are administered. Therefore any dentally used or prescribed drug with anticholinergic effects (e.g., scopolamine, amitriptyline) should be avoided.

Epilepsy, Seizures, and Convulsions

Epilepsy or grand mal seizures need to be identified and the degree of control of seizures determined. Specific etiologic factors of the seizures (e.g., odors, bright lights) should be identified and avoided. Some medications used to control seizures may affect dental treatment because of drug action or side effects. For example, gingival hyperplasia is a well-known side effect of diphenylhydantoin. Patients may discontinue use of antiseizure medication without their doctors' knowledge

and thus be susceptible to seizures during dental treatment. Therefore verification of patient's adherence to their medication needs is important. Removable intraoral appliances are ill-advised for patients with active seizures (see Chapter 22).

Psychiatric Treatment

Patients with a history of a psychiatric illness and the nature of the problem need to be identified. This information may help explain patients' behavioral patterns, problems, or complaints such as unexplainable or unusual conditions or pain. Additionally, some psychiatric drugs have the potential to interact adversely with vasoconstrictors in local anesthetics and produce oral side effects such as xerostomia. Some patients also may be excessively anxious or apprehensive about dental treatment requiring stress-reduction measures (Box 1-1, see Chapter 23).

GASTROINTESTINAL DISEASES

Stomach or Intestinal Ulcers, Gastritis, and Colitis

Patients with gastric conditions should not be given drugs that are directly irritating to the gastrointestinal tract, such as aspirin or nonsteroidal antiinflammatory drugs. Patients with colitis or a history of colitis may not be able to take certain antibiotics. Many antibiotics can cause a particularly severe form of colitis (i.e., pseudomembraneous colitis). Some drugs used to treat ulcers can cause dry mouth (see Chapter 11).

Hepatitis, Liver Disease, Jaundice, and Cirrhosis

Patients who have a history of viral hepatitis are of interest to dentistry because they may be asymptomatic carriers of the disease and transmit it unknowingly to dental personnel or other patients. Of the several types of viral hepatitis, only B, C, and D have carrier stages. Fortunately, laboratory tests are available to identify these patients. Patients also may have chronic hepatitis (B or C) or cirrhosis and, as a result, have impaired liver function. This can result in prolonged bleeding and an impaired ability to efficiently metabolize certain drugs, including local anesthetic and analgesics (see Chapter 10).

RESPIRATORY TRACT DISEASES

Allergies or Hives

Patients may be allergic to some drugs and materials used in dentistry. Common drug allergens include antibiotics and analgesics. Latex allergy also is common. For these patients, alternative materials such as vinyl or powderless gloves can be used to prevent an adverse reaction. True allergy to amide local anesthetics is uncommon. Dentists should procure an allergic history by specifically asking patients how they react to a substance. This will establish a diagnosis of allergy rather than an intolerance or adverse side effect that has been incorrectly identified as an allergy. True allergic symptoms include itching, urticaria (hives), rash, swelling, wheezing, angioedema, runny nose, and tearing eyes. Isolated symptoms such as nausea, vomiting, palpitations, and fainting are generally not of an allergic origin but rather examples of drug intolerance, side effects, and psychogenic reactions (see Chapter 18).

Emphysema

Patients with chronic pulmonary diseases such as emphysema and chronic bronchitis need to be identified to avoid use of medications or procedures that might further depress respiratory function or dry or irritate the airway. Chair position may be a factor; some patients cannot tolerate a supine position. Use of a rubber dam may not be tolerated because of a choking or smothering feeling (see Chapter 8). The use of high-flow oxygen may be contraindicated in some patients because it can decrease the respiratory drive.

Tuberculosis

Patients with a history of tuberculosis (TB) need to be identified for infection-control purposes and information concerning the diagnosis and appropriate treatment. History of the disease needs to be defined. A history of follow-up medical care is important to detect reactivation of the disease or inadequate treatment. The recent emergence of multidrug-resistant TB makes follow-up even more important. A positive skin test means that the person has been infected with TB but not that the patient has active disease. Positive skin testers may be placed on a chemophylaxis (eg., isonazid) to prevent active disease from developing. Active TB is diagnosed by chest x-ray, sputum culture, and clinical examination. Patients with AIDS have a high incidence of tuberculosis, and this relationship may need to be explored (see Chapter 8).

DERMAL, MUCOCUTANEOUS, AND MUSCULOSKELETAL DISEASES

Skin Rash and Dark Moles

Patients with skin lesions need to be identified and have the nature of these abnormalities defined. The dentist may uncover allergic manifestations or identify signs of autoimmmune, malignant, or infectious problems. The history of occurrence and behavior of the lesions are important. A mole that changes color, enlarges, or bleeds should be considered potentially malignant. The presence of oral lesions along with skin lesions may be a sign of a systemic disease.

Night Sweats

Night sweats is a nonspecific symptom of several serious illnesses such as AIDS, tuberculosis, bacterial endocarditis, and Hodgkin's disease.

Sore Muscles, Stiff Joints, and Arthritis

Patients with arthritis may be taking a variety of medications that could influence dental care. Nonsteroidal antiinflammatory drugs, aspirin, steroids, and cytotoxic drugs are examples. A tendency for bleeding and infection should be considered. Chair position may be a factor in physical comfort. Patients may have problems with manual dexterity and oral hygiene. In addition, patients with arthritis also may have involvement of the temporomandibular joints (see Chapter 24).

Artificial Joint

For patients with artificial joints, common clinical practices conflict with scientific data. Quite often these patients are told by their physicians that they should be given prophylactic antibiotics for dental treatment to prevent prosthetic infection. This practice is without scientific validity. Some patients who have artificial joints are potentially at increased risk for infection of these prostheses and may need to be provided with prophylactic antibiotics for dental care likely to result in bleeding. Patients included in this category are those with rheumatoid arthritis, diabetes mellitus, recent joint placement, hemophilia, and those who are immunosuppressed. Even for this at risk group, little data exist to support the need for prophylaxis. Patients with joint prostheses who do not fall into these at risk categories do not require antibiotic prophylaxis (see Chapter 24).

Fever Blister, Mouth Ulcers or Canker Sores, and Colored or Discolored Areas in the Mouth

Intraoral lesions can be benign conditions of the oral soft tissues but also may be infectious. Lesions can be manifestations of systemic problems such as AIDS and malignancies, or results from medication use.

ENDOCRINE DISEASES

Diabetes

Patients with diabetes mellitus need to be identified in terms of type of diabetes and control measure. Some patients with diabetes require insulin (type 1), whereas others usually do not require insulin (type 2) for control of their disease. However, more patients with type 2 diabetes are now treated with insulin than in the past. Those with type 1 diabetes have more severe disease with more complications and are of greater concern for management than are those with type 2 diabetes. Symptoms suggestive of diabetes are excessive thirst and hunger, frequent urination, weight loss, and frequent infections. Complications include blindness, hypertension, and kidney failure, which can affect dental management. Patients with diabetes typically do not handle infections very well and also may have exaggerated periodontal disease. Patients taking insulin are potentially prone to hypoglycemia in the dental office if normal meals are skipped (see Chapter 14).

Thyroid Disease

Patients with uncontrolled or unidentified hyperthyroidism are potentially hypersensitive to stress and sympathomimetics, and the use of vasoconstrictors is generally contraindicated. In rare cases, infection or surgery can initiate a thyroid crisis, a serious medical emergency. Patients with uncontrolled hyperthyroidism may be easily upset emotionally, intolerant of heat, and prone to tremors. Exophthalmos may be present. Patients with known hypothyroidism usually are taking a thyroid supplement and generally pose minimal concerns as long as the thyroid hormone level is not excessive (see Chapter 16).

URINARY TRACT AND SEXUALLY TRANSMITTED DISEASES

Urinary Frequency

Urinary frequency may be a sign of diabetes and should raise suspicion if present, especially if present with other symptoms. Drugs such as diuretics also may result in frequent urination.

Kidney and Bladder Problems

Patients with end-stage renal disease or a kidney transplant need to be identified. Potential for abnormal drug metabolism, immunosuppressive drug therapy, bleeding problems, hepatitis, infections, high blood pressure, and heart failure require management consideration (see Chapter 9).

Sexually Transmitted Diseases

A variety of sexually transmitted diseases such as syphilis, gonorrhea, and AIDS can have manifestations in the oral cavity because of oral-genital contact or hematogenous dissemination in the blood. The dentist may be the first to identify the conditions. In addition, some sexually transmitted diseases can be transmitted to the dentist via direct contact with oral lesions or infectious blood, including HIV, hepatitis B and C, and syphilis (see Chapter 12).

HIV-Positive and AIDS. The presence of oral lesions or other symptoms may be the first indication of the presence of the virus. Candidiasis, hairy leukoplakia, Kaposi's sarcoma, and necrotizing ulcerative gingivitis are some oral conditions commonly associated with AIDS (see Chapter 13).

OTHER CONDITIONS

Frequent Sore Throats and Enlarged Lymph Nodes
Patients who complain of frequent sore throats, enlarged lymph nodes, persistent diarrhea, chronic cough, breathing difficulties, mouth ulcers, or discolored areas in the mouth may have AIDS or other systemic disease. These symptoms may be the first indications that a patient has a disease.

Tobacco and Alcohol Use
Use of tobacco products is a risk factor associated with cancer, cardiovascular disease, pulmonary disease, and periodontal disease. Excessive use of alcohol is a risk factor for malignancies and heart disease and can cause liver disease.

Drug Addiction and Substance Abuse
Patients who have a history of intravenous drug use are at risk for infectious diseases such as hepatitis B or C, AIDS, and infective endocarditis. Antibiotic prophylaxis to prevent infective endocarditis for dental procedures likely to cause significant bleeding should be considered, although the American Heart Association does not include this as a risk category (see Chapter 3). Also, narcotics and sedatives should be prescribed cautiously or not at all for these patients. Vasoconstrictors should be used with caution in active cocaine users because of the possibility of precipitating arrhythmias.

Tumor and Cancer
Patients who have had cancer are at risk for recurrent disease; additional lesions or recurrences are always possible. Also, chemotherapeutic agents and radiation therapy can pose significant management considerations and may result in infection, gingival bleeding, oral ulcerations, mucositis, and impaired healing after invasive dental treatment (see Chapter 21).

Radiation or Cobalt Treatment and Chemotherapy
Patients with previous radiation treatment of the head, neck, or jaws with x-rays or cobalt need to be carefully evaluated because the radiation can permanently destroy the blood supply to the jaws and lead to osteoradionecrosis (a severe bone infection). Radiation treatment in the head and neck also can destroy salivary glands and result in decreased saliva, increased dental caries, and mucositis. Muscle fibrosis also can occur. Chemotherapy can produce many undesirable side effects, most commonly a severe mucositis (see Chapter 21).

CURRENT PHYSICIAN

During the medical history, information should be sought regarding the reason the patient is under medical care, diagnoses, and treatment received. If the reason for seeing a physician was for a physical examination only, the patient should be asked whether any abnormalities were discovered and the date of the examination. The name, address, and phone number of the patient's physician should be recorded for future reference. The patient who does not have a physician may need a more cautious approach than the person who sees one regularly. This is especially true for the patient who has not seen a physician in several years because of possible undiagnosed problems. The response to this question also may provide insight into the priorities the person assigns to health care.

DRUGS, MEDICINES, AND PILLS

Medications being taken for an illness may be the only clue to the patient's disorder. The patient may not have believed mentioning a problem was important but may include it as an answer to a question concerning the taking of medications. An example is the patient with chronic, stable angina pectoris who takes nitroglycerin but has not seen a physician regularly. Drugs may also cause untoward reactions during dental treatment. Thus dentists should identify the various drugs that patients may be taking and become familiar with their actions, side effects, and interactions. The dentist must be cautious not to administer any drug or medication that may interact adversely with the patient's medications. *Drug Information for the Health Care Professional* (USP DI), *Accepted Dental Therapeutics*, and the *Physicians' Desk Reference* (PDR) are examples of useful sources to aid in the identification of drugs and their actions and interactions. The PDR and other sources have pictorial sections helpful in the identification of unknown pills or capsules. The pill or capsule can be matched with pictures of various manufacturers' products. Once a pill is identified, the appropriate descriptive section can be consulted in the text or another drug reference. The questioner should stress "drugs, medicine, or pills of any kind" when questioning patients because frequently they will not list over-the-counter drugs or herbal medicines. For example, a patient taking several aspirin tablets or nonsteroidal antiinflammatory drugs a day for arthritis often answers "none" to this question.

Steroids

Corticosteroid usage is important because it can cause adrenal insufficiency and may render a patient unable to adequately respond to the stress of a dental procedure such as extractions or periodontal surgery. It also can result in a life-threatening situation. Cortisone and prednisone are common examples of steroids and are used in the treatment of many diseases. Generally, however, most routine dental procedures, except extractions or other surgery, do not require supplemental steroids.

Allergies and Reactions to Drugs or Medicines

Questions about allergies should not be limited to medications because patients are exposed to other allergens in the dental office, such as cements, tape, stains, latex, and iodine. Also, a person may be identified as an "allergic" individual because of existing allergies to numerous substances and thus would be at increased risk to be or become allergic to other medications or substances used in dentistry.

Operations or Hospitalizations

A history of hospitalizations can give a good record of past serious illnesses that may have current significance. For example, a patient may have been hospitalized for cardiac catheterization for ischemic heart disease. Another example is a patient hospitalized for hepatitis C. Both types of patients may never have received medical follow-up care for these problems, and the response to this question is the only indication of these past problems. Information about hospitalizations should include diagnosis, treatment, and complications. If a patient has undergone any operation, the reason for the procedures and any untoward events associated with them such as anesthetic emergencies, unusual postoperative bleeding, infections, and drug allergy should be addressed.

CARDIOVASCULAR OR PULMONARY SIGNS AND SYMPTOMS

Screening questions regarding limitation of activity, chest pain, and shortness of breath may identify underlying cardiovascular or respiratory diseases.

Diet

Information about diet may identify a patient who is on a special diet because of an underlying systemic problem such as diabetes, hyperthyroidism, or heart disease.

BLOOD CONTACT

The question of blood contact has significant implications because hepatitis, AIDS, syphilis, and other communicable diseases can be transmitted by contact with infectious blood or blood products. Thus blood contact is a risk factor for these diseases.

PREGNANCY

Women who are or may be pregnant may need special consideration in the taking of radiographs, administration of drugs, or timing of dental treatment.

SIGNATURE

The patient is requested to date and sign the questionnaire, attesting to the accuracy of the information provided. The dentist should also sign, indicating that the form has been reviewed.

VITAL SIGNS

Vital signs are obtained by direct measurement, such as blood pressure, pulse, and respiratory rate, and by questioning height and weight. This information may be important in a medical emergency to serve as a baseline and in the administration of emergency drugs, some of which are given on a milligram per kilogram (mg/kg) basis. Temperature is usually recorded only when indicated. Abnormal readings may require further investigation or referral.

AMERICAN SOCIETY OF ANESTHESIOLOGISTS CLASSIFICATION

The American Society of Anesthesiologists (ASA) classification is a subjective system of classifying patients according to the severity of their systemic disease and its affect on their daily lives. The purpose of the classification is to aid development of dental management decisions. Patients may change categories depending on control and stability of disease at a given time. The classification is as follows:

1. ASA I–Normal healthy patient; no dental management alterations required
2. ASA II–A patient with mild systemic disease that does not interfere with daily activity or who has a significant health risk factor (e.g., smoking, alcohol abuse, gross obesity); may or may not need dental management alterations

   Examples: Stage I or II hypertension, type 2 diabetes, heart murmur, asymptomatic rheumatic heart disease, allergy, well controlled asthma, well controlled epilepsy, hepatitis B surface antigen positive, HIV, mild chronic obstructive pulmonary disease, chronic stable angina
3. ASA III–A patient with moderate to severe systemic disease that is not incapacitating but may alter daily

activity; may have significant drug concerns; may require special patient care; would generally require dental management alterations

Examples: Type I diabetes, stage 3 hypertension, unstable angina pectoris, recent myocardial infarction, poorly controlled congestive heart failure, AIDS, chronic obstructive pulmonary disease, hemophilia

4. ASA IV–A patient with severe systemic disease that is a constant threat to life; definitely requires dental management alterations; best treated in special facility

Examples: Kidney failure, liver failure, advanced AIDS

HEALTH COMMENTS AND SUMMARY

This section is to allow comments on only those items to which the patient has positively responded *and* that have potential impact on the provision of dental care. It therefore provides a quick reference and a summary of the health status and treatment modifications required.

DENTAL HISTORY

A thorough dental history is important for any patient who is to be treated from a comprehensive standpoint. The history must include procedures that have been performed, dates of treatments, and the outcome of the previous treatment. This entails restorative procedures, prosthetic devices, surgical procedures, orthodontic treatment, endodontic therapy, periodontal treatment, and radiographs. Any complications with the treatment, anesthetic, or medications prescribed should be noted. Determination of the patient's view of dentists and any expectations also is helpful. Discussion of unpleasant past dental experiences is important. This may provide an explanation for a patient's fear or anxiety about dental treatment, which is important in risk assessment. Also, dental problems may occasionally serve as a clue to an underlying systemic disease. For example, a patient with severe, progressive periodontal disease may be found to have AIDS or diabetes.

PHYSICAL EXAMINATION

In addition to providing a comprehensive health history, the dental patient should be afforded the benefits of a simple, abbreviated physical examination. This should include assessment of general appearance, vital signs, body temperature (if appropriate), and an examination of the head and neck.

GENERAL SURVEY

Much can be learned about a patient and the state of health from a purposeful but tactful visual inspection. Careful observation can lead to an awareness and a recognition of abnormal or unusual features and conditions that may exist and could influence the provision of dental care. This survey consists of an assessment of the general appearance and inspection of specific exposed body areas, including skin, nails, face, eyes, nose, ears, and neck. Each visually accessible area may demonstrate peculiarities that can signal underlying systemic disease or abnormalities.

The outward appearance of a patient can give an indication of the general state of health and well-being. Examples of possible trouble include a wasted, cachectic appearance; lethargic demeanor; ill-kept, dirty clothing and hair; body odors; staggering or halting gait; extreme thinness or obesity; bent posture; and difficulty breathing. The dentist also should remain sensitive to breath odors such as acetone associated with diabetes, ammonia associated with renal failure, putrefaction of pulmonary infections, and alcohol possibly associated with alcohol abuse or subsequent liver disease.

Skin and Nails

The skin is the largest organ of the body, and usually large areas are exposed and available for inspection. Changes in the skin and nails frequently are associated with systemic disease. For example, cyanosis can indicate cardiac or pulmonary insufficiency, yellowing may be caused by liver diseases, pigmentation may be associated with hormonal abnormalities, and petechiae or ecchymoses can be signs of a blood dyscrasia or bleeding disorder (Fig. 1-3). Alterations in fingernails are usually caused by chronic disorders, such as clubbing (seen in cardiopulmonary insufficiency, Fig. 1-4), white

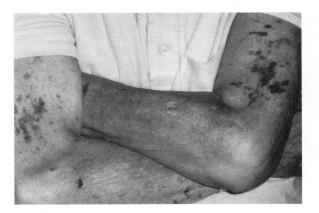

Fig. 1-3 Petechiae and ecchymosis in a patient that could signal a bleeding disorder. (Courtesy Robert Henry, Lexington, Ky.)

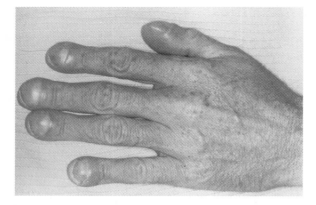

Fig. 1-4 Clubbing of digits and nails can be associated with cardiopulmonary insufficiency.

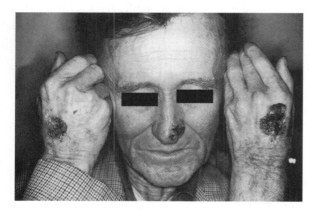

Fig. 1-5 Basal cell carcinomas of the dorsum of the hands and the bridge of the nose.

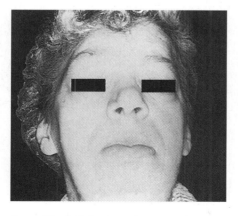

Fig. 1-6 Patient with acromegaly.

nails (seen in cirrhosis), yellowing of nails (from malignancy), and splinter hemorrhages (from bacterial endocarditis). The dorsal surfaces of the hands are common sites for actinic keratosis and basal cell carcinomas, as are the bridge of the nose, infraorbital regions, and ears (Fig. 1-5).

Face
The shape and symmetry of the face is abnormal in a variety of syndromes and conditions. Well-known examples include the coarse features of acromegaly (Fig. 1-6); pale, edematous features in nephrotic syndrome; moon facies in Cushing's syndrome (Fig. 1-7); the dull, puffy puffy facies of myxedema, and the unilateral paralysis of Bell's palsy (Fig. 1-8).

Eyes and Nose
The eyes can be sensitive indicators of systemic disease and therefore should be closely inspected. Patients who wear glasses should be requested to remove them during the examination of the head and neck. Hyperthyroidism can produce a characteristic lid retraction resulting in a wide-eyed stare (Fig. 1-9). Xanthomas of the eyelids are frequently associated with hypercholesterolemia (Fig. 1-10), as is arcus senilis in an older individual. Scleral yellowing can be caused by hepatitis. Reddened conjunctiva can be from the sicca syndrome, allergy, or iritis.

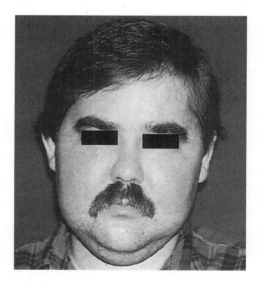

Fig. 1-7 Patient with cushinoid facies after several weeks of prednisone administration. (From Bricker SL, Langlais RP, Miller CS: *Oral diagnosis, oral medicine, and treatment planning*, ed 2, Philadelphia, 1994, Lea & Febiger.)

Ears

The ears should be inspected for gouti tophi in the helix or antihelix. Also, a lateral crease in the earlobe may be associated with an increased risk of coronary artery disease. Malignant or premalignant lesions (i.e., skin cancer) may be found on and around the ears (Fig. 1-11).

Neck

The neck should be inspected for enlargement and asymmetry. Depending on location and consistency, enlargement can be caused by goiter (Fig. 1-12), infection, cysts (Fig. 1-13), enlarged lymph nodes (Fig. 1-14), or vascular deformities.

VITAL SIGNS

The benefits of vital sign measurement during an initial examination are twofold. First, the establishment of baseline normal values ensures a standard of comparison in the event an emergency occurs during treatment. If an emergency occurs, knowledge of a patient's normal values is essential to determine the severity of the problem. For example, if a patient lost consciousness unexpectedly and blood pressure was 90/50 mm Hg, the concern would be entirely different for a patient whose blood pressure was normally 110/65 mm Hg than for the patient with hypertension whose blood pressure was normally 180/110 mm Hg. In the second example the patient may well be in a shock state.

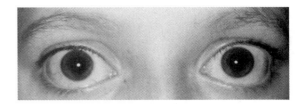

Fig. 1-9 Lid retraction from hyperthyroidism.

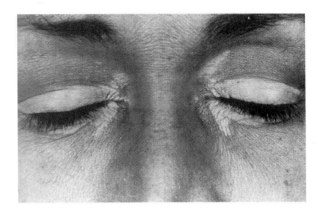

Fig. 1-10 Xanthomas of the eyelids can signal hypercholesterolemia.

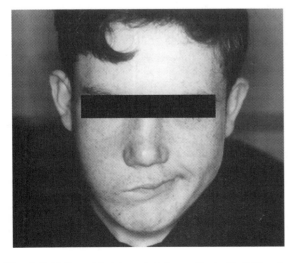

Fig. 1-8 Unilateral facial paralysis in a patient with Bell's palsy.

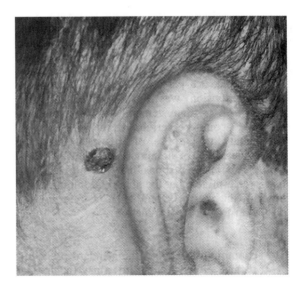

Fig. 1-11 Malignant melanoma posterior to the ear.

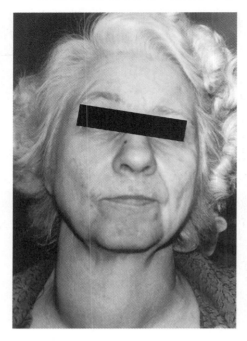

Fig. 1-12 Midline neck enlargement from a goiter.

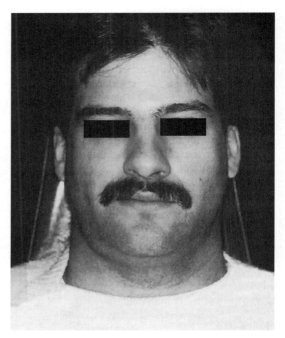

Fig. 1-14 Enlarged lymph node beneath the body of the mandible resulting from a salivary gland infection.

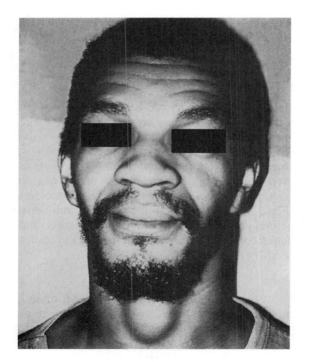

Fig. 1-13 Midline neck enlargement resulting from thyroglossal duct cyst.

A second benefit of vital sign measurement during an examination is screening to identify abnormalities, either diagnosed or undiagnosed. For example, if a person with severe, long-standing hypertension was not identified and treated with no management alteration, the consequences can be serious. The purpose of this examination is merely detection of an abnormality and not diagnosis. This is the responsibility of the physician. If the abnormal finding is deemed significant, the patient should be referred to a physician for further evaluation.

Pulse

The standard procedure to assess the pulse rate is to palpate either the carotid artery at the side of the trachea or the radial artery on the thumb side of the wrist (Figs. 1-15 and 1-16). Use of the carotid artery for pulse determination has some advantages. First, the carotid pulse is familiar because of CPR training of the dentist. Second, it is reliable because it is a central artery supplying the brain; therefore in emergency situations it may remain palpable when peripheral arteries are not. Finally, it is easily palpated because it is a large artery.

The carotid pulse can best be palpated along the anterior border of the sternocleidomastoid muscle at approximately the level of the thyroid cartilage. Dis-

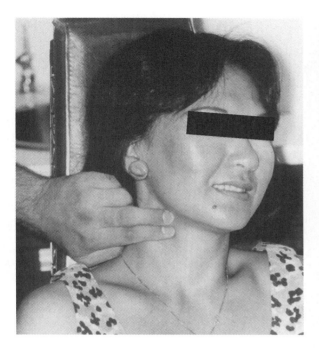

Fig. 1-15 Palpation of the carotid pulse.

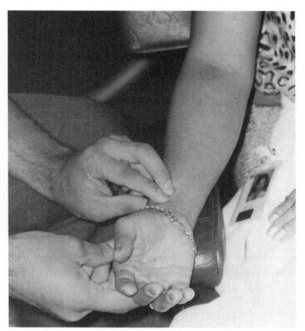

Fig. 1-16 Palpation of the radial pulse.

placement of the sternocleidomastoid muscle slightly posteriorly allows palpation of the pulse with the first and middle finger of the examiner, who monitors the pulse ideally for a full minute to detect irregular patterns.

Rate. The average pulse rate in normal adults is 60 to 100 beats per minute. A pulse rate greater than 100 beats per minute is termed *tachycardia*, whereas a slow pulse rate less than 60 beats per minute is called *bradycardia*. An abnormal pulse rate may be a sign of a cardiovascular disorder but also may be influenced by exercise, conditioning, anxiety, drugs, or fever.

Rhythm. The normal pulse is a series of rhythmic beats that follow at regular intervals. When the beats follow at irregular intervals, the pulse is termed *irregular, dysrhythmic,* or *arrhythmic.* One common benign arrythmia is a sinus arrhythmia, whereby the pulse rate varies with respiration. This type of rhythm is seen in younger adults and well-conditioned athletes.

Blood Pressure

Blood pressure is usually determined indirectly in the upper extremities with a blood pressure cuff and stethoscope (Fig. 1-17). The blood pressure cuff should be the correct width to give an accurate record-

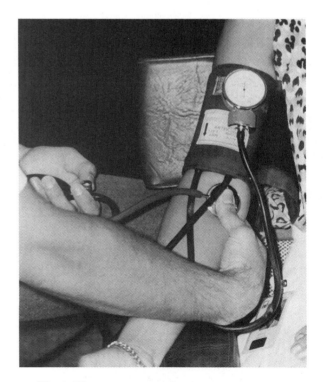

Fig. 1-17 Blood pressure cuff and stethoscope in place.

ing. The standard cuff width for an average adult arm is 12 to 14 cm. A cuff that is too narrow yields falsely elevated values, whereas a cuff that is too wide yields falsely low values. Narrower cuffs are available for use on children, and wider cuffs are available for use on obese or large patients. As an alternative on an obese patient, a standard-size cuff can be placed on the forearm below the antecubital fossa and the radial artery may be palpated to determine the systolic pressure only.[1]

The stethoscope should be of good standard quality. The bell end (cup) is preferred for auscultation of the brachial artery; however, the use of the diaphragm (flat) is common in practice and is acceptable.

The auscultation method of blood pressure measurement has gained universal acceptance. The technique, advocated by the American Heart Association, is described as follows.[1] The patient is in a standard sitting position and the cuff is placed on either bared arm. When the procedure must be repeated, the same position and arm should be used because blood pressure can vary between arms and positions. The cuff should be placed snugly above the elbow, with the lower border approximately an inch above the antecubital fossa. The standard cuff has arrows designating the location of the previously palpated brachial artery (at the medial aspect of the ten-

don of the biceps). A cuff that is too loose yields falsely elevated values. Clothing should not be left under the cuff because this too may yield incorrect readings.

The cuff is inflated until the radial pulse disappears and then inflated about an additional 30 mm Hg. The stethoscope is then placed over the previously palpated brachial artery at the bend of the elbow in the antecubital fossa (not under the cuff), and no sounds should be heard. The pressure is then slowly released 2 to 3 mm Hg per second, and as the needle falls, a point is noted when beats become audible. This is recorded as the systolic pressure.

As the needle continues to fall, the sound of the beats becomes louder, then gradually diminishes until a point is reached at which a sudden, marked diminution in intensity occurs. The weakened beats are heard for a few moments more and then disappear altogether (Fig. 1-18). The most reliable index of diastolic pressure is the point at which there is complete disappearance of sound. Occasionally, muffled sounds can be heard continuously far below the true diastolic pressure. When this occurs, the initial point of muffling is to be used as the diastolic pressure.

An "auscultatory gap" can be missed. Sounds may disappear between the systolic and diastolic pressures and then reappear. If the cuff pressure is raised only to the range of the gap, the systolic reading will be falsely low. This error is eliminated by previous determinination of the systolic level by the palpatory method.

In the average, healthy adult the normal systolic pressure varies between 90 and 140 mm Hg, generally increasing with age. The normal diastolic pressure varies between 60 and 90 mm Hg. Pulse pressure is the difference between the systolic and diastolic pressure, so hypertension in adults is defined as blood pressure being equal to or greater than 140/90 mm Hg[2] (Table 1-1). If the blood pressure is elevated, the procedure should be repeated once or twice during the appointment and the average taken as the final measurement.

Respiration

The rate and depth of respiration should be noted by careful observation of the movement of the chest and abdomen in the quietly breathing patient. The respiratory rate in a normal resting adult is approximately 12 to 16 breaths per minute. The respiratory rate in small children is higher than that of an adult.

Notice should be made of patients with labored breathing, rapid breathing, or irregular breathing patterns because all may be signs of systemic problems, especially cardiopulmonary disease.

A common finding in apprehensive patients is hyperventilation (rapid, prolonged, deep breathing or sighing), which can result in lowered carbon dioxide levels and

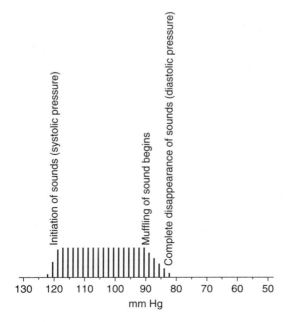

Fig. 1-18 Typical sound pattern obtained when recording blood pressure in a normotensive adult.

may cause disturbing symptoms, including perioral numbness, tingling in the fingers and toes, nausea, a "sick" feeling, and carpopedal spasms.

Temperature

Temperature is not usually recorded during a routine dental examination but rather when a patient has febrile signs or symptoms such as found with an abscessed tooth or a mucosal/gingival infection. Normal oral temperature is 98.6° F (37° C) but may vary as much as plus or minus 1° F over 24 hours and is usually highest in the afternoon. Rectal temperature is about 1° F higher than oral, and axillary temperature is about 1° F lower than oral.

Weight

Patients should be questioned about any recent unintentional gain or loss of weight. A rapid loss of weight may be a sign of malignancy, diabetes, tuberculosis, or other wasting diseases, whereas a rapid weight gain can be a sign of heart failure, edema, hyperthyroidism, or neoplasm.

Head and Neck Examination

An examination of the head and neck may vary in its comprehensiveness but should include inspection and palpation of the soft tissues of the oral cavity, maxillofacial region, and neck (Fig. 1-19) and an evaluation of cranial nerve function. (See standard texts on physical diagnosis for further descriptions.)

CLINICAL LABORATORY TESTS

Laboratory evaluation can be an important phase in determination of a patient's health status. Fortunately, most patients do not require laboratory screening; however, it can be a useful tool for those who do. The dentist should know the indications for ordering clinical laboratory tests, the procedure for ordering them from a clinical laboratory, and how to interpret the results. In dealing with a commercial laboratory, the dentist should take the time to visit the laboratory facilities and meet the pathologist in charge. At this time the dentist should find out which tests of interest are performed by the laboratory, what the costs are for these tests, and what the normal ranges are for test results. Copies of laboratory order sheets for these tests should also be obtained. If the patient is sent to the laboratory for collection of the sample to be tested (such as blood), the laboratory will send the results directly to the dentist for interpretation and will bill the patient. The dentist should inform the patient of the cost before referral to the laboratory.

TABLE 1-1

Classification of Blood Pressure for Adults Aged 18 Years and Older

Category	BLOOD PRESSURE mm HG		
	Systolic		Diastolic
Optimal*	< 120	and	< 80
Normal	< 130	and	< 85
High Normal	130-139	or	85-89
Hypertension			
Stage 1	140-159	or	90-99
Stage 2	160-179	or	100-109
Stage 3	≥ 180	or	≥ 110

From The Sixth Report of Joint National Committee on prevention, detection, evaluation, and treatment of high blood pressure. *Arch Int Med*, 157:2413-2444, 1997.
*Not taking antihypertensive medication.

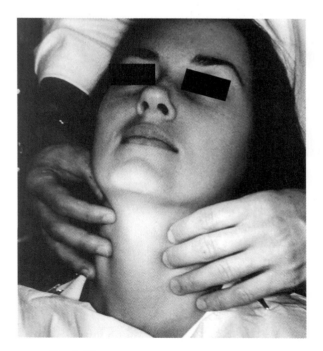

Fig. 1-19 Bimanual palpation of the anterior neck.

If the dentist does not want to become involved with ordering laboratory tests for the patients, then patients should be referred to a physician for medical and laboratory screening.

Tests such as biopsy, cytology, and culture and sensitivity are not included in this chapter but obviously are of great importance.

Clinical laboratory tests must be performed when indicated. Some indications for clinical laboratory testing in dentistry include the following:

1. Aiding in the diagnosis of suspected disease (e.g., diabetes, infection, bleeding disorders, leukemia, neutropenia)
2. Screening high-risk patients for undetected disease (e.g., hepatitis B, diabetes)
3. Establishing normal baseline values before treatment (e.g., anticoagulant status, chemotherapy, radiation therapy)
4. Addressing medicolegal considerations (e.g., possible bleeding disorders, hepatitis B infection)

It is beyond the scope of this text to discuss all laboratory tests that a dentist may order; however, Table 1-2 lists several common laboratory tests with the range of normal values. The following are examples of how clinical laboratory tests can be used in dental practice.

Case Studies

Case 1

A 38-year-old man was going to be treated for a periodontal condition that required surgery. During the history he mentioned that he had had a tooth extracted about 3 years earlier and had bled for several days after the extraction. He had gone to a physician, who had given him an injection of vitamin K, after which the bleeding stopped. Before the periodontal surgery this patient was screened for a possible bleeding condition through a commercial laboratory. A bleeding time, prothrombin time, partial thromboplastin time, and thrombin time were ordered. This battery of tests was necessary because no real insight into the possible cause of the bleeding problem, if indeed one existed, was evident. The possibilities to be ruled out included coagulation disorders, platelet abnormality, vascular wall defects, and defects of fibrinolysis. The laboratory results to the screening tests for this patient were all normal values, and he was treated with no complications. ■

Case 2

A 40-year-old man who had advanced periodontitis stated while giving his medical history that his mother had insulin-dependent diabetes mellitus. This situation placed the patient in a high-risk group for diabetes. A fasting glucose test was ordered for this patient, and the results were 150 mg/100 ml. This result was abnormally elevated, with suggested the possibility of diabetes, and the dentist recommended that the patient see his physician as soon as possible. ■

Case 3

A 30-year-old woman went to her dentist for routine care. During the discussion of her past medical history, she revealed that she had had hepatitis a few years before but did not know anything about the details of the disease and could not remember her physician's name. A screening test for hepatitis B surface antigen and antibodies to the hepatitis C virus was ordered to rule out the possibility of her being a carrier of hepatitis B or C. The test was positive for hepatitis B surface antigen, indicating that the patient was indeed a carrier of hepatitis B. She was referred to her physician for evaluation of her liver function before initiating any treatment, and plans were made to provide dental care with usual attention to asepsis, barrier techniques, and universal infection control procedures. ■

PHYSICIAN REFERRAL AND CONSULTATION

Based on the medical history, physical examination, laboratory screening, and dentist's level of training, contact with the patient's physician for consultation or referral purposes may be necessary. The usual methods are by phone, personal contact, or letter. Personal contact is common, particularly in a smaller community where physicians and dentists may informally discuss a mutual patient. The main drawback to this type of "sidewalk consultation" is its informality and the lack of a documented record of the consult. If this method is employed, a progress note should be entered in the patient's chart as soon as possible. A phone conversation also should have this type of formal follow-up documentation and confirmation. The principal advantage of the conversational approach is one of immediate information and the chance to gain additional information to questions that may not have been included in a letter (Figs. 1-20 through 1-22). The advantage of a letter or written consultation is having a permanent chart of the consultant's reply which can become a permanent part of the record. If a patient needs treatment without delay, a phone call to obtain the pertinent information from the physician allows the dentist to proceed; however, this should be followed-up with a chart entry.

TABLE 1-2

Clinical Laboratory Tests and Normal Values

Test	Range of Normal Values	Test	Range of Normal Values
Complete Blood Count		**Serum Chemistry**	
White blood cells	4,400-11,000	Glucose (fasting)	70-110 mg/dl
Red blood cells (male)	4.5-5.9 $10^6/\mu L$	Blood urea nitrogen	8-23 mg/dl
Red blood cells (female)	4.5-5.1 $10^6/\mu L$	Creatinine	0.6-1.2 mg/dl
Platelets	150,000-450,000/μL	Bilirubin, indirect (unconjugated)	0.1-1.0 mg/dl
Hematocrit (male)	41.5-50.4%	Bilirubin, direct (conjugated)	< 0.3 mg/dl
Hematocrit (female)	35.9-44.6%	Calcium	9.2-11 mg/dl
Hemoglobin (male)	14-17.5 g/dl	Magnesium	1.8-3.0 mg/dl
Hemoglobin (female)	12.3-15.3 g/dl	Phosphorus	2.3-4.7 mg/dl
Mean corpuscular volume	80-96 μm^3		
Mean corpuscular hemoglobin	27.5-33.2 pg	**Serum Electrolytes**	
Mean corpuscular hemoglobin concentration	33.4-35.5%	Sodium	136-142 mEq/l
		Potassium	3.8-5.0 mEq/l
Differential White Blood Cell Count (%)		Chloride	95-103 mEq/l
Segemented neutrophils	56	Bicarbonate	21-28 mmol/l
Bands	3		
Eosinophils	2.7	**Serum Enzymes**	
Basophils	0.3	Alkaline phosphatase	20-130 IU/l
Lymphocytes	34	Alanine aminotransferase	4-36 u/l
Monocytes	4	Aspartate aminotransferase	8-33 u/l
		Amylase	16-120 Somogyi units/dl
Hemostasis			
Bleeding time	2-8 minutes	Creatine kinase (male)	55-170 u/l
Prothrombin time	10-13 seconds	Creatine kinase (female)	30-135 u/l
Activated partial thrombo-plastin time	25-35 seconds		

Data compiled from Henry JB: *Clinical diagnosis and management by laboratory methods*, ed 19 Philadelphia, 1996, WB Saunders, pp 1450-1460.

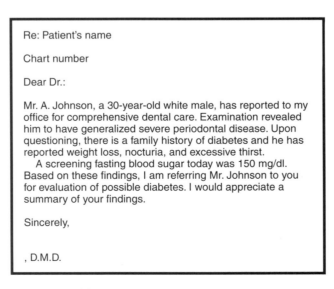

Re: Patient's name

Chart number

Dear Dr.:

Mr. A. Johnson, a 30-year-old white male, has reported to my office for comprehensive dental care. Examination revealed him to have generalized severe periodontal disease. Upon questioning, there is a family history of diabetes and he has reported weight loss, nocturia, and excessive thirst.

A screening fasting blood sugar today was 150 mg/dl. Based on these findings, I am referring Mr. Johnson to you for evaluation of possible diabetes. I would appreciate a summary of your findings.

Sincerely,

, D.M.D.

Fig. 1-20 Referral for evaluation of suspected diabetes.

Re: Patient's name

Chart number

Dear Dr.:

Mr. A. Smith, a 37-year-old white male, has reported to my office for comprehensive dental care. He reports a history of rheumatic fever at age 8 years but is unaware of any residual damage to his heart that would predispose to infective endocarditis. He denies any symptoms associated with heart disease and is a well-developed, well-nourished, athletic individual. We are planning to provide comprehensive dental care for Mr. Smith.

The purpose of this referral is to request an evaluation of his cardiac status to rule out the presence of rheumatic heart disease and the need for prophylactic antibiotics to prevent infective endocarditis or any additional medical problems of which I should be aware. If, Mr. Smith has valvular disease, I would plan to follow the current recommendations of the American Heart Association.

I would appreciate receiving a summary of your findings regarding his cardiac status at your earliest convenience.

Thank you for seeing this patient.

Sincerely,

, D.M.D.

Fig. 1-21 Referral to verify the presence of rheumatic heart disease.

Re: Patient's name

Chart number

Dear Dr.:

Mrs. A. Jones, a 50-year-old obese black female, has reported to my office for dental care. During the examination and history she reported frequent headaches and dizzy spells in addition to her eyes "bothering" her. She has not seen a physician for several years but remembers taking a "water pill" for blood pressure at one time. In my office today her blood pressure was 215/125 mm Hg, right arm, sitting, at the beginning of the appointment and 210/125 mm Hg at the termination of the appointment. At this point I have elected to postpone any dental work and have advised her to seek an immediate medical evaluation from you.

I would appreciate a summary of your findings of this patient, and I will plan to resume treatment when her blood pressure is controlled.

Thank you for seeing this patient.

Sincerely,

, D.M.D.

Fig. 1-22 Referral because of uncontrolled hypertension.

Date:_____

Patient Name:_____

Date of Birth:_____ Age:_____ Sex:_____

Dental Chart Number:_____

_____

To (Physician):_____

Physician's Address:_____

Physician's Phone#:_____

From (Dental Student):_____

Attending Dentist:_____

_____

Patient History:

Reason for Consult:

_____

Consultant Reply:

_____
Signature of Consultant

Fig. 1-23 Request for Medical Consultation form in use at University of Kentucky College of Dentistry.

A letter to a physician should be concise; only pertinent information should be included, and questions or the reasons the patient was referred should be specific.

An additional approach to the referral/consultation request is a printed form. Fig. 1-23 is the "Request for Medical Consultation" form in use at the University of Kentucky College of Dentistry. The advantage of this approach is that it simplifies and standardizes the procedure for the dentist and physician.

References

1. American Heart Association: *Human blood pressure determination by sphygmomanometry,* Publ. no. 70-1061(SA), Dallas, 1994, American Heart Association.
2. The sixth report of the Joint National Committee on Prevention, Detection, Evaluation, and Treatment of High Blood Pressure, *Arch Intern Med* 157:2413-2444, 1997.

Infective Endocarditis

2

CHAPTER

*I*nfective endocarditis (IE) is caused by microbial infection of the heart valves or endocardium and most often is related to congenital or acquired cardiac defects. A similar disease, infective endarteritis (IEA), involves a patent ductus arteriosus, coarctation of the aorta, surgical grafts of major vessels, and surgical arteriovenous shunts. Bacteria most often cause these diseases. However, in recent years, researchers have identified fungi and other microorganisms as the cause.

Dentists are most concerned with IE and IEA caused by bacteria. Thus the terms *bacterial endocarditis* (BE) and *bacterial endarteritis* (BEA) are used in this chapter to describe these infections (Table 2-1). A specific type of bacteria identified as the cause of the disease is referred to by such terms as *Streptococcus bovis* endocarditis, *Staphylococcus aureus* endocarditis, and so on. The American Heart Association uses this terminology in the recommendations it makes to the medical and dental professions for the prevention of endocarditis.[1-8]

The dentist must make every attempt to identify patients with congenital or acquired cardiovascular defects before performing any dental manipulations that could produce a significant transient bacteremia possibly resulting in BE or BEA. These infections were essentially 100% fatal before the antibiotic era. Even with the best of medical treatment, these diseases have approximately a 10% to 80% mortality rate.[9-14] Adequate prophylactic antibiotic therapy in many cases can prevent BE and BEA. This chapter deals primarily with BE and its prevention, but the same principles of prevention apply to BEA.

EPIDEMIOLOGY: INCIDENCE AND PREVALENCE

The characteristic lesion of BE is a vegetation that usually develops on a heart valve but occasionally appears elsewhere on the endocardium.[15] The incidence of BE is not positively known. A study by Porgrel and Welsby[16] in 1975 found 83 cases of bacterial endocarditis over a 15-year period from a population of approximately 500,000 persons served by the Aberdeen Royal Infirmary. This would suggest an incidence of much less than 1%. Mostaghim and Millard[17] reported 64 cases of BE treated at the University of Michigan Hospital over a 10-year period, also much less than 1%. Falace and Ferguson[9] reported 49 patients admitted to the University of Kentucky's University Hospital for BE between 1963 and 1975. During this period, 142,082 admissions to the hospital were recorded, or a 0.034% incidence. The worldwide incidence for BE has been estimated at 10 to 60 cases per 1 million persons per year. In the United States the rate is probably 1.6 to 6.0 cases per 100,000 persons per year. This would result in approximately 4000 to 15,000 cases of BE occuring per year in the United States.[15] In Delaware Valley, where the population includes a large number of intravenous drug users, the estimated rate is much higher: 11.6 cases per 100,000 persons per year.[15]

Based on these data, BE is relatively rare in the United States. However, when only the more susceptible portion of the population is considered, BE becomes a much more common problem. The Bland and Jones study of rheumatic fever[18] in 1951 found 10% of the deaths caused by BE. In that study 30 patients out of 1000 died of BE. No mention was made of the number of patients with the disease who lived. Patients on hemodialysis have a 2% to 6% risk for BE.[15] Patients with a previous history of endocarditis have approximately a 2% to 31% risk of another BE episode.[15,19]

Certain features of BE have changed during the past 20 to 30 years. It is now more common in men (1.5:1 ratio, increasing to 8:1 for patients over age 60), and the median age has increased from 30 to 50 years. The number of acute cases has increased and the proportion of streptococcal cases has decreased slightly. Cases caused by fungi and gram-negative bacteria have increased.

TABLE 2-1

Endocarditis Terminologies

Term	Abbreviation	Definition
Infective endocarditis	IE	Microbial infection of heart valves or endocardium
Infective endarteritis	IEA	Microbial infection of endothelium of arteries
Bacterial endocarditis	BE	Bacterial infection of heart valve or endocardium
Alpha-hemolytic streptococcus	—	Identification of infecting organism
Bacterial endarteritis	BEA	Bacterial infection of endothelium of arteries
Nonbacterial thrombotic endocarditis	NBTE	Sterile vegetation formed by platelets and fibrin at sites of endocardial damage
Acute bacterial endocarditis	ABE	Condition with sudden onset, fatal in less than 6 weeks if untreated, usually caused by *Staphylococcus aureus*, normal valves often involved
Subacute bacterial endocarditis	SBE	Condition with slower onset, fatal in months if not treated, most often caused by *Streptococcus viridans* infecting damaged valves
Native valve endocarditis	NVE	Infection of native heart valves
Prosthetic valve endocarditis	PVE	Infection of prosthetic heart valves
Nosocomial infective endocarditis	NSE	Hospital-acquired endocarditis

Cases in injected drug users have greatly increased. Some classic signs of advanced subacute endocarditis (SBE) such as Osler's nodes, finger clubbing, splenomegaly, and Roth's spots have shown a reduced incidence. Prosthetic heart valve infections have become much more numerous. The list of etiologic organisms has increased, with more cases being caused by various rare and unusual microbes. The concomitant infection with HIV and endocarditis has increased.[15]

BE remains uncommon in children and rare during infancy. No underlying cardiac disease is found in approximately 15% of children with endocarditis. The incidence of endocarditis appears to be increasing in smaller infants with cyanotic heart disease.[20] Endocarditis has become more common in the elderly. About 25% of all cases of endocarditis occur in patients over age 60. The annual risk for endocarditis is strongly age related, with the rate approximately five times higher in patients older than 80 years.[15]

Elderly dental patients are considered at risk for BE because of increased prevalence of cardiac valvular disease and impairment of the immune system. Those over age 60 have shown increases in aortic stenosis; degenerative calcification of the mitral valve ring develops in those over age 70. Men over age 60 with mitral valve prolapse and systolic hypertension are at risk of BE because of excessive hemodynamic load placed on the abnormal valve. This causes extensive stretching of cusps and loss of valve surface endothelium.[21]

The use of prophylactic antibiotics has not appeared to reduce the number of cases of BE being reported. This may be because fewer than one in five cases of SBE have been associated with medical or dental procedures, and very few of the acute cases are associated with medical or dental procedures.[15]

More than 200 cases of streptococcal endocarditis that followed dental and genitourinary tract procedures have been reported in the literature. In the vast majority of these cases symptoms of the disease occurred within 2 weeks of the procedure. A few patients have symptoms within 1 or 2 days afterwards. In cases wherein symptoms of BE do not occur within 2 weeks the suspected procedure probably was not the cause of the infection. However, the upper limit of the incubation period is not known with any certainty.[12,15,22]

ETIOLOGY

Endocarditis occurs when bacteria enter the bloodstream and infect damaged endocardium or endothelial tissue located near high-flow shunts between arterial and venous channels. Other microorganisms such as

TABLE 2-2

Conditions and Procedures Possibly Leading to Infective Endocarditis

Conditions and Procedures	Normal Heart	Cardiac Defect
IV drug abuse	Usually	Uncommon
Hemodialysis	Usually	Uncommon
Genitourinary tract manipulation		
Cystoscopy	Uncommon	Usually
Urethral catheterization	Uncommon	Usually
Prostatectomy	Uncommon	Usually
Septic abortion	Uncommon	Usually
Pelvic infection		
Intrauterine contraceptive device	Uncommon	Usually
Skin infections (staphylococcal)	Sometimes	Usually
Cancer of colon	Rare	Usually
Dental treatment and dental infection	Rare	Usually
Nosocomial		
Surgery	Sometimes	Sometimes
Intracardiac pressure—monitoring devices	Usually	Uncommon
Ventriculoatrial shunts	Usually	Uncommon
Hyperalimentation lines into right ventricle	Usually	Uncommon
Severe burns	Usually	Uncommon

fungi may rarely infect these sites. Other host factors must be important because a number of patients with congenital or acquired heart lesions did not develop BE after medical or dental procedures without antibiotic protection.

Mostaghim and Millard[17] suggested that drug addicts, with or without cardiac lesions, might be more susceptible to the disease. Recent reports[15,19,23] have confirmed the increased risk of BE in drug addicts. Intravenous drug abusers have a 30% risk for BE within 2 years of drug use.[24] Bacteria are either released directly into the bloodstream because of use of nonsterile needles or gain access to the bloodstream because an infection develops at the injection site. More than 50% of the cases of endocarditis in drug addicts are caused by S. *aureus*, and approximately 50% to 70% involve the right side of the heart, usually the tricuspid valve.[15,19,23] Septic pulmonary infarcts are a common finding in these patients. Other conditions that may lead to BE in patients with or without cardiac defects are shown in Table 2-2.

Mitral valve prolapse is a common cardiac condition, occurring in approximately 16 million people in the United States. Primary prolapsing mitral valves may be familial or nonfamilial and associated with myxomatous degeneration of the mitral valve leaflets such as occurs in Marfan's syndrome and other connective tissue disorders. Secondary forms may be associated with such entities as rheumatic fever (especially after commissurotomy) and coronary artery disease (in the presence of ruptured chordae tendineae) and with congenital conditions such as interatrial defect and primary cardiomyopathy with outflow tract obstruction. Late systolic murmur and midsystolic click both characterize prolapsing mitral valve. Approximately one fourth of mitral valve prolapse cases progress with mitral insufficiency. This group of patients is at increased risk for endocarditis. Approximately three fourths of patients with prolapsing mitral valve syndrome lead normal lives and do not appear to be at risk for endocarditis.[25]

Various agents can cause iatrogenic valve disease.[26] Mediastinal irradiation for various malignancies has been reported to cause cardiac valve damage. Valve injury has been reported after the use of both certain migraine medications (ergotamine and methysergide) and appetite suppressants. The appetite suppressants fenfluramine and dexfenfluramine have been reported to cause cardiac valvular damage. The use of these agents for 4 or more months has been associated with an increased risk for newly diagnosed cardiac valve disorders, particularly aortic regurgitation. Jick[27] reported 11 cases

TABLE 2-3

Approximate Frequencies of Major Preexisting Cardiac Lesions in Patients with Infective Endocarditis in the United States

Condition	Children Under 2 (%)	Children 2 to 15 (%)	Adults 15 to 50 (%)	Adults Over 50 (%)	Injecting Drug Abusers (%)
No known heart disease	50-70	10-15	10-20	10	50-60
Congenital heart disease*	30-50	70-80	25-35	15-25	10
Rheumatic heart disease	Rare	10	10-15	10-15	10
Degenerative heart disease	0	0	Rare	10-20	Rare
Previous cardiac surgery	5	10-15	10-20	10-20	10-20
Previous endocarditis	Rare	5	5-10	5-10	10-20

From Durack DT: In Alexander RW et al, editors: *Hurst's the heart, arteries, and veins*, ed 9, New York, 1998, McGraw-Hill, p 2207.
*Includes mitral valve prolapse.

of newly diagnosed idiopathic valvular disorders in more than 8,000 patients who had taken one of these drugs. No cases of idiopathic valve disorders were found in the matched control group.

A vena cava filter or umbrella is used to prevent thromboemboli from reaching the pulmonary vascular bed. To date, no evidence exists of an increased risk for BE in patients with these devices.

Endocarditis may occur in patients who do not have cardiac defects (Table 2-3). Approximately 50% to 70% of children under the age of 2 years with endocarditis have no history of cardiac defects. Between 50% and 60% of adult intravenous drug abusers with endocarditis have no history of previous cardiac defects.[15] Endocarditis in other adults may occur in normal hearts in 10% to 40% of the cases.[15,19] Approximately 25% of cases of BE occur in patients with rheumatic heart disease, 10% to 20% occur in patients with congenital heart disease, 10% to 20% in patients with prosthetic heart valves, and 10% to 33% in patients with mitral valve prolapse.[15,19]

Streptococci and staphylococci are responsible for approximately 80% of the cases of BE. However, the percentage caused by streptococci is decreasing. During the 1960s, gram-negative bacteria accounted for about 1.7% of cases of BE. These organisms now cause 5% to 7% of cases.[4,15,19,28,29] They account for 13% to 20% of cases in drug addicts and for 10% to 20% in patients with prosthetic heart valves[12,30,31] (Tables 2-4 and 2-5).

The primary risk factor for BE in individuals infected with HIV is the continued use of intravenous drugs. The severe cellular immunosuppression caused by HIV is not a major risk factor for endocarditis.[15] Valencia[32] investigated the influence of HIV infection on BE in intravenous drug users. Two groups of intravenous drug

addicts with BE were compared: those infected with HIV (117 patients) and those free of infection by the acquired immune deficiency syndrome (AIDS) virus (19 patients). The vegetations originated mainly on the tricuspid valve, and S. *aureus* was recovered from most blood cultures. The mortality rate was similar in both groups: 6% in the HIV-infected patients and 5% in the other. BE was reported in the early stages of HIV infection, and its presence had no apparent influence on the clinical course of BE.

Normal childbirth presents a low risk of endocarditis, even in the presence of preexisting valvular disease. However, bacteremias associated with perinatal infective complications such as endometritis, parametritis, septic thrombophlebitis in pelvic veins, and urinary tract infection can lead to endocarditis in mothers with cardiac defects. Septic abortion or pelvic infection related to intrauterine contraceptive devices can also be the source of bacteremia resulting in endocarditis.[15]

The risk of endocarditis occurring in an at-risk patient after receiving dental treatment is not known. The rate is estimated to vary from 0 to 1 in 533.[16,33] The number of patients susceptible to endocarditis has been estimated as high as 5% to 10% of the general population (or between 100 and 200 individuals susceptible to BE in a dental practice with 2,000 patients).[16] This includes individuals with conditions such as rheumatic heart disease and congenital heart disease and devices such as prosthetic heart valves (Box 2-1).

PATHOPHYSIOLOGY AND COMPLICATIONS

The lesions of BE are divided into three groups: cardiac, embolic, and general.

TABLE **2-4**

Types of Endocarditis

Causative organism	Most Common Location	Predisposing Defect	Mortality Rate
Native Valve Streptococci most common Streptococci and staphylococci, over 80% of cases When *Streptococcus bovis* found, look for carcinoma of colon	Mitral valve	Lesion, 60% to 68%	Streptococci, 10% Staphylococci, 40% Fungi, high
Prosthetic Valve *Staphylococcus epidermidis* most common Gram-negative bacilli and fungi, up to 25%	Aortic valve	Prosthetic device at suture line	Early PVE, 40% to 80% Late PVE, 20% to 40%
Drug Abusers *Staphylococcus aureus*, over 50% Gram-negative bacilli, about 15% of cases	Tricuspid valve	Most often on normal valves	Staphylococci, 10% (90% cure rate)

PVE, Prosthetic valve endocarditis.

TABLE **2-5**

Frequency of Organisms Causing Infective Endocarditis

Organism	NVE (%)	IV Drug Abusers (%)	Early PVE (%)	Late PVE (%)
Streptococci	60	< 15-25	5	35
Alpha-hemolytic	35	< 5-10	< 5	25
S. bovis	10	< 5	< 5	< 5
S. faecalis	10	10	< 5	< 5
Staphylococci	25	50	50	30
Coagulase-positive	23	50	20	10
Coagulase-negative	< 5	< 5	30	20
Gram-negative bacilli	< 5	< 5	20	10
Fungi	< 5	< 5	10	5
Culture-negative endocarditis	5 to 10	< 5	< 5	< 5

From Durack DT: In Alexander RW et al, editors: *Hurst's the heart, arteries, and veins*, ed 9, New York, 1998, McGraw-Hill, p 2208.
NVE, Native valve endocarditis.
PVE, prosthetic valve endocarditis.

BOX 2-1

Degree of Risk for Infective Endocarditis Posed by Various Cardiac or Vascular Lesions*

Relatively High-Risk
Prosthetic heart valve*
Previous infective endocarditis*
Cyanotic congenital heart disease
Aortic valve disease
Mitral regurgitation
Mitral stenosis with regurgitation
Patent ductus arteriosus
Ventricular septal defect
Coarctation of aorta

Intermediate Risk
Mitral valve prolapse with regurgitation
Pure mitral stenosis
Tricuspid valve disease
Pulmonary stenosis
Asymmetric septal hypertrophy
Hyperalimentation lines into right atrium

Intermediate Risk—cont'd
Degenerative valvular disease in elderly patients
Nonvalvular intracardiac prosthetic implants
Pressure monitoring lines into right atrium

Very Low or Negligible Risk
Mitral valve prolapse without regurgitation
Trivial valvular regurgitation by echocardiography without structural abnormality
Atrial septal defects, secundum type
Arteriosclerotic plaques
Coronary artery disease
Cardiac pacemaker
Surgically repaired intracardiac lesions, with minimal or no hemodynamic abnormality, more than 6 months after operation
Vena cava filter
Syphilitic aortitis

From Durack DT: In Alexander RW et al, editors: *Hurst's the heart, arteries, and veins*, ed 9. New York, 1998, McGraw-Hill, p 2207.
*Considered high risk by the American Heart Association.

Cardiac lesions are usually valvular, and the mitral valve is most often affected. Infection of the pulmonary valve is rare. Vegetative lesions occur on the line of contact of the damaged valve cusps and grow to cover the valve. Vegetations also can occur at the contact area of jet flow caused by certain cardiac lesions. They generally consist of an amorphous mass of fused platelets, fibrin, and bacteria (Fig. 2-1).

Sterile vegetations may develop before becoming infected with bacteria or other microorganisms. This condition is termed *nonbacterial thrombotic endocarditis* (NBTE). NBTE now is thought to precede most cases of native valve bacterial endocarditis[15,19] (Fig. 2-2). NBTE has been reported in approximately 50% of cases of systemic lupus erythematosus,[34] and it appears to increase the risk for BE in these patients.[35]

Embolic lesions are common because the vegetations are friable and easily detached. Petechial hemorrhages on skin and mucous membranes may result from these emboli (Fig. 2-3). Osler's nodes (small, raised, red, tender lesions) involving the skin of the extremities, usually in the tip (pulp) of the fingers, may arise from small, infected emboli in distal arterioles.

Splinter hemorrhages, linear subungual hemorrhages resembling tiny splinters of wood under the nails may be found in approximately 20% of patients with SBE. These lesions are probably caused by microembolization to linear capillaries. Septic emboli also may lodge in small vessels of the kidneys, brain, eyes, and other tissues.[15,19]

General lesions include an enlarged spleen, mycotic aneurysms, clubbing of the fingers, and arthritis. Clubbing of the fingers used to be a common finding in SBE, but with earlier diagnosis and treatment of BE clubbing is found in less than 5% of the cases. The pathogenesis of this lesion is not understood. Other conditions that may be present in patients with BE include cardiac failure, conduction abnormalities, neurologic disorders such as stroke and psychiatric symptoms, liver disease, renal failure and anemia. These effects may be a result of toxemia from the infection or secondary spread of the infection.[15]

As stated, patients with BE who do not receive antibiotic treatment have a mortality rate of 100%.[15] The mortality rate for treated patients varies from 10% to 80%.[14,15,19] The highest mortality rate of between 40% and

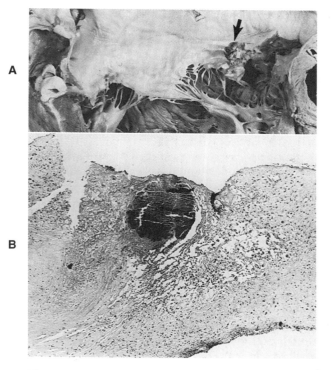

Fig. 2-1 A, Gross appearance of the vegetations of infective endocarditis of the mitral valve (arrow). **B,** Photomicrograph of the vegetations of bacterial endocarditis of the aortic valve. (**A** courtesy Jesse E. Edwards, St. Paul Minn.; **B** courtesy W. O'Connor, Lexington, Ky.)

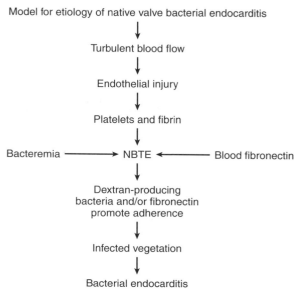

Fig. 2-2 Sequence of events in the formation of nonbacterial thrombotic endocarditis (NBTE).

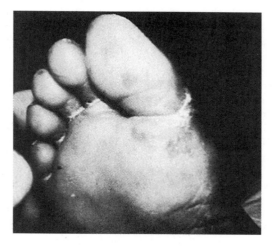

Fig. 2-3 Petechiae caused by septic emboli of bacterial endocarditis. (Courtesy H.D. Wilson, Lexington, Ky.)

80% is found in patients with early prosthetic valve endocarditis. The lowest mortality rate of between 2% and 10% is found in patients with native valve group A streptococcal endocarditis. The mortality rate (of about 40%) is higher for S. *aureus* endocarditis in nonaddicts and compared with the death rate of only 10% in drug addicts.[15,19,22]

The morbidity rate also is significant, with the average hospital stay ranging from 4 to 6 weeks. Patients who recover face many potential complications, including reinfection, congestive heart failure, renal disease, and cerebrovascular accident. Early and effective treatment decreases both the death rate and the number of complications. Patients who have recovered from native valve BE often will have a scarred valve that may be perforated or ruptured. The valve may be functionally altered, and the patient is at increased risk for reinfection, which occurs in 2% to 31% of the cases.[15,22]

CLINICAL PRESENTATION

SIGNS AND SYMPTOMS

The classic findings of BE included fever, anemia, positive blood culture, and heart murmur. These still may be found in many patients, but the clinical manifestations of the disease today often are more complex.

Furrer and Malinverni[36] described the clinical aspects and diagnosis of BE. The first step in the diagnosis of BE must be a high level of clinical suspicion. Every organ system can be involved by embolic or immunologic complications. Manifestations can be found on skin and mucosa, central nervous system, kidney, locomotor system, and lungs. The clinical spectrum has changed over the last decades. More elderly patients, patients with prosthetic heart valves, and intravenous drug users are affected. The clinical presentation of right-sided BE differs from that of the left-sided variant. A diagnosis of BE has to be considered in every patient with unexplained fever or a multisystem disease. Diagnosis involves the clinician and the echocardiography and microbiology laboratories.

The diagnostic triad of fever, cardiac murmur, and positive blood cultures is not always present. Elderly patients often have more nonspecific symptoms than do younger ones. BE should be considered in conditions dominated by the insidious onset of congestive heart failure, acute mental status and neurologic changes or the acute onset of arthralgias or myalgias.[14]

SBE progresses over a period of weeks to months, with an often insidious onset. Organisms of low virulence usually cause SBE. Alpha-hemolytic streptococci are the most common organisms causing SBE. The patient may be unable to pinpoint when the disease first started. However, symptoms usually can be identified to within 2 weeks of the precipitating event.[15,37]

Symptoms include weakness, weight loss, fatigue, fever, chills, night sweats, anorexia, and arthralgia. Emboli may produce paralysis, chest pain, abdominal pain, blindness, and hematuria. The fever may spike, with peaks often being noted in the afternoon or evening. Petechiae occur on the skin or mucosal tissues. Linear hemorrhages may be found under the nails in about 20% of the patients, and Osler's nodes may be found in various subcutaneous areas in 10% to 20% of the patients. Janeway lesions (flat, nontender, red spots), found on the palms and soles, are hemorrhagic and will blanch on pressure. Retinal hemorrhages can be found in 10% to 25% of patients.[15,19]

Anemia often is associated with endocarditis. In longstanding cases clubbing of the fingers may occur. Heart findings are related to the underlying cardiac disease, which usually is valvular. Thus almost all patients will have a murmur (Table 2-6). Heart failure is a most important finding and carries a poor prognosis. The spleen and liver may be enlarged. Neurologic symptoms occur in approximately 40% to 50% of the cases of BE and include confusional states, psychiatric manifestations, strokes, and cerebritis.[15,19]

Osteomyelitis is thought to occur as a complication of BE in as many as 6% of cases. Osteomyelitis may be difficult to diagnose in patients with endocarditis because symptoms such as fever, bone pain, and stiffness are common to both illnesses. Patients with endocarditis and persistent or localized musculoskeletal symptoms should be investigated to exclude osteomyelitis. Bone scans should be performed because plain radiographs can be normal in 50% of cases of osteomyelitis in the early stages or show only minor abnormalities.[38,39]

Acute bacterial endocarditis (ABE) develops over a period of days to 1 or 2 weeks. The clinical course is hectic. Complications develop quickly and, if untreated, will lead to death within 6 weeks. Highly pathogenic microorganisms such as *S. aureus* are the causative organisms for ABE, which frequently involves normal hearts. Severe suppurative infections often precede the onset of this type of endocarditis.[15,19] Mostaghim and Millard[17] suggested that the number of cases of this type of endocarditis might be increasing. More recent studies have shown that the total number of cases of endocarditis has not changed but that the proportion caused by staphylococci, fungi, and gram-negative bacilli has increased. The same studies have shown a decrease in the proportion of cases caused by streptococci.[15,19,22,40]

LABORATORY FINDINGS

Laboratory tests for the presence of active infection usually are positive in the patient with BE. Leukocytosis with neutrophilia is common; however, in some cases the leukocyte count is normal. The erythrocyte sedimentation rate is increased in approximately 90% of the cases, the C-reactive protein is usually positive, and serum immunoglobulins may be increased. A positive test for rheumatoid factor is found in 30% to 50% of the cases of SBE and is rare in ABE.[15,19]

Obtaining a blood culture is one of the most important steps in the diagnosis of BE and usually is taken before specific therapy for the infection is begun. Blood cultures should be obtained for all patients with fever and a heart murmur unless the cause is clear. In cases of suspected SBE, three samples of venous blood should be taken on the first day. Samples for cultures can be drawn at any time of day or body temperature. The person drawing the samples should allow at least 1 hour between the first and last venipuncture. Each blood sample is divided for aerobic and anaerobic culturing. If the cultures are negative after 3 days, two more samples of venous blood should be drawn for culture. Samples of arterial blood or bone marrow offer no advantage over venous blood.[15,19] Patients receiving penicillin to prevent recurrent attacks of rheumatic fever who develop BE may not show a positive blood culture for 7 or more days. The blood culture is positive in approximately

TABLE **2-6**

Clinical Manifestations of Endocarditis

	History	Signs and Symptoms	Findings
Systemic Infection	Fever, chills, rigors, sweats, malaise, weakness, lethargy, delirium, headache, anorexia, weight loss, backache, arthralgia, myalgia. Portal of entry: oropharynx, skin, urinary tract, drug addiction, nosocomial bacteremia	Fever, pallor, weight loss, asthenia, splenomegaly	Anemia, leukocytosis (variable), increased erythrocyte sedimentation rate, positive blood culture, findings abnormal cerebrospinal fluid levels
Intravascular Lesion	Dyspnea, chest pain, focal weakness, stroke, abdominal pain, cold and painful extremities	Murmurs, signs of cardiac failure, petechiae (skin, eye, mucosae), Roth's spots, Osler's nodes, Janeway lesions, splinter hemorrhages, stroke, mycotic aneurysm, ischemia or infarction of viscera or extremities	Blood in urine, abnormal chest radiography, echocardiography, arteriography, liver-spleen scan, lung scan, brain scan, CT scan, histology, culture of emboli
Immunologic Reactions	Arthralgia, myalgia, tenosynovitis	Arthritis, signs of uremia, vascular phenomena, finger clubbing	Proteinuria, hematuria, casts, uremia, acidosis, polyclonal increase in gamma globulins, rheumatoid factor, decreased complement, immune complexes in serum, antistaphylococcal teichoic acid antibodies

Modified from Durack DT: In Alexander RW et al, editors: *Hurst's the heart, arteries, and veins,* ed 9, New York, 1998, McGraw-Hill, p 2217.

95% of the patients with BE. These figures are from a single clinical and laboratory team experienced in evaluation of endocarditis. Hospitals generally report approximately 80% to 85% positive blood cultures. Most cases of BE caused by *Aspergillus* organisms are culture negative. At least 20% of the *Candida* cases are culture negative. SBE of long duration may be culture negative.[15,19]

Streptococcus viridans is the microorganism most commonly responsible for the form of endocarditis that has a slow onset (subacute). S. *aureus* is the most common cause of a sudden onset of the disease (acute). As stated, recent studies[15,19,23] have shown an increase in the num-

ber of cases caused by S. *aureus* and a reduction in the number caused by S. *viridans*.[15,19,23]

Electrocardiography

Electrocardiography studies are performed initially and repeated at intervals based on the patient's progress during treatment. A disturbance of conduction that develops during the course of endocarditis suggests extension of infection into the myocardium. Development of a prolonged PR interval, if caused by an abscess, often is an indication for valve replacement and a worse prognosis. Electrocardiograms also can show evidence of silent

myocardial infarction resulting from embolization to a coronary artery.[15]

Echocardiography

Echocardiographic studies are vitally important in the diagnosis of endocarditis. Properly defined positive echocardiographic findings constitute one of the two major criteria for its clinical diagnosis. They are of equal importance to blood culture findings. Transthoracic two-dimensional echocardiography (TTE) combined with color-flow Doppler imaging provides a great deal of information for the diagnosis and management of endocarditis. TTE detects vegetations, valvular perforations, and other abnormalities such as abscesses and pericarditis. It also aids in the assessment of ventricular function. Sensitivity for detection of vegetations is 60% to 75%. Sensitivity can be improved to better than 95% by use of transesophageal echocardiography (TEE). TEE also is much more sensitive than TTE for detection of abscess and valve perforation. TEE is better for evaluation of prosthetic valve endocarditis, especially involving the mitral valve.[15,19]

Other Imaging Studies

Results of the standard chest radiograph are used to evaluate evidence of early congestive heart failure. Multiple small patchy infiltrates in the lungs of an intravenous drug user with fever suggest septic emboli from right-sided endocarditis. Calcification of a cardiac valve may aid in localization of intravascular infection. Widening of the aorta suggests possible mycotic aneurysm.[15]

Computed tomography, magnetic resonance imaging, and angiography are helpful in establishing the cause of focal neurologic lesions in patients with endocarditis. These causes include infarction, hemorrhage from mycotic aneurysm, and brain abscess.[15]

Radionuclide Imaging

Gallium scintigraphy using single photon emission computed tomography has been shown to be a noninvasive method to demonstrate prosthetic valve endocarditis and associated valve ring abscess. Radionuclide imaging is used to confirm embolization to the liver or spleen.[41] Scintigraphic studies after injection of indium-111-labeled leukocytes have been used to detect intracardic abscesses.[15]

DIAGNOSIS

The major criteria for the diagnosis of endocarditis are positive blood culture, evidence of endocardial involve-

ment by echocardiogram findings, and new valvular regurgitation. An increase or change in preexisting murmur is not sufficient. The blood culture must show a typical microorganism for BE resulting from two separate blood cultures, or it must be persistently positive with recovery of a microorganism consistent with BE from cultures drawn more than 12 hours apart, or all of three or majority of four or more being positive with the first and last drawn at least 1 hour apart. Positive echocardiogram findings must show an oscillating intracardiac mass on a valve or supporting structures, in the path of regurgitant jets, or on implanted material; an abscess; new partial dehiscence of prosthetic valve; or new valvular regurgitation.[15]

The minor criteria for the diagnosis are the existence of a predisposing heart condition, intravenous drug use, fever, vascular phenomena (emboli, septic pulmonary infarcts, mycotic aneurysm, intracranial hemorrhage, Janeway lesions), immunologic phenomena (glomerulonephritis, Osler nodes, Roth spots, rheumatoid factor), isolated blood culture or serologic evidence of active infection, and echocardiogram findings consistent with endocarditis but not diagnostic of the disease.[15]

MEDICAL MANAGEMENT

Clinical observation, clinical trials, and animal studies have led to the current treatment options now available for endocarditis.[42] The basic principles for the treatment of patients with BE include the following: early intervention; therapy based on culture and sensitivity findings whenever possible; use of bactericidal agents and adequate doses of antibiotics; intravenous administration of antibiotics; and continuation of treatment for as long as needed[15,19] (Box 2-2). The best prognosis for patients with endocarditis is if they are young, have been diagnosed

---

BOX **2-2**

Medical Management for Infective Endocarditis—Principles of Treatment

1. Early treatment
2. Culture and sensitivity tests
3. Bactericidal agents
4. Adequate dosage
5. IV route
6. Long enough treatment

early, find that the causative agent is penicillin-sensitive streptococcus, and start treatment promptly.

Along with cultures and sensitivity testing, the minimum inhibitory concentration of relevant antibiotics can be determined for cases other than those caused by group A streptococci. Some organisms may be resistant to the tested antibiotic; others may be tolerant (inhibited but not killed) to the tested antibiotic. No definitive evidence exists in humans that tolerance determines treatment outcome. Thus minimum inhibitory concentration is not performed for most cases of endocarditis. The serum bactericidal titer was performed to monitor treatment of endocarditis. This is an in vitro study in which the patient's serum containing the administered antibiotic is titered against the causative organism. The antibiotic dosage was thought adequate when a serum concentration was considered bactericidal for the causative organism at a 1:8 dilution or greater. The serum bactericidal titer is difficult to perform and to standardize. After years of clinical use the clinical value of the titer remains

unproven. Today most experts in the field consider the serum bactericidal titer obsolete.[15]

Penicillin G is the drug of choice for most cases of endocarditis caused by S. *viridans*. An adequate starting dose for endocarditis caused by S. *viridans* is 4 million units intravenously every 6 hours. Duration of treatment usually is about four weeks (Table 2-7). In cases caused by relatively penicillin-resistant streptococci, gentamicin (1 mg/kg) is given twice a day intravenously in addition to the penicillin. In cases caused by penicillin-resistant streptococci, high doses of penicillin G (18 to 30 million units per day) and gentamicin, ampicillin plus gentamicin, or vancomycin plus gentamicin are used; all are administered intravenously. Treatment of penicillin-resistant streptococci may have to be extended to 6 weeks to be effective.[15,19]

For infections caused by S. *aureus*, the selection of antibiotics for treatment depends on several factors. When the infection does not involve prosthetic material and the staphylococci are methicillin susceptible, nafcillin (2 g)

TABLE **2-7**

Medical Treatment Regimens for Endocarditis*

	Treatment Regimen: Dose and Route	Duration (wk)	Comments
Penicillin-Sensitive Streptococci	Penicillin G 4 million units every 6 hours IV	4	Suitable for hospital patients but not for outpatient therapy
Relatively Penicillin-Resistant Streptococci	Penicillin G 4 million units IV every 4 hours plus gentamicin 1.0 mg/kg every 12 hours for first 2 weeks	4	For outpatient therapy ceftriaxone plus gentamicin
Penicillin-Resistant Streptococci	Penicillin G 18-30 million units per day IV continuously or in divided doses plus gentamicin every 8 hours	4 to 6	Susceptibility testing needed: do not use penicillin if strain produces beta-lactamase
Staphylococci (No Prosthetic Material)	**Methicillin-Susceptible** Nafcillin 2 g IV every 4 hours **Methicillin-Resistant** Vancomycin 15 mg/kg IV every 12 hours	4 to 6 4 to 6	Cefazolin or vancomycin may be substituted for nafcillin if necessary due to drug hypersensitivity
Staphylococci (Prosthetic Valve or Other Prosthetic Material)	**Methicillin-Susceptible** Nafcillin 2 g IV every 4 hours plus gentamicin 1.0 mg/kg IV every 8 h **Methicillin-Resistant** Vancomycin 15 mg/kg IV every 12 h plus gentamicin plus rifampin	6 weeks or longer 6 weeks or longer	Cefazolin or vancomycin may be substituted for nafcillin if necessary due to drug hypersensitivity

Modified from Durack DT: In Alexander RW et al, editors: *Hurst's the heart, arteries, and veins*, ed 9, New York, 1998, McGraw-Hill, p 2226 and 2227.
*Standard regimens only; special regimens are indicated for other variables, such as penicillin allergy or infection by other organisms.

intravenously every 4 hours is used as the standard regimen. Cefazolin (2 g) intravenously every 8 hours is used in some individuals with a history of allergy to penicillins. Vancomycin (15 mg/kg) intravenously every 12 hours is used in those patients with a history of allergy that precludes the use of penicillins or cephalosporins. Gentamicin (1 mg/kg) intravenously every 8 hours for the first 3 to 5 days may be added to any of these regimens. Treatment usually takes 4 to 6 weeks (see Table 2-7).

Infections associated with prosthetic materials by methicillin-susceptible staphylococci are treated with nafcillin (2 g) every 4 hours plus gentamicin (1.0 mg/kg) intravenously every 8 hours (see Table 2-7). Treatment usually takes 6 weeks or longer. Cefazolin or vancomycin may be substituted for nafcillin if necessary in cases of drug hypersensitivity. Patients with prosthetic materials infected by methicillin-resistant staphylococci are treated using vancomycin (15 mg/kg) intravenously every 12 hours plus gentamicin (1 mg/kg) intravenously every 8 hours and rifampin (300 mg) orally every 8 hours. Again, treatment usually takes 6 weeks or longer. The treatment of other organisms that may cause endocarditis such as haemophilus, actinobacillus, cardiobacterium, eikenella, kingella (HACEK) group, *Neisseria* species, *Pseudomonas aeruginosa*, other gram-negative bacilli, and various fungi is beyond the scope of this book and the reader is referred to chapters in other textbooks for this information.[15,19]

Anticoagulant therapy should be avoided if possible in patients with BE. If anticoagulants must be used, the physician should apply warfarin. Patients with prosthetic heart valves needing anticoagulant therapy should be kept at an International Normalized Ratio between 2.5 and 3.5. Heparin is contraindicated in patients with BE. Antibiotic treatment should not include an intramuscular regimen if the patient is on anticoagulant therapy.[15,19] Home therapy now is considered for selected patients with endocarditis. It is very cost effective and has been used successfully with stable, nonintravenous drug users who are highly motivated, able to administer the therapy, and living with someone else. Intravenous ceftriaxone has been used for streptococcal endocarditis and intravenous vancomycin for staphylococcal endocarditis. These antibiotics have long half-lives and permit once-daily administration at home.[15,19]

Surgical correction of infected valves is indicated when (1) severe, intractable heart failure is present, (2) systemic emboli recur, (3) the infecting organism is a fungus and the patient does not respond to medical therapy, and (4) endocarditis, particularly fungal infection, is superimposed on an artificial valve. Other patients likely for surgery are those with gram-negative infection of prosthetic valves, those with valve ring abscesses and aortic valve involvement, and non-drug addicts with staphylococcal infection. Patients with congenital heart defects and endocarditis are best managed by corrective surgery after successful medical treatment of the endocarditis (Fig. 2-4). However, if the infection cannot be controlled, surgical repair may be attempted.[15,19] Surgical approaches include insertion of a prosthetic valve, insertion of an aortic root homograft, use of the patient's pulmonary valve to replace the damaged aortic valve (replacement of the pulmonary valve with homograft), and debridement of vegetations combined with valvuloplasty to spare the native valve[15] (Table 2-8).

Results of a study by Aranki[43] indicates the risk with surgical treatment of endocarditis. In that study 200 patients underwent aortic valve replacement for endocarditis, with 132 (66%) having native valve endocarditis and 68 (34%) having prosthetic valve endocarditis. Surgery was required in 120 patients (60%) during the active phase of infection and in 80 patients (40%) during the healed phase of endocarditis. The main indication for surgery in both groups was congestive heart failure and sepsis in the patients with active endocarditis. Streptococcal infections predominated in native valve endocarditis, and staphylococcal in prosthetic valve endocarditis, and culture-negative endocarditis predominated in the healed group. Isolated aortic valve surgery was performed in 68% of the patients. The overall operative mortality rate was 12.5%. It was highest in patients with prosthetic valve endocarditis, 22% (33% in early PVE and 18% for late PVE). The operative mortality rate was 7.5% in patients with native valve endocarditis. It was 15% in patients with active endocarditis and 7% for patients with healed endocarditis. The authors sug-

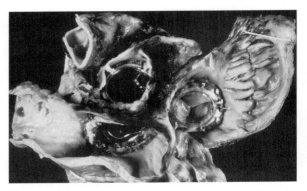

Fig. 2-4 Postmortem specimen from a patient with rheumatic heart disease who underwent surgical replacement of three valves. (Courtesy W. O'Conner, Lexington, Ky.)

TABLE **2-8**

Estimated Microbiologic Cure Rate (in Percent) for Various Forms of Endocarditis

	Antimicrobial Therapy (%)		Antimicrobial Therapy Plus Surgery (%)	
Native Valve Endocarditis (NVE)				
Alpha-hemolytic streptococci, group A streptococci, *Streptococcus bovis*, pneumococci, gonococci	98		98	
S. faecalis	90		> 90	
Staphylococcus aureus (young addicts)	90		> 90	
S. aureus (elderly patients)	50		70	
Gram-negative aerobic bacilli	40		65	
Fungi	< 5		50	
	Early (%)	**Late (%)**	**Early (%)**	**Late (%)**
Prosthetic valve endocarditis (PVE)				
Alpha-hemolytic streptococci, group A streptococci, *S. bovis* pneumococci, gonocci	Insufficient data	80	Insufficient data	90
S. faecalis	Insufficient data	60	Insufficient data	75
Staphylococcus aureus (young addicts)	25	40	50	60
S. aureus (elderly patients)	20	40	60	70
Gram-negative aerobic bacilli	< 10	20	40	50
Fungi	< 1	< 1	30	40

From Durack DT: In Alexander RW et al, editors: *Hurst's the heart, arteries, and veins*, ed 9, New York, 1998, McGraw-Hill, p 2229.

gested that for active endocarditis, surgery should be delayed to achieve a healed status provided immediate surgery is not needed. Patients with staphylococcal endocarditis, particularly on prosthesis, should be operated on sooner.[43]

Dacron and other prosthetic materials used in cardiovascular surgery to correct congenital or acquired lesions may become infected. Often under these circumstances, removal of the infected graft and replacement is the only option to obtain a cure. The surgical risk is high for these procedures in patients with endocarditis, but the alternative is a very high mortality rate.

Patients with exteriorized transvenous cardiac pacemakers sometimes develop an infection resembling endocarditis. For this condition the pacemaker and wire are replaced and moved to another location. The removed wire is cultured, and sensitivity tests are made from the cultured microorganisms. The patient is then treated as for endocarditis.

DENTAL MANAGEMENT

MEDICAL CONSIDERATIONS

The dentist's goal is to prevent BE from occurring in susceptible patients. Any dental procedure that causes injury to the soft tissue or bone resulting in bleeding can produce a transient bacteremia that in susceptible patients can result in endocarditis. Even minor dental manipulations such as the cleaning of teeth or the placement of a matrix band can result in a transient bacteremia (Table 2-9). In normal patients, the body's defenses handle these bacteremias and usually no serious problem develops. However, in the patient with a heart defect such as rheumatic heart disease the anatomy and function of the affected valve are altered because of the scarring that occurs after the acute rheumatic fever attack.[44] When bacteremias occur, the altered valvular tissue with NBTE provides an ideal location for attachment

TABLE **2-9**

Frequency of Bacteremia Associated with Various Dental Procedures and Oral Manipulations

Dental Procedure/ Oral Manipulation	Frequency
Extractions	51% to 85%
Periodontal surgery	88%
Periodontal scaling	8% to 80%
Dental prophylaxis	0% to 40%
Toothbrushing	0% to 40%
Chewing	17% to 51%
Random in patients with periodontal disease	11%
Random using anaerobic techniques	60% to 80%
Endodontic therapy (nonvital tooth)	0%
Wooden cleansing devices	20% to 40%
Irrigation devices	7% to 50%

Data from Bender IB et al: J Am Dent Assoc 109:415-420, 1984; and Pallasch: TJ, J Calif Dent Assoc 17(6):27-39, 1989.

and growth of bacteria. Thus in patients with rheumatic heart disease or those with other types of cardiovascular defects (see Box 2-1), endocarditis is possible during every period of significant bacteremia.

Transient bacteremias have been reported to occur after normal physiologic activities involving the mouth. These bacteremias usually clear within 10 minutes. The chewing of paraffin was found to introduce bacteria into the bloodstream in about 50% of subjects investigated. Tooth brushing resulted in transient bacteremias in 40%. Oral irrigation produced bacteremias in up to 50%, and random testing of individuals with periodontal disease showed the presence of bacteria in the blood in 11% of the cases.[12,45-48] Guntheroth[49] estimated that with normal physiologic use of the mouth, approximately 5376 minutes of transient bacteremia per month occurs in an individual (approximately 12% of the time).

Dental procedures resulting in injury to the oral tissues and bleeding can lead to transient bacteremias usually lasting 10 minutes or less. The risk of transient bacteremia has been estimated to be as high as 85% of the time when teeth are extracted, 88% with periodontal surgery, and less often for other procedures.[29,46,49] Shafer et al[50] reported in a summary of 15 studies on the frequency of transient bacteremias after various dental procedures. In 25% of the cases (302 of 1232), bacteria were released into the bloodstream.

Based on the high frequency of physiologic bacteremias and the low incidence of dental procedures preceding the onset of endocarditis, Guntheroth[49] suggested that the odds of any given case of endocarditis occurring from the physiologic "seeding" of oral bacteria was 1000 times greater than if it occurred after a given dental procedure. He stated, "Blaming the dentist for endocarditis would be like blaming the cardiologist for myocardial infarction."[49] Most cases of BE are not related in time to medical or dental procedures. Only 4% to 19% of cases of SBE follow a medical or dental procedure that might cause transient bacteremias. Even fewer cases of ABE are associated with such procedures.[30] In a study in the Netherlands, only 10.5% of patients with native valve endocarditis or late-onset prosthetic valve endocarditis had undergone a procedure needing prophylaxis within 30 days of the onset of symptoms.[51]

Van der Meer[52] calculated that only about 6% of cases of endocarditis in the Netherlands could have been prevented. This percentage represented the theoretic maximum of preventable cases. The actual number that could be prevented would be smaller. Based on those calculations, extensive use of optimal antibiotic prophylaxis in the United States could prevent at most 240 to 480 cases each year.[22]

Finch[53] estimated that less than 3% of 254 cases of SBE caused by oral bacteria could have been prevented by antibiotic prophylaxis. Other authors place this figure higher, but at best at only 15% to 20%. In a survey of 533 patients with valvular prostheses who underwent 677 dental or surgical procedures, Horstkotte et al found that 6 cases of prosthetic valve endocarditis occurred in the 229 patients who received no prophylaxis and none in the 304 that did.[54] Also, a review of nonstreptococcal and nonstaphylococcal cases of BE found that 32.4% of 330 cases reviewed reported dental treatment or dental disease associated with the onset of BE (Table 2-10). No estimate was made of the number of these cases that might have been prevented.[55]

Imperiale and Horwitz[56] reported findings from a case-control study that strongly supported antibiotic prophylaxis. This study involved 8 patients with high-risk lesions who developed BE within 12 weeks of a dental procedure and 24 control subjects matched for lesion and age. The authors estimated a 91% protective efficacy for antibiotic prophylaxis.[56] In contrast, Van der Meer[52] found in a similar case-control study of more than 438 patients that the efficacy for antibiotic prophylaxis was only about 49%.

A recent study by Strom[57] of patients with endocarditis suggested that antibiotic prophylaxis for dental treatment might be overkill. Cases of community-acquired endocarditis in 54 Philadelphia-area hospitals were studied during a 3-year period. It found 416 patients with endocarditis. Children, intravenous drug users, and pa-

TABLE 2-10

Nonstreptococcal and Nonstaphylococcal Bacterial Endocarditis: Relationship with Dental Treatment and Dental Disease

Organism	Total Cases	Related*
Haemophilus	81	28
Actinobacillus actinomyceternitans	88	26
Cardiobacterium hominis	60	6
Eikenella corrodens	24	7
Capnocytophaga ochracea	5	4
Kingella denitrifi cans	6	2
Kingella kingae	22	7
Neisseria subflava	7	2
Neisseria mucosa	7	4
Lactobacillus	30	21
	330	107 (32.4%)

From Barco CT: J *Periodontol* 6:55 1, 1991.
*Cases reported to be related to dental treatment or disease.

tients with incomplete medical or dental records were excluded. Thus the number of cases used in the study was 273. Appropriate matched controls (273) from community residents were identified. History of valvular disease was highly associated with endocarditis. Approximately 23% of both groups, including patients with endocarditis and the control patients, had dental treatment within the 3 months before the disease or initial contact. Risk for endocarditis was not increased by prior dental treatment. Of the total, 6 case and 2 control patients had received antibiotic prophylaxis 1 month before hospitalization. Extractions were the only dental procedure that approached being significant, but too few cases were involved with 6 case patients having extractions and none of the control patients. The authors concluded no link existed between dental procedures and endocarditis and stated, "Current policies for antibiotic prophylaxis for endocarditis prevention should be reconsidered."[57]

In an editorial that accompanied the Strom paper, Dr. David Durack,[15] a world expert in endocarditis and its prevention, suggested the number of dental patients given prophylaxis be greatly reduced. He indicated only those patients with high-risk cardiac conditions, prosthetic heart valves, or a history of endocarditis require antibiotic prophylaxis. He further suggested that only certain dental procedures, extractions, periodontal surgery, or dental implants would require prophylaxis in patients with high-risk conditions. According to Durack,[15] all other at-risk patients

do not need antibiotic prophylaxis for any type of dental treatment. Patients with high-risk cardiac conditions do not require prophylaxis for dental treatment other than extractions, periodontal surgery, or dental implants.

The American Heart Association Committee on Rheumatic Fever, Endocarditis, and Kawasaki Disease was asked to comment on the Strom study[57] and its implications. Dr. Kathryn Taubert[58] of the American Heart Association stated, "The Strom study and others will be assessed in conjunction with previously available data in future committee discussions regarding the updating of prophylaxis guidelines. The committee believes, however, that the American Heart Association's currently published guidelines *Prevention of Bacterial Endocarditis*[8] remain valid in the face of the results of the Strom study and does not recommend changes in practice or patient education at this time."[58]

In summary, only a small number of cases of endocarditis are associated with dental or surgical procedures. Limited data are available to demonstrate the effectiveness of prophylaxis in preventing endocarditis. The efficacy appears to fall between the extremes shown by the preceding two case-control studies: 49% to 91%. Thus, the total number of preventable cases applying maximal antibiotic prophylaxis is small.

ANTIBIOTIC PROPHYLAXIS

Antibiotics may prevent endocarditis by killing bacteria or damaging them so that they can be destroyed by host defenses. These effects could occur in the oral cavity, in the bloodstream, or after the bacteria adhere to the heart. Antibiotics also may prevent adherence. The primary mechanism by which antibiotics might prevent endocarditis has not been established.[22]

Antibiotic prophylaxis in general should be considered when the following three clinical situations exist[24]: (1) a complication is common but not fatal, (2) a complication is rare but has a high mortality rate, and (3) a single type of organism usually is involved. In practice, effective prophylaxis is complicated by several factors[24]: (1) often a number of different organisms may be involved, (2) organisms involved have variable virulence, (3) organisms may originate from multiple sites, (4) organisms may have varying sensitivity to given antibiotics, (5) random physiologic bacteremias may occur, and (6) no controlled studies exist to show the efficacy of antibiotic prophylaxis.

Several important general principles are involved in ideal antibiotic prophylaxis.[24] The specific organism involved should be known, and an antibiotic effective against that organism should be selected. The proper dosage of the antibiotic should be used, and the antibiotic should be given just before the procedure to provide maximum blood levels at the time of the injury. The antibiotic should be continued as long as bacteria can be

released, which is usually for a short duration. The benefit to risk ratio must be considered for each procedure; in other words, the dentist must determine whether the risk of developing a problem outweighs the risks involved by the use of the antibiotic.

The American Heart Association guidelines for the prevention of BE meet most of the preceding principles for effective prophylaxis.[8] BE, although a rare disease, has a significant mortality risk. Prophylaxis is designed against alpha-hemolytic streptococci. These organisms are by far the most common ones found in transient dental bacteremias. Amoxicillin is effective against these bacteria. High doses at the time of bacteremia are provided and continued for an adequate length of time. However, no clinical trials show that antibiotic prophylaxis prevents BE in humans. The risk to benefit ratio is questioned for lesions that have moderate to low risk. The use of prophylaxis for patients with moderate-risk lesions may not be cost effective. In addition, dental procedures may not be associated with the onset of endocarditis.[57]

When a dentist applies the preceding principles for effective prophylaxis the use of antibiotic prophylaxis for patients with organ transplants, blood dyscrasias, immune deficiencies, joint prostheses, or penile implants, and for those undergoing chemotherapy or radiation therapy is even more difficult to justify. This is true despite studies that show antibiotic prophylaxis at the time of surgery to reduce infectious complications of prosthetic heart valves, joint prostheses, penile implants, and organ transplants.[33,48,59,60]

An estimated 25% to 50% of antibiotic use in hospitals is for prophylaxis (typically at the time of surgery).[61] The complications associated with antibiotic use include toxicity, allergy, super infections, resistant bacteria, high costs, and in some cases, careless surgery. The problem with allergy alone is significant. About 5% to 10% of the patients who take penicillin have an allergic reaction.[61] A small number of these patients (0.04% to 0.14%) will develop an anaphylactic reaction, and 10% of these individuals will die. Anaphylactic deaths caused by penicillin account for 400 to 800 deaths per year in the United States.[48,61]

Several other problems must be considered with the current use of antibiotic prophylaxis against endocarditis. The risk of developing the disease in susceptible patients is not known. A number of different microorganisms are found to cause endocarditis; therefore no antibiotic is effective in preventing the disease. The duration of coverage is not known for oral wounds healing by secondary intention. Bacterial resistance during a coverage period is becoming a problem, as is the presence of resistant strains in the oral flora before antibiotic prophylaxis is initiated. If the antibiotic regimen is too complicated and expensive, the patient may be discouraged from seeking needed dental treatment. The failure of prophylaxis to protect a patient

TABLE 2-11

Estimated Death Rates Associated with Mitral Valve Prolapse with and without Penicillin Prophylaxis (10 Million Dental Patient Visits)

Status	Prophylaxis	No Prophylaxis
Number of infective endocarditis cases	5	47
Number of deaths by infective endocarditis	0	2
Number of allergy-related deaths	175	0
Total number of deaths	175	2

From Bor DH, Himmelstein DF: *Am J Med* 76:711-717, 1984.

(i.e., one who was given recommended antibiotic prophylaxis but still developed endocarditis) also has been reported. The benefit to risk ratio appears to differ depending on the nature of the underlying cardiac defect.[24,33,62,63]

Several studies that question the benefit of antibiotic prophylaxis when considering the number of endocarditis deaths prevented by antibiotic prophylaxis and the number of deaths caused by severe allergic reactions are considered.[24,33,62-65]

One study estimated that 47 cases of endocarditis would occur in 10 million dental visits by patients with mitral valve prolapse if no antibiotic prophylaxis were given.[62] A total of 2 deaths could be predicted in the 47 cases of endocarditis. If penicillin prophylaxis were given for each visit, the number of cases of endocarditis would be reduced to 5, with no deaths occurring. However, an estimated 175 deaths related to penicillin allergy would occur (Table 2-11).

Another study using rheumatic fever as the model estimated that about 26 deaths per year for a population of 100 million would be caused by endocarditis associated with dental treatment.[63] If the estimated 3.4 million individuals with rheumatic heart disease in this population each received one dental visit per year and were covered by penicillin prophylaxis, approximately 136 deaths would occur from anaphylactic shock (Table 2-12).

Based on the preceding studies, the use of antibiotic prophylaxis for noncomplicated mitral valve prolapse and other low-risk conditions does not appear to be supported. The efficacy of its use for moderate-risk conditions such as rheumatic heart disease also can be questioned. The models used in the previous studies—decision-tree analytic analysis—do show a benefit for

TABLE 2-12

Estimated Yearly Death Rate in a Population of 100 Million Caused by Infective Endocarditis of Dental Origin Versus Yearly Death Rate Attributable to Prophylactic Antibiotics in Patients with Rheumatic Heart Disease Receiving Dental Treatment

Status	Infective Endocarditis	Rheumatic Heart Disease
Prevalence or incidence	1900 (0.0019%)	3,400,000 (3.4%)
Known susceptible patients	1092 (57.5%)	3,400,000
Probability of infective endocarditis caused by dental care	39 (3.6%)	?
Patients with anaphylactic reaction	—	13650 (0.04%)
Deaths from anaphylactic shock	—	136 (10%)
Deaths from infective endocarditis of dental origin	26 (67%)	—

From Tzukert AA et al: *Oral Surg* 62:276-280, 1986.

high-risk groups such as patients with prosthetic heart valves or a previous history of endocarditis. These studies question the value in terms of risks to benefits for antibiotic prophylaxis in low to moderate at-risk patients. When the findings of the Strom study[57] are considered, the case for antibiotic prophylaxis for the moderate-risk conditions becomes even weaker.

Available data do not support the concept that prophylaxis is effective for this group of patients. However, the American Heart Association still recommends prophylaxis. Although the American Heart Association states that its guidelines are not intended to serve as a standard of care, they are interpreted to be the standards. The next guidelines issued by the American Heart Association are expected to reduce the number of medical conditions and dental procedures recommended for antibiotic prophylaxis.

The next question is to determine which dental procedures need to be covered. According to Durack,[66] only extractions, periodontal surgical procedures, and placement of dental implants require antibiotic prophylaxis in patients with high-risk conditions for endocarditis (prosthetic heart valves and history of endocarditis). Again, the American Heart Association has listed the dental procedures it feels require prophylaxis in the susceptible patient, which are much more inclusive than the three identified by Dr. Durack.

The cost-effectiveness of prophylaxis in dental practice to prevent infective endocarditis was investigated in Great Britain. Gould[67] used the annual death rate from BE in Great Britain (high-risk patients), number of high-risk dental procedures (extractions) performed without prophylaxis, and costs estimated based on health records of 63 patients with BE from 1980 to 1990. For every 10,000 extractions in at-risk patients, appropriate prophylaxis will prevent 5.7 deaths and a further 22.85 cases of nonfatal BE. This represents a saving in costs of hospital care of 289,600 pounds sterling ($438,107) for 10,000 extractions. Thus prophylaxis to prevent BE in at-risk patients undergoing dental extraction is highly cost effective. If the rate of patients at risk receiving prophylaxis for dental extraction were increased from the current 50% to 100%, an annual saving of 2.5 million pounds sterling ($3.782 million) and prevention of 50 deaths would result.[67]

Even when antibiotic prophylaxis is used, however, it is not 100% effective in preventing endocarditis.[68] In 1981 the American Heart Association formed a national registry to record prophylaxis failures for endocarditis.[29,47,68] As of 1983, 52 cases had been reported involving the development of endocarditis in patients given antibiotic prophylaxis. Most patients had cardiac lesions, and 10 had prosthetic heart valves. The vast majority had received dental treatment. They had been given either penicillin or erythromycin prophylaxis. However, only 6 of the 52 cases reported had received one of the standard regimens recommended by the American Heart Association.[29] These data highlight two aspects. First, the majority of failures received improper coverage. Second, 6 cases involved patients who were covered as recommended and still developed the disease. A number of questions remain unanswered concerning this topic.

Determining the real need for antibiotic prophylaxis may require a double-blind placebo study involving 6000 at-risk patients.[33] This has not been done because of the serious nature of the disease and the moral and ethical problems involved in conducting an investigation on human subjects. Wahl[69] in a recent paper suggested that such a study now might be considered because exposure of patients to the known risks of antibiotics without more evidence of their benefit in preventing endocarditis also is unethical.

Current practice involves the use of antibiotic prophylaxis in at-risk persons before certain dental procedures are performed that are likely to result in a significant transient bacteremia that could induce BE.

American Heart Association Recommendations
The problem of BE prevention has been the subject of eight sets of recommendations by the American Heart Association[1-8] (Table 2-13).

1955. In 1955 the American Heart Association[1] made the first of what proved to be a series of recommendations.

TABLE 2-13

American Heart Association Guidelines: 1955-1990

	Oral	Parenteral-Oral	Parenteral	Penicillin Allergy Protection	Special
1955	Low loading dose Low dosage Day before, day of, 4 days following	None	Single IM injection	None	None
1960	None	Oral, 2 days before, day of, 2 days following IM loading dose	IM injections (procaine) one on each of 2 days before and 2 days following IM loading dose (aqueous and procaine) on day of procedure	Erythromycin for penicillin allergy	None
1965	Start 1 hour before Low dosage 3 days	None	Single IM injection	Erythromycin for penicillin allergy	None
1972	Start 1 hour before Extra loading dose* Low dose 3 days following	None	Three IM injections, reduced aqueous dosage, 1 hour before and 2 days following	Erythromycin for penicillin allergy or patients on penicillin for rheumatic fever protection	None
1977	High-loading dose* Moderate dosage About 2 days	High IM loading dose* Moderate oral dose About 2 days	None	Erythromycin High loading dose Moderate following dose	IM penicillin and streptomycin plus oral penicillin IV or vancomycin plus oral erythromycin*
1984	High loading dose Single following dose* Less than 1 day	None	High IM loading dose followed by IM dose 6 hours later Only aqueous*	Erythromycin High loading dose Single following dose Less than 1 day	IM or IV ampicillin, gentamicin plus single-dose oral penicillin IV vancomycin only
1990	High loading dose Single following dose, less than 1 day	None	None	Clindamycin* or Erythromycin High loading dose Single following dose less than 1 day	IM or IV ampicillin, gentamicin plus single following dose oral penicillin IV vancomycin only

*Significant changes or new recommendations.

Its Committee on Prevention of Rheumatic Fever and Bacterial Endocarditis consisted of seven members, all physicians. The original recommendations were for either an oral or a parenteral route using penicillin G. The oral regimen consisted of 250,000 units of penicillin G given four times on the day before the procedure, 250,000 units of penicillin G given four times on the day of the procedure, and an additional 250,000 units of penicillin G given just before the procedure, followed by administration of the same dose four times a day on each of the 4 days after the procedure. The parenteral regimen (which was preferred) consisted of a single intramuscular injection of 600,000 units of aqueous penicillin G plus 600,000 units of procaine penicillin G given 30 minutes before the procedure.

1960. The American Heart Association[2] made its next recommendations in 1960. Committee members were not identified; however, dentistry did not appear to be represented. Recommendations were modified by (1) eliminating the oral regimen; (2) extending the parenteral regimen to include injections 2 days before, on the day of, and 2 days after the dental procedure; and (3) introducing a combined oral and parenteral regimen (500,000 units of penicillin V four times a day 2 days before, on the day of, and 2 days after the procedure, with an intramuscular injection of 600,000 units of aqueous penicillin G given 1 hour before the procedure). In addition, the committee recommended for the first time that erythromycin should be used if a history of penicillin allergy was found.

1965. In 1965 the American Heart Association[3] changed its recommendations to again include an oral regimen and reduced the parenteral regimen to a single intramuscular injection of 600,000 units of aqueous penicillin G and 600,000 units of procaine penicillin G given 1 hour to 2 hours before the dental procedure. The oral regimen consisted of 250 mg of penicillin V starting 1 hour before the dental procedure and continuing on a four-times-a-day basis for the rest of that day and the next 2 days. Starting with 250 mg given 1 hour before the dental procedure and continuing on a four-times-a-day basis for the rest of that day and the next 2 days modified the erythromycin regimen for patients allergic to penicillin. The committee membership had been expanded to 12, with dentistry still not represented.

1972. In 1972 the American Heart Association[4] made its next recommendations. The committee for the first time had a dentist, Dr. Dean Millard, as a member representing the American Dental Association. The oral regimen was modified by increasing the initial dose of penicillin to 500 mg given 1 hour before the dental procedure. The parenteral regimen was once again extended to include injections on each of the 2 days after the dental procedure. Decreasing the aqueous component from 600,000 to 200,000 units of penicillin G reduced the dose for each of the three injections. Increasing the initial dose to 500 mg modified the erythromycin regimen for patients allergic to penicillin. However, the committee for the first time recommended that this regimen be used for patients on continual oral penicillin prophylaxis for prevention of rheumatic fever. (The low dose is ineffective in endocarditis prevention and penicillin-resistant bacteria are present in the oral flora.) Past committees had suggested increasing the penicillin dose or using other antibiotics for patients on penicillin prophylaxis for rheumatic fever prevention.

1977. In 1977 the American Heart Association[5] made major changes in the recommendations for endocarditis prevention. These changes were based on the results of studies in animals.[30,70,71] The animal studies had shown that endocarditis could be prevented by very high blood levels of antibiotics if present before the release of bacteria into the bloodstream and if maintained for at least 9 hours. Therefore, the initial dose of all regimens was greatly increased. In addition, a regimen was recommended for patients considered to be at greatest risk—those with recent open-heart surgery, a history of endocarditis, and prosthetic heart valves.

The oral penicillin regimen recommended consisted of 2 g of penicillin V given 30 to 60 minutes before the procedure, followed by 500 mg of penicillin V every 6 hours for eight doses. A combined parenteral-oral regimen also was suggested using 1 million units of aqueous penicillin G and 600,000 units of procaine penicillin G intramuscularly given 30 to 60 minutes before the dental procedure. That was to be followed by 500 mg penicillin V every 6 hours for eight doses. The committee preferred this regimen. However, others recommended selection of the oral route whenever possible. The reason is when penicillin is given by injection 1% to 2% of the patients will develop an allergy to the drug. When it is given by the oral route, however, the rate of developing an allergy is reduced to 0.1% to 0.2%. Hence with reliable patients, the oral regimen was preferable (see Chapter 18).

Patients at high risk (e.g., those with prosthetic heart valves) were recommended to be given a special regimen for prophylaxis. Those not allergic to penicillin were to be given a parenteral-oral regimen consisting of 1 million units of aqueous penicillin G and 600,000 units of procaine penicillin G intramuscularly 30 to 60 minutes before the dental procedure along with 1 g of streptomycin intramuscularly followed by 500 mg penicillin V orally every 6 hours for eight doses. High-risk patients allergic to penicillin were to be given 1 g of vancomycin by intravenous infusion over a 30-minute period just before the dental procedure, followed by 500 mg of erythromycin orally every 6 hours for eight doses.

1984. The American Heart Association next made recommendations in December 1984.[6] These included several important changes. A clear preference was suggested for the use of an oral regimen for low to moderate at-risk patients. The other major change was to reduce the duration of coverage after the dental procedure. The standard regimen recommended for most patients consisted of 2 g of penicillin V orally 1 hour before the dental procedure, followed 6 hours later by 1 g penicillin V (i.e., 6 hours after the loading dose). Patients allergic to penicillin, those on a low dose of oral penicillin for prevention of rheumatic fever, or those taking penicillin for other reasons were given 1 g of erythromycin orally 1 hour before the procedure, followed by 500 mg erythromycin 6 hours later. (Dentists should allow 1 to 2 hours to elapse after the loading dose to ensure maximum blood levels of erythromycin.) For the few patients at low to moderate risk for endocarditis who could not take oral penicillin, the committee recommended 2 million units of aqueous penicillin G intramuscularly 30 to 60 minutes before the dental procedure, followed by 1 million units of aqueous penicillin G intramuscularly 6 hours later.

For patients at high risk of developing endocarditis (e.g., prosthetic heart valves) the committee recommended a special regimen. Those patients not allergic to penicillin were given 1 to 2 g of ampicillin intramuscularly or intravenously and in a separate dose gentamicin 1.5 mg/kg intramuscularly or intravenously 1 hour before the dental procedure, followed by 1 g penicillin V orally 6 hours later. Patients allergic to penicillin were given, as recommended in 1977, 1 g of vancomycin by intravenous infusion over the 60 minutes before the dental procedure. However, the erythromycin administered after this dose was eliminated. The committee made no mention of the high-risk patient taking anticoagulation medication. Parenteral injection may be contraindicated in these patients.

1990. The 1990 American Heart Association recommendations[7] demonstrated that organization's concerns regarding the low compliance rate reported for the 1984 special regimens among high-risk patients. As a result, the 1990 recommendations suggested the use of an oral amoxicillin regimen as the standard regimen for all at-risk patients. A two-dose oral regimen was recommended, 3 g one hour before the procedure followed by 1.5 g 6 hours later.[7,72] The American Heart Association preferred using a two-dose oral regimen of erythromycin or clindamycin in patients who were allergic to penicillin. Two forms of erythromycin were suggested: erythromycin ethylsuccinate, 800 mg initial oral dose followed 6 hours later by 400 mg, and erythromycin stearate, 1 g initial oral dose followed 6 hours later by 500 mg. The time of the initial or loading dose was extended to 2 hours before the dental procedure. Patients allergic to penicillin and unable to tolerate erythromycin were given clindamycin, 300 mg initial oral dose 1 hour before the procedure followed 6 hours later by 150 mg. Patients taking penicillin for prevention of rheumatic fever or who were being treated with penicillin for other reasons could have been protected with erythromycin or clindamycin. High-risk patients who were allergic to amoxicillin were given clindamycin if an oral regimen was selected.[7,72]

Dental patients undergoing general anesthesia for surgical treatment were given IM ampicillin according to the 1990 American Heart Association guidelines.[1] The next dose is given with IM ampicillin if the patient is not yet awake. Oral amoxicillin is suggested if the patient is awake. Clindamycin is recommended for patients undergoing general anesthesia if they are allergic to penicillin.[7,72]

Parenteral-oral regimens were still available for use in selected patients. Also penicillin V was still available for use as an alternative oral regimen. The American Heart Association did not speak directly to the issue of changing the regimen for patients taking oral penicillin V to amoxicillin. The following statement was made[7,72]: *"The choice of the 1984 penicillin V oral regimen for standard-risk patients against alpha-hemolytic streptococcal bacteremia following dental and oral procedures was still rational and acceptable."*

Current AHA Guidelines—1997. The American Heart Association published its most recent guidelines in June 1997.[8] The committee's recommendations reflected analyses of relevant literature regarding procedure-related endocarditis, in vitro susceptibility data of pathogens causing endocarditis, results of experimental animal models on prophylaxis, and retrospective analyses of human endocarditis cases in terms of antibiotic prophylaxis usage patterns and apparent prophylaxis failures.

The committee reported that no randomized and carefully controlled human trials in patients with structural heart disease show the effectiveness of antibiotic prophylaxis during bacteremia-inducing medical and dental procedures. It pointed out that most cases of endocarditis are not attributable to invasive medical or dental procedures. The committee also stated that a reasonable approach for endocarditis prophylaxis should consider level of risk, risk for bacteremia, adverse reaction risk with the antibiotic selected, and the cost-benefit aspects of the recommended prophylactic regimen. The committee stated that this guideline for prevention of bacterial endocarditis is not intended as the standard of care or as a substitute for clinical judgment.[8]

BOX 2-3

Conditions Considered by the American Heart Association for Antibiotic Prophylaxis for Endocarditis Prevention

Antibiotic Prophylaxis Recommended
High-Risk Conditions
Prosthetic cardiac valves
Bioprosthetic
Homograft
Previous bacterial endocarditis
Complex cyanotic congenital heart disease (tetralogy of Fallot)
Surgically constructed systemic-pulmonary shunts

Moderate-Risk Conditions
Most other congenital cardiac malformations (other than above and those listed below)
Acquired valvar dysfunction (e.g., rheumatic heart disease)
Hypertrophic cardiomyopathy

Mitral valve prolapse with valvar regurgitation and/or thickened leaflets

Antibiotic Prophylaxis Not Recommended
Low or Negligible Risk Conditions
Isolated secundum atrial septal defect
Surgical repair without residua beyond 6 months
    Ventricular septal defect
    Patent ductus arteriosus
Previous coronary artery bypass graft surgery
Mitral valve prolapse without valvar regurgitation
Physiologic, functional, or innocent heart murmurs
Previous Kawasaki disease without valvar dysfunction
Previous rheumatic fever without valvar dysfunction (RHD)
Cardiac pacemakers and implanted defibrillators

From *Circulation* 96:358-366, 1997.

Box 2-3 shows the ranking of cardiac conditions in regard to the risk for endocarditis, including severity of the disease in terms of morbidity and mortality rates. Individuals with the conditions listed in the high-risk group are at a much higher risk for developing severe infection that is often associated with high morbidity and mortality rates even though the risk for endocarditis is not much greater for some conditions such as prosthetic heart valves when compared with some conditions listed in the moderate-risk group.

Mitral valve prolapse is a common problem, and the need for prophylaxis for patients with that condition is controversial. Patients with documented murmur of mitral regurgitation are recommended for prophylaxis. Also, men over age 45 with thickened mitral leaflets were recommended for prophylaxis. Referral for cardiac evaluation is recommended in patients with mitral valve prolapse where the presence or absence of mitral regurgitation is unknown or unestablished. This evaluation should include auscultation, echocardiogram, and Doppler examination for murmur and regurgitation. When these tests are negative, no prophylaxis is indicated. If the dentist must provide emergency treatment for a patient with a history of mitral valve prolapse who is unaware of the presence or absence of murmur and regurgitation antibiotic prophylaxis should be provided.[8]

Conditions listed in Box 2-3 under the heading low- or negligible-risk category do not require prophylaxis. Conditions not recommended for prophylaxis include previous coronary artery bypass graft surgery, previous rheumatic fever without valvar dysfunction, and mitral valve prolapse without valvar regurgitation.[8]

Box 2-4 shows the dental procedures for which the committee recommends prophylaxis. Prophylaxis is still recommended for periodontal probing, recall maintenance, and cleaning of teeth or implants where bleeding is anticipated. Not recommended for prophylaxis are restorative dentistry with or without retraction cord, placement of rubber dams, postoperative suture removal, taking of oral impressions, and placement of removable prosthodontic or orthodontic appliances.[8]

The committee stated that individuals at risk for developing bacterial endocarditis should establish and maintain the best possible oral health to reduce potential sources of bacterial seeding. Antiseptic mouth rinses applied just before dental procedures may reduce the incidence and magnitude of bacteremia. Agents include chlorhexidine and povidone-iodine. Gingival irrigation is *not* recommended as it had been in 1990. In addition,

BOX 2-4

American Heart Association Recommendation Regarding Dental Procedures and Antibiotic Prophylaxis for Endocarditis Prevention

Endocarditis Prophylaxis Recommended	**Endocarditis Prophylaxis Not Recommended**
Dental extractions	Restorative dentistry* (operative and prosthodontic) with or without retraction cord†
Periodontal surgery, scaling, root planning, probing, and recall maintenance	Local anesthetic injections (nonintraligamentary)
Placement of dental implants	Intracanal endodontic treatment, post placement, and crown buildup
Reimplantation of avulsed teeth	Placement of rubber dams
Endodontic instrumentation or surgery only beyond the apex of teeth	Postoperative suture removal
Subgingival placement of antibiotic fibers/strips	Placement of removable prosthodontic or orthodontic appliances
Initial placement of orthodontic bands but not brackets	Taking of oral impressions
Intraligamentary local anesthetic injections	Fluoride treatments
Prophylactic cleaning of teeth or implants where bleeding is anticipated	Taking of oral radiographs
	Orthodontic appliance adjustment
	Shedding of primary teeth

From *Circulation* 96:358-366, 1997.
*Includes restoration of decayed teeth and replacement of missing teeth.
†Clinical judgment may indicate antibiotic use in selected circumstances that may 'create significant bleeding.

sustained or repeated frequent interval use of these agents is not indicated because this may result in the selection of resistant microorganisms.[8]

Antibiotic prophylaxis for patients at risk is recommended for dental procedures likely to cause bacteremia (see Box 2-4). If unanticipated bleeding occurs with a procedure not recommended for prophylaxis, the dentist can give antimicrobial prophylaxis within the first 2 hours with the belief that it will be effective based on data from experimental animal models.[8,73] Antibiotics given more than 4 hours after the procedure probably will have no prophylactic benefit. If a series of dental appointments is required, an interval of 9 to 14 days between appointments may be prudent.[8,74] A combination of procedures should be planned for each appointment.

Edentulous patients may develop bacteremia from ulcers caused by ill-fitting dentures. When new dentures are inserted, the patient should return to the dentist to correct any problems that could cause mucosal ulceration. Denture wearers should be encouraged to return to the practitioner if discomfort develops.[8]

Practitioners must exercise their own clinical judgment in determining the choice of antibiotics and the number of doses that are to be administered in individual cases or special circumstances. Endocarditis may

occur in spite of appropriate antibiotic prophylaxis. Thus the dentist should maintain a high index of suspicion regarding any unusual clinical events after dental procedures in patients who are at risk for developing bacterial endocarditis.[8] These unusual clinical events include unexplained fever, night chills, weakness, myalgia, arthralgia, lethargy, and malaise.

The recommended standard prophylactic regimen is a single 2-g dose of oral amoxicillin given 1 hour before the dental procedure. The pediatric dose is 50 mg/kg not to exceed the adult dose (Box 2-5). For patients who are unable to take or unable to absorb oral medications, intramuscular or intravenous ampicillin sodium is recommended (Box 2-6). Individuals allergic to penicillin should be treated with alternative oral regimens.[8]

Clindamycin, azithromycin, clarithromycin are recommended alternative oral regimens.[8] Also, first-generation cephalosporins (cephalexin and cefadroxil) can be used in patients provided they have not had an immediate local or systemic immunoglobulin E mediated (type I) allergic reaction to penicillin[8] (Box 2-7). The newer azalides, azithromycin and clarithromycin, are more expensive than the other regimens.

Clindamycin phosphate is recommended when parenteral administration is needed for a patient with a his-

American Heart Association Recommended Standard Prophylactic Regimen for Dental Procedures*

Adults
Amoxicillin 2 g, orally, 1 hour before procedure

Children
Amoxicillin 50 mg/kg, orally, 1 hour before procedure†

From *Circulation* 96:358-366, 1997.
*Used *in* all at-risk patients, including those with prosthetic heart valves.
†Children's doses should not exceed adult dose.

Alternate Prophylactic Regimen for Patients Given General Anesthesia for Oral Surgical or Dental Procedures or Who Are Unable to Use Oral Medications

Not Allergic to Penicillin

Adults
Ampicillin 2 g IV or IM 30 minutes before procedure

Children
Ampicillin 50 mg/kg IV or IM 30 minutes before procedure

Allergic to Penicillin

Adults
Clindamycin 600 mg/kg IV 30 minutes before procedure

Children*
Clindamycin phosphate 10 mg/kg 30 minutes before procedure

From *Circulation* 96:358-366, 1997.
*Total pediatric dose should not exceed total adult dose.

Alternate Prophylactic Regimens to Prevent Endocarditis for Dental Procedures in Patients Allergic to Penicillin

Adults
Clindamycin 600 mg orally 1 hour before procedure
or
Cephalexin or Cefadroxil 2.0 g orally 1 hour before procedure
or
Azithromycin or Clarithromycin 500 mg orally 1 hour before procedure

Children*
Clindamycin 10 mg/kg 1 hour before procedure, then half dose 6 hours after initial dose
or
Cephalexin or Cefadroxil 50 mg/kg orally 1 hour before procedure
or
Azithromycin or Clarithromycin 15 mg/kg orally 1 hour before procedure

From *Circulation* 96:358-366, 1997.
*Children's doses should not exceed adult doses.

tory of penicillin allergy. Parenteral cefazolin may be used in the patient who did not have an immediate type I hypersensitivity reaction to penicillin (see Box 2-7). Erythromycin is no longer recommended because of gastrointestinal upset and complicated pharmacokinetics. However, dentists who have successfully used erythromycin for prophylaxis in individual patients may choose to continue with this antibiotic.[8]

Patients taking oral penicillin for secondary prevention of rheumatic fever or for other purposes such as acute infection may have viridans streptococci in their oral cavities that are relatively resistant to amoxicillin or ampicillin. In these cases the dentist should select clindamycin, azithromycin, or clarithromycin.[8] Because of possible cross-resistance with the cephalosporins, this class of antibiotics should be avoided. In patients being treated for a short time such as for acute infection, the dental procedure could be delayed until at least 9 to 14 days after completion of the antibiotic. Then amoxicillin or ampicillin can be used as the oral flora is reestablished.

Intramuscular injections for endocarditis prophylaxis should be avoided in patients receiving anticoagulants such as heparin or warfarin sodium. Oral or intravenous regimens should be used for these patients whenever possible.[8]

A careful preoperative dental evaluation is recommended for all patients undergoing cardiac surgery. All required dental treatment should be completed before cardiac surgery. These procedures may decrease the incidence of late postoperative endocarditis.[8] A study

by Hakeberg[75] involving two groups of patients planned for heart valve surgery investigated the impact of dental status on the early postoperative rate of infection. One group of 149 patients was examined for its oral health status and received necessary dental treatment 3 to 6 months before heart valve surgery. The oral health status of a second group of 104 patients was examined before surgery, but no dental treatment was rendered. Infections were recorded for all patients during the first 3 weeks after valve surgery and correlated to the dental status at the time of surgery. The results did not support the contention that dental intervention before valve surgery decreases the rate of early postoperative infection. However, needed dental treatment should be completed before cardiac surgery whenever possible.

Reparative cardiac procedures may not modify the patient's long-term risk for endocarditis. In the case of prosthetic valve replacement, the risk of endocarditis increases postoperatively. In other conditions, such as closure of ventricular septal defect or patent ductus arteriosus without residual leak, the risk of endocarditis diminishes to the level of the general population after a 6-month healing period. No evidence exists that coronary artery bypass graft surgery or stents introduces a risk for endocarditis. Synthetic vascular grafts may merit antibiotic prophylaxis for the first 6 months after implantation.[8]

Insufficient data exist to support recommendations for patients who have had heart transplants. The combination of intermittent valve dysfunction and immunosuppression leads most transplant physicians to administer prophylaxis according to regimens for the moderate-risk category.[8]

A case of endocarditis perceived as result of failure to administer a recommended prophylactic regimen requires careful analysis.[8] The following factors should be considered: the time period (performance of the procedure and time before onset of symptoms), the bacteria causing endocarditis, the possibility that the procedure would have resulted in bacteremia, and awareness by the patient of the underlying lesion and communication of this to the treating dentist before the procedure. Most cases of procedure-related endocarditis occur with a short incubation period of approximately 2 weeks or less after the procedure.[37] The vast majority of endocarditis cases caused by oral organisms are not related to dental treatment procedures. A recent case-control study was unable to demonstrate any independent risk for endocarditis attributable to prior dental treatment.[57]

Comments. A number of significant changes were made from the 1990 American Heart Association guidelines. From a practical standpoint the most important changes for the dentist were using an oral regimen for all at-risk patients; decreasing the standard regimen amoxicillin loading dose from 3 to 2 g; dropping the second dose from all regimens (single-dose regimens now being recommended); dropping erythromycin as an alternate regimen; increasing the dosage for the now single dose alternative clindamycin regimen from 300 mg to 600 mg; adding azithromycin, clarithromycin, cephalexin, and cefadroxil as alternative regimens; and adding the following dental procedures to the list that do not require prophylaxis: restorative dentistry, placement of rubber dams, postoperative suture removal, taking of impressions, and placement of removable appliances.

Little benefit is seen in the new suggested regimens of azithromycin, clarithromycin, cephalexin, and cefadroxil. The azalides, azithromycin and clarithromycin, are more expensive than the other oral regimens. Clindamycin can be used rather than these more expensive drugs. The cephalosporins, cephalexin and cefadroxil, have a limited use in patients with a history of penicillin allergy. They should not be used in patients with a history of: a severe type I hypersensitivity reaction or any recent type I reaction to penicillin. Most dentists likely will use the alternative regimen of clindamycin for patients with a history of penicillin allergy.

The 1997 American Heart Association report provided the reader with a discussion of mitral valve prolapse and identified those patients with the condition it believes require prophylaxis. Patients with mitral valve regurgitation are recommended for prophylaxis. In addition, men over age 45 with thickened or redundant mitral valves were recommended for prophylaxis.[8]

The committee listed the various cardiac lesions in terms of their risks for endocarditis. Lesions in the high- and moderate-risk categories require prophylaxis for the dental procedures indicated by the committee. Those in the low- or negligible-risk category do not require prophylaxis.

An important addition to the 1997 guidelines was a discussion of cases of endocarditis perceived as a result of failure to administer a recommended prophylactic regimen. If the onset of BE symptoms is longer than 2 weeks after the dental procedure, the likelihood that the procedure was the cause of the endocarditis is significantly reduced.

In cases in which the dental procedures performed were not recommended for prophylaxis but significant unanticipated bleeding occurred, the committee recommends that antimicrobial prophylaxis be administered within 2 hours after the procedure. Experimental animal models suggest that this administration can still result in effective prophylaxis.

Several areas of confusion were noted in the new guidelines. In one location the committee referred to two studies that indicated an interval of 9 to 14 days should elapse between treatment appointments. In another section of the report it states, "If possible, one could delay the procedure until at least 9 to 14 days after completion of the antibiotic." In most cases 7 days is sufficient to allow the oral flora to be reestablished.[76]

The committee dropped the 1990 recommendation to use sucular irrigation with chlorhexidine before extraction and periodontal surgery. No rationale was given. In addition, committee members stated that sustained or repeated frequent interval use of chlorhexidine is not indicated. They failed to explain the way they defined "sustained" or "repeated intervals." Chlorhexidine has been used for patients with severe periodontal disease and a cardiac lesion at risk for endocarditis. At the first appointment, with the standard American Heart Association regimen for prophylaxis in place, the teeth can be cleaned using a cavitron. The patient is sent home and directed to rinse with chlorhexidine once a day and to return in about 7 days. At the second appointment, with the patient on the standard American Heart Association regimen for endocarditis prevention, the teeth can be cleaned of calculus using instruments and the patient introduced to tooth brushing and flossing. The chlorhexidine is stopped after the second appointment. This approach is designed to reduce patient-caused bacteremias resulting from brushing and flossing while gross gingival disease is present.

Although the 1997 American Heart Association recommendations for the prevention of BE are by far the simplest, some physicians and dentists still do not comply with them. One reason is that many clinicians rely on myths of dental-induced endocarditis prevention. To educate clinicians on endocarditis and its prevention, Wahl formalized the myths of dental-induced endocarditis prevention[69]:

Myth 1—For the most part physicians and dentists are aware of and comply with American Heart Association guidelines on antibiotic prophylaxis for prevention of infective endocarditis.

Myth 2—Most cases of bacterial endocarditis of oral origin are caused by dental procedures.

Myth 3—American Heart Association antibiotic regimens give almost total protection against endocarditis after dental procedures.

Myth 4—Antibiotics should be administered for any dental procedure that causes bleeding.

Myth 5—If a patient is receiving antibiotic therapy for an infection before the dental procedure, the dentist does not need to change the patient to another antibiotic before the dental procedure.

Myth 6—The risk of endocarditis is almost always greater than the risk of toxic effects of the antibiotic.

Myth 7—Parenteral antibiotics before dental procedures are preferable for most patients with high-risk conditions (e.g., prosthetic heart valves and previous history of endocarditis).

Myth 8—All patients with mitral valve prolapse should routinely receive antibiotic prophylaxis for dental procedures.

Myth 9—Clinicians should err on the positive side of antibiotic prophylaxis to prevent lawsuits.

All clinicians need to be aware of the falseness of these myths to best protect their patients from BE.

PREVENTION OF MEDICAL COMPLICATIONS

Current dental management for the prevention of endocarditis involves the identification of at-risk patients and the use of antibiotic prophylaxis before dental procedures according to the 1997 American Heart Association recommendations.[8] Excellent oral hygiene, the prevention of dental disease, and the treatment of existing disease in susceptible patients are the best means of preventing endocarditis.

PATIENT IDENTIFICATION

The first step in management is the identification of susceptible patients. A careful health history identifies most of these patients (see Boxes 2-1 and 2-3). Medical consultation should be used to clarify or confirm a patient's current status and the need for antibiotic prophylaxis. Two groups of patients present the greatest problem to the dentist in trying to determine susceptibility to endocarditis: those with a history of rheumatic fever and those who state that they have a heart murmur (see Chapter 3).

A single attack of rheumatic fever now results in residual heart damage (rheumatic heart disease) in about 20% of the cases. Approximately 40 years ago the rate was about 66%. If the patient has had more than one attack of rheumatic fever, the chance that rheumatic heart disease is present is nearly 100% (see Chapter 3).

A patient with a history of a single episode of rheumatic fever who needs emergency dental care must be assumed to have rheumatic heart disease unless the heart clearly was not damaged or the patient's current status can be confirmed by a telephone consultation with the physician. If the patient is not sure of the current status, and medical consultation does not substantiate the absence of rheumatic heart disease, prophylactic antibiotics should be given for the procedure.

Patients needing routine dental care who have a history of a single attack of rheumatic fever should have a medical consultation to establish the presence of rheumatic heart disease. Referral to an internist or cardiologist for evaluation is indicated for those not aware of their current status and not under the care of a physician. The evaluation includes auscultation, an echocardiogram, an electrocardiogram, and an anteroposterior chest radiograph. If the patient is found to be free of rheumatic heart disease, no antibiotic coverage is recommended for future dental treatment.

A patient needing routine dental care who has a history of more than one attack of rheumatic fever can be assumed to have rheumatic heart disease. However, as a matter of professional courtesy, consultation with the patient's physician to confirm the current status and need for prophylaxis is recommended. Such patients nearly always require antibiotic prophylaxis for dental treatment.

A patient may report having a heart murmur but not know whether it is functional or pathologic. The murmur must be considered pathologic until proved otherwise. Thus the patient needing emergency dental care who has a history of murmur should be given prophylactic antibiotics unless the functional nature of the murmur is confirmed or a telephone consultation establishes that the murmur is functional.

Medical consultation should be initiated for the patient needing routine dental care who gives a history of having a murmur. If the murmur is found to be functional, no antibiotic prophylaxis is needed. The most common "cause" of functional murmurs is growth of the individual during childhood and adolescence, and pregnancy. In both examples the murmur is transient. Prophylactic antibiotics for designated bacteremia-producing dental treatment should be given to a patient with a pathologic or an organic murmur as recommended by the American Heart Association.

Intravenous drug users have an increased risk for endocarditis. The prevalence of occult valvular pathology in this group of patients has not been established. Levitt[77] found that both non-intravenous drug users and intravenous drug users have occult valvular pathology. An increased thickening of the tricuspid and mitral valves was found in the intravenous drug users. The prevalence of valvular regurgitation was small for both groups, with no statistical difference noted. This observation and the causative agent of S. *aureus* for most cases of endocarditis in intravenous drug users, which is a rare finding in dental bacteremias, do not support the routine use of antibiotic prophylaxis for this group of individuals.

The American Heart Association states that patients with hypertrophic cardiomyopathy are at moderate risk for endocarditis after certain invasive dental procedures.[8]

Most literature on endocarditis in hypertrophic cardiomyopathy is confined in large part to case reports. The risk of endocarditis in this group of patients is not well defined. Spirito et al[78] found 10 cases of endocarditis occurred in 810 patients with hypertrophic cardiomyopathy from 1970 to 1997. They concluded that endocarditis in hypertrophic cardiomyopathy is virtually confined to patients with outflow obstruction and more common in those patients with both obstruction and atrial dilation. Thus they suggested that antibiotic prophylaxis is required only in patients with obstructive hypertrophic cardiomyopathy. The dentist should rely on medical consultation before deciding to recommend prophylaxis for this group of patients.

Patients with systemic lupus erythematosus have been reported to have an increased prevalence of functionally impaired cardiac valves resulting from sterile thrombi (Libman-Sacks lesions). The risk for endocarditis in this group of patients has not been well established but appears to be increased. In a review of records from two health care facilities Miller et al[35] found 275 records that met the 1982 American Rheumatism Association criteria for systemic lupus erythematosus. A clinically detectable heart murmur found in 18.5% of the patients required further investigation to determine its significance. Approximately 4% of the patients had cardiac valve abnormalities that placed them in the moderate-risk group for endocarditis. However, no cases were found that demonstrated an association between endocarditis and diagnosed systemic lupus erythematosus. Based on current American Heart Association guidelines, the 4% of the patients with confirmed valvular disease should receive antibiotic prophylaxis for designated bacteremia-producing dental procedures. The dentist should rely on medical consultation to identify these patients.

PREVENTIVE DENTISTRY, DENTAL REPAIR, AND ANTIBIOTIC PROPHYLAXIS

The major means by which endocarditis can be minimized in the susceptible dental patient is to reduce the probability of bacteremia, reduce its magnitude when it occurs, and use the most effective antibiotic in the proper dosage for prophylaxis when indicated.[8,24,63,79]

Patients with no active dental disease experience fewer physiologic bacteremias from brushing, flossing, chewing, and other oral functions. The magnitude of any bacteremia occurring in patients with healthy, clean mouths is minimal. Therefore the primary goal of the physician and dentist dealing with patients susceptible to endocarditis is to encourage excellent dental repair and effective preventive dental procedures including regular dental checkups, fluoridation, diet modification to

reduce the risk of caries and periodontal disease, and daily oral hygiene (with effective brushing and flossing of the teeth).[8,24,63,79]

Patients with active dental or periodontal disease who are susceptible to endocarditis should be encouraged to upgrade the general health of their gingival tissues by improved oral hygiene procedures before having elective dental procedures performed. By helping a patient reduce the amount of gingival inflammation, the dentist can lower the risk for bacteremias associated with dental treatment procedures. In addition, when bacteremias occur their magnitude also should be reduced.[47,63,79]

The preceding approach for preventing endocarditis in susceptible dental patients is widespread. However, general agreement has not existed for some other suggested methods used to reduce the risk of endocarditis in susceptible dental patients. These methods include (1) using an antibacterial mouth rinse,[80,81] (2) using sulcular irrigation with antibacterial solutions,[47] (3) using an antibiogram[79] of the individual's oral flora for the selection of antibiotics to be used in prophylaxis, and (4) performing a minimum amount of dental treatment during each coverage period.[47,79]

Antibacterial mouth rinses have been shown to reduce the frequency and possibly the magnitude of dental bacteremias, but their use in the past has not generally been accepted. In addition, some authors recommend both antibacterial mouth rinses and sulcular irrigation before extraction of teeth or periodontal therapy.[47,79-81] A 1% povidone-iodine solution has been suggested for rinsing and sulcular irrigation.[47] A 0.2% or 1% solution of chlorhexidine also has been recommended.[79] However, no direct evidence shows that these procedures reduce the risk of endocarditis in susceptible patients. Nevertheless, the logic of their use is understandable.

The 1990 American Heart Association guidelines[7,72] for the first time suggested the use of antibacterial mouth rinses before invasive dental procedures in high-risk patients and patients with poor oral hygiene. The 1990 American Heart Association guidelines also suggested sulcular irrigation with chlorhexidine or 1% providone-iodine solution prior to extraction of teeth. The current AHA guidelines (1997) still suggest antibacterial mouth rinses but dropped the recommendation of sulcular irrigation.[8]

Tzukert et al[79] recommended an antibiogram (antibiotic sensitivity testing) of the individual patient's oral flora be used as the basis of selection of prophylactic antibiotics. The antibiogram is an in vitro method for the determination of susceptibility of bacterial samples to specific antibiotics. For most patients requiring antibiotic prophylaxis, the use of an antibiogram does not seem cost effective, nor does it alter the decision that the

most appropriate antibiotic is amoxicillin in most cases. In the management of high-risk patients in hospital settings, the antibiogram may be useful for identifying patients with resistant bacteria and thus alter the selection of antibiotics to be used for prophylaxis. However, current practice in the United States does not include the use of an antibiogram when patients susceptible to endocarditis are managed in the dental office.

In certain high-risk patients, this procedure can be considered. The patient, physician, and dentist should discuss the advantages and disadvantages involved with the incorporation of this procedure into the management plan.

Several authors have recommended a limited amount of dental treatment be planned for each prophylactic coverage period.[47,79] The assumption is that the larger the magnitude of the bacteremia, the greater the risk for endocarditis. However, this point has not been proved by any clinical investigations involving humans. The more coverage periods needed, the greater the risk for allergic reactions and development of resistant bacterial strains. In addition, the cost and difficulty for the patient to obtain needed dental treatment increase. The 1997 American Health Association guidelines[8] suggested the maximal amount of dental treatment be performed during each coverage period.

The dental procedures recommended for prophylaxis in patients at risk for endocarditis has been greatly modified by the most recent AHA guidelines.[8] The most significant change from the 1990 AHA recommendations was the dropping of all restorative and prosthodontic procedures from the list suggested for prophylaxis. Gingival bleeding associated with dental procedures is no longer a valid criterion indicating the need for prophylaxis. The amount of tissue damage that results from a given procedure and the frequency and magnitude of the resulting bacteremia bleeding appear to be the new criteria to determine which dental procedures require prophylaxis. Thus only those dental procedures causing significant bacteremia require antibiotic prophylaxis. The American Health Association recommends prophylaxis for invasive dental procedures known to induce significant gingival or mucosal injury—including extractions, periodontal surgical procedures, placement of dental implants, professional cleaning of the teeth, and intraligamentary injections. It does not recommend antibiotic prophylaxis for dental procedures less likely to injure these tissues, such as simple adjustment of orthodontic appliances, placement of matrix bands or rubber dam clamps, infiltration or block anesthesia injections, and restorative and prosthodontic procedures. If the findings of the Strom study[57] that dental procedures are not associated with the onset of endocarditis can be

supported by additional investigations, major changes in the next American Heart Association guidelines can be expected in this area. Until that time the dentist is best advised to follow the current AHA guidelines. The British have held the position for some time that only extractions and various periodontal procedures excluding professional cleaning are being recommended for antibiotic prophylaxis.[82]

Based on the current American Heart Association recommendations, dental procedures recommended for prophylaxis should be performed once the loading dose has been given and the appropriate waiting time has elapsed. The next 1 to 2 hours of the coverage period (period of time patient is taking antibiotics) can be used to perform treatment needing antibiotic prophylaxis and other procedures. During this period the patient is best protected. If additional coverage periods are needed, at least 1 week should elapse before another coverage period is initiated. This allows the oral flora to return to normal.

Several studies[83,84] have suggested that resistant bacteria may remain as long as 6 months after the use of penicillin. Other studies have shown that penicillin V and ampicillin had no effect on the oral, throat, and fecal flora.[85,86] In one study the agents were given for 10 days and the various flora examined each day and for 19 days after termination of the antibiotics. No resistant strains were found; both aerobic and anaerobic testing was done.[85]

A study demonstrated that individuals given penicillin V prophylaxis on three consecutive Mondays developed resistant oral streptococci.[76] These organisms represented only 0.0003% to 0.41% of the total cultivable streptococcal population. The authors concluded that the use of penicillin V prophylaxis on three consecutive occasions 1 week apart should not result in the development of clinically significant levels of resistance among oral streptococci.[76] The elapse of 9 days or longer between coverage periods is adequate to prevent a problem with resistant bacteria that could have developed as a result of the preceding prophylaxis. A dentist concerned about the presence of resistant bacteria may use clindamycin rather than amoxicillin in the next coverage period. If at least 9 days has elapsed before the next coverage period is started, the alternative use of clindamycin is not necessary.

Patients needing complete dentures should receive antibiotic coverage when preprosthetic surgery is performed. The current American Heart Association guidelines[8] do not recommend antibiotic coverage during the construction of dentures or to cover the susceptible patient during denture insertion. The patient should be seen on the next day, and any irritations or ulcerations caused by overextended areas of the denture should be corrected. All denture patients who are at risk for IE should be rescheduled if any sore spots develop any time after the insertion period.

A possible situation in a busy dental practice is both the patient and dentist discovering after a dental procedure that antibiotic prophylaxis had not been taken. Although this situation should be avoided, the American Heart Association recommends that antibiotics be administered within 2 hours of the procedure. Another situation that can occur in a patient at risk is a procedure being performed not recommended for prophylaxis but complicated by excessive tissue damage and bleeding. The dentist may give the patient the appropriate antibiotic regimen at that time or arrange for it to be taken within the next 2 hours. To provide this type of service, the dentist can consider keeping amoxicillin and clindamycin tablets in the office.

Dens in dente has been reported to be associated with the development of BE. Whyman and MacFadyen[87] described an episode of endocarditis in an 11-year-old patient caused by a strain of nutritionally deficient streptococci. Endocarditis developed after the occurrence of a dental abscess associated with dens in dente affecting the maxillary left lateral incisor. A prolonged period of hospitalization was required to control the disease. This case underlines the need to consider sealants for all at-risk patients and to treat all acute infection in patients at risk for endocarditis in a rapidly effective manner.

Patients having orthodontic bands adjusted do not require prophylactic coverage, and patients undergoing exfoliation of their deciduous teeth do not need coverage. Children requiring endocarditis prophylaxis because of conditions such as congenital heart defects should not routinely be given antibiotics for initial or periodic dental examinations. The examination, radiographs, and fluoride treatment can be done without antibiotic coverage. When dental prophylaxis or other treatment procedures are indicated, antibiotic prophylaxis should be used as indicated[88] (see Boxes 2-3 and 2-4).

TREATMENT PLANNING CONSIDERATIONS

Patients at risk for BE (see Table 2-1) who are in good general health can receive any indicated dental care as long as they are protected by antibiotics against BE for those procedures that may cause significant bleeding. If the general health is compromised the patient may need special management depending on the nature of the systemic illness. (For example, patients with congestive heart failure should be managed as described in Chapter 7.) Antibiotic prophylaxis still would be indicated for the at-risk patient based on the dental procedures planned. The most important aspects of dental care are dental ed-

ucation, preventive dentistry procedures, and the maintenance of good dental repair. Active gingival disease should be treated, and good periodontal health obtained before extensive restorative procedures are undertaken. Complex restorative treatment should be encouraged when indicated. The dentist should plan to do as much treatment as possible during each coverage period (the time a patient is taking antibiotics) so the patient's dental treatment will not be spread over too long a time and thus the number of necessary coverage periods can be kept to a minimum. Nine days to two weeks or more should elapse between coverage periods.

References

1. American Heart Association: Prevention of rheumatic fever and bacterial endocarditis through control of streptococcal infection, *Circulation* 11:317-20, 1955.
2. American Heart Association: Prevention of rheumatic fever and bacterial endocarditis through control of streptococcal infection, *Circulation* 21:151-55, 1960.
3. American Heart Association: Prevention of rheumatic fever and bacterial endocarditis through control of streptococcal infection, *Circulation* 31:953-55, 1965.
4. American Heart Association: Prevention of bacterial endocarditis, *Circulation* 46(suppl):3-5, 1972.
5. American Heart Association: Prevention of bacterial endocarditis, *Circulation* 56:139A-43A, 1977.
6. American Heart Association: Prevention of bacterial endocarditis, *Circulation* 70:1123A-27A, 1984.
7. Dajani AS et al: Prevention of bacterial endocarditis: recommendations by the American Heart Association, *JAMA* 264:2919-22, 1990.
8. Dajani AS et al: Prevention of Bacterial Endocarditis: Recommendations by the American Heart Association, *JAMA* 22(June 11):1794-801, 1997.
9. Falace D, Ferguson T: Bacterial endocarditis, *Oral Surg* 40:189-95, 1976.
10. Murrah VA et al: Compliance with guidelines for management of dental school patients' susceptible to infective endocarditis, *J Dent Educ* 51(5): 229-32, 1987.
11. Watanakunakorn C, Burkert T: Infective endocarditis at a large community teaching hospital, *Medicine* 72(2):90-102, 1993.
12. Durack DT: Infective and Noninfective Endocarditis. In Alexander RW et al, editors: *Hurst's the heart, arteries and veins.* ed 8, New York, 1994, McGraw-Hill.
13. Kaye D: Infective endocarditis. In Isselbacher KJ et al, editors: *Harrison's principles of internal medicine*, New York, 1994, McGraw-Hill.
14. Matthews D: The prevention and diagnosis of infective endocarditis: The primary care provider's role, *Nurse Pract* 19(8):53-60, 1994.
15. Durack DT: Infective Endocarditis. In Alexander RW et al, editors: *Hurst's the heart, arteries and veins*, ed 9 New York, 1998, McGraw-Hill.
16. Porgrel MA, Welsby PD: The dentist and prevention of infective endocarditis, *Br Dent J* 139:12-16,1975.
17. Mostaghim D, Millard HO: Bacterial endocarditis: a retrospective study, *Oral Surg* 40:219-34, 1975.
18. Bland EF, Jones TD: Rheumatic fever and rheumatic heart disease, *Circulation* 4:836-43,1951.
19. Kaye D: Infective endocarditis. In: Fauci AS et al, editors: *Harrison's principles of internal medicine*, ed 14 New York, 1998, McGraw-Hill.
20. Brook MM: Pediatric bacterial endocarditis: Treatment and prophylaxis, *Pediatr Clin North Am* 46(2):275-87, 1999.
21. Friedlander AH, Marshall CE: Pathogenesis and prevention of native valve infective endocarditis in elderly dental patients, *Drugs & Aging* 4(4):325-30, 1994.
22. Durack DT: Prevention of infective endocarditis, *N Engl J Med* 332(1):38-44, 1995.
23. Mathew J et al: Results of surgical treatment for infective endocarditis in intravenous drug users, *Chest* 108(1):73-7,1995.
24. Pallasch TJ: Antibiotic prophylaxis: theory and reality. *J Calif Dent Assoc* 17(6):27-39,1989.
25. Chapman DW: The cumulative risks of prolapsing mitral valve: 40 years of follow-up, *Tex Heart Inst J* 21(4):267-71, 1994.
26. Edwards WD: Valvular heart disease, concise review: the changing spectrum of valvular heart disease pathology. In: Fauci AS et al, editors: *Harrison's principles of internal medicine*, ed 14, New York, 1998, McGraw-Hill.
27. Jick H et al: A population-based study of appetite-suppressant drugs and the risk of cardiac-valve regurgitation, *N Engl J Med* 339:719-24,1998.
28. Cohen PS, Maguire JH, Weinstein L: Infective endocarditis caused by gram-negative bacteria: a review of the literature, 1945-1977, *Prog Cardiovasc Dis* 22(4):205-42,1979.
29. Durack DT: Infective and non-infective endocarditis. In: Hurst JW, editor: *The heart, arteries, and veins*, ed 5, New York, 1983, McGraw-Hill.
30. Durack DT: Infective and noninfective endocarditis. In: Hurst JW, editor: *The heart, arteries, and veins*, ed 7, New York, 1990, McGraw-Hill.
31. Kaye D: Infective endocarditis. In: Wilson JD et al, editors. *Harrison's principles of internal medicine*, New York, 1991, McGraw-Hill.
32. Valencia ME et al: Study of 164 episodes of infectious endocarditis in drug addicts: comparison of HIV positive and negative patients (see comments), *Rev Clin Esp* 194(7):535-9, 1994.
33. Pallasch TJ: Principles of antibiotic therapy: prevention of infective endocarditis, *Dent Drug Serv Newsletter* 4 (January):1, 1983;.
34. Bulkley BH, Humphries JO: The heart and collagen vascular disease. In: Hurst JW, editor, *The heart, arteries, and veins*, ed 6, New York, 1986, McGraw-Hill.
35. Miller CS et al: Prevalence of infective endocarditis in patients with systemic lupus erythematosus. *J Am Dent Assoc* 130(3):387-92, 1999.
36. Furrer H, Malinverni R: Clinical aspects and diagnosis of infectious endocarditis, *Schweiz Rundsch Med Prax* 83(47): 1309-15, 1994.

37. Starkebaum M, Durack D, Beeson P: The incubation period of subacute bacterial endocarditis, *Yale J Biol Med* 50:49-58, 1977.

38. Speechly-Dick ME, Swanton RH: Osteomyelitis and infective endocarditis, *Postgrad Med J* 70(830):885-90, 1994.

39. Speechly-Dick ME, Vaux EC, Swanton RH: A case of osteomyelitis secondary to endocarditis, *Br Heart J* 72(3):298, 1994.

40. Mathew J et al: Clinical features, site of involvement, bacteriologic findings, and outcome of infective endocarditis in intravenous drug users, *Arch Intern Med* 155(15):1641-8,1995.

41. O'Brien K et al: Gallium-spect in the detection of prosthetic valve endocarditis and aortic ring abscess, *J Nucl Med* 70(2):1791-93, 1991.

42. Carbon C: Animal models of endocarditis. *Int J Biomed Comput* 36(1-2):59-67, 1994.

43. Aranki SF et al: Aortic valve endocarditis. Determinants of early survival and late morbidity, *Circulation* 90(5 Pt 2):175-82, 1994.

44. Stollerman GH: Rheumatic fever. In: Thorm GW et al, editors: *Harrison's principles of internal medicine*, ed 8 New York, 1977, McGraw-Hill.

45. Okell CC, Elliott SD: Bacteraemia and oral sepsis, with special reference to the aetiology of subacute endocarditis, *Lancet* 2:869-72, 1935.

46. Murray M, Moosnick F: Incidence of bacteremia in patients with dental disease, *J Lab Clin Med* 26:801, 1941.

47. Bisno AL et al: Failure of prophylaxis for bacterial endocarditis: American Heart Association Registry, *J Fam Pract* 19:16-20, 1980.

48. Pallasch TJ: A critique of antibiotic prophylaxis, *Can Dent Assoc J* 52:28-36, 1986.

49. Guntheroth WG: How important are dental procedures as a cause of infective endocarditis? *Am J Cardiol* 54:797-801, 1984.

50. Shafer WG, Hine MK, Levy BM: Oral Infections. In: Shafer WG, Hine MK, Levy BM, editors, *Textbook of oral pathology*, ed 4, Philadelphia: 1983, WB Saunders.

51. Vuille C et al: Natural history of vegetations during successful medical treatment of endocarditis, *Am Heart J* 128(6 Pt 1):1200-9, 1994.

52. Van der Meer JT et al: Efficacy of antibiotic peophylaxis for prevention of native-valve endocarditis, *Lancet* 339(8786):135-39, 1992.

53. Finch R: Chemoprophylaxis of infective endocarditis. *Scand J Infect Dis* (suppl) 70:102-10, 1990.

54. Horstkotte D et al: Contributions for choosing the optimal prophylaxis of bacterial endocarditis, *Eur Heart J* (S-suppl) J:379-81, 1987.

55. Barco CT: Prevention of infective endocarditis: a review of the medical and dental literature, *J Periodontol*, 6:510-23, 1991.

56. Imperiale TF, Horwitz RI: Does prophylaxis prevent post dental infective endocarditis? A controlled evaluation of protective efficacy, *Am J Med* 88(2):131-36, 1990.

57. Strom BL et al: Dental and cardiac risk factors for infective endocarditis: a population-based, case-control study, *Ann Intern Med* 129(10):761-69, 1998.

58. Taubert K, Bayer A: Dental endocarditis prophylaxis: American Heart Association (AHA) *Comments*, CID *Hot Page* (April):1, 1999.

59. Dascomb HE: The current status of prophylaxis against infective endocarditis, *J La State Med Soc* 132:91-99, 1980.

60. Kaye D: Infective endocarditis. In: Rose LF KD, editor: *Internal medicine for dentistry*, St Louis, 1983, CV Mosby.

61. Requa-Clark B, Holroyd SV: *Antimicrobial agents*, ed 3, St Louis, 1983, CV Mosby.

62. Bor DH, Himmelstein DV: Endocarditis prophylaxis for patients with mitral valve prolapse: a quantitive analysis, *Am J Med* 76:711-17, 1984.

63. Tzukert AA et al: Analysis of the American Heart Association's recommendations for the prevention of infective endocarditis, *Oral Surg*, 62:276-80, 1986.

64. Clemens JD, Ransohoff J: A quantitive assessment of predental antibiotic prophylaxis for patients with mitral valve prolapse, *J Chronic Dis* 37:531-44, 1984.

65. Devereux RB et al: Cost-effectiveness of infective endocarditis prophylaxis for mitral valve prolapse with or without a mitral regurgitant murmur, *Am J of Cardio*, 74(10):1024-29, 1994.

66. Durack DT: Antibiotics for prevention of endocarditis during dentistry: time to scale back? *Ann Intern Med* 129(10):829-30, 1998.

67. Gould IM, Buckingham JK: Cost effectiveness of prophylaxis in dental practice to prevent infective endocarditis, *Brit Heart J* 70(1):79-83, 1993.

68. Kaplan EL: *Personal communications*, 1986.

69. Wahl MJ: Myths of dental-induced endocarditis, *Arch Intern Med* 154(2):137-44, 1994.

70. Garrison PK, Freedman LR: Experimental endocarditis: I. Staphylococcal endocarditis in rabbits resulting from placement of a polyethylene catheter in the right side of the heart, *Yale J Biol Med* 42:394-410, 1970.

71. Scheld WM, Sande MA: Endocarditis and intravascular infections. In: Mandell GL et al, editors: *Principles and practice of infectious disease*, New York, 1979, John Wiley & Sons.

72. American Dental Association: Preventing bacterial endocarditis: a statement for the dental profession, *J Am Dent Assoc* 122:87-92, 1991.

73. Berney P: Successful prophylaxis of experimental streptococcal endocarditis with single-dose amoxicillin administered after bacterial challenge, *J Infect Dis* 161:281-85, 1990.

74. Leviner E et al: Development of resistant oral viridans streptococci after administration of prophyalctic antibiotics: time management in the dental treatment of patients susceptible to infective endocarditis, *Oral Surg Oral Med Oral Pathol* 64:417-20, 1987.

75. Hakeberg M et al: The significance of oral health and dental treatment for the postoperative outcome of heart valve surgery, *Scand Cardiovasc J* 33(1):5-8, 1999.

76. Fleming P et al: The development of penicillin-resistant oral streptococci after repeated penicillin prophylaxis, *Oral Surg* 70:440-44, 1990.

77. Levitt MA et al: Prevalence of cardiac valve abnormalities in afebrile injection drug users, *Acad Emerg Med* 6(9):911-5, 1999.

78. Spirito P et al: Infective endocarditis in hypertrophic cardiomyopathy: prevalence, incidence, and indications for antibiotic prophylaxis, *Circulation* 99(16):2132-7, 1999.
79. Tzukert AA, Leviner E, Sela M: Prevention of infective endocarditis: not by antibiotics alone, *Oral Surg* 62:385-89, 1986.
80. Scopp IW: *Gingival degermining: bacteremia reduction in dental procedures,* Chicago, 1977 American Heart Association.
81. Scopp IW, Orvietto LD: Gingival degerming by povidone-iodine irrigation: bacteremia reduction in extraction procedures, *J Am Dent Assoc* 83:1294-96, 1971.
82. Simmons NA et al: Antibiotic prophylaxis of infective endocarditis: recommendations from the endocarditis working party of the British Society for Antimicrobial Chemotherapy, *Lancet* 335:88-89, 1990.
83. Sprunt K: *Role of antibiotic resistance in bacterial endocarditis,* Dallas, 1977, American Heart Association.
84. Enffmeyer JE: Penicillin allergy, *Clin Rev Allergy* 4:171-86, 1986.
85. Hermdah IA, Nord CE, Weilander K: Effect of phenoxymethylpenicillin, bacampicillin and clindamycin on the oral, throat, and colon microflora of man, *Swed Dent J* 4:39-52, 1980.
86. Istre GR, et al: Susceptibility of group A beta-hemolytic streptococcus isolates to penicillin and erythromycin, *Antimicrob Agents Chemother* 20:244-46, 1981.
87. Whyman RA, MacFadyen EE: Dens in dente associated with infective endocarditis, *Oral Surg Oral Med Oral Pathol* 78(1):47-50, 1994.
88. Crespi PV, Friedman RB: Dental examination guidelines for children requiring infective endocarditis prophylaxis, *J Am Den Assoc* 7:931-33, 1985.

Cardiac Conditions Associated with Endocarditis

3

CHAPTER

acterial endocarditis (BE) occurs most often on or adjacent to a congenital or an acquired valvular defect. The defect causes a narrowing in the path of blood flow.[1] This results in an increase in flow velocity upstream from the defect with low velocity blood flow and turbulence downstream from it. Endocarditis tends to develop in the area of turbulence and low flow (Fig. 3-1). The American Heart Association (AHA) has identified conditions that pose a risk for the development of BE and recommends guidelines for the provision of antibiotic prophylaxis[2] (Box 3-1). The designations of *high*, *moderate*, and *negligible risk* refer to both the likelihood of infection developing and the morbidity and mortality rates of the infection. This chapter examines the risk conditions for BE as identified by the AHA as well as some additional conditions and situations that are not included in the current guidelines.

HIGH RISK CONDITIONS

PROSTHETIC VALVES

Replacement of diseased or abnormal cardiac valves with prosthetic valves began in the early 1960s and has become commonplace. Two basic classes of prosthetic valves are used: mechanical and biological or tissue. Mechanical valve types include reciprocating ball (Fig. 3-2), tilting disk, and semicircular hinged leaflets. The reciprocating or caged ball and tilting disk types are the most common ones used today. Tissue valves are usually porcine valves treated with glutaraldehyde and mounted on a prosthetic stent (Fig. 3-3). The glutaraldehyde destroys the antigenicity of the tissue and allows placement without the danger of rejection.

Although valve replacement is usually successful, many complications can occur. Approximately 60% of

prosthetic valve recipients develop a serious prosthesis-related problem within 10 years after surgery.[3] These problems include structural deterioration of the valve, non-structural dysfunction, valve thrombosis, thromboembolism, anticoagulant-related hemorrhages, and prosthetic valve endocarditis (PVE).[4]

Patients who have a prosthetic cardiac valve are at risk for developing PVE (Fig. 3-4). The risk is 3% during the first year after placement and 0.5% each year thereafter.[4] PVE typically is classified as *early* (within the first 2 months after placement) or *late* (longer than 2 months after placement). Researchers believe perioperative infection causes early PVE and that bacteremias from other sources cause the late category.

The microbiologic factors of PVE differ from early or late occurrences.[5] In early PVE streptococci are found in only 5% of infections (S. *viridans* less than 5%) and staphylococci in 50% of infections. In the late occurrence, however, streptococci account for 35% of infections (*Streptococcus viridans* 25%) and staphylococci account for 30% of infections. Thus bacteremias of oral origin can be the source of late PVE, the majority of those cases still caused by bacteria of nondental origin. The risk of occurrence for endocarditis is the same for both mechanical and tissue valves. However, the mortality rate of PVE is significantly higher than that for native valve endocarditis. The 6-month survival rate after early PVE is 37% and 65% with late occurrence.[6]

PREVIOUS BACTERIAL ENDOCARDITIS

Repeat infections of BE are fairly common and found in from 2% to 31% of cases after initial BE.[5] Patients remain permanently at risk for reinfection after cure of BE because of residual valve damage superimposed on the original defect. Patients who have had native valve endocarditis are also at higher risk to develop prosthetic valve endocarditis.[7]

COMPLEX CYANOTIC CONGENITAL HEART DISEASE

Several diseases have cyanosis as a sign of their congenital disorder. Cyanosis is a bluish tinge of the skin caused by the presence of at least 3 g/dl of reduced hemoglobin.[8] In this group of diseases, cyanosis results from the mixing of unoxygenated blood in the systemic circulation caused by intracardiac shunting of the blood from the right side of the heart to the left. All these congenital disorders require immediate perinatal diagnosis with medical and surgical treatment to sustain life. They all involve multiple, complex abnormalities of the heart and blood vessels. All the numer-

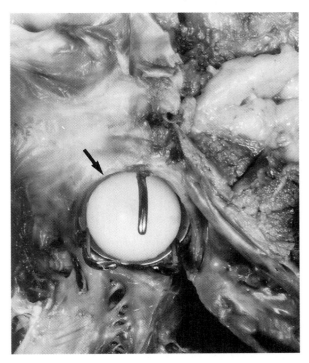

Fig. 3-2 Mechanical prosthetic valve *(arrow)*. (Courtesy Jesse E. Edwards, St. Paul, Minn.)

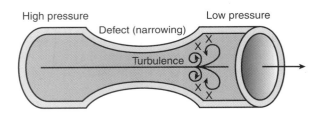

Fig. 3-1 Altered flow across a defect with *(x)* indicating the areas most prone to endocarditis.

BOX 3-1

Cardiac Conditions Associated with Endocarditis

Endocarditis Prophylaxis Recommended

High-risk category

Prosthetic cardiac valves, including bioprosthetic and homograft valves

Previous bacterial endocarditis

Complex cyanotic congenital heart disease (e.g., single ventricle states, transposition of the great arteries, tetralogy of Fallot)

Surgically constructed systemic pulmonary shunts or conduits

Moderate-risk category

Most other congenital cardiac malformations (other than above and below)—uncorrected

Acquired valvular dysfunction (e.g., rheumatic heart disease)

Hypertrophic cardiomyopathy without flow obstruction

Mitral valve prolapse with valvular regurgitation and/or thickened leaflets

Endocarditis Prophylaxis Not Recommended

Negligible-risk category (no greater risk than the general population)

Isolated secundum atrial septal defect

Surgical repair of atrial septal defect, ventricular septal defect, or patent ductus arteriosus (without residua beyond 6 mo)

Previous coronary artery bypass graft surgery

Mitral valve prolapse without valvular regurgitation

Physiologic, functional or innocent heart murmurs

Previous Kawasaki disease without valvular dysfunction

Previous rheumatic fever without valvular dysfunction

Cardiac pacemakers (intravascular and epicardial) and implanted defibrillators

From Dajani AS et al: Prevention of bacterial endocarditis. Recommendations by the American Heart Association. JAMA 1997;277: 1794-1801.

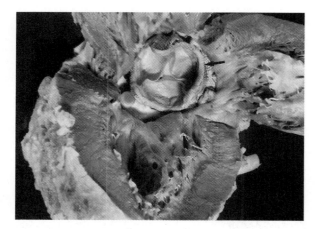

Fig. 3-3 A porcine tissue valve *(arrow)*. (Courtesy Jesse E. Edwards, St. Paul, Minn.)

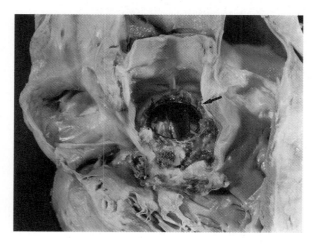

Fig. 3-4 Mechanical prosthetic heart valve with prosthetic valve endocarditis *(arrow)*. (Courtesy Jesse E. Edwards, St. Paul, Minn.)

ous treatment modalities used require surgical repair to redirect the unoxygenated blood from the systemic circulation into the pulmonary circulation (systemic-pulmonary shunt or conduit) to allow oxygenation in the lungs. Patients with these disorders are at high risk for BE even after repair and establishment of a systemic-pulmonary shunt.

In addition to being alert to the patient's risk of developing BE with cyanotic congenital heart disease, the dentist also should be aware of other effects of cyanosis and hypoxemia. A variety of abnormalities occur when cyanosis and hypoxemia are chronic and not corrected. These abnormalities include hematologic, neurologic, renal, and rheumatic conditions. Of particular importance in dentistry are the hematologic effects seen in 20% of cyanotic patients. These include erythrocytosis, iron deficiency, various clotting factor deficiencies, leukopenia, and both qualitative and quantitative platelet disorders.[9]

Single Ventricle States

Single ventricle is a relatively rare condition in which one ventricle (usually the left) develops while the other does not. The two atria subsequently empty into the common single ventricle, resulting in the mixture of oxygenated and unoxygenated blood. Pulmonary stenosis is common and requires systemic pulmonary arterial shunting.[8] Patients who do not undergo this procedure die in infancy or childhood. Repair usually consists of creation of an anastomosis between the systemic venous and pulmonary circulations. Patients whose surgery is successful have a 10-year survival rate of 60% to 70%.[9]

Transposition of the Great Arteries

Transposition of the great arteries is a relatively common congenital cyanotic condition in which an anatomic reversal of the positions of the aorta and the pulmonary artery exists. Thus the aorta arises from the right ventricle instead of the left and the pulmonary artery arises from the left ventricle instead of the right. In addition, other abnormalities coexist, such as a patent foramen ovale, patent ductus arteriosus, and ventricular septal defect.[8] Surgery that includes systemic-pulmonary shunting via arterial switching is required in the first few weeks of life. Successful patients have a 20-year survival rate of 70%.[9]

Tetralogy of Fallot

Tetralogy of Fallot is the most common of the congenital cardiac defects that cause cyanosis. Four basic abnormalities are associated with this disorder: (1) biventricular origin of the aorta, (2) large ventricular septal defect, (3) obstructed pulmonary blood flow, and (4) right ventricular hypertrophy[8] (Fig. 3-5). The disorder requires early diagnosis and surgical correction that includes systemic-pulmonary shunting to adequately oxygenate the blood. Patients who have not had the defect repaired through surgery rarely survive beyond childhood. After complete surgical repair the prognosis for these patients is generally excellent, with 30-year survival rates as high as 85%.[9]

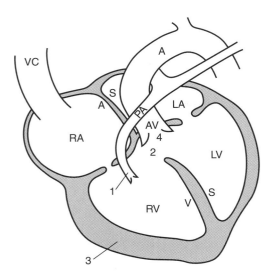

Fig. 3-5 Anatomic relationships in tetralogy of Fallot. *1)* Obstructed pulmonary blood flow caused by stenosis, *2)* large ventricular septal defect, *3)* right ventricular hypertrophy, and *4)* aorta positioned over septum communicating with both ventricles.

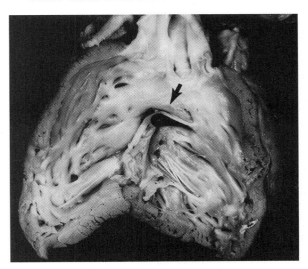

Fig. 3-7 Ventricular septal defect *(arrow).*

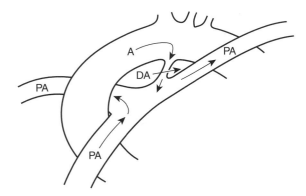

Fig. 3-6 Patent ductus arteriosus. The ductus *(DA)* connects with the aorta *(A)* and the pulmonary artery *(PA).*

MODERATE RISK CONDITIONS

PATENT DUCTUS ARTERIOSUS

Patent ductus arteriosus represents a persistence of the fetal connection of the pulmonary artery to the aorta (Fig. 3-6). In the fetus the ductus arteriosus is necessary to allow blood to flow through the placenta, where it is oxygenated, thus bypassing the nonfunctional lungs. At birth, this flow pattern abruptly changes, allowing blood from the pulmonary artery to flow to the lungs for oxygenation. The umbilical cord is clamped, thus removing the placenta from the circulation and from its function as the oxygenating organ. The ductus arteriosus then closes within 2 to 3 days and becomes the ligamentum arteriosum. The foramen ovale, which was a fetal shunt from the right atrium to the left atrium, also closes.[8]

The hemodynamic significance of a patent ductus arteriosus is determined by its size and resistance. Large connections with low resistance allow free blood flow with significant left to right shunting and must be repaired quickly; otherwise patients will develop pulmonary vascular obstruction, pulmonary hypertension, and cyanosis. Small, high-resistance cases of patent ductus arterious allow minimal shunting of blood with insignificant hemodynamic effects and may not be repaired in infancy. However, patients are at risk for infective endarteritis.[9] Ligated or repaired cases of patent ductus arteriosus pose minimal risk for endarteritis and do not require antibiotic prophylaxis if more than 6 months have passed since the repair and no residual shunting exists.[2,10] Patients with an unrepaired patent ductus arteriosus have a 30% lifetime risk of endarteritis and such patients do require antibiotic prophylaxis.[8]

VENTRICULAR SEPTAL DEFECT

A ventricular septal defect is an opening in the septum that separates the two ventricles and is a common form of congenital heart disease (Fig. 3-7). It constitutes about

10% of the congenital cardiac malformations found among adults.[11] The opening allows a left to right shunting of blood, the extent and consequence depending on the size of the opening. Small ventricular septal defects are generally of little physiologic consequence. However, the larger the opening, the more shunting occurs. This equalizes ventricular systolic pressures and increases pulmonary arterial pressure with resulting severe congestive heart failure.

Surgical closure of the defect is necessary for moderate or large openings and usually is performed before the patient is 2 years old. Smaller defects often do not require surgery if minimal effect on ventricular and arterial pressures exists. Approximately 75% of small ventricular septal defects close spontaneously by the time the patient is 10 years old.[12] Even large defects tend to decrease in size, but complete closure is unlikely. The risk of infective endocarditis in patients with an uncomplicated, unrepaired ventricular septal defect is between 4% and 10% for the first 30 years of life.[13] All patients with unrepaired ventricular septal defects require endocarditis prophylaxis. Patients with a surgically repaired ventricular septal defect do not require antibiotic prophylaxis if more than 6 months have passed since the repair and no residual shunting exists.[2]

ATRIAL SEPTAL DEFECT

An atrial septal defect is an opening in the septum between the two atria of the heart that is distinct from a patent foramen ovale (Fig. 3-8). The communication allows a left to right shunt; however, usually no significant pressure differences are detected between the atria. The classification of atrial septal defect depends on the anatomic location of the defect. The most common type of atrial septal defect is at the fossa ovalis (ostium secundum), which accounts for 70% of these defects.

Children often show no symptoms. With age, symptoms increase and by age 40 the majority of individuals display symptoms of the defect.[15] Surgical closure of the atrial septal defect generally is performed before the child enters school. Infective endocarditis is rare in patients with an unrepaired atrial septal defect; therefore antibiotic prophylaxis is not required for an unrepaired secundum atrial septal defect or for one that has been surgically repaired if more than 6 months have passed since the repair and no residual shunting occurs.[2,8]

COARCTATION OF THE AORTA

Coarctation of the aorta is a narrowing of the aortic arch that occurs in the area distal to the attachment of the fetal ductus arteriosus. The coarctation causes increased resistance to blood flow with resulting left ventricular hypertrophy. Development of extensive collateral circulation compensates for the ensuing decreased blood flow to the lower extremities. Patients develop hypertension in the upper extremities that can lead to congestive failure, stroke, aortic rupture, valvular disease, and atherosclerosis. The average age of death of adults with unrepaired coarctation of the aorta is 34 years.[16] Surgical repair usually is accomplished by resection of the narrowed segment with end-to-end anastomosis. Occasionally, a tubular vascular prosthesis is used. Unrepaired coarctation conveys a risk of endarteritis at the site of narrowing and endocarditis of the aortic and mitral valves.[8] Thus patients with unrepaired coarctation require antibiotic prophylaxis. The risk of endocarditis or endarteritis is negligible for repaired coarctation, which does not require antibiotic prophylaxis if more than 6 months have passed after repair unless a residual valvular disease such as a bicuspid aortic valve is present.[2]

BICUSPID AORTIC VALVE

The aortic valve normally comprises three leaflets or cusps (tricuspid). However, a congenital defect can result in biscuspid aortic valve, in which only two leaflets or cusps are present. This is the most common congenital cardiac abnormality in adults and occurs in about 2% of the general population.[8] The condition frequently is found in association with other forms of congenital heart disease such as coarctation of the aorta. Common complications of bicuspid aortic valve include stenosis, regurgitation, an association with aortic root dilitation and dissection, and infective endocarditis.[17] Patients with un-

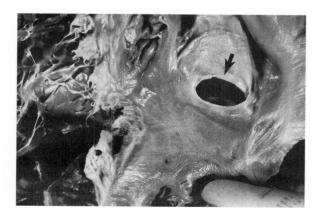

Fig. 3-8 Large atrial septal defect *(arrow)*. (Courtesy W. O'Conner, Lexington, Ky.)

complicated bicuspid aortic valve show no symptoms; the condition often is discovered incidentally in otherwise normal individuals. Approximately 20% of patients eventually require surgical intervention.[9] Patients in whom the valve has become stenotic or regurgitant are susceptible to infective endocarditis and require antibiotic prophylaxis.

ACQUIRED VALVULAR DYSFUNCTION AND CONNECTIVE TISSUE DISEASE

Rheumatic Heart Disease

Rheumatic heart disease is a sequelae of acute rheumatic fever and associated with valvular stenosis and regurgitation that predisposes to BE. The incidence of acute rheumatic fever (ARF) has decreased markedly over the past several decades. In the 1940s and 1950s, the incidence of ARF in the United States was between 20 and 50 in every 100,000 persons, but by the mid 1970s the rate had dropped to 1 in every 100,000 persons.[18,19] In developing countries, however, the rate has remained high. In the mid-1980s, for reasons not understood, a resurgence of ARF in the United States seemed to concentrate in various geographic areas of the country.[20]

ARF occurs as a result of a group A beta-hemolytic streptococcal infection of the upper respiratory tract (pharyngitis) (Fig. 3-9). Streptococcal pharyngitis is predominately a disease of childhood. Approximately 3% of patients who have not had the infection treated with antibiotics subsequently develop ARF one or more weeks later. The exact pathogenesis of ARF is unclear. A plausible hypothesis is that it is caused by an abnormal immune response to the streptococci resulting in an autoimmune-like reaction in specific tissues or organs.[20]

The diagnosis of ARF is based on the presence of major and minor criteria (Jones Criteria).[21] Major criteria include carditis, polyarthritis, chorea, erythema marginatum, and subcutaneous nodules. Minor criteria are arthralgia, fever, an increased erythrocyte sedimentation rate, increased C-reactive protein levels, and prolonged P-R interval on the electrocardiogram. A diagnosis of ARF requires the existence of either two major criteria or one major and two minor criteria in addition to evidence of a previous upper respiratory streptococcal infection.

Carditis is the most serious manifestation of ARF and can result in permanent damage to the heart valves, usually the mitral valve (rheumatic heart disease) (Fig. 3-10). From various series the incidence rate of carditis in patients with rheumatic fever is an estimated 40% to 50%.[22] Approximately 50% of patients with rheumatic carditis develop rheumatic heart disease with a persistent heart murmur.[20] Thus many individuals with a history of rheumatic fever will not have rheumatic heart disease.

If patients are unfortunate enough to contract subsequent streptococcal pharyngitis, the sequence can repeat itself with inevitable additional cardiac damage. Patients who have had ARF are highly susceptible to repeat streptococcal pharyngitis and thus frequently placed on long-term, low-dose antibiotic prophylaxis to prevent its recurrence (secondary prophylaxis). Prophylaxis is given as intramuscular penicillin G (1.2 million units monthly), oral penicillin (250 mg twice a day), oral sulfadiazine (1 g daily), or oral erythromycin (250 mg twice a day).[20]

Approximately 70% of those who developed a murmur of mitral regurgitation at the time of the acute attack lose the murmur if secondary prophylaxis is implemented effectively. This type of secondary antibiotic prophylaxis for streptococcal pharyngitis is inadequate for prevention of BE because of the low dosages and the development of

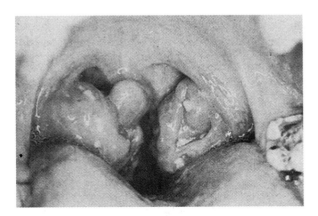

Fig. 3-9 Hypertrophied tonsils with purulent exudate.

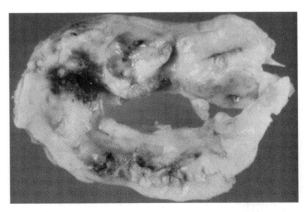

Fig. 3-10 Severely stenotic mitral valve of rheumatic heart disease.

resistant oral bacteria[2] (see Chapter 2). Patients with rheumatic heart disease are susceptible to BE and require antibiotic prophylaxis. Patients with a history of ARF but without rheumatic heart disease do not require antibiotic prophylaxis.

Systemic Lupus Erythematosis

Systemic lupus erythematosis is an autoimmune, inflammatory connective tissue disease that affects multiple organs, including skin, joints, kidneys, brain, and heart. It occurs most commonly in black women of childbearing age.

Approximately one fourth of patients with systemic lupus erythematosis have cardiac involvement, including valvular disease.[24] The most common of the valve abnormalities is mitral valve prolapse with the formation of sterile vegetations on the valve leaflets, composed of fibrin and platelets called *Libman-Sacks verrucae*. These verrucae also are called *nonbacterial thrombotic endocarditis*. The verrucae can cause the valves to thicken and become dysfunctional with resulting regurgitation. Libman-Sacks verrucae can embolize and also become infected, resulting in BE.[25] A recent study of a group of 275 patients with systemic lupus erythematosis showed 18.5% with a heart murmur that would have required consultation with a physician before dental treatment.[26] Endocarditis prophylaxis is indicated if evidence indicates that valvular dysfunction is present.

Ankylosing Spondylitis

Ankylosing spondylitis is the most common inflammatory connective tissue disease of the spine and can cause back pain, kyphosis, and ultimately fusion and immobilization of the spine. The condition is found most commonly in young men aged 20 to 30 and follows a chronic progressive course.[27] The cardiac lesion associated with ankylosing spondylitis is sclerotic inflammation of the aortic root area and aortic valve that results in aortic regurgitation in approximately 5% of patients.[24,28] This predisposes them to BE. Thus patients with a murmur of regurgitation should have endocarditis prophylaxis.

Rheumatoid Arthritis

Rheumatoid arthritis is the most common connective tissue disease, causing severe deformation of the joints, especially of the hands, wrist, and feet, and is found most commonly in women. Among the many systemic manifestations of the disease are subcutaneous rheumatoid nodules. Rheumatoid nodules rarely may infiltrate the heart, including the cardiac valves. This results in regurgitation, usually aortic.[29] The incidence of such valvular infiltration is estimated at 1% to 2% in autopsy studies of patients with rheumatoid arthritis.[24] Patients with this type of valvular dysfunction are susceptible to BE and should receive endocarditis prophylaxis.

Hypertrophic Cardiomyopathy

The principle feature of hypertrophic cardiomyopathy is left ventricular hypertrophy with a nondilated ventricular cavity. The cause is unknown, but approximately 50% of patients have a positive family history of the disease.[14] Accompanying left ventricular hypertrophy is an asymptomatic ventricular septal hypertrophy with apposition of the anterior mitral valve leaflet against the septum during systole. This results in a dynamic outflow obstruction in approximately 20% of patients.[30] Other pathophysiologic features of hypertrophic cardiomyopathy include diastolic dysfunction, myocardial ischemia, and a variety of arrhythmias.[31]

Patients with hypertrophic cardiomyopathy often show no symptoms, with sudden death being the first indication that the disorder existed. This is especially true for children and young adults. Hypertrophic cardiomyopathy is the most common cause of sudden death in young, competitive athletes.[31] Death is most likely caused by ventricular arrhythmias. A holosystolic murmur is usually present in patients with obstruction to outflow and results from mitral regurgitation. Infective endocarditis occurs in less than 10% of patients with the obstructive form of hypertrophic cardiomyopathy.[30] Therefore patients with hypertrophic cardiomyopathy *and* outflow obstruction should be provided endocarditis prophylaxis.[32] If the patient's status is not known, the dentist has two options: (1) assume the patient has outflow obstruction and provide antibiotic prophylaxis if immediate treatment is necessary or (2) delay dental treatment and refer to a physician for cardiac evaluation.

Mitral Valve Prolapse

In mitral valve prolapse a myxomatous degeneration of the mitral valve leaflets occurs and results in thickened, redundant valves that prolapse or balloon back into the left atrium during systole (Fig. 3-11). The valves may remain competent and function normally, or they may become dysfunctional and allow regurgitation of blood back into the atrium. This most common form of valve disease is found in from 3% to 8% of the population,[33] mostly in young women. It usually remains asymptomatic. The cause of most mitral valve prolapse cases is unknown; however, it is associated with the heritable connective tissue disorders including Marfan's syndrome, Ehlers-Danlos syndrome, and osteogenesis imperfecta.[34] In some cases, mitral valve prolapse is part of a symptom complex of syncope, palpitation, chest pain, and autonomic dysfunction. A relatively small percentage of patients experience the complication of BE. However, only

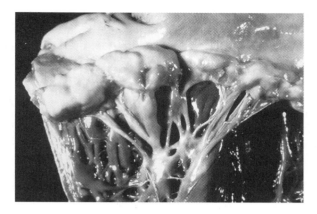

Fig. 3-11 Thickened, redundant, ballooning valve leaflets in mitral valve prolapse.

mitral valve prolapse accompanied by a regurgitant murmur is considered a risk condition for BE, and patients with this condition should be provided endocarditis prophylaxis.[2] In the absence of a murmur, antibiotic prophylaxis is not required. An exception to this is men older than 45 years with mitral valve prolapse without a consistent systolic murmur who may warrant prophylaxis because of their increased risk of BE.[35]

MISCELLANEOUS CONDITIONS

Heart Murmur of Unknown Significance

Heart murmurs are sounds or vibrations caused by turbulent blood flow across the heart valves or through the chambers of the heart. Turbulence may be caused by physiologic factors or pathologic factors. Physiologic factors include the viscosity of blood, the velocity of blood flow, and the volume of blood. Examples of pathologic factors include stenotic or narrowed valves, incompetent or dysfunctional valves, and deformities in the walls or septa of the heart. Murmurs caused by physiologic factors are termed *innocent*, or *functional*, and do not place patients at risk for BE. Thus these patients do not require antibiotic prophylaxis. Conversely, murmurs caused by pathologic factors are termed *pathologic*. They most often do constitute a risk for BE and these patients require antibiotic prophylaxis.

One common problem a dentist faces is treating a patient who reports a history of a heart murmur without any contributing history to explain its presence or significance. Further, the murmur may have been detected years earlier and the patient does not know whether the condition still exists. Common practice once was to routinely provide antibiotic prophylaxis for these patients to be "safe rather than sorry." Today, however, this approach is inappropriate with the growing problem of antibiotic resistance and the adverse effects of antibiotics such as allergy and side effects.

Most dentists are not trained to detect and evaluate heart murmurs. Therefore they usually must rely on the physician to perform this task. The dentist may be able to identify from the patient's history two examples of innocent or functional murmurs. The first is a murmur that develops during pregnancy and disappears soon after delivery. This murmur is caused mainly by an increase in blood volume (physiologic) and is not a risk for BE (see Chapter 17). The second is a murmur detected only during early childhood but not since. This is a common innocent (physiologic) murmur that merely reflects normal changes in growth or vascular physiologic functioning. Many young children have this condition but see it disappear by adolescence. This type does not represent a pathologic murmur and is not a risk for BE; thus antibiotic prophylaxis is not indicated.

The dentist needs to consult a physician if the type or significance of a murmur cannot be determined by the patient's history. When a consultation cannot be obtained quickly enough, the dentist should consider the murmur potentially pathologic and has two choices: If the patient requires immediate treatment, antibiotic prophylaxis should be provided for dental treatment that produces significant bleeding, and then the patient should be referred to a physician for consultation. For elective procedures, treatment should be deferred and the patient referred for consultation before further treatment.

Intravenous Drug Use

The current AHA guidelines do not address the issue of BE with intravenous drug use; however, it constitutes a significant risk condition for BE. The true incidence rate for BE with intravenous drug use is difficult to determine because of the often clandestine nature of the habit and its practitioners' unpredictable use of the health care system. However, available data estimate that incidence rates of BE in intravenous drug users range from 2% to 5% per year, which is significantly higher than that for those with rheumatic heart disease or for those with a prosthetic valve.[36] *Staphylococcus aureus* is responsible for more than 50% of BE intravenous drug users. However, *S. viridans* affects 5% to 13% of patients.[1,37] This reflects the probability that the causative organisms usually originate from the skin rather than the mouth. Most cases of BE in intravenous drug users occur on normal valves and the right side of the heart; however, 20% to 40% of patients are estimated to have predisposing valvular disease, usually of the mitral or aortic valves. The microbiologic finding is similar to that in nonintravenous drug

users, although S. *aureus* is probably disproportionately involved in users.[1,36] Some valve abnormalities may be the result of previous infections of BE. In an autopsy study of intravenous drug users who had died from drug overdose, 48% were found to have signs of past or present infective endocarditis.[38]

A recent study of intravenous drug users who did not display symptoms, however, questions some previous assumptions and estimates.[39] The study compared a group of 98 intravenous drug use patients with one of 99 nonintravenous drug use patients. Both groups were found to have occult valvular pathologic conditions, with an increased prevalence in intravenous drug users of tricuspid and mitral valve thickening. However, the prevalence of valvular regurgitation was small and the affected valves were not statistically different between the two groups.

Thus from the evidence, intravenous drug use does constitute a risk factor for endocarditis. However, that risk may be less than previously thought. Patients should be questioned about the presence of a heart murmur or valvular disease. If their status is unknown, referral to a physician for evaluation is recommended. When this is not possible or practical the patient may have valvular disease and need antibiotic prophylaxis if invasive treatment is necessary. The AHA is expected to address this issue in the next update of recommendations.

Coronary Artery Bypass Graft

Patients who have had coronary artery bypass graft surgery are not at risk for BE after the first few weeks of surgery and do not require antibiotic prophylaxis.[2] If invasive dental treatment is necessary in the immediate postoperative period prophylaxis may be considered (see Chapter 5).

Cardiac Pacemakers and Implanted Defibrillators

Patients who have either a cardiac pacemaker or an implanted defibrilator are at a negligible risk for BE, and prophylaxis is not recommended[2] (see Chapter 2).

Kawasaki Disease

Kawasaki disease or syndrome is of unknown etiology of early childhood, most commonly affecting children of Japanese ethnicity. Its symptoms include a general vasculitis, fever, palmar and plantar erythema with desquamation, rash, conjunctivitis, oral erythema, dry cracked lips, strawberry tongue, and cervical lymphadenopathy. Multiple-organ systems are involved, the most serious of which is the cardiovascular system. Many patients develop myocarditis or pericarditis, and approximately 20% of patients develop severe coronary artery abnormalities including aneurysms with narrowing, tortuosity, and

thrombosis. Valvulitis and papillary muscle dysfunction also can occur, resulting in mitral regurgitation in approximately 1% of patients, which usually disappears. Treatment consists of administration of intravenous gamma-globulin and aspirin.[40] Residual valvular dysfunction is uncommon; however, if a regurgitant murmur is present, endocarditis prophylaxis is indicated.[2]

Coronary Artery Stents

Coronary artery stents are not discussed in the current AHA guidelines. Intraluminal stents placed in coronary arteries to maintain patency after balloon angioplasty are rapidly covered with endothelium, generally within 2 to 4 weeks.[41,42] If emergency invasive dental procedures are needed during the first several weeks after placement of a stent, prophylaxis can be considered. Once endothelialized, they should not constitute a risk for BE and would not appear to need antibiotic prophylaxis (see Chapter 5).

NONCORONARY VASCULAR GRAFTS

Synthetic vascular grafts are used to replace segments of major arteries such as the aorta that have developed defects such as aneurysms (Fig. 3-12). The current AHA guidelines do not make any definitive statement concerning these types of grafts except to say that they "may merit antibiotic prophylaxis for the first 6 months after implantation."[2] This may be excessively cautious because of the causative microorganisms for these infections being overwhelmingly S. *aureus*, coagulase-negative Staphylococci and S. *epidermidis*, none of which are usual oral microflora.[43,44] In addition, current techniques of encouraging endothelial cell growth to rapidly cover graft surfaces result in decreased complications of infection and thrombosis.[45] The AHA should clarify this issue in the next set of guidelines.

Vena Cava Filters

Vena cava filters are devices implanted in the inferior vena cava in patients with deep vein thrombosis of the lower extremities. Their purpose is to interrupt and filter venous blood flow from the lower extremities to prevent venous clots that have embolized from reaching the pulmonary circulation. The treatment of choice for patients with deep vein thrombosis is anticoagulation using heparin and warfarin sodium. However, the vena cava filter is an alternative form of treatment used when anticoagulant-induced bleeding or hemorrhagic complications or failure of anticoagulant therapy exists.[46] The AHA's published statement for health care professionals on the management of deep vein thrombosis and pulmonary embolism is a discussion of the vena cava filter

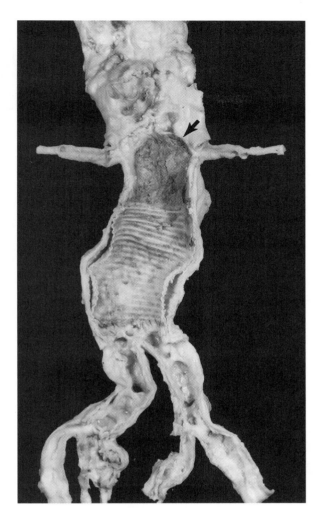

Fig. 3-12 Dacron arterial graft sutured in place (*arrow* points to edge of graft). (Courtesy Jesse E. Edwards, St. Paul, Minn.)

including complications and does not mention infections of these devices.[47] Other sources summarizing the use of these filters likewise do not mention infections as a complication.[46,48] Therefore antibiotic prophylaxis is not indicated for patients with a vena cava filter. The dentist should, however, be aware that a patient with one of these devices may be on chronic anticoagulant therapy.

Exposure to Fenfluramine or Dexfenfluramine

In 1997 an association between heart disease and the appetite-suppressant drugs fenfluramine and dexfenfluramine was reported. As many as 32% of individuals exposed to these drugs developed valvular disease.[49] This resulted in the U.S. Food and Drug Administration's removing these drugs from the market. Subsequent reports have confirmed this association but with varying degrees of incidence.[50] This variation may be related to dose and length of time of exposure. The lower the dose and the shorter the time of exposure, the less likely valvular disease will be present.

In 1998 a joint task force of the American College of Cardiology and the AHA recommended that all patients who had been exposed to these drugs should be seen by a physician for a careful history and thorough cardiovascular examination.[51] The task force recommended that a patient found not to have evidence of valvular disease be reevaluated in 6 to 8 months because of the possibility of later development.

Based on the foregoing, dental patients should be asked about exposure to either fenfluramine or dexfenfluramine. Those who have had an exposure should be referred to a physician for a thorough cardiovascular evaluation. If valvular disease is present, these patients should be considered at risk for endocarditis and antibiotic prophylaxis should be provided according to the 1997 American Heart Association guidelines. If valve disease is not present, antibiotic prophylaxis is not indicated.

References

1. Levison ME: Infective Endocarditis. In Goldman L, Bennett JC, editors: *Cecil's textbook of medicine*, vol 2, Philadelphia, 2000, WB Saunders.
2. Dajani AS et al: Prevention of bacterial endocarditis: recommendations by the American Heart Association, *Clin Infect Dis* 25:1448-58, 1997.
3. Hammermeister KE et al: A comparison of outcomes in men 11 years after heart valve replacement with a mechanical valve or bioprosthesis, *N Engl J Med* 328:1289-1301, 1993.
4. Grunkemeier GL, Starr A, Rahimtoola SH: Clinical performance of prosthetic heart valves. In Alexander RW, et al, editors: *Hurst's the heart, arteries and veins*, vol 2. New York, 1998, McGraw-Hill.
5. Durack DT: Infective endocarditis. In Alexander RW et al, editors: *Hurst's the heart, arteries and veins*, vol 2, New York, 1998, McGraw-Hill.
6. Lu V, et al: Prosthetic valve endocarditis: Superiority of surgical valve replacement versus medical therapy only, *Ann Thorac Surg* 58:1073-1077, 1994.
7. Ivert TS, Dismukes WE, Cobbs CG, et al: Prosthetic valve endocarditis, *Circulation* 69:223-32, 1984.
8. Freed MD, Plauth WH: The pathology, pathophysiology, recognition, and treatment of congenital heart disease. In Alexander RW, et al, editors: *Hurst's the heart, arteries and veins*, vol 2, New York, 1998, McGraw-Hill.

9. Marelli AJ: Congenital heart disease in adults. In Goldman L, Bennett JC editors: *Cecil's Textbook of Medicine*, vol 1, Philadelphia, 2000, WB Saunders.

10. Freed MD: Infective endocarditis in the adult with congenital heart disease, *Cardiol Clin* 11:589-602, 1993.

11. Engle MA, Kline SA, Borer JS: Ventricular septal defect. In Roberts WC, editor: *Adult congenital heart disease*, Philadelphia, 1987, Davis.

12. Alpert BS, et al: Spontaneous closure of small ventricular defects: ten-year follow-up, *Pediatrics* 63:204-206, 1979.

13. Gersony WM, Hayes CJ: Bacterial endocarditis in patients with pulmonary stenosis, aortic stenosis or ventricular septal defect, *Circulation* 56:184-187, 1977.

14. Edwards JE: Classification of congenital heart disease in the adult. In Roberts WC, editor: *Congenital heart disease in adults: cardiovascular clinical series*, Philadelphia, 1979, Davis.

15. Hamilton WT, et al: Atrial septal defect secundum: clinical profile with physiologic correlates. In Roberts WC editor: *Adult congenital heart disease*, Philadelphia, 1987, Davis.

16. Campbell M: Natural history of coarctation of the aorta, *Brit Heart J* 32:633-640, 1970.

17. Braverman AC: Bicuspid aortic valve and assorted aortic wall abnormalities, *Curr Opin Cardiol* 11:501-503, 1996.

18. Land MA, Bisno AL: Acute rheumatic fever: a vanishing disease, *JAMA* 249:895-898, 1983.

19. Odio A: The incidence of acute rheumatic fever in a suburban area of Los Angeles: a ten-year study, *West J Med* 144:179-184, 1986.

20. Kaplan EL: Acute rheumatic fever. In Alexander RW, editor: *Hurst's the heart, arteries and veins*, vol 2, New York, 1998, McGraw-Hill.

21. Special Writing Group of the Committee on Rheumatic Fever: Guidelines for the diagnosis of rheumatic fever: Jones criteria, *JAMA* 268:2069-2073, 1992.

22. Bisno AL: Rheumatic fever. In Goldman L, Bennett JC, editors: *Cecil's textbook of medicine*, vol 2, ed 21, Philadelphia, 2000, WB Saunders.

23. Thompkins DG, Boxerbaum B, Liebman J: Long term prognosis of rheumatic fever patients with regular intramuscular benzathine penicillin, *Circulation* 45:543-551, 1972.

24. Schlant RC, Gonzalez EB, Roberts WC: The connective tissue diseases. In Alexander RW et al, editors: *Hurst's the heart, arteries and veins*, vol 2, New York, 1998, McGraw-Hill.

25. Roldan CA, Shively BK, Crawford MH: An electrocardiographic study of valvular heart disease associated with systemic lupus erythematosis, *N Engl J Med* 335:1424-1430, 1996.

26. Miller CS, et al: Prevalence of infective endocarditis in patients with systemic lupus erythematosis, *J Am Den Assoc* 130:387-392, 1999.

27. Julkunen H: Rheumatoid spondylitis-clinical and laboratory study of 149 cases compared with 182 cases of rheumatoid arthritis, *Acta Rheumatoliga Scandinavia* 172:1-116, 1962.

28. Bulkley BH, Roberts WC: Ankylosing spondylitis and aortic regurgitation: description of the characteristic cardiovascular lesion from study of eight necropsy patients, *Circulation* 48:1014-1027, 1973.

29. Roberts WC, Dangel JC, Bulkley BH: Non-rheumatic valvular cardiac disease: a clinicopathologic survey of 27 different conditions causing valvular dysfunction, *Cardiovasc Clin* 5:333-446, 1973.

30. Wayne J, Braunwald E: The cardiomyopathies and myocarditides. In Fauci AS et al, editors: *Harrison's principles of internal medicine*, vol 1, ed 14, New York, 1998, McGraw-Hill.

31. Maron BJ: Hypertrophic cardiomyopathy. In Alexander RW et al, editors: *Hurst's the heart, arteries and veins*, vol 2, ed 9, New York, 1998, McGraw-Hill.

32. Spirito P et al: Infective endocarditis in hypertrophic cardiomyopathy: prevalence, incidence, and indications for antibiotic prophylaxis, *Circulation* 99:2132-2137, 1999.

33. O'Rourke RA: Mitral valve prolapse. In Alexander RW et al, editors: *Hurst's the heart, arteries and veins*, vol 2, ed 9, New York, 1998, McGraw-Hill.

34. Braunwald E: Valvular heart disease. In Fauci AS et al, editors: *Harrison's principles of internal medicine*, vol 1, ed 14, New York, 1998, McGraw-Hill.

35. Devereux RB et al: Cost effectiveness of infective endocarditis prophylaxis for mitral valve prolapse with and without a mitral regurgitant murmur, *Am J Cardiol* 74:1024-1029, 1994.

36. Sande MA et al: Endocarditis in intravenous drug users. In Kaye D et al, editors: *Infective endocarditis*, ed 2, New York, 1992, Raven Press.

37. Weinstein L, Brusch JL: *Infective endocarditis*, Oxford, 1996, Oxford University Press.

38. Dressler FA, Roberts WG: Mode of death and type of cardiac disease in opiate addicts: analysis of 169 necropsy cases, *Am J Cardiol* 64:909-920, 1989.

39. Levitt MA, Snoey ER, Tamkin GW: Prevalence of cardiac valve abnormalities in afebrile injection drug users, *Academic Emergency Medicine* 6:911-915, 1911.

40. Fukusahige J, Nihill NR: Kawasaki disease. In Garson A Jr et al, editors: *The science and practice of pediatric cardiology*, vol 2, ed 2, Baltimore, 1998, Williams and Wilkins.

41. Sigwart U et al: Intravascular stents to prevent occlusion and restenosis after transluminal angioplasty, *N Engl J Med* 316:701-706, 1987.

42. Rogers GP: The coronary artery response to implantation of a balloon-expandable flexible stent in the aspirin and non-aspirin treated swine model, *Am Heart J* 122:640-647, 1911.

43. Bandyk DF et al: In situ replacement of vascular prosthesis infected by bacterial biofilms, *J Vasc Surg* 13:575-583, 1991.

44. Vinard E et al: Human vascular graft failure and frequency of infection, *J Biomed Mater Res* 25:499-513, 1991.

45. Deutsch M et al: Cinical autologous in vitro endothelialization of infrainguinal ePTFE grafts in 100 patients: a 9-year experience. *Surgery* 126:847-855, 1999.

46. Dodson TF, Smith RB: Surgical treatment of peripheral vascular disease. In Fuster V et al, editors: *Hurst's the heart, arteries and veins*, vol 2, ed 10, New York, 2001, McGraw-Hill.

47. Hirsh J, Hoak J: Management of deep vein thrombosis and pulmonary embolism: a statement for healthcare professionals, *Circulation* 93:2212-2245, 1996.

48. Greenfield LJ, Proctor MC: Twenty-year clinical experience with the Greenfield filter, *Cardiovasc Surg* 3:199-205, 1995.

49. Prevention Centers for Disease Control: Cardiac valvulopathy associated with exposure to fenfluramine of dexfenfluramine: US Department of Health and Human Services: interim public health recommendation, MMW *Morb Mortal Wkly Rep* 46:1061-1066, 1997.

50. Pallasch TJ: Current status of fenfluramine/dexfenfluramine-induced cardiac valvulopathy, J *Calif Dent Assoc* 27:400-404, 1999.

51. Bonow RO et al: Guidelines for the management of patients with valvular heart disease, Executive summary: a report of the American College of Cardiology/American Heart Association Task Force on practice guidelines, committee on management of patients with valvular heart disease, *Circulation* 98:1949-1984, 1998.

Hypertension

CHAPTER 4

*H*ypertension is an abnormal elevation of arterial pressure that can be fatal if sustained and untreated. People with hypertension may not display its symptoms for a long time but could experience damage with resultant symptoms in several target organs, including kidneys, heart, brain, and eyes. In adults a sustained diastolic blood pressure of 90 mm Hg or greater and a sustained systolic blood pressure of 140 mm Hg or greater are abnormal.[1] (Table 4-1). The Sixth Report (1997) of the Joint National Committee on Prevention, Detection, Evaluation, and Treatment of High Blood Pressure revised previous guidelines for blood pressure detection and treatment strategies.[1] These guidelines are intended to assist dentists and other health care providers to better identify and manage patients with high blood pressure. The new guidelines include an updated classification and rationale for treatment and use of antihypertensive medications. Diagnostic and treatment decisions had been based primarily on diastolic pressures. However, recent data underscore the importance of systolic and diastolic pressures in addition to medical and lifestyle risk factors in decisions about diagnosis and therapy.[1] The diagnosis of hypertension is rather straightforward, but the decision of when to initiate drug therapy frequently is unclear, especially in patients with stage 1 or 2 hypertension. Treatment decisions are made individually and consider factors such as the absolute value of the blood pressure, physical and laboratory findings, family history, race, diet, lifestyle, age, and patient reliability. Generally, healthy people maintain blood pressure readings close to the normal range.

The dentist can play a significant role in the detection of hypertension and the monitoring of its effective control. The dentist may be the first to detect in a patient an elevation of blood pressure or symptoms of hypertensive disease. Patients aware of their conditions and receiving treatment often may not be controlled adequately because of poor compliance or inappropriate selection of drug therapy. The dentist can provide a valuable monitoring service for those patients. The Joint National Committee on Detection, Evaluation, and Treatment of High Blood Pressure[1] specifically encourages the active participation of health care professionals in the detection of hypertension and the surveillance of treatment compliance. Only the physician diagnoses hypertension and makes decisions on its treatment. The dentist, however, must make determinations of abnormal readings, which then become the basis for physician referral.

The dental patient with hypertension poses some significant management considerations. These include identification, monitoring, stress and anxiety reduction, prevention of drug interactions, awareness and management of drug side effects such as orthostatic hypotension, and management of drug effects on the oral tissues.

GENERAL DESCRIPTION

INCIDENCE AND PREVALENCE

Researchers estimate that more than 58 million people in the United States have high blood pressure (HBP) or are taking antihypertensive medication.[1,2] This translates to 15% to 20% of the Caucasian population and 20% to 25% of the African American population of the United States.[1] This was a 16% decrease over a 10-year period.[3] The National High Blood Pressure Education Program began in 1972, and in a little more than two decades the number of people with HBP aware of their condition has increased from 51% to 73%. The percentage of those taking medication for HBP has increased from 36% to 49%. Concomitant with the increased awareness and treat-

TABLE **4-1**

Classification of Blood Pressure for Adults*

Category	Systolic (mm Hg)		Diastolic (mm Hg)
Optimal†	<120	and	<80
Normal	<130	and	<85
High normal	130-139	or	85-89
Hypertension‡			
Stage 1	140-159	or	90-99
Stage 2	160-179	or	100-109
Stage 3	>180	or	>110

Sixth Report of the Joint National Committee on Detection, Evaluation, and Treatment of High Blood Pressure, *Arch Int Med* 157:154-183, 1997.
*Applies to adults who are not taking antihypertensive medication and who are not acutely ill. When the systolic blood pressure and diastolic blood pressure fall into different categories, the higher value should be used.
†Optimum blood pressure with respect to risk of cardiovascular complications <120/80. However, unusually low blood pressure measurements should be evaluated for clinical significance.
‡Based on an average of two or more blood pressure measurements taken at each of two or more visits.

BOX **4-1**

Cardiovascular Risk Groups

Risk Group A
No risk factors, no target organ damage or clinical cardiovascular disease

Risk Group B
At least one risk factor, not including diabetes; no target organ damage or clinical cardiovascular disease

Risk Group C
Target organ damage, diabetes, clinical cardiovascular disease, presence or absence of other risk factors

ment has been a significant decline in mortality from coronary heart disease (50%) and stroke (57%).*

One third of people with HBP, however, are not aware of it and more than half of those with HBP do not take medication appropriately.[2,4] A clear relationship exists between HBP at any level and an increase in morbidity and mortality rates from stroke and coronary heart disease.[5] Dentistry can play a significant role in the detection of patients with HBP and monitoring of control efforts. Therefore dentists should be concerned with three groups of patients with hypertension: those who are undiagnosed, those who are noncompliant, and those being medically treated.[2]

Important steps in the overall management of HBP are the patient's awareness, willingness to adhere to treatment recommendations, and compliance with treatment. Unfortunately, recent evidence indicates increases in target organ damage (i.e., end-stage renal disease and congestive heart failure, both serious complications from long-term hypertension).[4]

The prevalence for hypertension increases with age, is greater in men and blacks, and in both blacks and whites

is greater in the less educated.[1] The prevalence in blacks and whites is higher in the southeastern United States than in other parts of the country.[6] In a 1999 study by Hennessy et al,[7] 12.05% of all active-duty military personnel over age 40 at Fort Hood, Texas, were taking antihypertensive medications compared with only 0.24% under age 30 who were taking antihypertensive medications, a fiftyfold difference in a similar population with age as the primary variable.

ETIOLOGY

Age, ethnicity (African American) and gender (male) are all risk factors for hypertension. With other risk factors such as hypercholesterolemia, cigarette smoking, abnormal glucose tolerance, and left ventricular hypertrophy, hypertension becomes a major determinant for cardiovascular complications. Hypertension in approximately 5% of individuals can be explained by the existence of an underlying, associated condition. This form of hypertension is called *secondary hypertension*. The most common cause of secondary hypertension in women is use of oral contraceptives. The majority of conditions that cause secondary hypertension, such as renal disease, endocrine disorders, and neurogenic problems, lead to an elevation of both diastolic and systolic blood pressure. The other 95% of individuals with hypertension have what is termed *essential hypertension*, the exact cause of which is undetermined.[1]

Lifestyle also can play a role in the severity and progression of hypertension, with excess body fat, excessive alcohol, excessive dietary sodium, and physical inactivity being significant contributing factors.[8] Cardiovascular risk assessment of the patient, which relates to the relative risk of complications from hypertension (Box 4-1) is

---

considered an important strategy in the medical and dental management of hypertension.[9,10]

Patients who have secondary hypertension resulting from unilateral renal disease such as renal artery obstruction or pyelonephritis can be cured of the hypertension by surgical correction of the defect or removal of the diseased kidney. In a few patients with secondary hypertension, a pheochromocytoma tumor of the adrenal medulla has been found responsible. This lesion is surgically treatable. Hyperfunction of the adrenal gland caused by a tumor of the adrenal cortex or cortical hyperplasia may cause secondary hypertension in a few cases. These conditions also are amenable to surgery. Weight gain has been demonstrated to cause an increase in blood pressure.[11]

PATHOPHYSIOLOGY AND COMPLICATIONS

Blood pressure is measured by the use of a sphygmomanometer (Fig. 4-1). The diastolic pressure represents the total resting resistance in the arterial system after passage of the pulsating force produced by contraction of the left ventricle. The pulsating force is modified by the degree of elasticity of the walls of larger arteries and the resistance of the arteriolar bed. The pressure at the peak of ventricular contraction is the systolic blood pressure. The difference between the diastolic and systolic pressures is termed *pulse pressure.*

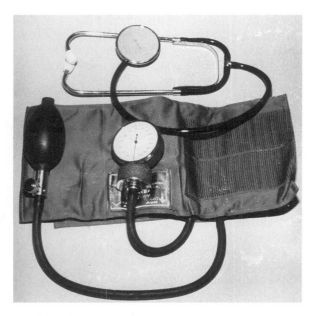

FIG. 4-1 Standard sphygmomanometer and stethoscope.

Many factors may have a transient effect on blood pressure. Increased viscosity of the blood can cause an elevation of blood pressure as a result of an increase in the resistance to flow. A decrease in blood volume or tissue fluid volume reduces blood pressure. Conversely, an increase in blood volume or tissue fluid volume increases blood pressure. Increased cardiac output associated with exercise, fever, and thyrotoxicosis increases blood pressure. In sustained hypertension, however, the basic underlying defect is a failure in the regulation of vascular resistance. Control of vascular resistance is multifactorial, and abnormalities may exist in one or more areas. Mechanisms of control include neural reflexes and ongoing maintenance of sympathetic vasomotor tone; neurotransmitters such as norepinephrine, extracellular fluid, and sodium stores; the renin-angiotensin-aldosterone pressor system; and locally active hormones and substances such as prostaglandins, kinins, adenosine, and hydrogen ions (H^t). In the isolated systolic hypertension commonly seen in the elderly the underlying defect is loss of elasticity of the aorta.[9,12]

Blood pressure increases normally with age from under 110/75 mm Hg in children less than 6 years of age to 140/90 mm Hg in adults (see Table 4-1 and Box 4-1). A sustained blood pressure in excess of 140/90 mm Hg in adults is considered abnormal. In about one third of the population, a transient period of increased blood pressure may occur in early adulthood. On an individual basis such increases may be of little significance, but data based on large numbers of people indicate that occasional rises in the resting blood pressure are associated with shortened life span. Researchers have estimated that untreated hypertension reduces life span by 10 to 20 years. Even mild hypertension that has not been treated for 7 to 10 years increases the risks of complications such as stroke and heart attack.[3,9,10,13]

Both the diagnosis and treatment of hypertension once were based largely on elevation of diastolic blood pressure. Recently, however, the significance of systolic hypertension has been recognized. Patients with systolic hypertension may be at greater risk for serious cardiovascular events than are patients with elevated diastolic pressure. A few systemic conditions result only in an increase of the systolic blood pressure, including aortic regurgitation, thyrotoxicosis, arteriovenous fistula, and patent ductus arteriosus.[10]

Hypertension precedes the onset of vascular changes in the kidney, heart, brain, and retina that then lead to such clinical complications as renal failure, cerebrovascular accident, coronary insufficiency, myocardial infarction, congestive heart failure, and blindness. Approximately 1% of patients with hypertension develop malignant hyperten-

sion, a medical emergency characterized by severe blood pressure elevation, papilledema, retinal hemorrhages, exudates, and frequently encephalopathy. This condition requires immediate medical treatment.[7]

CLINICAL PRESENTATION

SIGNS AND SYMPTOMS

Most cases of essential hypertension are chronic. Elevated blood pressure measurements may be the only sign present for a number of years. Patients with intermittently elevated blood pressures are said to have *labile hypertension*. Isolated diastolic hypertension is rare and found in children or young adults. Isolated systolic hypertension generally is found in older patients.[12,14] The early symptoms of hypertension are occipital headache, vision changes, ringing ears, dizziness, and weakness and tingling of the hands and feet.[10,11] Other signs and symptoms related to these organ systems appear if significant kidney, brain, heart, or eye involvement develops (Box 4-2).

Funduscopic examination of the eyes may show early changes of hypertension consisting of hemorrhages, narrowed arterioles, exudate, and papilledema in more advanced cases. Also, in more advanced cases the left ventricle may be enlarged and a tapping left ventricular apical beat often can be observed in thin individuals. Renal involvement can result in hematuria, proteinuria, and renal failure. Persons with hypertension may complain of fatigue and coldness of the legs as a result of peripheral artery changes that occur in advanced hypertension.[10,11]

These findings may be seen for patients with essential or secondary hypertension. However, additional signs or symptoms may be present in secondary hypertension that are associated with the underlying disease.

LABORATORY FINDINGS

The Sixth Report of the Joint National Committee on Detection, Evaluation, and Treatment of High Blood Pressure[1] recommends that patients who have sustained hypertension be screened using urinalysis, a complete blood count, and potassium, calcium, creatinine, cholesterol, triglyceride, fasting glucose, and uric acid measurements. Performing an electrocardiogram also is suggested. These tests serve as baseline laboratory values that the physician should obtain before initiating therapy. Additional tests should be ordered if clinical and laboratory findings suggest the presence of an underlying cause for the hypertension.

MEDICAL MANAGEMENT

The management of a patient with hypertension necessarily begins with detection. Because hypertension is generally asymptomatic for many years, the only sign of trouble may be an elevated blood pressure. The Joint National Committee on Detection, Evaluation, and Treatment of High Blood Pressure recommends that efforts be directed toward maintenance and surveillance in persons with hypertension and in high-risk groups (i.e., blacks, obese individuals, and blood relatives of those with hypertension). Standard measurement of blood pressure should be accomplished with a relaxed patient (see Chapter 1). The dentist should not make a diagnosis of hypertension but should tell the patient who has elevated blood pressure that its numeric value is abnormal and that a physician should evaluate the condition.

The physician compiles a medical history about the patient, including family history, identification of risk factors, a list of associated disorders, and history of known hypertension and its treatment. A thorough physical examination by a physician emphasizes the identification of the causes of secondary hypertension and the discovering of evidence of target organ changes caused

---

BOX 4-2

Signs and Symptoms of Hypertensive Disease

Signs
Early
Increase blood pressure readings
Narrowing of retinal arterioles
Retinal hemorrhages

Advanced
Papilledema
Cardiac enlargement of the left ventricle
Hematuria
Proteinuria
Congestive heart failure
Angina pectoris
Renal failure

Symptoms
Occipital headache
Failing vision
Ringing ears
Dizziness
Weakness
Tingling of hands and feet

by hypertension (e.g., eyes, kidneys, brain, heart). A few simple laboratory tests previously mentioned are included. Additional tests may be warranted based on clinical judgment. For example, some physicians advocate 24- to 48-hour monitoring of blood pressure for definitive diagnosis.

Physicians often are uncertain when to initiate pharmacologic treatment of hypertension. Data now unequivocally demonstrate that drug treatment of mild to moderate hypertension is effective in preventing cardiovascular complications. Adequate therapy also may reverse cardiac and retinal changes. Effective drugs with minimal side effects are available to treat hypertension.[1,13,14]

Factors exist that complicate drug treatment of patients with essential hypertension. Drugs are expensive, some medications have significant side effects, and therapy is difficult when severe renal damage is present and may be dangerous if significant cerebral or coronary artery disease exists.[1,13,14]

The decision to begin treatment is made by the physician and patient based on the absolute blood pressure value and the presence of risk factors and physical complications, which includes target organ damage (Box 4-1 and Table 4-2). Nonpharmacologic measures generally are begun first that may be definitive or used in addition to drug therapy. The goal of antihypertensive therapy is to achieve and maintain the diastolic blood pressure lower than 90 mm Hg and the systolic pressure below 140 mm Hg.

Nonpharmacologic measures include weight loss for obese patients, restriction of dietary sodium, moderation of alcohol intake, reduction of dietary saturated fats and cholesterol, avoidance of smoking, participation in regular aerobic exercise, and initiation of relaxation therapy and stress reduction.[1] These measures alone may prove effective in the control of high normal and mild hypertension for long periods. However, moderate and severe hypertension almost always requires additional drug therapy to effectively decrease the blood pressure. Isolated systolic hypertension is seen in middle-aged and older patients and usually is caused by atherosclerosis of the aorta and its major branches. Recent data suggest definite benefit to the pharmacologic treatment of this entity.[7,15,16] Although some controversy exists regarding initiation of the pharmacologic treatment for high blood pressure between 90 and 94 mm Hg, the benefits of drug therapy clearly outweigh the risks.[14,15]

The amount of drugs prescribed in the United States for hypertension rank second only to those prescribed for respiratory disease. Drug therapy initiated to control hypertension usually is chosen and administered according to a stepped-care approach as suggested by the Joint National Committee on Detection, Evaluation, and Treatment of High Blood Pressure.[1] This stepped-care approach begins by initiating therapy with a small dose of an antihypertensive drug, increasing the dosage of that drug, then adding or substituting one drug after another in gradually increasing doses as needed until the blood pressure goal is reached, side effects become intolerable, or the maximum dose of each drug is reached. Once drug therapy becomes necessary, it usually is continued for the rest of the patient's life (see Table 4-2).

The Sixth Report of the Joint National Committee on Detection, Evaluation, and Treatment of High Blood Pressure recommends individualized drug therapy for the patient depending on associated medical conditions and risk factors (Table 4-3):[1]

Step 1. Initial therapy is begun with a diuretic or beta blocker. Angiotensin-converting enzyme inhibitors, calcium antagonists, alpha-receptor blockers, and alpha-beta blockers also are effective and acceptable

---

TABLE **4-2**

Medical Management of Hypertension Based on Cardiovascular Risk Groups

	Risk Group A	Risk Group B	Risk Group C
High Normal (130-139/85-89)	Lifestyle modification	Lifestyle modification	Lifestyle modification and drug therapy
Stage 1 Hypertension (140-159/90-99)	Lifestyle modification up to 12-month trial	Lifestyle modification up to 6-month trial	Lifestyle modification and drug therapy
Stages 2 and 3 Hypertension (>160/>100)	Lifestyle modification and drug therapy	Lifestyle modification and drug therapy	Lifestyle modification and drug therapy

Sixth Report of the Joint National Committee on Detection, Evaluation, and Treatment of High Blood Pressure, *Arch Int Med* 157:154-183, 1997.

TABLE 4-3

Antihypertensive Drugs and Dental Management Considerations

Class	Mode of Action	Vasoconstrictor Interaction	Oral Manifestations	Other Considerations
Diuretics				
Thiazides	Reduce plasma volume and extracellular fluid by increasing excretion of sodium	None	Dry mouth Lichenoid reactions	Orthostatic hypotension Prolonged use of nonsteroidal antiinflammatory drugs (NSAIDs) possibly reducing antihypertensive effects
Hydrochlorthiazide (HCTZ, Esidrix)				
Chlorothiazide (Diuril)				
Loop				
Furosemide (Lasix)				
Potassium-sparing				
Spironolactone (Aldactone)				
Triamterene (Dyrenium)				
Combination				
Aldactazide, Dyazide				
Beta-Adrenergic Blockers				
Nonselective	Block beta-adrenergic receptor sites and probably have direct effects on the myocardium	Nonselective— Potential (use maximum of 0.036 mg epinephrine or 0.20 mg levonordefrin) Cardioselective —Normal use	Altered taste Lichenoid reactions	Orthostatic hypotension Prolonged use of NSAIDs possibly reducing antihypertensive effects Possible increase in serum levels of lidocaine (reduced hepatic clearance)
Propanolol (Inderal)				
Timolol (Blocadren)				
Nadolol (Corgard)				
Pindolol (Visken)				
Penbutolol (Levatol)				
Carteolol (Cartrol)				
Cardioselective				
Metoprolol (Lopressor)				
Acebutolol (Sectral)				
Atenolol (Tenormin)				
Betaxolol (Kerlone)				
Bisoprolol (Zebeta)				
Direct Vasodilators				
Hydralazine (Apresoline)	Cause direct dilation of arteries (mechanism unclear)	Possible decrease in effectiveness of epinephrine and levonordefrin	Lupuslike oral and skin lesions Lymphadenopathy	Prolonged use of NSAIDs possibly reducing antihypertensive effects Orthostatic hypotension
Minoxidil (Loniten)				

Continued

TABLE 4-3

Antihypertensive Drugs and Dental Management Considerations—cont'd

Class	Mode of Action	Vasoconstrictor Interaction	Oral Manifestations	Other Considerations
Angiotensin-Converting Enzyme (ACE) Inhibitors				
Benazepril (Lotensin) Captopril (Capoten) Enalapril (Vasotec) Fosinopril (Monopril) Lisinopril (Prinivil; Zestril) Quinapril (Accupril) Ramipril (Altace)	Block conversion of angiotensin I to angiotensin II	None	Cough Angioedema of lips, face, tongue Loss of taste	Prolonged use of NSAIDs possibly reducing antihypertensive effects Neutropenia, thrombocytopenia
Calcium Channel Blockers				
Diltiazem (Cardizem) Verapamil (Calan) Amlodipine (Norvasc) Felodipine (Plendil) Isradipine (DynaCirc) Nicardipine (Cardene) Nifedipine (Procardia)	Inhibit calcium-ion influx into cardiac and vascular smooth muscle cells	None	Gingival hyperplasia Dry mouth	

as alternate choices if diuretics and beta blockers have proved unacceptable or ineffective. Angiotensin-converting enzyme inhibitors may be used as a first-line drug for patients with hypertension who also have diabetes with proteinuria, congestive heart failure, or postmyocardial infarction. Beta-blockers also may be used for patients with postmyocardial infarction. Diuretics may be used with patients who have congestive heart failure. The new angiotensin II antagonists also have been shown to be effective.[15]

Step 2. If control has not been achieved after 1 to 3 months, one of three options is recommended: (1) increasing dosage of first drug, (2) adding an agent from a different class, or (3) substituting a drug from another class.

Step 3. If control has not been achieved, a second or third drug or diuretic is added if not already prescribed. Supplemental antihypertensives include vasodilators, alpha2 agonists, and peripherally acting adrenergic neuron antagonists.

Because lack of compliance is a major problem in the treatment of patients with hypertension, periodic monitoring of patients is important. Health care professionals are encouraged to measure the blood pressure at each patient visit.

DENTAL MANAGEMENT

MEDICAL CONSIDERATIONS

The stress and anxiety associated with dental procedures may raise a patient's already elevated blood pressure to dangerous levels and result in a cerebrovascular accident or myocardial infarction. In addition, the dentist may use an excessive amount of local anesthetic containing a vasoconstrictor, which can result in a significant rise in blood pressure. The dentist also may use a concentrated vasoconstrictor to control gingival bleeding or to retract gingival tissues in preparation for taking impressions. This can result in a significant elevation of the blood pressure that could be life threatening in an undetected or uncontrolled patient with hypertension.

The first task of the dentist is to identify through history and measurement of blood pressure those patients who

Detection of Hypertension

History
Past diagnosis of hypertension
Signs and symptoms
Medications
   Physicians' Desk Reference
   Drug Information for the Health Care Professional
   Physician, pharmacist
Blood pressure measurement
   Baseline for emergency management
   Screen for hypertensive disease
   Medicolegal necessity

may have elevated blood pressure (Box 4-3). A complete medical history should be obtained from each patient (see Chapter 1). Included in the history are questions concerning the presence of signs or symptoms associated with hypertension and its sequelae. The duration and level of the high blood pressure and history of treatment for it must be determined. Many patients known to have hypertension may be receiving medical treatment for complications of hypertensive disease, such as congestive heart failure, cerebrovascular disease, myocardial infarction, renal disease, peripheral vascular disease, and diabetes mellitus. These problems must be identified because they may necessitate modification of the dental management plan.[18]

Another important way to assist in the determination of hypertensive disease and risk is through the use of a family history. A family history of congestive heart failure, cerebrovacular disease, myocardial infarction, renal disease, peripheral vascular disease, and diabetes mellitus, should be elicited and contributes to the overall status of the patient.

Patients should be asked whether they are or should be taking any medications and the duration and history of the treatment. If the patient does not know the name of the drug, a pictorial section of a pharmaceutical reference such as the *Physicians' Desk Reference* can be used to identify the drug, or the pharmacist may be consulted. The dentist should identify patients being treated with antihypertensive medications. Many of these drugs have significant side effects, and some may interact with vasoconstrictors or have oral manifestations (see Tables 4-2 and 4-3).

At least two or three blood pressure recordings separated by several minutes should be taken on all patients with an elevated blood pressure during the first dental appointment and the results averaged. The first measurement should not be taken immediately after the patient enters the office but after the patient has had time to become accustomed to the surroundings to avoid erroneous results. This average figure represents the blood pressure for that appointment. The blood pressure is recorded for three reasons. First, it serves as a baseline from which to make decisions for the emergency management of the patient should an untoward reaction occur during dental treatment. Second, it is used to screen patients (along with a medical history) to identify those who have or may have hypertension and to monitor compliance. Finally, it is a medicolegal necessity.

Once a patient has been referred to a physician for evaluation, diagnosis, and treatment, the dentist should determine the current medications, lifestyle modifications, and level of control. Blood pressure should be remeasured periodically and control confirmed. If the blood pressure has not returned to an acceptable level, the physician should be contacted.

Once an initial evaluation has been made, several dental management recommendations should be considered (Table 4-4). The dentist should attempt to develop an approach to the management of all patients that will reduce the stress and anxiety associated with dental treatment as much as possible. This is of particular importance in dealing with the patient with hypertension. A critical factor in providing an anxiety-free situation is the relationship established among the dentist, office staff, and patient. Patients should be encouraged to express and discuss their fears, concerns, and questions about dental treatment.

Anxiety can be reduced for many patients by premedication with a short-acting benzodiazepine such as triazolam (Halcion), oxazepam (Serax), or diazepam (Valium). An effective approach is to prescribe a dose at bedtime the night before and another dose 1 hour before the dental appointment. The dose is dictated by the age and size of the patient and prescribing guidelines for the agent selected. Nitrous oxide plus oxygen inhalation sedation is an excellent intraoperative anxiolytic for use in patients with hypertension. Care should be used to ensure adequate oxygenation at all times and especially at the termination of nitrous oxide administration. Hypoxia is to be avoided because of the resultant elevation of blood pressure that can occur.

Long or stressful appointments are best avoided. If the patient becomes anxious or apprehensive during the appointment, it should be terminated and scheduled for another day (Box 4-4).

Because many antihypertensive agents tend to produce orthostatic hypotension, sudden changes in chair

TABLE **4-4**

Dental Management of Hypertension: Follow-up and Treatment Recommendations*

Blood Pressure Category	Medical Referral	Dental Treatment
Optimal† <120/<80	Check in 2 years	All procedures
Normal <130/<85	Check in 2 years	All procedures
High Normal 130-139/85-89	Check in 1 year	All procedures OK
Hypertension‡ Stage 1: 140-159/90-99	Check in 2 months (next dental visit)	Most procedures
Stage 2: 160-169/100-109	Check in 1 month (next dental visit)	Some limitations
Stage 3: >180/>110	Refer immediately	No treatment

Sixth Report of the Joint National Committee on Detection, Evaluation, and Treatment of High Blood Pressure, *Arch Int Med* 157:154-183, 1997.

*Applies to adults who are not taking antihypertensive medication and who are not acutely ill. When the systolic blood pressure and diastolic blood pressure fall into different categories, the higher value should be used.

†Optimum blood pressure with respect to risk of cardiovascular complications is <120/80. However, unusually low blood pressure measurements should be evaluated for clinical significance.

‡Based on an average of two or more blood pressure measurements taken at each of two or more visits.

BOX **4-4**

Reduction of Stress and Anxiety

Establish honest, supportive relationship with patient
Discuss patient's questions, concerns, fears
Avoid long or stressful appointments
Use premedication as needed (benzodiazepines)
Use nitrous oxide as needed (avoid hypoxia)
Provide gradual changes of position to prevent postural hypotension
Avoid stimulating gag reflex
Dismiss patient if stress appears excessive

position during dental treatment routinely should be avoided. When the dentist has concluded treatment for that appointment, the dental chair should be returned to an upright position slowly and the patient physically supported while getting out of it until the patient has obtained good balance and stability.

Ambulatory (outpatient) general anesthesia administered in the dental office is generally recommended only for patients in the classifications by the American Society of Anesthesiologists (ASA) of ASA-I (healthy, normal patient) or ASA-II (mild systemic disease). This excludes some patients whose blood pressure is being controlled by drugs or whose blood pressure is greater than 109 mm Hg diastolic or 179 mm Hg systolic.

Vasoconstrictors and Local Anesthetic

One of the most common concerns encountered when dental treatment for patients with hypertension or other cardiovascular disorders is being planned is the use of a vasoconstrictor in the local anesthetic. Vasoconstrictors delay systemic absorption of the solution, which increases duration and depth of anesthesia and decrease the chances of toxicity, and provide local hemostasis, which enhances working conditions in the operative field. These properties allow for enhanced quality and duration of pain control and markedly facilitate the technical procedures to be performed. Without these advantages, the local anesthetic is of much shorter duration, and less effective and is absorbed more quickly, thus enhancing the possibilities of toxicity. In addition, the anesthetic solution itself often has mild vasodilatory properties that can result in increased

$\alpha_1 \Rightarrow$ 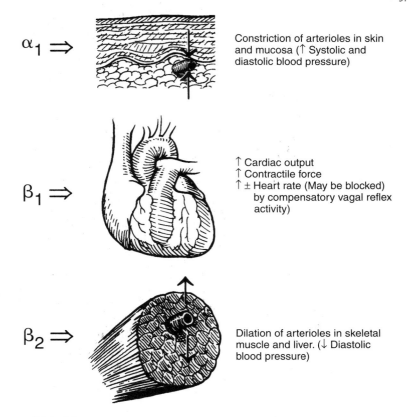 Constriction of arterioles in skin and mucosa (↑ Systolic and diastolic blood pressure)

$\beta_1 \Rightarrow$ ↑ Cardiac output
↑ Contractile force
↑ ± Heart rate (May be blocked) by compensatory vagal reflex activity)

$\beta_2 \Rightarrow$ Dilation of arterioles in skeletal muscle and liver. (↓ Diastolic blood pressure)

FIG. 4-2 The effect of adrenergic stimulation on the heart and blood vessels.

bleeding into the operative field. Therefore the advantages of including a vasoconstrictor in the local anesthetic are obvious.

The potential danger in administering a local anesthetic containing epinephrine or other vasoconstrictor to a patient with hypertension or other cardiovascular disease, is an untoward increase in the blood pressure or development of an arrhythmia. In most cases, the amount of epinephrine administered ranges from 0.018 mg to 0.036 mg (with 1 to 2 cartridges of 2% lidocaine containing 1:100,000 epinephrine).

To make rational decisions concerning the use of vasoconstrictors in patients who are hypertensive or otherwise medically compromised, the dentist should first understand the effect of those vasoconstrictors on adrenergic receptors. Two basic types of adrenergic receptors are alpha and beta. These are divided into two subtypes: alpha$_1$ and alpha$_2$, and beta$_1$ and beta$_2$. These receptors are found throughout the body in most tissues and organs; however, usually one type predominates. For example, alpha$_1$ receptors predominate in peripheral arterioles, alpha$_2$ and beta$_1$ receptors predominate in the heart, and beta$_2$ receptors predominate in arterioles in skeletal muscle and bronchiolar smooth muscle. Stimulation of each receptor produces different effects on various organs and tissues of the body. Of particular interest are the effects on blood vessels and the heart (Figs. 4-2 and 4-3).

Drugs that stimulate adrenergic receptors are called *sympathomimetic drugs*. Vasoconstrictors are examples of this type of drug and include epinephrine, norepinephrine, and levonordefrin. These drugs stimulate the adrenergic receptors to varying degrees and are dose dependent. Epinephrine is a potent stimulator of both alpha and beta receptors with a predominance of beta$_2$ activation. Large doses of epinephrine can cause a significant rise in blood pressure (systolic greater than diastolic) and heart rate; however, minute doses (0.1 μg/kg) may cause the pressure to fall because of the preponderance of action of the beta$_2$ receptors with a decrease in diastolic

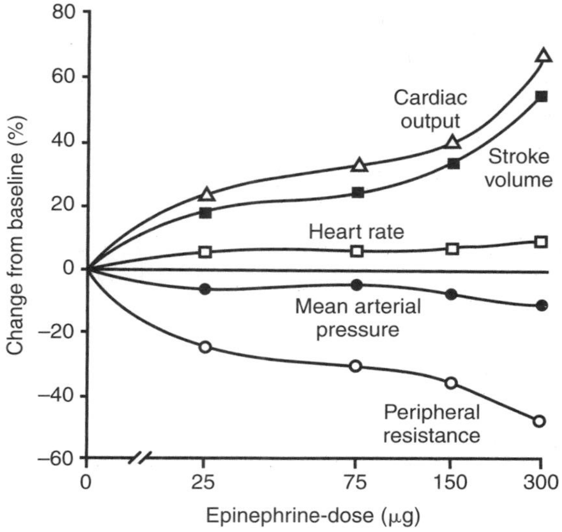

FIG. 4-3 Cardiovascular effects of epinephrine when used in regional anesthesia. (From Jastak JT, Yagiela JA, Donaldson D: *Local anesthesia of the oral cavity,* Philadelphia, 1995, WB Saunders.)

TABLE **4-5**

Actions of Epinephrine, Norepinephrine, and Levonordefrin on Adrenergic Receptors

	Activity on Alpha Receptors (%)	**Activity on Beta Receptors (%)**	**Relative Potency**
Epinephrine	50	50	1.25
Norepinephrine	90	10	0.25
Levonordefrin	75	25	0.15

Data from Malamed SF: *Handbook of local anesthesia,* ed 4, St Louis, 1997, Mosby.

pressure.[19] Norepinephrine is a potent stimulator of alpha$_1$ and beta$_1$ receptors but has little effect on beta$_2$. As a result, norepinephrine can cause a significant rise in both systolic and diastolic blood pressures. Levonordefrin is similar to norepinephrine in action but with somewhat less alpha$_1$ potency and slightly more beta$_2$ potency (Table 4-5).

Once the basic actions of adrenergic receptors are understood, definition of the normal baseline levels of endogenous epinephrine in patients and the response to injected epinephrine in patients who are healthy and compromised becomes necessary. Jastak et al[20] performed a metaanalysis on several clinical studies and determined that the normal resting venous plasma epinephrine concentration is 39 pg/ml. An earlier study investigated the threshold plasma epinephrine levels that were required to produce hemodynamic changes and found an increase in heart rate required 50 to 100 pg/ml

(1.5 to 2 times normal) and an increase in systolic blood pressure required 75 to 125 pg/ml (2 to 3 times normal).[6] In addition the mean resting secretion rate of epinephrine from the adrenal medulla of a 70-kg adult is 0.544 μg/min (0.009 μg/kg/min) with a range of 0.052 to 0.644 μg/min.[30] The amount of epinephrine in a single Carpule of 2% lidocaine with 1:100,000 epinephrine (18 μg) is about 36 times what the resting adrenal medulla secretes per minute.

Several clinical investigations have been evaluating changes in plasma epinephrine concentration and hemodynamic parameters in healthy patients after dental injections of 2% lidocaine with 1:100,000 epinephrine. After injection of 1.8 ml (one cartridge), plasma levels increased twofold to threefold but without any significant changes in heart rate or blood pressure.[4,5,21] With 5.4 ml of solution (three cartridges), however, plasma levels increased fivefold to sixfold and were accompanied by a

significant increase in both heart rate and systolic blood pressure but with no adverse symptoms or sequelae.[8,20] The critical question is how does a patient with hypertension or other cardiovascular disease react to these dose challenges of epinephrine?

This question was addressed empirically in 1955 by the New York Heart Association, which recommended that a maximum of 0.2 mg of epinephrine (11 cartridges of 1:100,000 epinephrine with procaine) be used at one session in dental patients with heart disease.[22] In 1964, a Working Conference of the American Dental Association and the American Heart Association[23] concluded, "Concentrations of vasoconstrictors normally used in dental local anesthetic solutions are not contraindicated in patients with cardiovascular disease when administered carefully and with preliminary aspiration."

Contrary to these recommendations, Abraham-Inpijn et al[24] found that patients with hypertension undergoing dental extractions had a greater increase in blood pressure than did patients thought to be normotensive after injection of 2% lidocaine with 1:80,000 epinephrine. In addition, 7.5% of the patients with hypertension developed significant arrythmias. In a similar study, however, comparing the response of patients who were normotensive and hypertensive to lidocaine plain, with 1:100,000 epinephrine and 1:20,000 norepinephrine during extractions, no significant differences were noted in heart rate or blood pressure between plain lidocaine and lidocaine with epinephrine. However, lidocaine with norepinephrine produced a significant increase in blood pressure and a decreased heart rate.[25]

A study of dental patients undergoing surgery found no difference in the blood pressure of patients with hypertension who received 2% lidocaine with 1:80,000 epinephrine.[26] A study evaluating epinephrine infusion as a stress test for 39 patients suspected of having coronary artery disease involved a series of increasing levels of epinephrine from 2.1 to 21.0 μg per minute injected intravenously over a 30 minutes.[27] (The 21.0-μg dose is roughly equivalent to the 18 μg in one cartridge of 1:100,000 epinephrine.) Of the 24 patients subsequently found not to have coronary artery disease, none developed electrocardiographic changes, and none had symptoms over the course of 30 minutes. Of the 15 patients diagnosed with coronary artery disease, however, 7 developed significant arrythmias, 7 had chest pain, and 4 had shortness of breath or other symptoms. In spite of the symptoms and hemodynamic changes, no test had to be terminated and all symptoms subsided after the test without sequelae.

From the preceding studies, one and probably two cartridges of 2% lidocaine with 1:100,000 epinephrine (0.18 to 0.036 mg epinephrine) are of little clinical signif-

icance in most patients with hypertension or other cardiovascular disease; the benefits far outweigh any potential disadvantages or risks. Using more than this amount is associated with an increased risk for adverse hemodynamic changes and should be approached cautiously. Norepinephrine and levonordefrin should not be used for patients with hypertension because of their excessive alpha$_1$ stimulation. Relative contraindications to the use of vasoconstrictors include patients with severe uncontrolled hypertension, refractory arrhythmias, recent myocardial infarction (less than one month), recent stroke (fewer than 6 months), unstable angina, recent coronary artery bypass graft (fewer than 3 months), uncontrolled congestive heart failure, and uncontrolled hyperthyroidism.[28,29] Vasoconstrictors should not be used in these patients under most circumstances.

An additional concern when patients with hypertension are treated is the potential for adverse drug interactions between vasoconstrictors and antihypertensive drugs, specifically the adrenergic-blocking agents. The basis for concern with nonselective beta-adrenergic-blocking agents (e.g., propranolol) is that the normal compensatory vasodilation of skeletal muscle vasculature mediated by beta$_2$ receptors is inhibited by these drugs and an injection of epinephrine, levonordefrin, or any other pressor agent can result in an uncompensated peripheral vasoconstriction because of stimulation of alpha$_1$ receptors. This can cause a significant elevation of blood pressure.[16,30] Adverse interactions are less likely to occur in patients taking cardioselective beta blockers.[20] The peripheral adrenergic antagonists, such as reserpine and guanethidine, also present the potential for adverse interaction with vasoconstrictors because of the enhanced receptor sensitivity to direct-acting sympathomimetics, resulting in reports of enhanced systemic response to vasoconstrictors.[31]

The potential exists for adverse interactions between vasoconstrictors and some of the adrenergic-blocking agents, but clinical experience suggests that the cautious use of epinephrine in small doses (0.018 to 0.036 mg) can be used safely in most patients. Jastak et al[20] suggest giving a small test dose (1 ml of the 1:100,000 epinephrine solution) and monitoring the blood pressure every minute for at least 5 minutes in patients taking a nonselective beta blocker or a peripheral adrenergic antagonist. If no significant change in blood pressure is noted during that period, epinephrine can be used after the previous recommendations.

Although not considered antihypertensive drugs, monoamine oxidase inhibitors occasionally have been used to treat hypertension. Some medical professionals have been concerned about the interaction between

monoamine oxidase inhibitors and vasoconstrictors, especially epinephrine. This concern for the most part is unfounded. Epinephrine and levonordefrin are not greatly potentiated by monoamine oxidase inhibitors because these exogenous agents are primarily metabolized by catechol-O-methyltransferase and not by monoamine oxidase; therefore the inhibition of monoamine oxidase has minimal effect on the metabolism or action of epinephrine and levonordefrin.[20]

Topical vasopressors generally should not be used to control local bleeding in the patient with hypertension. When performing crown and bridge procedures for patients with hypertension, the dentist should avoid using gingival retraction cord that contains epinephrine. One study, however, reported that tetrahydrozoline (Visine), oxymetazoline (Afrin), and phenylephrine (Neo-Synephrine) could be used to soak the cord with minimal systemic effects.[2]

Several drug interactions are of concern with antihypertensive agents and dentistry. Some antihypertensive agents can predispose patients to orthostatic hypotension and potentiate the actions of barbiturates or other sedatives. These drugs still can be used for patients taking antihypertensive medications; however, their usual dosage should be reduced. In addition, sedative medications may cause hypotensive episodes for patients taking antihypertensive agents and must be used with care. The activity of most antihypertensive drugs can be decreased by the prolonged use of nonsteroidal antiflammatory drugs and should be considered if these drugs are used for analgesia, although the use of nonsteroidal antiinflammatory drugs for a few days is of little practical concern.[32] Once again, the specific antihypertensive drug or drugs a patient is taking should be evaluated, significant side effects and drug interactions noted, and the appropriate action taken. Some antihypertensive agents can produce a tendency for nausea and vomiting. Excessive stimulation of the gag reflex during dental treatment of patients taking these drugs may precipitate nausea and vomiting and should be avoided. Another concern is for patients who may be using cocaine. In a study by Johnson et al,[33] both alcohol and cocaine use had an effect on blood pressure (increased) during oral surgery.

Blood pressure is subject to variation by circadian rhythms. Nichols[34] found by monitoring once every minute the blood pressure of dental patients undergoing various procedures that blood pressure varied significantly for nearly all individual patients. In several studies using continuous chronobiologic monitoring of blood pressure (every 15 minutes for 48 to 148 hours) in dental patients[35-38] a significant variation in blood pressure sometimes occurs during certain times of the day and week that may alter the patient's susceptibility to an adverse experience and should be considered in treatment planning and dental management. Chronobiology is the science of life in time and it recognizes that many features of the environment have become genetic adaptations. The biologic built-in day, week, month, and year are examples. The health care-related aspect of this particular science, termed *chronomedicine*, has a new impetus from physiologic monitors that automatically measures many dynamic body functions, blood pressure in particular, for 24 hours or longer. The data collected can be analyzed using computer methods of time series analysis.[36] These data allow for the identification of patients with hypertension and also can aid in the best timing for medications used to treat hypertension. Up to 31% of patients thought to be normotensive by casual, episodic blood pressure measurements have been found to actually be hypertensive when blood pressure is chronobiologically monitored.[37] Dental patients with elevated circadian hyper-amplitude-tension have experienced serious cardiovascular and cerebrovascular problems.[38]

TREATMENT PLANNING MODIFICATIONS

No elective dental procedures should be performed for the patient who has severe or uncontrolled hypertension (stage 3), according to the recommendation of the Sixth Report of the Joint National Committee on Detection, Evaluation, and Treatment of High Blood Pressure.[1] Patients receiving good medical management and under good control with no systemic complications can receive any indicated dental treatment. The treatment plan may be modified as needed where complications exist[18] (see Tables 4-2 and 4-4).

Oral Complications and Manifestations

Few oral complications are associated with hypertension itself. Patients with malignant hypertension have been reported to occasionally develop facial palsy.[39] Patients with severe hypertension have been reported to bleed excessively after surgical procedures or trauma; however, excessive bleeding in patients with hypertension is not common and controversial.[40,41]

Patients taking antihypertensive drugs, especially diuretics, may complain of dry mouth. The mercurial diuretics may cause oral lesions on an allergic or toxic basis. Lichenoid reactions have been reported with thiazides, methyldopa, propranolol, and labetalol. Angiotensin converting enzyme inhibitors can cause neutropenia, resulting in delayed healing or gingival bleeding. Angioedema is seen infrequently with angiotensin converting enzyme inhibitors. All calcium an-

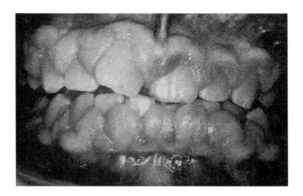

FIG. 4-4 Gingival hyperplasia caused by administration of nifedipine. (Courtesy Terry Wright, Lexington, Ky.)

tagonists and especially nifedipine can cause gingival hyperplasia (Fig. 4-4, see Table 4-3).

References

1. Sixth Report of the Joint National Committee on Detection, Evaluation, and Treatment of High Blood Pressure, *Arch Int Med* 157:154-183, 1997.
2. Little JW: The impact on dentistry of recent advances in the management of hypertension, *Oral Surg Oral Med Oral Pathol Oral Radiol Endo* 90:591-599, 2000.
3. Burt VL, Harris T: The Third National Health and Nutrition Examination Survey: contributing data on aging and health, *Gerontologist* 34:386-390, 1994.
4. McInnnes GT: Integrated approaches to management of hypertension: promoting treatment acceptance, *Am J Heart* 138:252-255, 1999.
5. Cioffi GA et al: The hemodynamic and plasma catecholamine responses to routine restorative dental care, *J Am Dent Assoc* 111:67-70, 1985.
6. Clutter WB et al: Epinephrine plasma metabolic clearance rates and physiologic thresholds for metabolic and hemodynamic actions in man, *J Clin Invest* 66:94-101, 1980.
7. Hennessy BJ, Kerns DG, Davies WG: The incidence of active duty dental patients taking antihypertensive medications, *Mil Med* 164:740-745, 1999.
8. Beilin LJ, Puddey IB, Burke V: Lifestyle and hypertension, *Am J Hypertension* 12:934-935, 1999.
9. Dionne RA, Goldstein DS, Wirdzeh PR: Effects of diazepam premedication and epinephrine-containing local anesthetic on cardiovascular and plasma catecholamine response in oral surgery, *Anesth Analg* 63:640-646, 1984.
10. Kaplan NM: Arterial hypertension. In Stein JH, editor: *Internal medicine*, ed 5, St. Louis, 1997, Mosby.
11. MacMahon S et al: Blood pressure, stroke and coronary heart disease. Part I. Prolonged differences in blood pressure: prospective observational studies corrected for the regression dilution bias, *Lancet* 335:765-774, 1990.
12. Smith WM: The case for treating hypertension in the elderly, *Am J Hypertens* 1:1735-1785, 1988.
13. Hypertension Detection and Follow-up Program Cooperative Group: Five-year findings of the Hypertension Detection and Follow-up Program. I. Reduction in mortality of persons with high blood pressure, including mild hypertension, *JAMA* 242:2562-2571, 1979.
14. Neaton JD et al: Treatment of mild hypertension study. Final results, *JAMA* 270:713-724, 1993.
15. Jagroop IA , Mikhailidis DP: Angiotensin II can induce and potentiate change in human platelets: effect of losartan, *J Hum Hypertens* 14:581-585, 2000.
16. SHEP Cooperative Research Group: Prevention of stroke by antihypertensive drug treatment in older persons with isolated systolic hypertension, *JAMA* 265:3255-3264, 1991.
17. Kaplan NM: Hypertension in the population at large. In: Kaplan NM: *Clinical hypertension*, ed 7, Baltimore, 1998, Williams and Wilkins.
18. Glick M: New guidelines for prevention, detection, evaluation and treatment of high blood pressure, *J Am Dent Assoc* 129:1589-1594, 1998.
19. Hoffman BB, Lefkowitz RJ: Catecholamines and sympathomimetic drugs. In Gilman AG, et al, editors: *Goodman and Gilman's the pharmacological basis of therapeutics*, ed 8, New York, 1990, Pergammon.
20. Jastak JT, Yagiela JA, Donaldson D: *Local anesthesia of the oral cavity*, Philadelphia, 1995, WB Saunders.
21. Tolas AG, Pflug AE, Hatler JB: Arterial plasma epinephrine concentrations and hemodynamic responses after dental injection of local anesthetic with epinephrine, *J Am Dent Assoc* 104:41-43, 1982.
22. Special Committee of the New York Heart Association: Use of epinephrine in connection with procaine in dental procedures, *J Am Dent Assoc* 50:108, 1955.
23. Working Conference of American Dental Association and American Heart Association on Management of Dental Problems in Patients with Cardiovascular Disease, *J Am Dent Assoc* 68:333-342, 1964.
24. Abraham-Inpijn L, Borgneijer-Hoelen A, Gortzak RAT: Changes in blood pressure, heart rate and electrocardiogram during dental treatment with use of local anesthesia, *J Am Dent Assoc* 116:531-536, 1988.
25. Meyer F-U: Hemodynamic changes of local dental anesthesia in normotensive and hypertensive subjects, *Int J Clin Pharmacol Ther Toxical* 24:477-481, 1986.
26. Meechan JG: Plasma potassium changes in hypertensive patients undergoing oral surgery with local anesthetics containing epinephrine, *Anesthesia Prog* 44:106-109, 1997.
27. Schecter E, Wilson MF, Kong Y-S: Physiologic responses to epinephrine infusion: the basis for a new stress test for coronary artery disease, *Am Heart J* 105:554-560, 1983.
28. Malamed SF: *Handbook of local anesthesia*, ed 4, St Louis, 1997, Mosby.
29. Paaerusse R, Goulet J-P, Turcotte J-Y: Contraindications to vasoconstrictors in dentistry, Part I. *Oral Surg Oral Med Oral Pathol* 74:679-686, 1992.
30. Mito RS, Yagiela JA: Hypertensive response to levonordefrin in a patient receiving propanolol: report of case, *J Am Dent Assoc* 116:55-57, 1988.

31. Hansten PD: Drug interactions affecting the cardiovascular response to sympathomimetics, *Drug Interact Newsletter* 1:21-26, 1981.

32. Oates JA et al: Clinical implications of prostaglandin thromboxane A formation, N *Engl J Med* 319:689-698, 761-767, 1988.

33. Johnson CD, Lewis VA, Brown RS: The relationship between chronic cocaine or alcohol abuse in black men during uncomplicated tooth extraction, *J Oral Maxillofac Surg* 56:323-329, 1998.

34. Nichols C: Dentistry and hypertension, *J Am Dent Assoc* 128:1557-1562,1997.

35. Little JW et al: Longitudinal chronobiological blood pressure monitoring for assessing the need and timing of antihypertensive treatment, *Prog Clin Biol Res* 20:245-250, 1990.

36. Rhodus NL et al: Chronobiological versus conventional blood pressure monitoring of dental patients, *J Dent Res* 77:255, 1998.

37. Raab F et al: Interpreting vital sign profiles for maximizing patient safety during dental visits, *J Am Dent Assoc* 129: 461-469, 1998.

38. Katinas GS et al: Individualized combination chronotherapy of coexisting CHAT and MESOR-hypertension including Diltiazem HCL, *Scripta Medica* 73:95-104, 2000.

39. Scully C, Clawson RA: Cardiovascular disease. In: *Medical problems in dentistry*, London, 1982, Wright PSG.

40. Knoll-Kauchler E et al: Changes in plasma epinephrine concentrations after dental infiltration anesthesia with different doses of epinephrine, *J Dent Res* 68:1098-1101, 1989.

41. Houben H, Thien T, van Laar A: Effect of low-dose epinephrine infusion on hemodynamics after selective and nonselective blockers in hypertension, *Clin Pharmacol Ther* 31:685-690, 1982.

Ischemic Heart Disease

CHAPTER 5

Coronary atherosclerotic heart disease is a major health problem in the United States and other industrialized nations. Atherosclerosis is the thickening of the intimal layer of the arterial wall caused by the accumulation of lipid plaques. The atherosclerotic process results in a narrowed lumen and diminished blood flow and oxygen supply. Atherosclerosis is the most common underlying cause of not only coronary heart disease (angina and myocardial infarction [MI]) but also cerebrovascular disease (stroke) and peripheral arterial disease (intermittent claudication).

Symptomatic coronary atherosclerotic heart disease is referred to as *ischemic heart disease*. Ischemic symptoms are the result of oxygen deprivation caused by reduced perfusion of a portion of the myocardium. Other conditions such as embolism, coronary ostial stenosis, coronary artery spasm, and congenital abnormalities may cause ischemic heart disease.

INCIDENCE AND PREVALENCE

Approximately 20 million Americans (8% of the population) are estimated to have some form of heart disease, with coronary artery disease affecting 13.7 million persons.[1] The mortality rate per year from cardiovascular diseases as a group has been declining since 1940. From 1970 to 1994, mortality from coronary heart disease decreased 53.2% and from stroke 59%.[2] In spite of this decline, cardiovascular diseases continue to be the most serious threat to health in America; 1 of every 3 men and 1 of every 10 women will develop significant cardiovascular disease before age 60.[1] Coronary heart disease is still the leading cause of death after age 40 years in men and 65 years in women. It causes about 800,000 new heart attacks each year and 450,000 recurrent attacks; more than 500,000 persons will die from these attacks.[3]

The incidence and severity of coronary heart disease increases with age in both men and women. Studies on autopsies in the United States have shown that nearly 20% of patients between the ages of 30 and 39 years have more than 50% occlusion of one or more coronary arteries.[4-7] Between the ages of 40 and 49 years the rate of occlusion increases to more than 40% of patients.

ETIOLOGY

The cause of coronary atherosclerosis is not known; however, research indicates the disease is related to a variety of risk factors. Men are more at risk than women of childbearing age. Other major risk factors include a family history of the disease and the presence of hyperlipidemia, hypertension, cigarette smoking, and diabetes mellitus.[8,9] The incidence of coronary atherosclerosis increases with age but this increase may be more the result of other risk factors acting for a longer time than the direct effects of aging.

The fact that men are much more prone to the clinical manifestations of coronary atherosclerosis is accentuated in nonwhite populations. Between ages 35 and 44 years, the risk is five times higher for men than women.[1] MI and sudden death are rare in premenopausal women; however, after menopause rapid reduction occurs in this gender difference.

Recent studies have confirmed that individuals with either parents or siblings affected by coronary atherosclerotic heart disease have a greater risk of developing the disease at a younger age than do those without such a history.[9-11] This risk may be as high as 5 times greater.

Elevation of serum lipid levels is a major risk factor for atherosclerosis. Increased levels of low-density lipoprotein cholesterol carry the greatest risk for coronary atherosclerosis, whereas increased levels of high-density lipoprotein cholesterol have been shown to reduce the risk.[11] Individuals with elevated triglyceride or

beta-lipoprotein levels have an increased risk for the disease. A diet rich in total calories, saturated fats, cholesterol, sugars, and salts also increases the risk. Other risk factors for the development of atherosclerosis include elevated levels of fibrinogen and plasminogen-activator inhibitor. Elevated levels of homocysteine also may promote thrombosis, but the exact mechanism of this is unclear.[8]

Increased blood pressure appears to be one of the most significant risk factors in coronary atherosclerotic heart disease. The Framingham Study showed that angina, MI, and nonsudden death were all significantly correlated with elevated blood pressure (more than 140/90 mm Hg).[4] Sudden death in men was related only to elevation in systolic blood pressure, and no correlation of sudden death in women was found with increased blood pressure. Hypertension affects primarily the rate of development of coronary atherosclerosis rather than being a primary cause in its development.[12]

The risk of developing coronary atherosclerotic heart disease in cigarette smokers is approximately twice that of nonsmokers. The increased risk appears to be proportional to the number of cigarettes smoked per day. In a 5-year study of 4165 smokers with coronary atherosclerotic heart disease, the death rate was reduced for individuals who stopped smoking.[13] The death rate was 22% for the 2675 individuals who continued smoking and 15% for the 1490 who stopped. In the Framingham Study,[14] participants who discontinued smoking lowered their risk of MI within 2 years. Pipe and cigar smoking apparently carries little risk for developing heart disease.

Patients with diabetes mellitus have a greater incidence of coronary atherosclerotic heart disease and more extensive lesions. They also develop the condition at an earlier age than persons who do not have diabetes.[8,9] The exact mechanism to explain this association with macroangiopathy, however, is not clear. In overt diabetes the mortality associated with coronary atherosclerosis definitely is increased. In the First National Health and Nutrition Examination Survey[15] the age-adjusted death rates for men and women with diabetes were twice those seen in those without the disease. Of the excess mortality among men with diabetes, 75% was caused by coronary artery disease. Minor risk factors are obesity, sedentary living pattern, personality type, and psychosocial tensions. Several studies have suggested an association between periodontal disease and cardiovascular disease, raising the question of whether periodontal disease is a risk factor for cardiovascular disease.[16-19] One hypothesis has been proposed to explain this relationship: Certain individuals appear to have a genetic predisposition to hyperrespond to inflammation, and periodontal infections may result in an unregulated inflammatory response to

these infections.[20] Thus periodontal infections may directly contribute to the pathogenesis of atherosclerosis and thromboembolic events by providing repeated systemic vascular challenges with lipopolysaccharide and proinflammatory cytokines. Other investigations are underway to define this relationship more clearly.[21]

No single risk factor is responsible for the development of coronary atherosclerosis, but many factors contribute to its development. Evidence suggests that modification of those risk factors that can be controlled such as cigarette smoking, hypertension, hyperlipidemia, and diabetes can reduce or modify the clinical effects of the disease.

PATHOPHYSIOLOGY AND COMPLICATIONS

The pathogenesis of atherosclerosis involves an inflammatory repair response of the arterial intima invoked by lipids.[22] The exact mechanism of atherogenesis is not completely understood, but the American Heart Association[23,24] has suggested ways of possible plaque evolution and a nomenclature for the various stages of plaque formation (Fig. 5-1).

A stage I lesion occurs with the adherence of monocytes to injured or altered endothelial surface of the

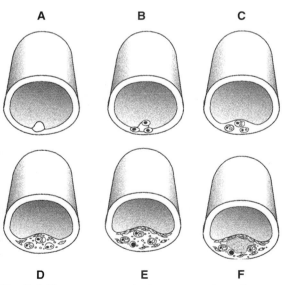

Fig. 5-1 The progression of atheromatous plaque formation. **A,** Area of endothelial injury. **B,** Adherence of monocytes to the endothelial surface and migration into the intima. **C,** Fatty streak with macrophages ingesting lipid. **D,** Extracellular pools of lipid. **E,** Appearance of smooth muscle cells and formation of lipid core. **F,** Formation of fibrous capsule over and around lipid core.

artery and the eventual migration of these monocytes into the intima of the vessel. Stage II is the "fatty streak" that occurs when the monocytes within the intima are transformed into macrophages and ingest lipid, thus becoming foam cells. These foam cells produce a variety of inflammatory cytokines. Stage III is marked by the appearance of small extracellular pools of lipid in the intima. Stage IV is noted by the appearance of smooth muscle cells beneath the endothelium, along with the coalescence of the small extracellular lipid pools into a larger pool or lipid core. Stage V is the deposition of connective tissue and the formation of a fibrous capsule surrounding the lipid pool, creating a fibrous cap overlying the lipid pool that extends into the lumen of the artery.

The plaque may grow and proliferate either away from the lumen of the artery or into the lumen. If it proliferates inwardly, the size of the lumen is reduced and blood flow may be chronically decreased. Ischemic symptoms may be produced when occlusion reaches 75% to 80% of the cross-sectional area of the artery[25] (Fig. 5-2).

Blood flow may be disrupted acutely by the formation of a thrombus. Thrombus formation occurs as a result of focal erosion of the endothelial surface overlying the plaque or more commonly by the rupture of a plaque. With focal erosion, underlying connective tissue is exposed, which leads to platelet adhesion and thrombi. Thrombi may be small, producing no symptoms, or large with occlusion and resulting ischemic symptoms.

Up to three fourths of major coronary thrombi are caused by plaque rupture.[24] In a plaque rupture the fibrous plaque cap tears, which allows arterial blood to enter the lipid core where tissue factor and collagen induces platelet adhesion, aggregation, and activation. Thrombus formation then occurs within the core and expands into the lumen causing obstruction (Fig. 5-3).

Atherosclerosis is usually a focal disease commonly occurring in certain areas or regions of arteries while sparing others.[8] For example, the proximal left anterior descending coronary artery is a common area of atherosclerosis as are the proximal portions of the renal arteries. In contrast, the internal mammary artery is rarely involved. The lumen of an affected artery may be circumferentially narrowed evenly or eccentrically depending on the location and extent of the plaque.

The outcome of the atherosclerotic process shows extreme variability. Some lesions never progress past the fatty streak phase; however, in most Western societies the presence of frank plaques are the norm. Even so, most atheromatous plaques produce no symptoms and may never cause clinical manifestations.[8] Several factors may be responsible, including arterial remodeling, in which the plaque grows outward away from the lumen with a compensatory increase in the diameter of the vessel. In addition, collateral circulation can develop to compensate for diminished blood flow.

For those lesions that do produce symptoms, flow-limiting intact plaques usually produce symptoms such as chest pain (angina) when oxygen need exceeds demand, as during exercise. However, plaque rupture produces acute or unstable symptoms such as rest angina, MI, or sudden death. Not all plaques have the same propensity to rupture and risk depends on the physical and biochemical characteristics of the plaque.

The intraarterial complications of coronary atherosclerosis are luminal narrowing, intramural hemorrhage, thrombosis, embolism, and aneurysm. Intramural hemorrhage occurs because of a weakening of the intimal tissues and may lead to thrombosis. It also may serve as an irritant and cause a reflex reaction that results in spasm

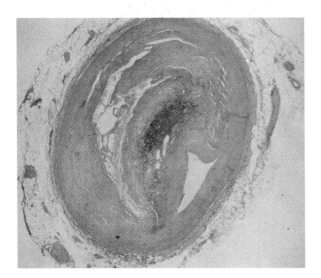

Fig. 5-2 Photomicrograph of a cross section of a coronary artery partially occluded as a result of coronary atherosclerotic disease. (Courtesy W. O'Conner, Lexington, Ky.)

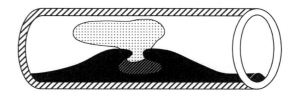

Fig. 5-3 A ruptured plaque with thrombus formation.

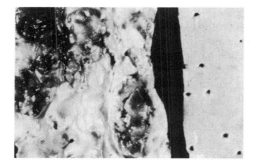

Fig. 5-4 Postmortem specimen demonstrating atherosclerotic plaques on the wall of the aorta on the left side. The specimen on the right is unaffected.

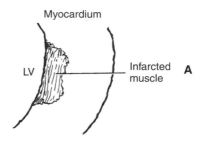

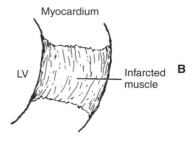

Fig. 5-5 Myocardial infarction. **A,** Subendocardial, **B,** Transmural. LV, left ventricle.

of the collateral vessels. Coronary thrombosis usually is found in the segment of the artery that contains an advanced atherosclerotic lesion. Once formed, a thrombus may become encapsulated and undergo fibrous organization and recanulization. The atherosclerotic process is not limited to the coronary arteries but is found throughout other arteries of the body (Fig. 5-4).

If the degree of ischemia resulting from coronary atherosclerosis is significant and prolonged, the area of myocardium supplied by that vessel can undergo necrosis. The reduced blood flow may result from thrombosis in the affected artery, a hypotensive episode, an increased demand for blood, or emotional stress. The infarction, or area of necrosis, may be subendocardial or transmural (Fig. 5-5), the latter involving the entire thickness of the myocardium.

Complications of MI include weakened heart muscle resulting in acute congestive heart failure, postinfarction angina, infarct extension, cardiogenic shock, pericarditis, and arrhythmias. The causes of death in patients who have had an acute MI (AMI) include ventricular fibrillation, cardiac standstill, congestive heart failure, embolism, and rupture of the heart wall or septum.[26]

CLINICAL PRESENTATION

SYMPTOMS

Chest pain is the most important symptom of coronary atherosclerotic heart disease. The pain may be brief, as in angina pectoris resulting from temporary ischemia of the myocardium, or it may be prolonged, as in MI. Ischemic myocardial pain results from an imbalance between the oxygen supply and oxygen demand of the muscle. Atherosclerotic narrowing of the coronary arteries is an important cause of this imbalance. The exact mechanism or agents involved in producing the cardiac pain are not known.

Ischemic myocardial pain that is brief (angina pectoris) usually is described as an aching, heavy, squeezing pressure or tightness in the midchest region. The pain typically is precipitated by eating, exercise, or stress. The area of discomfort often is described to be approximately the size of the fist and may radiate into the left or right arm to the neck or lower jaw. In rare cases it may be present in only one of these distant sites and the patient will be free of central chest pain. The pain usually is brief in duration, lasting only 1 to 5 minutes if the provoking stimulus is reduced or stopped.[25] Patients with initial pain, progressive pain, or pain at rest are described as having an *unstable angina*. Patients with chest pain that has not changed in frequency, severity, or duration over an extended period have *stable angina*. Patients with brief pain caused by myocardial ischemia and a stable pattern of attacks have a relatively good prognosis. Patients with unstable angina have a poor prognosis and often develop MI within a short period. A relatively uncommon form of angina, *Prinzmetal's variant angina*, occurs at rest and is caused by focal spasm of a coronary artery, usually with varying amounts of atherosclerosis.[25] Angina also can occur in individuals with normal coronary vessels.

Patients with coronary atherosclerosis who develop prolonged pain resulting from myocardial ischemia usually are having a MI. Objective clinical evidence of infarction may not exist. The pain resulting from infarction usually is more severe and lasts longer than 15 minutes but has the same character as that described for angina. Its location is the same and it may radiate in the same pattern as the brief pain resulting from temporary myocardial ischemia. The administration of vasodilators or the cessation of activity does not relieve the pain caused by infarction. Neither brief nor prolonged pain resulting from myocardial ischemia is aggravated by deep breathing. People with diabetes can develop "silent" MIs without pain.[27]

Sudden cardiac death accounts for 300,000 to 500,000 deaths annually in the United States and is the first symptom of coronary heart disease in 10% of all coronary events.[28] At autopsy some type of underlying heart disease is found in about 60% to 70% of the cases of sudden death. Predominant symptoms that most often precede sudden death include chest pain, cough, shortness of breath, fainting, dizziness, palpitations and fatigue. Pathologic examination of patients who died outside a hospital of sudden cardiac death have shown acute coronary occlusion and demonstrable AMI to be uncommon but signs of old subendocardial infarctions are common. The most common cause of sudden death is ventricular fibrillation, a form of abnormal electrical activity resulting from interruption of the electric conduction system.[29]

Palpitations of the heart may be present in patients with coronary atherosclerotic heart disease. The rhythm may be normal or abnormal. The complaint (disagreeable awareness of the heartbeat) is not directly related to the seriousness of the underlying cardiac problem. Syncope, a transient loss of consciousness resulting from inadequate cerebral blood flow, also may occur in patients with coronary atherosclerotic heart disease.

The symptoms of congestive heart failure experienced as a complication of coronary atherosclerotic heart disease include dyspnea, orthopnea, paroxysmal nocturnal dyspnea, edema, hemoptysis, fatigue, weakness, and cyanosis. Fatigue and weakness may be present early in the course of the disease before the onset of congestive failure (see Chapter 7).

SIGNS

The clinical signs of coronary atherosclerotic heart disease are few, and the patient may appear entirely normal. Conditions such as corneal arcus and xanthomas of the skin are related to hyperlipidemia and hypercholesterolemia. Blood pressure may be elevated, and abnormalities in the rhythm of the arterial pulse may occur. Diminished peripheral pulses in the lower extremities may be seen along with bruits in the carotid arteries. Panoramic radiographs of the jaws may occasionally demonstrate carotid calcifications in the area of C_3 and C_4 (see Chapter 22). Retinal changes are common in hypertensive disease and diabetes mellitus. Signs associated with advanced coronary atherosclerotic heart disease usually reflect the presence of congestive heart failure. Distention of neck veins, peripheral edema, cyanosis, ascites, and enlarged liver may be found.

LABORATORY FINDINGS

Laboratory tests used to evaluate patients with symptoms of angina pectoris include resting electrocardiogram, exercise stress testing, ambulatory (Holter) electrocardiography, stress thallium-201 perfusion scintigraphy, exercise echocardiography, ambulatory ventricular function monitoring, and cardiac catheterization.[30]

Serum enzyme determinations are often most helpful in establishing the presence of an AMI and the extent of infarction. The two enzymes routinely used for the diagnosis of AMI are creatine phosphokinase (CK) and an isoenzyme, MB-CK. CK levels becomes elevated within 4 to 8 hours after an AMI and return to normal within 48 to 72 hours. CK-MB reaches its peak level at approximately 20 hours. The difference between these two markers is in their specificity. CK is released not only with myocardial damage but also from skeletal muscle disorders or trauma. CK-MB, however, is more specific for the myocardium. In practice, both enzymes are measured, and the CK-MB/CK ratio is calculated with a ratio greater than or equal to 2.5%, suggesting a myocardial rather than skeletal muscle source.[27,28]

Two new serum markers for MI are troponin T and troponin I. They are cardiac-specific enzymes and similar to CK-MB in their specificity and sensitivity.[31] The two serum markers are especially useful in detecting damage to cardiac muscle because skeletal muscle disorders do not affect either enzyme.

MEDICAL MANAGEMENT

ANGINA PECTORIS

The patient with coronary atherosclerotic heart disease with a history of stable brief pain (angina pectoris) is managed medically by a combination of approaches (Box 5-1). A physician should explain the disease and reassure the patient about being able to lead a productive life. Management may include general lifestyle measures such as an exercise program; weight control; restriction of salt, cholesterol, and saturated fatty acids; cessation of

BOX 5-1

**Medical Management of Patients
with Angina Pectoris**

Explanation and reassurance
Lifestyle changes and reduction of risk factors
Elimination or control of coexisting illness (e.g., hypertension, diabetes)
Drug therapy
   Nitrates
   Beta-blockers
   Calcium channel blockers
   Antiplatelet agents
Revascularization
   Percutaneous transluminal coronary angioplasty or stents
   Coronary artery bypass grafting

smoking; and control of exacerbating conditions such as anemia, hypertension, and hyperthyroidism. Drug therapy includes nitrates (nitroglycerin or long-acting nitrates), beta-adrenergic blockers, calcium channel blockers, and antiplatelet agents[25,30] (Table 5-1).

The nitrates are vasodilators, predominantly venodilators, and are the cornerstone in the pharmacologic management of angina. The mechanism of action is unknown; however, researchers believe it may be caused by a decrease in cardiac load, resulting in decreased oxygen demand. Nitrates also may alleviate coronary artery spasm. Nitroglycerin comes in a variety of forms and can be sprayed or placed under the tongue; nitrates are taken orally as a long-acting agent, ointment may be applied to the skin, or long-acting transdermal nitrate patches can be applied. Nitrates are used to reduce symptoms of angina but do not slow, alter, or reverse the progression of coronary artery disease. They can be used to relieve an attack of angina pectoris or prophylactically before activities that predictably precipitate episodes of angina pectoris.

TABLE 5-1

Drugs Used in the Management of Angina

Drug	Mode of Action	Vasoconstrictor Interactions	Oral Manifestations	Other Considerations
Nitrates				
Nitroglycerin	Venous and arterial dilation, reduction of oxygen demand	Possible decrease in effectiveness of epinephrine and levonordefrin	Dry mouth	Orthostatic hypotension, headache
Nitrogard				
Nitrolingual				
Nitro-Bid				
Nitroject				
Nitrostat				
Nitroglyn				
Nitrol				
Tridil				
Nitrong				
Nitro-Dur				
Transderm-Nitro				
Minitran				
Erythrityl tetranitrate				
Cardilate				
Pentaerythritol tetranitrate				
Duotrate				
Peritrate				
Isosorbide dinitrate				
Dilatrate				
Isordil				
Isonate				

NS, Nonselective; CS, cardioselective; ADP, adenosine diphosphate.

TABLE 5-1

Drugs Used in the Management of Angina—cont'd

Drug	Mode of Action	Vasoconstrictor Interactions	Oral Manifestations	Other Considerations
Nitrates—cont'd				
Isosorbide dinitrate—cont'd				
Sorbitrate				
Isorbid				
Isorbid mononitrate				
Monoket				
Imdur				
Beta-Adrenergic Blockers				
Propanolol (Inderal) (NS)	Competition with catecholamines for beta-adrenergic receptors, NS (blockade of β_1 and β_2 receptors)	NS, increase in blood pressure possible with sympathomimetics, cautious use recommended (maximum 0.036 mg epinephrine, 0.20 mg levonordefrin)	Not significant	Orthostatic hypotension
Nadolol (Corgard) (NS)				
Carteolol (Cartrol) (NS)				
Oxprendolol (Trasicor) (NS)				
Timilol (Blocadren) (NS)				
Pembutalol (Levatol) (NS)				
Pindolol (Visken) (NS)				
Sotalol (Betapace) (NS)				
Metoprolol (Lopressor) (CS)	CS (blockade of β_1 receptors in heart)	CS, minimal effect with sympathomimetics, normal use		None
Atenolol (Tenormin) (CS)				
Acebutolol (Sectral) (CS)				
Labetalol (Normodyne, Trandate) (CS)				
Calcium Channel Blockers				
Bepridil (Vascor)	Block calcium entry into cardiac and vascular smooth muscles, vascular dilation, decreased heart rate and myocardial contractibility	None	Gingival hyperplasia, dry mouth, lichenoid eruptions (rare)	None
Diltiazem (Cardizem)				
Felodipine (Plendil)				
Isradipine (DynaCirc)				
Nifedipine (Adalat, Procardia)				
Verapamil (Calan, Isoptin, Verelan)				
Nicardipine				
Platelet Aggregation Inhibitors				
Aspirin	Inhibition of cycloxygenase 1 and 2	None	None	Increased bleeding time
Clopidogrel (Plavix)	Inhibition of ADP binding to platelets	None	None	Increased bleeding time
Ticlopidine (Ticlid)	Inhibition of ADP binding of fibrinogen to platelets	None	None	Increased bleeding time, possible blood dyscrasia
Dipyridamole (Persantine)	Not defined	None	None	Increased bleeding time

NS, Nonselective; CS, cardioselective; ADP, adenosine diphosphate.

Beta-blockers are effective in the treatment of many patients with angina. The beta-blockers compete with catecholamines for beta-adrenergic receptor sites, resulting in decreased heart rate and myocardial contractility and reducing myocardial oxygen demand. Nonselective beta-blockers block the β_1 and β_2 receptors, whereas the cardioselective beta-blockers preferentially block the β_1 receptors at normal therapeutic doses. Nonselective beta blockers can cause unwanted effects. These include increasing the tone of vascular smooth muscle and causing both vasoconstriction of peripheral vessels and contraction of bronchial smooth muscle. Thus nonselective beta-blockers are not prescribed for patients with a history of asthma. Injections of sympathomimetic drugs such as epinephrine or levonordefrin can result in significant elevation of blood pressure in patients taking nonselective beta-blockers.

Calcium channel blockers are effective in the treatment of chronic stable angina either alone or in combination with beta-blockers and nitrates.[30] These drugs decrease intracellular calcium, resulting in vasodilitation of coronary, peripheral, and pulmonary vasculature, and decreased myocardial contractibility and heart rate.

In unstable angina, antiplatelet therapy is a significant part of treatment. Aspirin has been shown to be beneficial in large randomized trials and decreases the incidence of fatal and nonfatal MI.[32] Aspirin is also beneficial for patients with chronic stable angina. Ample evidence exists to support the routine use of daily aspirin for patients with stable angina and those with a prior MI.

Other antiplatelet agents such as ticlopidine and clopidogrel produce effects equivalent to aspirin and are commonly prescribed for use in unstable angina. A new approach to platelet aggregation inhibition has been developed in the form of an antagonist for the platelet membrane receptor glycoprotein IIb/IIIa.[33] The prototype drug for this group of inhibitors is abciximab, which is administered intravenously, usually along with heparin.

Revascularization is also an option for patients with either stable or unstable angina. Available procedures for revascularization include percutaneous transluminal coronary angioplasty, stents, and coronary artery bypass grafts.

Percutaneous transluminal coronary angioplasty, also known as *balloon angioplasty*, employs a small inflatable balloon catheter over a thin guidewire threaded through the occluded segment of the artery. Once in place the balloon is inflated and compresses the plaque and thrombus against the arterial wall, increasing the lumen of the vessel (Fig. 5-6). This results in an immediate increase of blood flow and provides symp-

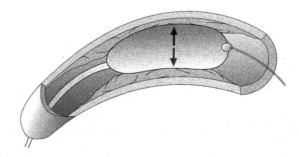

Fig. 5-6 Percutaneous transluminal coronary angioplasty.

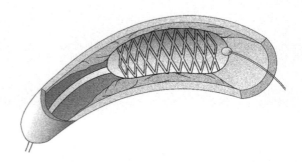

Fig. 5-7 Use of an expandable metallic stent in conjunction with percutaneous transluminal coronary angioplasty.

tomatic relief for ischemia. However, restenosis recurs within 6 months in approximately 30% of patients with a return of symptoms.[33]

A method to decrease the occurrence of restenosis with percutaneous transluminal coronary angioplasty involves the use of a thin, expandable, metallic mesh stent positioned by the balloon and expanded against the plaque and vessel wall then left in place. It functions as a permanent scaffold to help maintain vessel patency (Fig. 5-7). Stents become covered by endothelium within 2 to 4 weeks after placement.[34,35] The use of stents decreases the incidence of restenosis and the return of ischemic symptoms.[36] Recently even greater success has been achieved by stenting combined with the use of abciximab, a platelet inhibitor.[37] Other nonballoon angioplasty methods are rotational atherectomy and the use of lasers.

Coronary artery bypass graft surgery is an effective means of the control of symptoms for the management of unstable angina and can improve the long-term survival rate in certain subsets of patients. It also is effective in controlling symptoms in patients whose pain

persists despite medical control. Many patients with coronary artery disease are candidates for either angioplasty or bypass surgery. The decision can be difficult. The mortality and infarction rates associated with percutaneous transluminal coronary angioplasty is similar to bypass surgery.

Occlusion of the graft vessel is a major postoperative concern. Two primary sources of graft donor sites are used: the saphenous vein and internal mammary artery. Of the two the internal mammary artery graft is sturdier and much less susceptible to graft atherosclerosis and occlusion than vein grafts. They are preferred for the first bypass procedure when possible. Reoperation is difficult because of surgical site scarring and limited supply of graft donor material.

Rest is an important part of therapy. If activity brings on chest pain, the patient is instructed to stop and rest for several minutes or longer until the pain goes away. Nitroglycerin also may be taken. Patients who have significant angina are encouraged to avoid long hours of work, take rest periods during the working day, obtain adequate rest at night, use mild sedatives, take frequent vacations, and in some cases, change their occupation or retire.

Patients who have coronary atherosclerotic heart disease should avoid the precipitating factors that may bring on cardiac pain such as cold weather, hot and humid weather, big meals, emotional upsets, cigarette smoking, and drugs (e.g., amphetamines, caffeine, ephedrine, cyclamates, alcohol).

MYOCARDIAL INFARCTION

Patients with an AMI should be hospitalized as soon as possible (Box 5-2). The basic management goal is to minimize the size of the infarction and prevent death from lethal arrhythmias. The size and extent of the infarct is critical in the determination of outcome. Early administration of aspirin is recommended, with 160 to 325 mg being chewed and swallowed.[26]

The early management of AMI has undergone significant changes in the past several years with the recognition that thrombolytic therapy can result in a significant reduction of morbidity and mortality. The greatest benefit is realized if patients receive thrombolytic drugs within the first 1 hour to 3 hours after infarction; however, modest benefit is possible even up to 12 hours after the event.[27] The early use of thrombolytic drugs can decrease the extent of necrosis and myocardial damage and dramatically improve the outcome and prognosis. Fibrinolytic drugs approved by the U.S. Food and Drug Administration for use in treatment of AMI include recombinant plasminogen activator, retaplase (variant of recombinant tissue-

---

BOX 5-2

Medical Management of Patients with Acute Myocardial Infarction

Rapid hospitalization
Thrombolytic therapy
    Recombinant plasminogen activator
    Retaplase
    Streptokinase
    Anisoylated plasminogen streptokinase activator
Early revascularization
    Percutaneous transluminal coronary angioplasty or stent
    Coronary artery bypass grafting
Pharmacologic therapy
    Beta-adrenergic blockers
    ACE inhibitors
    Antiplatelet drugs
    Anticoagulants
    Nitrates
    Morphine
    Sedatives/hypnotics
    Oxygen

ACE, Angiotensin-converting enzyme.

---

type plasminogen activator) streptokinase, and anisoylated plasminogen streptokinase activator complex.

Early revascularization often is performed in addition to or in place of early thrombolytic therapy. Percutaneous transluminal coronary angioplasty and stenting are alternatives to thrombolytic therapy and compare favorably in outcome. Primary revascularization also is accomplished by coronary artery bypass graft. Adjunctive pharmacologic therapy includes the use of beta-adrenergic blockers and angiotensin-converting enzyme inhibitors. Antiplatelet drugs are significant in decreasing morbidity and mortality, and aspirin is the drug of choice. Daily doses of 160 to 325 mg are recommended. Clopidogrel (Plavix), ticlopidine (Ticlid), and dibpybridamole (Persantine) are other antiplatelet aggregating drugs that may be used. The use of anticoagulants is controversial; nevertheless, both heparin and warfarin sodium (Coumadin) are used in the management of AMI. Nitrates and other arterial vasodilators are essential in the treatment of AMI.

Pain relief is an important part of the early medical management of patients with an AMI, with morphine sulfate as the drug of choice. Sedatives and anxiolytic

medications also are used. Oxygen administered by nasal cannula is used during the acute period to increase the oxygen saturation of the blood and keep the heart workload at a minimum. However, high-flow oxygen is avoided because it may diminish the respiratory drive, cause hypoxia, and reduce coronary blood flow. The development of arrhythmias in patients who have had an AMI constitutes an emergency that must be treated aggressively. During the first several weeks after an infarction, the conduction system of the heart may be unstable and patients are prone to serious arrhythmias and reinfarction. A pacemaker may be used with severe myocardial damage and resultant heart failure.

The purpose of a rehabilitation program for patients who have had an AMI is to return them to as normal a life as possible. If this cannot be accomplished because of medical restrictions an attempt is made to alter the patient's lifestyle in a way that is consistent with that person's cardiac reserve but still allows full use of physical and emotional capacities.

DENTAL MANAGEMENT

RISK ASSESSMENT

Risk assessment for the dental management of patients with ischemic heart disease has three components: (1) the severity and stability of the disease, (2) the emotional or psychologic status of the patient, and (3) the type and magnitude of the dental procedure being planned. All must be factored into a dental management plan to arrive at a rational and safe decision, specifically to determine whether a patient can safely tolerate a planned procedure. Recently the American College of Cardiology and the American Heart Association have published risk stratification guidelines for patients with various types of heart disease who are undergoing various noncardiac surgical procedures. These can be of significant value in the determination of both surgical and nonsurgical dental procedures (Boxes 5-3 and 5-4).

BOX 5-3

Clinical Predictors of Increased Perioperative Cardiovascular Risk (Myocardial infarction, congestive heart failure, death)

Major
Unstable coronary syndromes
 Recent myocardial infarction* with evidence of important ischemic risk by clinical symptoms or noninvasive study
 Unstable or severe† angina (Canadian Class III or IV)‡
Decompensated congestive heart failure
Significant arrhythmias
 High-grade atrioventricular block
 Symptomatic ventricular arrhythmias in the presence of underlying heart disease
 Supraventricular arrhythmias with uncontrolled ventricular rate
Severe valvular disease

Intermediate
Mild angina pectoris (Canadian Class I or II)
Prior myocardial infarction by history or pathologic Q waves
Compensated or prior congestive failure
Diabetes mellitus

Minor
Advanced age
Abnormal electrocardiogram (left ventricular hypertrophy, left bundle branch block, ST-T abnormalities)
Rhythm other than sinus (e.g., atrial fibrillation)
Low functional capacity (e.g., inability to climb one flight of stairs with a bag of groceries)
History of stroke
Uncontrolled systemic hypertension

From Eagle KA, et al: Guidelines for perioperative cardiovascular evaluation for noncardiac surgery. Report of the American College of Cardiology/American Heart Association Task Force (Committee on Perioperative Cardiovascular Evaluation for Noncardiac Surgery), J Am Coll Cardiol 27(4):910-948, 1996.
*The American College of Cardiology National Database Library defines *recent* MI as more than 7 days but less than or equal to 1 month (30 days).
†May include "stable" angina in patients who are unusually sedentary.
‡Data from Campeau L: Grading of angina pectoris, *Circulation* 54:522-523, 1976.

Recent MI and unstable angina are classified as clinical predictors of major risk for perioperative complications. Stable or mild angina or a past history of an MI are identified as clinical predictors of intermediate risk for perioperative complications. The types of planned procedure must be considered, in addition to the perioperative risk conveyed by the diseases themselves. Most oral surgical procedures fall within the low-risk superficial procedures category of less than 1% risk. Nonsurgical dental procedures are likely to be even less of a risk. Some oral and maxillofacial surgical procedures, however, are included in the intermediate cardiac risk category under head and neck procedures. They carry a risk of less than 5%. The procedures with the highest risk involve major surgical procedures and are performed under general anesthesia; they have the potential for significant blood and fluid loss with resultant adverse hemodynamic effects.

BOX 5-4

Cardiac Risk* Stratification for Noncardiac Surgical Procedures

High (Reported cardiac risk of >5%)
Emergent major operations, particularly in elderly
Aortic and other major vascular
Peripheral vascular
Anticipated prolonged surgical procedures associated with large fluid shifts or blood loss

Intermediate (Reported cardiac risk of <5%)
Carotid endarterectomy
Head and neck
Intraperitoneal and intrathoracic
Orthopedic
Prostate

Low† (Reported cardiac risk of <1%)
Endoscopic procedures
Superficial procedures
Cataract
Breast

From Eagle KA, et al: Guidelines for perioperative cardiovascular evaluation for noncardiac surgery. Report of the American College of Cardiology/American Heart Association Task Force (Committee on Perioperative Cardiovascular Evaluation for Noncardiac Surgery), J Am Coll Cardiol 27(4):910-948, 1996.
*Combined incidence of cardiac death and nonfatal myocardial infarction.
†Do not generally require further preoperative cardiac testing.

These cardiac risk stratification guidelines can be applied to various dental management scenarios. For example, a patient with unstable angina or recent MI is classified as a major cardiac risk. However, if the dental procedure planned is limited to a routine clinical examination with radiographs (considered extremely low risk) and the patient is not fearful or anxious, the risk to the patient is not significant and thus the alterations in the dental management of this patient for this procedure would be minimal. Conversely, a patient with stable angina or a past history of MI classified as an intermediate cardiac risk who is scheduled to undergo a long, extensive periodontal surgery (low to intermediate risk) and is fearful or anxious poses a more significant risk and may require a more complex dental management plan.

ANGINA PECTORIS

A determination should be made about the severity and stability of angina. A patient with stable angina characteristically describes the occurrence of chest pain relatively infrequently. Pain predictably is precipitated by physical activity such as exercising, mowing the lawn, or climbing stairs and subsides with rest or the use of nitroglycerin. Pain occurs in a chronic, unchanging pattern for months or years and has minimal impact on activity. These patients pose an intermediate cardiac risk and are classified as either ASA II or ASA III depending on the restriction of activity and effect on daily routine.

A patient with unstable angina conversely describes a history of progressively worsening chest pain that occurs with physical exertion or at rest. Typically, a pattern of increasing severity, frequency, or duration of pain occurs. Pain occurring at rest or during sleep is particularly ominous. Patients with unstable angina should be considered a major cardiac risk and placed in an ASA IV category.

Based on the assessment of medical risk, type of planned dental procedure, and anxiety level of the patient, general management strategies for low- to intermediate-risk patients may include the following: short appointments in the morning, comfortable chair position, pretreatment vital signs, availability of nitroglycerin, oral or inhalation sedation, use of local anesthesia, limit on the amount of vasoconstrictor, avoidance of epinephrine-impregnated retraction cord, avoidance of anticholinergics, and use of effective postoperative pain control (Box 5-5).

Elective care should be postponed, however, for patients with a major risk. Necessary dental treatment should be performed as conservatively as possible and directed primarily toward pain and infection control. Consultation with the physician is advised. If treatment

BOX 5-5

Dental Management Considerations for Patients with Angina Pectoris or History of Myocardial Infarction*

Morning appointments
Short appointments
Comfortable chair position
Pretreatment vital signs
Nitroglycerin readily available
Stress-reduction measures:
  Good communication
  Oral sedation (e.g., triazolam 0.125-0.25 mg night before and 1 hour before appointment)
  Intraoperative N_2O/O_2
  Excellent local anesthesia
Limited use of vasoconstrictor (maximum 0.036 mg epinephrine, 0.20 mg levonordephrine), also applicable if patient taking a nonselective beta-blocker
If coronary artery stent in place and more than 2-4 weeks after placement, antibiotic prophylaxis not necessary[4-6]
Avoidance of epinephrine impregnated retraction cord, possible use of Afrin or Visine on plain cord
Avoidance of anticholinergics (e.g., scopolamine and atropine)
Adequate postoperative pain control

*Stable angina or longer than 1 month since myocardial infarction.

becomes necessary, additional management recommendations may include establishing and maintaining an intravenous line, continuously monitoring the electrocardiogram and vital signs, using a pulse oximeter, and administering nitroglycerin prophylactically just before the initiation of treatment. These measures may require the patient be treated in a special patient care facility or hospital dental clinic.

The use of vasoconstrictors in local anesthetic poses potential problems for patients with ischemic heart disease because of the possiblities of precipitating cardiac tachycardias, arrhythmias, and increases in blood pressure. Local anesthetic without vasoconstrictor can be used as needed. If vasoconstrictor is necessary, patients with low to intermediate risk and those taking nonselective beta-blockers can safely be given up to 0.036 mg epinephrine (2 cartridges containing 1:100,000 epi) or 0.20 mg levonordefrin, 2 cartridges containing 1:20,000 levo); intravascular injections are avoided. Greater quan-

tities of vasoconstrictor increase the risk of adverse cardiovascular effects. For patients at higher risk, the use of vasoconstrictors should be discussed with the physician. Studies have shown that modest amounts of vasoconstrictor can be used safely in high-risk patients when accompanied by oxygen, sedation, nitroglycerin, and excellent pain-control measures.[38-40]

For patients at all levels of cardiac risk, the use of gingival retraction cord impregnated with epinephrine should be avoided because of the rapid absorption of a high concentration of epinephrine and the resulting adverse cardiovascular effects. As an alternative, plain cord saturated with either tetrahydrozoline HCl, 0.05% (Visine), or oxymetazoline HCl, 0.05% (Afrin), provides the equivalent gingival effects of epinephrine without the adverse cardiovascular effects.[41]

A question as to the necessity for antibiotic prophylaxis for bacterial endocarditis or endarteritis often arises for patients who have undergone revascularization procedures, specifically percutaneous transluminal coronary angioplasty with placement of a stent or coronary artery bypass graft surgery. In its 1997 recommendations for the prevention of bacterial endocarditis, the American Heart Association[42] concluded that antibiotic prophylaxis was not recommended for patients with previous coronary artery bypass graft surgery. Coronary artery stents were not addressed. However, a recent article by three members of the American Heart Association Committee on Bacterial Endocarditis[43] suggested that antibiotic prophylaxis was not necessary if 6 months or longer had elapsed since the surgery. This 6-month period may be overly conservative in that stents become covered with endothelium within about 2 to 4 weeks; therefore the risk of endocarditis or endarteritis is greatly diminished after this period. A more reasonable approach may be to postpone elective dental care for 4 to 6 weeks after percutaneous transluminal coronary angioplasty and stent placement after which time antibiotics are not indicated.

Patients taking aspirin or another platelet aggregation antagonist can expect some increase in bleeding, but this is generally not clinically significant and the bleeding can be controlled with local measures. Discontinuation of these agents before dental treatment generally is unnecessary.[44-48] Bleeding time or platelet aggregation studies can be performed before invasive procedures if desired.

MYOCARDIAL INFARCTION

Patients who have had an MI have some degree of residual damage to the heart. The condition depends on the extent and location of the damage and its effect on the

function of the heart. Damage may be minimal, with little effect on the patient's daily activity. The patient also may receive a good prognosis. Patients who have had an MI within the previous month with residual ischemic symptoms or signs are classified as a *major cardiac risk* (ASA IV). Patients with a past history of an MI longer than 1 month who are clinically stable are classified as being an *intermediate cardiac risk* (ASA II or III) and, in most cases are at minimal risk for routine dental treatment. However, myocardial damage may be extensive, resulting in cardiac instability and an inability of the heart to function properly (i.e., heart failure). These patients are classified as a *major cardiac risk* (ASA IV) and pose a significant risk for the provision of routine dental care. The management recommendations also are applicable to patients with a past history of an MI (see Box 5-5).

The dentist should know when the patient had an MI because for several weeks after the incident the risk for cardiac instability, arrhythmias, and reinfarction may be increased. These effects decrease with time, assuming the electric conduction system of the heart has not been seriously damaged. In the past most authorities suggested not providing elective dental care for the first 6 months after an MI because of the above-cited risks. This recommendation stems from three studies from the late 1960s and 1970s that examined the reinfarction rates for patients who had had an MI and were undergoing emergency or elective surgery under general anesthesia.[49-51] These studies reported reinfarction rates of 27% to 37% during the first 3 months, 11% to 26% during the next 3 to 6 months, and 4% to 5% for 6 months and longer. These cases involved general surgery, including abdominal and thoracic procedures, under general anesthesia. Subsequent studies[50,52] of similar patients under similar conditions have reported much lower reinfarction rates of approximately 4% to 6% for the first 3 months, 0% to 2% for 3-6 months, and 2% to 6% for 6 months and longer. Currently the American College of Cardiology National Database Library[53] defines *recent* MI as longer than 7 days but less than or equal to 1 month (30 days).

An examination of the reinfarction rate when only local anesthesia is used finds the risk reduced further. Backer[54] reported on 195 patients with past MIs of various time periods who underwent ophthalmic surgery under local anesthetic. None of these patients were reported to have developed perioperative or postoperative reinfarction. Three studies have described the performance of a variety of dental procedures using local anesthesia on 129 patients with either recent MI or unstable angina, with no significant adverse effects.[38-40] Local anesthesia with vasoconstrictor was used in conjunction with sedation and close monitoring in all cases. Thus many patients recovering from a recent MI or who have unstable

angina can undergo dental treatment if necessary. Delaying elective treatment for at least 1 month after an uncomplicated MI is recommended. Again, risk assessment must be made as a precursor to decision making. Consultation with the physician is advisable. Patients with post-infarction disability or heart failure face significant risk and should delay elective care. If care becomes necessary, it should be provided (Box 5-6).

Patients taking aspirin or another platelet aggregation antagonist can expect some increase in bleeding. This effect generally is not clinically significant, and bleeding can be controlled with local measures. Discontinuation of these agents before dental treatment generally is unnecessary. Bleeding time or platelet aggregation studies can be performed before invasive procedures if desired. Patients taking Coumadin for anticoagulation need current International Normalized Ratio or values before any invasive procedure. Most dental procedures, including minor surgery, may be performed safely without altering the Coumadin dosage as long as the International Normalized Ratio is 3.5 or less, or the prothrombin time is 2.5 or less.[55,56] Local hemostatic measures generally are adequate to control bleeding. More extensive procedures associated with potentially more significant blood loss should be discussed with the patient's physician.

ORAL COMPLICATIONS AND MANIFESTATIONS

No lesions or oral complications are the direct result of coronary atherosclerotic heart disease. Drugs used in the treatment of this disease and its complications, however,

may result in oral changes such as dry mouth, taste changes, and stomatitis. Patients taking Dicumarol or aspirin can have increased bleeding after trauma or surgical procedures.

In rare cases patients with coronary atherosclerotic heart disease with angina may have pain referred to the lower jaw or teeth. The pattern of the onset of pain caused by physical activity and its disappearance with rest usually will serve as clues to its cardiac origin.

References

1. Thom TJ, et al: Incidence, prevalence, and mortality of cardiovascular diseases in the United States. In Alexander RW, et al, editors: *Hurst's the heart, arteries and veins*, vol 1, ed 9, New York, 1998, McGraw-Hill.
2. Joint National Committee on Prevention Detection, Evaluation, and Treatment of High Blood Pressure: The sixth report of the Joint National Committee on Prevention, Detection, Evaluation, and Treatment of High Blood Pressure, *Arch Intern Med* 157:2413-2444, 1997.
3. National Heart, Lung, and Blood Institute US Department of Health and Human Services: Morbidity and mortality chartbook on cardiovascular, lung, and blood diseases/1996, *Morb Mort Chart Cardio Dis*, 1996.
4. Gordon R, Kannel WB: Premature mortality from coronary artery heart disease: the Framingham study, *JAMA* 215:1617-1625, 1971.
5. Pitt B, et al: Myocardial infarction. In Harvey A, editor: *Osler's principles and practice of medicine*, ed 19, New York, 1976, Appleton-Century-Crofts.
6. Silber EM, Katz LM: *Heart disease*, New York, 1975, McMillan.
7. Strong J, Solberg L, Restrepo C: Atherosclerosis in persons with coronary heart disease, *Lab Invest* 18:527-537, 1968.
8. Libby P: Atherosclerosis. In Fauci AS, et al, editors: *Harrison's principles of internal medicine*, vol 1, ed 14, New York, 1998, McGraw-Hill.
9. Ross R: Factors influencing atherogenesis. In Alexander RW, et al, editors: *Hurst's the heart, arteries and veins*, vol 1, ed 9, New York, 1998, McGraw-Hill, 1998.
10. Becker DM, Becker LC, Pearson TA: Risk factors in siblings of people with premature coronary heart disease, *J Am Coll Card* 12:1273-1280, 1988.
11. Jorde LB, Williams RR: Relation between family history of coronary heart disease and coronary risk variables, *Am J Cardiol* 62:708-713, 1988.
12. Sinaiko AR, Wells TG: Childhood hypertension. In Laragh JH, Brenner BM, editors: *Hypertension*, vol 2, New York, 1990, Raven Press.
13. Vliestra RE, et al: Effect of cigarette smoking on survival of patients with angiographically documented coronary artery disease, *JAMA* 255:1023-1027, 1986.
14. Kannel WB: Hypertension, blood lipids, and cigarette smoking as co-risk factors for coronary heart disease, *Ann NY Acad Sci* 304:128-139, 1978.
15. Kleinman JC, et al: Mortality among diabetics in a national health sample, *Am J Epidemiol* 128:389-401, 1988.
16. DeStefano F, et al: Dental disease and risk of coronary heart disease and mortality, *BMJ* 306:688-691, 1993.
17. Mattila KJ, et al: Dental infection and the risk of new coronary events, *Clin Infect Dis* 20:588-592, 1995.
18. Joshipura KJ, et al: Poor oral health and coronary heart disease, *J Dent Res* 75:1631-1636, 1996.
19. Beck JD, et al: Periodontal disease and cardiovascular disease, *J Periodontol* 67:1123-1137, 1996.
20. Beck JD, et al: Dental infections and atherosclerosis, *Am Heart J* 138:S528-S533, 1999.
21. Chambless L, et al: Association of coronary heart disease incidence with carotid arterial wall thickness and major risk factors: the atherosclerosis risk in communities (ARIC) study, 1987-1993, *Am J Epidemiol* 146:483-494, 1997.
22. Ross R: The pathogenesis of atherosclerosis: a perspective for the 1990's, *Nature* 362:801-809, 1993.
23. Stary HC, et al: A definition of advanced types of atherosclerotic lesions and a histologic classification of atherosclerosis: a report from the Committee on Vascular Lesions of the Council on Atherosclerosis, *Circulation* 92:1355-1374, 1995.
24. Davies MJ: Pathology of coronary atherosclerosis. In Alexander RW, et al, editors: *Hurst's the heart, arteries and veins*, vol 1, New York, 1998, McGraw-Hill.
25. Selwyn AP, Braunwald E: Ischemic heart disease. In Fauci AS, et al, editors: *Harrison's principles of internal medicine*, vol 1, ed 14, New York, 1998, McGraw-Hill.
26. Alexander RW, Pratt CM, Roberts R: Diagnosis and management of patients with acute myocardial infarction. In Alexander RW, et al, editors: *Hurst's the heart, arteries and veins*, vol 1, New York, 1998, McGraw-Hill.
27. Antman EM, Braunwald E: Acute myocardial infarction. In Fauci AS, et al, editors: *Harrison's principles of internal medicine*, vol 1, ed 14, New York, 1998, McGraw-Hill.
28. Engelstein ED, Zipes DP: Sudden cardiac death. In Alexander RW, et al, editors: *Hurst's the heart, arteries and veins*, vol 1, ed 14, New York, 1998, McGraw-Hill.
29. Myerburg RJ, Castellanos A: Cardiovascular collapse, cardiac arrest, and sudden death. In Fauci AS, et al, editors: *Harrison's principles of internal medicine*, vol 1, ed 14, New York, 1998, McGraw-Hill.
30. Schlant RC, Alexander RW: Diagnosis and management of patients with chronic ischemic heart disease. In Alexander RW, et al, editors: *Hurst's the heart, arteries and veins*, vol 1, ed 9, New York, 1998, McGraw-Hill.
31. Roberts R, et al: Multicenter blinded trial utilizing multiple diagnostic markers to exclude myocardial infarction in patients presenting consecutively to the ER with chest pain (abstract), *Circulation* 94:I-322, 1996.
32. Theroux P, Waters D: Diagnosis and management of patients with unstable angina. In Alexander RW, et al, editors: *Hurst's the heart, arteries and veins*, vol 1, ed 9, New York, 1998, McGraw-Hill.
33. Baim DS, Grossman W: Coronary angioplasty and other therapeutic applications of cardiac catheterization. In Fauci AS, editor: *Harrison's principles of internal medicine*, vol 1, ed 14, New York, 1998, McGraw-Hill.

34. Sigwart U, et al: Intravascular stents to prevent occlusion and restenosis after transluminal angioplasty, N *Engl* J *Med* 316:701-706, 1987.

35. Rogers GP, et al: The coronary artery response to implantation of a balloon-expandable stent in the aspirin and non-aspirin treated swine model, *Am Heart* J 122:640-647, 1991.

36. Sirnes PA, et al: Sustained benefit of stenting chronic coronary occlusion: long-term clinical follow-up of the stenting in chronic coronary occlusion (SICCO) study, J *Am Coll Cardiol* 32:305-310, 1998.

37. Lincoff AM, et al: Complimentary clinical benefits of coronary artery stenting and blockade of platelet glycoprotein IIb/IIIa receptors: evaluation of platelet IIb/IIIa inhibition in stenting investigations, N *Engl* J *Med* 341:319-327, 1999.

38. Cintron G, et al: Cardiovascular effects and safety of dental anesthesia and dental interventions in patients with recent uncomplicated myocardial infarction, *Arch Int Med* 146:2203-2204, 1986.

39. Findler M, Galili D, Meidan Z: Dental treatment in very high risk patients with active ischemic heart disease, *Oral Surg Oral Med Oral Pathol* 76:298-300, 1993.

40. Niwa H, Sato Y, Matsuura H: Safety of dental treatment in patients with previously diagnosed acute myocardial infarction or unstable angina pectoris, *Oral Surg Oral Med Oral Pathol Oral Radiol Endod* 89:35-41, 2000.

41. Bowles WH, Tardy SJ, Vahadi A: Evaluation of new gingival retraction agents, J *Dent Res* 70:1447-1449, 1991.

42. Dajani AS, et al: Prevention of bacterial endocarditis: recommendations by the American Heart Association, *Clin Infect Dis* 25:1448-1458, 1997.

43. Pallasch TJ, Gage TW, Taubert KA: The 1997 prevention of bacterial endocarditis recommendations by the American Heart Association: questions and answers, J *Calif Dent Assoc* 27:393-399, 1999.

44. Alexander RE: Eleven myths of dentoalveolar surgery, J *Am Dent Assoc* 129:1271-1279, 1998.

45. Pawlak DF, et al: Clinical effects of aspirin and acetaminophen on hemostasis after exodontics, J *Oral Sur* 36:944-947, 1978.

46. Ferraris VA, Swanson E: Aspirin usage and perioperative blood loss in patients undergoing unexpected operations, *Surg Gynecol Obstet* 156:439-442, 1983.

47. Amrein PC, Ellman L, Harris WH: Aspirin-induced prolongation of bleeding time and perioperative blood loss, JAMA 245:1825-1828, 1981.

48. Sharis PJ, Cannon CP, Loscalzo J: The antiplatelet effects of ticlopidine and clopidogrel, *Ann Intern Med* 129:394-405, 1998.

49. Tarhan S, et al: Myocardial infarction after general anesthesia, JAMA 220:1451-1454, 1972.

50. Rao TLK, Kurt HJ, El-Etr AA: Reinfarction following anesthesia in patients with myocardial infarction, *Anesthesiology* 59:499-505, 1983.

51. Steen PA, Tinker JH, Tarhan S: Myocardial reinfarction after anesthesia and surgery, JAMA 239:2566-2570, 1978.

52. Shah KB, et al: Reevaluation of perioperative myocardial infarction in patients with prior myocardial infarction undergoing noncardiac operations, *Anesth Anal* 71:231-235, 1990.

53. Eagle KA, et al: Guidelines for perioperative cardiovascular evaluation for noncardiac surgery, J *Am Coll Cardiol* 27:910-948, 1996.

54. Backer CL, et al: Myocardial reinfarction following local anesthesia for ophthalmic surgery, *Anesth Anal* 59:257-262, 1980.

55. Wahl MJ: Myths of dental surgery in patients receiving anticoagulant therapy, J *Am Dent Assoc* 131:77-81, 2000.

56. Campbell JH, Alvarado F, Murray RA: Anticoagulation and minor oral surgery: should the anticoagulation regimen be altered? J *Oral Maxillofac Surg* 58:131-135, 2000.

Cardiac Arrhythmias

CHAPTER 6

Various forms of cardiac arrhythmias are present in a significant percentage of the population seeking dental treatment.[1-5] Some arrhythmias are of little concern to the patient or dentist; however, many can produce symptoms and a few can be life threatening, These include arrhythmias that occur because of anxiety associated with dental care.[6] Therefore patients with significant arrhythmias must be identified before undergoing dental treatment.

Cardiac arrhythmias may be found in normal, healthy individuals; those taking various medications; and those with certain cardiovascular conditions as well as other systemic diseases. The arrhythmias may be asymptomatic and even life threatening[1-6] (Box 6-1).

INCIDENCE AND PREVALENCE

A cardiac arrhythmia is any variation in the normal rhythm of the heartbeat. Cardiac arrhythmias may be disturbances of rhythm, rate, or conduction of the heart. They may be found in healthy individuals and those with various forms of cardiovascular disease[2-5] (Table 6-1).

A survey by Bialy et al[7] reported that 10.6% of all patients admitted to hospitals were diagnosed with a cardiac arrhythmia (Fig. 6-1). One of the most prevalent types is atrial fibrillation. The prevalence of atrial fibrillation in the United States is approximately 2.2 million people.[8] Little et al[4,5] found the prevalence of cardiac arrhythmias in a large population of general dental patients (more than 10,000) to be 17.2%, with more than 4% of those serious, life-threatening cardiac arrhythmias. Simmons et al[9] reported in a study of more than 2300 dental healthcare professionals the prevalence of 15.6% and just more than 4% as serious arrhythmias. In a study of dental and dental hygiene students, Rhodus and Little[10] found similar figures, with the prevalence of 15.3% and 1.7% with serious, life-threatening cardiac arrhythmias.

Furberg et al[3] estimate the overall prevalence of cardiac arrhythmia in the United States to be approximately 10% based on data from the 1993 Cardiovascular Health Study from the National Heart, Lung, and Blood Institute.

Various drugs may cause cardiac arrhythmias.[2,6,11] Digitalis, morphine, beta-blockers, and calcium channel blockers can induce sinus bradycardia. Atropine, epinephrine, nicotine, and caffeine can cause sinus tachycardia. Alcohol, tobacco, digitalis, tricyclic antidepressants, and coffee may precipitate premature atrial beats in normal individuals. Digitalis, alcohol, epinephrine, and amphetamines may cause ventricular extrasystoles in healthy individuals. Digitalis, quinidine, procainamide, potassium, and sympathetic amines may induce ventricular tachycardia in patients with cardiovascular disease.

Cardiac arrhythmias may be associated with various systemic diseases (Table 6-2). Pathologic sinus bradycardia may be found in patients with febrile illnesses, myxedema, obstructive jaundice, increased intracranial pressure, and myocardial infarction. Pathologic sinus tachycardia may be found in patients with fever, infection, hyperthyroidism, and anemia. Atrial extrasystoles may occur in patients with congestive heart failure, coronary insufficiency, and myocardial infarction. Supraventricular

---

BOX 6-1

Causes of Cardiac Arrhythmias

Primary cardiovascular disease
Pulmonary disorders
Autonomic disorders
Systemic diseases
Drug-related side effects
Electrolyte imbalances

TABLE 6-1

Incidence of Cardiac Arrhythmias in Healthy Individuals

Type of Arrhythmia	Population Group	Number	Percentage
Sinus bradycardia	Healthy children (7-11 years)	45,000	1.0
	Aviators (20-30 years)	380	38
	6014 Air Force personnel	902 to 1683	15-28
Sinus tachycardia	1000 Aviators (20-30 years)	3	0.3
Paroxysmal atrial tachycardia	98 Healthy men and women (60-85 years)	13	13.3
Atrial flutter	98 Healthy men and women (60-85 years)	1	1.0
	67,000 Air Force personnel	1	0.001
Atrioventricular block (first-degree)	19,000 Air crew applicants	59	0.3
	67,000 Air Force personnel	350	0.5
Atrial and ventricular extrasystoles	300 Men (middle aged)		62
	Boys (10-13 years)		13-26
	Women (22-28 years)		54-64
	Men and women (60-85 years)		80
Ventricular tachycardia	67,000 Air Force personnel	1	0.001
	98 Healthy men and women (60-85 years)	4	4.0

Data from Marriott H, Myerberg RJ: Recognition, clinical assessment, and management of arrhythmias. In Hurst JW, editor: *The heart, arteries, and veins*, ed 6, New York, 1986, McGraw-Hill.

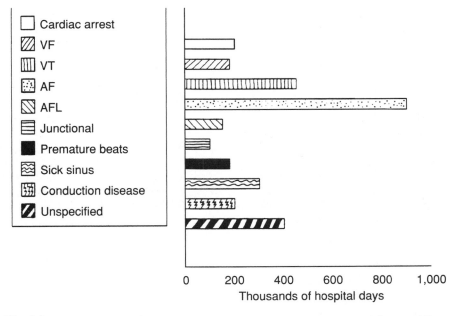

Fig. 6-1 Estimated number of hospital days with cardiac arrhythmia as the principal diagnosis. *VF*, ventricular fibrillation; *VT*, ventricular tachycardia; *AF*, atrial fibrillation; *AFL*, atrial flutter. (From Bialy D et al: Hospitalization for arrhythmias in the United States: importance of atrial fibrillation *J Am Coll Cardiol* 19:41, 1992.)

TABLE 6-2

Cardiac Arrhythmias Associated with Various Systemic Diseases

Arrhythmia	Systemic Condition
Sinus bradycardia	Infectious diseases, hypothermia, myxedema, obstructive jaundice, increased cranial pressure, myocardial infarction
Atrial extrasystoles	Congestive heart failure, coronary insufficiency, myocardial infarction
Sinoatrial block	Rheumatic heart disease, myocardial infarction, acute infections
Sinus tachycardia	Febrile illness, infections, anemia, hyperthyroidism
Atrial tachycardia	Obstructive lung disease, pneumonia, myocardial infarction
Atrial flutter	Ischemic heart disease, mitral stenosis, myocardial infarction, open-heart surgery
Atrial fibrillation	Myocardial infarction, mitral stenosis, ischemic heart disease, thyrotoxicosis, hypertension
Atrioventricular block	Rheumatic heart disease, ischemic heart disease, myocardial infarction, hyperthyroidism, Hodgkin's disease, myeloma, open heart surgery
Ventricular extrasystole	Ischemic heart disease, congestive heart failure, mitral valve prolapse
Ventricular tachycardia	Mitral valve prolapse, myocardial infarction, coronary atherosclerotic heart disease
Ventricular fibrillation	Blunt cardiac trauma, mitral valve prolapse, anaphylaxis, cardiac surgery, rheumatic heart disease, cardiomyopathy, coronary atherosclerotic heart disease

tachycardias have been reported in about 6% of individuals with mitral valve prolapse and may be found in patients with pneumonia or acute myocardial infarction.[6] Atrial flutter may be found in patients with ischemic heart disease and complicates 2% to 5% of myocardial infarction cases.[8] Atrial fibrillation may be found associated with rheumatic mitral disease, hypertension, ischemic heart disease, or thyrotoxicosis.[11]

Ventricular extrasystoles are the most common form of rhythm disturbance found in patients with ischemic heart disease and congestive heart failure. They also occur in approximately 45% of individuals with mitral valve prolapse.[11] Ventricular tachycardia almost always is associated with a diseased heart and has been reported in 6% of patients with mitral valve prolapse and 28% to 46% of monitored patients with myocardial infarction.[8] Ventricular fibrillation is a terminal arrhythmia unless rapid and effective therapy is given. It may be precipitated by coronary atherosclerotic heart disease, cardiomyopathy of any origin, rheumatic heart disease, blunt cardiac trauma, mitral valve prolapse, cardiac surgery, and cardiac catheterization.[2,6,11]

ETIOLOGY

The primary pacemaker for the heart is the sinoatrial (SA) node, a crescent-shaped structure 9 to 15 mm long lo-

cated at the junction of the superior vena cava and the right atrium. The SA node regulates the functions of the atria and results in the production of the P wave on the electrocardiogram (ECG). Impulses generated by the SA node result in a normal rhythm of 60 to 100 beats per minute. Secondary pacemakers are present and include atrial, atrioventricular (AV), and ventricular escape pacemakers.[2,10-14]

The impulse generated by the SA node usually is conducted in the following sequence: (1) SA node, (2) AV node, (3) bundle of His, (4) bundle branches, and (5) subendocardial Purkinje network (Fig. 6-2). The ECG is a record of the electrical activity of the heart (Figs. 6-3, 6-4, and 6-5).

The AV node serves as a gate, preventing too many atrial impulses from entering the ventricle. It also slows the conduction rate of impulses generated in the SA node. Normal cardiac function depends on cellular automaticity (impulse formation), conductivity, excitability, and contractility. Disorders in automaticity and conductivity form the basis of the vast majority of cardiac arrhythmias. Under normal conditions the SA node is responsible for impulse formation; however, other cells in the conduction system can generate impulses. Under abnormal conditions, ectopic pacemakers can emerge outside the conduction system. After the generation of a normal impulse and its discharge, the cells of the SA node need time for recovery

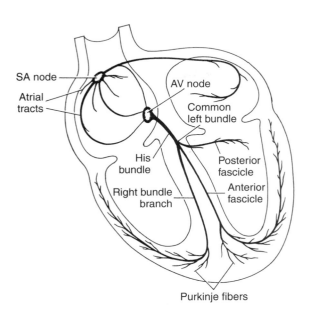

Fig. 6-2 The conduction system. (From Hurst C: *Dysrhythmia interpretation based on cardiac suppression and irritability*, Philadelphia, JB Lippincott, 1986.)

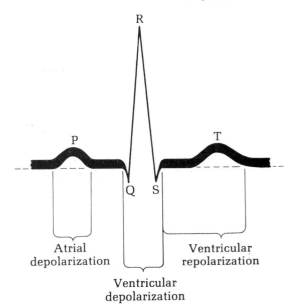

Fig. 6-3 Normal electrocardiographic deflections. The normal electrocardiogram consists of a P wave, representing atrial depolarization; a QRS complex representing ventricular depolarization, and a T wave representing rapid repolarization of the ventricles. (From Conover MB: *Understanding electrocardiography: arrhythmias and the 12-lead ECG*, ed 6, St Louis, 1992, Mosby.)

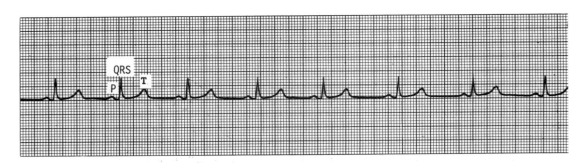

Fig. 6-4 Cardiac cycle. The basic P-QRS-T cycle repeats. (From Goldberger AL, Goldberger E: *Clinical electrocardiography: a simplified approach*, ed 4, St Louis, 1990, Mosby.)

in what is termed *refractoriness*. Complete refractoriness results in a block and partial refractoriness in a delay of conductivity.[2,6,12-15]

Disorders of conductivity (block or delay) paradoxically can lead to a rapid cardiac rhythm through the mechanisms of reentry. The type of arrhythmia may suggest the nature of its cause. For example, paroxysmal atrial tachycardia with block suggests digitalis toxic-

ity.[1,10] However, many cardiac arrhythmias are not specific for a given cause. In these patients a careful search is made to identify the etiology of the arrhythmia. The most common causes include primary cardiovascular disorders, pulmonary disorders (embolism, hypoxia), autonomic disorders, systemic disorders (thyroid disease), drug-related side effects, and electrolyte imbalances (see Box 6-1).

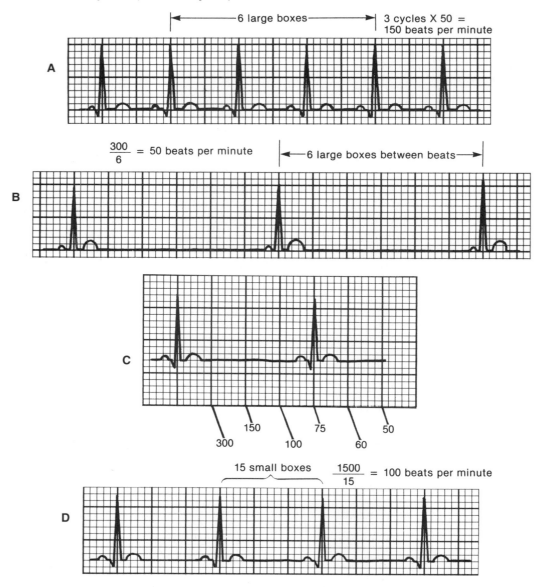

Fig. 6-5 Methods of determining heart rate. The rates shown (in beats per minute) are **A,** 150; **B,** 50; **C,** 75; **D,** 100. (From Johnson R, Swartz MH: *Simplified approach to electrocardiography,* Philadelphia, 1986, WB Saunders.)

PATHOPHYSIOLOGY AND COMPLICATIONS

Arrhythmias may be asymptomatic and cause no hemodynamic changes. However, some can affect cardiac output by producing insufficient forward flow because of a slow cardiac rate, reducing forward flow because of insufficient diastolic filling time with a rapid cardiac rate, and decreasing flow because of poor sequence in AV activation with direct effects on ventricular function.[2,16]

The effect of an arrhythmia often depends on the physical condition of the patient. For example, a young healthy person with paroxysmal atrial tachycardia may have minimal symptoms whereas an elderly patient who has heart disease with the same arrhythmia may develop shock, congestive heart failure, or myocardial ischemia.[2,3,4,12,17]

Types of Cardiac Arrhythmias

Isolated ectopic beats
  Premature atrial beats
  Premature atrioventricular beats
  Premature ventricular beats
Bradycardias
  Sinus bradycardia
  Sinoatrial heart block
  Atrioventricular heart block
Tachycardias
  Sinus tachycardia
  Atrial tachycardia

Atrial flutter
Atrial fibrillation
Ventricular tachycardia
Preexcitation syndrome
Cardiac arrest
  Ventricular fibrillation
  Ventricular asystole
  Agonal rhythm

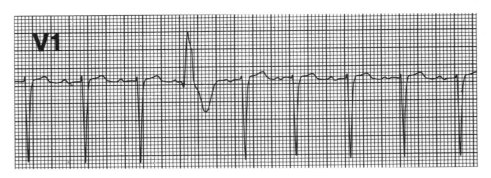

Fig. 6-6 Ventricular premature contraction. Note that this wide complex comes prematurely compared with the next sinus P wave. (From Johnson R, Swartz MH: *A simplified approach to electrocardiography,* Philadelphia, 1986, WB Saunders.)

Evidence indicates that patients with certain types of cardiac arrhythmias (e.g., atrial fibrillation) are more susceptible to ischemic events in the dental office.[18]

Arrhythmias can be classified into the following: isolated ectopic beats, bradycardias, tachycardias, preexcitation syndrome, and cardiac arrest (Box 6-2). They also may be categorized according to the site of origin (i.e., atrial, supraventricular, ventricular).

ISOLATED ECTOPIC BEATS

Isolated ectopic beats include the following forms:
Premature atrial beats—Premature impulses arising from ectopic foci anywhere in the atrium may result in premature atrial beats. They are common in conditions associated with dysfunction of the atria such as congestive heart failure.
Premature AV beats—Premature AV beats are less common than premature atrial or premature ventricular ectopic beats. Impulses can spread toward either the

atria or the ventricles. When they are present, digitalis toxicity should be suspected.
Premature ventricular beats—Premature ventricular beats are the most common form of arrhythmia, regardless of whether heart disease exists. In one study[11] more than 50% of middle-aged men and up to 80% of people between ages 60 and 85 were found to have premature ventricular beats. Approximately 80% of patients with myocardial infarction have premature ventricular beats.[2] They also are common with digitalis toxicity and hypokalemia. Late premature ventricular beats can lead to ventricular tachycardia or fibrillation in the presence of ischemia. More than 6 late premature ventricular beats per minute may be an indication of cardiac instability (Fig. 6-6).

BRADYCARDIAS

Bradycardias can be classified into the following:
Sinus bradycardia—A sinus rate of less than 60 beats

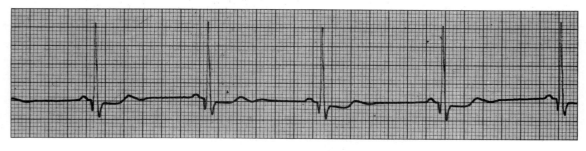

Fig. 6-7 Sinus bradycardia. In this tracing, the sinus rate is 50 beats per minute. (From Conover MB: *Understanding electrocardiography: arrhythmias and the 12-lead ECG*, ed 6, St Louis, 1992, Mosby.)

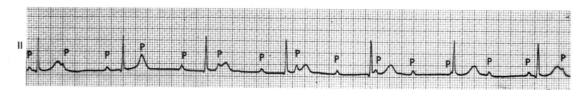

Fig. 6-8 Complete heart block is characterized by independent atrial *(P)* and ventricular *(QRS)* activity. The atrial rate is always faster than the ventricular rate. PR intervals are completely variable. Some P waves fall on the T wave, distorting the shape of the T wave. Others fall in the QRS complex and are "lost." Note that the QRS complexes are of normal width, indicating that the ventricles are being paced from the AV junction. (From Goldberger AL, Goldberger E: *Clinical electrocardiography: a simplified approach*, ed 4, St Louis, 1990, Mosby.)

per minute is defined as *bradycardia*.[2,6,11] Bradycardia is a normal finding in young, healthy adults and well-conditioned athletes and can occur secondary to medication use. Medications with parasympathetic effects such as digoxin and phenothiazines may slow the heart rate. In addition, medications that suppress the excitability of the heart such as beta-adrenergic blockers (e.g., propranolol, metoprolol) may cause bradycardia.[13,14] A sinus bradycardia that persists in the presence of congestive heart failure, pain, or exercise and follows atropine administration is considered abnormal. Sinus bradycardia is a common finding early in myocardial infarction. It also may occur in infectious diseases, myxedema, obstructive jaundice, and hypothermia (Fig. 6-7).

SA heart block—SA heart block is relatively uncommon. Most cases are caused by rheumatic heart disease, myocardial infarction, acute infection, or drug toxicity (digitalis, atropine, salicylates, quinidine). The block may occur in stages or degrees; in first-degree block an impulse takes undue time to enter the atrium; in second-degree block one or more impulses fail to emerge from the SA node; and in complete block no impulses emerge from the SA node.

AV heart block—Rheumatic fever, ischemic heart disease, myocardial infarction, hyperthyroidism, and drugs (digitalis, propranolol, potassium, quinidine) may cause AV heart block. Approximately 50% of the cases are associated with congenital heart disease.[5] AV block also occurs in degrees: the first-degree stage features slow impulses with increased conduction time; in second-degree block some impulses fail to reach the ventricles; and no impulses reach the ventricles in third-degree or complete heart block. Sarcoidosis, Hodgkin's disease, myeloma, and open-heart surgery (aortic valve, ventricular septal defects) also may result in complete heart block (Fig. 6-8).

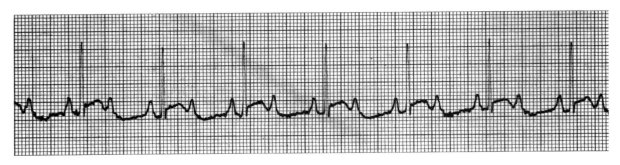

Fig. 6-9 Atrial tachycardia with 2:1 AV conduction. (From Conover MB: *Understanding electrocardiography: arrhythmias and the 12-lead ECG,* ed 6, St Louis, 1992, Mosby.)

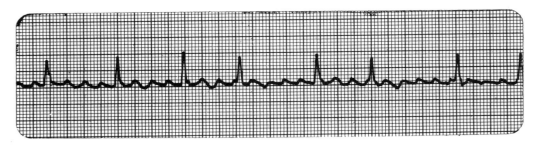

Fig. 6-10 Variable ventricular rate of a patient with atrial flutter. (From Goldberger AL, Goldberger E: *Clinical electrocardiography: a simplified approach,* ed 4, St Louis, 1990, Mosby.)

TACHYCARDIAS

Tachycardias consist of the following types:

Sinus tachycardia—A sinus rate greater than 100 beats per minute is defined as *sinus tachycardia*.[2,6,11] The condition is caused most often by a physiologic response to exercise, anxiety, stress, and emotions. Pharmacologic causes of sinus tachycardia include atropine, epinephrine, nicotine, and caffeine. Pathologic causes are fever, hypoxia, infections, anemia, and hyperthyroidism.

Atrial tachycardia—In atrial tachycardia, ectopic impulses may result in atrial rates of 150 to 200 per minute.[2] Often some degree of AV block with ectopic atrial tachycardia occur in approximately 75% of cases, digitalis toxicity or hypokalemia is present.[11] Atrial tachycardia also is seen in some cases of chronic obstructive lung disease, advanced pathology of the atria, acute myocardial infarction, pneumonia, and drug intoxications (alcohol, catechols)[2,6,11] (Fig. 6-9).

Atrial flutter—A rapid, regular atrial rate of 220 to 360 beats per minute is defined as *atrial flutter*, which is rare in healthy individuals and most often associated with ischemic heart disease in people over age 40.[2] It complicates approximately 2% to 5% of the cases of myocardial infarction and is a rare complication of digitalis intoxication.[11] Atrial flutter also is seen as a complication in patients with mitral stenosis or cor pulmonale and after open-heart surgery. It may result when patients with atrial fibrillation have been treated with quinidine or procainamide (Fig. 6-10).

Atrial fibrillation—Atrial fibrillation is a common arryhthmia characterized by an extremely rapid atrial rate of 400 to 650 beats per minute with no discrete P waves on the ECG tracing.[1,2] The ventricular response is irregular because only a portion of the impulses pass through the AV node. Atrial fibrillation may be found in healthy individuals, although the condition usually is associated with rheumatic heart disease, hypertension, ischemic heart disease, or thyrotoxicosis. It is more common than the other forms of atrial tachyarrhythmias and occurs in between 7% and 16% of patients with myocardial infarction. It also is found in approximately 90% of people with mitral stenosis who have had peripheral emboli.[1,11]

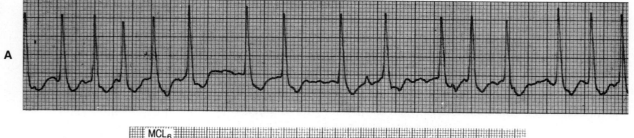

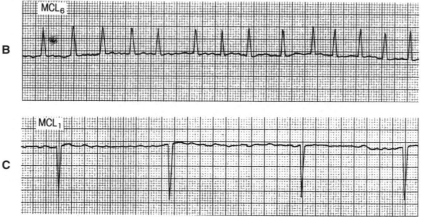

Fig. 6-11 A, Atrial fibrillation with an uncontrolled ventricular response and a fine fibrillatory line. (From Conover MB: *Understanding electrocardiography: arrhythmias and the 12-lead ECG,* ed 6, St Louis, 1992, Mosby.) **B,** Atrial fibrillation with a rapid ventricular response. **C,** Atrial fibrillation with a slow ventricular response. Chaotic atrial activity is demonstrated by the undulating baseline. (**B** and **C** from Guzzetta CE, Dossey BM: *Cardiovascular nursing: holistic practice,* ed 2, St Louis, 1992, Mosby.)

Two major hemodynamic events occur with atrial fibrillation: (1) poor atrial transport of blood and (2) generation of impulses that excite rapid and irregular ventricular response. A secondary complication of poor atrial transport of blood is peripheral or pulmonary emboli. In individuals with long-standing atrial fibrillation, 30% experience at least one embolic episode. Atrial fibrillation can precipitate congestive heart failure in patients with a history of heart disease [2,6,11] (Fig. 6-11).

Ventricular tachycardia—Three or more ectopic ventricular beats occurring at a rate of 100 or more per minute is defined as *ventricular tachycardia.* This arrhythmia almost always occurs in diseased hearts. Certain drugs such as digitalis, sympathetic amines (epinephrine), potassium, quinidine, and procainamide may induce ventricular tachycardia. On rare occasions it may be found in young, healthy adults. Ventricular tachycardia may be nonsustained or sustained, or may degenerate into ventricular fibrillation [2,6,11] (Fig. 6-12).

WOLFE-PARKINSON-WHITE PREEXCITATION SYNDROME

Three events are involved in the Wolfe-Parkinson-White preexcitation syndrome. First, an accessory AV pathway allows the normal conduction systems to be bypassed. Second, this accessory pathway allows rapid conduction and short refractoriness, with impulses being passed rapidly from atrium to ventricle. Third, the parallel conduction system provides a route for reentrant tachyarrhythmias. This pattern constitutes a syndrome when patients display symptoms from paroxysmal supraventricular tachycardia. Paroxysmal atrial fibrillation and flutter also may occur, leading to ventricular fibrillation and death. [2,6,11]

CARDIAC ARREST

Ventricular fibrillation, ventricular asystole, and agonal rhythm are the three types of arrhythmias associated with

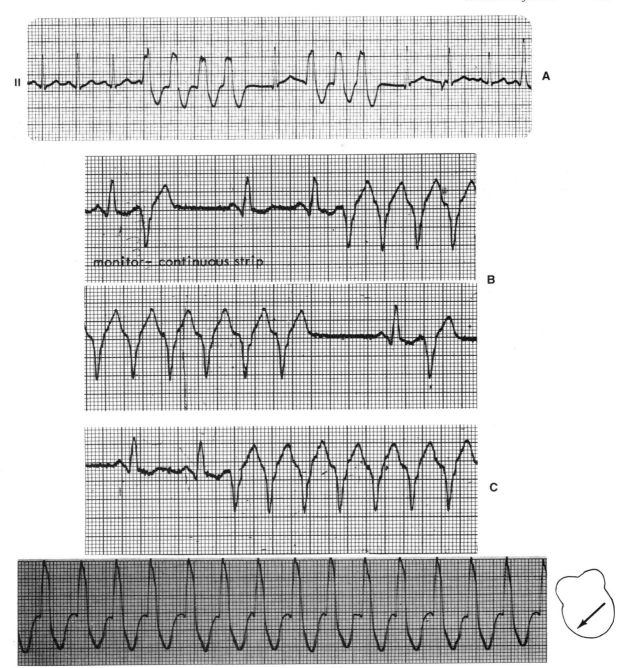

Fig. 6-12 A, Two short bursts of ventricular tachycardia, defined as three or more consecutive premature ventricular contractions. **B,** The monitor lead shows bursts of ventricular tachycardia. (**A** and **B** from Goldberger AL, Goldberger E: *Clinical electrocardiography,* ed 4, St Louis, 1990, Mosby.) **C,** Ventricular tachycardia. (**C** from Conover MB: *Understanding electrocardiography: arrhythmias and the 12-lead ECG,* ed 6, St Louis, 1992, Mosby.)

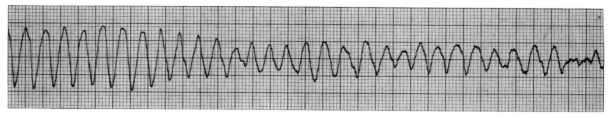

A

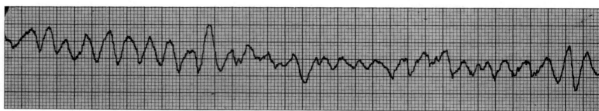

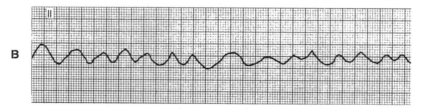

B

Fig. 6-13 A, Ventricular flutter deteriorating into ventricular fibrillation (continuous strip). (**A** from Conover MB: *Understanding electrocardiography: arrhythmias and the 12-lead ECG,* ed 6, St Louis, 1992, Mosby.) **B,** Ventricular fibrillation. **B** from Guzzetta CE, Dossey BM: *Cardiovascular nursing: holistic practice,* ed 2, St Louis, 1992, Mosby.)

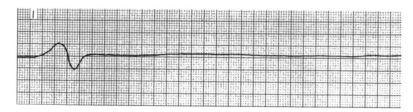

Fig. 6-14 Ventricular standstill. Note the agonal beat at the beginning of the strip. (From Guzzetta CE, Dossey BM: *Cardiovascular nursing: holistic practice,* ed 2, St Louis, 1992, Mosby.)

cardiac arrest. All are lethal. Patients with these conditions require immediate therapy for survival.

Ventricular Fibrillation
Ventricular fibrillation is represented as chaotic activity on the ECG, with the ventricles contracting rapidly but ineffectively. This usually is lethal unless therapy is administered rapidly. Coronary atherosclerosis is the most common form of heart disease predisposing to ventricular fibrillation. Other causes of this arrhythmia include rheumatic heart disease, anaphylaxis, blunt cardiac trauma, mitral valve prolapse, cardiac surgery, digitalis intoxication, and cardiac catheterization. Ventricular fibrillation is rare in young, healthy adults[2,6,11] (Fig. 6-13).

Ventricular Asystole. In ventricular asystole, cardiac standstill occurs when no impulses are conducted to the ventricles (ECG registering a flat line) and no muscular activity takes place. The conditions causing ventricular fibrillation also can lead to ventricular asystole (Fig. 6-14).

TABLE 6-3

Signs and Symptoms of Cardiac Arrhythmias

Signs	Symptoms
Slow heart (<60 beats/min)	Palpitations Fatigue Dizziness
Fast heart rate (>100 beats/min)	Syncope Congestive heart failure Angina
Irregular heart rate	Cardiac arrest

Symptoms listed can be found with any arrhythmia.

Agonal Rhythm

In agonal rhythm, effective ventricular contraction ceases. Although impulse conduction takes place, the ECG shows wide distorted complexes with no mechanical activity in the ventricles.[2,6,11,19]

CLINICAL PRESENTATION

SIGNS AND SYMPTOMS

Cardiac arrhythmias may be asymptomatic but detected because of a change in the rate or rhythm of the pulse. A slow pulse may indicate a form of bradycardia, and a fast pulse may indicate a tachyarrhythmia. Electrocardiographic monitoring is needed to identify the true nature of many cardiac arrhythmias.[2,12-16,20]

The impact of an arrhythmia on the circulation is more important than the arrhythmia itself. Symptoms that may indicate the presence of an arrhythmia include fatigue, dizziness, syncope, congestive heart failure, angina, and cardiac arrest. The patient may complain of heart palpitations.[2,6,11,12] (Table 6-3).

LABORATORY TESTS

The ECG is most helpful in identifying and diagnosing cardiac arrhythmias. Electrode catheter techniques now allow for intracavitary recordings of the specialized conducting systems, which aids greatly in the diagnosis of arrhythmias. Stress testing with monitoring commonly is used to assess an individual's cardiac status.[2]

MEDICAL MANAGEMENT

The management of cardiac arrhythmias involves medications, pacemakers, surgery, or cardioversion. Patients with asymptomatic arrhythmias usually require no therapy; those with symptomatic arrhythmias usually are treated first with medications. Generally, the molecular targets for optimal action of the drugs involve channels in the cellular membranes through which ions (Na^+, Ca^{++}, and K^+) are diffused rapidly. Various types of arrhythmias and degrees of severity are affected differently with different medications.[7] Patients who do not respond to medications then may be treated by an implanted pacemaker or cardioversion. Surgery may be attempted if both medications and pacing fail to control the arrhythmia. Cardioversion is indicated for any tachyarrhythmias that compromise hemodynamics or life. Cardiac arrest also is treated by cardioversion.[2,6,11,15,21]

Patients with atrial fibrillation often are prescribed warfarin sodium (Coumadin) to prevent atrial thrombosis. For these patients a consultation with the physician is necessary to determine the prothrombin time. If the prothrombin time ratio is 2.5 or less or the international normalized ratio is 3.5 or less, most dental treatment including minor oral surgery usually can be performed safely. However, each case must be evaluated before dental procedures that cause bleeding are performed. This involves medical consultation, possible modification of warfarin sodium dosage by the physician, and a prothrombin time test to verify that anticoagulation values are within the acceptable range (see Chapter 19).

Patients with arrhythmias medicated with digitalis are susceptible to digitalis toxicity, particularly the elderly and those who have hypothyroidism renal dysfunction, dehydration, hypokalemia hypomagnesemia, or hypocalcemia. Patients with electrolyte imbalances are more susceptible to digitalis toxicity because of the heightened sensitivity of the heart to these changes accompanying certain arrhythmias. (The clinical manifestations of digitalis toxicity are covered in Chapter 7.) Therapeutic doses of digitalis are 0.5 to 2.0 ng/ml. Levels greater than 2.5 ng/ml may result in digitalis toxicity. The dentist should monitor carefully patients' medications and dosage levels and watch for signs and symptoms of digitalis toxicity, which are found in three systems: gastrointestinal, neurologic, and cardiovascular (nearly any type of arrhythmia and cardiac conduction problems).[22]

ANTIARRHYTHMIC DRUGS

The toxic/therapeutic ratio with many antiarrhythmic drugs is narrow; therefore dosage for a patient must be individualized. Measurement of plasma levels of the medication is often an important part of therapy. The following medications are used for control of arrhythmias: digoxin, digitoxin, quinidine, procainamide, disopyramide, lidocaine, propranolol, verapamil and sotalol[2,6,11,15,22] (Table 6-4).

TABLE **6-4**

Drugs Used to Treat Cardiac Arrhythmias

Agent	Actions	Dosage	Side Effects
Digoxin	Improves the mechanical efficiency of the myocardium by slowing conduction in the AV node, prolonging refractoriness in the AV node, and decreasing the refractoriness of atrial tissue; is useful in treatment of supraventricular tachycardias, atrial flutter, and atrial fibrillation	PO 0.125-0.5 mg/day	Cardiac arrhythmias Conduction disturbances Gastrointestinal disturbances
Quinidine	Depresses automaticity arising from abnormal or ectopic locations; increases the threshold of excitability of the atrium and ventricle, slows conduction (except in the AV node, where it increases condition), and prolongs refractoriness; is used for supraventricular and ventricular arrhythmias, including atrial and ventricular premature beats, atrial flutter, and atrial fibrillation	200-600 mg every 6 hours	Diarrhea Nausea and vomiting Tinnitus Hearing loss Vertigo Thrombocytopenia Possible precipitation of ventricular tachycardia or fibrillation
Procainamide	Has same actions as Quinidine; is more effective in the treatment of ventricular arrhythmias	PO 250-750 mg every 3-4 hours	Nausea and vomiting Rarely diarrhea
Sotalol	Is a nonselective beta-blocker used to treat ventricular premature contractions and other ventricular arrhythmias; has possible additive effects with other drugs that prolong the QT interval, such as terfenadine (Seldane) and astemizole (Hismanal)	PO 80 mg twice per day	Fatigue Bradycardia Dyspnea
Propranolol	Is a nonselective beta-blocker that slows conduction and prolongs refractoriness in the AV node; is used to treat supraventricular arrhythmias	PO 20-80 mg every 6 hours	Hypotension Pulmonary vasoconstriction in patients with asthma or obstructive lung disease Possible precipitation of severe arrhythmias with sudden withdrawal in patients with ischemic heart disease, such as angina and myocardial infarction
Disopyramide	Has actions similar to Quinidine; requires caution in patients with prostatic hypertrophy or congestive heart failure and older patients with significant myocardial ischemia; is contraindicated in patients with glaucoma	PO 100-300 mg every 6 hours	Dry mouth Blurred vision Constipation
Lidocaine	Is used for emergency management of patients with serious ventricular arrhythmia, is effective in abolishing ventricular reentry impulses and has minimal effect on atrial tissues	IV 20-50 mg/min to total dose of 5 mg/kg	Dizziness Paresthesias Confusion Muscle tremors Seizures

TABLE 6-4

Drugs Used to Treat Cardiac Arrhythmias—Cont'd

Agent	Actions	Dosage	Side Effects
Verapamil	Is the drug of choice for paroxysmal atrioventricular junction tachycardias; is not used with propranolol, Disopyramide, or quinidine; possible heart block in patients with underlying abnormalities in atrioventricular node	PO 200-400 mg every 6 hours	Ankle edema Headache Palpitations Flushing Hypotension
Coumadin	Is an adjunctive drug used in patients with cardiac arrhythmias to prevent thrombosis, interference with the vitamin K dependent clotting factors (II, VII, IX, X), is particularly useful in individuals with atrial fibrillation	International normalized ratio of 2.0 to 3.0	Bleeding Skin necrosis (rare)

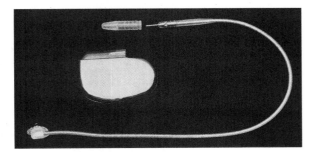

Fig. 6-15 One type of implantable pacemaker (pulse generator). This device usually is implanted subcutaneously in the right anterior side of the chest below the clavicle. (From Phipps WJ, editor: *Medical-surgical nursing,* ed 4, St Louis, 1991, Mosby.)

PACEMAKERS

In 1984 approximately 500,000 people in the United States had permanent pacemakers. That figure has more than doubled. More than 1.5 million pacemakers are in use worldwide. Approximately 100,000 new implants are performed each year. Today's pacemakers are smaller, lighter, more reliable, and longer lasting than those available 10 to 15 years ago.[14,16,20]

A pacing system consists of a generator that produces an electric impulse transmitted by a lead to an electrode in contact with endocardial or myocardial tissue. A variety of pacing systems are available. For example, the atrium and ventricle may be paced; transvenous or transmediastinal leads may be used; demand, asynchronous, or programmable pulse generators (Fig. 6-15) are available; and active or passive electrodes can be placed.[14,16,20]

Pacemakers are useful in the management of several conduction system abnormalities, including symptomatic sinus bradycardia, symptomatic AV block, and tachyarrhythmias refractory to drug therapy. The most common pacing system in use is the demand ventricular pacemaker with a lithium-powered generator and transvenous leads.[20] This pacemaker has a sensing circuit that can detect the patient's natural heartbeat and prevent competitive pacemaker firing. In addition, dual-chambered pacemakers can sense and pace both atria and ventricles. The newer units contain pacing circuits that allow for programming, memory, and telemetry.[1,14,16,20]

A classification code for modes of pacing has been developed.[12] The code shows the chamber that is paced and sensed and the mode of response. It also shows programmable functions (e.g., rate modification) and the system used for tachyarrhythmias found in the more complex pacemakers.[12] The most common pacemaker in use today has a code of VVI, which means it paces the ventricle, senses the ventricle, and is inhibited by the patient's own ventricular activity.[12]

A piezoelectric crystal bonded to the inner surface of the pulse generator detects patient movement. Increased activity causes increased pacing.[12] Some side effects can result from pacemakers. Infection at the generator site and thrombosis of the leads or electrodes are uncommon but do occur. Infective endocarditis rarely may occur. Skeletal muscle may be stimulated if insulation is lost around the lead or the generator rotates. In rare cases, myocardial burning can occur.[15,20] Some

Sources of Electromagnetic Interference

Television set	Electrocautery unit
Radio transmitter	Boat or automobile motor
Radar transmitter	Any electric motor
Arc welder	Cavitron
Microwave oven	Electric pulp tester
Diathermy unit	

patients become depressed; suicide attempts have been reported.[15,20]

Electromagnetic interference from noncardiac electrical signals may interfere temporarily with the function of a pacemaker by mimicking the frequency of spontaneous heartbeats, which causes inappropriate pacemaker inhibition. Transmission from high-powered television sets, radio and radar transmitters, arc welders are examples. Other forms of electrical signals can cause revision of the pacemaker mode to a fixed rate of transmission. Microwave ovens, ultrasonic scalers (e.g., Cavitron), certain pulp testers, diathermy and electrocautery units, defibrillators, any electric motor, and direct-contact pulse generators in boat or automobile motors can cause revision[15,20] (Box 6-3).

In a study by Miller et al[23] the only devices causing significant electromagnetic interference with pacemakers in the dental office were electrosurgery units, ultrasonic bath cleaners and ultrasonic scaling devices. Amalgamators, electric pulp testers, curing lights, handpieces, electric toothbrushes, microwave ovens, x-ray units, and sonic scalers did not cause any significant electromagnetic interference with pacemakers in the dental office. Internal shielding has been increased on the newer generators to minimize the adverse effects of electromagnetic interference. These units now are protected against adverse effects from microwave oven signals.

Certain patients with ventricular fibrillation or unstable ventricular tachycardias are candidates for an automatic implantable cardioverter-defibrillator (AICD). The AICD is a self-contained diagnostic-therapeutic system that monitors the heart. When it detects fibrillation or tachycardia of the ventricle it sends a correcting electric shock to restore normal rhythm.[10,12-17] By 1996 more than 100,000 patients worldwide had had an AICD surgically implanted (see Chapter 5).

The AICD is 99% reliable in detecting ventricular fibrillation and 98% reliable in detecting ventricular tachycardias. Its conversion effectiveness is excellent. Usually one 25-joule (J) discharge converts the arrhythmia.[12] The American Heart Association does not recommend antibiotic prophylaxis for patients with either a cardiac pacemaker or an AICD.[13-16]

CARDIOVERSION

Direct-current cardioversion to convert atrial and ventricular arrhythmias was first described in 1962.[2] Cardioversion can be effective for treatment of reentrant arrhythmias such as atrial flutter, atrial fibrillation, ventricular tachycardia, and ventricular fibrillation. Tachyarrhythmias that result in hemodynamic collapse, prolonged angina pectoris, or pulmonary edema should be treated promptly with direct-current cardioversion. The countershock simultaneously depolarizes the entire myocardium, allowing synchronous repolarization and the resumption of sinus rhythm.[2,6,11,15,21]

A defibrillator is an electrical device that sends a pulse of current through the heart to arrest several types of arrhythmias (Fig. 6-16). The pulse is applied to electrodes placed on the thorax. One electrode is placed on the left chest over the region of the apex and the other on the right side of the chest just to the right of the sternum and below the clavicle. Usually a damped sine wave defibrillator is used that can store 400 J of energy and deliver about 350 J into a 50-ohm resistor. Either multiple low-energy shocks (2 J/kg) or a single high-energy first shock (4 J/kg) is used. A dose concept should be developed so that the strength of the shock required is related to the size of the subject's heart. The practice of turning the output control to maximum and delivering a full jolt to all adults can be dangerous. Defibrillation usually is instantaneous and cardiac pumping resumes within a few seconds. It may have to be repeated if defibrillation is unsuccessful (i.e., regular heartbeat not occurring). Cardiopulmonary resuscitation must be used until defibrillation has been successful. When defibrillation is attempted all rescue personnel must stand clear of the patient except the individual holding the electrodes.[2,7,11,15,22]

Several types of automated external defibrillator (AED) devices can be purchased for use in the dental office. These AED devices include the Heartstream FR-2 AED, the Laerdal AED, the Medtronic Physio-control AED, and the Survivalink AED. The use of AEDs is even being taught in cardiopulmonary resuscitation courses and encouraged for public use by the American Heart Association. A brief training course should be helpful. These devices are simple, easy to use, and inexpensive,

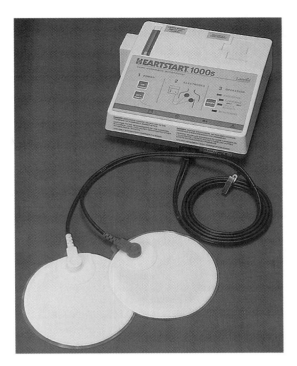

Fig. 6-16 The automated external defibrillator is connected to two pads that are applied to the patient's chest. The automated external defibrillator generally is not used for patients under 12 years of age or weighing less than 90 pounds. From Stoy WA: Mosby's EMT basic textbook, St. Louis, 1996, Mosby.

and may be helpful in the management of serious cardiac arrhythmias in the dental office.[24]

DENTAL MANAGEMENT

MEDICAL CONSIDERATIONS

Stress associated with dental treatment or excessive amounts of injected epinephrine may produce life-threatening cardiac arrhythmias in susceptible dental patients. Patients with an existing arrhythmia are at risk in the dental environment. In addition, patients at risk for developing an arrhythmia also may be in danger in the dental office if they are not identified and measures are not taken to minimize stressful situations that can precipitate an arrhythmia. Other patients may have their arrhythmias under control by drugs or a pacemaker but require special considerations when receiving dental treatment. The key to the dental management of patients prone to de-

---

BOX 6-4

Dental Management of the Patient with a Cardiac Arrhythmia—Medical Consultation

Refer for diagnosis and management any patient identified as having signs and symptoms suggesting the presence of cardiac arrhythmia.

Establish the current status for a patient with an arrhythmia under medical treatment and the type and severity of the arrhythmia.

For patients with pacemakers, determine the following:
Type of pacemaker being used
Type of arrhythmia being treated
Need for prophylactic antibiotics
Degree of shielding provided for generator and types of electrical equipment that should be avoided

Establish whether the patient with atrial fibrillation is being treated with warfarin sodium (Coumadin) to prevent atrial thrombosis and determine the way the dosage should be altered by the physician.

Establish the presence and current status of any underlying condition that may be the cause of arrhythmia.

---

veloping a cardiac arrhythmia and those with an existing arrhythmia is identification and prevention. Even under the best of circumstances, however, a patient may develop a cardiac arrhythmia that requires immediate emergency measures.

PREVENTION OF MEDICAL COMPLICATIONS

Identification of patients with an existing arrhythmia and those prone to developing one is most important for the dentist, who must obtain a medical history and evaluate the vital signs (pulse rate and rhythm, blood pressure, respiratory rate) for all patients desiring dental treatment (see Table 6-3). Several studies[4,5,9,10] have documented the benefit of using a 3-lead ECG unit to screen dental patients for arrhythmias.

Patients with a history of palpitations, dizziness, angina, dyspnea, or syncope may have a cardiac arrhythmia and should be evaluated by a physician before a dentist performs treatment. Patients with an irregular cardiac rhythm (even without symptoms) should be referred for medical evaluation. Elderly patients with a regular heart rate that varies in intensity with respiration should be referred for evaluation of possible sinus arrhythmias and sinus node disease[15,25] (Box 6-4).

Dental Management of the Patient with a Cardiac Arrhythmia—Patient Identification

Undetected arrhythmia
    Rapid or slow pulse rate
    Irregular pulse rhythm
    Associated symptoms:
        Palpitations
        Dizziness
        Syncope
        Angina
        Dyspnea
Susceptibility to development of arrhythmia during
    dental treatment
    History of ischemic heart disease
    History of valvular heart disease
    History of thyroid disease
    History of obstructive pulmonary disease
Under medical treatment for arrhythmia
    Antiarrhythmic medication use
    Implanted pacemaker

Risk of Types of Cardiac Arrhythmias*

Low risk—no medication use, infrequent symptoms
    Atrial arrhythmias
    Premature ventricular beats
    Young, active individuals with sinus bradycardia
Moderate risk—chronic medication use, asymptomatic
    Atrial arrhythmias
    Ventricular arrhythmias
    Medications known to affect function of sinus node
    Pacemaker
High risk
    Display of symptoms
    Pulse greater than 100 or less than 60 with another
        type of arrhythmia
    Irregular pulse rhythm
    Irregular pulse and bradycardia
    Bradycardia with cardiac pacemaker

*Medical consultation is recommended to help establish the risk for each patient.

Patients with a history of significant heart, thyroid, or chronic pulmonary diseases must be detected. Their medical status must be determined and medical consultation obtained regarding their current status and risk for developing a cardiac arrhythmia. In addition, patients taking antiarrhythmic medication and those with a pacemaker must be identified through their medical history and their current status established by medical consultation (Box 6-5).

The dentist can prevent many cardiac arrhythmia-related medical emergencies by being aware of the high-risk patients (Box 6-6) and taking appropriate precautions during dental treatment (Box 6-7). In the rare case when a life-threatening cardiac arrhythmia occurs during dental treatment the dentist and staff must be prepared to take immediate action (Box 6-8).

Precautions include the following:

1. *Consider the type of underlying cardiovascular disorder.* Patients with underlying cardiac disease must be identified carefully and managed as indicated by the nature of the cardiac problem (e.g., those susceptible to endocarditis, ischemic heart disease, congestive heart failure, hypertrophic cardiomyopathy, etc.).[15,25]

2. *Reduce patient anxiety.* Any increase in sympathetic tone can precipitate an arrhythmia. Premedication

with a short-acting benzodiazepine (e.g., triazolam [Halcion] 0.125-0.25 mg, diazepam [Valium] 5 mg, or oxazepam [Serax] 5 mg) on the night before the appointment and 5 mg one hour before the appointment may be used. Nitrous oxide-oxygen inhalation sedation can be initiated. An open, honest approach with the patient to explain the procedure is important.

3. *Minimize stressful situations.* Patients with coronary atherosclerotic heart disease, ischemic heart disease, or congestive heart failure should be managed to prevent or minimize acute exacerbation of these conditions that might trigger significant arrhythmias (see Chapters 1, 4, 5, and 7 for general stress reduction protocols).

4. *Avoid excessive amounts of vasoconstrictive agents and local anesthetic considerations.* Vasoconstrictors in appropriate concentration in the local anesthetic are beneficial. The need to achieve profound local anesthesia and hemostasis far outweighs the very slight risk of using these agents in small amounts (e.g., 1:100,000 epinephrine). However, the use of more than two cartridges (3.6 ml) of anesthetic (containing 0.036 mg of epinephrine) is not advised for any given appointment (see Chapter 4). In patients with severe arrhythmias and for short appointments use of a

---

BOX 6-7

Dental Management of the Patient at Risk for a Cardiac Arrhythmia—Precautions

Reduce anxiety:
  Premedication
  Open and honest communication
  Morning appointments
  Short appointments
  Nitrous oxide–oxygen inhalation
Avoid excessive amounts of epinephrine:
  1:100,000 in local anesthetic, except for patients
    with severe arrhythmias
  Long-acting local anesthetic without epinephrine
    for patients with severe arrhythmias, confirma-
    tion by medical consultation
  No more than two cartridges of anesthetic
  No epinephrine in gingival packing
  No epinephrine to control local bleeding
Avoid general anesthesia
Avoid use of electrical equipment that may interfere
  with functioning of the pacemaker
Manage underlying problem such as rheumatic heart
  disease as indicated (e.g., antibiotic prophylaxis for
  endocarditis prevention)

BOX 6-8

Dental Management of the Patient with a Life-Threatening Arrhythmia*

Stop the procedure.
Evaluate vital signs: pulse rate and rhythm, blood pres-
  sure, and mental alertness of patient.
Call for medical assistance if indicated.
Administer oxygen.
Place patient in Trendelenburg position (to reduce hy-
  potension).
Give nitroglycerin if indicated (chest pain).
Perform vagal maneuver (carotid massage) in cases of
  hypotension with tachycardia.
Initiate cardiopulmonary resuscitation as indicated for
  cardiac arrest.

*A patient with cardiac arrest requires cardioversion and other advanced life-support measures as soon as possible. In most cases these measures are provided as medical assistance becomes available or when the patient has been transported to the hospital.

---

local anesthetic without epinephrine may be the optimal choice. Vasoconstrictors must not be used in gingival packing material for crown impressions or to control local bleeding. Intraosseous and periodontal intraligamentary injections of local anesthetics containing vasoconstrictors should be avoided. Additionally, caution should be exercised when using local anesthetics containing vasoconstrictors with patients taking digitalis.

5. *Avoid general anesthesia.* Patients susceptible to developing significant cardiac arrhythmias should not be given general anesthesia in the dental office.
6. *Be careful when using electrical equipment.* During the medical consultation for patients with a pacemaker, the risk for electromagnetic interference from electrical equipment used in the dental office should be discussed. Patients with a new, well shielded generator are at low risk. However, patients with poor shielding may be at high risk for complications in pacing because of electromagnetic interference. Although studies have identified certain types of equipment that may be safe, pulp testers, motorized dental chairs, belt-driven handpieces, and ultrasonic scalers all may cause pacemaker malfunction in a patient with poor shielding in the pacemaker generator. Electrosurgery units can be a risk to all patients with pacemakers, and their use in these patients is not recommended.
7. *Alter anticoagulant regimen when necessary.* Patients with arrhythmias may be receiving anticoagulant therapy and therefore clinicians must determine the prothrombin time ratio or the international normalized ratio levels before surgery. The anticoagulant regimen need not be altered for most dental procedures. If the prothrombin time ratio is 2.5 or less or the international normalized ratio is 3.5 or less, most dental procedures (including minor oral surgery) can be performed without alteration of the anticoagulant regimen and use of only local methods of hemostasis (see Chapter 19).
8. *Monitor for digitalis intoxication.* Patients at risk for digitalis toxicity should be monitored carefully. Patients with arrhythmias medicated with digitalis may be susceptible to digitalis toxicity if they are elderly or have hypothyroidism, renal dysfunction, dehydration, hypokalemia, hypomagnesemia, or hypocalcemia. Patients with electrolyte imbalances are more susceptible to digitalis toxicity because of

TABLE **6-5**

Oral Complications of Antiarrhythmic Drugs*

Drug	Complication
Procainamide	Mucosal ulcerations
	Drug-induced lupus erythematosus
Propranolol	Mucosal ulcerations
	Petechiae
Disopyramide	Xerostomia
Quinidine	Mucosal ulcerations
Verapamil	Gingival hyperplasia

*When findings are noted, the patient's physician should be contacted and informed.

the heightened sensitivity of the heart to these changes accompanying certain arrhythmias.

Therapeutic doses of digitalis are 0.5 to 2.0 ng/ml. Levels greater than 2.5 ng/ml may result in digitalis toxicity. Patients' medications and dosage levels should be monitored. Patients should be watched for signs and symptoms of digitalis toxicity, which are found in three systems: gastrointestinal, neurologic and cardiovascular (nearly any type of arrhythmia and cardiac conduction problems).[22]

TREATMENT PLANNING CONSIDERATIONS

A patient susceptible to cardiac arrhythmias can receive virtually any indicated dental procedure once identified and the steps just described are taken. Complex dental procedures should be spread over several appointments to avoid overstressing the patient.

ORAL COMPLICATIONS AND MANIFESTATIONS

The only significant oral complications found in patients with an arrhythmia are those occurring as side effects to the medication used to control the arrhythmia. Procainamide can cause agranulocytosis secondary to drug toxicity affecting the bone marrow. Mucosal ulcerations may occur in the mouth from agranulocytosis. Patients taking procainamide who develop oral ulcerations should be evaluated for possible bone marrow suppression. Procainamide also has been reported to produce a lupuslike syndrome in some patients. Quinidine can cause a similar reaction leading to oral ulceration. Because of its anticholinergic effect, disopyramide may cause xerostomia. If the xerostomia becomes severe

medical consultation is indicated to see whether another antiarrhythmic agent can be used in place of the disopyramide. Propranolol may produce bone marrow suppression resulting in agranulocytosis or thrombocytopenia. In these patients, oral ulcers and petechiae may be found[15,25] (Table 6-5; see Appendix B).

References

1. DiMarco JP, Prystowsky EN, editors: *Atrial arrhythmias*, American Heart Association Monograph, Armonk, NY, 1995, Futura Pub.
2. Gallagher JJ: Cardiac arrhythmias. In Wyngaardin JB, Smith LH, editors: *Cecil textbook of medicine*, ed 20, Philadelphia, 1996, WB Saunders.
3. Furberg CD et al: Prevalence of atrial fibrillation in elderly subjects: initial finding of the Cardiovascular Health Study, JAMA 269(2):214-215, 1993.
4. Little JW et al: Evaluation of an ECG system for the dental office, *Gen Dent* 38:278-282, 1990.
5. Little JW et al: Dental patient reaction to ECG screening, *Oral Surg* 70:433-439, 1990.
6. Luck JC, Engel TR: Cardiac arrhythmias. In Rose LF, Kaye D, editors: *Internal medicine for dentistry*, ed 2, St Louis, 1990, Mosby-Year Book.
7. Bialy D et al: Hospitalization for arrhythmias in the United States: importance of atrial fibrillation, *J Am Coll Cardiol* 19:41,1992 (abstract 716-4).
8. Feinberg WM et al: Prevalence, age distribution and gender of patients with atrial fibrillation: analysis and implications, *Arch Int Med.* 155:469-473, 1995.
9. Simmons MS et al: Screening dentists for risk factors associated with cardiovascular disease, *Gen Dent* 42:440-446, 1994.
10. Rhodus NL, Little JW: The prevalence of cardiac arrhythmias in dental and dental hygiene students, *California Institute of Continuing Education in Dentistry* 5:23-26, 1998.
11. Marriott HJ, Myerberg RJ: Recognition of arrhythmias and conduction abnormalities. In Hurst JW, editor: *The heart, arteries, and veins*, ed 9, New York, 1998, McGraw-Hill.
12. Mond HG, Sloman JG: The indications for and types of artificial cardiac pacemakers. In Hurst JW, editor: *The heart, arteries, and veins*, ed 9, New York, 1998, McGraw-Hill.
13. Mond HG, Strathmore NF: The technique of using cardiac pacemakers: implantation, testing, and surveillance. In Hurst JW, editor: *The heart, arteries, and veins*, ed 9, New York, 1998, McGraw Hill.
14. Moraes, JC: Effects of electronic autodefense on cardiac pacemakers, *Artif Organs* 19:238-240, 1995.
15. Riegel B et al, editors: *Dreifus pacemaker therapy: an interprofessional approach*, Philadelphia, 1986, FA Davis.
16. Mond HG, Sloman JG: Artificial cardiac pacemakers. In Hurst JW, editor: *The heart, arteries, and veins*, ed 9, New York, 1998, McGraw-Hill.

17. Mirowski M: The implantable cardioverter-defibrillator. In Hurst JW, editor: *The heart, arteries, and veins*, ed 9, New York, 1998, McGraw-Hill.

18. Matsuura H: The systemic management of cardiovascular risk patients in dental practice, *Anesth Pain Contr Dent* 3:49-61, 1999.

19. Smith MB, Wallace AG: Management of arrhythmias and conduction abnormalities. In Hurst JW, editor: *The heart, arteries, and veins*, ed 9, New York, 1998, McGraw-Hill.

20. Rose LF, Godfrey P, Steinberg BJ: Dental correlations: arrhythmia. In Rose LF, Kaye D, editors: *Internal medicine for dentistry*, St Louis, 1983, Mosby.

21. Sonis ST, Frazio RC, Fang L, editors: *Principles and practice of oral medicine*, ed 2, Philadelphia, 1990, WB Saunders.

22. Tasota FJ, Tate J: Assessing digoxin levels, *J Nursing* 20(1):24-25, 2000.

23. Miller CS, Leonelli FM, Latham E: Selective interference with pacemaker activity by electrical dental devices, *Oral Surg Oral Med Oral Pathol Oral Radiol Endo* 1998, 85(1):33-36.

24. Alexander RE: The AED: a lifesaving device for medical emergencies, JADA 130(8):1162, 1999.

25. Smith MB, Gallagher JJ: Mechanisms of arrhythmias and conduction abnormalities. In Hurst JW, editor: *The heart, arteries, and veins*, ed 9, New York, 1998, McGraw-Hill.

Congestive Heart Failure

7

CHAPTER

Congestive heart failure (CHF) is much like anemia in that it represents a symptom complex that can be caused by a number of specific diseases (Box 7-1). CHF represents the end-stage of many of the underlying types of cardiovascular disease that ultimately lead to heart failure. CHF may be defined as a systemic syndrome produced by a failing myocardium or a significant increase in left-ventricular end-diastolic pressure despite normal cardiac function. Stated differently, CHF is the syndrome in which cardiac output is unable to meet the metabolic demands of the body.[1] Patients with untreated heart failure or poorly managed response to it are at high risk during dental treatment for such complications as infection, cardiac arrest, cerebrovascular accident, and myocardial infarction. The dentist must be able to detect these patients, based on history and clinical findings, refer them for medical diagnosis and management, and work closely with the physician to develop a dental management plan that will be effective and safe for the patient.

GENERAL DESCRIPTION

INCIDENCE AND PREVALENCE

CHF affects between 1 million and 2 million persons in the United States, with approximately 400,000 new cases each year.[1,2] It represents the most common diagnosis-related group category for Medicare expense. Approximately 700,000 Americans are in this category.[1] CHF is especially common in the elderly and is the most common hospital discharge diagnosis in patients over age 65. In all age groups CHF represents the fourth-most-common diagnosis.[3] The most common underlying causes of CHF in the United States are coronary artery disease, hypertension, cardiomyopathy, and valvular heart disease.[4]

More than 75% of CHF patients have a long-standing history of hypertension.[1] A large proportion of patients who have had a myocardial infarction develop ischemic cardiomyopathy. The second-most-common presentation of CHF, especially in younger patients, is primary dilated cardiomyopathy. The causes of primary dilated cardiomyopathy are alcohol abuse, hereditary cardiomyopathies, adriamycin and radiation therapy (especially in women), and viral infections.[1] The rates of rheumatic heart disease and congenital heart disease (both potential causes of CHF) in the United States have leveled off, although the incidence is still high in developing countries.[1] Although the mortality rate from myocardial infarction and stroke are declining, CHF continues to be a major cause of morbidity.[1] The incidence of CHF is the only cardiovascular condition increasing: hospitalizations for CHF quadrupled between 1970 and 1995.[3] More than 1 million hospital admissions each year are caused by CHF.[3] The overall 5-year mortality rate for CHF is 50%. For severe CHF the 1-year mortality rate is 50% to 60%.[3,4]

Heart failure is caused by the inability of the heart to function efficiently as a pump, which results in either an inadequate emptying of the ventricles during systole or an incomplete filling of the ventricles during diastole. This in turn results in an inadequate volume of blood being supplied to the tissues or a backup of blood, causing systemic congestion. Thus heart failure may be defined as a state in which cardiac dysfunction results in a diminished functional capacity and an impaired quality of life.[3]

Congestive heart failure may involve failure of one or both ventricles. Most of the acquired disorders that lead to congestive heart failure result in failure of the left ventricle. This often is followed by failure of the right ventricle. Initial failure of the right side of the heart is much less common and is associated with certain congenital heart defects or with emphysema. By the time most pa-

BOX 7-1

Most Common Causes of Congestive Heart Failure

Coronary heart disease and its sequelae
Hypertension
Valvular heart disease
Myocarditis
Cardiomyopathy
Infective endocarditis
Congenital heart disease
Pulmonary hypertension
Pulmonary embolism
Endocrine disease

BOX 7-2

Signs of Congestive Heart Failure

Rapid, shallow breathing
Cheyne-Stokes respiration (hyperventilation alternating with apnea)
Inspiratory rales
Heart murmur
Gallop rhythm
Increased venous pressure
Cardiac enlargement on chest radiograph
Pulsus alternans
Distended neck veins
Large, tender liver
Jaundice
Peripheral edema
Ascites
Cyanosis
Weight gain
Clubbing of fingers

BOX 7-3

Symptoms of Congestive Heart Failure

Fatigue and weakness
Dyspnea (breathlessness)
Orthopnea (dyspnea in recumbent position)
Paroxysmal nocturnal dyspnea (dyspnea awakening patient from sleep)
Hyperventilation followed by apnea
Low-grade fever
Anorexia, nausea, vomiting, constipation
Liver pain
Cough
Insomnia
History of weight gain
History of increased body girth
History of sweating
Dizziness, confusion

tients are seen for medical treatment, failure of both sides of the heart usually has occurred.

PATHOPHYSIOLOGY AND COMPLICATIONS

Heart failure appears when the heart no longer functions properly as a pump. Congestive heart failure is the end-stage of a disproportion between the required hemodynamic load and the capacity of the heart to handle the load. This imbalance can occur with chronic increase in the load or damage to the myocardium. In most cases a combination of these two factors is involved. Chronic congestive heart failure usually evokes compensatory adjustments consisting of increased peripheral resistance, redistribution of blood flow to the heart and brain, and an increased efficiency of oxygen utilization by the tissues.

Heart failure usually occurs in stages.[5] The first stage involves ventricular dysfunction with the development of a gallop rhythm. The second stage consists of congestive failure with dyspnea, pulmonary congestion, and peripheral edema. The third stage, termed *compensated heart failure*, is the control or elimination of the clinical signs and symptoms of congestion by medical therapy (Box 7-2 and Box 7-3).

Failure of the heart most often begins with left ventricular failure brought on by increased workload or disease of the heart muscle. The increased workload may result from a variety of entities, including aortic valve disease and arterial hypertension. Direct effects on the myocardium may be a result of infections, rheumatic fever, or infarction. The outstanding symptom of left ventricular failure is dyspnea, which results from blood accumulation in the pulmonary vessels. Acute pulmonary edema often is associated with left ventricular failure. Left-sided heart failure leads to pulmonary hypertension, which increases the work of the right ventricle pumping against the increased pressure and often leads to right-sided heart failure. The most common cause of right-sided heart failure is preceding failure of the left ventricle. An important feature of left ventricular failure is the retention of sodium and water and

TABLE 7-1

Comparison of Left-Sided vs. Right-Sided Heart Failure

Left Ventricular Failure	Right Ventricular Failure
Early	Respiratory distress
Exertional dyspnea	Peripheral edema
Paroxysmal nocturnal	Nausea, anorexia
dyspnea	Dyspnea
Orthopnea	Dependent edema
Fatigue	Right upper quadrant
Nonproductive cough	discomfort
Increased BP	Fatigue
	Hepatojugular reflux
Later	Hepatomegaly
Decreased functional	Ascites
capacity	Weight gain
Cognitive impairment	Heart murmurs
Hypoxemia	Pleural effusion
S-3 or S-4 heart sound	Jugular vein distension
Heart murmurs	Nocturia
Tachypnea	
Tachycardia	
Anxiety	
Pulsus alternans	
Pleural effusion	
Arrhythmias	
Severe respiratory	
distress	
Pallor or cyanosis	
Diaphoresis	
Productive cough	
Crackles	

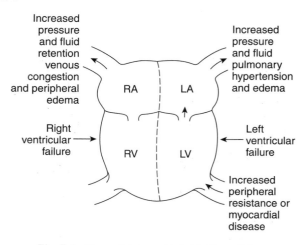

Fig. 7-1 Effects of right- and left-sided heart failure.

contraction. This leads to dyspnea, orthopnea, and pulmonary edema[6] (Fig. 7-2).

The natural history of severe congestive heart failure is that it worsens. From 50% to 60% of patients with severe symptoms die within 1 year; of those with less severe symptoms, 50% will die in 3 to 5 years.[6] The prognosis is better if the underlying cause can be treated. Patients who respond to the initial attempts of medical treatment have a better prognosis. Sudden death caused by ventricular fibrillation is common in patients with severe congestive heart failure.[7]

CLINICAL PRESENTATION

SIGNS AND SYMPTOMS

Patients with congestive heart failure may have rapid, shallow breathing or alternating cycles of hyperventilation with apnea, called *Cheyne-Stokes respirations*.[3] Percussive evidence may be present of pleural effusion as well as inspiratory rales.

Cardiac examination often reveals a laterally displaced apical impulse caused by left ventricular hypertrophy. A murmur of mitral regurgitation may be heard as well as an S_3 or S_4 gallop.[6] Pulsus alternans is pathognomonic of left ventricular failure but is not present in most patients with heart failure.[6] Central venous pressure increases. The chest radiograph may reveal enlargement of specific cardiac chambers or

insufficient emptying of the left ventricle during systole[6] (Table 7-1).

Failure of the right side of the heart alone is uncommon. The most common cause of pure right-sided heart failure is emphysema. When this occurs, the condition is called *cor pulmonale*. The major results are systemic venous congestion and peripheral edema (Fig. 7-1).

Ventricular failure will lead to dilation and hypertrophy of the ventricle as it attempts to compensate for its inability to keep up with the workload. Venous pressure and myocardial tone increase along with the increase in blood volume. The net effect is diastolic dilation, to increase the force and volume of the subsequent systolic

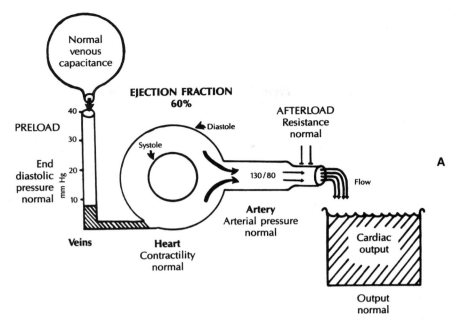

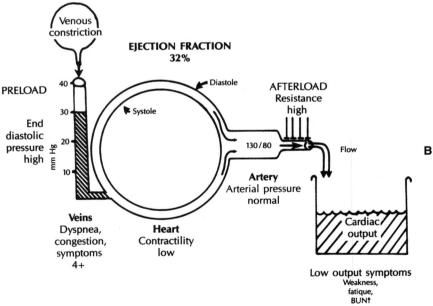

Fig. 7-2 A, Diagram of the normal heart and circulation. **B,** Diagram of the failing heart and circulation, showing the effects of Starling mechanisms (diastolic cardiac dilation, causing increased force and volume of the subsequent systolic contraction and ejection), increased venous pressure, and increased peripheral resistance in the attempt to maintain central blood pressure and allocate limited cardiac output to vital areas such as the brain and heart. (From Spann JF: In Hurst JW, editor: *The heart, arteries, and veins,* ed 7, New York, 1990, McGraw-Hill, p 420.)

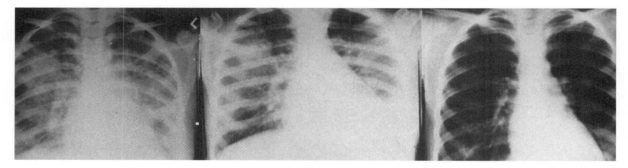

Fig. 7-3 Chest radiographs demonstrate the resolution of pulmonary edema (*left to right*). (Courtesy J. Noonan, Lexington, Ky.)

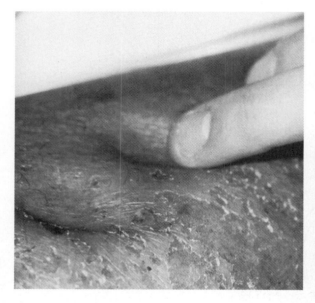

Fig. 7-4 Pitting pretibial edema in a patient with congestive heart failure. (Courtesy N. Wood, Alberta, Canada.)

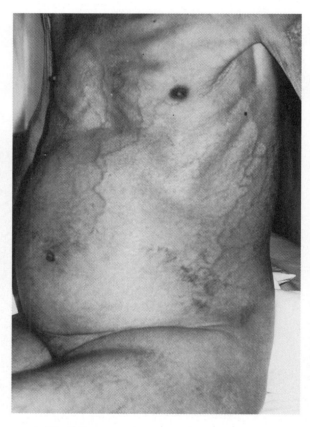

Fig. 7-5 Ascites. (Courtesy P. Akers, Evanston Ill.)

abnormalities of the pulmonary vasculature.[3] Evidence of interstitial fluid or pleural effusion may be seen (Fig. 7-3).

Evidence of systemic venous congestion may be detected by the presence of distended neck veins, a large tender liver, peripheral edema (Fig. 7-4), and ascites (Fig. 7-5). The retention of fluid will cause weight gain and may increase body girth. On occasion patients with chronic CHF may show clubbing of the fingers (Fig. 7-6, see Box 7-2).

Exertional dyspnea and fatigue in a patient suggest the possibility of beginning left-sided heart failure. Symptoms of overt heart failure include orthopnea (shortness of breath when supine), paroxysmal nocturnal dyspnea (patient wakes gasping for breath), Cheyne-Stokes respi-

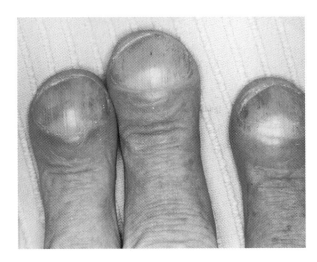

Fig. 7-6 Clubbing of the fingers in a patient with congestive heart failure.

TABLE **7-2**

Laboratory Tests for Congestive Heart Failure

Test	To Evaluate
Chest x-ray	Heart size, shape and pulmonary congestion
ECG	Myocardial ischemia, infarction, other arrhythmias
Echocardiogram	Chamber size, wall thickness, valve shape and motion
Serum electrolyte levels	Imbalances in sodium and potassium
Multiple gated acquisition scanning	Cardiac function, ejection fraction, wall motion abnormalities
Serum albumin levels	Edema
Hemodynamic pulmonary artery monitoring	Cardiac output, pulmonary capillary wedge pressure (left ventricular pressure, right ventricular pressure, right atrial pressure, systemic vascular resistance, pulmonary vascular resistance
Arterial blood gas levels	Hypoxia and acid-base balance
Radionuclide angiography (scintigraphy)	Severity of ventricular dysfunction
Liver function studies	ALT, AST levels (severity of liver dysfunction)
Exercise stress test	Activity tolerance and severity of ischemic heart disease
Cardiac catheterization	Cardiac abnormalities and underlying cardiovascular disease

ration, and weakness. The patient may have a low-grade fever[6] (see Box 7-3).

LABORATORY FINDINGS

A variety of specialized tests are used to diagnose and monitor congestive heart failure, depending on the etiology. Among these are chest radiograph, electrocardiogram, echocardiography, radionuclide angiography or ventriculography, exercise stress test, ambulatory electrocardiogram (Holter) monitoring, and cardiac catheterization[6] (Table 7-2).

Measurement of plasma hormone levels of norepinephrine, plasma atrial natriuretic peptide, and plasma renin have possible prognostic value but usually are not helpful clinically.[4] Several blood chemistry tests may be abnormal in patients with CHF.[8] These blood chemistry tests include elevated liver enzymes (aspartate amino-

Medical Management of Congestive Heart Failure

Nonpharmacologic (Conservative) Treatment
Weight loss, sodium restriction, alcohol reduction, smoking cessation, regular exercise, adequate rest, balanced diet

Pharmacologic Treatment
NYHA class I CHF (ejection fraction >40%; asymptomatic patient)
Long-acting ACE inhibitor
NYHA class II, III, IV CHF (ejection fraction <40%; symptomatic patient)
Digoxin (loading dose 0.75-1.25 mg; maintenance dose adjusted with age, lean body mass and renal function)
plus,
Furosemide (20-120 mg; watch for hypokalemia and gout)
Long-acting ACE inhibitors (enalapril 5-10 mg twice daily)
Potassium chloride supplementation (>4.0 mEq/L)
Metozalone, 5-10 mg every other day may be added when furosemide dose exceeds 160 mg/day

transferase-AST and alanine aminotransferase-ALT) and bilirubin secondary to liver congestion. Urinalysis may reveal proteinuria and a high specific gravity indicating renal involvement. Blood urea nitrogen also may be elevated.[8]

MEDICAL MANAGEMENT

The medical management of CHF involves three basic aspects. First, the identification of all causative factors and their correction or stabilization is addressed. This includes such factors as the control of hypertension, correction or control of coronary artery disease, and repair of diseased heart valves.

Second, lifestyle modification is necessary and includes smoking cessation, strict salt restriction, loss of weight for the obese patient, reduction of risk factors for coronary artery disease, mild aerobic exercise, adequate rest and moderate use of alcohol for those who use it (Box 7-4).

Drug therapy is the third aspect of treatment (Table 7-3). In the past few years, the pharmacologic management of CHF has undergone significant changes, the most important of which is the use of the angiotensin-converting enzyme (ACE) inhibitors as the primary drugs for the treatment of CHF.[9] This is based on the finding

TABLE 7-3

Drugs Commonly Used in the Management of Congestive Heart Failure

Drug	Mode of Action	Vasoconstrictor Interaction	Oral Manifestations	Other Considerations
Angiotensin-Converting Enzyme (ACE) Inhibitors				
Enalapril maleate (Vasotec)	Block conversion of angiotensin I to angiotensin II	None	• Cough • Angioedema of lips, face, tongue • Oral ulceration • Burning pain of oral mucosa	• Prolonged use of nonsteroidal antiinflammatory drugs (NSAIDs) can reduce effectiveness • Neutropenia and thrombocytopenia
Captopril (Capoten)				
Lisinopril (Prinivil; Zestril)				
Quinapril hydrochloride (Accupril)				
Thiazide Diuretics				
Hydrochlorthiazide (HCTZ; Esidrix)	Reduce plasma volume and extracellular fluid by increasing excretion of sodium and urine output	None	• Dry mouth • Lichenoid reactions	• Orthostatic hypotension • Prolonged use of NSAIDs can reduce effectiveness
Chlorthalidone (Diuril)				

TABLE **7-3**

Drugs Commonly Used in the Management of Congestive Heart Failure—cont'd

Drug	Mode of Action	Vasoconstrictor Interaction	Oral Manifestations	Other Considerations
Thiazide-Related Diuretics				
Metolazone; Zaroxolyn	Reduce plasma volume and extracellular fluid by increasing excretion of sodium and urine output	None	• Dry mouth • Lichenoid reactions	• Orthostatic hypotention • Prolonged use of NSAIDs can reduce effectiveness
Loop Diuretics				
Furosemide (Lasix) Bumetanide (Bumex) Ethacrynic acid (Edecrin)	Reduce plasma volume and extracellular fluid by increasing excretion of sodium and urine output	None	• Dry mouth • Lichenoid reactions	• Orthostatic hypotention • Prolonged use of NSAIDs can reduce effectiveness
Potassium-Sparing Diuretics				
Spironolactone (Aldactone) Triamterene (Dyrenium) Amiloride hydrochloride (Midamor)	Reduce plasma volume and extracellular fluid by increasing excretion of sodium and urine output	None	• Dry mouth • Lichenoid reactions	• Orthostatic hypotention • Prolonged use of NSAIDs can reduce effectiveness
Digitalis Glycosides				
Digoxin (Lanoxin)	Increase force and velocity of myocardial contractions and decrease conduction rate of atrioventricular (AV) node	Use of epinephrine or levonordefrin may precipitate arrhythmia—avoid	• Increased gag reflex—prone to nausea and vomiting	• Erythromycin can cause digoxin toxicity—avoid
Long-Acting Nitrates				
Isosorbide dinitrate (Isordil; Isorbid)	Venous and arterial dilation, reduces work load on heart	May decrease effectiveness of epinephrine and levonordefrin	• Dry mouth	• Orthostatic hypotension
Vasodilators				
Hydralazine (Apresoline) Prazosin (Minipres)	Direct dilitation of arteries; mechanism unclear	May decrease effectiveness of epinephrine and norepinephrine	• Lupus-like lesions • Dry mouth	• Prolonged use of NSAIDs can reduce effectiveness • Orthostatic hypotension

Continued

TABLE 7-3

Drugs Commonly Used in the Management of Congestive Heart Failure—cont'd

Drug	Mode of Action	Vasoconstrictor Interaction	Oral Manifestations	Other Considerations
Beta-Adrenergic Agonists				
Dobutamine	Selectively stimulates beta-adrenergic receptors to increase myocardial contractibility, stroke volume, and cardiac output	Tachycardias, asthmatic episodes, other arrhythmias	• Dry mouth	• Orthostatic hypotension
Alpha Nonselective Beta-Blocker				
	Decreases systematic blood pressure, pulmonary artery pressure, right arterial pressure, systematic vascular resistance and heart rate while increasing stroke volume			

BOX 7-5

Clinical Manifestations of Digitalis Intoxication

CNS-stimulated anorexia, nausea, vomiting
Premature ventricular beats
AV block
Nonparoxysmal atrial tachycardia
Vision changes—blurred, color changes
Fatigue, malaise, drowsiness
Headache
Ventricular tachycardias
Neuralgias
Weight loss
Gynecomastia
Delirium
Salivation

From Braunwald E: In Wilson JD, et al, editors: *Harrison's principles of internal medicine*, ed 12, New York, 1991, McGraw-Hill; and from Lathers CM: In Smith CM, Reynard AM, editors: *Textbook of Pharmacology*, Philadelphia, 1992, WB Saunders.

that enlapril maleate reduces mortality in mild, moderate, and severe CHF.[7,10] Enalapril also has been shown to reduce mortality more than the conventional use of isosorbide dinitrate and hydralazine.[8] Enalapril, captopril, lisinopril, and quinapril are the ACE inhibitors that are FDA approved for management of CHF.[3] For mild CHF, an ACE inhibitor alone may provide adequate relief; however, they most often are used in combination with a diuretic.[3,6] Other commonly used vasodilators include long-acting nitrates (isosorbide dinitrate) and hydralazine.

Diuretics are used to treat orthopnea, dyspnea, and edema as well as to normalize the central venous pressure.[6] The minimum dose is used because of side effects such as hypokalemia and the precipitation of ventricular arrhythmias. Diuretics and ACE inhibitors usually are used concomitantly. In moderate to severe CHF, loop diuretics are necessary (e.g., furosemide).[6]

The digitalis glycosides (digoxin) have been the cornerstone of treatment for CHF for 200 years[9] (see Table 7-3). Currently, however, their use is questioned because of unresolved issues regarding dose and the effect of these agents on arrhythmic sudden death and disease progression.[11] Nevertheless, convincing evidence exists for their beneficial effects, especially in patients with se-

BOX 7-6

Dental Management of the Patient with Congestive Heart Failure

1. Evaluate patient
   a. For patient with untreated or uncontrolled CHF-avoid elective dental care
   b. For patients under medical care for CHF
      (1) Confirm status with patient or physician
      (2) Consider routine dental care for NYHA-class I and II patients
      (3) For NYHA class III patients, require consultation with physician and consider treatment in outpatient setting or special care facility (hospital dental clinic)
      (4) Treat NYHA class IV patients conservatively in special care setting
2. Identify underlying causative factors (i.e., coronary artery disease, valvular disease, hypertension) and manage appropriately
3. Consider drug usage
   a. For patients taking digitalis, use epinephrine or levonordefrin cautiously (maximum 0.036 mg epinephrine or 0.20 mg levonordefrin); avoid gag reflex; also avoid erythromycin, which can increase the absorption of digitalis and lead to toxicity.
   b. For patients with NYHA class III and IV CHF, avoid use of vasoconstrictors
   c. See Table 7-3 for drug considerations and side effects
4. Use semisupine or upright chair position as per patient comfort
5. Watch for orthostatic hypotension, make position or chair changes slowly, and assist in and out of chair.
6. Watch for signs of digitalis toxicity (i.e., tachycardia, hypersalivation, visual disturbances, etc.)
7. Schedule short, stress-free appointments

vere failure as well as in patients with mild to moderate CHF who do not respond to ACE inhibitors and diuretics.[2,9,12] A significant problem with digitalis glycosides is their narrow therapeutic range and the resulting toxicity that easily can occur (Box 7-5). Other drugs used to treating CHF unresponsive to ACE inhibitors include direct vasodilators, alpha₁-adrenergic blockers and centrally acting alpha agonists.

DENTAL MANAGEMENT

MEDICAL CONSIDERATIONS

The New York Heart Association (NYHA) has devised a functional classification of heart disease that grades the severity of CHF.[3] The classification is useful in following the course of disease and assessing the effects of therapy (Box 7-6). It also can be used to aid in the dental management of patients.

Class I: No limitation of physical activity. No dyspnea, fatigue, or palpitations with ordinary physical activity.

Class II: Slight limitation of physical activity. These patients have fatigue, palpitations, and dyspnea with ordinary physical activity but are comfortable at rest.

Class III: Marked limitation of activity. Less than ordinary physical activity results in symptoms, but patients are comfortable at rest.

Class IV: Symptoms are present at rest, and any physical exertion exacerbates the symptoms.

Patients with untreated or uncontrolled congestive heart failure are not a candidate for elective dental care and should be referred to their physician for immediate care. Once the congestive heart failure is under control, they should be encouraged to return for the resumption of dental care. Confirmation of the status of CHF should be made through discussion with the patient or preferably by consultation with the physician. Patients who are NYHA class I and II can receive routine outpatient dental care. Many class III patients may receive treatment in an outpatient setting after approval by their physician. Some class III patients and all class IV patients are best treated in a special care facility such as a hospital dental clinic.

Current medications should be identified as should underlying causative conditions such as rheumatic heart disease, myocardial infarction, and hypertension. Appropriate management adjustment for these conditions should be made. An assessment of the patient's cardiac stability and the presence of complications or drug side effects should be made (see Box 7-6 and Table 7-3).

Patients under good control with no complications can receive routine dental care. Short, stress-free appointments are advised. Patients with class II through IV CHF may not tolerate a supine chair position because of pulmonary edema and will need a semisupine or upright chair position. Patients taking a digitalis glycoside (digoxin) should be given epinephrine or levonordefrin cautiously as the combination can potentially precipitate arrhythmias. A maximum of 0.036 mg epinephrine (two cartridges of 2% lidocaine with 1:100,000 epinephrine) is recommended (see Chapter 4). Patients should be observed for signs of digitalis toxicity. In patients who are NYHA class III or IV, vasoconstrictors should be avoided. Nitrous oxide plus oxygen sedation can be used if adequate O_2 flow (at least 30%) is maintained (see Box 7-6 and Table 7-3).

TREATMENT PLANNING MODIFICATIONS

In general, patients with congestive heart failure who are under good medical management can receive any indicated dental treatment as long as the dental management plans deal effectively with the problems presented by the heart failure, its underlying cause, and the effects of the medications. Patients with unstable CHF present a definite challenge that mandates specific management considerations (see Box 7-6).

ORAL COMPLICATIONS AND MANIFESTATIONS

Oral complications are usually not directly related to congestive heart failure. However, drugs used to manage CHF can cause xerostomia and oral lesions (including lichenoid reactions). Digitalis may exaggerate the patient's gag reflex (see Table 7-3).

References

1. Hess ML: Congestive heart failure. In Hess ML: *Heart disease in primary care*, Baltimore, 1999, Williams and Wilkins.
2. Schocken DD et al: Prevalence and mortality rate of congestive heart failure in the United States, J Am Coll Cardiol 20:310, 1992.
3. McCall D: Congestive heart failure. In Stein JH, editor: *Internal medicine*, ed 5, St Louis, 1997, Mosby.
4. Kloner RA, Fowler MB, Dzau V: Heart failure. In Kloner RA, editor: *The guide to cardiology*, ed 3, Greenwich, 1995, Le Jacq Communications.
5. Schlant RC, Sonnenblick EH: Pathophysiology of heart failure. In Schlant RC, Alexander RW, editors: *Hurst's the heart, arteries and veins*, ed 9, vol 1, New York, 1998, McGraw-Hill.
6. Cohn JN, Sonnenblick EH: Diagnosis and therapy of heart failure. In Schlant RG, Aleander RW, editors: *Hurst's the heart, arteries and veins*, ed 9, vol 1, New York, 1998, McGraw-Hill.
7. CONSENSUS Trial Study Group: Effects of enalapril on mortality in severe congestive heart failure, N Engl J Med 316:1429-1435, 1987.
8. Cohn JN, et al: A comparison of enalapril with hydralazine-isosorbide dinitrate in the treatment of chronic congestive heart failure, N Engl J Med 325:303-310, 1991.
9. Baker DW, et al: Management of heart failure. I. Pharmacologic treatment, JAMA 272:1361-1366, 1994.
10. SOLVD Investigators: Effect of enalapril on survival in patients with reduced left-ventricular ejection fractions and congestive heart failure, N Engl J Med 325:293-302, 1991.
11. Smith, TW: Digoxin in heart failure, N Engl J Med 329:51-53, 1993.
12. Packer M, et al: Withdrawal of digoxin from patients with chronic heart failure treated with angiotensin-converting enzyme inhibitors: RADIANCE Study Group, N Engl J Med 329:1-7, 1993.
13. Jaeschke R, Oxman AD, Guyatt GH: To what extent do congestive heart failure patients in sinus rhythm benefit from digoxin therapy? A systematic overview and meta-analysis, Am J Med 88:279-286, 1990.

Pulmonary Disease

8

CHAPTER

Many types of pulmonary disorders may influence routine dental care and require special management of the patient. The more commonly encountered pulmonary diseases include chronic obstructive pulmonary disease (COPD), asthma, and tuberculosis.

■ CHRONIC OBSTRUCTIVE PULMONARY DISEASE ■

DEFINITION

COPD is a general term for pulmonary disorders characterized by chronic irreversible obstruction of airflow from the lungs. The two most common diseases classified as COPD are chronic bronchitis and emphysema. The basis for obstructed airflow in these two diseases is different. Chronic bronchitis is a condition associated with excessive tracheobronchial mucus production sufficient to cause cough with expectoration for at least 3 months of the year for more than 2 consecutive years. Emphysema is defined as distention of the air spaces distal to the terminal bronchioles because of destruction of alveolar walls (septa).[1] These diseases can be described as individual entities but often represent the progression of disease. Thus patients may have overlapping symptoms, making differentiation difficult.

EPIDEMIOLOGY

COPD is the fourth-leading cause of death in the United States and estimated to affect 16 million people—14.2 million with chronic bronchitis and 1.8 million with emphysema.[2] COPD affects approximately 6% of adults, more commonly men, and is second only to arthritis as the leading cause of long-term disability and functional impairment. Prevalence, incidence, and mortality rates increase with age and are highest in white men.[1,3] Emphysema, which can be definitively diagnosed only through autopsy, is found to some degree in two thirds of men and one fourth of women. Most of those affected, however, have no recognized dysfunction.[4]

ETIOLOGY

The most important etiologic factor in COPD is cigarette smoking. Approximately 12.5% of current smokers and 9% of former smokers have COPD.[5] Smoking also accounts for 80% to 90% of COPD mortality in both men and women. The risk of COPD is dose related and increases as the number of cigarettes smoked per day and duration of smoking increase.[6] The risk of COPD is 8.8 times higher in male smokers and 5.9 times higher in female smokers compared with nonsmokers of the same gender.[7] Despite the increased risk, only about one in six chronic smokers develops COPD.[1] This suggests that genetic susceptibility to the production of inflammatory mediators (i.e., cytokines) in response to smoke plays an important role. In addition to cigarette smoking, chronic exposure to occupational and environmental pollutants and the absence of alpha₁-antitrypsin are etiologic factors that contribute to COPD.

PATHOPHYSIOLOGY AND COMPLICATIONS

Although chronic bronchitis and emphysema both lead to obstruction of airflow, the pathophysiologic responses of each is distinct. In chronic bronchitis the pathologic changes consist of thickened bronchial walls with inflammatory cell infiltrate, an increase in size of the mucous glands, and goblet cell hyperplasia. Obstruction is caused by narrowing of small airways, mucous plugging, and collapse of peripheral airways from a loss of surfactant.[1] Obstruction is present on inspiration and expiration.

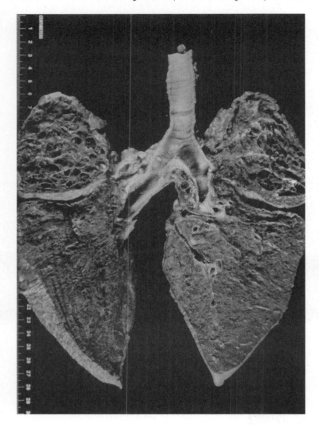

Fig. 8-1 Gross lung specimen from a patient with emphysema. (Courtesy Peggy Falace, Lexington, Ky.)

In emphysema, by contrast, smoke injures alveolar epithelium and causes a release of inflammatory mediators that attract activated neutrophils. The neutrophils release enzymes (elastase) that destroy the alveolar walls, resulting in enlarged air spaces distal to the terminal bronchioles and loss of elastic recoil of the lungs. Obstruction is caused by the collapse of these unsupported and enlarged air spaces on expiration (Fig. 8-1). No obstruction exists during inspiration.[4] A deficiency in alpha1-antitrypsin increases the susceptibility to developing emphysema because when present at normal levels, alpha1-antitrypsin neutralizes neutrophil elastase.

The course of COPD is one of deterioration unless intervention is performed early in its onset. The types of complications that develop vary depending on the predominance of either chronic bronchitis or emphysema. With continued exposure to primary etiologic factors (cigarette smoking, environmental pollutants), COPD usually results in progressive dyspnea and hypercapnia to the point of severe debilitation. Recurrent pulmonary infections with *Haemophilus influenzae*, *Morbaxella catarrhalis*, and *Streptococcus pneumoniae* are especially common with bronchitis. These acute exacerbations are managed with antibiotics. Pulmonary hypertension can develop, leading to cor pulmonale (right-sided heart failure) in chronic bronchitis, whereas patients with emphysema more frequently experience enlarged air space, thoracic bullae, and pneumothorax. Poor quality of sleep because of nocturnal hypoxemia is common with both types of COPD. Although emphysema and chronic bronchitis are irreversible processes for which no cure exists, avoidance of pulmonary irritants can be of significant benefit in the decrease of the morbidity and mortality rates of both diseases.

CLINICAL PRESENTATION

SIGNS AND SYMPTOMS

The onset phase of COPD takes many years in most patients. Individuals who have chronic bronchitis often have a chronic cough with copious sputum production. Patients tend to be sedentary, overweight, cyanotic, edematous, and breathless—leading to the term "blue bloaters."

Patients with emphysema exhibit severe exertional dyspnea with a minimal, nonproductive cough. Their chest walls enlarge and they become "barrel chested" while losing weight as the disease progresses. Cyanosis usually is not seen, and these patients are labeled "pink puffers." Expiration often is accompanied by patients pursing their lips to forcibly remove air from their lungs. The clinical presentation of chronic bronchitis is distinct from emphysema until progression to emphysema occurs (Box 8-1).

LABORATORY FINDINGS

Diagnosing COPD in its early stages can be difficult. The hallmark feature of COPD is reduced maximal expiratory flow rate. Clinical symptoms of dyspnea, cough, and sputum production and blood gas and chest radiograph abnormalities are additional features of COPD.[8] The forced expiratory volume in 1 second (FEV_1) on spirometry is used to determine pulmonary function. The term COPD is used when patients have pulmonary symptoms and a FEV_1 of less than 70% of the predicted volume (forced vital capacity, [FVC]) in the absence of any other pulmonary disease. The term *end-stage* COPD is used when the FEV_1/FVC is less than 50%.

BOX 8-1

Predominant Clinical Features of Patients with Chronic Bronchitis or Emphysema

Chronic Bronchitis	Emphysema
Onset ~50 years	Onset ~60 years
Frequently overweight	Thin, barrel-chested
Chronic productive cough	Cough not prominent
Copious mucopurulent sputum	Scanty sputum
Mild dyspnea	Severe dyspnea
Frequent respiratory infections	Few respiratory infections
Elevated Pco_2	Normal Pco_2
Decreased Po_2 (hypoxia)	Decreased Po_2 (hypoxia)
Elevated hematocrit value	Normal hematocrit value
Hypoxia	No hypoxia

In addition, patients with chronic bronchitis have an elevated Pco_2 and decreased Po_2 (as measured by arterial blood gases), leading to erythrocytosis, an elevated hematocrit value, and compensated respiratory acidosis. Total lung capacity usually is normal, with a moderate elevation of residual volume. Patients with emphysema have a relatively normal Pco_2 and a decreased Po_2, which maintains normal hemoglobin saturation, thus avoiding erythrocytosis. These patients have a normal hematocrit value. The total lung capacity and residual volume are markedly increased. The ventilatory drive of hypoxia also is reduced in both types of patients with COPD.

Chest radiographs of patients with chronic bronchitis demonstrate increased bronchovascular markings at the base of the lungs. In emphysema the films demonstrate a persistent and marked overdistention of the lungs, flattening of the diaphragm, and emphysematous bullae.

MEDICAL MANAGEMENT

No cure exists for COPD. However, much can be done to improve the quality of life for these patients and to prevent progression of the disease. The cornerstone of management is early intervention. Smoking cessation and elimination of exposure to environmental pollutants and irritants are critical to limit the progression of the disease. Other recommended palliative measures include regular exercise, good nutrition, prevention of respiratory infections with annual pneumococcal and influenza vaccinations, aggressive treatment of pulmonary infections with antibiotics, adequate daily hydration, and low-flow oxygen therapy.[9]

Bronchodilators such as methylxanthines and beta-adrenergic stimulators are useful in many patients to relieve symptoms. In addition, corticosteroids, anticholinergics, and nonsteroid antiinflammatory agents also are used (Table 8-1). Until recently theophylline was the most widely used methylxanthine bronchodilator for the treatment of COPD. It relaxes bronchial smooth muscle cells weakly by blocking adenosine receptors and inhibiting the formation of cyclic adenosine monophosphate. Theophylline also appears to have immunomodulating effects.[10] Theophylline has a narrow therapeutic range. Numerous factors and medications can displace the protein-bound fraction of the drug in the bloodstream, causing toxicity. Because of the likelihood of obtaining adverse effects in the elderly, theophylline has been replaced over the last few years with beta$_2$-adrenergic agonists that dilate the bronchial airways and have fewer side effects. Anticholinergics (e.g., ipratropium) that block acetylcholine and bronchoconstriction are added when needed. Theophylline is recommended when inhaled bronchodilators are inadequate. Corticosteroids are used in some patients generally as a systemic drug for 1 to 2 weeks during acute periods and in combination with beta agonists in persons with end-stage disease who are steroid responsive. Low-flow oxygen therapy is used for severe COPD.[11]

DENTAL MANAGEMENT

PREVENTION OF POTENTIAL PROBLEMS

Most patients with COPD have a history of smoking tobacco. Dental health providers can take an important step in the management of patients with COPD by encouraging those who smoke to quit. By providing knowledge of the diseases associated with smoking, dental health providers may help patients to start thinking seriously about giving up the habit. Many interventive approaches are available (e.g., nicotine replacement, bupropion), and providers should use the method with which they feel most comfortable[12] (see Chapter 23).

Before initiating dental care clinicians should assess the severity of the patient's disease and its control. A patient coming to the office for routine dental care who displays shortness of breath at rest, a productive cough, upper respiratory infection, or an oxygen saturation of

TABLE 8-1

Drugs Used in the Outpatient Management of COPD and Asthma

Category and Generic Name	Product Name
Antiinflammatory Drugs	
Corticosteroids—inhaled	
Beclomethasone dipropionate	Vanceril, Beclovent
Budesonide	Pulmicort
Dexamethasone	Decadron
Flunisolide	AeroBid
Fluticasone propionate	Flonase
Triamcinolone acetonide	Azmacort
Corticosteroids—systemic	
Prednisone	Deltasone or generic
Prednisolone	Delta-Cortef
Methylprednisolone	Solu-Medrol
Antileukotrienes	
5-Lipoxygenase inhibitor	Zileuton (Zylfo)
Leukotriene D_4 receptor antagonists	Zafirlukast (Accolate), Montelukast (Singulair)
Nonsteroidal—chromones	
Cromolyn sodium	Intal inhaler
Nedocromil	Tilade inhaler
Beta-Adrenergic Bronchodilators	
Fast-acting nonselective beta agonist inhalers	
Epinephrine*	Primatene Mist, Bronkaid (available parenteral also)
Ephedrine†	Eted II
Intermediate-acting nonselective beta agonist inhalers (3 to 6 hours)	
Isoproterenol‡	Isuprel
Isoetharine	Bronkosol
Metaproterenol§	Alupent, Metaprel, and others
Beta$_2$ selective agonist inhalers	
Albuterol‡	Proventil, Ventolin
Bitolterol mesylate	Tornalate
Pirbuterol	Maxair, Maxair Autohaler
Terbutaline‡	Brethaire, Bricanyl
Fenoterol	Not available in U.S., restricted availability in New Zealand

*Inhalation and parenteral.
†Oral and parenteral.
‡Inhalation, oral, and parenteral.
§Inhalation and oral.

TABLE **8-1**

Drugs Used in the Outpatient Management of COPD and Asthma—cont'd

Category and Generic Name	Product Name
Long-acting beta$_2$ selective agonist inhalers (>12 hours)	
Salmeterol (slow onset, long duration)	Serevent
Formoterol (rapid onset, long duration)	Not available in United States
Methylxanthines	
Theophylline	Theo-Dur
Quaternary Ammonium Derivative of Atropine (Anticholinergic Bronchodilator)	
Ipratropium bromide	Atrovent
Tiotropium (not yet approved by the U.S. Food and Drug Administration)	
Experimental Antiasthmatic Drugs	
Inhaled heparin, inhaled indomethacin	

less than 91% (as determined by pulse oximetry) is unstable, and staff should reschedule the appointment. If the patient is stable and the breathing is adequate, efforts should be directed toward the avoidance of anything that could further depress respiration (Box 8-2). Patients should be placed in a semisupine or upright chair position for treatment, rather than the supine position, to prevent orthopnea and the feeling of respiratory discomfort. Pulse oximetry monitoring is advised. Humidified low-flow oxygen, generally between 2 and 3 liters per minute, can be provided and should be considered for use when the oxygen saturation is less than 95%.

No contraindication exists to the use of local anesthetic. However, use of bilateral mandibular blocks or bilateral palatal blocks can cause an unpleasant airway constriction sensation in some patients. This may be more important when managing a severe COPD patient with a rubber dam or when medications are administered that dry mucous secretions. Humidified low-flow oxygen can be provided to alleviate the unpleasant airway feeling produced by nerve blocks, use of a rubber dam, and medications.

If sedative medication is required, low-dose oral diazepam (Valium) may be used. Nitrous oxide-oxygen inhalation sedation should be used with caution in patients with mild to moderate chronic bronchitis. It should not be used in patients with severe COPD and emphysema because the gas may accumulate in air

BOX **8-2**

Dental Management of the Patient with COPD

Review history for evidence of concurrent heart disease, take appropriate precautions if heart disease present

Avoid treating if upper respiratory infection present

Treat in upright chair position

Use local anesthetic as usual

Avoid use of rubber dam in severe disease

Use pulse oximetry to monitor oxygen saturation

Consider low-flow (2 to 3 L/min) supplemental oxygen is helpful when oxygen saturation drops below 95%; may be necessary when oxygen saturation drops 91%

Avoid nitrous oxide-oxygen inhalation sedation with severe COPD and emphysema

Consider low-dose oral diazepam or other benzodiazepine; may cause oral dryness

Avoid use of barbiturates, narcotics, antihistamines, and anticholinergics

May need supplemental steroids if patient taking steroids and invasive procedure planned

Avoid erythromycin, macrolide antibiotics, and ciprofloxacin for patient taking theophylline

Do not use outpatient general anesthesia

spaces of the diseased lung. If used in the patient with chronic bronchitis, flow rates should be reduced to an overall rate of no greater than 3 liters per minute, and the clinician should anticipate approximately twice as long induction and recovery times with N_2O than with healthy patients.[13] Narcotics and barbiturates should not be used because of their respiratory depressant properties. Anticholinergics and antihistamines generally should not be used because of their drying properties and the resultant increase of mucous tenacity.

Patients with COPD often have hypertension and coronary heart disease (see Chapters 4 and 5). Patients taking corticosteroids may require supplementation for major surgical procedures because of adrenal suppression (see Chapter 15). Macrolide antibiotics (e.g., erythromycin and azithromycin) and ciprofloxacin hydrochloride should be avoided for patients taking theophylline because these antibiotics can retard the metabolism of theophylline, resulting in theophylline toxicity. The dentist should be aware of the manifestations of theophylline toxicity. Symptoms include anorexia, nausea, nervousness, insomnia, agitation, thirst, vomiting, headache, cardiac arrhythmias, and convulsions. Outpatient general anesthesia is contraindicated for most patients with COPD.

TREATMENT PLANNING MODIFICATIONS

No technical treatment planning modifications are required of patients with COPD.

ORAL COMPLICATIONS AND MANIFESTATIONS

Patients with COPD who are chronic smokers have an increased likelihood of developing halitosis, extrinsic tooth stains, nicotine stomatitis, periodontal disease, and oral cancer. In rare instances, theophylline has been associated with the development of Stevens-Johnson syndrome.

■ ASTHMA ■

DEFINITION

Asthma is a chronic inflammatory respiratory disease consisting of recurrent episodes of dyspnea, coughing, and wheezing resulting from hyperresponsiveness of the tracheobronchial tree. The bronchiole lung tissue of patients with asthma is particularly sensitive to a variety of stimuli. Overt attacks may be provoked by allergens, upper respiratory tract infections, exercise, cold air, certain medications (salicylates, nonsteroidal anti-inflammatory drugs, cholinergic drugs, and beta-adrenergic blocking drugs), chemicals, smoke, and highly emotional states such as anxiety, stress and nervousness.

EPIDEMIOLOGY

INCIDENCE AND PREVALENCE

Asthma is a worldwide problem. In Japan the prevalence has more than doubled since the 1960s, from 1.2% to 3.1%.[14] The prevalence in the United States from 1980 to 1994 increased 75%, from 3.5% to 4.9% (13.7 million) of the general population. Asthma is a disease primarily of children, with 10% of children affected.[15] Young persons with asthma most often are male, whereas adults who contact the disease more frequently are women. However, the disease occurs in all races, with a slightly higher prevalence in African-Americans (58 persons per 1000 population) than other races (49 persons per 1000 population).[15] Based on these figures, the average dental practice is predicted to have up to 100 patients who have asthma.

ETIOLOGY

Asthma is a multifactorial disease whose exact etiology is not well defined. Five types of asthma have been described: extrinsic (allergic or atopic), intrinsic (idiosyncratic, nonallergic, or nonatopic), drug induced, exercise induced, and infectious.

Allergic or *extrinsic* asthma is the most common form and accounts for approximately 35% of all adult cases. It is triggered by inhaled seasonal allergens such as pollens, dust, house mites, and animal danders and usually is seen in children and young adults.[16] A dose-response relationship exists between allergen exposure and immunoglobulin E (IgE)-mediated sensitization, positive skin testing to various allergens, and associated family history of allergic diseases in these patients. During an attack, allergens interact with IgE antibodies affixed to mast cells along the tracheobronchial tree. The complex of antigen with antibody causes mast cells to degranulate and secrete vasoactive autocoids and cytokines such as bradykinins, histamine, leukotrienes, and prostaglandins.[10] Histamine causes bronchoconstriction and increased vascular permeability. Leukotrienes produce smooth muscle spasm, increase vascular permeability, and attract eosinophils into the airway.[17] The release of platelet-activating factor sustains bronchial hyperresponsiveness. Release of E-selectin and endothelial cell

adhesion molecules, neutrophil chemotactic factor, and eosinophilic chemotactic factor of anaphylaxis is responsible for recruitment of leukocytes to the airway wall, which increases tissue edema and mucous secretion. T lymphocytes prolong the inflammatory responses.

Intrinsic asthma accounts for about 30% of asthma cases and seldom is associated with a family history of allergy or with a known cause. Patients usually are nonresponsive to skin testing and demonstrate normal IgE levels. This form of asthma generally is seen in middle-aged adults, and its onset is associated with endogenous causes such as emotional stress (implicated in at least 50% of persons with asthma), gastroesophageal acid reflux, or vagal-mediated responses.[16,18]

Ingestion of drugs (aspirin, nonsteroidal antiinflammatory drugs, beta-blockers, angiotensin-converting enzyme inhibitors), and some food substances (nuts, shellfish, strawberries, milk, tartrazine food dye and color yellow no. 5) can trigger asthma. Aspirin causes bronchoconstriction in about 10% of patients with asthma, and sensitivity to aspirin occurs in 30% to 40% of people with asthma who have pansinusitis and nasal polyps (*triad asthmaticus*).[19] The ability of aspirin to block the cyclooxygenase pathway appears causative. The buildup of arachidonic acid and leukotrienes via the lipoxygenase pathway results in bronchial spasm.[20]

Metabisulfite preservatives of foods and drugs (local anesthetics containing epinephrine) may cause wheezing when metabolic levels of the enzyme sulfite oxidase are low.[21] Sulfur dioxide is produced in the absence of sulfite oxidase.[22] The buildup of sulfur dioxide in the bronchial tree precipitates an acute asthma attack.[22]

Exercise-induced asthma is stimulated by exertional activity. Although the pathogenesis of this form of asthma is unknown, thermal changes during inhalation of cold air provoke mucosal irritation and airway hyperactivity. Children and young adults are more severely affected because of their high level of physical activity.

Patients with infectious asthma develop bronchial constriction and increased airway resistance because of the inflammatory response of the bronchi to infection. Causative agents often are viruses, bacteria, dermatologic fungi (*Trichophyton*), and *Mycoplasma* organisms. Treatment of the infection usually improves control of the pulmonary constriction.

PATHOPHYSIOLOGY AND COMPLICATIONS

The obstruction of airflow in asthma is the result of bronchial smooth muscle spasm, inflammation of bronchial mucosa, mucous hypersecretion, and sputum plugging. The most striking macroscopic finding in the asthmatic lung is occlusion of the bronchi and bron-

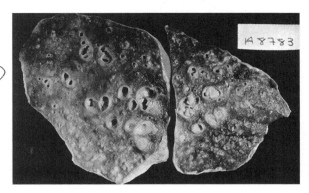

Fig. 8-2 Section of a lung with the bronchioles occluded by mucous plugs. (Courtesy A. Golden, Lexington, Ky.)

chioles by thick, tenacious mucous plugs (Fig. 8-2). Characteristic histologic findings include (1) thickened basement membrane (because of collagen deposition) of the bronchial epithelium, (2) edema, (3) hypertrophy of the mucous glands, (4) hypertrophy of the bronchial wall muscle, and (5) mast cell and inflammatory cell infiltrate.[23] These changes result in decreased diameter of the airway, and contribute to increased airway resistance and difficulty in expiration.

Asthma is relatively benign in terms of morbidity. Most patients can expect a reasonably good prognosis, especially those in whom the disease develops during childhood. In many young children, the condition resolves spontaneously after puberty. However, a small percentage of patients can progress to emphysema and respiratory failure or will develop *status asthmaticus*, the most serious manifestation of asthma. Status asthmaticus is a particularly severe and prolonged asthmatic attack (one lasting longer than 24 hours) that is refractory to usual therapy. Signs include increased dyspnea, jugular venous pulsation, cyanosis, and *pulsus paradoxus* (a fall in systolic pressure with inspiration). S. *asthmaticus* often is associated with a respiratory infection and can cause exhaustion, severe dehydration, peripheral vascular collapse, and death. Although death directly attributable to asthma is relatively uncommon, the disease causes more than 5000 deaths per year in the United States.

CLINICAL PRESENTATION

SIGNS AND SYMPTOMS

Asthma attacks often occur at night, for reasons that are unclear, but also may follow exposure to an allergen, exercise, respiratory infection, and emotional upset and

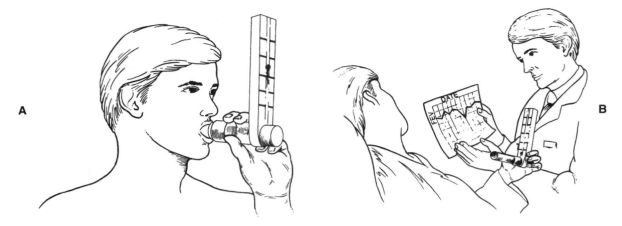

Fig. 8-3 A, Measure of forced expiratory volume by spirometry. **B,** Discussion of daily spirometry results with physician.

excitement. The typical symptoms of asthma consist of reversible episodes of breathlessness (dyspnea), chest tightness, wheezing, cough that is worse at night, and flushing. Onset usually is sudden. Respirations become difficult and are accompanied by expiratory wheezing. Tachypnea and prolonged expiration are characteristic. The termination of an attack is commonly accompanied by a productive cough with thick, stringy mucus. Episodes usually are self-limiting though severe episodes may require medical assistance.[24]

LABORATORY FINDINGS

Diagnostic testing by a physician is important in the differentiation of asthma from COPD. Clinical judgment is required, as laboratory tests for asthma are relatively nonspecific and any test alone is not diagnostic. Commonly ordered tests include chest radiographs (for hyperinflation), skin testing (for specific allergens), histamine or methacholine chloride challenge testing, sputum smears, blood counts (for eosinophilia), arterial blood gases, antibody-based enzyme-linked immunosorbent assay (ELISA) for measurement of environmental allergen exposure, and spirometry (a peak expiratory flowmeter that measures pulmonary function) before and after administration of a short-acting bronchodilator.[25] This latter test is important as the diagnosis of asthma requires airflow obstruction be episodic and at least partially reversible. Accordingly, decreased pulmonary function (i.e., FEV_1) as measured by spirometry is a feature of the disease. A recent drop in FEV_1 can be interpreted as a prediction of an asthma attack (Fig. 8-3).

CLASSIFICATION

Patients with chronic asthma are classified as *mild* (intermittent or persistent), *moderate*, or *severe* according to the frequency of acute attacks and lung function (Box 8-3). Persons with mild asthma have symptoms only when exposed to a condition that triggers asthma and their FEV_1 is greater than 80%. Symptoms last less than an hour and occur less than twice a week. Patients with moderate asthma have FEV_1 greater than 80% and symptoms more than twice a week that affect sleep and activity level, occur over several days, and on occasion require emergency care. Asthma is severe when patients have less than 60% FEV_1 which results in ongoing symptoms that limit normal activity. Attacks are frequent, at night, and occasionally result in emergency hospitalization.

MEDICAL MANAGEMENT

The goals of asthma therapy are to limit exposure to triggering agents, allow normal activities, restore and maintain normal pulmonary function, prevent adverse effects from medications, and minimize frequency and severity of attacks.[26] These goals can be achieved by educating patients, preventing or eliminating precipitating factors, establishing an intervention plan for self-management, and providing regular follow-up care. Educating the patient with known allergies about the importance of avoidance of allergens is the first step in preventing attacks. This can be emphasized by monitoring allergen levels (tobacco smoke and pollutants) in the patient's house, providing desensitization intradermal in-

BOX 8-3

Classification of Asthma

Mild Intermittent

Intermittent wheezing less than 2 days per week, exacerbations that are brief, asymptomatic between exacerbations, nocturnal symptoms less than 2 times a month, relatively good exercise tolerance, FEV_2 more than 80% predicted, less than 20% variability

Mild Persistent

Wheezing 2-5 days per week (occurs over several days), exacerbations that affect activity and sleep, nocturnal asthma attacks more than 2 times a month, limited exercise tolerance; rare ER visit, FEV_1 more than 80% predicted, 20-30% variability

Moderate Persistent

Daily symptoms of wheezing (occur over several days), daily use of short-acting beta-agonist, exacerbations that affect activity and sleep and may last for days, nocturnal asthma attacks at least 1 time a week, limited exercise tolerance, ER visit, FEV_1 60-80% predicted, 20-30% variability

Severe Persistent

Frequent/daily exacerbations, continual symptoms, frequent (more than 4 times a month) nocturnal asthma, exercise intolerance, FEV_1 less than 60%, more than 30% variability, often resulting in hospitalization

Mild Intermittent Asthma
As needed use of bronchodilator

↓

Mild Persistent Asthma
Anti-inflammatory drug
Low dose inhaled corticosteroid or cromolyn, or Zafirlukast (Accolate), Montelukast (Singulair), or Zileuton (Zyflo)

↓

Moderate Persistent Asthma
One medium dose inhaled corticosteroid, or Two daily medications: Low to medium dose inhaled corticosteroid and long-acting bronchodilator (e.g., Salmeterol [Serevent], sustained-released theophylline or long-acting β_2 agonist tablets)

↓

Severe Persistent Asthma
Daily medications: High-dose inhaled corticosteroid + Long-acting bronchodilator (Salmeterol [Serevent], sustained-released theophylline or long-acting β_2 agonist tablets) + oral corticosteroid (usually 2mg/kg; total dose <60 mg)

Asthma Attack
Short-acting bronchodilator

Fig. 8-4 Algorithm for management of asthma.

jections, and monitoring their pulmonary function zone based on daily peak flowmeter results (spirometry). Unfortunately, poor control of asthma often is related to low socioeconomic status (e.g., the patient cannot afford medication), increased anxiety, poor compliance, and poor home environment.

The selection of an antiasthmatic drug is based on the type and severity of asthma and whether the drug is to be used as a prophylactic or as therapy.[23] Chronic asthma once was controlled with the use of beta$_2$-adrenergic agonists and theophylline; however, current guidelines recommend a "step care" approach with the use of inhaled antiinflammatory agents (corticosteroids, nonsteroidal drugs and leukotriene inhibitors) for the prophylaxis of chronic asthma (Fig. 8-4).[10,27] Beta-adrenergic agonists, methylxanthines, and anticholinergic drugs are secondary agents added when antiinflammatory drugs are inadequate. Current national guidelines[23] recommend adding long-acting beta$_2$ agonists or an antileukotriene to low-dose inhaled corticosteroids before increasing corticosteroids. Antileukotrienes are most useful in mild to moderate asthma and in blocking aspirin-induced asthmatic responses.[28]

For persistent asthma, inhaled corticosteroids are recommended over beta-adrenergic agonists because steroids provide better overall control of asthma and less likelihood of a sudden overwhelming attack.[29,30] Steroids act by reducing the inflammatory response and preventing the formation of cytokines, adhesion molecules and inflammatory enzymes. Aerosol dosage is two (for mild to moderate disease) to four times daily (severe asthma). The onset of action is usually 2 hours, and peak effects occur 6 hours later. Long-term use of steroid inhalers rarely is associated with systemic side effects—provided the maximum recommended dose of 1.5 mg per day of inhaled beclomethasone dipropionate (Beclovent, Vanceril) or equivalent is not exceeded. Use of systemic steroids is reserved for asthma unresponsive to inhaled corticosteroids and bronchodilators, and during the recovery phase of a severe acute attack. Corticosteroid sparing agents (cyclosporine, methotrexate) are used in severe asthma to minimize the adverse effects of high

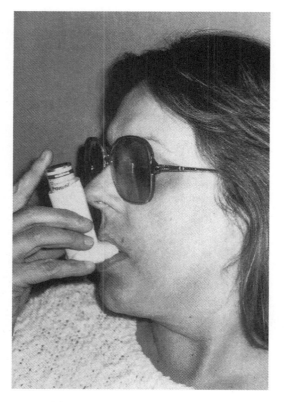

Fig. 8-5 Use of an inhaler by a patient.

dose systemic steroids but have their own set of adverse effects. Recombinant monoclonal antibody against human IgE is a newer agent that appears to be the treatment of persons with moderate to severe allergic asthma.[31]

Inhaled beta$_2$-adrenergic agonists are the drugs of choice for the fastest and greatest bronchodilation and smooth muscle relaxation required for relief of acute asthma attacks (Fig. 8-5). These agonists produce bronchodilatation by activating beta$_2$ receptors on airway smooth muscle cells.[10] Inhalation corticosteroids and cromolyn sodium are used infrequently for this purpose because of slow onset of action. Beta$_2$-adrenergic agonists (administered by a metered-dose inhaler) and cromolyn sodium (Intal) may be used in preventing exercise-induced bronchospasm. They are taken about 30 minutes before exposure to physical activity. Cromolyn sodium decreases airway hyperresponsiveness by stabilizing the membrane of mast cells so mediators are not released when challenged by exercise or cold air.

DENTAL MANAGEMENT

PREVENTION OF POTENTIAL PROBLEMS

The goal of management for dental patients with asthma must be to prevent an acute asthma attack (Box 8-4). The first step in achieving this goal is to identify patients with asthma by history, learn as much as possible about their problem, and prevent precipitating factors.

Through a good history, the dentist should be able to determine the severity and stability of disease. Questions should be asked that ascertain the type of asthma (e.g., allergic, nonallergic), the precipitating substances, the frequency and severity of attacks, the time of day attacks occur, whether this is a current or past problem, how attacks usually are managed, and whether the patient has received emergency treatment of an acute attack. The clinician must realize that severe disease is associated with frequent exacerbations, exercise intolerance, FEV$_1$ less than 60%, use of several medications, and a history of visits to an emergency facility for treatment of acute attacks (see Box 8-3).

The stability of the disease can be assessed by clinical and laboratory measures. Features such as shortness of breath, wheezing, increased respiration rate (more than 50% above normal), FEV$_1$ below 80% of peak FEV$_1$, an eosinophil count elevated above 50 per mm,[3] and emergency department visits within the previous three months suggest inadequate treatment and poor stability. Also, the use of more than 1.5 canisters of a beta-agonist inhaler per month (more than 200 inhalation per month) or a doubling of the monthly use indicates high risk of a severe asthma attack.[32] For severe and unstable asthma, consultation with the patient's physician is advised. Routine dental treatment should be postponed until better control is achieved.

Modifications in the preoperative and operative phases of dental management of a patient with asthma can minimize the likelihood of an attack. Patients who have nocturnal asthma should be scheduled for late-morning appointments, when attacks are less likely. Operatory odorants (e.g., methyl methacrylate) should be reduced before the patient is treated. Patients should be instructed to bring their inhalers (bronchodilators) to each appointment and inform the dentist at the earliest sign or symptom of an asthma attack. Prophylactic inhalation of a patient's bronchodilator at the beginning of the appointment is a valuable method of preventing an asthma attack. Alternatively, patients may be advised to bring their spirometer and daily expiratory record to the office. The dentist can request that the patient exhale into the spirometer and record

BOX 8-4

Dental Management of the Patient with Asthma

1. Identification and assessment by history
   a. Type of asthma (mild, moderate, or severe)
   b. Precipitating factors
   c. Age at onset
   d. Frequency, time of day, and severity of attacks
   e. How usually managed
   f. Medications being taken (how often quick-relief medication used) and taken correctly the day of appointment
   g. Necessity of emergency care
   h. Baseline FEV_1 stable (not decreasing)
2. Avoidance of known precipitating factors
3. Medical consultation for severe, active asthmatic
4. Patient to bring medication inhaler to every appointment and keep it available; used prophylactically in persons with chronic moderate to severe disease
5. Drug considerations
   a. Avoidance of aspirin-containing medications (use acetaminophen)
   b. Avoidance of nonsteroidal antiinflammatory drugs (NSAIDs) (see Table 16-3)
   c. Avoidance of barbiturates and narcotics (histamine-releasing drugs)
   d. Avoidance of erythromycin and macrolide antibiotics in patients taking theophylline
   e. Discontinuance of cimetidine 24 hr before intravenous sedation in patients taking theophylline
6. Local anesthetic considerations (may elect to avoid solutions containing epinephrine or levonordefrin because of sulfite preservative)
7. Patients taking chronic corticosteroid medications may require supplementation (see Chapter 15)
8. Provision of stress-free environment through establishment of rapport and openness
9. If sedation required, nitrous oxide-oxygen inhalation sedation and/or small doses of oral diazepam recommended
10. Recognition of signs and symptoms of a severe asthma attack
    a. Inability to finish sentences with one breath, ineffectiveness of bronchodilators to relieve dyspnea, tachypnea equal to or greater than 25 breaths per minute, tachycardia equal to or greater than 110 beats per minute, diaphoresis, accessory muscle usage, paradoxic pulse
    b. Administering of fast-acting bronchodilator (Note: corticosteroids have delayed onset of action), oxygen and if needed subcutaneous 0.3 to 0.5 ml of epinephrine (1:1000)

---

the expired volume. A significant drop in lung function (below 80% of peak FEV_1) compared with previous recordings would indicate that prophylactic use of the inhaler or a referral to a physician is needed.[33] The use of a pulse oximeter also is valuable for determining oxygen saturation of the patient. Healthy patients should remain between 97% and 100%, whereas a drop to 90% or below indicates poor oxygen exchange and the need for intervention.

Because stress is implicated as a precipitating factor in asthma attacks and dental treatment can result in decreased lung function,[34] the dental staff should make every effort to identify patients who are anxious and provide a stress-free environment through establishment of rapport and openness. Preoperative and intraoperative sedation may be desirable. If sedation is required, nitrous oxide-oxygen inhalation is best. Nitrous oxide is not a respiratory depressant nor an irritation to the tracheo-bronchial tree. Oral premedication may be accomplished with small doses of a short-acting benzodiazepine. Reasonable alternatives with children include the use of hydroxyzine (Vistaril) for its antihistamine-sedative properties or ketamine, which causes bronchodilation. Barbiturates and narcotics, particularly meperidine, are histamine-releasing drugs and can provoke an attack. Outpatient general anesthesia generally is contraindicated for patients with asthma.

The selection of the local anesthetic may require alteration. In 1987 the U.S. Food and Drug Administration[21] warned that drugs containing sulfites were a cause of allergic-type reactions in susceptible individuals. Sulfite preservatives are found in local anesthetic solutions containing epinephrine or levonordefrin, albeit the amount of sulfite in a local anesthetic cartridge is less than the amount commonly found in certain foods. Although rare, at least one case of an acute asthma attack precipitated

by exposure to sulfites has been reported.[35] Thus the use of local anesthetic without epinephrine or levonordefrin may be advisable for patients with moderate to severe disease. As the data remain limited concerning this problem, dentists should discuss past responses to local anesthetic and allergy to sulfites with the patient and consult with the physician. As an alternative, local anesthetics without vasoconstrictor can be used in at-risk patients.

Patients with asthma who are chronically medicated with systemic corticosteroids may require supplementation for major dental procedures (see Chapter 15). However, long-term use of inhaled corticosteroids rarely causes adrenal suppression unless the dosage exceeds 1.5 mg beclomethasone dipropionate daily.[10]

Administration of aspirin-containing medication or other nonsteroidal antiinflammatory drugs to patients with asthma is not advisable because aspirin ingestion is associated with the precipitation of asthma attacks in a small percentage of patients. Likewise, barbiturates and narcotics are best not used as they also may precipitate an asthma attack. Antihistamines have beneficial properties but should be used cautiously because of their drying effect. Patients taking theophylline preparations should not be given macrolide antibiotics (i.e., erythromycin and azithromycin) or ciprofloxacin hydrochloride as this may result in a toxic blood level of theophylline. To prevent serious toxicity the dentist should ask the patient who takes theophylline whether the dosage is being monitored based on serum theophylline levels (recommended to be less than 10 μg/ml). Approximately 3% of patients taking zileuton experience elevated alanine transaminase levels and liver dysfunction that could affect the metabolism of dentally administered drugs.[36]

MANAGEMENT OF POTENTIAL PROBLEMS: ASTHMA ATTACK

An acute asthma attack requires immediate therapy. The signs and symptoms (see Box 8-4) should be recognized quickly and an inhaler provided rapidly. A short-acting beta$_2$-adrenergic agonist inhaler (Ventolin, Proventil) is the most effective and fastest-acting bronchodilator. It should be administered at the first sign of an attack. Long-lasting beta$_2$ agonist drugs like salmeterol (Serevent) and corticosteroids do not act quickly and are not given for an immediate response, but they can provide a delayed response. In cases of a severe asthma attack, use of subcutaneous injection of epinephrine (0.3 to 0.5 ml, 1:1000) or inhalation of epinephrine (Primatene Mist) is the most potent and fastest-acting method for

relieving an asthma attack. Supportive treatment includes providing positive-flow oxygenation, repeating bronchodilator doses as necessary, monitoring vital signs (including oxygen saturation, if possible), and activating the emergency medical system, if needed.

TREATMENT PLANNING MODIFICATIONS

No specific treatment planning modifications are required of the patient with asthma.

ORAL COMPLICATIONS AND MANIFESTATIONS

Nasal symptoms, allergic rhinitis and mouth breathing are common with extrinsic asthma. Mouth breathers with asthma can have altered nasorespiratory function that can result in increased upper anterior and total anterior facial height, higher palatal vaults, greater overjets, and a higher prevalence of crossbites.[37]

The medications patients with asthma take also can cause oral disease. For example, beta$_2$ agonist inhalers decrease salivary flow by 20% to 35%, decrease plaque pH,[38] and are associated with increased prevalence of gingivitis and caries in patients with moderate to severe asthma.[39-41] Gastroesophageal acid reflux is common in patients with asthma and is exacerbated by the use of beta agonists and theophylline.[18] The reflux can contribute to erosion of enamel. Oral candidiasis (acute pseudomembranous type) occurs in approximately 5% of patients using inhalation steroids chronically at high dose or frequency.[42] However, this is rare if a "spacer" or aerosol-holding chamber is attached to the metered-dose inhaler and the mouth is rinsed with water after each use.[43] The condition readily responds to local antifungal therapy, such as nystatin or clotrimazole. Patients should receive instructions on the proper use of their inhaler and the need for oral rinsing. Headache is a frequent side effect of antileukotrienes and theophylline. The clinician should be aware of this adverse effect when diagnosing patients with myofascial pain complaints.

■ TUBERCULOSIS ■

DEFINITION

Tuberculosis (TB) is a major global health problem caused by an infectious and communicable organism, *Mycobacterium tuberculosis*. The disease is spread by inhalation of infected droplets and usually demonstrates a pro-

longed quiescent period. M. *tuberculosis* replication leads to a host inflammatory and granulomatous response and classic pulmonary and systemic symptoms. Although M. *tuberculosis* is by far the most common causative agent in this human infection, other species of mycobacteria are occasionally encountered, such as M. *avium complex*, M. *kansasii*, M. *abscessus*, M. *xenopi*, M. *bovis*, and M. *africanum*. These mycobacterium can cause systemic disease (pulmonary, lymphadenitis, cutaneous or disseminated) which are termed *"mycobacteriosis."*

EPIDEMIOLOGY

INCIDENCE AND PREVALENCE

TB kills more adults worldwide each year than any other single pathogen.[44,45] In contrast to the world picture, the occurrence of TB in the United States has steadily decreased during the last century and dropped at a rate of 5% per year during the past 40 years. Around the turn of the 20th century approximately 500 new cases of active TB per 100,000 population were identified every year in the United States. In 1985 a rate of 9.3 per 100,000 population was reported to the Centers for Disease Control (CDC).[46] This figure rose to 10.6, or 26,000 cases,[47,48] in 1993, mostly because of adverse social and economic factors, the AIDS epidemic, and the immigration of foreign-born persons who have TB. In 1998, 18,361 cases of TB were reported, a rate of 6.8 per 100,000.[49] That was the lowest rate reported during the past century. Although the figures are encouraging, the disease continues to exist in every state of the United States. Moreover, approximately 40% of new U.S. cases occur in foreign-born persons who migrate or travel to the United States.[50]

Although the present rate for the United States as a whole is low, minority residents of inner-city ghettos, the elderly urban poor, persons living in congregate settings (prisons and shelters), and persons with AIDS have occurrence rates several times the national average (Box 8-5). Approximately 7% of the U.S. population and 50% of the world's population have been infected with TB, and a higher risk for the disease exists with human HIV-positive persons (a 8% chance of developing TB per year).[51-53] TB is diagnosed most often in men (1.6 to 1 woman) and persons between 25 and 64 years of age.[49]

Important factors in reducing the spread of TB in the United States during the past century have been improved sanitation and hygiene measures and the use of effective antituberculous drugs. Unfortunately, failure in completing a course of therapy (which occurs in more than 20% of patients) and improper drug selection have

---

BOX 8-5

High-Risk Groups for Tuberculosis

Close contacts of persons having TB
Persons infected with HIV
Injecting drug users
Persons with medical risk factors
Residents and employees of congregate settings (prisons, nursing homes, mental institutions, shelters)
Healthcare workers who serve high-risk persons
Foreign-born persons (and migrant workers) from countries that have a high TB incidence or prevalence
Medically underserved persons
High-risk racial or ethnic minority populations

---

contributed to the persistence of this disease and the rise in the percentage of cases of multidrug-resistant TB, from 0.5% in 1982 to about 9% in 1998.[54,55]

ETIOLOGY

In the majority of cases of human TB the causative agent is M. *tuberculosis*, an acid-fast, nonmotile, intracellular rod that is an obligate aerobe. Because M. *tuberculosis* is an aerobe, it exists best in an atmosphere of high oxygen tension; therefore it most commonly infects the lung.

The typical mode of transmission of the bacteria is by way of infected airborne droplets of mucus or saliva that have been forcefully expelled from the lungs, most commonly by a cough but also by sneezing and talking. The quantity and size of the expelled droplets influence transmission. The smaller droplets evaporate readily, leaving the bacteria and other solid material as floating particles that are easily inhaled. The larger droplets quickly settle to the ground. Transmission by way of fomites rarely occurs.[52,56] Transmission by ingestion (e.g., of contaminated milk) also rarely occurs because of the use of pasteurized milk. A secondary mode of transmission, by ingestion, can occur when a patient coughs up infected sputum and inoculates oral tissues. Oral lesions of TB may be initiated through this mechanism.

The interval from infection to development of active TB is widely variable, ranging from a few weeks to decades. Most cases of TB result from reactivation of a tubercle; only 10% of cases result from the initial infection. The number of organisms inhaled and the level of immunocompetency determine largely whether the disease is contracted.

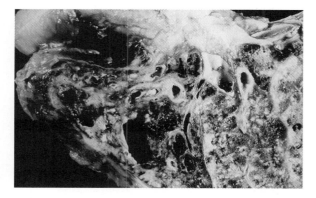

Fig. 8-6 Gross specimen of a tuberculous lung, demonstrating cavitation. (Courtesy R. Powell, Lexington, Ky.)

PATHOPHYSIOLOGY AND COMPLICATIONS

TB can affect virtually any organ of the body, though the lung is the most common site of infection. The typical infection of primary pulmonary TB begins with the inhalation of infected droplets. The droplets are carried into the alveoli, where the bacteria are engulfed by macrophages and begin to multiply. The infection progresses locally and may involve regional (hilar) lymph nodes. Distant dissemination through the bloodstream can occur if the infection is not controlled locally; however, the vast majority of disseminated bacteria are destroyed by natural host defenses. Approximately 2 to 8 weeks after infection a delayed hypersensitivity to the bacteria develops that is mediated by T (CD4+) helper lymphocytes. The condition is manifested by conversion of the tuberculin skin test (purified protein derivative [PPD]) from negative to positive. Subsequently, a chronic granulomatous inflammatory reaction develops involving activated epithelioid macrophages and granuloma formation. These natural host defenses usually control and contain the primary pulmonary TB infection. If they are not contained, the nidus of infection (granuloma) may become a productive tubercle with central necrosis and caseation. Cavitation may occur, resulting in the dumping of organisms into the airway for further dissemination either into other lung tissue or the outside by means of forceful expulsion (Fig. 8-6).

The limitation and local containment of the infection may be caused by a variety of factors, including host resistance, host immune capabilities, and virulence of the mycobacterium. Once the infection is successfully interrupted, the lesion heals spontaneously then undergoes inspissation, hardening, encapsulation, and calcification. Though the lesion is "healed," some bacteria may remain in a dormant state. If the infection is not interrupted, dis-

semination of bacilli can occur through the lung parenchyma, resulting in extensive pulmonary lesions and lymphohematogenous spread. A widespread infection with multiple organ involvement is termed *miliary tuberculosis*.

Primary pulmonary TB is seen most often in infants and children; however, cavitation is rare in these age groups. The majority of children produce no sputum and usually swallow the sputum even if some bacilli are present in the bronchi. The expression of the disease differs somewhat in teenagers and adults in that lymph node involvement and lymphohematogenous spread are not prominent features. However, cavitation commonly occurs. The usual form of disease found in adults is termed *secondary* or *reinfection* TB. This occurs with the reactivation of persistent dormant viable bacilli and probably represents a relapse of a previous infection. This form of the disease usually is confined to the lungs, and cavitation is common. The reasons for relapse are inadequate treatment of the primary infection and influences of illness, immunosuppressive agents, and age. AIDS is responsible for a growing number of cases of reactivation TB.

Some of the more common sequelae of TB include progressive primary TB, cavitary disease, pleurisy and pleural effusion, meningitis, and disseminated or miliary TB. Isolated organ involvement other than of the lung can occur and commonly affects the pericardium, peritoneum, kidneys, adrenal glands, and bone (known as *Pott's disease* when it affects the spine).[57,58] The tongue and other tissues of the oral cavity also are involved infrequently.

Approximately 5% to 10% of persons who develop TB die of the disease.[59] However, the death rate attributable to TB is much larger (54%) in young persons who have AIDS.[59] The advent of effective chemotherapy undoubtedly has been the most significant reason for the lower mortality rate seen in nonimmunosuppressed, TB-infected persons.

CLINICAL PRESENTATION

SIGNS AND SYMPTOMS

A characteristic feature in most people who have TB is the relative lack of definitive signs and symptoms until the lesions have become extensive. Exceptions to this are a positive skin test and radiographic findings. Once symptoms become apparent they usually are nonspecific and could be associated with any infectious disease. They include lassitude and malaise, anorexia, weight loss, night sweats, and fever. Temperature elevation commonly occurs in the evening or during the night and is accompanied by profuse sweating.

Specific local symptoms of the disease are dependent on the organ involved. Persistent cough is associated with pulmonary TB although it may be late in appearance. The condition is commonly seen with cavitary disease. Sputum produced is characteristically scanty and nonpurulent, and hemoptysis (blood in sputum) is common. Dyspnea also is seen in advanced pulmonary disease.

Manifestations of extrapulmonary disease occur in about 10% to 20% of cases and may include localized lymphadenopathy with development of sinus tracts, back pain over the affected spine, gastrointestinal disturbances (in intestinal TB), dysuria and hematuria (in renal involvement), heart failure, and neurologic deficits.[56] Physical examination may be inconclusive.

LABORATORY FINDINGS

The tuberculin skin test (Mantoux) is the most useful and reliable method of determining whether a person has been infected with M. *tuberculosis*. However, the test is neither 100% sensitive nor 100% specific. A positive test presumptively means a person has been infected.[60,61] It does not mean a person has clinically active TB. This is determined by physical examination and identification tests for M. *tuberculosis*.

Tuberculin is a standardized PPD (PPD-S) of culture extract from M. *tuberculosis*. Specifically, PPD-S is used as the international testing standard. The test is administered by an intradermal injection of 0.1 ml of PPD containing 5 tuberculin units into the volar or dorsal surface of the forearm. The test is read 48 to 72 hours later and evidence of induration is noted. An area of induration measuring 5 mm or less is considered a negative result. An area of induration measuring greater than 5 mm is considered positive if the patient has had close contact with an infectious person, an abnormal chest radiograph consistent with TB, or is suspected or known to be HIV positive. An area of induration measuring 10-mm or greater is considered positive if significant medical risk factors are present (i.e., diabetes, end-stage renal disease, immunosuppressed condition), and if the patient is a foreigner, medically underserved, alcoholic, intravenous drug abuser, a resident of a congregate setting such as a nursing home, or a child or adolescent exposed to adults in high-risk categories. Induration of at least 15 mm is considered positive for everyone.[48] A positive test necessitates a physical examination, radiographic evaluation, and, if necessary, sputum culture to rule out active disease. Without treatment, approximately 5% of skin test converters develop TB within 2 years and another 5% develop it later.[62] Thus individuals at risk for TB—including dentists—should obtain a tuberculin skin test annually.

Although radiographic findings of TB are not pathognomic, chest radiographs are extremely helpful in the diagnosis of TB. Multinodular infiltration in the apical posterior segments of upper lobes, cavitation, and infiltrates are common findings in active TB. Healed primary lesions leave a calcified peripheral nodule and a calcified hilar lymph node (Ghon complex).[61]

For a preliminary diagnosis, microscopic examination of sputum smear for acid-fast bacilli is advocated because the process is inexpensive and can produce results within 24 hours. The definitive diagnosis of TB is based on culture or direct molecular tests that identify M. *tuberculosis* or other species from body fluids and tissues, usually sputum. Multiple specimens should be obtained for culturing to ensure positive results. Traditional culture techniques take several weeks to grow mycobacteria on solid medium; however, the use of selective broth (Bactec-R, Becton-Dickson, Townson Md.), or similar systems reduce the time to about 1 week.[53,56] Cultures should be accompanied by antimicrobial susceptibility testing for all isolates of M. *tuberculosis* because of the rising incidence of drug resistance. Antibiotic sensitivity testing takes about 7 to 10 days. Molecular tests (nucleic acid amplification and probe kits) are advantageous because they provide results within 24 hours.[63] The previously mentioned tests (skin testing, sputum smears, cultures, and chest films) are less reliable when the patient has HIV infection.

MEDICAL MANAGEMENT

The Advisory Council for the Elimination of Tuberculosis recommends[64] treatment begin as soon as TB is diagnosed and the case be reported to the local health department. Within 1 week, an initial treatment plan should be developed that addresses the medical regimen, monitoring for clinical and bacteriologic response and toxicity, patient education, and assessment of the patient's social and behavioral needs that may affect compliance and completion of therapy, including personal contacts at risk of the disease.

Effective chemotherapy of TB is dependent on (1) patient education and compliance, (2) appropriate selection of drugs, (3) multiple drug use, and (4) drug administration continuance for a sufficient time. The selection of a treatment regimen is dictated by the health of the patient and the presence or likelihood of drug-resistant strains (initially based on community infectivity rates, subsequently based on laboratory tests). If a patient is determined to harbor fully susceptible organisms and the community drug resistance rate is less than 4%, isoniazid, rifampin, and pyrazinamide are given for 8 weeks

---

BOX 8-6

Common Drug Regimens for the Treatment of Tuberculosis

Non–drug-resistant TB

3 drugs for 2 months (isoniazid + rifampin + pyrazinamide), followed by two drugs for 4 months (isoniazid and rifampin without pyrazinamide); 6 months total treatment time

Drug resistance suspected or confirmed to one antituberculous drug, or diagnosis made in a region that has more than 4% resistance to antituberculosis drug

4 drugs for 2 months (isoniazid + rifampin + pyrazinamide + either ethambutol or streptomycin)

Determination of resistance again; if resistant only to isoniazid: rifampin + pyrazinamide + either

ethambutol or streptomycin for 6 months *or* rifampin + ethambutol continued for 12 months

Immunosuppressed patients to receive treatment for at least 9 months

Confirmed multiple-drug resistance

3 to 7 drugs (isoniazid + rifampin + pyrazinamide + ethambutol, an aminoglycoside, or capreomycin, ciprofloxacin, or ofloxacin and either cycloserine, ethionamide, or aminosalicylic acid) to which the organism is susceptible and continued for 12 to 24 months after the culture becomes negative

Adapted from Bass JB Jr, Farer LS, Hopewell, PC: Treatment of tuberculosis and tuberculosis infection in adults and children. American Thoracic Society and The Centers for Disease Control and Prevention. Am J *Respir Crit Care Med* 149:1359-1374, 1994. Rifapentine is available for substitution with rifampin. Dosing is twice weekly.

---

followed by isoniazid and rifampin (without pyrazinamide) for the next 4 months to complete 6 months of therapy.[65] A larger combination of drugs and increased duration of treatment are recommended when drug-resistant strains are present, the community drug resistance rate is greater than 4%, or the patient is infected with HIV (Box 8-6).[64]

Protection measures also have been introduced to control the spread of disease. For example, hospitalized patients with potentially infectious TB may be placed in isolation rooms with negative pressure during treatment.[45,64,66] In addition, many regional health departments in the United States have implemented "directly observed therapy" to ensure that patients with TB take the appropriate medicine and dose on schedule.

Following the initiation of chemotherapy, reversal of infectiousness is dependent on proper drug selection and patient compliance. Within 3 to 6 months, approximately 90% of patients become noninfectious and their sputum cultures convert to negative.[64,67] Patients are allowed to return to normal public contact based on the reversal of infectiousness and provided they continue chemotherapy.

Sputum cultures should be tested for drug-resistant bacteria, the most threatening feature of the disease, which occurs in approximately 9% of cases in the United States and more than 30% of cases in parts of Southeast Asia.[55] Most drug-resistance cases (90%) develop in HIV-infected persons, and most mycobacterial strains are resistant to

the two best anti-TB drugs (isoniazid and rifampin).[68] Transmission of drug-resistant TB has occurred between patients, patients and healthcare workers, and patients and family members. Multi-drug resistant TB is more common in foreign-born persons[69] and the outcome is quite serious. Mortality rates range from 70% to 90%, and the period to death has been 4 to 16 weeks from diagnosis.

The patient who has had a negative skin test result and on retesting has it converted to positive is considered infected with M. *tuberculosis*. Once physical examination, radiographs, and sputum culturing establish that the disease is not active, the patient may be given a course of chemoprophylaxis to prevent clinical disease from developing. Not all patients with positive skin tests are placed on chemoprophylaxis. Those most likely to receive chemoprophylaxis are the young, household contacts of patients with TB, patients who have converted to positive within the past 2 years, and others at high risk for development of the disease (AIDS, immunosuppression, renal failure). Many patients with infectious disease, including TB, cannot be clinically or historically identified; therefore all patients should be treated as though they are potentially infectious and universal precautions for infection control strictly followed (see Appendix A). Most commonly, chemoprophylaxis is provided by the oral administration of isoniazid (INH), 300 mg daily for 6 to 12 months (10 mg/kg; 9 months for children).[64] A higher dose of INH or the addition of ethambutol is recommended for tuberculin-positive persons exposed

BOX 8-7

Dental Management of the Patient with a History of Tuberculosis

1. Active sputum-positive tuberculosis
   a. Consult with physician before treatment
   b. Perform urgent care only; palliate urgent problems with medication if contained facility in hospital environment not available
   c. Perform urgent care requiring use of handpiece (older than 6 years) only in hospital setting with isolation, sterilization (gloves, mask, gown), special ventilation
   d. Treat these underage 6 years as normal patients (noninfectious after consultation with physician to verify status)
   e. Treat patient producing consistently negative sputum as normal patient (noninfectious—verify with physician)
2. History of tuberculosis
   a. Approach with caution; obtain good history of disease and its treatment duration; making appropriate review of systems mandatory
   b. Obtain from patient history of periodic chest radiographs and physical examination to rule out reactivation or relapse
   c. Consult with physician and postpone treatment if there is
      (1) Questionable history of adequate treatment time
      (2) Lack of appropriate medical follow-up since recovery
      (3) Sign or symptom of relapse
   d. Treat as normal patient if present status is free of clinically active disease
3. Recent conversion to positive tuberculin skin test
   a. Verify if evaluated by physician to rule out active disease
   b. Verify if receiving isoniazid 6 months to 1 year for prophylaxis
   c. Treat as normal patient
4. Signs or symptoms suggestive of tuberculosis
   a. Refer to physician and postpone treatment
   b. Treat as in 1 above if treatment necessary

to patients infected with organisms resistant to INH alone. Even though this usually prevents active disease from occurring, the person retains hypersensitivity to the tuberculin test and will remain positive when skin tested. Major efforts towards developing a TB vaccine are under way.[70]

DENTAL MANAGEMENT

MEDICAL CONSIDERATIONS

The implementation of infection control measures for patients with TB includes updating each patient's medical history, recognizing the signs and symptoms of TB, and following the CDC guidelines for infection control[71] (see Appendix A). The CDC places most dental facilities in the minimal risk category for potential occupational exposure to TB. Based on this risk category it recommends each dental facility have a written TB control protocol that includes instrument reprocessing and operatory cleanup, and protocols for identifying, managing, and referring patients with active TB, and educating and train-

ing staff.[72] Moreover, the CDC recommends that periodic screening of dental care workers with PPD be provided to document any recent exposure, and protocols be available that explain how the office evaluates, manages and investigates dental staff with positive PPD tests.

When managing patients with TB, decisions regarding care are based on the potential infectivity of the patient. The four infectivity categories are (1) active TB, (2) a history of TB, (3) a positive tuberculin test, and (4) signs or symptoms suggestive of TB (Box 8-7).

Patients with Clinically Active Sputum-Positive TB
Patients with recently diagnosed clinically active TB and positive sputum cultures should not be treated on an outpatient basis. Treatment is best rendered in a hospital setting with appropriate isolation, sterilization (mask, gloves, gown), and special engineering control (ventilation) systems and filtration masks.[72] The clinician should refer to the CDC recommendations which can be found at: http://www.cdc.gov/mmwr/PDF/RR/RR4313.pdf for greater detail. Also, because of the risk of transmission, treatment in the isolation room should be limited to urgent care only and a rubber dam used to minimize aerosolization

of oropharyngeal microbes. After receiving chemotherapy for several weeks and confirmed by a physician to be non-infectious and lacking any complicating factors, the patient can be treated on an outpatient basis in the same manner as any normally healthy individual.

A child with active TB receiving chemotherapy usually can be treated as an outpatient because bacilli are found only rarely in the sputum of young children. The child should be considered noninfectious unless a positive sputum culture has been obtained.[64] This should be verified with the physician. The reasons that a child with TB is considered noninfectious are the rarity of cavitary disease in children and their inability to cough up sputum effectively. Defining exactly what age constitutes a "child" in this instance is difficult. As a general rule, children under age 6 years can be confidently treated. Over age 6 some degree of concern may exist. The physician should be consulted before treatment is begun. Of greater concern in this case are the family contacts of the patient because the disease most likely was contracted from an infected adult. On being questioned, all family members who have had contact with the child should give a history of skin testing and chest radiograph to rule out the possibility of active disease. If such assurances are not obtained, the physician or health department should be contacted to ensure that proper preventive action is taken.

Patients with a Past History of TB

Fortunately, relapse is rare in patients who have received adequate treatment for the initial infection. However, this is not the case in patients who have not received adequate treatment and those who are immunosuppressed. Regardless of what type of treatment the patient received, any individual with a history of TB should be approached with initial caution. The dentist should obtain a medical history, including diagnosis and dates and type of treatment. Treatment duration of less than 18 months if treated in past decades, or less than 9 months if treated recently, would require consultation with the physician to determine the patient's status. Patients should give a history of periodic physical examinations and chest radiographs to check for evidence of reactivation of the disease. Consultation with the physician is advisable to verify the current status. The patient found free of active disease and immunosuppression may be treated without special precautions. A good review of systems is important with these patients, and referral to a physician is indicated if questionable signs or symptoms are present.

Patients with a Positive Tuberculin Test

A person with a positive skin test for TB should be viewed as having been infected with mycobacterium. The patient should give a history of being evaluated for active disease by physical examination and chest radiograph. In the absence of clinically active disease, a regimen of prophylactic isoniazid may be started for 6 months to a year to prevent clinical disease. These patients are not infectious and can be treated in a normal manner. Special precautions are not required.

Patients with Signs or Symptoms Suggestive of TB

Any time a patient demonstrates unexplained, persistent signs or symptoms that may be suggestive of TB (dry nonproductive cough, pleuritic chest pain, fatigue, fever, dyspnea, hemoptysis, weight loss), dental care should not be rendered, and the patient should be referred to a physician for evaluation. If TB exposure occurs to a health care provider, the person should be evaluated for skin test conversion. Converters should receive prompt intervention with isoniazid.[73]

DRUG ADVERSE EFFECTS

Isoniazid and rifampin therapy can cause hepatotoxicity and elevations of serum aminotransferases (Table 8-2). When serum aminotransferases are elevated in patients taking isoniazid, acetaminophen-containing medications should be avoided because of an increased potential for hepatotoxicity. With use of rifampin, the clearance of diazepam, clarithromycin (Biaxin), ketoconazole (Nizoral), itraconazole (Sporanox), and fluconazole (Diflucan) is likely to be accelerated, thus decreasing their effect. In addition, rifampin can cause leukopenia and thrombocytopenia, resulting in an increased incidence of infection, delayed healing, and gingival bleeding. Patients being administered streptomycin should not be given aspirin because of the potential for increased ototoxicity.[74]

TREATMENT PLANNING MODIFICATIONS

Treatment planning modifications are not required of these patients.

ORAL COMPLICATIONS AND MANIFESTATIONS

TB manifests infrequently in the oral cavity. Oral lesions can occur at any age but are most frequently seen in men about 30 years old and children. The classic mucosal lesion is a painful, deep, irregular ulcer on the dorsum of the tongue. The palate, lips, buccal mucosa, and gingival also can be affected.[75,76] Mucosal lesions have been reported to be granular, nodular or leukoplakic and sometimes painless.[77] Extension into the jaws can cause osteomyelitis. The cervical and submandibular lymph nodes can become infected with TB, which is termed *scrofula*. The nodes are

TABLE 8-2

Dental Considerations of Antituberculosis Drugs

Generic Drug (Trade Drug)	Adverse Effects	Dental Considerations
Isoniazid (INH, Laniazid, Nydrazid, Tubizid)	Hepatotoxic, elevation of serum aminotransferase activity in 10% to 20% of patients*	Avoid acetaminophen
Rifampin (Rifadin, Rimactane)	Hepatotoxic, gastrointestinal (GI) disturbances, flulike symptoms, thrombocytopenia, rash, turns urine red orange	Increased incidence of infection, delayed healing, gingival bleeding; decreases metabolism of diazepam, clarithromycin (Biaxin), ketoconazole (Nizoral), itraconazole (Sporanox), and fluconazole (Diflucan)
Pyrazinamide (generic)	Arthralgias, hyperuricemia, GI disturbance, and hepatitis	—
Ethambutol (Myambutol)	Optic neuritis (rare)	—
Streptomycin (generic)	Ototoxicity, vestibular disturbances, infrequent renal toxicity	Avoid concurrent use of aspirin
Amikacin (Amikin), kanamycin (Kantrex), capreomycin (Capastat)	Nephrotoxicity and ototoxicity	Avoid concurrent use of aspirin
Ofloxacin (Floxin), ciprofloxacin (Cipro)	GI disturbances, inhibits bone plate growth	Avoid in children <16 years of age
Aminosalicylic acid (PAS, Teebacin)	GI disturbances	—

*Greater risk of liver damage in persons over 35 years of age.
Vitamin B$_6$ is recommended to counteract the adverse effect profile of INH.

enlarged and painful (Fig. 8-7), and abscesses may form and drain.[78] Involvement of salivary glands is rare.[79]

Biopsy in addition to culture can be diagnostic if acid-fast bacilli are found. Resolution of the infectious oral lesion is secondary to treatment of the TB with antituberculous drugs. Pain is managed symptomatically (see Appendix B).

OCCUPATIONAL SAFETY AND HEALTH ASSOCIATION

Dentists should be aware that the Occupational Safety and Health Association (OSHA) issued an enforcement guidance policy in 1993 to protect workers against exposures to M. *tuberculosis*. The policy obligates employers to provide safe, healthful workplaces and allows for inspection of occupational exposure to TB in health care settings when complaints are received from public sector

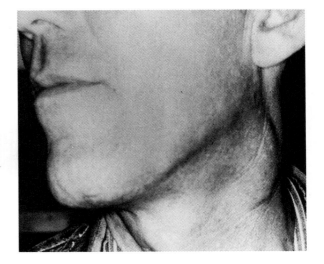

Fig. 8-7 Tuberculosis of the cervical lymph nodes.

employees. Employers found in violation of the requirements can be fined.

In 1997 OSHA proposed an additional policy based on the CDC guidelines. This newer proposal requires dentists to prepare a written exposure control plan, provide baseline skin tests and medical history, make medical management available after an exposure incident, provide medical removal protection if necessary, provide information and training to employees with exposure potential, and comply with record-keeping requirements. Periodic medical surveillance and respiratory protection would not be required if the dental facility does not admit or treat persons with active TB, has had no confirmed cases of infectious TB within the past year, and is in a county with no cases of active TB within the past 2 years. By contrast, more strict guidelines (i.e., isolation rooms for suspected or confirmed infectious TB patients and ventilation equipment) are required when employees have potential for exposure to the exhaled air of an individual with suspected or confirmed TB, or were exposed to a high hazard procedure performed on an individual who may have TB and which has the potential to generate potentially infectious airborne respiratory secretions. Dentists may visit the OSHA website at http://www.osha-slc.gov/FedReg_osha_data/FED19971017.html to better familiarize themselves with their legal responsibilities.

References

1. Rodarte J: Chronic bronchitis and emphysema. In Bennett JC, Goldman L, editors: *Cecil textbook of medicine*, Philadelphia, 2000, WB Saunders.
2. American Lung Association: Minority Lung Disease Data-Chronic Obstructive Pulmonary Disease, *http://www.lungusa.org/pub/minority/copd.html* 2000.
3. Centers for Disease Control: Mortality patterns-United States, 1989, MMWR 41:121-125, 1992.
4. Ingram RJ: Chronic bronchitis, emphysema, and airway obstruction. In Wilson JD et al, editors: *Harrison's principles of internal medicine*, 1991, New York, McGraw-Hill.
5. Mannino D et al: Obstructive lung disease and low lung function in adults in the United States: data from the National Health and Nutrition Examination Survey, 1988-1994, *Arch Intern Med* 160:1683-1689, 2000.
6. US Department of Health and Human Services: *Chronic obstructive lung disease: the health consequences of smoking. A report of the Surgeon General*, Public Health Service, Publication 84-50205, 1984.
7. Lee P, Fry J, Forey B: Trends in lung cancer, chronic obstructive lung disease, and emphysema death rates for England and Wales 1941-1985 and their relation to trends in cigarette smoking, *Thorax* 5:657-665, 1990.
8. American Thoracic Society: Standards for the diagnosis and care of patients with chronic obstructive pulmonary disease, *Am J Respir Crit Care Med* 152:S77-S121, 1995.
9. Ferguson G: Recommendations for the management of COPD, *Chest* 117:23S-28S, 2000.
10. Barnes P: Molecular mechanisms of antiasthma therapy, *Ann Med* 27:531-535, 1995.
11. Bellamy D: Progress in the management of COPD, *Practitioner* 244:24,27-28,30, 2000.
12. Crews K et al: Tobacco cessation: a practical dental service, *Gen Dent* 47:476-483, 1999.
13. Vichitvejpaisal H et al: Effect of severity of pulmonary disease on nitrous oxide washin and washout characteristics, *J Med Assoc Thai* 80:378-383, 1997.
14. Akiyama K: Review of epidemiological studies on adult bronchial asthma in Japan, *Nippon Kyobu Shikkan Gakkai Zasshi* 32:S200-S210, 1994.
15. Centers for Disease Control: Surveillance for asthma-United States, 1960-1995, MMWR 47(SS-1):1-28, 1998.
16. McFadden EJ: Asthma. In Wilson JD et al, editors: *Harrison's principles of internal medicine*, New York, 1991, McGraw-Hill.
17. Ford-Hutchinson A, Evans J: Leukotriene B_4: biologic properties and regulation of biosynthesis. In Piper P, editor: *The leukotrienes: their biological significance*, 1986, New York, Raven Press.
18. Rumbak M, Self T: A diagnostic approach to 'difficult' asthma, *Postgrad Med* 92:80-90, 1992.
19. Mathison D, Stevenson D, Simon R: Precipitating factors in asthma: aspirin, sulfites, and other drugs and chemicals, *Chest* 87(suppl 1):50-54S, 1985.
20. Babu K, Salvi S: Aspirin and asthma, *Chest* 118:1470-1476, 2000.
21. US Department of Health and Human Services: Warning on prescription drugs containing sulfites, FDA *Drug Bull* 17:2-3, 1987.
22. Stevenson D, Simon R: Sulfites and asthma, *J Allergy Clin Immunol* 74:469-472, 1984.
23. National Asthma Education and Prevention Program (National Heart, Lung, and Blood Institute): Second Expert Panel on the Management of Asthma: *Expert panel report 2: guidelines for the diagnosis and management of asthma*, Publication no. 97-4051, 1997, Bethesda, Md.: National Institutes of Health. Retrieved January 2001 from http://www.nhlbi.nih.gov/guidelines/asthma/asthgdln.pdf.
24. Malamed SF: *Medical emergencies in the dental office*, ed 5, 2000, St Louis, Mosby.
25. Centers for Disease Control: Asthma-United States, 1982-1992, MMWR 43:952-953, 1995.
26. Lalloo U et al: Guideline for the management of chronic asthma in adults-2000 update, S *Afr Med J* 90:540-541, 544-552, 2000.
27. Kleerup E, Tashkin D: Outpatient treatment of adult asthma, *West J Med* 163:49-63, 1995.
28. O'Byrne P, Israel E, Drazen J: Antileukotrienes in the treatment of asthma, *Ann Intern Med* 127:472-480, 1997.
29. Ernst P et al: Risk of fatal and near-fatal asthma in relation to inhaled corticosteroid use, JAMA 269:3462-3464, 1992.

30. Sears M: Changing patterns in asthma morbidity and mortality, J Investig Allergol Clin Immunol 5:66-72, 1995.

31. Milgrom H et al: Treatment of allergic asthma with monoclonal anti-IgE antibody, N Engl J Med 341:1966-1973, 1999.

32. Suissa S, Ernst P: Albuterol in mild asthma, N Engl J Med 336:729, 1997.

33. Ulrik C, Frederiksen J: Mortality and markers of risk of asthma death among 1,075 outpatients with asthma, Chest 108:10-15, 1995.

34. Mathew T et al: Effect of dental treatment on the lung function of children with asthma, J Am Dent Assoc 129:1120-1128, 1998.

35. Schwartz H et al: Metabisulfite sensitivity and local dental anesthesia, Annals of Allergy 62:83-86, 1989.

36. Elnabtity MN, et al: Leukotriene modifiers in the management of asthma, JAOA 7:S1-S6, 1999.

37. Bresolin D et al: Mouth breathing in allergic children: its relationship to dentofacial development, Am J Orthod 83:334-340, 1983.

38. Kargul B et al: Inhaler medicament effects on saliva and plaque pH in asthmatic children, J Clin Pediatr Dent 22:137-140, 1998.

39. Ryberg M, Moller C, Ericson T: Effect of beta 2-adrenoceptor agonists on saliva proteins and dental caries in asthmatic children, J Dent Res 66:1404-1406, 1987.

40. Ryberg M, Moller C, Ericson T: Saliva composition and caries development in asthmatic patients treated with beta 2-adrenoceptor agonists: a 4-year follow-up study, Scand J Dent Res 99:212-218, 1991.

41. McDerra E, Pollard MA, Curzon MEJ: The dental status of asthmatic British school children, Pediatr Dent 20:281-287, 1998.

42. Barnes P: Efficacy and safety of inhaled corticosteroids: new developments, Am J Respir Crit Care Med 157(Suppl):S1-S53, 1998.

43. Drugs for ambulatory asthma, Med Lett Drugs Ther 33:9-12, 1991.

44. Sudre P, ten Dam G, Kochi A: Tuberculosis: a global overview of the situation today, Bull World Health Organ 70:149-159, 1992.

45. Sbarbaro J: Tuberculosis in the 1990s: epidemiology and therapeutic challenge, Chest 108:58S-62S, 1995.

46. Centers for Disease Control: Tuberculosis-United States, 1985, MMWR 35:699-703, 1986.

47. Centers for Disease Control: Summary of notifiable diseases, United States, 1990, MMWR 39:1-29, 1990.

48. Centers for Disease Control: Expanded tuberculosis surveillance and tuberculosis morbidity-United States, 1993, MMWR 43:361-366, 1994.

49. Centers for Disease Control and Prevention: Summary of Notifiable Diseases, United States, 1998, MMWR 47(53):1-93, 1999.

50. Centers for Disease Control: Tuberculosis morbidity-United States, 1997, MMWR 47:253-257, 1998.

51. Centers for Disease Control: Guidelines for preventing the transmission of tuberculosis in health-care settings, with special focus on HIV-related issues, MMWR 39:1-29, 1990.

52. Centers for Disease Control: Tuberculosis morbidity in the United States: final data, 1990, MMWR 23-26:23-26, 1991.

53. Haas D, Des Prez R: Tuberculosis and acquired immunodeficiency syndrome: a historical perspective on recent developments, Am J Med 96:439-450, 1994.

54. Snider D, Roper W: The new tuberculosis, N Engl J Med 326:703-705, 1992.

55. Bradford W, Daley C: Multiple drug-resistant tuberculosis, Infect Dis Clin North Am 12:157-172, 1998.

56. Weir M, Thornton G: Extrapulmonary tuberculosis: experience of a community hospital and review of the literature, Am J Med 79:467-478, 1985.

57. Fowler N: Tuberculous pericarditis, JAMA 266:99-103, 1991.

58. Von Lichtenberg F: Infectious disease: viral, chlamydial, rickettsial, and bacterial diseases. In Cottran RS, Kumar V, Robbins S, editors: Robbins' pathologic basis of disease, 1989, Philadelphia, WB Saunders.

59. Braun M, Cote T, Rabkin C: Trends in death with tuberculosis during the AIDS era, JAMA 269:2865-2868, 1993.

60. American Thoracic Society: The tuberculin skin test, Am Rev Respir Dis 124:356-363, 1981.

61. Daniel T: Tuberculosis. In Wilson JD et al, editors, Harrison's principles of internal medicine, 1991, New York, McGraw-Hill.

62. Centers for Disease Control and Prevention: Epidemiology of tuberculosis. In Self-study modules on tuberculosis, Atlanta, National Center for Prevention Services, Division of Tuberculosis Elimination, 1995.

63. Salfinger M, Hale Y, Driscoll J: Diagnostic tools in tuberculosis: present and future, Respiration, 65:163-170, 1998.

64. American Thoracic Society: Treatment of tuberculosis and tuberculosis infection in adults and children, Am J Respir Crit Care Med 149:1359-1374, 1994.

65. Centers for Disease Control: Initial therapy for tuberculosis in the era of multidrug resistance: Recommendations of the Advisory Council for the Elimination of Tuberculosis, MMWR 42(RR-7):1-8, 1993.

66. Ravikrishnan K: Tuberculosis: how can we halt its resurgence? Postgrad Med 91:333-338, 1992.

67. Centers for Disease Control: Bacteriologic conversion of sputum among tuberculosis patients-United States, MMWR 34:747-750, 1985.

68. Antonucci G et al: Risk factors for tuberculosis in HIV-infected persons: a prospective cohort study, JAMA 274:143-148, 1995.

69. Centers for Disease Control and Prevention: Recommendations for prevention and control of tuberculosis among foreign-born persons, MMWR 47(RR-16):1-26, 1998.

70. Centers for Disease Control and Prevention: Development of new vaccines for tuberculosis, MMWR 47:1-6, 1998.

71. Centers for Disease Control: Recommended infection-control practices for dentistry, 1993, MMWR 42(RR-8): http://www.cdc.gov/mmwr/preview/mmwrhtml/00021095.htm, 1993.

72. Centers for Disease Control: Guidelines for preventing the transmission of tuberculosis in health-care facilities, MMWR 43(RR-13):1-132; http://www.cdc.gov/mmwr/PDF/RR/RR4313.pdf, 1994.

73. Stead W: Management of health care workers after inadvertent exposure to tuberculosis: a guide for the use of preventive therapy, Ann Intern Med 122:906-912, 1995.

74. *Drug information for the health care professional* ed 20, 2000, Rockville, Md., United States Pharmacopeial Convention.

75. Dimitrakopoulos I et al: Primary tuberculosis of the oral cavity, *Oral Surg* 72:712-715, 1991.

76. Shafer W, Hine M, Levy B: A *textbook of oral pathology*, ed 4, 1983, Philadelphia, WB Saunders.

77. Kolokotronis A et al: Oral tuberculosis, *Oral Dis* 2:242-243, 1996.

78. Florio S, Ellis EI, Frost D: Persistent submandibular swelling after tooth extraction, *J Oral Maxillofac Surg* 55:390-397, 1997.

79. Bhargava S et al: Case report: tuberculosis of the parotid gland-diagnosis by CT, *Br J Radiol* 69:1181-1183, 1996.

Chronic Renal Failure and Dialysis

9

CHAPTER

The kidneys regulate fluid volume and acid-base balance of the plasma, excrete nitrogenous waste, synthesize erythropoietin, 1,25-dihydroxy-cholecalciferol and renin, and are responsible for drug metabolism. The kidneys also are the target organ for parathormone and aldosterone. Progressive disease of the kidney can result in decreased function and manifestations in several organ systems. As a result, the practice of dentistry can be impacted by the resulting anemia, abnormal bleeding, electrolyte and fluid imbalance, hypertension, drug intolerance, and skeletal abnormalities. In addition, patients who have severe and progressive disease may require artificial filtration of the blood by dialysis or transplantation of a kidney (see Chapter 25).

DEFINITION

End-stage renal disease (ESRD) is a bilateral, progressive, and chronic deterioration of nephrons, the functional unit of the kidney. The disease results in uremia and can lead to death. ESRD manifests when 50% to 75% of the approximately 2 million nephrons lose function. Under normal physiological conditions, 25% of the circulating blood perfuses the kidney each minute. The blood is filtered through a complex series of tubules and glomerular capillaries. Ultrafiltrate, the precursor of urine, is produced at a rate of about 125 ml/min in the nephrons.

Nephron deterioration leads to ESRD through successive laboratory and clinical stages. The first stage, termed *diminished renal reserve*, is usually asymptomatic. This stage is characterized by a mildly elevated creatinine level and slight glomerular filtration rate (GFR) decline (10% to 20% change from normal). Progression leads to *renal insufficiency*, a term used when the GFR is mild to moderately diminished (20% to 50% of normal) and nitrogen products begin to accumulate in the blood. In the third stage, called *renal failure*, the kidney's ability to per-

form excretory, endocrine, and metabolic functions has deteriorated beyond compensatory mechanisms. This indicates inability of the kidneys to maintain normal homeostasis. The resulting clinical syndrome—caused by renal failure, retention of excretory products, and interference with endocrine and metabolic functions—is called *uremia*. Sequelae involve multi-organ systems, including cardiovascular, hematological, neuromuscular, endocrine, gastrointestinal, and dermatological manifestations. The rate of destruction and the severity of disease depend on the underlying causative factors; however, in many cases the cause remains unknown.

EPIDEMIOLOGY

INCIDENCE AND PREVALENCE

Approximately 8 million people in the United States have some form of kidney disease. Of these, more than 360,000 have irreversible ESRD.[1] Each year approximately 79,000 new cases of ESRD are diagnosed, a rate of 1.3 in 10,000 persons. The disease is increasing by approximately 9% per year, most rapidly in patients over age 65, and in those who have diabetes and hypertension.[1,2] ESRD occurs more commonly in men, African-, Native- and Asian-Americans, and those between the ages of 45 and 64 years. More than 90% of ESRD patients will be over the age of 18 years.[4] Approximately 58,000 Americans die annually as a result of ESRD, with related cardiovascular disease being the cause of death for most.[3] An average dental practice of 2000 patients can expect to have 2 patients with ESRD.

ETIOLOGY

ESRD is caused by any condition that destroys nephrons. The three most common known causes of

ESRD are diabetes mellitus (34%), hypertension (25%), and chronic glomerulonephritis (16%).[5] Other common causes include polycystic kidney disease, systemic lupus erythematosus, neoplasms and AIDS nephropathy. Hereditary and environmental factors such as amyloidosis, congenital diseases, hyperlipidemia, immunoglobulin A nephropathy, and silica exposure also are contributory to the disease.[6-8]

PATHOPHYSIOLOGY AND COMPLICATIONS

Deterioration and destruction of functioning nephrons are the underlying pathologic processes of renal failure. The nephron includes the glomerulus, tubules, and vasculature. Various diseases affect different segments of the nephron at first, but the entire nephron eventually is affected. For example, hypertension affects the vasculature first, whereas glomerulonephritis affects the glomeruli first. Once lost, nephrons are not replaced. However, because of a compensatory hypertrophy of the remaining nephrons, normal renal function is maintained for a time. This is a period of relative renal insufficiency during which homeostasis is preserved. The patient remains asymptomatic and demonstrates minimal laboratory abnormalities such as a diminished GFR.[9] Normal function is maintained until about 50% to 75% of the nephrons are destroyed.[10] Subsequently, compensatory mechanisms are overwhelmed, and the signs and symptoms of uremia appear. In terms of morphology, the end-stage kidney is markedly reduced in size, scarred, and nodular (Fig. 9-1).

A patient with early renal failure may remain asymptomatic, but physiologic changes occur invariably as the disease progresses. These changes occur because of the loss of nephrons. Renal tubular malfunction causes the sodium pump to lose its effectiveness and sodium excretion occurs. Along with sodium, excess amounts of dilute urine also are excreted, which accounts for the polyuria commonly encountered.[10]

Patients with advanced renal disease develop uremia, which is uniformly fatal if not treated. The failing kidneys are unable to concentrate and filtrate the intake of sodium, which contributes to the development of fluid overload, hypertension, and risk for cardiac disease. This in part contributes to the fact that approximately 50% of the annual mortality of patients with ESRD is the result of cardiovascular-related events.

Loss of the glomerular filtration function results in buildup of nonprotein nitrogen compounds in the blood, mainly urea, and is called *azotemia*. The level of azotemia is measured as blood urea nitrogen (BUN). Acids also accumulate because of the tubular impairment. The combination of waste products results in metabolic acidosis, the

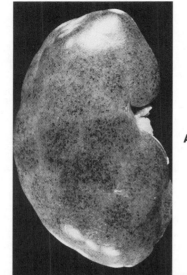
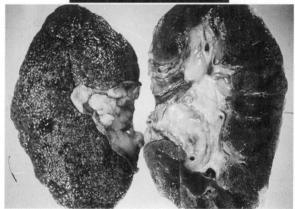

Fig. 9-1 Morphology of **A,** a normal kidney and, **B,** a kidney in end-stage renal disease. (Courtesy A. Golden, Lexington, Ky.)

major result of which is ammonia retention. In the later stages of renal failure, acidosis causes nausea, anorexia, and fatigue. Patients may tend to hyperventilate to compensate for the metabolic acidosis. In the patient with ESRD and acidosis, adaptive mechanisms already are taxed beyond normal and any increase in demand can lead to serious consequences. For example, sepsis or a febrile illness can lead to a profound acidosis and be fatal.

Severe electrolyte disturbances occur in renal failure. Sodium depletion and hyperkalemia develop as azotemia progresses, urine output falls, and acid-base balance continues to deteriorate. Patients with ESRD demonstrate several hematologic abnormalities, including ane-

mia, leukocyte and platelet dysfunction, and coagulopathy. Anemia is one of the most familiar manifestations of ESRD, caused by decreased erythropoietin production by the kidney, inhibition of red blood cell production and hemolysis, bleeding episodes, and shortened red cell survival. Most of these effects result from unidentified toxic substances in uremic plasma and other factors.[11,12]

Host defense is compromised because of nutritional deficiencies and changes in the production and function of white blood cells. The latter is caused by reduced bioavailability of interleukin 2, downregulation of phagocyte adhesion molecules, increased production of interleukin 1, interleukin 6, and tumor necrosis factor, cell-mediated immune defects, and hypogammaglobulinemia that lead to diminished granulocyte chemotaxis, phagocytosis, and bactericidal activity.[13] Accordingly, individuals with these conditions are more susceptible to infection.

Hemorrhagic diatheses, characterized by a tendency to abnormal bleeding and bruising, are common in patients with ESRD and attributed primarily to abnormal platelet aggregation and adhesiveness, decreased platelet factor 3, and impaired prothrombin consumption. Defective platelet production also may play a role.[11,12] Platelet factor 3 enhances the conversion of prothrombin to thrombin by activated factor X.

The cardiovascular system is affected by a tendency to develop congestive heart failure or pulmonary edema, sometimes both. The most common complication, however, is arterial hypertension, caused by NaCl retention, fluid overload, and inappropriately high renin levels.[10] Hypertrophy of the left ventricle also occurs and may compromise blood supply by way of the coronary vessels. This condition is worsened by anemia. A tendency exists for accelerated atherosclerosis to develop in patients with ESRD, and pericarditis is common.[11]

A variety of bone disorders are seen in ESRD, collectively referred to as *renal osteodystrophy*.[10] Decreased glomerular filtration occurs with decreasing nephron function, which results in decreased 1,25 dihydroxyvitamin D production by the kidney, decreased calcium absorption by the gut, and an increased level of serum phosphate. Because phosphate is the driving force of bone mineralization, the excess phosphate tends to cause serum calcium to be deposited in bone (osteoid), leading to a decreased serum calcium level and weak bones. In response to low serum calcium, the parathyroid glands are stimulated to secrete parathormone (PTH), which results in a secondary hyperparathyroidism. The function of PTH is to (1) inhibit the tubular reabsorption of phosphate, (2) stimulate the renal production of the vitamin D necessary for calcium metabolism, and

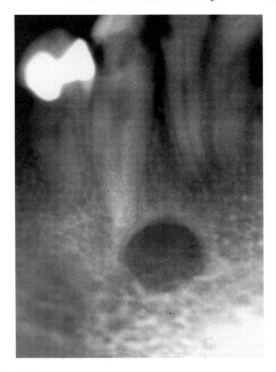

Fig. 9-2 Lytic lesion in the anterior mandible of a patient with hyperparathyroidism. (Courtesy L.R. Bean, Lexington, Ky.)

(3) enhance vitamin D absorption from the intestine. However, high levels of PTH are sustained because in ESRD the failing kidney does not synthesize 1,25-dihydroxycholecalciferol, the active metabolite of vitamin D; thus calcium absorption in the gut is inhibited. PTH, tumor necrosis factor, and interleukin 1 activate bone remodeling and mobilize calcium from the bones as well as promote the excretion of phosphate, which can lead to renal and metastatic calcifications.[14] The progression of osseous changes are osteomalacia (increased unmineralized bone matrix), followed by osteitis fibrosa (bone resorption lytic lesions and marrow fibrosis) (Fig. 9-2), and finally osteosclerosis in varying degrees (enhanced bone density) (Fig. 9-3). With renal osteodystrophy impaired bone growth occurs in children as well as a tendency for spontaneous fractures with slow healing, myopathy, aseptic necrosis of the hip, and extraosseous calcifications.[11] The incidence of osteomalacia is decreasing because of the identification that its etiology most commonly is linked to intoxication by aluminum and other heavy metals associated with dialysis treatment of ESRD. Dialysate fluids currently have reduced levels of these intoxicants.[14]

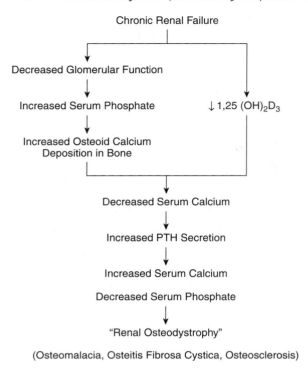

Fig. 9-3 Summary of changes that result in renal osteodystrophy.

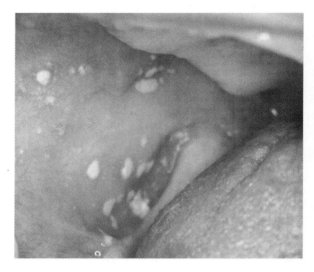

Fig. 9-4 Oral candidiasis in a patient with end-stage renal disease.

CLINICAL PRESENTATION

SIGNS AND SYMPTOMS

Patients with renal failure appear ill and anemic and also develop nocturia. The anemia produces pallor of the skin and mucous membranes and contributes to the symptoms of lethargy, listlessness, and dizziness. The widespread effects cause multiorgan system involvement. Hyperpigmentation of the skin is characterized by a brownish-yellow appearance caused by the retention of carotene-like pigments normally excreted by the kidney. These pigments also may cause profound pruritus. An occasional finding is a whitish coating on the skin of the trunk and arms produced by residual urea crystals left when perspiration evaporates ("uremic frost").

Patients with renal failure may demonstrate a variety of gastrointestinal signs such as anorexia, nausea, and vomiting, generalized gastroenteritis, and peptic ulcer disease. Uremic syndrome commonly causes malnutrition and diarrhea. Patients demonstrate mental slowness or depression and become psychotic in later stages. They also may show muscular hyperactivity.

Convulsion is a late finding directly correlated with the level of azotemia. Stomatitis manifested by oral ulceration and candidiasis can occur (Fig. 9-4). Parotitis may be seen and a urinelike odor to the breath may be detected.

Because of the bleeding diatheses that accompany ESRD, hemorrhagic episodes are not uncommon, particularly occult gastrointestinal bleeding. However, patients who receive dialysis have improved control of uremia and less severe bleeding. Manifestations include ecchymoses, petechiae, purpura, and gingival or mucous membrane bleeding (epistaxis).

Cardiovascular manifestations of ESRD include hypertension, congestive heart failure (shortness of breath, orthopnea, dyspnea on exertion, peripheral edema), and pericarditis.

LABORATORY FINDINGS

Several tests are used to monitor the progress of ESRD, including urinalysis, BUN, serum creatinine, creatinine clearance, electrolyte measurements, and protein electrophoresis. The most basic test of kidney function is uri-

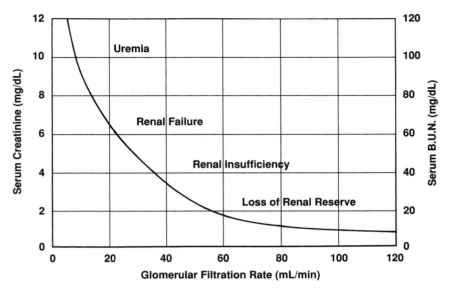

Fig. 9-5 Relationship of renal function with serum enzymes.

TABLE **9-1**

Primary Laboratory Values for the Assessment of Renal Function and Failure

Laboratory Test	Reference Value	Indicator of Renal Insufficiency	Indicator of Renal Failure
Urine			
Creatinine clearance	85-125 ml/min (women) 97-140 ml/min (men)	50-90 ml/min	10-50 ml/min (moderate); <10 ml/min (severe)
Glomerular filtration rate	100-150 ml/min	50-90 ml/min	10-50 ml/min (moderate); <10 ml/min (severe)
Serum			
Blood urea nitrogen	8 to 18 mg/dL (3 to 6.5 mmol/L)	20-30 mg/dL	30 to 50 mg/dL (moderate); >50 mg/dL (severe)
Creatinine	0.6 to 1.20 mg/dL	2 to 3 mg/dL	3 to 6 mg/dL (moderate); >6 mg/dL (severe)

Secondary indicators of renal function. Normal reference values: Calcium 8.2 to 11.2 mg/dL; Chloride 95 to 103 mmol/L; Inorganic phosphorous 2.7 to 4.5 mg/dL; Potassium 3.8 to 5 mmol/L; Sodium 136 to 142 mmol/L; Total carbon dioxide for venous blood 22 to 26 mmol/L.
Adapted in part from Zachee P, Vermylen J, Boogaerts MA: *Ann Hematol* 69:33-40, 1994, and De Rossi SS, Glick M, *JADA* 127:211-219, 1996.

nalysis, with special emphasis on the specific gravity and the presence of protein. Fig. 9-5 illustrates laboratory features of the four pathophysiologic stages of chronic renal failure. Table 9-1 lists specific lab values indicative of renal function and dysfunction. Of these tests, three are used primarily to assess renal function: creatinine clearance, serum creatinine and GFR. Creatinine is a measure of muscle breakdown and filtration capacity of the nephron. It is proportional to the glomerular filtration and tubular excretion rate and commonly is used as the

index of clearance (creatinine clearance) in a 24-hour urine collection. The BUN is a common indicator of kidney function but is not as specific as creatinine clearance or serum creatinine level.

As renal failure develops, the patient often remains asymptomatic until the GFR drops below 20 mL/min, the creatinine clearance drops below 20 mL/min, and the BUN is above 20 mg/dL. For example, uremic syndrome is rare before the BUN concentration exceeds 60 mg/dL.[10] Other serum tests are used to monitor serum electrolytes involved in acid-base regulation and calcium-phosphate metabolism that are affected by renal disease (see Table 9-1).

Protein and blood in the urine are two predictors of end-stage renal disease[15] and have been used in screening large populations. These tests are used in ruling out renal disease in the elderly and persons with diabetes, hypertension, and unexplained fatigue.

MEDICAL MANAGEMENT

CONSERVATIVE CARE

Once the diagnosis of ESRD is made, the goals of treatment are to retard the progress of disease and preserve the patient's quality of life. A conservative approach is the first step and may be adequate for prolonged periods. Conservative care is designed to slow the progression of renal disease and involves decreasing the retention of nitrogenous waste products, and controlling hypertension, fluids, and electrolyte imbalances. This is accomplished by dietary modification—restricting protein and monitoring fluid, sodium, and potassium intake. Any treatable associated condition such as diabetes, hypertension, congestive heart failure, infection, volume depletion, urinary tract obstruction, secondary hyperparathyroidism, and hyperuricemia is corrected or controlled. In particular, secondary hyperparathyroidism is treated with low-phosphate diet, use of nonaluminum phosphate binders (i.e., calcium carbonate), calcitriol and other vitamin D preparations to decrease serum parathyroid hormone levels.[16] Conservative care includes the avoidance of nephrotoxic drugs or agents metabolized principally by the kidney.

Anemia that occurs in renal failure usually is treated with the use of recombinant human erythropoietin.[12] Subcutaneous doses 50 to 75 IU/kg triweekly normalize hemoglobin levels within 3 months in most patients. Adverse effects are infrequent and include seizures, hypertension, and thrombosis. A small percentage of

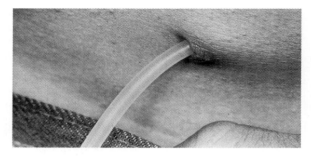

Fig. 9-6 Chronic ambulatory peritoneal dialysis catheter site in the abdominal wall. (Courtesy Dialysis Center, Lexington, Ky.)

patients develop resistance to recombinant human erythropoietin.[12]

DIALYSIS

Dialysis is a medical procedure that artificially filters blood. Dialysis becomes necessary when the number of nephrons diminishes to the point that azotemia is unpreventable or uncontrollable. The initiation of dialysis is an individual patient decision that becomes important when the serum creatinine is chronically above 3 mg/dL and the creatinine clearance is below 20 mL/min.[17,18] More than 250,000 individuals receive dialysis in the United States at a cost of more than $7 billion a year.[19,20] The procedure can be accomplished either by peritoneal dialysis or hemodialysis.

Peritoneal dialysis is performed on more than 26,000 Americans.[1] It is accomplished by either continuous cyclic (CCPD) peritoneal dialysis or chronic ambulatory peritoneal dialysis (CAPD). Both instill a hypertonic solution into the peritoneal cavity via a permanent peritoneal catheter. After a period of time the solution and dissolved solutes (e.g., urea) are drawn out. The older method, CCPD, uses a machine at night to perform seven to eight dialysate exchanges while the patient sleeps. During the day, excretory fluids fill in the abdomen of the patient until the dialysis is repeated that evening.

A newer and more commonly used method of peritoneal dialysis is CAPD. Dialysis by this method (Fig. 9-6) is performed with shorter exchange periods of 30 to 45 minutes, 4 to 5 times per day usually around breakfast, lunch, dinner, and before bedtime. The dialysis exchanges are performed manually with 2 to 3 liters of the dialysate instilled into the peritoneal cavity. The catheter is sealed, and every 4 to 6 hours the dialysate is allowed to drain into a bag strapped to the patient and new dialysate instilled. CAPD allows the patient more free-

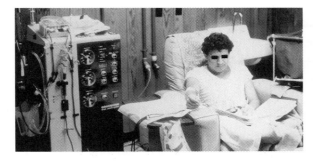

Fig. 9-7 Patient undergoing hemodialysis. (Courtesy Dialysis Center, Lexington, Ky.)

dom than CCPD. However, both methods allow patients to perform routine functions between exchanges (e.g., walking and working).

The advantages of peritoneal dialysis are its relatively low cost, ease of performance, reduced likelihood of infectious disease transmission, and lack of anticoagulation. Disadvantages include the need for frequent sessions, risk of peritonitis (approximately 1 per patient every 1.5 years) abdominal hernia, and its significantly lower effectiveness than hemodialysis. Its principal use is for patients in acute renal failure or who require only occasional dialysis.

Most dialysis patients (90%) receive hemodialysis.[1,21] Hemodialysis is the method of choice when azotemia occurs and dialysis becomes chronic. Treatments are performed every 2 or 3 days, depending on need. Usually 3 to 4 hours are required for each session (Fig. 9-7). Hemodialysis consumes an enormous amount of the patient's time and is extremely confining. However, daily nocturnal home hemodialysis likely will become available. Between dialysis sessions, patients lead a relatively normal lifestyle.[17]

More than 80% of the approximately 220,000 people who receive hemodialysis in the United States do so through a permanent and surgically placed arteriovenous graft or fistula, usually placed in the forearm.[19] Access is achieved by cannulation of the fistula with a large-gauge needle (Fig. 9-8). Approximately 18% of patients receive dialysis through a temporary or permanent central catheter, as permanent access is healing or when all other access options have been exhausted.[19] Patients are "plugged in" to the hemodialysis machine at the fistula/graft site, and blood is passed through the machine, filtered, and returned to the patient. Heparin is usually administered during the procedure to prevent clotting.

Although hemodialysis is a lifesaving technique, dialysis provides only about 15% of normal renal function and

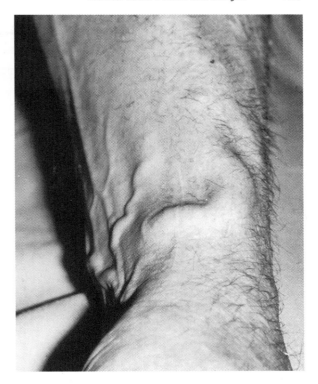

Fig. 9-8 Site of a surgically created arteriovenous fistula, with subsequent dilation and hypertrophy of the veins. (Courtesy Dialysis Center, Lexington, Ky.)

complications develop as a result of the procedure.[21] Serum calcium concentrations require close regulation that is achieved with calcium supplements, calcitriol (active form of vitamin D) or use of dialysate containing calcium. Improper blood levels contribute to muscle tetany and oversecretion of parathyroid hormone. Anemia is a common feature of renal failure and dialysis; however, use of recombinant human erythropoietin has virtually eliminated this problem.[17] In addition, the risk of hepatitis B, hepatitis C, and HIV infections is present because dialyzers usually are disinfected–not sterilized–between reuse and patients usually have multiple blood exposures.[19] Risk for transmission of viruses from hemodialysis increases when screening hepatitis tests are not performed, hepatitis B vaccine has not been administered to patients, and separate machines and staff members are not used in the treatment of patients who are carriers of the hepatitis B virus or hepatitis C virus.[19] A 1997 national survey reported that among chronic hemodialysis patients the prevalence of hepatitis B surface antigen positivity (carriers of hepatitis B) was 0.9%, for hepatitis C 9.3%, and for

BOX 9-1

Dental Management of the Patient with End-Stage Renal Disease (including emergency dental care)

Under Conservative Care

Consult with physician advised

Avoid dental treatment if disease is unstable (poorly controlled or advanced)

Screen for bleeding disorder before surgery (bleeding time, platelet count, hematocrit, hemoglobin)

Monitor blood pressure closely

Pay meticulous attention to good surgical technique

Avoid nephrotoxic drugs (acetaminophen in high doses, acyclovir, aspirin, nonsteroidal antiinflammatory drugs)

Adjust dosage of drugs metabolized by the kidney (see Table 9-2)

Manage orofacial infections aggressively with culture and sensitivity test and antibiotics

Consider hospitalization for severe infection or major procedures

Receiving Hemodialysis

Same as conservative care recommendations

Beware of concerns of arteriovenous shunt

Consult with physician about low risk for infective endarteritis or endocarditis

Avoid blood pressure cuff and IV medications in arm with shunt

Avoid dental care on day of treatment (especially within first 6 hours afterward); best to treat on day after

Assess status of liver function and presence of opportunistic infection in these patients because of increased risk for carrier state of hepatitis B, C viruses and HIV

HIV 1.3%.[19] Although all three viruses constitute a reservoir of potential infection, only hepatitis B virus and hepatitis C virus have been reported to be transmitted nosocomially in dialysis centers in the United States.

Infection of the arteriovenous fistula is an ongoing concern and can result in septicemia, septic emboli, infective endarteritis, and infective endocarditis. *Staphylococcus aureus* is the most common cause of vascular access infections and related bacteremia in these patients.[22] The risk of fistula infection from surgical procedures (e.g., urogenital, oral surgical, dental) is not precisely known but considered low. A related concern is risk for infection and antibiotic-resistant infections. Chronic hemodialysis patients have a higher rate of tuberculosis and of vancomycin- and methicillin-resistant infections than does the general public.[19]

As with all patients with ESRD, drugs that are metabolized primarily by the kidney or that are nephrotoxic must be avoided by patients receiving dialysis.

A final problem associated with dialysis is that of abnormal bleeding. As mentioned, patients with ESRD have bleeding tendencies because of altered platelet aggregation and decreased platelet factor III. With hemodialysis the additional problem exists of platelet destruction by mechanical trauma of the procedure. Aluminum contamination of the diasylate water may interfere with heme synthesis and contributes to the development of osteomalacia.[14] Another report[47] suggests that hemodialysis

may activate prostaglandin I_2, which can reduce platelet aggregation. However, prostaglandin I_2 has a half-life of 1 to 3 minutes and its adverse effects may not be demonstrable by routine laboratory tests.

The 1-year survival rate of patients on dialysis is 78%. The 5-year survival rate is 28%. An alternative to long-term dialysis is renal transplantation (see Chapter 25). This has obvious advantages but also a significant number of problems.

DENTAL MANAGEMENT

PATIENT UNDER CONSERVATIVE CARE

Medical Considerations

Consultation with the patient's physician is suggested before dental care is provided to patients under care for ESRD. Problems generally do not occur in providing outpatient dental care if the patient's disease is well controlled and conservative medical care is being provided. However, if the patient is in the advanced stages of failure or has another systemic disease common to renal failure (e.g., diabetes mellitus, hypertension, or systemic lupus erythematosus), or electrolyte imbalance is present, dental care may best be provided after physician consultation and in a hospital-like setting. Deferral of treatment may be required until adequate control is obtained (Box 9-1).

If the person is to be treated as an outpatient, blood pressure should be closely monitored before and during the procedure (see Chapters 4, 7). Because of the potential for bleeding problems, these patients should receive pretreatment screening for bleeding disorders, including bleeding time and platelet count. A hematocrit level and a hemoglobin count also should be obtained to assess the status of anemia. Any abnormal values should be discussed with the physician. Few problems are encountered with nonhemorrhagic dental procedures when the hematocrit level is above 25%. If bleeding is anticipated hematocrit levels can be raised with the use of erythropoietin. A less desirable option would be red blood cell transfusion, which has the risk of sensitization and blood-borne infections. If an orofacial infection exists, aggressive management is necessary using culture and sensitivity tests and appropriate antibiotics.

When surgical procedures are undertaken, meticulous attention to good surgical technique is necessary to decrease the risks of excessive bleeding and infection. The dentist should consult with the physician to determine the need for antibiotics when invasive procedures are planned. Alteration in drug dosage may be needed based on the amount of kidney function present.

One of the major problems in treating a patient with ESRD is that of drug therapy. Of concern are drugs excreted primarily by the kidney, or that are nephrotoxic. As a general rule, drugs excreted by the kidney are eliminated twofold less efficiently when the GFR drops to 50 ml/min and thus may reach toxic levels at lower GFR. In these circumstances, drug dosage needs to be reduced and timing of administration needs to be prolonged. Nephrotoxic drugs such as acyclovir, aminoglycosides, aspirin, nonsteroidal antiinflammatory drugs, and tetracycline require special dosage adjustments. Acetaminophen also is nephrotoxic and can cause renal tubular necrosis at high doses but is probably safer than aspirin in these patients because it is metabolized in the liver.

The frequency and dosage of dental drug administration requires adjustment during uremia for reasons besides nephrotoxicity and renal metabolism. For example, (1) a low serum albumin value reduces the number of binding sites for circulating drugs, thus enhancing drug effects, (2) uremia can modify hepatic metabolism of drugs (increasing or decreasing clearance), (3) antacids can affect acid-base or electrolyte balance, further complicating uremic effects on electrolyte balance, and (4) aspirin and nonsteroidal antiinflammatory drugs potentiate uremic-platelet defects, thus these antiplatelet drugs should be avoided (Table 9-2).

Although nitrous oxygen-oxide and diazepam are antianxiety drugs that require little modification for use in pa-

tients with ESRD, the hematocrit or hemoglobin concentration should be measured before intravenous sedation to ensure adequate oxygenation. Also, drugs that depress the central nervous system (barbiturates, narcotics) are best avoided in the presence of uremia because the blood-brain barrier may not be intact and excessive sedation may result. General anesthesia is not recommended for patients with ESRD, when the hemoglobin concentration is below 10 g/100 ml.

The risk of bleeding diathesis in patients with uremia dictates that the dentist have local (topical thrombin, microfibrillar collagen, suture) or systemic (desmopressin 0.3 µg/kg over 30 minutes) hemostatic agents available during surgical procedures. Conjugated estrogens are helpful when longer duration of action is required; however, 1 week of therapy usually is needed to guarantee efficacy. Cryoprecipitate (a plasma derivative rich in factor VIII, fibrinogen, and fibronectin) is a less frequently used hemostatic alternative, because of risk of disease transmission. Platelet transfusions are used infrequently because of risk of immunogenic sensitization.

Treatment Planning Modifications

The goal of dental care for patients receiving conservative treatment for ESRD is to restore the mouth to the healthiest condition possible and to eliminate possible sources of infection. Oral physiotherapy training is important for the maintenance of long-term oral health. Recall appointments may need to be more frequent when salivary flow rates are diminished to reduce the development of oral infections and periodontal disease. Once an acceptable level of oral hygiene has been established, no contraindication exists to routine dental care.

Oral Complications and Manifestations

Several oral changes are seen with chronic renal failure. One of the most common is pallor of the oral mucosa secondary to anemia. Red-orange discoloration of the cheeks and mucosa caused by pruritus and deposition of carotene-like pigments occurs when renal filtration is decreased.[23] Diminished salivary flow also may occur, resulting in xerostomia and parotid infections.[24] Candidiasis is more frequent when salivary flow is diminished. Patients frequently complain of an altered or metallic taste, and the saliva may have a characteristic ammonia-like odor resulting from a high urea content.[24]

In severe failure, uremic stomatitis may be present, characterized early by red, burning mucosa covered with a gray exudates and later as frank ulceration. White patches termed *uremic frost* caused by urea crystal deposition are more common on the skin but may be seen on the oral mucosa. These mucosal changes are generally associated with BUN levels greater than 55 mg/dL.[25]

TABLE 9-2

Drug Adjustments in Chronic Renal Disease

Drug	Route of Elimination and Metabolism	Removed by Dialysis	DOSAGE ADJUSTMENT FOR RENAL FAILURE				Supplement Dose Following Hemodialysis
			Method	GFR, ml/min			
				> 50	10-50	< 10	
Analgesic							
Aspirin	Liver (kidney)	Yes	I	q4h	q6h	Avoid	Yes
Acetaminophen	Liver	Yes (HD); No (PD)	I	q4h	q6h	q8h	No
Ibuprofen (Motrin)	Liver	No	—		No adjustment		No
Propoxyphene* (Darvon)	Liver (kidney)	No	DR	100%	100%	Avoid	No
Codeine	Liver	?	DR	100%	75%	50%	No
Meperidine* (Dermerol)	Liver	?	DR	100%	75%	50%	No
Anesthetic							
Lidocaine (Xylocaine)	Liver (kidney)	No	—		No adjustment		N/A
Antimicrobial							
Acyclovir (Zovirax)	Kidney	Yes	I & DR	q8h	q12-24 h	50% q24-48 h	Yes
Amoxicillin, Penicillin V	Kidney (liver)	No	I	q8h	q8-12h	q24h	Yes
Cephalexin (Keflex)	Kidney	Yes	I	q8h	q12h	q12h	Yes; 50% of usual dose after HD
Clindamycin (Cleocin)	Liver	No	—	100%	100%	100%	No
Erythromycin	Liver	No	DR	100%	100%	50-75%	No
Ketoconazole (Nizoral)	Liver	No	—	100%	100%	100%	No
Metronidazole (Flagyl)	Liver (kidney)	Yes	DR	100%	100%	50%	Yes (HD); No (PD)
Tetracycline (Doxycycline)	Kidney (liver)	No	I	q8-12h	q12-24th	q24h	No
Benzodiazepine							
Diazepam (Valium); Triazolam (Halcion)	Liver	?	—		No adjustment		No
Corticosteroid							
Dexamethasone	Local site and liver		—		No adjustment		No

Adapted from Bennett WM, et al: Drugs prescribing in renal failure: dosing guidelines for adults, ed 3, Philadelphia, PA, 1994, American College of Physicians, and Cutler RE, Forland SC, St. John Hammon PG: Drugs in renal failure. In Massry SG, Glassock RJ, editors: Massry and Glassock's textbook of nephrology, Vol. 2, ed 3, Baltimore, MD, 1995, Williams and Wilkins.

DR = Dosage Reduction; I = Increase Interval between doses; GFR = glomerular filtration *rate*; HD = Hemodialysis; PD = peritoneal dialysis.

*Have toxic metabolites that can build up in severe ESRD.

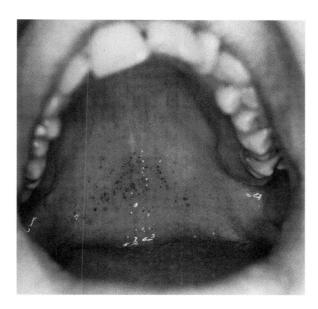

Fig. 9-9 Palatal petechiae in a patient with end-stage renal disease.

Bleeding tendencies are evident as petechiae and ecchymoses on the labial and buccal mucosa, soft palate and margins of the tongue as well as gingival bleeding (Fig. 9-9).

Enamel hypoplasia has been documented in patients with ESRD whose disease began at an early age.[24,26] In the developing dentition, red-brown discoloration and delayed or altered eruption also have been reported. Tooth erosion also can be seen, resulting from persistent vomiting. Caries, however is not a feature because salivary urea inhibits the metabolic end products of bacterial plaque and increases the buffering capacity of saliva, thus preventing a drop in pH sufficient to attain cariogenic levels.[24,27,28]

Specific osseous changes of the jaws accompany chronic renal failure. The most classically described osseous change is the triad of loss of lamina dura, demineralized bone ("ground-glass"), and localized radiolucent jaw lesions (central giant cell granulomas; "brown tumor"). The lytic bone lesions are the result of hyperparathyroidism. Other osseous findings include widened trabeculations, loss of cortication, calcified extraction sites ("socket sclerosis"), and metastatic calcifications within the skull.[29]

PATIENT RECEIVING DIALYSIS

Medical Considerations

Peritoneal dialysis presents no additional problems in dental management. However, this is not the case with patients receiving hemodialysis (see Table 9-1). Research in dogs[30] and humans[31] has shown that the surgically cre-

ated arteriovenous fistulas are potentially susceptible to infection (endarteritis) and are a source of bacteremia that can cause infective endocarditis. The infective endocarditis that develops in patients undergoing hemodialysis occurs even when preexisting cardiac defects are absent.[32] Although the factors that place these patients at risk for infective endocarditis have not been established fully, altered host defenses, altered cardiac output and mechanical stresses,[33] and bacterial seeding and growth on the shunt are important factors.[34]

Infective endocarditis occurs in 2% to 9% of patients receiving hemodialysis. This rate is significantly higher than the incidence in persons with rheumatic heart disease.[32,34,35] The majority of these infections are caused by staphylococcal infections that develop at the site of the graft, fistula, or catheter. Approximately 10% to 17% of cases are caused by organisms that can arise from the oral cavity (*Streptococcus viridans*, lactobacillus).[34-36] Patients with the following devices—dual-lumen cuffed venous catheters and polytetrafluoroethylene grafts, newly placed grafts[37] and long-term catheters—are at increased risk for bacterial seeding compared with patients with primary arteriovenous fistulae.[36]

The most recent American Heart Association guidelines,[38] based on an apparent low risk, do not include a recommendation for prophylactic antibiotics before invasive dental procedures for patients with intravascular access devices. Despite this, several investigators[33,34,39-42] suggest that prophylactic antibiotics are prudent for hemodialysis patients with arteriovenous shunts/grafts when invasive dental procedures are performed. While

controversy exists[43] antibiotic prophylaxis should be provided for patients on hemodialysis who have known cardiac risk factors (e.g., previous history of infective endocarditis, prosthetic cardiac valves, cardiac malformations, acquired valvular dysfunction, hypertrophic cardiomyopathy, mitral valve prolapse with regurgitation, and congestive heart failure—which is often associated with valvular regurgitation) that places them at increased risk for infective endocarditis when invasive dental procedures are planned. For patients undergoing hemodialysis who do not have known cardiac risk factors, consultation regarding the need for antibiotic prophylaxis should be obtained from the managing physician/nephrologist. When prophylaxis is selected, the standard regimen of the current American Heart Association's guidelines should be used[38] (see Chapter 2).

The clinician should be aware of other cardiovascular considerations of patients undergoing hemodialysis. For example, the arm containing the arteriovenous shunt should be protected from application of the blood pressure cuff, blood drawing, and the introduction of intravenous medications. An inflated blood pressure cuff or tourniquet could collapse the shunt and render it useless. Likewise, the complication of phlebitis from intravenous medications could produce a clot that could jeopardize the shunt.

Approximately 40% of patients on dialysis have congestive heart failure, and 9% of them die of cardiovascular complications each year.[44] These patients often take several medications to control hypertension, congestive heart failure, or hypercoagulability (i.e., anticoagulation). Dental care must be provided when the patient is medically stable, and with an understanding of these medications and the needed appropriate dental precautionary measures (see Chapters 3, 4, 7 and 19).

Hemodialysis tends to aggravate bleeding tendencies through physical destruction of platelets and the use of heparin. Thus determining the status of hemostasis is important before oral surgery is performed. A battery of screening tests, including bleeding time and platelet count, should be ordered. Patients at higher risk are those who have elevated laboratory values (e.g., PT equal to or greater than 2.5 times the control) and a history of a gastrointestinal bleeding. While increased risk for bleeding is anticipated for these patients, the clinician can perform several management modifications that will reduce the risk. These include:

- Providing dental treatment at the optimum time, usually the day after hemodialysis since on the day of dialysis patients are generally fatigued and could have a bleeding tendency. The activity of heparin is 3 to 6 hours after infusion and delay of treatment is prudent until that medication is eliminated from the bloodstream.
- Obtaining primary closure and use of, as needed, pressure and hemostatic agents such as thrombin, oxidized cellulose, desmopressin, tranexamic acid (see Chapter 19).
- Performing major surgical procedures on the day after the end of the week of hemodialysis treatment to provide additional time for clot retention before dialysis is resumed. For example, on a Monday-Wednesday-Friday weekly hemodialysis regimen, surgery performed on Saturday allows for an additional day for clot stabilization before hemodialysis is resumed on Monday of the following week.
- Contacting, when necessary, the nephrologist and requesting that the heparin dose be reduced or eliminated during the first hemodialysis session after the surgical procedure. Note: hemodialysis can be performed without heparin when hemostasis and clot retention are important.[45]
- Administering protamine sulfate (usually done by a physician) if immediate care is necessary; doing so will block the anticoagulation effect of heparin.

Patients dependent on chronic dialysis, especially patients with diabetes, are prone to infection. Such patients also have a higher rate of tuberculosis[46] and vancomycin- and methicillin-resistant infections than does the general public.[19] Thus efforts should be made to identify orofacial manifestations of these infections and eliminate oral sources of infection. Patients with active tuberculosis should not be treated until the disease is rendered inactive (see Chapter 8). The selection of antibiotics for hemodialysis patients with oral infections should be prudent and based on appropriate criteria.

Patients undergoing hemodialysis also can benefit from periodic testing for hepatitis viruses and HIV since vaccination or antiviral agents can be administered to reduce the risk of complications of these diseases. The dentist should be aware that a negative test result in the past is not predictive of a carrier state because patients may have acquired the disease since last tested or may be carriers of other infectious viruses (e.g., Epstein-Barr virus, cytomegalovirus) that can cause hepatic injury (see Chapter 10) or immune deficiency. Accordingly, all patients should be treated using universal infection control procedures.

Patients who are carriers of hepatitis viruses from infections during hemodialysis could have altered hepatic function. Liver function should be assessed before hemorrhagic procedures.

The dentist should be aware that hemodialysis removes certain drugs from the circulating blood, which may shorten

the effect of prescribed medications. The chance that a given drug will dialyze is governed by four factors: (1) the molecular weight and size, (2) degree of protein binding, (3) volume of drug distribution, and (4) endogenous drug clearance.[47] For example, drugs with molecular weights above 500 daltons are poorly dialyzed. Drugs removed during hemodialysis are those with low binding capacity to plasma proteins.[48] However, uremia may greatly alter the normal degree of protein binding. A drug such as phenytoin that normally has high protein binding exhibits lower plasma protein binding during uremia and is available to a greater extent for dialysis removal. Drugs with high lipid affinity have high tissue binding and are not available for dialysis removal. Lastly, efficient liver clearing of a drug greatly reduces the effect of dialysis treatment. Dosage amounts and intervals should be adjusted with advice from the patient's physician (see Table 9-2).

Oral Complications and Manifestations
Hemodialysis reverses many of the severe oral manifestations associated with ESRD. However, uremic odor, dry mouth, taste change, tongue and mucosal pain are symptoms that persist in many of these patients. Petechiae, ecchymosis, higher plaque and calculus indices, and lower salivary secretion occur among patients undergoing hemodialysis more frequently than healthy patients.[24,49]

RENAL TRANSPLANT PATIENT

Patients who have a transplanted kidney may have special management needs including the need for supplemental corticosteroids or antibiotic prophylaxis, and management of oral infections and gingival overgrowth secondary to cyclosporine therapy (see Chapter 25).

References

1. United States Renal Data System 1999, annual data report, National Institute of Diabetes and Digestive and Kidney Diseases. http://www.med.umich.edu/kidney/usrds/index.htm. 1999: Human Health Services.
2. Agodoa L, Jones C, Held P: End-stage renal disease in the USA: data from the United States renal data system, Am J Nephrol 16:7-16, 1996.
3. Culleton B et al: Cardiovascular disease and mortality in a community-based cohort with mild renal insufficiency, Kidney Int 59:2214-2219, 1999.
4. VIII: Pediatric End-Stage Renal Disease, Am J Kidney Dis 32:S98-S108, 1998.
5. Brancati F et al: Risk of end-stage renal disease in diabetes mellitus. A prospective cohort study of men screened for MRFIT, JAMA 278:2069-2074, 1997.
6. Freedman B, Bowden D: The role of genetic factors in the development of end-stage renal disease, Curr Opin Nephrol Hypertens 4:230-234, 1995.
7. Goldsmith J, Goldsmith D: Fiberglass or silica exposure and increased nephritis or ESRD (end-stage renal disease), Am J Ind Med 23:873-881, 1993.
8. Krolewski A, Warram J, Christlieb A: Hypercholesterolemia: a determinant of renal function loss and deaths in IDDM patients with nephropathy, Kidney Int 45:S125-S131, 1994.
9. Preuss H, Podlasek S, Henry J: Evaluation of renal function and water, electrolyte, and acid-base balance. In Henry J, editor: Clinical diagnosis and management of laboratory methods, 1991, Philadelphia, WB Saunders.
10. Luke R: Chronic renal failure. In Goldman L, Bennett J, editors: Cecil textbook of medicine, 2000, Philadelphia, WB Saunders.
11. Brenner B, Lazarus J: Chronic renal failure. In Wilson J et al, editors: Harris's principles of internal medicine, 1991, New York, McGraw-Hill.
12. Zachee P, Vermylen J, Boogaerts M: Hematologic aspects of end-stage renal failure, Ann Hematol 69:33-40, 1994.
13. Descamps-Latscha B: The immune system in end-stage renal disease, Curr Opin Nephrol Hypertens 2:883-891, 1993.
14. Hruska K, Teitelbaum S: Renal osteodystroph, N Eng J Med 333:166-174, 1995.
15. Iseki K, Iseki C, Ikemiya Y et al: Risk of developing end-stage renal disease in a cohort of mass screening, Kidney Int 49:800-805, 1996.
16. Monier-Faugere M, Malluche H: Calcitriol pulse therapy in patients with end-stage renal failure, Curr Opin Nephrol Hypertens 3:615-619, 1994.
17. Uribarri J: Past, present and future of end-stage renal disease therapy in the United States, Mt Sinai J Med 66:14-19, 1999.
18. Bonomini V, Vangelista A, Stefoni S: Early dialysis in renal substitutive programs, Kidney Int 8(Suppl):S112-S116, 1978.
19. Tokars J, Miller ER, Alter MJ et al: National surveillance of dialysis-associated diseases in the United States, 1997, Semin Dial 13:75-85, 2000.
20. Green I: Laboratory tests in end-stage renal disease patients undergoing dialysis, Health Technol Assess 2:1-12, 1994.
21. Curtis J: Treatment of irreversible renal failure. In Goldman L. and Bennett J, editors: Cecil textbook of medicine, 2000, Philadelphia, WB Saunders.
22. Kaplowitz L et al: A prospective study of infections in hemodialysis patients: patient hygiene and other risk factors for infection, Infect Control Hosp Epidemiol 9:534-541, 1988.
23. Shoop K: Pruritus in end stage renal disease, ANNA J 21:147-153, 1994.
24. Kho H-S et al: Oral manifestations and salivary flow rate, pH, and buffer capacity in patients with end-stage renal disease undergoing hemodialysis, Oral Surg Oral Med Oral Pathol Oral Radiol Endod 88:316-319, 1999.
25. Hovinga J, Roodvoets A, Gaillard J: Some findings in patients with uremic stomatitis, J Maxillofac Surg 3:125-127, 1975.

26. Bottomley W, Cioffi R, Martin A: Dental management of the patient treated by renal transplantation: preoperative and postoperative considerations, J Am Dent Assoc 85:1330-1335, 1972.

27. Obry F et al: Low caries activity and salivary pH in youngsters dialyzed for chronic renal failure (Fiable activite carieuse et pH salivaire de jeunes dialyses renaux chroniques). J Biol Buccale 12:181-186, 1984.

28. Peterson S, Woodhead J, Crall J: Caries resistance in children with chronic renal failure: plaque pH, salivary pH, and salivary composition, Pediatr Res 19:796-799, 1985.

29. Molpus W et al: The radiographic spectrum of renal osteodystrophy. Am Fam Phys 43:151-158, 1991.

30. Lillehei C, Bob J, Visscher M: The occurrence of endocarditis with valvular deformities in dogs with arteriovenous fistulas, Ann Surg 32:544-577, 1950.

31. Goodman J et al: Bacterial endocarditis as a possible complication of chronic hemodialysis, N Eng J Med 280:876-877, 1969.

32. Leonard A, Raij L, Shapiro FL: Bacterial endocarditis in regularly dialyzed patients, Kidney Int 4:407-422, 1973.

33. Manton S, Midda M: Renal failure and the dental patient: a cautionary tale, Br Dent J 160:388-390, 1986.

34. Reid C, Rahimtoola S: Infective endocarditis in chronic renal failure. In O'Rourke R, editor: The heart and renal disease, New York, 1984, Churchill Livingstone.

35. Cross A, Steigbigel R: Infective endocarditis and access infections in patients on hemodialysi, Medicine 55:453-466, 1976.

36. Robinson D et al: Bacterial endocarditis in hemodialysis patients, Am J Kid Dis 30:521-524, 1997.

37. Goldstone J, Moore W: Infection in vascular prostheses: Clinical manifestations and surgical management, Am J Surg 128:225-233, 1974.

38. Dajani A et al: Prevention of bacterial endocarditis: recommendations by the American Heart Association, Clin Infect Dis 25:1448-1458, 1997.

39. Naylor G, Hall E, Terezhalmy G: The patient with chronic renal failure who is undergoing dialysis or renal transplantation: another consideration for antimicrobial prophylaxis, Oral Surg Oral Med Oral Pathol 65:116-121, 1988.

40. Werner C, Saad T: Prophylactic antibiotic therapy prior to dental treatment for patients with end-stage renal disease, Spec Care Dent 19:106-111, 1999.

41. DeRossi S, Glick M: Dental considerations for the patient with renal disease receiving hemodialysis, J Am Dent Assoc 127:211-219, 1996.

42. Tong D, Rothwell B: Antibiotic prophylaxis in dentistry: a review and practice recommendations, J Am Dent Assoc 131:366-374, 2000.

43. Pallasch T, Slots J: Antibiotic prophylaxis and the medically compromised patient, Periodontology 2000 10:107-138, 1996.

44. Foley R, Parfre P, Sarnak M: Cardiovascular disease in chronic renal disease. Clinical epidemiology of cardiovascular disease in chronic renal disease, Am J Kidney Dis 32:S112-S119, 1998.

45. McKeown JW, personal communication, 2000.

46. Mitwalli A: Tuberculosis in patients on maintenance dialysis, Am J Kidney 18:579-582, 1991.

47. Kaplan A: Maintenance haemodialysis: prescription and management. In Briggs J et al, editors: Renal dialysis, 1994, London, Chapman & Hall Medical.

48. Daugirdas J, Ing T, editors: Handbook of dialysis, 1988, Boston, Little and Brown.

49. Gavalda C et al: Renal hemodialysis patients: oral, salivary, dental and periodontal findings in 105 adult cases, Oral Dis 5:299-302, 1999.

Liver Disease

*P*atients with liver disorders are of significant interest to the dentist because the liver plays a vital role in metabolic functions, including the secretion of bile needed for fat absorption, conversion of sugar to glycogen, and excretion of bilirubin, a waste product of hemoglobin metabolism. Impairment of liver function can lead to abnormalities of the metabolism of amino acids, ammonia, protein, carbohydrates, and lipids (triglycerides and cholesterol). Many biochemical functions performed by the liver, such as synthesis of coagulation factors and drug metabolism, may be adversely affected. Viral hepatitis and alcoholic liver disease are two of the more common liver disorders.

DEFINITION

Hepatitis is inflammation of the liver that can result from infectious or noninfectious causes. Examples of hepatitis with infectious causes are viral hepatitis, infectious mononucleosis, secondary syphilis, and tuberculosis. Noninfectious hepatitis can result from excessive or prolonged use of toxic substances (acetaminophen, alcohol, halothane, ketoconazole, methyldopa, and methotrexate).

ETIOLOGY

Acute viral hepatitis is the most common form of infectious hepatitis. Five distinct viruses—types A, B, C, D, and E—are associated with this disease (Table 10-1). These viruses each belong to a different family with distinct antigenic properties. They have little in common except for the target organ they infect and some epidemiologic characteristics. Hepatitis A was called "infectious hepatitis," and hepatitis B was termed "serum hepatitis." Hepatitis D (also known as "delta") occurs only in association with hepatitis B. Hepatitis C and hepatitis E were known as "non-A non-B hepatitis" (NANB). They were distinguished by the route of transmission. The parenterally acquired form now is known as *hepatitis* C, and the community-acquired form and enteric subtypes (found in India, Southeast Asia, and Central America) is termed *hepatitis* E.

In up to 20% of cases of hepatitis, a standard virus cannot be identified, and the disease is not associated with toxic, metabolic, and genetic conditions. Viruses may be causative. The term *hepatitis* non-A-E is used to describe these conditions. Hepatitis F virus, hepatitis G virus, and the transfusion transmitted virus (TTV) are candidate viruses associated with hepatitis non-A-E. Definitive evidence that these viruses play a pathogenic role in liver disease is lacking.[1]

Hepatitis A

Hepatitis A virus (HAV) is a 28 nm ribonucleic acid (RNA) virus of the Picornaviridae family that replicates in the liver, is excreted in the bile, and shed in the stool. HAV has been isolated from feces, grown in culture, and examined by electron microscopy. One serotype and seven genotypes have been identified. Serologic tests for HAV and its antibodies—anti-HAV, immunoglobulin M (IgM), and anti-HAV immunoglobulin G (IgG)—are readily available.

Hepatitis B

Hepatitis B virus (HBV) is a deoxyribonucleic (DNA) virus of the Hepadnaviridae family first identified in 1965. The virus replicates predominately in hepatocytes and to a lesser extent in stem cells in the pancreas, bone marrow, and spleen.[2] Electron microscopy has determined several virus-associated particles related to hepatitis B infection. The intact HBV, or *Dane particle*, is composed of an outer shell and an inner core. The outer shell is the hepatitis B surface antigen (HBsAg). It circulates in the blood as both 22-nm spherical and tubular particles for up to 6 months after infection, depending on resolution of

TABLE 10-1

Features of Hepatitis Viruses

	Hepatitis A	Hepatitis B	Hepatitis C	Hepatitis D	Hepatitis E
Old Terminology	Infectious hepatitis	Serum hepatitis	Post-transfusion hepatitis non-A-non-B	Delta hepatitis	Hepatitis non-A non-D
Family and Types	Picornavirus 1 serotype, 7 genotypes	Hepadnavirus	Flavivirus 6 major genotypes (40 related subtypes)	Satellite 3 genotypes	Calicivirus 3 genotypes
Virion Structure	28 nm RNA non-enveloped virus	42 nm DNA enveloped virus; enveloped (Dane particles), spherical and tubular particles	30-80 nm ss+RNA enveloped virus	35-40 nm defective RNA non-enveloped virus (uses HBsAg for viral envelope)	32-34 nm non-enveloped RNA virus
Incubation	15-50 days $\overline{X}$ = 25 days	45-180 days $\overline{X}$ = 75 days	14-180 days $\overline{X}$ = 50 days	15-150 days $\overline{X}$ = 35 days	15-60 days $\overline{X}$ = 40 days
Main Route of Transmission	Fecal-oral route	Parenteral, sexual contact*	Parenteral, sexual contact* (low risk)	Parenteral, sexual contact*	Fecal-oral route
Diagnosis†‡	Anti-HAV IgG (recovery)	HBsAg (infectious) Anti-HBsAg (recovery) Anti-HBc (acute, persistently infected, or previously infected non-protective) HBeAg (infectious) Anti-HBeAg (clearing/cleared infection)	Anti-HCV (previous infection) HCV RNA (infectivity)	Anti-HDV HD-Ag	Anti-HEV

Chronic Carrier State	No	Yes, 90% risk of becoming carrier if infected as neonate; 25-50% risk of becoming carrier if infected as infant; 5-10% risk of becoming carrier if infected as adult	Yes, risk of becoming carrier is 80-90%	Yes, carrier state in 20-70%	No
Complications§ of the Liver	Rare	Yes, increased risk of liver cirrhosis and hepatocellular carcinoma (HCC) after 25-30 years of infection	Yes, 10-fold increased risk of liver cirrhosis within 20 yrs; 1-5% of carriers develop HCC by 20 years—the risk of HCC with chronic HCV exceeds risk with chronic HBV.	Yes	Rare morbidity and mortality except in pregnant women
Associated Clinical Syndromes		Yes	Yes		
Immunization Passive	Immune globulin IG (0.02 ml/kg)	Hepatitis B immune globulin (HBIG) (0.06 ml/kg)	Not available	Not available	Not available
Active	Harivax, Vaqta and Twinrix	Recombivax, Engerix‖ and Twinrix	None (difficult development because of the many genotypes)	Yes; protected with Recombivax, Engerix‖, and Twinrix	Genetech has applied for vaccine patent

*Risk groups include: IDUs, HCWs, hemodialysis patients, low socioeconomic level, sexual/household contacts of infected persons, persons with multiple sex partners, history of transfusion prior to 1991. $\overline{X}$ = mean. HCC = hepatocellular carcinoma.

†Diagnostic markers of viral hepatitis include: elevation of AST, ALT, GGT, WBC count and PT.

‡Preicteric phase: anorexia, nausea, vomiting, fatigue, myalgia, malaise, fever.

Icterus: Jaundice, discolored stool, dark urine, hepatosplenomegaly, bleeding disorder. Serum sickness like features (arthralgia, rash, angioedema) in 5% to 10%.

§Risk for complications and severe liver disease increases with co-infection of HBV and HCV and chronic alcohol consumption.

‖Immunization recommended for dental personnel.

infection. The antibody responsible for clearing the infection is anti-HBs, signaling long-term immunity. The inner core of the particle is the hepatitis B core antigen (HBcAg), with corresponding IgG antibodies anti-HBc and IgM anti-HBc (indicating recent infection). A third particle is the hepatitis B early antigen (HBeAg), an antigenic component derived from cleavage of the core antigen. It is related to hepatitis B infectivity. Its corresponding antibody is anti-HBe. Serologic tests are available for all these antigen-antibody systems except the HBcAg, which is retained in hepatocytes.

Hepatitis C
Hepatitis C virus (HCV) is a 30- to 80-nm diameter, single-stranded RNA virus of the Flaviviridae family, identified in 1989. HCV is related to the flaviviruses and the pestiviruses and was previously known as one of the non-A non-B hepatitis viruses. HCV has six major genotypes. It causes the most common chronic bloodborne infection in the United States. Serologic tests for both the viral antigen and its antibody (anti-HCV) became available in 1991.[3]

Hepatitis D
Hepatitis D virus (HDV), first described in 1977,[4] is a defective, negative strand RNA virus 35 to 40 nm in diameter. HDV requires HBsAg for its viral envelope and transmissibility but once inside a permissive cell replicates without the helper HBV. HDV occurs only in patients with HBV infection, either as a coinfection or superinfection. The hepatitis D antigen (HDAg) and its antibody (anti-HDV) can be detected with serologic testing.

Hepatitis E
Hepatitis E virus (HEV) is a 32- to 34-nm, nonenveloped RNA-type virus that resembles viruses of the Caliciviridae family. Three genotypes have been detected. This virus is responsible for enterically transmitted (formerly "NANB") hepatitis, a disorder clinically similar to hepatitis A infection. HEV was recognized first in 1983 and genetically analyzed in 1990.[5] Outbreaks have been documented in developing countries with poor sanitation, such as India, northern Africa, Mexico, and Southeast Asia. Infection by HEV is more common in men than women. The virus was cloned in 1990, and serologic tests for both antigen and antibody recently became available.[2]

Hepatitis Non-A-E
Cases of acute hepatitis that appear to have a viral etiology but cannot be attributed to any known virus are referred to as *hepatitis non*-A-E. This category includes unknown viruses and emerging viruses associated with hepatitis, such as hepatitis F virus,[6] hepatitis G viruses,[7] and the TTV virus.[8]

EPIDEMIOLOGY

INCIDENCE AND PREVALENCE
Hepatitis is a worldwide health problem with more than 5 million new cases occurring annually and more than 300 million persons across the globe carrying the viruses. Regional incidence rates are lowest in the Western Hemisphere and northern regions and highest in the Eastern Hemisphere and tropical regions. In the United States viral hepatitis ranks 7th behind chlamydia, gonorrhea, varicella, AIDS, salmonellosis, and syphilis in reportable infectious diseases. More than 4 million Americans are chronic carriers of hepatitis viruses.[9]

Hepatitis A occurrence declined for several years; 32,859 cases were reported in 1966 in the United States, whereas 21,532 cases were reported in 1983. Since 1983 a slight increase in reported cases has occurred, with the latest report showing 23,229 cases in 1998.[9] Overall, the Centers for Disease Control (CDC) estimates that between 125,000 and 200,000 cases of hepatitis A occur annually.[10] Approximately 47% of acute viral hepatitis cases reported in the United States are caused by HAV.[11]

Between 140,000 and 320,000 new HBV infections occur in the United States annually, with 10,258 cases reported in 1998.[9,12] This represents approximately 27% of the reported cases of acute hepatitis[1] and more than a 50% decrease in the number of cases reported during the past decade. This downward trend likely will continue as a national strategy for eliminating HBV transmission is implemented. Approximately half the reported cases required hospitalization, and more than 100 infected persons (0.2% to 2%) die annually of fulminant disease. Most infections occur in young adults, with 10% of cases occurring in infants and young children.[13] Many transfusion recipients and hemophiliacs who received factor replacement during the 1960s and 1970s are infected with HBV. The current prevalence of volunteer blood donations in the United States that are antibody positive against HBV is 0.2%.[17] Health professionals estimate 1.25 million persons are chronic HBV carriers in the United States.[12]

HCV is a major cause of acute and chronic hepatitis worldwide.[14] Since diagnostic testing was implemented, the rate of new infections has declined from an estimated 240,000 in the 1980s to 36,000 reported annually in the United States in the late 1990s.[15,16] Carrier rates for HCV range from 0.2% to 2.2% in developed countries (0.4% of volunteer blood donations in the United States are antibody positive to HCV).[3,17] Higher rates (2% to 10%) are found in developing nations and inner cities. The prevalence in dialysis patients ranges from 0.5% to

approximately 40%,[3,18,19] and rates approach 90% in organ recipients following donation of a HCV-RNA positive organ. Health professionals estimate that 3.5 million to 4 million Americans have chronic HCV infection,[20] making this disease the most common bloodborne infection in the United States. Approximately 10,000 persons die each year in the United States because of HCV-related liver disease.[20,21] Current estimates predict that mortality rates caused by chronic hepatitis C infection will triple in the United States in the next 10 years, rivaling that of HIV.[22]

The incidence of HDV infection correlates directly with the worldwide rate of chronic HBV infection. Countries with low rates of chronic HBV infection have low prevalence of HDV infection. In contrast, countries with high endemicity for HBV infection (Southeast Asia and China) have a greater prevalence of HDV infection.[23] HDV accounts for approximately 7,500 infections in the United States annually. The prevalence of HDV infection among HBsAg-positive patients is low in the general population (1.4% to 8% in blood donors). The prevalence of HDV infection is highest in persons who are injection drug users (20% to 53%) and have hemophilia (48% to 80%).[23] Hepatitis D has a mortality rate of 2% to 20%.

The exact prevalence of HEV in the United States is not known but considered between 1% and 5%.[5] Reported cases of HEV in the United States have been isolated and from people who recently traveled to endemic regions (Asia, India, Southeast Asia, Middle East, Central America and Mexico).[24] HEV is not a significant factor in the United States, though it has produced a 20% fatality rate in pregnant women in the third trimester of pregnancy. HEV is not considered a problem in developed countries.

TRANSMISSION

Hepatitis A
Transmission of HAV occurs almost exclusively by fecal contamination of food or water.*

Common sources include contaminated wells or water supplies, restaurants, and raw shellfish. Because the reservoir for infection is frequently a common food or water source, an occurrence of hepatitis A often becomes an epidemic. Transmission is enhanced by poor personal hygiene, which places school-age youngsters, food handlers, daycare workers, and travelers in developing countries at greater risk for contracting the disease. Transmission by contaminated blood products is rare, occurring

---

*A small number of cases of transmission of HAV through clotting factor concentrates also has been reported. Centers for Disease Control: MMWR 45:29-32, 1996.

early during the course of the infection when titers in blood can be high and the patient is most infectious.

Hepatitis A is a common disease, with serologic evidence of infection in approximately 40% of urban populations in the United States.[2] Its incubation period ranges from 15 to 50 days and averages 25 days. Persons of any age may be infected; however, the disease occurs primarily in children and young adults. Hepatitis A tends to be of mild severity, lasting a couple of weeks and often goes undiagnosed. No carrier state is known to exist for it, and recovery usually conveys immunity against reinfection. In 1995 the first of three vaccines was developed as a form of immunized protection.

Hepatitis B
Hepatitis B is transmitted efficiently by percutaneous and permucosal exposures, with the most frequent route of transmission in the United States being sexual activity.[25,26] Exposures that can cause HBV infection include (1) direct percutaneous inoculation, transfusion of infective blood or blood products (serum, plasma, factor concentrates),* needle sharing, tattooing, and body piercing; (2) indirect percutaneous introduction of infective serum or plasma through minute skin cuts or abrasions; (3) absorption of infective serum or plasma through mucosal surfaces of the mouth or eye; (4) absorption of infective secretions, such as saliva or semen through mucosal surfaces, as might occur following heterosexual or homosexual contact; and (5) transfer of infective serum or plasma via inanimate environmental surfaces or possibly vectors.[27] Experimental data[28,29] indicate that fecal transmission of HBV does not occur and airborne spread is not of epidemiologic importance. The incubation period ranges from 45 to 180 days and averages 75 days.

The lifetime risk of hepatitis B occurrence among the general population is low; however, certain groups have a much higher risk. Included among these are dental personnel and other healthcare workers, refugees from Indochina and Haiti, residents of mental institutions and prisons, hemodialysis patients, users of illicit drugs, men who have sex with men, heterosexuals with multiple partners, and recipients of blood transfusions (Box 10-1). The risk of infection is directly related to exposure to blood, resulting in a reported prevalence rate of past infection among general dentists in the 1980s ranging from 13% to

---

*The Food and Drug Administration requires that all donated whole blood, transusable components, and plasma for human blood use in the United States be subjected to serologic tests for syphilis, HBsAg, anti-HBc, anti-HCV, and anti-HIV. The current incidence of posttransfusion hepatitis B is approximately 0.002% per transfusion recipient.

BOX 10-1

Persons at Substantial Risk for Hepatitis B Who Should Receive Vaccine

Individuals with occupational risk
    Healthcare workers
    Public-safety workers
    Clients and staff of institutions for the developmentally disabled
Hemodialysis patients
Recipients of certain blood products
Household contacts and sex partners of HBV carriers
Adoptees from countries where HBV infection is endemic
International travelers
Illicit drug users
Sexually active homosexual and bisexual men
Sexually active heterosexual men and women (who have multiple partners)
Inmates of long-term correctional facilities

From Centers for Disease Control: MMWR 40:14-16, 1991.

30%. Among oral surgeons the prevalence rate was as high as 38%.[30-33] More recent reports[24,34] cite the prevalence for general dentists at 7.8 to 8.9% and oral surgeons at 21%. This reduction presumably reflects the effectiveness of vaccination and infection control measures.

Although hepatitis B can occur at any age, statistics indicate the condition is unusual in persons under the age of 15 years. Of the 10,258 cases of type B hepatitis reported to the CDC in 1998,[9] only 282 were in patients under age 15 years (2.8%). Compared with hepatitis A, hepatitis B tends to cause greater morbidity and mortality, especially in the very young and older patients.

Hepatitis C

HCV is similar to HBV in behavior and characteristics. The incubation period of HCV ranges from two weeks to six months, with a median of 50 days. Approximately 60% to 90% of HCV cases are transmitted by blood and blood products, with approximately 90% of posttransfusion hepatitis cases being attributed to HCV until routine screening of blood was implemented in 1992.[35] The current risk for posttransfusion hepatitis C in the United States is estimated at 1 in 103,000 patients.[36] Those at greatest risk for this disease are injecting drug users and those with large or repeated percutaneous exposures. Injection drug users account for more than 60% of acute HCV infections, and HCV infection is four times more common than HIV in this population.[14,37,38] Others at increased risk are patients on he-

modialysis, persons who have multiple sexual partners or sexual contacts with those who have chronic HCV, healthcare workers exposed to blood, and recipients of whole blood, blood cellular components, or plasma.[20] The risk of vertical transmission of HCV from infected mother to infant is low, accounting for 5% of cases.[2] Approximately 1% of sexual partners of HCV-infected persons are infected per year.[38,39] In approximately 30% to 40% of HCV infections, the means of transmission is not determined.[23]

Hepatitis D

Hepatitis D occurs only as a coinfection with acute hepatitis B or as a superinfection in carriers of hepatitis B. HDV is transmitted parenterally and sexually like HBV. HDV is seen primarily in drug addicts and persons with hemophilia and frequently is associated with more severe fulminant infections than is infection with hepatitis B alone.[3,40] HDV produces extraordinarily high titers in the blood of infected persons. The incubation period ranges from 15 to 150 days and averages 35 days.

Hepatitis E

Hepatitis E resembles hepatitis A and is transmitted similarly via fecal-oral contamination. The incubation period ranges from 15 to 60 days with an average incubation of 40 days. Viremia occurs during the incubation phase, but the infectious titer has not been determined.

Occupational Transmission

Little to no risk exists of transmission of HAV, HEV, and non-A-E hepatitis viruses from occupational exposure of dental health care workers to persons infected with these viruses. In contrast, risk exists for transmission of HBV and a lesser risk is present for HCV following occupational exposure to infected blood or bodily fluids containing infected blood. HCV is less infectious and less efficient in transmission compared with HBV. Following percutaneous or other sharp injury of healthcare workers to contaminated blood, the risk of contracting HBV is reported to range from 6% to 30%,[41,42] with potential infectiousness correlating with HBeAg in the serum (i.e., serum with HBeAg and HBsAg may be 10 times more infectious than serum with HBsAg alone).[43] Moreover, HBV can survive for at least one week in dried blood on environmental surfaces and contaminated needles and instruments. In contrast, the seroconversion rate of an accidental blood exposure to HCV is between 2% and 8%.[38,44] For comparison purposes, the risk of contracting HIV after a percutaneous or other sharp injury is 0.3%.[42]

The role of saliva in HBV transmission,[45] except by percutaneous or permucosal routes, does not appear to be significant.[46] Observations reported to the Centers for Disease Control[47] suggest that transmission of hepatitis B to humans after surface oral contact with HBsAg-

positive saliva is unlikely. Another study[32] reported that out of 19 dental professionals who had cutaneous contact with saliva containing HBsAg and HBeAg, none developed serologic evidence of hepatitis B. Transmission has been reported,[48] however, as a result of a human bite. Permucosal or percutaneous inoculation of infectious saliva is necessary for transmission of hepatitis B. HCV has been detected in saliva.[49] However, HCV is less infectious than HBV and does not appear to be spread by contact with saliva. Spread of HCV rarely has been reported after a human bite[50] and blood splash to the conjuctiva.[51]

During the past 30 years, HBV transmission has been documented to occur from 9 dental health care workers to dental patients (see Dental Management). Although HCV has not been reported to occur from DHCW to patient, HCV has been reported to be transmitted from 2 cardiac surgeons to several of their patients.[52,53] Current data indicate about 0.7% to 2.0% of general dentists and 2% of oral surgeons are positive for anti-HCV.[34,54]

PATHOPHYSIOLOGY AND COMPLICATIONS

Hepatitis viruses replicate in hepatocytes and ultimately damage the host cell. HBV infection produces high serum titers reaching 10^8 to 10^{11} virions/ml. In contrast, HAV produces a viremia that may reach 10^5 virions/ml in blood but 10^6 to 10^{10} genomes per gram of stool.[2]

No single histopathologic lesion is characteristic of viral hepatitis, but the appearances of types A, B, C, D, and E hepatitides are similar and are described together. Commonly, acute viral hepatitis is characterized by ballooning degeneration and necrosis of liver cells (hepatocytes). The entire liver lobule is inflamed and consists of lymphocytes and mononuclear phagocytes.

Icterus (jaundice) is associated with hepatitis in approximately 70% of cases of HAV, approximately 30% of cases of HBV infection, and approximately 25% of cases of HCV and HEV. The cause is an accumulation of bilirubin in the plasma, epithelium, and urine. Bilirubin is a degradation product of hemoglobin, one of the major constituents of bile, and yellowish. Bilirubin normally is transported to the liver by way of the plasma. In the liver it conjugates with glucuronic acid then is excreted into the intestine where it aids in the emulsification of fats and stimulates peristalsis. When liver disease is present, bilirubin tends to accumulate in the plasma because of decreased liver metabolism and transport. Jaundice usually will become clinically apparent when the plasma level of bilirubin approaches 2.5 mg/100 ml (normal is less than 1 mg/100 ml).[23] If the plasma bilirubin does not reach this level, the patient is anicteric (without jaundice), thus explaining nonicteric hepatitis.

Most cases of viral hepatitis, especially types A and E, resolve without any complications. HBV, HCV, and HDV can persist and replicate in the liver when the virus is not completely cleared from the organ. The consequences of hepatitis include recovery, persistent infection (or carrier state), dual infection, chronic active hepatitis, fulminant hepatitis, cirrhosis, hepatocellular carcinoma, and death. Dual infections and the chronic consumption of alcohol lead to more severe disease. Approximately 16,000 people die annually because of complications related to hepatitis infection.

Fulminant Hepatitis

A serious complication of acute viral hepatitis is fulminant hepatitis, characterized by massive hepatocellular destruction and a mortality rate of approximately 80%. The condition occurs more commonly among the elderly and those with chronic liver disease. Coinfection or superinfection of HBV and HDV or infection by a single hepatitis virus can cause fulminant disease. Mutant strains of these viruses have been proposed to be causative. In the United States each year more than 100 persons die of fulminant hepatitis A and E, and approximately 350 persons die of HBV–HDV-associated fulminant disease. HCV rarely causes fulminant hepatitis.

Chronic Infection

Chronic infection (carrier state) is characterized by the persistence of low levels of virus in the liver and serum viral antigens (HBsAg, HBeAg, and HCVAg) for longer than 6 months without signs of liver disease. Individuals with this condition potentially are infectious to others. The rate of carrier establishment varies based on the virus, age, and health of patient.[23,24] For example, approximately 50% to 90% of infected infants, 25% of infected children, and 6% to 10% of adults infected with HBV become carriers. In contrast, 70% to 90% of adults infected with HCV develop a persistent carrier state.[20] With both viruses, men and immunosuppressed persons are more commonly affected. Approximately 0.1% to 0.5% of the general population in the United States (more than 4 million persons) are carriers of HBV and/or HCV, whereas 5% to 15% of the populations of China, Southeast Asia, sub-Saharan Africa, most Pacific Islands, and the Amazon Basin are HBV carriers.[55] This marked difference reflects the endemicity of hepatitis B in these latter countries. The carrier rate of dentists in the United States has decreased, but the risk still is estimated to be 3 to 10 times that of the general population.[24] The highest HCV carrier rates are found among injection drug users and persons with hemophilia (20%). Healthcare workers show approximately a 1% to 2% prevalence.[23,54] The lowest rates of anti-HCV are found among blood donors with about 0.5% to 1.0% being positive.[23] Approximately 2% to 5% of acute co-infections of HBV and HDV result in chronic infections. Superinfections are more frequent than co-infections and result in more than 70% of persons becoming chronic carriers.[23]

The carrier state may persist for decades or cause liver disease by progressing to chronic active hepatitis. Chronic active hepatitis is characterized by active virus replication in the liver, HBsAg and HBeAg, or HCVAg in the serum, signs and symptoms of chronic liver disease, persistent hepatic cellular necrosis, and elevated liver enzymes for longer than 6 months.[3,23] Approximately 3% to 5% of patients infected with HBV, 25% of HBV carriers, and 40% to 50% of those infected with HCV develop chronic active hepatitis.

HBV- and HCV-related chronic liver destruction and the resulting fibrosis lead to cirrhosis in approximately 20% of cases of chronic hepatitis. Approximately 1% to 5% of these patients develop primary hepatocellular carcinoma. An estimated 4000 persons die each year from HBV-related cirrhosis, 10,000 die from HCV-related cirrhosis and more than 800 die from HBV- and HCV-related liver cancer. The relationship with liver cancer is 30 times to 100 times higher for chronic carriers compared with uninfected persons and particularly strong in some selected Asian populations.[24]

CLINICAL PRESENTATION

SIGNS AND SYMPTOMS

After an incubation phase that varies with the infecting virus, approximately 10% of hepatitis A, 60% to 70% of hepatitis C and 70% to 90% of hepatitis B cases are asymptomatic. When manifestations occur, the clinical features of acute viral hepatitis are similar and are discussed together.[23] Many of the signs and symptoms are common to many viral illnesses and may be described as flulike. This is especially true of the early, or prodromal, phase. Patients classically exhibit three phases of acute illness.

The prodromal (preicteric) phase usually precedes the onset of jaundice by 1 or 2 weeks and consists of abdominal pain, anorexia, intermittent nausea, vomiting, fatigue, myalgia, malaise, and fever. With hepatitis B, 5% to 10% of patients demonstrate serum sickness-like manifestations including arthralgia or arthritis, rash, and angioedema.[23]

The icteric phase is heralded by the onset of clinical jaundice, a yellow-brown cast of the eyes, skin, oral mucosa, and urine. Many of the nonspecific prodromal symptoms may subside, but gastrointestinal symptoms (e.g., anorexia, nausea, vomiting, and right upper quadrant pain) may increase, especially early in the phase. Hepatomegaly and splenomegaly frequently are seen. This phase lasts 2 to 8 weeks and is experienced by at least 70% of patients infected with HAV, 30% of those acutely infected with HBV, and 25% to 30% of patients acutely infected with HCV.[23]

During the convalescent or recovery (posticteric) phase, symptoms disappear, but hepatomegaly and abnormal liver function values may persist for a variable period. This phase can last for weeks or months, with recovery time for hepatitis B and C generally being longer. The usual sequence is recovery (clinical and biochemical) within approximately 4 months after the onset of jaundice.[23] HBV infrequently is associated with clinical syndromes, including polyarteritis nodosa, glomerulonephritis, and leukocytoclastic vasculitis. Coagulopathy, encephalopathy, cerebral edema, and fulminant hepatitis are rare.

Chronic hepatitis is associated with liver abnormalities but is often asymptomatic for 10 to 30 years. Nonspecific symptoms of chronic hepatitis C (loss of weight, easy fatigue, sleep disorder, difficulty in concentrating, right upper quadrant pain, and liver tenderness) may not appear until hepatic fibrosis, cirrhosis, or hepatocellular carcinoma are present. The hepatic damage is caused by both the cytopathic effect of the virus and inflammatory changes secondary to immune activation. Extrahepatic immunologic disorders associated with chronic HCV infection result from the production of autoantibodies and include immune complex-mediated disease (vasculitis, polyarteritis nodosa), autoimmune disorders (rheumatoid arthritis, glomerulonephritis, thrombocytopenic purpura, thyroiditis, pulmonary fibrosis), and two immunologic disorders: lichen planus and Sjögren's-like syndrome (lymphocytic sialadenitis).[56] If these diseases or signs of advanced liver disease (bleeding esophageal varices, ascites, jaundice, spider angioma, dark urine) develop, testing for chronic hepatitis is recommended.

HDV infection often results in severe acute hepatitis or rapidly progressive chronic liver disease. Coinfection usually results in transient and self-limiting disease, whereas super-infection more often results in severe clinical disease indicated by sudden exacerbation in a chronic carrier of HBV.

LABORATORY FINDINGS

The serum transaminases (aspartate aminotransferase [AST], serum glutamate oxaloacetate transaminase, alanine aminotransferase [ALT], serum glutamate pyruvate transaminase) are sensitive indicators of liver injury and acute viral hepatitis, with ALT being a more specific indicator.[57] Also useful in the diagnosis of hepatitis are elevated levels of serum bilirubin, alkaline phosphatase (heat fraction) level, gamma-glutamyl transpeptidase, lactate dehydrogenase, white blood cell count, and prothrombin time. Antigen-antibody serologic tests are required for identifying the viral agent and in distinguishing acute, resolved, and chronic infections.

The serum transaminase levels become elevated from damage to infected liver cells. Normal levels are less than 30 to 40 U/L. The AST and ALT become elevated usually before elevation of the serum bilirubin occurs. The highest levels often correspond to the peak of the icteric

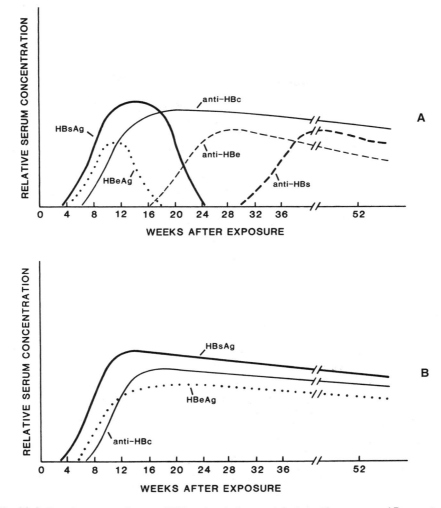

Fig. 10-1 Typical sequence of various HBV markers in **A,** acute infection with recovery and **B,** acute infection resulting in a chronic carrier state.

phase and gradually subside during the convalescent phase. Jaundice becomes clinically evident as the serum bilirubin level approaches 2.5 mg/100 ml. An elevated bilirubin level may persist after the transaminase level begins to fall. The serum alkaline phosphatase level may be mildly elevated or normal; however, this is a relatively nonspecific test.

An increase in the white blood cell count usually occurs, with a relative lymphocytosis. Atypical lymphocytes are seen that are identical to those observed in infectious mononucleosis. Monitoring the prothrombin time is important because it may be elevated, especially in more extensive disease that results in hepatic cellular destruc-

tion. Abnormal hemostasis may occur if the prothrombin time is severely elevated.

Hepatitis A is diagnosed by the presence of IgM anti-HAV rising 2 to 4 weeks during the acute phase of the infection, and later by a rise in IgG anti-HAV indicative of the convalescent phase. IgG anti-HAV persists in blood and confers lifelong protection, whereas IgM anti-HAV tends to disappear by the sixth month.

The serologic relationships that occur during hepatitis B virus infection are shown in Fig. 10-1 and are summarized as following:

- The first markers to appear in blood are HBsAg, HBeAg, and HBV DNA followed by antibodies

against the core antigen (IgM anti-HBc and IgG anti-HBc). The IgM antibodies are markers of the acute infection.

- IgG antibodies contribute to control of disease and indicate immunity.
- Presence of the virus surface antigen (HBsAg) indicates acute or chronic hepatitis B; the patient is infectious.
- Antibody against the surface antigen (anti-HBs) indicates either previous exposure to HBV, HBV vaccination, or HBIG prophylaxis. It connotes recovery and immunity to HBV. If HBsAg is present with anti-HBs, the antibody is ineffective and the patient has chronic hepatitis.
- A window between the 24th and 28th weeks exists where neither HBsAg nor anti-HBs may be present.
- The hepatitis B virus core antigen (HBcAg) is present in liver, is not secreted during acute or chronic disease but elicits an antibody response.
- HBeAg is a truncated form of HBcAg secreted into the blood. The presence of HBeAg correlates with high infectivity. Antibody to HBeAg (anti-HBe) is an indicator of decreased infectivity and recovery.
- The diagnostic markers that most accurately predict acute hepatitis B are HBsAg and IgM anti-HBc.

Screening for HCV is performed by (1) anti-HCV enzyme-linked immunosorbent assay and recombinant immunoblot assay-1 that detect antibodies against recombinant proteins of nonstructural and core regions of the viral genome, and (2) reverse transcriptase PCR testing for HCV RNA. Anti-HCV are detected in approximately 90% of patients within 3 months after onset of infection. The presence of anti-HCV is an indication of infectivity; it does not confer recovery or immunity.[3,24,58] During chronic HCV infection, ALT levels often are elevated or fluctuate from normal to elevated levels, HCV RNA is detected in blood, and liver disease is evident in a biopsy of tissue. Screening for HCV infection is recommended for high prevalence groups such as injection drug users, recipients of transfusions, and recipients of solid organ transplants before 1992, recipients of clotting factor concentrate before 1987, persons with persistently elevated ALT levels, and those receiving long-term hemodialysis.[59]

Enzyme immunoassay for antibody against HDV (anti-HDV) and anti-HEV tests are available in the United States. The amount of virus in the blood (viral load of HDV RNA and HEV RNA) can be assessed in laboratories using hybridization techniques and the polymerase chain reaction.

A biopsy of liver tissue is reserved to confirm the diagnosis of chronic hepatitis and rule out other causes of liver damage. The histopathologic report is provided in terms of cause, inflammatory activity and location, and degree of fibrosis.

MEDICAL MANAGEMENT

PREVENTION THROUGH ACTIVE IMMUNIZATION

Risk for viral hepatitis is reduced by receiving active immunization. Currently 2 vaccines are available for HAV, 2 vaccines are available for HBV, 1 vaccine (Twinrix)[60] is available for combination hepatitis A and B, and 1 vaccine (COMVAX)[61] is available for combination hepatitis B, Haemophilus influenzae type b conjugate vaccine for infants. The hepatitis A vaccine was first approved for use in the United States in 1995. Harivax and Vaqta are the formalin-inactivated whole virus vaccines used specifically to prevent HAV infection. The hepatitis A virus vaccines are safe, highly immunogenic, and recommended for persons 2 years of age and older.

Hepatitis B vaccines have evolved from first development in 1982. The vaccine originally was derived from pooled donor plasma; however, this form no longer is available. The two vaccines licensed for prevention of HBV infection (Engerix-B and Recombivax HB) are produced by recombinant DNA technology. These vaccines are administered in three doses over a 6-month period and produce an effective antibody response in more than 90% of adults and 95% of infants, children, and adolescents.[62] The conversion rate is based on injections given in the deltoid muscle because injections administered in the buttocks resulted in only 81% of recipients developing effective antibody titers.[55] Individuals who have received the vaccine in the buttocks should have serologic confirmation of their antibody titer status. Adverse effects of all three vaccines include soreness at the injection site, fever, chills, flulike symptoms, arthralgia, and rarely neuropathy. No risk exists of developing viral infection with the vaccines, including the original plasma derived vaccine.[63]

The duration of immunity and need for booster doses remain controversial. Current information based on experience with the plasma-derived HBV vaccine[62] and a study by Mahoney[64] indicates that immunity remains effective for more than 10 years. Current guidelines of the CDC's Advisory Committee on Immunization Practices only recommends booster doses for persons who did not respond to the primary vaccine series.[65]

TABLE 10-2

Recommendations Following Accidental Exposure to Blood of a Person Infected with Hepatitis Virus*

SOURCE Persons is	Unvaccinated HCW	Vaccinated HCW† Known Responder	Vaccinated HCW Known Non Responder	Vaccinated HCW Response Unknown
HBsAg positive	1 dose of hepatitis B immune globulin (HBIG 0.06 ml/kg IM) as soon as possible preferably within 24 hrs + initiate hepatitis B vaccine series	No treatment	Administer 1 dose of HBIG + hepatitis B vaccine, or 2 doses of HBIG with second dose 1 month after the first	Test exposed worker for anti-HBsAg If inadequate (<10 mIU/mL) 1 dose HBIG + hepatitis B vaccine booster dose
HBsAg negative	Initiate hepatitis B vaccine series	No treatment	No treatment	No treatment
If unknown, not tested	Initiate hepatitis B vaccine series	No treatment	If known high-risk source, consider treating as if source is HBsAg positive	Test exposed worker for anti-HBsAg If inadequate, initiate revaccination

*Adapted from Centers for Disease Control and Prevention: Immunization of Health-Care Workers: Recommendations of the Advisory Committee on Immunization Practices and the Hospital Infection Control Practices Advisory Committee (HICPAC). MMWR 46[RR-18]:1-42, 1997.

Following a percutaneous or permucosal exposure, the blood of the source (and exposed) person should be tested for HBsAg, anti-HCV and HIV antibody. Testing should be done in accordance with state laws and where appropriate pre- and post-test counseling is available. Currently no treatment is available or recommended for occupational postexposure to HCV, HEV, and non-A-E hepatitis viruses. (Centers for Disease Control Morbidity and Mortality Weekly Report: Recommendations for Follow-Up of Health-Care Workers After Occupational Exposure to Hepatitis C Virus. 46[26]:603-606, 1997.)

Also, current data suggest that an HAV percutaneous or permucosal exposure in an occupational setting is unlikely to result in transmission of HAV. Unvaccinated individuals (> 2 years of age) recently exposed to HAV, are advised to receive a single 0.02 mL/kg intramuscular injection of immune globulin according to the Advisory Committee on Immunization Practices's recommendations. (Centers for Disease Control and Prevention: Prevention of hepatitis A through active or passive immunization: Recommendation of the advisory committee on immunization practice. MMWR 48[RR-12]:1-31, 1999.)

†Exposed worker vaccinated against hepatitis B virus

During the decade after vaccine licensure, vaccination of target populations who were at high risk for contracting HBV was recommended (Table 10-2). Healthcare workers, including dentists, are at the top of the list and are recommended strongly to be inoculated with the vaccine. A post-testing strategy is important for determining those who are non-responders.

A strategy to interrupt HBV transmission in all age groups was developed in 1991 and updated in 1995.[62] The current strategy includes (1) prevention of perinatal HBV infection, (2) routine vaccination of all infants, and (3) vaccination of selected adolescents and adults not vaccinated as infants.[66,67] Implementation of this strategy also eventually should control hepatitis D in parallel with control of hepatitis B.

PREVENTION THROUGH PASSIVE IMMUNIZATION

Treatment of viral hepatitis can be accomplished by administering early postexposure immune globulins or postexposure hepatitis B vaccine (see Active Immunization, page 170). Immune serum globulin (IG) is a pool of antibodies collected from human plasma that is free of HBsAg, HCV, and HIV. This sterile solution contains antibodies against both hepatitis A and hepatitis B. Another type of IG is called *hepatitis B immune globulin* (HBIG). It is specially prepared from preselected plasma that is high in titers of anti-HBs. Administration of both IG and HBIG is safe, but they interact adversely with live attenuated vaccines (i.e., measles, mumps, rubella [MMR] vaccine) if given within 5 months of each other (Table 10-2).[23,68]

TREATMENT

As with many viral diseases, therapy basically is palliative and supportive. Bed rest and fluids may be prescribed, especially during the acute phase. A nutritious and high-calorie diet is advised. Alcohol and drugs metabolized by the liver are not to be ingested. Viral antigen and ALT levels should be monitored for 6 months to determine whether the hepatitis is resolving.

Chronic hepatitis rarely resolves spontaneously. Standard therapy for patients with chronic hepatitis is interferon (IFN) alfa-2b (3 to 10 million units) administered three times weekly for six months to one year. Newer modalities have used the pegylated form of IFN with better sustained virologic response.[69] IFN therapy normalizes ALT levels in up to 17% of patients infected with HDV, 30% of those infected with HCV, and 40% of those infected with HBV and reduces the risk for development of hepatocellular carcinoma.[70] Response is better when IFN is initiated early in the course of the disease.[71] Treatment costs, however, are high, and only 10% to 30% of patients achieve long-term remission. Adverse effects (fatigue, flu-like symptoms, and bone marrow suppression) are common, and up to 15% experience significant side effects that result in the discontinuation of treatment. The addition of lamuvidine (a nucleoside analogue active against HBV) or ribavirin (a guanosine analogue active against HCV) gains a virologic response in an additional 15% to 25%.[72] Corticosteroids are usually reserved for fulminant hepatitis. Liver transplantation is a last resort for patients who develop cirrhosis (see Chapter 25).

DENTAL MANAGEMENT

MEDICAL CONSIDERATIONS

The identification of potential or actual carriers of HBV, HCV, and HDV is problematic because in most instances carriers cannot be identified by history. The inability to identify potentially infectious patients extends to HIV infection and other sexually transmitted diseases. Therefore all patients with a history of viral hepatitis must be managed as though they are potentially infectious.

The recommendations for infection-control practice in dentistry published by the CDC and the American Dental Association have become the standard of care to prevent cross infection in dental practice (see Appendix A).[55,73] These organizations strongly recommend that all dental health care workers who provide patient care receive vaccination against hepatitis B virus and implement universal precautions during the care of all dental pa-

---

BOX 10-2

Dental Drugs Metabolized Primarily by the Liver

Local anesthetics (appear safe for use during liver
disease when used in appropriate amounts)
  Lidocaine (Xylocaine)
  Mepivacaine (Carbocaine)
  Prilocaine (Citanest)
  Bupivacaine (Marcaine)
Analgesics
  Aspirin*
  Acetaminophen (Tylenol, Datril)b
  Codeine†
  Meperidine (Demerol)†
  Ibuprofen (Motrin)*
Sedatives
  Diazepam (Valium)†
  Barbiturates†
Antibiotics
  Ampicillin
  Tetracycline
  Metronidazole‡
  Vancomycin‡

*Limit dose or avoid if severe liver disease (acute hepatitis and cirrhosis), or hemostatic abnormalities present.
†Limit dose or avoid if severe liver disease (acute hepatitis and cirrhosis), or encephalopathy present, or taken with alcohol.
‡Avoid if severe liver disease (acute hepatitis and cirrhosis) present.

---

tients.[26,24,74] In addition, the U.S. Occupational Safety and Health Administration's standards require employers to offer hepatitis B vaccine for free to employees occupationally exposed to blood or other potentially infectious materials.[75,76] No recommendations exist for immunization against the other hepatitis viruses.

Patients with Active Hepatitis

No dental treatment other than urgent care (absolutely necessary work) should be rendered for a patient with active hepatitis unless the patient is clinically and biochemically recovered. Urgent care should be provided only in an isolated operatory while adhering to strict universal precautions (see Appendix A). Aerosols should be minimized and drugs metabolized in the liver avoided as much as possible (Box 10-2). If surgery is necessary, a preoperative prothrombin time and bleeding time should be obtained and abnormal results discussed with the

physician. The dentist should refer the patient who has acute hepatitis for medical diagnosis and treatment.

Patients with a History of Hepatitis

Most carriers HBV, HCV, and HDV are unaware they have had hepatitis. An explanation is that many cases of hepatitis B and hepatitis C apparently are mild, subclinical, and nonicteric. These cases may be essentially asymptomatic or resemble a mild viral disease and therefore go undetected. Studies of dental school patients who were carriers of hepatitis B[77] found that up to 80% did not give a history of hepatitis infection. Thus these patients are not identifiable by medical history. Routine laboratory screening of every patient would be required to identify the estimated more than 1 million hepatitis carriers in the United States, which would not be practical. The only practical method of protection from these individuals, and other patients with undetected infectious diseases, is to adopt a strict program of clinical asepsis for all patients (see Appendix A). In addition, use of the hepatitis B vaccine further decreases the threat of hepatitis B infection. Inoculation of all dental personnel with hepatitis B vaccine is strongly urged.

For those patients who provide a positive history of hepatitis, additional historical information occasionally can be of some help in determining the type of disease. For instance, an infection that occurred while the person was under age 15 years or was caused by contaminated food or water would suggest hepatitis A. Disease acquired in a Third World country may indicate hepatitis E. Unfortunately, this approach will not reveal a person who has had infection with both type A and type B or C in which the HBV or HCV infection was subclinical or undiagnosed.

An additional consideration in patients with a history of hepatitis of unknown type is to use the clinical laboratory to screen for the presence of HBsAg or anti-HCV. This may be indicated even in patients who specifically indicate which type of hepatitis they had, because studies[77] have shown that historically provided information of this type is unreliable 50% of the time.

Patients at High Risk for HBV or HCV Infection

Several groups are at unusually high risk for HBV and HCV infection (see Box 10-1). Screening for HBsAg and anti-HCV is recommended for individuals who fit into one or more of these categories unless they are already known to be seropositive. Even if a patient is found to be a carrier, no modifications in treatment approach theoretically would be necessary. However, this information still may be of benefit in certain situations. If a patient is found to be a carrier, the information could be of extreme importance for the modification of lifestyle. In addition, the patient might have undetected chronic active hepatitis, which could lead to bleeding complications or drug metabolism problems. Finally, if an accidental needlestick or puncture wound occurs during treatment and the dentist is not vaccinated (or antibody titer status is unknown), knowing whether the patient was HBsAg or HCV positive would be of extreme importance in determining the need for HBIG, vaccination, and follow-up medical care.

Patients Who are Hepatitis Carriers

If a patient is found to be a hepatitis B carrier (HBsAg positive) or have a history of hepatitis C, universal precautions (see Appendix A) are to be followed to prevent transmission of infection. In addition, some hepatitis carriers may have chronic active hepatitis, leading to compromised liver function and interference with hemostasis and drug metabolism. Physician consultation and laboratory screening of liver function are advised to determine current status and future risks.

Patients with Signs or Symptoms of Hepatitis

Any patient who has signs or symptoms suggestive of hepatitis should not be given elective dental treatment but instead referred immediately to a physician. Necessary emergency dental care should be provided by using an isolated operatory and minimizing aerosol production.

Dentists Who are Hepatitis Virus Carriers

A question also arises concerning dentists who are carriers of HBsAg or HCV. As of this writing, 9 outbreaks of hepatitis B traceable to carrier dentists or oral surgeons have been reported since 1974. No cases of HCV transmission from dentist to patient were reported. In each instance of HBV transmission, the practitioner was found to be seropositive for HBsAg and (if tested) HBeAg and did not use gloves during dental or surgical procedures. None of the practitioners were aware of their chronic infections. As a result of these infections 2 patients died.[78] No additional outbreaks have been reported since 1987, which is a result of increased awareness of blood-borne pathogens and the implementation of vaccinations and infection-control measures in dentistry.

After the discovery of a carrier state and the documented transmission of disease, some HBsAg-carrier dentists have been forced to quit practice and others have faced lengthy periods of discontinuance until they have undergone seroconversion. The CDC suggests that health care professionals who perform invasive procedures should know their infectivity status; if found positive for a blood transmissible virus, they should not

perform exposure-prone procedures unless they have sought counsel from an expert review panel in their state of practice.[79] If after discussion with this panel a carrier dentist elects to continue practice, professional ethics and practice guidelines recommend aggressive efforts to prevent potential transmission by adherence to strict aseptic technique, periodic retesting of HBsAg and HCV RNA, and informed consent from patients.

CDC Guidelines for Exposures to Blood

To reduce the risk of transmission of hepatitis viruses, the CDC has published postexposure protocols for percutaneous or permucosal exposures to blood. Implementation of the protocol is dependent on the virus present in the source person and the vaccinated state of the exposed person (e.g., a dental healthcare worker) (see Table 10-2).

Briefly, a vaccinated individual who sustains a needlestick or puncture wound contaminated with blood from a patient known to be HBsAg positive should be tested for an adequate titer of anti-HBs if those levels are unknown. If the levels are inadequate, the individual immediately should receive an injection of HBIG and a vaccine booster dose.[74] The risk of contracting HBV from a sharps injury in health care workers from HBV carriers may approach 30%.[80] If the antibody titer is adequate, nothing further is required. If an unvaccinated individual sustains an inadvertent percutaneous or permucosal exposure to hepatitis B, immediate administration of HBIG and initiation of the vaccine are recommended.[74]

Although no post-exposure protocol or vaccine is available yet for HCV infection, current CDC guidelines recommend (1) the source person receive baseline testing for anti-HCV, (2) the exposed persons receive baseline and follow-up testing at six months for anti-HCV and liver enzyme activity, (3) RIBA confirmation of anti-HCV enzyme immunoassay positive results, (4) postexposure prophylaxis be avoided with immunoglobulin or antiviral agents, (5) healthcare workers be educated regarding the risk and prevention of blood-borne infections.[74]

Exposure-Control Plan

With respect to hepatitis viruses, the U.S. Occupational Safety and Health Administration mandates that all employers maintain an exposure-control plan and protect their employees from the hazards of bloodborne pathogens by using universal precautions and providing the following as a minimum: (1) hepatitis B vaccinations to employees, (2) post-exposure evaluation and follow-up, (3) recordkeeping of exposures, (4) generic bloodborne pathogens training, and (5) personal protective equipment at no cost to employees. All dentists should be familiar with the agency's compliance directive CPL 2-2.69—

Enforcement Procedures for the Occupational Exposure to Bloodborne Pathogens which at the time of printing could be found at http://www.osha-slc.gov/OshDoc/Directive_data/CPL_2-2.69.html.[76]

DRUG ADMINISTRATION

No special drug considerations are needed for a patient who has completely recovered from viral hepatitis. However, if a patient has chronic active hepatitis or is a carrier of HBsAg or HCV and has impaired liver function, drugs metabolized by the liver should have the dosage decreased or avoided if possible as advised by the physician. As a guideline, drugs metabolized in the liver should be considered for diminished dosage when 1 or more of the following are present: (1) aminotransferase levels are elevated greater than 4 times normal, (2) serum bilirubin is elevated above 35 μM/l or 2 mg/dl, (3) serum albumin levels are less than 35 g/l, (4) signs are present of ascites, encephalopathy, and malnutrition (Table 10-3). Many drugs commonly used in dentistry are metabolized principally by the liver, but in other than the most severe cases of hepatic disease these drugs can be used, although in limited amounts (see Box 10-2). A measurement of 3 cartridges of 2% lidocaine (120 mg) is considered a relatively limited amount of drug.

TREATMENT PLANNING MODIFICATIONS

Treatment planning modifications are not required for the patient who has recovered from hepatitis.

ORAL MANIFESTATIONS AND COMPLICATIONS

Abnormal bleeding is associated with hepatitis and significant liver damage is abnormal bleeding. This can be the result of abnormal synthesis of blood clotting factors, abnormal polymerization of fibrin, inadequate fibrin stabilization, excessive fibrinolysis, or thrombocytopenia associated with splenomegaly that accompanies chronic liver disease. Before any surgery is performed, the platelet count should be obtained and the prothrombin time checked to ensure it is 2.5 times or less times the normal measurement of 11 to 14 seconds and that the international normalized ratio is 3.5 or less (see Chapter 19). If the international normalized ratio is greater than 3.5, the potential for severe postoperative bleeding exists. In this case, extensive surgical procedures should be postponed. If surgery is necessary, an injection of vitamin K usually will correct the problem and should be discussed with the physician. The bleeding time and platelet function analysis (see Chapter 19) can be performed to

TABLE 10-3

Dental Management of the Patient with Alcoholic Liver Disease

1. Detection by such methods as:
   History
   Clinical examination
   Alcohol odor on breath
   Information from family members or friends
2. Referral or consultation with physician to ascertain the following:
   Verify history
   Check current status
   Check medications
   Check laboratory values
   Discuss suggestions for management
3. Laboratory screening (if not available from physician) to record the following:
   CBC with differential
   AST, ALT
   Bleeding time
   Thrombin time
   Prothrombin time
4. Assessment of risk of adverse outcome associated with invasive procedure or infection using prognostic formula (i.e., Child-Pugh Classification found in table below)

Parameter	1	2	3
Ascites	None	Moderate	Severe
Encephalopathy	None	Mild	Severe
Nutritional status	Good	Mild malnutrition	Severe malnutrition
Serum bilirubin	< 35 μM/l; < 2 mg/dl	35-50 μM/l; 2-3 mg/dl	> 50 μM/l; > 3 mg/dl
Serum albumin	> 35 g/l	30-35 g/l	< 30 g/l

Patients are scored by adding the value obtained from each row, then categorized as either **class A** (mild disease) = score 5 or 6; **class B** (moderate disease) = score of 7 to 9; or **class C** (severe disease) = score of 10-15.
Albers I: Superiority of the Child-Pugh classification to quantitative liver function tests for assessing prognosis of liver cirrhosis. *Scand J Gastroenterol* 24:269-276, 1989.

5. Minimizing of drugs metabolized by liver (see Box 10-2)
6. If screening tests abnormal, for surgical procedures consideration given to thrombin, gelfoam, antifibrinolytic agents, fresh frozen plasma, Vitamin K, platelets—with help of physician or PharmD.

determine whether platelet replacement may be required before surgery and should be discussed with the patient's physician.

Chronic viral hepatitis increases the risk for hepatocellular carcinoma. This malignancy rarely metastasizes to the jaw (less than 30 cases had been reported in the jaws as of this writing). However, the incidence of hepatocellular carcinoma is on the rise in the United States.[81] Oral metastases primarily present as hemorrhagic expanding masses located in the premolar and ramus region of the mandible.

■ ALCOHOLIC LIVER DISEASE ■

DEFINITION

Alcoholism is the chronic addiction to ethanol in which a person craves and consumes ethanol uncontrollably, becomes tolerant to its intoxicating effects, and has symptoms of alcohol withdrawal when drinking stops.[82] The Diagnostic and Statistical Manual of Mental Disorders (DSM)-IV defines *alcohol dependence* as repeated alcohol-related difficulties in at least three of seven areas of

functioning. These include any combination of (1) tolerance, (2) withdrawal, (3) the taking of larger amounts of alcohol over longer periods than intended, (4) an inability to control use, (5) the giving up of important activities to drink, (6) the spending of a great deal of time associated with alcohol use, and (7) the continued use of alcohol despite physical or psychological consequences.[83] *Alcohol abuse* is the harmful use of alcohol. Individuals who drink alcohol excessively without evidence of dependence have an *alcohol abuse disorder*. A form of alcohol abuse associated with excessive heavy drinking is "binge drinking." This form of consumption is associated with an increased risk of death due to injury. Alcohol abuse and dependence are not limited to any particular group. All ages and races, both sexes, and all socioeconomic levels are affected. The stereotypical picture of the skid row vagrant applies to only a small percentage of cases.

Alcohol abuse is known to cause or exacerbate many physical conditions. The economic impact of alcohol abuse and dependence in the United States is estimated to cost $100 billion annually.[84] The wide use of alcohol makes it no surprise that alcohol has been implicated as the leading cause of accidental deaths and work-related accidents in the United States. Motor vehicle accidents are the major cause of injury-related deaths, and alcohol is involved in at least half of them. Many behavioral and physical disorders are associated with alcohol abuse and require the dentist to be knowledgeable of this topic.[85]

EPIDEMIOLOGY

INCIDENCE AND PREVALENCE

Nearly two thirds of Americans older than 14 years drink alcoholic beverages, 44% of adults are current drinkers while 22% are former drinkers.[86] The prevalence of alcohol abuse and dependence in the United States is 7.4% to 9.7%, with a lifetime prevalence of 13.7% to 23.5%.[87,88] Men are 2 times to 5 times more likely to have pervasive alcoholism than females[82] although less of a difference exists in the younger age groups.

Drinking patterns vary by gender and age. For both genders, the prevalence of drinking is highest among persons in the 21- to 34-year-old range. Recent studies project that between 7% and 17% of college students have alcohol-drinking problems.[89] Overall, 14 million persons in the United States are dependent on alcohol.[90] Based on these figures, the average dental practice having 2000 adult patients is predicted to have 170 to 200 patients who have a problem with alcohol. Whereas problem drinking primarily is seen in adults, the prevalence among teenagers is alarmingly high. One

study[31] reported that an estimated 3.3 million persons aged 14 to 17 years could be classified as problem drinkers. Alcoholism among the elderly also is a significant problem, with prevalence estimates varying between 1% and 10%.[91]

The lack of treatment of alcohol abuse leads to significant morbidity and mortality rates. Current figures indicate that 105,000 persons die annually in the United States because of alcohol abuse[90] and more than 20% of hospital admissions are alcohol-related.[92] Cirrhosis is a sequela of alcohol abuse and the 10th-leading cause of death among adults in the United States[93] In addition, ethanol alone or with other drugs such as benzodiazepines is probably responsible for more toxic overdose deaths than any other agent.[83]

ETIOLOGY

Alcohol consumption in large or chronic amounts contributes to disease and injury. In contrast, moderate consumption of alcohol (2 to 6 drinks per week) is associated with decreased mortality and cardiovascular disease rates.[94] The quantity and duration of alcohol ingestion required to produce cirrhosis are not clear. However, the typical alcoholic with cirrhosis has a history for at least 10 years of daily consumption of a pint or more of whiskey, several quarts of wine, or an equivalent amount of beer.[95]

A relationship exists between excessive alcohol ingestion and liver dysfunction, leading to cirrhosis. However, the exact effect of alcohol on the liver was not known until researchers demonstrated that alcohol is hepatotoxic[96] and its metabolite, acetylaldehyde, is fibrinogenic.[97] Chemokines also are implicated in the pathogenesis of alcoholic liver disease. Alcohol-induced influx of endotoxin (lipopolysaccharides) from the gut into the portal circulation can activate Kupffer cells, which leads to enhanced chemokine release.[98] Chemokines, in turn, directly and indirectly damage liver hepatocytes. Curiously, only 10% to 15% of heavy alcohol users ever develop cirrhosis, a fact probably explained by hereditary, nutrition, and biochemical differences among individuals.[95,99]

PATHOPHYSIOLOGY AND COMPLICATIONS

Alcohol has a deleterious effect on neural development, the corticotropin-releasing hormone system, metabolism of neurotransmitters, and the function of their receptors. As a result, the acetylcholine and dopaminergic systems are affected, causing sensory and motor disturbances (e.g., peripheral neuropathies).[100] Prolonged abuse of alcohol contributes to malnutrition (folic acid deficiency), anemias, and decreased immune function.[101] Increased

mortality rates exist among men who consume more than three drinks daily.[102,103]

The pathologic effects of alcohol on the liver are expressed by 1 of 3 disease entities.[95] These conditions may exist alone but commonly appear in combination. The earliest change seen in alcoholic liver disease is a fatty infiltrate. The hepatocytes become engorged with fatty lobules and distended, with enlargement of the entire liver. No other structural changes usually are noted. These changes may be seen after only moderate usage of alcohol for a brief time; however, they are considered completely reversible.

A second and more serious form of alcoholic liver disease is alcoholic hepatitis. This is a diffuse inflammatory condition of the liver characterized by destructive cellular changes, some of which may be irreversible. The irreversible changes can lead to necrosis. Nutritional factors may play a significant role in the progression of this disease. For the most part, alcoholic hepatitis is considered a reversible condition; however, it can be fatal if damage is widespread.

The third and most serious form of alcoholic liver disease is cirrhosis, which is generally considered an irreversible condition characterized by progressive fibrosis and abnormal regeneration of liver architecture in response to chronic injury or insult (i.e., prolonged and heavy use of ethanol) (Fig. 10-2). Cirrhosis results in the progressive deterioration of the metabolic and excretory functions of the liver and ultimately leads to hepatic failure. Hepatic failure is manifested by myriad of health problems.[95] Some of the more important of these are esophagitis, gastritis, and pancreatitis, which contribute to generalized malnutrition, weight loss, protein deficiency (including coagulation factors), impairment of urea synthesis and glucose metabolism, endocrine disturbances, encephalopathy, renal failure, portal hypertension, and jaundice. Accompanying portal hypertension is the development of ascites and esophageal varices[95] (Fig. 10-3). In some patients with cirrhosis, blood from bleeding ulcers and esophageal varices is incompletely metabolized to ammonia, which travels to the brain and contributes to encephalopathy. In addition, chronic large consumption of ethanol can result in dementia and psychosis (Wernicke's and Korsakoff's syndromes), cerebellar degeneration, upper alimentary tract cancer and liver cancer, and hematopoietic changes.

Bleeding tendencies are a significant feature in advanced liver disease. The basis for the diathesis is in part a deficiency of coagulation factors, especially the prothrombin group (factors II, VII, IX, and X). These all rely on vitamin K as a precursor for production. Vitamin K is absorbed from the large intestine and stored in the liver, where it is converted into an enzymatic cofactor for the carboxylation of prothrombin complex proteins. Widespread hepatocellular destruction as seen in cirrhosis decreases the liver's storage and conversion capacity of vitamin K, leading to deficiencies of the prothrombin-dependent coagulation factors. In addition to these deficiencies, thrombocytopenia may be caused by hypersplenism secondary to portal hypertension and to bone marrow depression. Anemia and leukopenia also may be present because of toxic effects of alcohol on the bone marrow and nutritional deficiencies. Accelerated fibrinolysis also is seen.[95,96,104]

The combination of hemorrhagic tendencies and severe portal hypertension sets the stage for episodes of gastrointestinal bleeding, epistaxis, ecchymoses, or ruptured esophageal varices. Most patients with advanced cirrhosis die of hepatic coma, often precipitated by massive hemorrhage from esophageal varices or intercurrent infection.[95]

Ethanol abuse predisposes the individual to infection by the several mechanisms.[101] The liver's resident cell population, in patients with alcoholism, is exposed to high concentrations of ethanol. The Kupffer cells, representing more than 80% of tissue macrophages in the body, become impaired because of alcohol bathing of the liver sinusoids. Alcohol-induced impairment of Kupffer cell function and T-cell responses result in increased risk of infection. Although cirrhosis is generally considered to be an end-stage condition, some evidence suggests that at least partial reversibility of the process is possible with complete and permanent removal of the offending agent during the early phase of cirrhosis.

CLINICAL PRESENTATION

SIGNS AND SYMPTOMS

The behavioral and physiologic effects of alcohol depend on the amount of intake, its rate of increase in plasma, the presence of other drugs or medical problems, and the past experience with alcohol. Chronic use of heavy alcohol intake can result in clinically significant cognitive impairment (even when the person is sober) or distress. The pattern displayed is usually one of intermittent relapse and remission. If allowed to progress untreated, many individuals develop other psychiatric problems (anxiety, antisocial behavior, and affective disorders), whereas some develop alcohol amnestic disorder and are unable to learn new material or to recall known material. Alcoholic blackouts may occur. In some individuals alcohol-induced dementia and severe personality changes develop.

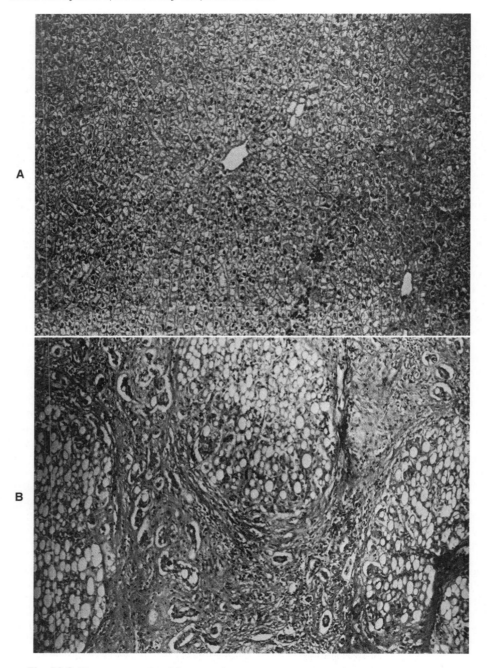

Fig. 10-2 Photomicrographs of **A,** normal liver architecture and **B,** liver architecture in alcoholic cirrhosis. (Courtesy A. Golden, Lexington, Ky.)

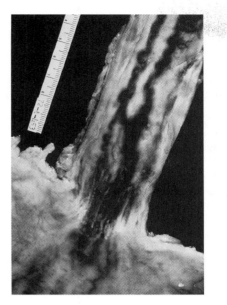

Fig. 10-3 Gross section of esophageal varices from an alcoholic patient. (Courtesy A. Golden, Lexington, Ky.)

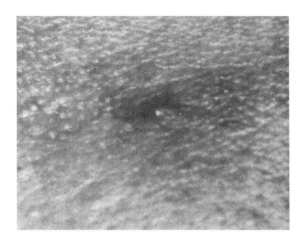

Fig. 10-4 Spider angioma.

Clinically, with the possible exception of enlargement, no visible manifestations of a fatty liver are present, and the diagnosis usually is made incidentally in conjunction with another illness. The clinical presentation of alcoholic hepatitis often is nonspecific and may include features such as nausea, vomiting, anorexia, malaise, weight loss, and fever. More specific findings include hepatomegaly, splenomegaly, jaundice, ascites, ankle edema, and spider angiomas. With advancing disease, encephalopathy and hepatic coma may ensue, ending in death.

Alcoholic cirrhosis may remain asymptomatic for many years until sufficient destruction of the liver parenchyma exists to produce clinical evidence of hepatic failure. Ascites, spider angiomas (Fig. 10-4), ankle edema, or jaundice may be the earliest signs, but frequently hemorrhage from esophageal varices is the initial sign. The hemorrhagic episode may progress to hepatic encephalopathy, coma, and death. Other less specific signs of alcoholic liver disease include anemia, purpura, ecchymoses, gingival bleeding, palmar erythema, nail changes, and parotid gland enlargement (known as sialadenosis).

Laboratory Findings

Laboratory findings in alcoholic liver disease vary from minimal abnormalities caused by a fatty liver to manifestations of alcoholic hepatitis and cirrhosis. Liver abnormalities cause elevations of bilirubin, alkaline phosphatase, AST, ALT, gamma-glutamyl transpeptidase, amylase, uric acid, triglyceride, and cholesterol. Leukopenia (or leukocytosis) or anemia often is present.[95] For these reasons, a simple screen for alcoholism comes from a sequential mult-analyzer-20 and complete blood cell count with differential. Elevated blood levels of gamma-glutamyl transpeptidase and mean corpuscular volume are highly suggestive of alcoholism, whereas an AST/ALT ratio of at least 2 is 90% predictive of alcoholic liver disease.[57,105,106,107] The carbohydrate-deficient transferrin test is also used to screen for and monitor alcohol-dependent patients.[108,109]

Alcoholic liver disease also leads to deficiencies of clotting factors reflected as elevations in the prothrombin time and partial thromboplastin time. Thrombocytopenia may be present owing to hepatosplenomegaly, causing a decreased platelet count and increased bleeding time. Increased fibrinolytic activity may be evident by an increased bleeding time, prolonged thrombin time, or decreased euglobulin clot lysis time (see Chapter 19).

MEDICAL MANAGEMENT

Treatment of patients with alcoholism consists of three basic steps. The first is identification and intervention. A thorough physical examination is performed to evaluate

organ systems that could be impaired. This includes a search for evidence of liver failure, gastrointestinal bleeding, cardiac arrhythmia, and glucose or electrolyte imbalance. Hemorrhage from esophageal varices and hepatic encephalopathy require immediate treatment. Ascites mandates measures to control fluids and electrolytes, alcoholic hepatitis is often treated with glucocorticoids, and infection or sepsis is managed with antimicrobial agents. During this phase, the patient may refuse to accept the diagnosis and deny that a problem exists.

The second step is withdrawal from alcohol, or in cases of severe dependence reduction of alcohol consumption. Abrupt alcohol withdrawal results in loss of appetite, tachycardia, anxiety, insomnia, and delirium tremens (DT)—characterized by hallucinations, disorientation, impaired attention and memory, and extreme agitation. Physical findings include severe sweating, elevated blood pressure, and tachycardia. Management goals are to minimize the severity of withdrawal symptoms. Strict dietary modifications are required including a high-protein, high-calorie, low-sodium diet and possibly fluid restriction. Patients should receive adequate nutrition and rest, oral multiple B vitamins, including 50 to 100 mg of thiamine daily for at least a week or two, and iron replacement and folic acid supplementation as needed to correct any anemia present.

The third step is to manage the central nervous system depression caused by the rapid removal of the ethanol. Administration of a benzodiazepine, such as diazepam or chlordiazepoxide, gradually decreasing the level of the drug over a 3- to 5-day period alleviates alcohol withdrawal symptoms.[83] Beta-blockers, clonidine and carbamazepine, have been recent additions to the pharmacotherapeutic management of withdrawal.[108]

Once treatment of withdrawal has been completed, the patient with alcoholism is educated about alcoholism. This includes teaching the family and friends to stop protecting the patient from the problems caused by alcohol. Attempts are made to help the patient with alcoholism achieve and maintain a high level of motivation toward abstinence. Steps also are taken to help the patient with alcoholism readjust to life without alcohol and to reestablish a functional lifestyle. The drug disulfiram has been used for some patients during alcohol rehabilitation. Disulfiram inhibits aldehyde dehydrogenase causing accumulation of acetaldehyde blood levels and thus sweating, nausea, vomiting, and diarrhea when taken with ethanol. Naltrexone (an opioid antagonist) and acamprosate (an inhibitor of the γ-aminobutyric acid system) may be used to decrease the amount of alcohol consumed or shorten the period during which alcohol is used in cases of relapse.[83] Untreated disease that progresses to cirrhosis requires alcohol withdrawal and management of the complica-

tions that are present. End-stage cirrhosis can not be reversed and is only remedied by liver transplantation (see Chapter 25).

DENTAL MANAGEMENT

MEDICAL CONSIDERATIONS

The dentist has an excellent opportunity to assist patients at risk for or with alcohol-abuse problems. Unfortunately, patients with alcoholism are poorly recognized by healthcare providers in healthcare settings unless they have medical complications.[108,110] Areas of assistance include (1) screening for alcohol risks and abuse, (2) providing alcohol prevention information, (3) directing patients with abuse problems to healthcare providers for assessment or treatment, (4) supporting dependent patients during the recovery period, and (5) minimizing relapse in recovering patients.[111]

SCREENING

The patient with chronic alcoholism can be recognized from examination of health problems and behaviors, such as medical signs and symptoms, noncompliance, exacerbated anxieties and fears, failure to fulfill obligations, and emotional fluctuations. During the medical history, the dentist should obtain information from all adolescent and adult patients about the type, quantity, frequency, pattern of alcohol use, consequences of use, and family history of alcoholism. The questioning should be done in a nonjudgmental manner and aided by using the standardized questionnaire, such as the CAGE or CUGE. The 4-question CAGE questionnaire, the most widely studied and best known instrument, focuses on impaired control (Cut down), use despite consequences (Annoyed by criticism, experiencing Guilt) and dependence (Eye-opener in the morning) (Box 10-3). The CUGE replaces the second CAGE question with a question of being Under the influence when driving a car or riding a bike.

Family members also may be a source of information when interviews are granted in confidence. A high index of suspicion should be followed by clinical examination and a series of laboratory tests for screening purposes regardless of whether the patient admits to the heavy use of alcohol (chronic consumption of more than 14 alcoholic drinks per week for men or more than 4 drinks per occasion and more than 7 drinks per week for women or more than 3 drinks per occasion).[112] Signs suggestive of alcohol abuse, such as enlargement of the parotid glands (Fig. 10-5) or a distinctive breath odor may be detectable. Other signs are suggestive of the disease (Box 10-4).

CAGE and CUGE Questionnaires for Screening of Alcohol Abuse

C	Have you ever felt the need to cut down on your drinking
A	Have you ever felt annoyed by criticism of your drinking?
U	Have you often been under the influence of alcohol in a situation where it increased your chances of getting hurt, for example, when riding a bicycle or driving a car?
G	Have you ever felt guilty about your drinking?
E	Have you ever taken a drink (eye-opener) first thing in the morning?

Mayfield D, McLeod G, Hall P: The CAGE questionnaire: validation of a new alcoholism screening instrument. *Am J Psychiatry* 131:1121-1123, 1974. Buntinx BA, et al: The value of the CAGE, CUGE, and AUDIT in screening for alcohol abuse and dependence among college freshmen. Alcoholism: *Clin Exp Res* 24:53-57, 2000.

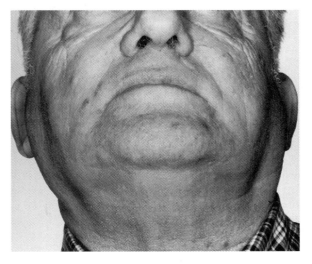

Fig. 10-5 Painless enlargement of the parotid glands associated with alcoholism. (Courtesy Valerie Murrah, Chapel Hill, NC.)

BOX 10-4

Features Suggestive of Advanced Alcoholic Liver Disease

Systemic Complications
Traumatic or unexplained injuries (driving under the influence, bruises, cuts, scars, broken teeth)
Attention and memory deficits
Slurred speech
Spider angiomas
Jaundice (sclerae, mucosa)
Peripheral edema (edematous puffy face, ankle edema)
Ascites
Palmar erythema, white nails or transverse pale band on nails
Ecchymoses, petechiae, or prolonged bleeding
Failure to fulfill role obligations at work, school, home (e.g., missed dental appointments)
Increased levels of bilirubin, aminotransferases, alkaline phosphates, γ-glutamyl transpeptidase and mean corpuscular volume

Oral Complications
Poor oral hygiene
Oral neglect—caries, gingivitis, periodontitis
Glossitis
Angular or labial cheilosis
Candidiasis
Gingival bleeding
Oral cancer
Petechiae
Ecchymoses
Jaundiced mucosa
Parotid gland enlargement
Alcohol (sweet musty) breath odor
Impaired healing
Bruxism
Dental attrition
Xerostomia

Alcoholism transcends the age, gender, and socioeconomic spectrum, and many of these patients are great at masquerading their dependence.

Providing Preventive Information

If the dentist suspects a patient to be abusing alcohol, a spouse or significant other can be interviewed to gather additional diagnostic information. If the suspicions are confirmed, preventive information should be provided to the patient in a nonthreatening manner. Treatment success depends on motivating the patient to enter treatment and breaking down denial.

Directing Patient for Assessment or Treatment and Supportive Care

Assisting a patient into a treatment program requires that the dentist share concerns obtained from the medical assessment. The dentist can point out destructive patterns of alcohol use and discuss future problems expected if alcohol use continues. Discussions should include the possibilities and successes of treatment. This requires that the dentist be familiar with treatment options within the local community such as detoxification, inpatient programs, outpatient programs, halfway houses, and continuing care. Active communication and expression of concern from the dentist with the patient and the patient's family during therapy and recovery, along with group meetings, are supportive measures that improve the chances of successful rehabilitation.

Minimizing Relapse

To minimize relapse, the dentist should avoid the use of psychoactive drugs, narcotics, sedatives, and alcohol-containing medications in patients who are recovering from alcoholism (Table 10-4). If a potentially mood-altering drug is required, the patient's primary care physician (or substance abuse advisor) should be consulted about its use. If approved for use, the drug should be prescribed only in the amount needed without refills. Designating a family member to fill and dispense the drug can minimize the risk of abuse.

Treatment Considerations

In addition to the above mentioned considerations, three major dental treatment considerations exist for a patient with alcoholism: (1) bleeding tendencies, (2) unpredictable metabolism of certain drugs, and (3) risk or spread of infection. A complete blood cell count with differential, AST and ALT, bleeding time, thrombin time, and prothrombin time are sufficient to screen for potential problems. Abnormal laboratory values, accompanied by abnormal clinical examination or positive history, are the basis for referral to a physician for positive

TABLE 10-4

Alcohol Content of Over-the-Counter Medications

	Alcohol (%)
Mouthwash and gargle	
Scope	14.3-15
Signal	14.5
Cepacol	14
Listerine	26.5
Listermint	0
Tom's of Maine	0
Antiplaque rinse	
Peridex, Periogard	11.6
Plax	8.7
Peroxyl	6
Fluoride rinse	
ACT	0
Sore throat spray and liquid	
Chloraseptic	12.5
Toothache drops and gel	
Orajel Maximum Strength Liquid	44.2
Anbesol Maximum Strength	60
Decongestant and cough suppressant	
NyQuil	10
Robitussin Alcohol Free	0
Dimetapp Elixir Alcohol Free	0

diagnosis and treatment. A patient with untreated alcoholic liver disease is not a candidate for elective, outpatient dental care and should be referred to a physician. Once the patient is managed medically, dental care may be provided after consultation with the physician.

If a patient provides a history of alcoholic liver disease or alcohol abuse, the physician should be consulted to verify the patient's current status, medications, laboratory values, and contraindications for medications, surgery, or other treatment. In cases where the patient has not been seen by a physician within the past several months, screening laboratory tests should be ordered, including CBC with differential, AST and ALT, platelet count, thrombin time, and prothrombin time before invasive procedures. Precautionary measures should be taken to minimize the risk for bleeding (see Chapter 19) including a PT test that is particularly sensitive to deficiency of factor VII. Bleeding diatheses should be managed in conjunction with the physician and may entail using local hemostatic agents, fresh frozen plasma, vitamin K, platelets, and antifibrinolytic agents. Hemostatic measures are particularly important

when major invasive or traumatic procedures are performed in a patient who has been assigned an ASA category of III or greater and has signs of jaundice, ascites, clubbing of fingers or has been classified as a Child-Pugh class B or C.

A second area of concern in patients with alcoholic liver disease is the unpredictable metabolism of drugs. The concern is twofold. In mild to moderate alcoholic liver disease, significant enzyme induction is likely to have occurred, leading to an increased tolerance of local anesthetics, sedative and hypnotic drugs, and general anesthesia. Thus larger than normal doses of these medications may be required to obtain the desired effects.

Also, with more advanced liver destruction, drug metabolism may be markedly diminished and can lead to an increased or unexpected effect. For example, if acetaminophen is used in usual therapeutic doses in chronic alcoholism, or if acetaminophen is taken with alcohol and a fasting state, severe hepatocellular disease with mortality has resulted.[113] The dentist should use the drugs listed in Box 10-2 with caution when treating patients with chronic alcoholism and consider adjusting their doses (e.g., half the dose if cirrhosis or alcoholic hepatitis is present) or avoid their use as advised by the patient's physician. Once again, more than one of the following findings, aminotransferase levels elevated greater than 4 times normal, serum bilirubin level elevated above 35 μM/l (2 mg/dl), serum albumin level less than 35 g/l, and signs of ascites, encephalopathy or malnutrition (see Table 10-3) are suggestive that drug metabolism will be impaired.

A third area of concern is risk of infection or spread of infection in the patient who has alcoholic liver disease. Risk increases with surgical procedures or trauma, as oral microorganisms can be introduced into the blood circulation and may not be efficiently eliminated by the reticuloendothelial system. Although patients who have alcoholic liver disease have reduced reticuloendothelial capacity and altered cell-mediated immune function,[101] studies do not indicate that antibiotic prophylaxis should be provided before invasive dental procedures in the absence of an ongoing infection. Despite the lack of evidence, recommendations exist in the literature for the use of antibiotic prophylaxis for these patients.[114,115] Antibiotic prophylaxis is not needed if oral infection is absent. A greater concern is the risk of spread of an ongoing infection, as bacterial infections are more serious and sometimes fatal in patients with liver disease.[116] To determine those at risk for responding poorly to invasive procedures and infections, clinicians should consider using one of the assessment formulas for staging liver disease (i.e., Child-Pugh classification scheme,[117] see Table 10-3) as well as identifying whether a history of bacterial infections (e.g., spontaneous bacterial peritonitis, pneumonia, bacteremia) exists. Consultation with the patient's physician regarding the use of antibiotics should be considered for persons with moderate to severe disease—Child-Pugh Class B or C—(i.e., ascites, encephalopathy, elevated bilirubin levels or SBP). Antibiotics should be provided when infection is present and unlikely to resolve without it.

TREATMENT PLANNING MODIFICATIONS

Patients with cirrhosis tend to have more plaque, calculus, and gingival inflammation than patients without the condition. This seems to be the case in any patient who is a substance abuser and is related to oral neglect rather than any inherent property of the abused substance. Based on the degree of neglect, caries, and periodontal disease, the dentist should not provide extensive care until the patient demonstrates an interest in and ability to care for their dentition.

Liver enzyme induction and central nervous system effects of alcohol in patients with alcoholism can require increased amounts of local anesthetic or additional anxiolytic procedures to be used. Appointments with these patients may therefore require more time if this manifestation was not anticipated.

ORAL COMPLICATIONS AND MANIFESTATIONS

Poor hygiene and neglect (caries) are prominent oral findings in patients with chronic alcoholism. In addition, a variety of other abnormalities may be found[96,118,119] (see Box 10-4). Patients with cirrhosis have been reported to have impaired gustatory function[122] and are malnourished. Nutritional deficiencies can result in glossitis and loss of tongue papillae along with angular or labial cheilitis, which is complicated by concomitant candidal infection. Vitamin K deficiency, disordered hemostasis, portal hypertension, and splenomegaly (causing thrombocytopenia) can result in spontaneous gingival bleeding, mucosal ecchymoses and petechiae. In some instances unexplained gingival bleeding has been the initial complaint of alcoholic patients.[119,120] Also, a sweet, musty odor to the breath is associated with liver failure, as is jaundiced mucosal tissue.

A bilateral, painless hypertrophy of the parotid glands (sialadenosis) is a frequent finding in patients with cirrhosis. The enlarged glands are soft and nontender and are not fixed to the overlying skin.[120,121] The condition appears to be caused by a demyelinating polyneuropathy that results in abnormal sympathetic signaling, abnormal acinar protein secretion and acinar cytoplasmic

swelling.[121,122] Because of the etiology, the parotid ducts remain patent and produce clear salivary flow.

Alcohol abuse and tobacco use are strong risk factors for the development of oral squamous cell carcinoma, and the dentist must be aggressive (as with all patients) in the detection of unexplained or suspicious soft-tissue lesions (especially leukoplakia, erythroplakia, or ulceration) in chronic alcoholics. High-risk sites for oral squamous cell carcinoma include the lateral border of the tongue and the floor of the mouth (see Chapter 21).

References

1. Alter MJ et al: Acute non-A-E hepatitis in the United States and the role of hepatitis G virus infection, N Engl J Med 336:741-746, 1997.
2. Hoofnagle JH LK: Acute viral hepatitis. In: Goldman L BJ, editor: *Cecil textbook of medicine*, ed 21, Philadelphia, 2000, WB Saunders.
3. Centers for Disease Control: Public Health Service interagency guidelines for screening disorders of blood, plasma, organs, tissues, and semen for evidence of hepatitis B and hepatitis C, MMWR 40(RR-4):6-17, 1991.
4. Rizzetto M et al: Immunofluorescence detection of new antigen-antibody system (delta/anti-delta) associated to hepatitis B virus in liver and in serum of HBsAg carriers, Gut 18:997-1003, 1977.
5. Purcell R: Hepatitis viruses: changing patterns of human disease, Proc Natl Acad Sci USA 91:2401-2406, 1994.
6. Deka N, Sharma MD, Mukerjee R: Isolation of the novel agent from human stool samples that is associated with non-A, non-B hepatitis, J Virol 68:7810-7815, 1994.
7. Konomi N et al: Epidemiology of hepatitis B, C, E, and G virus infections and molecular analysis of hepatitis G virus isolates in Bolivia, J Clin Microbiol 37:3291-3295, 1999.
8. Nishizawa T et al: A novel DNA virus (TTV) associated with elevated transaminase levels in posttransfusion hepatitis of unknown etiology, Biochem Biophys Res Commun 241:92-97, 1997.
9. Centers for Disease Control and Prevention: Summary of Notifiable Disease in the United States, 1998, MMWR; 47(53):1-93, 1999.
10. Centers for Disease Control and Prevention: Hepatitis A fact sheet. Available at: http://www.cdc.gov/ncidod/diseases/hepatitis/a/fact.htm. Accessed Nov. 25, 2000.
11. Alter MJ, Mast ME: The epidemiology of viral hepatitis in the United States, Gastroenterol Clin N Am 23:437-455, 1994.
12. Centers for Disease Control and Prevention: Hepatitis B fact sheet. Available at: http://www.cdc.gov/ncidod/diseases/hepatitis/b/fact.htm. Accessed Nov. 25, 2000.
13. West DJ, Margolis HS: Prevention of hepatitis B virus infection in the United States: a pediatric perspective, Pediatr Infect Dis J 11:866-874, 1992.
14. Wasley A, Alter JM: Epidemiology of hepatitis C: geographic differences and temporal trends, Sem Liver Dis 2:1-16, 2000.
15. Centers for Disease Control: Summary of notifiable diseases, United States, 1994, MMWR 43:1-8, 1995.
16. Centers for Disease Control: Hepatitis C fact sheet. Available at: http://www.cdc.gov/ncidod/diseases/hepatitis/c/fact.htm. Accessed Nov. 25, 2000.
17. Glynn SA et al: Trends in incidence and prevalence of major transfusion-transmissible viral infections in the US blood donors, 1991 to 1996. JAMA 284:229-235, 2000.
18. Seelig R, Bottner C, Seelig HP: Hepatitis C virus infections in dialysis units: prevalence of HCV-RNA and antibodies to HCV, Ann Med 26:45-52, 1994.
19. Dussol B et al: Hepatitis C virus infection among chronic dialysis patients in the south of France. A collaborative study, Am J Kidney Dis 25:399-404, 1995.
20. Alter MJ et al: The prevalence of hepatitis C virus infection in the United States, 1988 through 1994, N Engl J Med 342:556-562, 1999.
21. NIH Consensus Development Conference on Management of Hepatitis C, March 24-26, Bethesda, Md., 1997, National Institutes of Health.
22. Patrick L: Hepatitis C: epidemiology and review of complementary/alternative medicine treatments, Altern Med Rev 4:220-238, 1999.
23. Vinayek R, Rakela J: Acute and Chronic Hepatitis. In: Stein JH, editor: Internal medicine, ed 2, St. Louis, 1998, Mosby.
24. Cottone J: Recent developments in hepatitis: new virus, vaccine, and dosage recommendations, J Am Dent Assoc 120(5):501-508, 1990.
25. London TW, Evans AA: The epidemiology of hepatitis viruses B, C, and D, Clin Lab Med 16:251-271, 1996.
26. Centers for Disease Control: Hepatitis B virus: A comprehensive strategy for eliminating transmission in the United States through universal childhood vaccination: Recommendations of the immunization practices advisory committee (ACIP), MMWR 40 (RR-13):1-25, 1991.
27. Centers for Disease Control: Inactivated hepatitis B virus vaccine: recommendations of the Immunization Practices Advisory Committee, MMWR 31:318-328,1982.
28. Centers for Disease Control: Immune globulins for protection against viral hepatitis, MMWR 30:423-435, 1981.
29. Centers for Disease Control: Protection against viral hepatitis: recommendations of the Immunization Practices Advisory Committee (ACIP), MMWR 39:5-22, 1990.
30. Bass BD et al: Quantitation of hepatitis B viral markers in a dental school population, J Am Dent Assoc 104:629-632,1982.
31. Mosley JW et al: Hepatitis B viruses infection in dentists, N Engl J Med 293:729-734, 1975.
32. Sywassink JM, Lutwick LLI: Risk of hepatitis B in dental care providers: a contact study, J Am Dent Assoc 106(2):182-184, 1983.
33. Weil RB et al: A hepatitis serosurvey of New York dentists, NY State Dent J 43:587-590, 1977.
34. Thomas DL et al: Occupational risk of hepatitis C infections among general dentists and oral surgeons in North America, Am J Med 100:41-45, 1996.
35. Smith JL et al: From the Center for Disease Control: comparative risk of hepatitis B among physicians and dentists, J Infect Dis 13:705-706, 1976.

36. Schreiber GB et al: The risk of transfusion-transmitted viral infection, N Engl J Med 334:1685-1690, 1996.

37. Garfein RS et al: Viral infections in short-term injection drug users: the prevalence of the hepatitis C, hepatitis B, human immunodeficiency and human T-lymphotropic viruses, Am J Public Health 86:655-661, 1996.

38. Cleveland JL et al: Risk and prevention of hepatitis C virus infection: implications for dentistry, JADA 130:641-647, 1999.

39. Piazza M et al: Sexual transmission of the hepatitis C virus and efficacy of prophylaxis with intramuscular immune serum globulin. A randomized controlled trial, Arch Intern Med 157:1537-1544, 1997.

40. Centers for Disease Control: Hepatitis B among parenteral drug users–North Carolina. MMWR 35:481-482, 1986.

41. Gerberding J: Management of occupational exposures to blood-borne viruses, N Engl J Med 332:444-451, 1995.

42. Lanphear B: Trends and patterns in the transmission of bloodborne pathogens to health care workers, Epidemiol Rev 16:437-450, 1994.

43. Werner BG, Grady GF: Accidental hepatitis B surface antigen positive inoculations: use of e antigen to estimate infectivity, Ann Intern Med 97:367-369, 1982.

44. Lanphear B et al: Hepatitis C virus infection in healthcare workers: risk of exposure and infection, Infect Control Hosp Epidemiol 15:745-750, 1994.

45. Wong ML, Lehmann NI, Gust ID: Detection of hepatitis B surface antigen in the saliva of patients with acute hepatitis B, and of chronic carriers, Med J Aust 2:52-55, 1976.

46. Tullman MJ et al: The threat of hepatitis B from dental school patients: a one year study, Oral Surg 49:214-216, 1980.

47. Centers for Disease Control: Lack of transmission of hepatitis B to humans after oral exposure to hepatitis B surface antigen-positive saliva, MMWR 27:247, 1978.

48. MacQuarrie MB, Forghani B, Wolochow DA: Hepatitis B transmitted by a human bite, JAMA 230:723-724, 1974.

49. Chen M et al: Detection of hepatitis G virus (GB virus C) RNA in human saliva, J Clin Microbiol 35:973-975, 1997.

50. Dusheiko GM, Smith M, Scheuer PJ: Hepatitis C virus transmitted by human bite (letter), Lancet 336:503-504, 1990.

51. Sartori M et al: Transmission of hepatitis C via blood splash into conjunctiva (letter), Scand J Infect Dis 25:270-271, 1993.

52. Esteban J et al: Transmission of hepatitis C virus by a cardiac surgeon, N Engl J Med 334:555-560, 1996.

53. Duckworth GJ, Heptonstall J, Aitken C: Transmission of hepatitis C virus from a surgeon to a patient: the incident control team, Commun Dis Public Health 2:188-192, 1999.

54. Klein RS et al: Occupational risk for hepatitis C virus infection among New York City dentists, Lancet 338:1539-1542, 1991.

55. Centers for Disease Control: Recommended infection-control practices for dentistry, 1993. MMWR 41(RR-8):1-12,1993.

56. Pawlotsky J-M, Dhumeaux D, Bagot M: Hepatitis C virus in dermatology: a review, Arch Dermatol 131:1185-1193, 1995.

57. Pratt D, Kaplan M: Evaluation of abnormal liver-enzyme results in asymptomatic patients. N Engl J Med 342:1266-1271, 2000.

58. Smith D: Hepatitis C update. New answers, new questions, Postgrad Med 90(8):199-206, 1991.

59. Centers for Disease Control and Prevention: recommendations for prevention and control of hepatitis C virus (HCV) infection and HCV-related chronic disease, MMWR 47:1-38, 1998.

60. Thoelen S et al: The first combined vaccine against hepatitis A and B: an overview, Vaccine 17:1657-1662, 1999.

61. From the Centers for Disease Control and Prevention: FDA approval for infants of a Haemophilus influenzae type b conjugate and hepatitis B (recombinant) combined vaccine, JAMA 277:620-621, 1997.

62. Centers for Disease Control: Update toward the elimination of hepatitis B virus–United States, MMWR 44:574-575, 1995.

63. Centers for Disease Control: Hepatitis B vaccine: evidence confirming lack of AIDS transmission, MMWR 33:685-686, 1984.

64. Mahoney F et al: Progress toward the elimination of hepatitis B virus transmission among health care workers in the United States, Arch Intern Med 157:2601-2605, 1997.

65. Centers for Disease Control: Immunization of health-care workers: recommendations of the advisory committee on immunization practices (ACIP) and the hospital infection control practices advisory committee (HICPAC), MMWR 46(RR-18):1-44, 1997

66. Guidelines for hepatitis B virus screening and vaccination during pregnancy. ACOG Committee opinion: Committee on Obstetrics: Maternal and Fetal Medicine Number 78–January 1990, Int J Gynaecol Obstet, Aug:35(4):367-369, 1991.

67. American Academy of Pediatrics: Red book: report of the Committee on Infectious Diseases, ed 23 Elk Grove Village, Illinois, 1994, American Academy of Pediatrics.

68. Centers for Disease Control: Prevention of hepatitis A through active or passive immunization: Recommendation of the advisory committee on immunization practice. MMWR 48(RR-12):1-31, 1999.

69. Zeuzem S et al: Peginterferon alfa-2a in patients with chronic hepatitis C, N Engl J Med 343:1666-1672, 2000.

70. Yoshida H et al: Interferon therapy reduces the risk for hepatocellular carcinoma: national surveillance program of cirrhotic and noncirrhotic patients with chronic hepatitis C in Japan, Ann Intern Med 131:174-181, 1999.

71. Camma C, Almasio P, Craxi A: Interferon as treatment for acute hepatitis C: a meta-analysis, Dig Dis Sci 41:1248-55, 1996.

72. Pianko S MJ: Treatment of hepatitis C with interferon and ribavirin, J Gastroenterol Hepatol 15:581-586, 2000.

73. ADA Council on Scientific Affairs, ADA Council on Dental Practice: Infection control recommendations for the dental office and the dental laboratory, JADA 127:672-680, 1996.

74. Advisory Committee on Immunization Practices (ACIP) and the Hospital Infection Control Practices Advisory Committee (HICPAC): Immunization of health-care workers: recommendations of the Advisory Committee on Immunization Practices (ACIP) and the Hospital Infection Control Practices Advisory Committee (HICPAC), MMWR 46(RR-18):1-42, 1997.

75. U.S. Department of Labor: Bloodborne pathogens: the standard, *Federal Register* 60:64175-64182, 1991.

76. U.S. Department of Labor: OSHA Directives, CPL 2-2.44D–Enforcement Procedures for the Occupational Exposure to Bloodborne Pathogens, accessed at *http://www.osha-slc.gov/OshDoc/Directive_data/CPL_2-2_44D.html*.

77. Goebel W: Reliability of the medical history in identifying patients likely to place dentists at an increased hepatitis risk, *J Am Dent Assoc* 98(6):907-913, 1979.

78. Goodman RA, Soloman SL: Transmission of infectious diseases in outpatient health care settings, *JAMA* 265:2377-2381, 1991.

79. Center for Disease Control: Recommendations for preventing transmission of human immunodeficiency virus and hepatitis B virus to patients during exposure-prone invasive procedures, *MMWR* 40:1-8, 1991.

80. Seeff LB et al: Type B hepatitis after needle-stick exposure: prevention with hepatitis B immune globulin, *Ann Intern Med* 88:285-293, 1978.

81. El-Serag H, Mason AC: Rising incidence of hepatocellular carcinoma in the United States, *N Engl J Med* 340:745-751, 1999.

82. Diamond I, Jay C: Alcoholism and Alcohol Abuse. In: Goldman L BJ, editor: *Cecil textbook of medicine*, 21 ed, Philadelphia, 2000, WB Saunders.

83. Schuckit MA et al: The clinical course of alcohol-related problems in alcohol dependent and nonalcohol dependent drinking women and men, *J Stud Alcohol* 59:581-590, 1998.

84. Secretary of Health and Human Services: *Ninth special report of the U.S. Congress on alcohol and health*, Washington, DC, Government Printing Office, 1997.

85. Bergman B, Brismar B: Characteristics of violent alcoholics, *Alcohol Alcohol* 29:451-457, 1994.

86. Dawson DA et al: Subgroup aviation in U.S. drinking patterns: results of the 1992 National Longitudinal Alcohol Epidemiologic Study, *J Subst Abuse* 7:331-344, 1995.

87. Kessler RC et al: Lifetime and 12-month prevalence of DSM-III-R psychiatric disorders in the United States: results from the National Comorbidity Survey, *Arch Gen Psychiatry* 51:8-19, 1994.

88. Grant BF et al: Prevalence of DSM-III-R alcohol abuse and dependence–United States, 1988. *Alcohol Health Res World* 15(1):91-96, 1991.

89. Kuzel AJ et al: A survey of drinking patterns during medical school, *South Med J* 84:9-12, 1991.

90. McGinnis JM, Foege WH: Mortality and morbidity attributable to use of addictive substances in the United States, *Proc Assoc Am Physicians* 111(2):109-118, 1999.

91. Brody J: Aging and alcohol abuse, *J Am Geriatr Soc* 30:123-126, 1982.

92. Muller A: Alcohol consumption and community hospital admissions in the United States: a dynamic regression analysis, 1950-1992, *Addiction* 91:321-342, 1996.

93. Hoyert DL, Kochanek KD, Murphy SL: Deaths: final data for 1997, *Natl Vital Stat Rep* 47:1-104, 1999.

94. Hanna EZ, Chou SP, Grant BF: The relationship between drinking and heart disease morbidity in the United States: results from the National Health Interview Survey. *Alcohol Clin Exp Res* 21:111-118, 1997.

95. Podolsky DK, Isselbacher KJ: Cirrhosis of the liver. In: Wilson JD BE et al, editors: *Harrison's principles of internal medicine*, ed 12, New York, 1991, McGraw-Hill.

96. Leonard R: Alcohol, alcoholism and dental treatment, *Compendium* 12(4):274-283, 1991.

97. Greenwel P: Acetaldehyde-mediated collagen regulation in hepatic stellate cells, *Alcohol Clin Exp Res* 23:930-933, 1999.

98. Bautista A: Impact of alcohol on the ability of Kupffer cells to produce chemokines and its role in alcoholic liver disease, *J Gastroenterol Hepatol* 15:349-356, 2000.

99. Bassendine MF, Day CP: The inheritance of alcoholic liver disease, *Baillieres Clin Gastroenterol* 12:317-335, 1998.

100. Kuriyama K, Ohkuma S: Alteration in the function of cerebral neurotransmitter receptors during the establishment of alcohol dependence: neurochemical aspects, *Alcohol Alcohol* 25:239-249, 1990.

101. Watson RR et al: Alcohol, immunomodulation, and disease, *Alcohol Alcohol* 29:131-139, 1994.

102. Camargo CA Jr et al: Prospective study of moderate alcohol consumption and mortality in US male physicians, *Arch Intern Med* 157:79-85, 1997.

103. Boffetta P, Garfinkel L: Alcohol drinking and mortality among men enrolled in an American Cancer Society prospective study, *Epidemiology* 1:342-348, 1990.

104. Lieber CS, Rubin E: Ethanol: a hepatotoxic drug, *Gastroenterology* 54:642-646, 1968.

105. Harasymiw JW, Vinson DC, Bean P: The early detection of alcohol consumption (EDAC) score in the identification of heavy and at-risk drinkers from routine blood tests, *J Addict Dis* 19:43-59, 2000.

106. Glick M: Medical considerations for dental care of patients with alcohol-related liver disease, *Jour Am Den Assoc* 128:61-70, 1997.

107. Cohen J, Kaplan M: The SGOT/SGPT ratio–an indicator of alcoholic liver disease, *Dig Dis Sci* 24:835-838, 1979.

108. O'Connor PG, Schottenfeld RS: Patients with alcohol problem, *N Engl J Med* 338:592-602, 1998.

109. Mundle G et al: Sex differences of carbohydrate-deficient transferrin, gamma-glutamyltransferase, and mean corpuscular volume in alcohol-dependent patients, *Alcohol Clin Exp Res* 24:1400-1405, 2000.

110. McQuade WH LS et al: Detecting symptoms of alcohol abuse in primary care setting, *Arch Fam Med* 9:814-821, 2000.

111. Sammon P: Personal communication, 1995.

112. National Institute on Alcohol Abuse and Alcoholism: The Physicians' Guide to Helping Patients with Alcohol Problems, Washington D.C.: 1995, Government Printing Office.

113. Seeff LB et al: Acetaminophen hepatotoxicity in alcoholics: a therapeutic misadventure, *Ann Intern Med* 104:399-404, 1986.

114. Demas PN, McClain JR: Hepatitis: implications for dental care, *Oral Surg Oral Med Oral Pathol Oral Radiol Endod* 88:2-4, 1999.

115. Douglas LR et al: Oral management of the patient with end-stage liver disease and the liver transplant patient, *Oral Surg Oral Med Oral Pathol Oral Radiol Endod* 86:55-64, 1998.

116. Wyke R: Bacterial infections complicating liver disease, *Baillieres Clin Gastroenterol* 3:187-210, 1989.

117. Albers I et al: Superiority of the Child-Pugh classification to quantitative liver function tests for assessing prognosis of liver cirrhosis, *Scand J Gastroenterol* 24:269-276, 1989.

118. Friedlander AH, Mills MJ, Gorelick DA: Alcoholism and dental management, *Oral Surg* 62:42-46, 1987.

119. Galili D et al: A modern approach to prevention and treatment of oral bleeding in patients with hepatocellular disease, *Oral Surg* 54:277-280, 1982.

120. Rauch S, Gorlin RJ: Diseases of the salivary glands. In: Gorlin RJ GH, editor: *Thomas' oral pathology*, ed 6, St Louis, 1970, CV Mosby.

121. Mandel L, Hamele-Bena D: Alcoholic parotid sialadenosis, *JADA* 128:1411-1415, 1997.

122. Madden AM, Bradbury W, Morgan MY: Taste perception in cirrhosis: its relationship to circulating micronutrients and food preferences, *Hepatology* 26:40-48, 1997.

Gastrointestinal Disease

Gastrointestinal diseases such as peptic ulcer disease, inflammatory bowel disease, and pseudomembranous colitis are common and may affect the delivery of dental care. A patient who has one of these conditions presents several areas of concern to the dental practitioner. The dentist must be cognizant of the patient's condition, monitor for symptoms indicative of initial disease or relapse, and be aware of drugs that interact with gastrointestinal medications or may aggravate their condition. In addition, oral manifestations of gastrointestinal disease are not rare; thus the dentist must be familiar with the oral patterns of disease.

■ PEPTIC ULCER DISEASE ■

DEFINITION

A peptic ulcer is a well-defined break in the gastrointestinal mucosa (greater than 3 mm in diameter as defined by many industry-sponsored studies) that results from chronic acid-pepsin secretions and the destructive effects of and the host response to *Helicobacter pylori*. Peptic ulcers develop principally in regions of the gastrointestinal tract that are proximal to acid-pepsin secretions (Fig. 11-1). The first portion of the duodenum is the location of approximately 80% of ulcers, with the rest generally occurring in the stomach.[1] The upper jejunum rarely is involved. Peptic ulcer disease usually is chronic and focal; only approximately 10% of patients have multiple ulcers.

EPIDEMIOLOGY

INCIDENCE AND PREVALENCE

Peptic ulcer disease is one of the most common human ailments, once affecting up to 15% of the population in industrialized countries. Current estimates suggest that 5% to 10% of the world population is affected, and 500,000 new cases occur in the United States annually.[2,3] The incidence of peptic ulceration peaked between 1900 and 1950 and progressively decreased thereafter. The reasons for the decline in Northern Europe and the United States may be the result of decreased cigarette and aspirin consumption, increased use of vegetable cooking oils (a rich source of raw materials for synthesis of prostaglandins, which have cytoprotective properties), and better sanitation.[4] The disease affects 5% to 7% of Northern Europeans and accounts for more than 400,000 hospitalizations annually in the United States. Peptic ulcers are rare in Greenlander Eskimos, southwestern Native Americans, Australian aborigines, and Indonesians.[2]

Peak prevalence of peptic ulceration occurs in young adulthood (age 30 to 50 years).[5] Until the 1980s, the male/female ratio in the United States was 2:1, but current figures approximate the ratio at 1:1.[6] (The male/female ratio is 2:1 in England, Denmark, and Wales.[2]) First-degree relatives have a threefold higher risk of the disease.[5] Persons who smoke and are heavy drinkers of alcohol are more prone to the disease. An association with blood type O exists. A higher prevalence is seen in patients with hyperparathyroidism and conditions associated with increased gastrin levels (i.e., renal dialysis, Zollinger-Ellison syndrome, mastocytosis). Use of nonsteroidal antiinflammatory drugs (NSAIDs) for more than one month is associated with gastrointestinal bleeding or ulcer complication in 2% to 4% of patients per year who ingest these drugs.[7]

The disease is rare in children, with only 1 in 2500 pediatric hospital admissions attributable to peptic ulceration.[8] When a peptic ulcer is diagnosed in a child younger than 10 years of age, the condition most often is associated with an underlying systemic illness, such as a severe burn or major trauma.[9] The majority of the deaths that

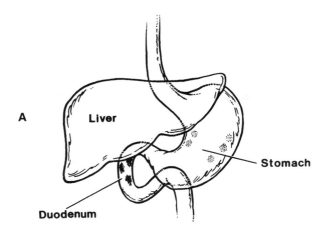

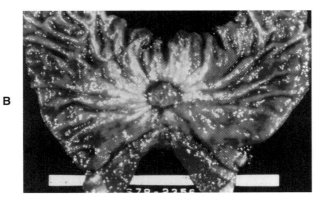

Fig. 11-1 A, Location of peptic ulceration (shaded areas). Darker stipulations are higher-risk sites. **B,** Appearance of a benign peptic ulcer on the lesser curvature of the stomach with sharp flat margins. (Courtesy R Estensen, Minneapolis, Minn.)

occur from peptic ulcer disease occur in patients older than 65 years. An average dental practice of 2000 adult patients is predicted to have about 100 patients with peptic ulcer disease.

ETIOLOGY

Until recently, medical dogma held that excess acid in the stomach was the cause of peptic ulcer disease. However, acid hypersecretion is not uniformly found in patients with peptic ulceration.[10] Current evidence supports a complex interaction between aggressive factors that are potentially destructive to the mucosa and defensive factors that are protective of the mucosa. The primary aggressive factor appears to be H. *pylori* (formerly *Campylobacter pylori*). This organism is

present in more than 90% of duodenal ulcers.[11] Other aggressive factors include acid hypersecretion, cigarette smoking, use of NSAIDs and psychological and physical stress.[12]

H. *pylori* is a microaerophilic, gram-negative, spiral-shaped bacillus with 4 to 6 flagella.[13] H. *pylori* was first reported to reside in the antral mucosa by Marshall and Warren.[14,15] The organism is an adherent but noninvasive bacterium that lives at the interface between the surface of gastric epithelium and the overlying mucous gel. It produces a potent urease that hydrolyses urea to ammonia and carbon dioxide. The urease may protect the bacteria from the immediate acidic environment by increasing local pH while damaging mucosa via the generation of its byproduct, ammonia. Chemotaxis of neutrophils and the antibody response are involved in the local tissue damage that subsequently occurs.

Humans are the only known host of H. *pylori*. The bacteria display a 0.5% infection rate of adults per year.[16] H. *pylori* is acquired primarily during childhood, possibly as a result of entrance from the oral cavity via contaminated food and poor sanitary habits. The organism has been shown to reside in the oral cavity,[17] from which it probably descends to colonize the gastric mucosa. H. *pylori* can persist in the stomach indefinitely and remains clinically silent in most persons who are infected.[18] The rate of H. *pylori* acquisition is higher in developing than in developed countries.[19] In developing countries, 80% of the population carries the bacterium by the age of 20 years, whereas only 20% of 20-year-olds are infected in the United States. The prevalence of infection in blacks and Hispanics is twice that seen in whites in the United States.[20] Infection is correlated with poor socioeconomic status, contaminated drinking water, and familial overcrowding, especially during childhood. Approximately 20% of those infected go on to develop peptic ulcer disease,[12] suggesting that other physiological and psychological (stress) factors[21] are required for presentation of this disease.

NSAIDs also are associated with 15% to 20% of peptic ulcers as a result of their ability to directly damage mucosa, reduce mucosal prostaglandin production, and inhibit mucous secretion. Ulcers caused by NSAIDs more often are located in the stomach than the duodenum. Risk with NSAID use increases with age older than 60 years, high dosage-chronic therapy, NSAIDs with long plasma half-lives (i.e., piroxicam) compared with those having short half lives (i.e., ibuprofen), and concomitant use of alcohol, corticosteroids, anticoagulants, or aspirin. Use of bisphosphonate drugs (aledronate, risedronate) for treatment osteoporosis also are associated with esophageal and gastric ulcer.[22]

Aggressive factors

Tobacco
Alcohol
Stress
NSAIDs
Debilitating illness

Defensive factors

Mucus gel
Bicarbonate
Prostaglandins
Mucosa blood flow

Helicobacter pylori

- → (Mucosa)

(Ammonia, lipopolysaccharide, urease, toxins)

Nutrients

Inflammation

Suppressor mechanisms

Inflammatory mediators

Renal dialysis
Hyperparathyroidism

Gastrin secretion
Parietal cell function

Atrophy

Chronic superficial gastritis
Duodenal ulcer
Gastric ulcer

Lymphoma

Carcinoma

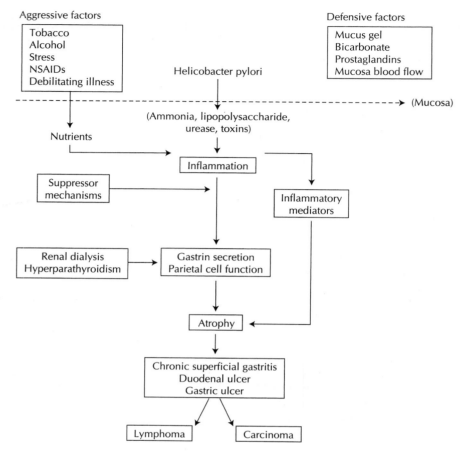

Fig. 11-2 Complex interplay of aggressive and defensive factors involved in the formation of peptic ulcer disease.

PATHOPHYSIOLOGY AND COMPLICATIONS

Ulcer formation is the result of a complex interplay of aggressive and defensive factors (Fig. 11-2). Resistance to acidic breakdown is provided normally by mucosal resistance, mucous and prostaglandin production, blood flow, bicarbonate secretion, and ion-carrier exchange. Additional resistance is gained from antibacterial proteins such as lysozyme, lactoferrin, interferon, and defensin/cryptdin.

Under normal circumstances, food stimulates gastrin release, gastrin stimulates histamine release by the enterochromaffin-like cells in the stomach, and the parietal cells secrete hydrogen ions and chloride ions (hydrochloric acid). Vagal nerve stimulation, caffeine, and histamine also are stimulants of parietal cell se-

cretion of hydrochloric acid.[23] Aggressive factors include vagal over activity and factors that enhance the release of pepsin, gastrin, and histamine. Physical and emotional stress, obsessive-compulsive behavior, parasitic infections, and drugs such as caffeine, high-dose corticosteroids, and phenylbutazone enhance hypersecretion of stomach acid. Alcohol and NSAIDs are directly injurious to gastric mucosa. Alcohol alters cell permeability and can lead to cell death. NSAIDs and aspirin disrupt mucosal resistance by impairing prostaglandin production, denaturating mucous glycoproteins and promoting degranulation of mast cells. Hyperparathyroidism enhances gastrin secretion, and renal dialysis inadequately removes circulating gastrin. Smoking tobacco and family history are risk factors independent of gastric acid secretion for peptic ulcer dis-

ease.[6,24] The mechanism by which tobacco smoke affects gastric mucosa is unknown.

H. *pylori* is associated strongly with peptic ulcer disease; however, the mechanism whereby infection with H. *pylori* results in peptic ulcer disease is not completely understood. H. *pylori* clearly causes inflammation of the gastric mucosa and is responsible for most cases of etiologic gastritis. The bacterium has been implicated in promoting acute gastritis by its ability to disrupt mucosal resistance. The process may involve H. *pylori*'s induction of increased gastrin release by G cells[19,25,26] and inflammatory mediators (cytokines) and cells that respond to H. *pylori* antigens, ammonia, and vacuolating toxin.[27-29] H. *pylori*-associated antral gastritis is found in 90% to 100% of patients with duodenal ulcers.[30-31] However, no correlation between H. *pylori* and acid hypersecretion exists. In fact, acid secretion in patients with peptic ulcer is similar to that in patients without ulcers,[10] and H. *pylori* alone has been unable to injure stomach mucosa (ex vivo and in vitro).[32] This suggests that the inflammatory response causes the mucosal breakdown.[28]

Complications associated with peptic ulcer disease depend on the degree of destruction of the gastrointestinal epithelium and supporting tissues. Superficial ulcers are characterized by necrotic debris and fibrin. Beneath this layer are numerous polymorphonuclear leukocytes, scattered macrophages, and eosinophils. Below is active granulation tissue and fibrosis. A chronic or aggressive ulcer can penetrate through the fibrotic tissue into the muscular layer (muscularis mucosa). The muscularis layer, weakened by scar tissue, can result in perforation into the peritoneal cavity (peritonitis) or into the head of the pancreas. Arteries or veins in the muscularis layer may be eroded by ulcers, giving rise to hemorrhage (a bleeding ulcer), anemia, and potential shock. Untreated ulcers often heal by fibrosis, which can lead to pyloric stenosis, gastric outlet obstruction, dehydration, and alkalosis. Complications are more common in the elderly.

H. *pylori* is associated with the development of a low-grade gastric mucosa-associated lymphoid tissue lymphoma.[33] Accordingly, H. *pylori* has been classified as a definite (Class I) human carcinogen by the World Health Organization.[34]

Peptic ulcers rarely undergo carcinomatous transformation. Ulcers of the greater curvature of the stomach have a greater propensity for malignant degeneration than do those of the duodenum. Atrophic gastritis associated with chronic proton pump inhibitor use (see *Medical Management*) also increases the risk for stomach cancer.[35]

CLINICAL PRESENTATION

SIGNS AND SYMPTOMS

Although many patients with active peptic ulcer have no ulcer symptoms, most develop epigastric pain that is long-standing (several hours) and sharply localized. The pain is described as "burning" or "gnawing" but may be "ill-defined" or "aching." The discomfort of a duodenal ulcer manifests most commonly on an empty stomach, usually 90 minutes to 3 hours after eating, and frequently awakens the patient in the middle of the night. The ingestion of food, milk, or antacids provides rapid relief in most cases. Patients with gastric ulcers, however, are less predictable in their response to food and may develop abdominal pain from eating. Symptoms associated with peptic ulceration tend to be episodic and recurrent. Epigastric tenderness often accompanies the condition.

Changes in the character of pain may indicate the development of complications. For example, increased discomfort, loss of antacid relief, or pain radiating to the back may signal deeper penetration or perforation of the ulcer. Protracted vomiting a few hours after a meal is a sign of gastric outlet (pyloric) obstruction. Melena (bloody stools) or black tarry stools indicate blood loss due to gastrointestinal hemorrhage.

Laboratory Findings

A peptic ulcer is diagnosed primarily by fiberoptic endoscopy in combination with double-contrast barium radiographs and laboratory tests for H. *pylori*. Endoscopy affords the opportunity for visualization, access for biopsy, and therapeutic procedures if bleeding is present. Of the variety of laboratory tests, urea breath tests (UBTs) and serology are most widely used. UBTs are advantageous because they measure indirectly the presence of H. *pylori* before treatment and eradication after treatment. Serology is useful in determining current or past infection but is limited in documenting the eradication of H. *pylori* because antibody titers persist after elimination of the organism.[5]

UBTs involve the ingestion of urea labeled with carbon-13 or carbon-14. Degradation of urea by the bacillus releases ^{13}C or ^{14}C in the expired breath. A ^{13}C test can be performed in the office, but ^{14}C tests must be performed in nuclear medicine facilities. Breath tests are advantageous in that they are noninvasive, highly accurate, and highly sensitive.[36]

A biopsy of the marginal mucosa adjacent to the ulcer is performed during endoscopy to confirm the diagnosis and rule out malignancy. During endoscopy, the rapid

urease test can be performed. Microscopic analysis of the biopsied tissue with Giemsa, acridine orange, and Warthin-Starry stains are effective in the microscopic detection of H. *pylori* (Fig. 11-3). The urease test involves direct inoculation of a portion of the gastric mucosal biopsy into a gel medium containing urea and phenol red. If the organism is present, the gel is metabolized to ammonia (pH greater than or equal to 6.0) that causes

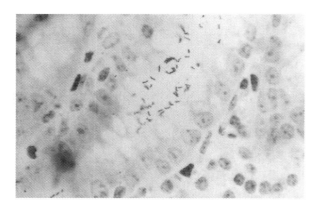

Fig. 11-3 *Helicobacter pylori* (dark rods) evident in the lumen of the intestine. (Warthin-Starry stain, courtesy Eun Lee, Lexington, Ky.)

the gel to change from yellow to pink. Culture of the organism is reserved for when antimicrobial resistance is suspected, as the technique is tedious, difficult, and no more sensitive than routine histologic analysis.

MEDICAL MANAGEMENT

Most patients with peptic ulcer disease suffer for several weeks before going to a doctor for treatment. If the peptic ulcer is confined and uncomplicated and H. *pylori* is not present, antisecretory drugs are administered (Table 11-1). If the patient is infected with H. *pylori*, inhibitors of gastric acid secretion and antimicrobial agents are recommended.[36] Combination therapy is recommended because antisecretory drugs provide rapid relief of pain and accelerate healing. Antibiotics are used because they are efficient in eradicating H. *pylori*, accelerating healing and producing an ulcer-free state in 92% to 99% of treated patients.[38,39]

For those with a peptic ulcer and H. *pylori* infection, current first-line therapy is the administration of at least 2 antibiotics and 1 antisecretory drug. This is known as "triple" or "quadruple" therapy (Box 11-1). The antibiotics most commonly used are tetracycline and metronidazole, or amoxicillin and clarithromycin. These usually are combined with 1 antisecretory drug, either a proton-pump inhibitor (PPI) or bismuth subsalicylate.[40] Therapy gener-

TABLE 11-1

Antisecretory Drugs

Class	Generic Drug	Trade Name	Daily Treatment Dose	Dental Management Considerations
H$_2$-histamine antagonist	Cimetidine	Tagamet	600 to 1000 mg	Delayed liver metabolism of benzodiazepines; reversible joint symptoms with preexisting arthritis
	Ranitidine	Zantac	300 mg	—
	Famotidine	Pepcid	20 to 40 mg	Anorexia, dry mouth
	Nizatidine	Axid	300 mg	Potential increased serum salicylate levels with concurrent aspirin use
Proton-pump inhibitor	Omeprazole	Prilosec	20 to 80 mg	May reduce absorption of ampicillin, ketoconazole and itraconazole
	Lansoprazole	Prevacid	15 to 30 mg	
	Pantoprazole	Protonix, Protium	40 to 80 mg	
	Esomeprazole	Nexium	20 to 40 mg	
Prostaglandin*	Misoprostol	Cytotec	200 mg	Diarrhea, cramps

*Not a first-line drug for treating peptic ulcers. Used in the prevention of peptic ulcer and in NSAID users.

ally is given for 10 days to 2 weeks, with 2 weeks producing greater success.[41,42]

In the past, more than 50% of patients with peptic ulcer disease experienced recurrences. This was because antisecretory drugs alone were the treatment of choice, and these drugs alone do not eradicate H. *pylori* infection and are noncurative of peptic ulcer disease. Eradication of H. *pylori* with antibiotic treatment reduces the rate of recurrence of peptic ulceration by 85% to 100%.[19,41,43-46] Reemergence of an ulcer usually is traced to the persistence of H. *pylori* after treatment because of inappropriate drug choice, discontinuance of drug therapy, and lack of behavior modification.

In all patients undergoing peptic ulcer therapy, ulcerogenic factors, (i.e., continued use of alcohol, aspirin, NSAIDs, corticosteroids–along with foods that aggravate symptoms and stimulate gastric acid secretion, and stress) should be eliminated to accelerate healing and limit relapses. Patients appear to benefit from smoking cessation, as perforation rates are higher in smokers and continued smoking results in a higher rate of relapse after treatment and lower eradication rates of H. *pylori*.[47,48] However, when H. *pylori* is successfully eradicated, cigarette smoking does not appear to increase the risk of recurrence.[49]

BOX 11-1

Antimicrobial Regimens for the Treatment of *Helicobacter pylori* Infection in Peptic Ulcer Disease

Triple therapy:
Proton pump inhibitor plus Clarithromycin (250-500 mg) plus Metronidazole (500 mg)*
Proton pump inhibitor plus Clarithromycin (500 mg) plus Amoxicillin (1 g)*
Bismuth subsalicylate (Pepto-Bismol), 2 tablets qid plus Metronidazole (Flagyl), 250 mg qid (or 500 mg tid) plus Tetracycline (or amoxicillin), 500 mg qid
Ranitidine (Zantac) 400 mg bid plus Clarithromycin (500 mg bid) plus Tetracycline (or amoxicillin), 500 mg qid for 2 weeks

Quadruple therapy:
Bismuth subsalicylate (Pepto-Bismol), 2 tablets qid plus Metronidazole (Flagyl), 500 mg tid (or Clarithromycin 500 mg tid) plus Tetracycline, 500 mg qid plus Proton pump inhibitor

*Medications are given twice daily for 10 to 14 days. Above listed therapies provide ~90% efficacy.

Elective surgical intervention (e.g., dissection of the vagus nerves from the gastric fundus) largely has been abandoned in management of peptic ulcer disease. Today, surgery is reserved primarily for complications of peptic ulcer disease such as significant bleeding (when unresponsive to coagulant endoscopic procedures), perforation, and gastric outlet obstruction. On the occasion that peptic ulcer disease is associated with hyperparathyroidism and parathyroid adenoma, surgical removal of the affected gland is the treatment of choice. Resolution of gastrointestinal disease occurs secondary to termination of abnormal endocrine function. Several prototype protein-based vaccines against H. *pylori* have shown promising results; however, they have not been proven to resolve infection and prevent reinfection.[50]

DENTAL MANAGEMENT

MEDICAL CONSIDERATIONS

The dentist must identify intestinal symptoms from a careful history before the initiation of dental treatment because many gastrointestinal diseases, despite being chronic and recurrent, go undetected for long periods of time. This includes a careful review of medications (i.e., aspirin, NSAIDs, oral anticoagulants) and alcohol consumption that can result in gastrointestinal bleeding. If gastrointestinal symptoms are suggestive of active disease, a medical referral is needed. Once the patient returns from the physician and the condition is under control, the dentist should update current medications in the dental record, including the type and dosage, and follow the guidelines outlined in the following material. Further, periodic physician visits should be encouraged to afford early diagnosis and cancer screenings for at-risk patients.

Of primary importance are the impact and interactions of certain drugs prescribed to patients with peptic ulcer disease. In general, the dentist should avoid prescribing aspirin, aspirin-containing compounds, and NSAIDs to patients with and history of peptic ulcer disease because of the irritative effects of these drugs on the gastrointestinal epithelium. Acetaminophen and compounded acetaminophen products are recommended instead. If NSAIDs are used, a COX-2 selective inhibitor (rofecoxib [Vioxx]; celecoxib [Celebrex])[51] in combination with a proton pump inhibitor or misoprostol (Cytotec, 200 μg 2-3 times daily)–a prostaglandin E1 analogue–is advised to reduce the risk of gastrointestinal bleeding.[52] Analgesic selection should consider patient risk factors (prior gastrointestinal bleeding, age, use of alcohol, anticoagulants or steroids) and provide the lowest dose for the shortest period to achieve the

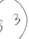

desired affect. H_2-antagonists and sucralfate are not beneficial selections as they do not appear to protect patients from NSAID-induced complications.[53,54]

Acid-blocking drugs, such as cimetidine, decrease the metabolism of certain dentally prescribed drugs (i.e., diazepam, lidocaine, tricyclic antidepressants) and enhance the duration of action of these medications (see Table 11-1). Under such circumstances, dosing of anesthetics, benzodiazepines, and antidepressants that are metabolized in the liver may require dosing adjustment. Antacids also impair the absorption of tetracycline, erythromycin, oral iron, and fluoride, and impair optimal blood levels of these drugs. To avoid this problem, antibiotics and dietary supplements should be taken 2 hours before or 2 hours after the ingestion of antacids.

Routine dental treatment during medical therapy for peptic ulceration can be provided; however, the decision should be based on patient comfort and convenience. Should antibiotics become necessary to treat a dental infection during the course of peptic ulcer disease therapy, the choice of antibiotics may be altered by the patient's current medications. For example, tetracycline or metronidazole are not appropriate choices for most odontogenic infections, and amoxicillin or clarithromycin can be substituted with the approval of the patient's physician.

TREATMENT PLANNING MODIFICATIONS

H. *pylori* is found in dental plaque and may serve as a reservoir of infection and reinfection along the alimentary tract.[17,55] Good oral hygiene measures and periodic scaling and prophylaxis may be useful for reducing the spread of this organism. Rigorous hygiene measures should be discussed with the patient and consideration given to detecting oral organisms in patients who have a history of peptic ulcer disease and are symptomatic or experiencing recurrences. Routine dental care requires no other modifications in technique for patients with peptic ulcer disease.

ORAL COMPLICATIONS AND MANIFESTATIONS

The use of systemic antibiotics for peptic ulcer disease can result in fungal overgrowth (candidiasis) in the oral cavity. The dentist should be alert to identify oral fungal infections, including median rhomboid glossitis, in this patient population (Fig. 11-4). A course of antifungal agents (see Appendix B) should be prescribed to resolve the fungal infection.

Two less-common oral manifestations of peptic ulcer disease are (1) vascular malformations of the lip and (2) enamel erosion. The former have been reported to range

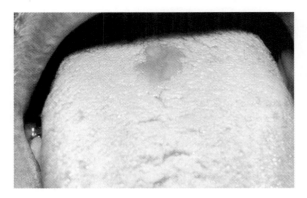

Fig. 11-4 Median rhomboid glossitis as a result of antibiotic use.

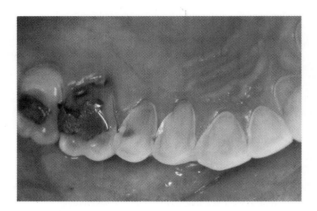

Fig. 11-5 Perimylolysis. Destruction of palatal enamel of maxillary incisors in a patient with persistent regurgitation. (From Neville, Damm, Allen, et al: Oral and Maxillofacial Pathology, ed 2, Philadelphia, WB Saunders, 2002.)

from a small macule (microcherry) to a large venous pool and occur in older men with peptic ulcer disease.[56] The latter finding is the result of persistent regurgitation of gastric juices into the mouth when pyloric stenosis occurs (Fig. 11-5). The finding of enamel erosion with the history of reflux dictates that the patient be evaluated by a physician.

Medications taken by patients for the treatment of peptic ulcer disease can produce oral manifestations. Proton-pump inhibitors can alter taste perception. Cimetidine and ranitidine can have a toxic effect on bone marrow and infrequently cause anemia, agranulocytosis, or thrombocytopenia. Mucosal ulcerations may be a sign of agranulocytosis, whereas anemia may present as mucosal pallor and thrombocytopenia as gingival bleeding or petechiae. Xerostomia has been associated with the use of famotidine and anticholinergic drugs, such as propantheline (Pro-Banthine). A chronic dry mouth ren-

ders the patient susceptible to bacterial infection (caries and periodontal disease) and fungal disease (candidiasis). Erythema multiforme has been associated with use of cimetidine and ranitidine.

■ INFLAMMATORY BOWEL DISEASE ■

DEFINITION

Inflammatory bowel disease (IBD) describes two idiopathic diseases of the gastrointestinal tract, ulcerative colitis and Crohn's disease. The main criteria that separate the two diseases are the site and extent of tissue involvement; thus they are discussed together. Ulcerative colitis is a mucosal disease limited to the large intestine and rectum. In contrast, Crohn's disease is a transmural process (affects entire wall of the bowel) that may produce focal ulcerations along any point of the alimentary canal from the mouth to the anus but most commonly involves the terminal ileum.

EPIDEMIOLOGY

Incidence and Prevalence

The incidence and prevalence of IBD varies widely by race and geographic location. Occurrence is much higher among Jews and whites than in blacks, and considerably higher in the United States and Europe than in Asia and Africa. Approximately 4 to 8 new cases per 100,000 persons are diagnosed annually in the United States and Europe.[57] Approximately 200,000 to 400,000 persons in the United States are affected.[58] Peak age of onset is young adulthood (20 to 40 years of age). However, a second incidence peak of Crohn's disease occurs in persons over age 60 years. Children also have been known to develop IBD. The predilection for ulcerative colitis in men and women is equal, whereas Crohn's disease has a slight predilection for women. A tenfold increased risk of disease in first-degree relatives of patients suggests strongly that genetic factors are involved.[59] The mode of inheritance is unclear. The environment is a contributory factor, as Crohn's disease occurs more often in nonsmokers, and smoking protects against ulcerative colitis. Breast-feeding also appears to reduce the risk of developing IBD.[60] In the average general dentistry practice having 2000 adult patients, approximately 5 adults are predicted to have IBD.

ETIOLOGY

Ulcerative colitis and Crohn's disease are inflammatory diseases of unknown etiology. Although several factors including allergy, destructive enzymes, bacterial and viral infection, psychological disturbance, and immunologic factors have been suggested as etiologic, no infectious agent has been identified. Atypical mycobacteria have been identified in a minority of Crohn's patients.[58]

PATHOPHYSIOLOGY AND COMPLICATIONS

Ulcerative Colitis

Ulcerative colitis is an inflammatory reaction of the large intestine characterized by remissions and exacerbations. The disease starts in the colon-rectum region and may spread proximally to involve the entire large intestine and the ileum. Pathologic findings include edema, vascular congestion, distorted cryptic architecture, and monocellular infiltration. Persistent disease causes epithelial erosions and hemorrhage, pseudopolyp formation, crypt abscesses, and submucosal fibrosis. Chronic deposition of fibrous tissue may lead to fibrotic shortening, thickening, and narrowing of the colon.

Ulcerative colitis usually is lifelong, and progression to its more severe forms predisposes the patient to toxic dilatation (toxic megacolon) and dysplastic changes (carcinoma) of the intestine. Toxic megacolon is the result of disease extension through deep muscular layers. The colon dilates because of weakening of the wall, and intestinal perforation becomes more likely. Fever, electrolyte imbalance, and volume depletion are present. Carcinoma of the colon is 10 times more likely in patients with ulcerative colitis than in the general population.[61] Likelihood of malignant transformation increases with the proximal extension of the disease and long-standing disease (greater than 8 to 10 years, at rate of 0.5% to 2% per year).[62]

Crohn's Disease

Crohn's disease is a chronic and relapsing idiopathic disease characterized by segmental distribution of intestinal ulcers (skip lesions) intervened by normal-appearing mucosa. Although the distal ileum and proximal colon are affected most frequently, any portion of the bowel may be involved. The rectum is involved in up to 80% of patients, much more often than that of ulcerative colitis. Macroscopically, the intestine displays a thickened bowel wall, irregular glandular openings, mucosal fissuring, ulcerations, erosions, and benign strictures (Fig. 11-6). In chronic disease, the intestinal mucosa takes on a nodular or "cobblestoned" appearance as a result of dense inflammatory infiltrates and submucosa thickening. Transmural involvement of the intestinal wall and noncaseating epithelioid granulomas of the intestine and mesenteric lymph nodes are classic features of the disease.

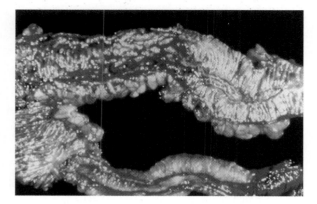

Fig. 11-6 Crohn's disease resulting in segmental edema and thickening of the bowel wall known as *skip lesions* that can lead to obstruction, ulceration and fistula. (Courtesy R. Estensen, Minneapolis, Minn.)

At the microscopic level, ulcerative colitis and Crohn's disease are characterized by infiltrative lesions of the bowel wall that contain activated inflammatory cells (neutrophils, macrophages) and immune-based cells (lymphocytes and plasma cells). These cells appear to be attracted to the region as a result of increased levels of interleukin 1 (IL-1) that stimulates the production of prostaglandins, leukotrienes, and other cytokines (e.g., tumor necrosis factor).[63-65] Mononuclear cells in the lamina propria of the bowel wall are the source of IL-1 and tumor necrosis factor release. Investigations are seeking to identify antigenic stimuli that provoke the release of IL-1.

Crohn's disease is characterized by remissions and relapses, with relapses more common in persons who smoke tobacco. Unremitting disease is complicated by small bowel stenosis and fistulas. The majority of patients who have Crohn's disease require at least one operation for their condition.[66] Long-standing disease also increases slightly the risk for the development of intestinal carcinoma.

CLINICAL PRESENTATION

SIGNS AND SYMPTOMS

Ulcerative Colitis
Patients with ulcerative colitis have three prominent symptoms: (1) attacks of diarrhea, (2) rectal bleeding (or bloody diarrhea), and (3) abdominal cramps. Onset may be sudden or insidious, but the disease continues in a chronic intermittent course in the majority of patients.

Dehydration, fatigue, weight loss, and fever frequently accompany the condition as a result of malabsorption of water and electrolytes. Extraintestinal manifestations may include arthritis, erythema nodosum or pyoderma gangrenosum, eye disorders like iritis and uveitis, and growth failure. While many patients have long periods of remission, less than 5% of patients remain symptom free over a 10-year period.[62]

Crohn's Disease
Signs and symptoms of Crohn's disease include recurrent or persistent diarrhea (often without blood), abdominal pain of the right lower quadrant, anorexia, unexplained fever, malaise, arthritis, uveitis, and weight loss. Symptoms vary from patient to patient according to the site and extent of involved alimentary tissue. For example, compromised intestinal lumen size can contribute to bowel obstruction and colicky pain that is aggravated by eating. In contrast, the patient may display rectal bleeding, a perirectal abscess or fistula, or dramatic weight loss. Variability in symptoms and the episodic pattern contribute to the average 3-year delay in diagnosis from onset of symptoms.[58] Complications of Crohn's disease include anemia, clubbing of the fingers, striking degrees of weight loss, and growth failure. Many of these findings result from malabsorption due to chronic inflammatory damage, transmural fibrosis, intestinal fissuring, fistulae, and abscess formation.

LABORATORY FINDINGS

The diagnosis of IBD is based primarily on the clinical findings, colonoscopy, biopsy, and histologic examination of intestinal mucosal. Intestinal radiographs (air-contrast barium enema), stool examinations, and electrolyte abnormalities are also supportive. Newer imaging techniques, including radiolabelled leukocyte scanning and computed tomography, are used to identify sites of activity and regions complicated by abscess and fistula formation.[67]

Ulcerative colitis produces friable, granular, erythematous and eroded mucosa with regions of edema and chronic inflammation upon endoscopic and microscopic inspection. Crohn's disease demonstrates patchy erosions and ulcerations with noncaseating granulomas. Blood tests in IBD may show anemia (deficiencies of iron, folate, or vitamin B_{12}) caused by malabsorption, decreased levels of serum total protein and albumin (as a result of malabsorption), and inflammatory activity (elevated erythrocyte sedimentation rate and C reactive protein) in conjunction with a negative microbial stool sample.

MEDICAL MANAGEMENT

Ulcerative colitis and Crohn's disease can be managed, but not cured, by an array of drugs. Antiinflammatory medications (sulfasalazine, 5-aminosalicylic acid, and corticosteroids) are generally first-line drugs. Immunosuppressive agents and antibiotics are used as second-line drugs. Third-line approaches for persons with Crohn's disease who are refractory to steroid treatment include monoclonal antibody (infliximab [Remicade]) against tumor necrosis factor,[68] or surgical resection to remove the diseased portion of the colon. Supportive therapy that includes bed rest, dietary manipulation, and nutritional supplementation are required with Crohn's disease to a greater degree than with ulcerative colitis. Dietary intervention with fish oil supplements may be beneficial to those with Crohn's disease.[69]

Over the past 20 years, sulfasalazine has been the cornerstone of therapy for patients with mild to moderate IBD. It is administered 4 g/day in divided doses for active disease and 1 g/day as a maintenance dose during remission.[70,71] Sulfasalazine is a conjugate of 5-aminosalicylic acid (5-ASA) and sulfapyridine linked by an azo bond.[72] After oral administration, the drug is cleaved by colonic bacteria into its 2 components. The therapeutic properties of sulfasalazine are primarily caused by the local effects of 5-ASA in the intestine. The adverse effects of sulfasalazine (nausea, headache, fever, arthralgia, rash, anemia, agranulocytosis, cholestatic hepatitis) have been ascribed to the sulfapyridine component and are dose-related and occur more often after long-term use. The side effect profile of sulfasalazine has contributed to its decreased popularity in recent years. Also, folic acid or iron supplementation is recommended during sulfasalazine therapy to combat the associated anemia.

The 5-ASA preparations are better tolerated and used more frequently in contemporary medicine. However, a problem with oral administration of 5-ASA by itself is that it is absorbed primarily in the proximal bowel and unable to reach the diseased colon. As a result, generic and controlled release oral formulations of 5-ASA (mesalamine [Asacol, Pentasa], olsalazine and balsalazide) have been developed that dissolve in the distal ileum and colon or are available as rectal suppository or enema.[62] Use of these drugs and rectally administered 5-ASA drugs are of great use in the management of ulcerative colitis when the disease is limited to distal segments (sigmoid) of the colon.[58] Renal function is monitored by the physician because 5-ASA drugs are potentially nephrotoxic.

Corticosteroids often are combined with sulfasalazine for patients who are moderately to severely ill. Steroids are not recommended for maintenance therapy of disease in remission because of adverse effects associated with long-term use. When severe attacks develop that produce abdominal tenderness, dehydration, fever, vomiting, and severe bloody diarrhea, the patient should be hospitalized and parenteral corticosteroids administered. After about 2 weeks, or once a satisfactory response is achieved, oral steroids are substituted for parenteral steroids. The dosage is gradually tapered every week so that the total steroid treatment course lasts only 4 to 8 weeks.

Second-line and third-line drugs are used in patients with progressive disease that is unresponsive to sulfasalazine and corticosteroids. Immunosuppressive agents, azathioprine (Imuran) and its metabolite 6-mercaptopurine are used only in conjunction with corticosteroids to reduce the amount of steroid needed and to limit steroid dose-dependent adverse effects. These immunosuppressives are limited by their side effects (agranulocytosis, pancreatitis, hepatitis and life-threatening infections). Cyclosporine, an immunosuppressant, also has been used intravenously to heal fistula caused by ulcerative colitis and Crohn's disease.[62] Bone marrow transplant has been associated with permanent remission.[73]

Methotrexate, an immunomodulator, and infliximab (anti-TNF monoclonal antibody) are used for severe disease and to maintain remission.[74] Infliximab is an expensive drug given specifically for Crohn's disease as a single two-hour infusion.[27] A single infusion induces remission in one third of patients within 4 weeks; however, relapses are likely after 3 months unless infusions are continued at 8- to 12-week intervals.[75]

Antibiotics (metronidazole or ciprofloxacin) have been used for active disease and to maintain remission. They also are used after surgery, if toxic colitis develops, or if fever and leukocytosis are present. Although opioids are used sometimes for their antidiarrheal effect, their use demands caution because these drugs can be addictive and detrimental to the course of therapy. Cromolyn sodium, a mast cell stabilizer, has been used in the rectum to diminish the release of inflammatory substances from mast cells and alter the course of disease. Supplemental iron is prescribed to some patients to control anemia. A clinical trial of growth hormone has been reported to reduce symptoms in patients with Crohn's disease.[76]

Surgery is recommended for severe cases of IBD when patients do not respond to corticosteroids or if complications develop (i.e., massive hemorrhage, obstruction, perforation, toxic megacolon, and carcinomatous transformation). A total proctocolectomy with ileostomy is the standard, but infrequent, operation for intractable ulcerative colitis. Approximately 70% of patients with Crohn's

disease require some form of surgery, and 40% of patients have recurrent disease requiring additional resections.[58]

DENTAL MANAGEMENT

MEDICAL CONSIDERATIONS

The use of a steroid drug by a patient with IBD is of concern to the dentist because corticosteroids can suppress adrenal function and reduce the ability of the patient to withstand stress. When a patient is taking corticosteroids, most routine dental care can be performed without the need for additional corticosteroids as long as adequate pain and anxiety control are obtained (Box 11-2). However, an adrenal crisis can be precipitated when a patient has recently discontinued the use of steroids and a particularly stressful or invasive procedure is performed that is associated with severe postoperative pain. In the latter circumstance, the need for supplemental corticosteroids should be determined according to the guidelines delineated in Chapter 15.

Immunosuppressors (AZA/6-MP) are associated with pancytopenia in approximately 5% of patients. Methotrexate is associated with hypersensitivity pneumonia and hepatic fibrosis, and cyclosporine can induce renal damage. Blood studies (complete blood count with differential, liver function and renal function studies) and coagulation studies should be obtained before invasive procedures are performed. For patients taking methotrexate, inquiries should be made as to the patient's breathing capacity. A review of the liver enzymes tests (assessed every 3 months) also should be performed. The presence of liver abnormalities dictates that management modifications be made based on the potential for altered drug metabolism and blood coagulation (see Chapter 10). In addition, a thorough head and neck examination should be performed on patients taking immunosuppressants because of increased the risk for lymphoma and infections (e.g., infectious mononucleosis, recurrent herpes). The development of fever for unknown reason in this select population dictates a prompt referral to the physician.

The criteria for analgesic selection is similar for patients with peptic ulcer disease and IBD. Aspirin and other NSAIDs are to be avoided. COX-2 inhibitors, acetaminophen alone or in combination with opioids may be used. A careful drug history should be obtained to avoid prescribing additional opioids to patients taking these medications to manage their intestinal pain.

TREATMENT PLANNING MODIFICATIONS

The severity, clinical course, and ultimate prognosis of patients with IBD are highly variable and can have an impact on routine dental care. Most patients with IBD have intermittent attacks, with asymptomatic remissions between attacks. Patients often require physical rest and emotional support throughout the disease as anxiety and depression may be severe. Only urgent dental care is advised during acute exacerbations of gastrointestinal disease. The clinician can assess the severity of the disease by assessing the patient's temperature and inquiring as to the number of diarrheal bowel movements occurring per day and whether blood is present in the stool.

Elective dental procedures should be scheduled during periods of remission when complications are absent and feelings of well being have returned. Flexibility in appointment scheduling may be required because of the unpredictability of the disease. When elective surgical procedures are scheduled for IBD patients taking sulfasalazine, the dentist should review preoperatively the patient's systemic health as well as obtain a complete blood count with differential and bleeding times. This can be important because, in addition to the immunosuppressive effects of their medications, sulfasalazine is associated with pulmonary, nephrotic, and hematologic abnormalities (i.e., variety of anemias, leukopenia, and thrombocytopenia).

ORAL COMPLICATIONS AND MANIFESTATIONS

Several oral complications have been associated with patients having IBD. Aphthous-like lesions affect up to 20% of patients with ulcerative colitis. Oral lesions erupt gen-

---

BOX 11-2

Pain and Anxiety Control Measures for Patients with Gastrointestinal Disease

1. Patients are advised to obtain proper rest the night before treatment.
   a. Benzodiazepine sedative (i.e., Dalmane) can be prescribed to be taken the night before treatment.
2. Appointments are tolerated best when they are scheduled in the morning and limited in duration.
3. Patients are advised to reduce business and social obligations the day of the appointment.
4. Intraoperative sedation by an oral, inhalation, or intravenous route can be provided.
5. Analgesic (COX-2 inhibitor, acetaminophen alone or in combination with opioid) should be provided during postoperative phase when needed.

erally during gastrointestinal flareups. The ulcers are mildly painful and may be of the major or minor variety. They affect alveolar, labial, buccal mucosa, soft palate, uvula and retromolar trigone, and may be difficult to distinguish from aphthous. Granularity or irregular margins may be helpful in the diagnosis (Fig. 11-7).

Pyostomatitis vegetans also can affect patients with ulcerative colitis and often aids in the diagnosis. To date, 37 cases have been reported in the literature.[77] This form of stomatitis produces raised, papillary, vegetative projections or pustules on an erythematous base of the labial mucosa, gingiva, and palate. The tongue rarely is involved. Without treatment, the initial erythematous appearance eventually degenerates into an ulcerative and suppurative mass. Treatment of both the aphthouslike lesions and pyostomatitis vegetans requires medical control of the colitis. Oral lesions that persist after anti-inflammatory drug therapy typically respond to repeated topical steroid applications. The vegetative growths can be eradicated by surgical means.

Unique oral manifestations of Crohn's disease occur in approximately 20% of patients and may precede the diagnosis of gastrointestinal disease by several years. Features include atypical mucosal ulcerations and diffuse swelling of the lips and cheeks. The ulcerations appear as linear mucosal ulcers with hyperplastic margins or papulonodular "cobblestone" proliferations of the mucosa. The proliferations often appear in the buccal vestibule and soft palate. Oral lesions are intermittent but chronically present. They become symptomatic when intestinal disease exacerbates. Like the oral lesions associated with ulcerative colitis, oral ulcerations of Crohn's disease resolve when the gastrointestinal state is medically controlled. Topical steroids are beneficial during symptomatic phases.

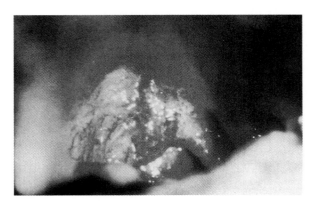

Fig. 11-7 Oral ulceration association with Crohn's disease. (Courtesy Robert P. Langlais, San Antonio, Tex.)

Use of sulfasalazine has been associated with a toxic effect on bone marrow, resulting in anemia, agranulocytosis, or thrombocytopenia. Corticosteroid use can result in osteopenia that may affect the alveolar bone. Methotrexate can cause oral mucositis and increase the frequency of recurrent oral herpes simplex virus infections. A discussion of the oral management of these abnormalities is found elsewhere in the text (see *Oral Complications, Peptic Ulcer Disease,* and Chapter 15).

■ PSEUDOMEMBRANOUS COLITIS ■

DEFINITION

Pseudomembranous colitis is a severe and sometimes fatal form of colitis that results from the overgrowth of *Clostridium difficile.* The overgrowth results from the loss of competitive anaerobic gut bacteria most commonly from use of broad-spectrum antibiotics, but can result from heavy metal intoxication and sepsis. *C. difficile* produces disease via potent enterotoxins that induce colitis and diarrhea.

EPIDEMIOLOGY

INCIDENCE AND PREVALENCE

Pseudomembranous colitis is the most common nosocomial infection of the gastrointestinal tract. The incidence of the disease is unknown. The reported incidence varies with type and frequency of antibiotic exposure. No gender predilection exists; however, the disease is more common in the elderly, patients in hospitals and nursing homes, and those who receive tube feeding.[78] Infants and young children rarely are affected.

ETIOLOGY

C. difficile is a gram-positive, spore-forming anaerobic rod that has been found in sand, soil, and feces. It colonizes the gut of 2% to 3% of asymptomatic adults and up to 50% of the elderly.[79] Risk of disease increases with prolonged use of broad-spectrum antibiotics that effectively eliminate commensal intestinal bacteria. As a result, *C. difficile* overgrows and produces an enterotoxin. The most frequently offending antimicrobial agents are those with greatest influence on the anaerobic flora of the colon. Highest risk is associated with lincomycin and clindamycin (2% to 20% of usage), ampicillin or amoxicillin (5% to 9% of usage), and cephalosporins (less than 2% of usage). Erythromycin, penicillins, sulfamethoxazole-trimethoprim (Bactrim, Septra), and tetracycline are

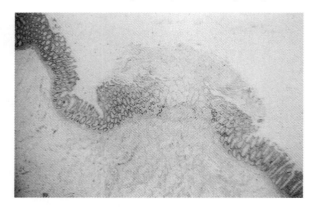

Fig. 11-8 Destruction of intestinal epithelium in pseudomembranous colitis. (Courtesy Deborah Powell, Lexington, Ky.)

involved less frequently, whereas aminoglycosides, antifungal agents, metronidazole, and vancomycin are rarely causative. In general, oral antibiotics are more often causative then parenteral antibiotics.[80]

PATHOPHYSIOLOGY

C. *difficile* produces enzymes that mediate tissue degradation, and toxins A and B that bind to intestinal mucosal cells resulting in cytoskeletal disaggregation and altered vascular permeability. As cells die, microscopic and macroscopic pseudomembranes form in the distal colon. Mild disease demonstrates punctate lesions, whereas severe disease demonstrates large coalescent plaques and extensive denuded areas. The microscopic composition of a pseudomembranous plaque is inflammatory cells, mucin, fibrin, and sloughed mucosal cells (Fig. 11-8).

CLINICAL PRESENTATION

SIGNS AND SYMPTOMS

Although the course of illness can be quite variable, diarrhea is the most common symptom. In mild cases, the stool is watery and loose. In severe cases, the bloody diarrhea is accompanied by numerous bowel movements, abdominal cramps and tenderness, and fever. Diarrhea often occurs within the first 4 to 10 days of antibiotic administration but may develop 1 day to 8 weeks after drug administration. Severe dehydration, metabolic acidosis, hypotension, peritonitis, and toxic megacolon are serious complications of untreated disease.

LABORATORY FINDINGS

Pseudomembranous colitis is associated with leukocytosis, leukocytic-laden stools, and a stool sample positive for C. *difficile* or one of its toxins as determined by enzyme immunoassay. Colonic, yellow-white pseudomembranes that are 5 to 10 mm in diameter are often visible upon sigmoidoscopy.

MEDICAL MANAGEMENT

Treatment of pseudomembranous colitis consists of discontinuing the use of the antimicrobial agent implicated as perturbing the intestinal flora, along with introducing an antibiotic that will eradicate the toxin-producing C. *difficile*. In patients with mild disease, cessation of the offending antibiotic is all that may be needed. In more severe cases, metronidazole (Flagyl, 250 mg four times a day for 7 to 10 days) by oral administration is the therapy of first choice. Vancomycin (125 to 500 mg four times a day for 7 to 10 days) is recommended for cases unresponsive to metronidazole. Both are active against all strains of C. *difficile*. However, C. *difficile* spores can survive treatment, and relapses occur in about 20% of patients. Intravenous fluids also are provided when electrolyte and fluid imbalances exist.

DENTAL MANAGEMENT

MEDICAL CONSIDERATIONS

The practitioner should be cognizant that the use of certain systemic antibiotics—especially lincomycin, clindamycin, ampicillin, and cephalosporins—is associated with a higher risk of pseudomembranous colitis in elderly, debilitated patients and in those with a previous history of pseudomembranous colitis. The decision to use an antibiotic should be based on sound, clinical judgment that these drugs are indeed necessary and should not be used in a cavalier manner. The dentist also should be aware that no reports exist of pseudomembranous colitis following short-term use of clindamycin in the American Heart Association prophylactic regimen.

TREATMENT PLANNING MODIFICATIONS

The dentist should delay elective dental care until after pseudomembranous colitis is resolved.

ORAL COMPLICATIONS AND MANIFESTATIONS

The use of systemic antibiotics for pseudomembranous colitis can result in fungal overgrowth (candidiasis) in the oral cavity.

References

1. Bouchier I et al: *Textbook of gastroenterology*, 1984, London, Bailliaere Tindall.
2. Lam S: Aetiological factors of peptic ulcer: perspectives of epidemiological observations this century, *J Gastroenterol Hepatol* 9:S93-S98, 1994.
3. Lam S: Differences in peptic ulcer between East and West, *Baillieres Best Pract Res Clin Gastroenterol* 14:41-52, 2000.
4. Hollander D, Tarnawaski A: Dietary essential fatty acids and the decline in peptic ulcer disease—a hypothesis, *Gut* 27:239-242, 1986.
5. Soll A, Isenberg J: Peptic ulcer disease: epidemiology, pathophysiology, clinical manifestations, and diagnosis. In Goldman L, editor: *Cecil textbook of medicine*, Philadelphia, 2000, WB Saunders Co.
6. Leoci C et al: Incidence and risk factors of duodenal ulcer: a retrospective cohort study, *J Clin Gastroenterol* 20:104-109, 1995.
7. McCarthy D: Nonsteroidal anti-inflammatory drug-related gastrointestinal toxicity: definitions and epidemiology, *Am J Med* 105:3S-9S, 1998.
8. Drumm B et al: Peptic ulcer disease in children: etiology, clinical findings, and clinical course, *Am J Meds* 82:410-414, 1988.
9. Sherman P: Peptic ulcer disease in children: diagnosis, treatment and implication of Helicobacter pylori, *Pediatr Gastroenterol* 23:707-725, 1994.
10. Euler A, Byrne W, Campbell M: Basal and pentagastrin-stimulated gastric acid secretory rates in normal children and in those with peptic ulcer disease, *J Pediatr* 103:766-768, 1983.
11. Walsh J, Peterson W: The treatment of *Helicobacter pylori* infection in the management of peptic ulcer disease, *N Engl J Med* 333:984-991, 1995.
12. Borum M: Peptic-ulcer disease in the elderly, *Clin Geriatr Med* 15:457-471, 1999.
13. Graham D: Helicobacter pylori infection in the pathogenesis of duodenal ulcer and gastric cancer: a model, *Gastroenterology* 113:1983-1991, 1997.
14. Marshall B, Warren J: Unidentified curved bacilli in the stomach of patients with gastritis and peptic ulceration, *Lancet* 1:1311-1315, 1984.
15. Warren J, Marshall B: Unidentified curved bacilli on gastric epithelium in active chronic gastritis, *Lancet* i:1273-1275, 1983.
16. Taylor D, Blaser M: The epidemiology of Helicobacter pylori infection, *Epidemiol Rev* 13:42-59, 1991.
17. Shames B et al: Evidence for the occurrence of the same strain of Campylobacter pylori in the stomach and dental plaque, *J Clin Microbiol* 27:2849-2850, 1989.
18. Dooley C et al: Prevalence of Helicobacter pylori infection and histologic gastritis in asymptomatic persons, *N Engl J Med* 321:1562-1566, 1989.
19. Graham D et al: Effect of triple therapy (antibiotics plus bismuth) on duodenal ulcer healing: a randomized controlled trial, *Ann Intern Med* 115:266-269, 1991.
20. Malaty H et al: Helicobacter pylori in Hispanics: comparison with blacks and whites of similar age and socioeconomic class, *Gastroenterology* 103:813-816, 1992.
21. Levenstein S: Peptic ulcer at the end of the 20th century: biological and psychological risk factors, *Can J Gastroenterol* 13:753-759, 1999.
22. Lanza F et al: Endoscopic comparison of esophageal and gastroduodenal effects of risedronate and alendronate in postmenopausal women, *Gastroenterology* 119:631-638, 2000.
23. Scott D et al: Actions of antiulcer drugs, *Science* 262:1453-1454, 1993.
24. Kikendall J, Evaul J, Honson L: Effect of cigarette smoking on gastrointestinal physiology and non-neoplastic digestive diesease, *J Clin Gastroenterol* 6:65-79, 1984.
25. Moss S, Calam J: Acid secretion and sensitivity to gastrin in patients with duodenal ulcer: effect of eradication of Helicobacter pylori, *Gut* 34:888-892, 1993.
26. Peterson W et al: Acid secretion and serum gastrin in normal subjects and patients with duodenal ulcer: the role of Helicobacter pylori, *Am J Gastroenterol* 88:2038-2043, 1993.
27. Wall G, Heyneman C, Pfanner T: Medical options for treating Crohn's disease in adults: focus on antitumor necrosis factor—a chimeric monoclonal antibody, *Pharmacother* 19:1138-1152, 1999.
28. Lehman E, Stalder G: Hypotheses on the role of cytokines in peptic ulcer disease, *Eur J Clin Invest* 28:511-519, 1998.
29. Wallace J et al: Secretagogue—specific effects of interleukin 1 on gastric acid secretion, *Am J Physiol Gastrointest Liver Physiol* 261:559-564, 1991.
30. Misiewicz J: Helicobacter pylori: past, present and future, *Scand J Gastroenterol* 27(suppl194):25-29, 1992.
31. Peterson W: Helicobacter pylori and peptic ulcer disease, *N Engl J Med* 324:1043-1048, 1991.
32. Saita H et al: Helicobacter pylori has an ulcerogenic action in the ischemic stomach of rats, *J Clin Gastroenterol* 141:S122-S126, 1992.
33. Zucca E et al: Molecular analysis of the progression from *Helicobacter pylori*-associated chronic gastritis to mucosa-associated lymphoid-tissue lymphoma of the stomach, *N Engl J Med* 338:804-810, 1998.
34. IARC Working Group on the evaluation of carcinogenic risks to humans: Schistosomes, liver flukes and *Helicobacter pylori*, *IARC Monogr Eval Carcinog Risks Hum* 61:1-241, 1994.
35. Hansson L: Risk of stomach cancer in patients with peptic ulcer disease, *World J Surg* 24:315-320, 2000.
36. Chiba N et al: *Helicobacter pylori* and peptic ulcer disease: current evidence for managment strategies, *Can Fam Phys* 44:1481-1488, 1998.
37. National Institutes of Health consensus development panel statement: Helicobacter pylori in peptic ulcer disease, *JAMA* 272:65-69, 1994.
38. Chiba N et al: Meta-analysis of the efficacy of antibiotic therapy in eradicating Helicobacter pylori, *Am J Gastroenterol* 87:1716-1727, 1992.
39. Bayerdorffer E et al: High dose omeprazole treatment combined with amoxicillin eradicates Helicobacter pylori, *Eur J Gastroenterol Hepato* 4:697-702, 1992.
40. Baggiolini M, Walz A, Kunkel S: Neutrophil-activating peptide-1/interleukin 8, a novel cytokine that activates neutrophils, *J Clin Invest* 84:1045-1049, 1989.

41. Hentschel E et al: Effect of ranitidine and amoxicillin plus metronidazole on the eradication of Helicobacter pylori and the recurrence of duodenal ulcer, N Engl J Med 328:308-312, 1993.

42. Labenz J et al: Amoxicillin plus omeprazole versus triple therapy for eradication of Helicobacter pylori in duodenal ulcer disease: a prospective, randomized, and controlled study, Gut 34:117-170, 1993.

43. Sonnenberg A, Townsen W: Costs of duodenal ulcer therapy with antibiotics, Arch Intern Med 155:922-928, 1995.

44. Forbes G et al: Duodenal ulcer treated with Helicobacter pylori eradication: seven-year follow-up, Lancet 343(258-260) 1994.

45. Falk G: Current status of Helicobacter pylori in peptic ulcer disease, Cleve Clin J Med 62:95-104, 1995.

46. Coghlan J et al: Campylobacter pylori and recurrence of duodenal ulcers–a 12-month follow-up study, Lancet 2:1109-1111, 1987.

47. Kornman M et al: Influence of cigarette smoking on healing and relapse in duodenal ulcer disease, Gastroenterology 85:871-874, 1983.

48. Svanes C: Trends in perforated peptic ulcer: incidence, etiology, treatment, and prognosis, World J Surg 24:277-283, 2000.

49. Borody T et al: Smoking does not contribute to duodenal ulcer relapse after Helicobacter pylori eradication, Am J Gastroenterol 87:1390-1393, 1992.

50. Morrow W, Hatzifoti C, Wren B: Helicobacter pylori vaccine strategies–triggering a gut reaction, Immunol Today 21:615-619, 2000.

51. Morrison B et al: The optimal analgesic dose of rofecoxib: overview of six randomized controlled trials, JADA 131:1720-1737, 2000.

52. Wolfe M, Lichtenstein D, Singh G: Gastrointestinal toxicity of nonsteroidal antiinflammatory drugs, N Engl J Med 340:1888-1899, 1999.

53. Nguyen A-MH et al: Nonsteroidal anti-inflammatory drug use in dentistry: gastrointestinal implications, Gen Dent 47:590-596, 1999.

54. Ehsanullah R et al: Prevention of gastroduodenal damage induced by nonsteroidal antiinflammtory drugs: controlled trial with ranitidine, Brit Med J 297:1017-1021, 1988.

55. Nguyen A-M, El-Zaatari F, Graham D: Helicobacter pylori in the oral cavity: a critical review of the literature, Oral Surg Oral Med Oral Pathol Oral Radiol Endod 76:705-709, 1995.

56. Gius J et al: Vascular formations of the lip and peptic ulcer, J Am Med Assoc 183:725-729, 1963.

57. Probert C et al: Epidemiological study of ulcerative protocolitis in Indian migrants and the indigenous population of Leicestershire, Gut 33:687-693, 1992.

58. Goldner F, Kraft S: Idiopathic inflammatory bowel disease I. In J. Stein, editor: Internal medicine, 1994, St Louis, Mosby.

59. Ogorek C, Fisher R: Differentiation between Crohn's disease and ulcerative colitis, Med Clin N Am 78:1249-1259, 1994.

60. Russel M, Stockbruegger R: Epidemiology of inflammatory bowel disease: an update, Scan J Gastroenterol 31:417-427, 1996.

61. The SSAT, AGA, ASLD, ASGE, AHPBA Consensus Panel: Ulcerative colitis and colon carcinoma: epidemiology, surveillance, diagnosis, and treatment, J Gastrointest Surg 2:305-306, 1998.

62. Ghosh S, Shand A, Ferguson A: Regular review: ulcerative colitis, BMJ 320:1119-1123, 2000.

63. Cominelli F et al: Regulation of eicosanoid production in rabbit colon by interleukin-1, Gastroenterology 97:1400-1405, 1989.

64. Rogler G, Andus T: Cytokines in inflammatory bowel disease, World J Surg 22:382-389, 1998.

65. Dinarello C, Wolff S: The role of interleukin-1 in disease, N Engl J Med 328:106-113, 1993.

66. Becker J: Surgical therapy for ulcerative colitis and Crohn's disease, Gastroenterol Clin N Am 28:371-390, 1999.

67. Rampton D: Management of Crohn's disease, BMJ 19:1480-1485, 1999.

68. D'Haens G: Infliximab (Remicade), a new biological treatment for Crohn's disease, Ital J Gastroenterol Hepatol 31:519-520, 1999.

69. Belluzi A et al: Effect of an enteric-coated fish-oil preparation on relapses in Crohn's disease, N Engl J Med 334:1557-1560, 1996.

70. Peppercorn M: Advances in drug therapy for inflammatory bowel disease, Ann Intern Med 112:50-60, 1990.

71. Ludwig D, Stange E: Treatment of ulcerative colitis, Hepato-Gastroenterol 47:83-89, 2000.

72. Hak S, Dukes G: Therapeutic advances in ulcerative colitis, Pharm Times Sept:110-120, 1991.

73. Kashyap A, Forman S: Autologous bone marrow transplantation for non-Hodgkin's lymphoma resulting in long-term remission of coincidental Crohn's disease, Br J Haematol 103:651-652, 1998.

74. Feagan B et al: A comparison of methotrexate with placebo for the maintenance of remission in Crohn's disease, N Engl J Med 342:1627-1632, 2000.

75. Rutgeerts P: Review article: efficacy of infliximab in Crohn's disease–induction and maintenance of remission, Aliment Pharmacol Therap 13 Suppl 4:9-15, 1999.

76. Slonim A et al: A preliminary study of growth hormone therapy for Crohn's disease, N Engl J Med 342:1633-1637, 2000.

77. Soriano M et al: Pyodermatitis-pyostomatitis vegetans: report of a case and review of the literature, Oral Surg Oral Med Oral Pathol Oral Radiol Endod 87:322-326, 1999.

78. Bliss D et al: Acquisition of Clostridium difficile and Clostridium difficile-associated diarrhea in hospitalized patient receiving tube feeding, Ann Intern Med 129:1012-1019, 1998.

79. Fekety R: Pseudomembranous colitis. In Goldman L, editor: Cecil textbook of medicine, Philadelphia, 2000, WB Saunders.

80. Brar H, Surawicz C: Pseudomembranous colitis: an update, Can J Gastroenterol 14:51-56, 2000.

Sexually Transmitted Diseases

12

CHAPTER

Sexually transmitted diseases (STDs) are a major health problem in the United States and the world and in many instances are on the increase. In the United States some of the highest rates of infection occur in adolescents and young adults. More than 25 STDs have been identified (Table 12-1). Current estimates predict that more than 65 million Americans are infected with one or more STDs, and 15 million new infections occur annually.[1] The morbidity and mortality rates of STDs vary from minor inconvenience or irritation to severe disability and death. The diagnosis of an STD also has psychosocial effects.

STDs have important implications for dentistry. First, many STDs have oral manifestations. Second, some STDs can be transmitted by direct contact with lesions, blood, and saliva. Because many patients may be asymptomatic, the dentist must approach all patients as though disease transmission were possible and adhere to universal precautions. Third, the presence of one STD is accompanied by additional STDs in approximately 10% of cases, and an STD-associated genital ulceration increases the risk for human immunodeficiency virus (HIV) infection.[2,3] Fourth, because STDs exhibit antimicrobial resistance, proper treatment is essential.[4] Fifth, dental healthcare workers can be an important component of STD control through diagnosis, education, and referral.

The prototypical STDs—gonorrhea, syphilis, genital herpes, and human papillomavirus infections—are of special interest or importance to dental practice and will serve to illustrate basic principles. Infectious mononucleosis also is discussed briefly; although not typically classified as an STD, it is transmitted by intimate contact (see Chapters 10 and 13).

■ GONORRHEA ■

DEFINITION

Gonorrhea is a worldwide sexually transmitted disease caused by *Neisseria gonorrhoeae*. It produces symptoms in men that usually cause them to seek treatment soon enough to prevent serious sequelae but may not be soon enough to prevent transmission to others. Infections in women often do not produce recognizable symptoms until complications have occurred. Because gonococcal infections among women often are asymptomatic, an important component of gonorrhea control in the United States continues to be the screening of women at high risk for STDs.

INCIDENCE AND PREVALENCE

Gonorrhea is the second-most-commonly reported infectious STD in the United States behind chlamydia, with 355,642 cases reported to the Centers for Disease Control and Prevention (CDC) in 1998.[5,6] Although the reported incidence has been decreasing since 1979, when more than 1 million cases were reported, cases are rising again among young people. Within the last 3 years, rates have increased among adolescents, gay and bisexual men, and blacks.[1] Incidence trends reflect increased awareness of disease transmission because of the AIDS epidemic with compensatory decreased awareness of other STDs. Clinicians should realize that the incidence figures of the CDC are an underestimation because of underreporting, and that approximately 600,000 new infections with gonorrhea occur each year in the United States. Humans are the only

TABLE 12-1

Sexually Transmitted Diseases

Disease	Organism
Acquired immune deficiency syndrome (AIDS)	Human immunodeficiency virus (HIV)
Amebiasis	*Entamoeba histolytica*
Bacterial vaginosis	*Bacteroides* spp., *Mobiluncus* spp.
Chancroid	*Haemophilus ducreyi*
Condyloma acuminatum (genital warts)	Human papillomavirus infection (HPV-6, [ql HPV-11)
Cytomegalovirus infection	Cytomegalovirus
Enterobiasis	*Enterobius vermicularis*
Epididymitis, mucopurulent cervicitis, lymphogranuloma venereum, nongonococcal urethritis, pelvic inflammatory disease, Reiter's syndrome	*Chlamydia trachomatis*
Epididymitis, gonorrhea, mucopurulent cervicitis, pelvic inflammatory disease	*Neiseria gonorrhoeae*
Genital herpes	Herpes simplex viruses (HSV-1, HSV-2)
Giardiasis	*Giardia lamblia*
Granuloma inguinale	*Calymmatobacterium granulomatis*
Hepatitis B	Hepatitis B virus (HBV)
Molluscum contagiosum	Poxvirus
Nongonococcal urethritis, nonspecific vaginitis	*Trichomoniasis vaginalis*
Nongonococcal urethritis	*Ureaplasma urealyticum*
Pediculosis	*Pediculus pubis*
Salmonellosis	*Salmonella* spp.
Shigellosis	*Shigella* spp.
Streptococcal infections	Streptococcal group B spp.
Syphilis	*Treponema pallidum*
Vulvovaginal candidiasis	*Candida* spp., *Torulopsis* spp.

natural host for this disease. The transmission of N. *gonorrhoeae* is almost exclusively via sexual contact—whether genital-genital, oral-genital, or rectal-genital. The primary sites of infection are the genitalia, anal canal, and pharynx.

Gonorrhea can occur at any age, though it is seen most commonly in the 15- to 29-year age group.[5] Rates of infections differ by racial background, with African-Americans having 2 to 5 times higher rates than whites and Hispanics.[5] Risk factors other than age include having a first sexual experience at a young age, multiple sexual partners, low education, low socioeconomic standing, and being an urban dweller.[7] Through the mid-1990s, cases were reported more commonly in men than in women; however, the 1998 CDC data indicate that reportable cases have increased in women (with a male-female ratio of 1.02:1).[2,5] At the current rate of 132.88/100,000 population, an average dental practice of 2000

adult patients can expect to have about 2 patients with gonorrhea.[5]

ETIOLOGY

N. *gonorrhoeae* is a gram-negative diplococcus commonly found within polymorphonuclear leukocytes. N. *gonorrhoeae* is an aerobe that requires high humidity and specific temperature and pH for optimum growth. It is a fragile bacterium readily killed by drying, so it is not easily transmitted by fomites. It develops resistance to antibiotics rather easily, and many strains have become resistant to penicillin and tetracycline as well as to other antibiotics.

PATHOPHYSIOLOGY AND COMPLICATIONS

The pathophysiology of gonorrhea is significant in that of N. *gonorrhoeae* is influenced by the type of host epithelium

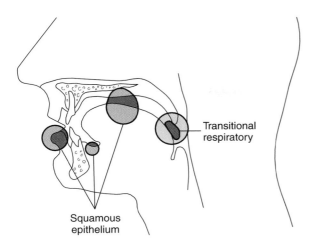

Fig. 12-1 Areas of relative epithelial susceptibility to infection by *Neisseria gonorrhoeae* within the oral cavity.

influences the invasiveness of the bacterium. Columnar epithelium (as found in the mucosal lining of the urethra and cervix) and transitional epithelium (as in the oropharynx and rectum) are highly susceptible to infection, whereas stratified squamous epithelium (skin and mucosal lining of the oral cavity) is generally resistant to infection.[8] This explains the occurrence of rectal, pharyngeal, and tonsillar infection and the relative infrequency of oral infection. Another indication of the resistance of skin to gonococcal infection is the fact that no reported cases exist of gonorrhea of the fingers. Fig. 12-1 depicts areas of relative epithelial susceptibility to N. *gonorrhoeae* infection in the oral cavity and oropharynx.

Infection in men usually begins in the anterior urethra. The bacteria invade subepithelial tissues and produce a purulent exudate. The infection may remain localized or extend to the posterior urethra, bladder, epididymis, prostate, or seminal vesicles and is spread by means of lymphatics and blood vessels. Gonococcemia, although present in only 1% to 2% of cases, may occur and cause dissemination of the disease to distant body sites.

Infection in women occurs most commonly in the cervix and urethra. The same subepithelial invasion with production of purulent exudate occurs. The infection tends to be less severe in women but may spread to the endometrium, fallopian tubes, ovaries, and pelvic peritoneum. Disseminated gonorrhea also can occur, with varying frequency. Many cases of pelvic inflammatory disease are a result of gonococcal infection. Both symptomatic and asymptomatic cases of pelvic inflammatory disease can result in tubal scarring that leads to infertil-

ity or ectopic pregnancy. Vertical transmission accounts for a small percentage of cases in the United States.

In both genders, gonorrhea of the rectum may occur after anal-genital intercourse or by direct anal contamination from genital lesions. Infection of the pharynx and oral cavity is seen predominantly in women and homosexual men following fellatio. It also is seen occasionally following cunnilingus. Gonococcemia can lead to widespread dissemination and result in a variety of disorders, including migratory arthritis, skin and mucous membrane lesions, endocarditis, meningitis, pelvic inflammatory disease, and pericarditis.

CLINICAL PRESENTATION

SIGNS AND SYMPTOMS

In men, symptoms usually occur after an incubation period of 2 to 5 days. The most common findings include a mucopurulent urethral discharge, pain on urination, urgency, and frequency. Tenderness and swelling of the meatus may occur. In women, a significant percentage of cases may be asymptomatic or only minimally symptomatic. Women who have a symptomatic infection may demonstrate vaginal or urethral discharge and dysuria with frequency and urgency. Backache and abdominal pain also may be present. Approximately 50% of women and 1% to 3% of men are asymptomatic or only mildly symptomatic.[9] These patients may not seek medical care for their problem and as a result constitute a large reservoir of infection.

Gonococcal infection of the anal canal is commonly less intense than genital infection. Similar symptoms can be noted, including a copious purulent discharge and pain.

Within the oral cavity, the pharynx is most commonly affected. Pharyngeal infection is found in 3% to 7% of heterosexual men, 10% to 20% of heterosexual women, and 10% to 25% of homosexual men.[9] The condition usually is seen as an asymptomatic infection with diffuse, nonspecific inflammation or as a mild sore throat. The likelihood of transmission of pharyngeal gonorrhea to the genitalia is much less than that of genital-genital transmission.[10,11] Of significance, however, is the fact that N. *gonorrhoeae* has been cultured from the expectorated saliva of two thirds of patients with oropharyngeal gonorrhea.[10]

Gonococcal stomatitis or oral gonorrhea is uncommon, although several case reports[9,12-15] confirm its existence. Many of the reported cases of oral gonorrhea, however, lack definitive laboratory identification of N. *gonorrhoeae* and are based on presumptive evidence. Chue[16] has presented a review of the varied and nonspecific manifestations of oral gonorrhea. These include

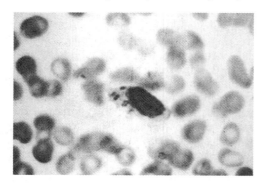

Fig. 12-2 Smear demonstrates gram-negative diplococci within a leukocyte. (Courtesy H.D. Wilson, Lexington, Ky.)

acute ulceration, diffuse erythema, necrosis of the interdental papillae, lingual edema, edematous tissues that bleed easily, vesiculations, and a pseudomembrane that is nonadherent and leaves a bleeding surface on removal. Lesions may be solitary or widely disseminated. Symptoms include burning or itching sensation, dryness, increased salivation, bad taste, fetid breath, fever, and submandibular lymphadenopathy. The lesions of oral gonorrhea may resemble closely the lesions of erythema multiforme, bullous or erosive lichen planus, or herpetic gingivostomatitis. In a separate report, Chue[17] describes acute temporomandibular joint arthritis caused by disseminated gonococcal infection from a genital site.

LABORATORY FINDINGS

Laboratory diagnosis of N. *gonorrhoeae* infection can be made presumptively in genital infection from finding gram-negative diplococci within polymorphonuclear leukocytes in a smear of purulent discharge (Fig. 12-2). However, culture is the gold standard for the diagnosis of N. *gonorrhoeae*. The use of DNA probes and ligase chain reaction assays are highly sensitive and specific for the organism[7] and can be used (e.g., GenProbe PACE system) to simultaneously test for C. *trachomatis*. In suspected cases of oropharyngeal gonorrhea, a smear and Gram stain are not as helpful because other species of *Neisseria* are normal inhabitants of the oral cavity. Therefore culturing with selective media or using ligase chain reaction is necessary.

MEDICAL MANAGEMENT

The CDC recommendation[18] provides several choices for the treatment of uncomplicated gonococcal infec-

tion of the cervix, urethra, and rectum. All are single dose regimens. They include oral Cefixime 400 mg orally in a single dose or injectable ceftriaxone 125 mg intramuscularly in a single dose, or a quinolone (ciprofloxacin [Cipro]); 500 mg orally single dose; or ofloxacin (Floxin) 400 mg orally single dose, plus coverage against the common coinfecting organism *Chlamydia trachomatis* with Azithromycin 1 g orally in a single dose, or doxycycline (100 mg orally two times a day for 7 days). For patients who cannot take ceftriaxone, spectinomycin (2 g intramuscularly) is the preferred alternative.[18] A notably low (0.9%) treatment failure rate with ceftriaxone-doxycycline exists in the United States, and follow-up cultures are not considered essential unless symptoms persist. Following the institution of antibiotic therapy, infectiousness is diminished rapidly within a matter of hours.[11,19] Infections detected after treatment are generally the result of reinfection from a sexual partner, not from treatment failure. Quinolone-resistant strains are sporadic in the United States but more common in the Far East[20]; thus the clinician must be aware of patient travel.[21] Because quinolone-resistant strains still comprise less than 1% of all N. *gonorrhoeae* strains isolated in sentinel North American cities, the fluoroquinolone regimens still are being recommended for use.

Because gonococcal pharyngitis is more difficult to eradicate than infections at urogenital and anorectal sites (few antigonococcal regimens reliably can cure such infections greater than 90% of the time) treatment duration may be longer. As with all STDs, sex partners of all patients who have N. *gonorrhoeae* infection should be evaluated and treated.

■ SYPHILIS ■

DEFINITION

Syphilis is an acute and chronic STD caused by *Treponema pallidum* that produces skin and mucous membrane lesions in the acute phase. In the chronic phase, bone, viscera, cardiovascular, and neurological disease are produced. The variety of systemic manifestations associated with the later stages of syphilis resulted in its being historically designated as the "great imitator" disease. As with gonorrhea, humans are the only known natural host for syphilis. The primary site of syphilitic infection is the genitalia, although primary lesions also occur extragenitally.[22] Syphilis remains an important infection in contemporary medicine because of the morbidity it causes and its ability to enhance the transmission of HIV.[23]

EPIDEMIOLOGY

INCIDENCE AND PREVALENCE

Syphilis is the fourth-most-frequently reported STD in the United States, surpassed only by chlamydia, gonorrhea, and AIDS. In 1990 the incidence of primary and secondary syphilis peaked at 50,223 cases.[10] The number of primary and secondary syphilis cases dropped to 20,627 by 1994.[6] A total of 6,657 primary and secondary syphilis cases were reported to the CDC in 1999.[1] During the past decade the rate of primary and secondary syphilis has declined 87%, from 20.3 cases per 100,000 population to 2.6 per 100,000.[5] The disease is at its lowest level since reporting began in 1941. Disproportionately high numbers of cases continue to occur in the South and among Hispanic and non-Hispanic black men and women. Syphilis remains most common in persons aged 20 through 40 years, with a greater incidence in males than females, by more than 2 to 1.[5]

The transmission of syphilis is predominantly sexual, including oral-genital and rectal-genital; however, transmission also can occur via nonsexual means such as kissing, blood transfusion, or accidental inoculation with a contaminated needle. Indirect transmission by fomites is possible but uncommon because the organism survives only a short time out of the body.[22] Congenital syphilis occurs when the fetus is infected in utero by an infected mother. In 1998 a total of 801 cases of congenital syphilis were reported to the CDC. This represents a rate of 20.6 per 100,000 live births, a sharp decline from a peak of 107.3 cases per 100,000 live births in 1991.[5]

ETIOLOGY

The etiologic agent of syphilis is *Treponema pallidum*, a slender, fragile, anaerobic spirochete. *T. pallidum* is easily killed by heat, drying, disinfectants, and soap and water. The organism is difficult to stain, except with certain silver impregnation methods. Demonstration is best done using dark-field microscopy with a fresh specimen.

PATHOPHYSIOLOGY

T. pallidum does not invade completely intact skin but can invade intact mucosal epithelium and gain entry via minute abrasions or hair follicles. Within a few hours after invasion, bacterial spread to the lymphatics and bloodstream occurs, resulting in early widespread dissemination of the disease. The early response to the bacterial invasion is an endarteritis and periarteritis.[22] Risk of

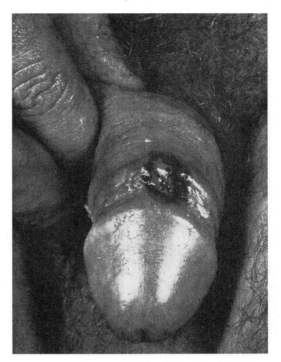

Fig. 12-3 Primary syphilis: chancre of the penis. (From Rudolph AH: In Top FH, Wehrle PF, editors: *Communicable and infectious diseases,* ed 8, St Louis, 1976, Mosby.)

transmission occurs during the primary, secondary, and early latent stages of disease but not in late syphilis.[24] Overall, patients are most infectious during the first 2 years of the disease.

CLINICAL PRESENTATION

SIGNS AND SYMPTOMS

The manifestations and descriptions of syphilis are classically divided into stages of occurrence, with each stage having its own peculiar signs and symptoms related to time and antigen-antibody responses. The stages are primary, secondary, latent, tertiary, and congenital.

Primary Syphilis

The classic manifestation of primary syphilis is the chancre, a solitary granulomatous lesion at the site of contact with the infectious organism. Accompanying the chancre are enlarged regional lymph nodes. The chancre usually occurs within 2 to 3 weeks after exposure (Fig. 12-3). Patients are infectious, however, before

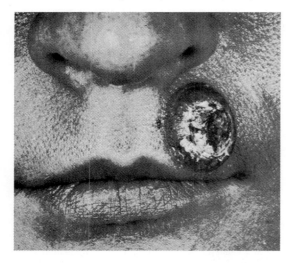

Fig. 12-4 Primary syphilis: extragenital chancre of the lip. (From Rudolph AH: In Top FH, Wehrle PF, editors: *Communicable and infectious diseases,* ed 8, St Louis, 1976, Mosby.)

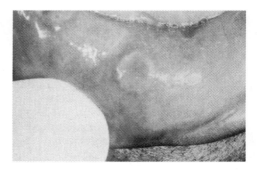

Fig. 12-6 Secondary syphilis: mucous patch of the lower lip.

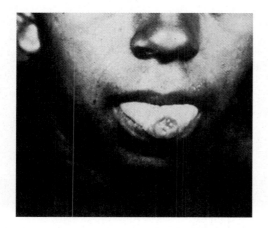

Fig. 12-5 Primary syphilis: extragenital chancre of the tongue.

one appears. The lesion begins as a small papule and enlarges to form a surface erosion or ulceration that commonly is covered by a yellowish hemorrhagic crust that teems with T. *pallidum*. It is commonly painless. Associated with the chancre are enlarged, painless, hard regional lymph nodes. The chancre usually subsides in 3 to 6 weeks, leaving variable scarring in the form of a healed papule.[22,25] The genitalia, oral cavity (lips, tongue), fingers, nipples, and anus are common sites for chancres (Figs. 12-4, 12-5).

Secondary Syphilis

The manifestations of secondary syphilis appear 6 to 8 weeks after initial exposure. The chancre may have completely resolved by this time. Symptoms and signs of secondary syphilis include fever, arthralgia and malaise, and generalized lymphadenopathy; 80% develop generalized eruptions of the skin and mucous membranes. The papules of the rash are well demarcated, have a coppery hue, and have a predilection for the palms and soles. Oral manifestations of secondary syphilis include pharyngitis, papular lesions, erythematous or grayish white erosions (mucous patches, Fig. 12-6), irregular linear erosions, and rarely parotid gland enlargement. The lesions of skin and mucous membranes are highly infectious.[22,25] However, even without treatment secondary syphilis ultimately resolves.

Latent Syphilis

Latent syphilis is the third stage of the untreated infection. Patients are seroreactive but asymptomatic and show no clinical evidence of disease. Latent syphilis is divided into early latent syphilis (acquired the disease within the preceding year) and late latent syphilis (more than 1 year). During the first 4 years of latent syphilis, patients may have mucocutaneous relapses and are considered infectious. After 4 years, relapses do not occur and patients are considered noninfectious (except for blood transfusions and pregnant women).[22] The latent stage may last for many years or for the remainder of the person's life. In some untreated patients, progression to tertiary syphilis will occur.

Tertiary Syphilis

The tertiary (late) stage occurs in 10% to 40% of untreated persons generally several years after onset of syphilis and is the destructive stage of the disease.[26] Patients are noninfectious. Any organ of the body (mucocutaneous, os-

seous, visceral or neural) may be involved. Signs and symptoms of this stage do not occur until years after the initial infection.

The gumma—the classic localized lesion of tertiary syphilis—may involve the skin, mucous membranes, bone, nervous tissue, and viscera. Researchers believe the condition to be the end result of a hypersensitivity reaction, basically an inflammatory granulomatous lesion with a central zone of necrosis that is not infectious.

All the other manifestations of tertiary syphilis are essentially vascular in nature and result from an obliterative endarteritis. Cardiovascular syphilis is most commonly seen as an aneurysm of the ascending aorta. Neurosyphilis can result in a meningitis-like syndrome, Argyll Robertson pupils (which react to accommodation but not to light), altered tendon reflexes, general paresis, or tabes dorsalis (degeneration of dorsal columns of the spinal cord and sensory nerve trunks).

The oral lesions of tertiary syphilis are a diffuse interstitial glossitis and the gumma. The interstitial glossitis should be considered a premalignant condition. The tongue may appear lobulated and fissured with atrophic papillae, resulting in a bald and wrinkled surface. Leukoplakia frequently is present. The oral gumma is a rare lesion that most commonly involves the tongue and palate. It appears as a firm tissue mass with central necrosis. Palatal gummas may perforate into the nasal cavity or maxillary sinus.

Congenital Syphilis

Syphilis and its sequelae occur in the newborn if the mother is infected while carrying the child. The disease is transmitted to the fetus in utero, usually after the 16th week, since before this time the placenta prevents transmission of bacteria. The disease persists worldwide because a substantial number of women do not receive syphilis serologic testing during pregnancy or receive the testing too late in pregnancy and often do not receive prenatal care.[27] Physical manifestations vary depending on the time of infection. The sequelae of early infection include osteochondritis, periostitis (frontal bossing of Parrot), rhinitis, rash, and ectodermal changes. Syphilis contracted during late pregnancy can involve bones, teeth, eyes, cranial nerves, viscera, skin, and mucous membranes. A classic triad of congenital syphilis known as Hutchinson's triad includes interstitial keratitis of the cornea, eighth nerve deafness and dental abnormalities (i.e., Hutchinson's incisors and mulberry molars [Fig. 12-7]).

LABORATORY FINDINGS

T. *pallidum* never has been cultured successfully on any kind of medium; therefore the definitive diagnosis of

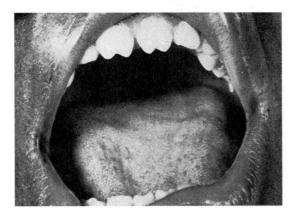

Fig. 12-7 Congenital syphilis: Hutchinsonian teeth. (From Rudolph AH: In Top FH, Wehrle PF, editors: *Communicable and infectious diseases,* ed 8, St Louis, 1976, Mosby.)

syphilis is made from a positive dark-field microscopic examination or direct fluorescent antibody tests on fresh lesion exudate. Dark-field examination is consistently positive only during primary and early secondary stages. Definitive diagnosis of oral lesions by this method is difficult because other *Treponema* species are indigenous to the oral cavity.

Although dark-field examination is the only way to make a definitive diagnosis of syphilis, the serologic test for syphilis furnishes presumptive evidence. These serologic tests are of two basic types (indirect and direct) and are differentiated by the type of antibodies they investigate.

Screening Serologic Tests for Syphilis

The standard screening tests for syphilis are the venereal disease research laboratory slide test (VDRL), the rapid plasma reagin (RPR) test, and the automated reagin test. These indirect, nontreponemal serological tests are designed to detect the presence of an antibody-like substance called reagin that is produced when T. *pallidum* reacts with various body tissues. The tests are equally valid. A disadvantage of reaginic tests is the occasional biologic false-positive result that can occur.

Nontreponemal tests produce titers (reported quantitatively as serologic dilutions, e.g., 1:2, 1:4, 1:8) that usually correlate with disease activity. Test results are consistently positive and yield the highest titers between 3 and 8 weeks after the appearance of the primary chancre. In primary syphilis, the nontreponemal tests usually revert to negative within 12 months after successful treatment. In secondary syphilis, up to 24 months may be required for the patient to become seronegative.

Occasionally patients will remain seropositive for the rest of their lives or test positive with an associated infection or condition (false-positive). With tertiary syphilis, many patients remain seropositive for life.[2]

Confirmatory Serologic Tests for Syphilis

Treponemal tests are designed to detect the specific antibody produced against treponemes, which cause syphilis, yaws, and pinta.[22] The tests are more specific than the reaginic tests but less sensitive. Thus they typically are performed after a positive VDRL slide test or RPR test. The T. *pallidum* immobilization test, fluorescent treponemal antibody test, fluorescent treponemal antibody absorption test, and microhemagglutination-assay for antibody to T. *pallidum* are examples.[2] The microhemagglutination-assay for antibody to T. *pallidum* and fluorescent treponemal antibody absorption tests are the most commonly used. Treponemal antibody titers wane over time but remain positive in approximately 80% of patients regardless of treatment. Thus they should not be used to assess response to treatment. Polymerase chain reaction for specific treponemal DNA sequences can be helpful in confirming the diagnosis when other studies are not helpful.[28]

MEDICAL MANAGEMENT

The current medical management of primary, secondary or early latent syphilis includes the use of parenteral long-acting benzathine penicillins (e.g., penicillin G, 2.4 million units intramuscularly in single dose). Alternate drugs for patients allergic to penicillin include oral doxycycline (100 mg orally two times a day for 2 weeks for the primary stage) and erythromycin (500 mg orally four times a day for 2 weeks for the primary stage) or ceftriaxone sodium intramuscularly injection.[18] Testing for HIV status also is recommended. After treatment, patients periodically should be retested serologically to monitor their conversion to negative. This conversion usually will occur within a year. A low failure rate exists in the treatment of syphilis. Noteworthy in the management of syphilis is that, as with gonorrhea, infectiousness is reversed rapidly, probably within a matter of hours on initiation of medical treatment.[19,22] The Jarisch-Herxheimer reaction, manifested by fever, chills, myalgias, and headache, occurs in more than 50% of patients after treatment for syphilis is initiated.

Congenital syphilis is managed best by implementation of preventive measures. This requires that all pregnant women be tested for syphilis by serology. If positive, the expectant mother should be treated with penicillin and retested at the 28th week and again at delivery. Infants born to seroreactive mothers should be evaluated with a nontreponemal serologic test and if positive treated with intravenous penicillin G for at least 10 days post-partum. Although treatment is recommended for congenital and tertiary stage of syphilis, response is limited by the extent of damage already incurred.

■ GENITAL HERPES ■

DEFINITION

Genital herpes is a recurrent, incurable viral infection of the genitalia caused by one of two closely related types of herpes simplex virus (HSV) types 1 and 2. Most genital herpes infections are caused by HSV-2. The disease has acute and recurrent phases, and is associated with high rates of subclinical infection and viral shedding. The prevalence of genital herpes has increased by 30% since the late 1970s.[29]

EPIDEMIOLOGY

INCIDENCE AND PREVALENCE

HSV-2 is an important STD in the United States as well as the world. Its exact incidence is unknown because it is not a reportable disease and most persons have not been diagnosed because their disease is mild or asymptomatic. Approximately 45 million persons, or 22% of persons 12 years and older, in the United States are infected.[18,29] Moreover, 750,000 people seroconvert annually in the United States.[30] The prevalence in developing countries is between 40% and 60%.[31] Many cases of genital herpes are acquired from persons who are asymptomatic at the time of sexual contact or do not know that they have genital herpes. Approximately 70% to 95% of first-episode cases of genital herpes are caused by HSV-2, whereas 5% to 30% are caused by HSV-1.[18] The prevalence is 46% in African-Americans and 18% in whites.[29]

ETIOLOGY

HSV belongs to the herpesviridae family, which also includes cytomegalovirus, Epstein-Barr virus, varicella-zoster virus, human herpesvirus type 6 (HHV-6), human herpesvirus type 7 (HHV-7), and Kaposi's sarcoma associated herpesvirus (HHV-8). HSV-1 is the causative agent of most herpetic infections that occur above the waist, especially on the mucosa of the mouth (herpetic gingivostomatitis, herpes labialis), nose, eyes, brain, and

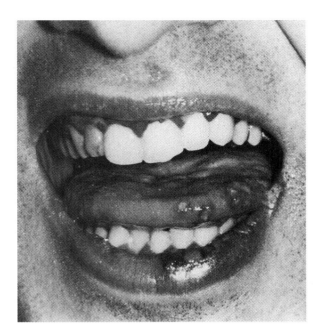

Fig. 12-8 Primary herpes simplex type 2 occurring in the oral cavity documented by laboratory testing. (Courtesy R.C. Noble, Lexington, Ky.)

skin. Infection with HSV-1 is extremely common; most adults demonstrate antibodies to this virus. Many primary infections with HSV-1 are subclinical and thus are never known to the infected person. Transmission is usually by close contact, such as touching or kissing and transfer of infective saliva. HSV-1 also is transmitted via sexual contact. Airborne droplet infection is not well demonstrated, although it is possible.[32] Autoinoculation to the face, fingers, eyes, and genitalia is a persistent clinical problem.

HSV-2 is the causative agent of most herpes infections that occur below the waist, such as in or around the genitalia (genital herpes). HSV-2 is transmitted predominantly by sexual contact but also may be passed nonsexually. Its primary mode of transmission is from an asymptomatic viral shedder. HSV-2 can be transmitted to a newborn from an infected mother. Although the primary site of occurrence of HSV-1 is above the waist and that of HSV-2 below the waist, each infection may occur in either site and can be inoculated from one site to the other[33] (Fig. 12-8). The type cannot be differentiated clinically.

PATHOPHYSIOLOGY

The pathologic process of herpesvirus infections of HSV-1 and HSV-2 are essentially identical, and as such the lesions of skin and mucous membranes are identical. The infection arises from intimate contact with a lesion or infective fluid (e.g., saliva). Epithelial cells are invaded and viral replication occurs. Characteristic cellular changes include ballooning degeneration, intranuclear inclusion bodies, and the formation of multinucleated giant cells. With cellular destruction comes inflammation and increasing edema, which results in a papular formation and fluid-filled vesicles. The vesicles rupture, leaving an ulcerated or crusted surface.

Lymphadenopathy and viremia are prominent features. In normal individuals, the infection is contained by usual host defenses. However, spreading to other epidermal sites (i.e., herpetic whitlow—infection of the fingers, eyes [keratoconjunctivits], pharynx and neonates during childbirth) has been documented. In rare cases infants and immunosuppressed persons can develop systemic meningitis and widespread infection that can result in significant morbidity and death.

As the infection runs its course, usually in 10 to 20 days, the viruses enter the ends of local peripheral neurons and migrate up the axon to the regional ganglion (HSV-1 primarily in the trigeminal, and HSV-2 primarily in the sacral), where they reside latently. After stimulation such as trauma, sunlight, menses, or intercourse the virus reactivates, migrates down the axon, and produces a recurrent infection with lesions similar to the primary but less severe in nature and more localized. Of the two HSV serotypes that can infect the sacral ganglia, HSV-2 is more efficient in reactivating and producing recurrent genital lesions.

CLINICAL PRESENTATION

SIGNS AND SYMPTOMS

Approximately 60% of cases of primary HSV-2 infection are asymptomatic,[30] with newly acquired cases being asymptomatic more frequently in men than in women. After an incubation period of 2 to 7 days, lesions (papules, vesicles, ulcers, crusts and fissures) of primary genital herpes can appear. In women, both internal and external genitalia may be involved as may the perineal region and skin of the thighs and buttocks. In men, the external genitalia may be involved as may the skin of the inguinal area. Lesions in moist areas tend to ulcerate early, are painful, and can cause dysuria. Lesions on exposed dry areas tend to remain pustular or vesicular then crust over (Fig. 12-9). Painful regional lymphadenopathy accompanies the infection with headache, malaise, myalgia, and symptoms of fever. These subside in about 2 weeks, with healing in 3 to 5 weeks.[33]

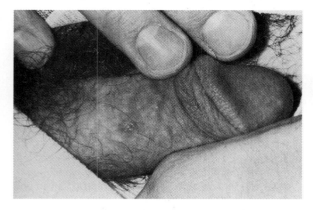

Fig. 12-9 Solitary herpetic lesion on the shaft of the penis. (Courtesy R.C. Noble, Lexington, Ky.)

Recurrent genital herpes is generally a less severe infection than the primary infection and is frequently precipitated by menses or intercourse. A prodrome of localized itching, tingling, pain, and burning may be noted and is followed by a vesicular eruption. Healing occurs in 10 to 14 days. Constitutional symptoms are generally absent. Between recurrences infected persons shed virus intermittently in the genital tract.

HSV-1 and HSV-2 lesions are highly infectious and therefore can be transmitted to other individuals or other sites on the patient. Oro-genital contact can result in spread from the source to the oral cavity or genitals of the sexual partner. The infectious period of herpetic lesions is of uncertain length, but positive viral cultures are detected mostly from stages before crusting.[34] Therefore one should assume that all herpetic lesions (i.e., papular, vesicular, pustular, ulcerative) before complete crusting are infectious.

LABORATORY FINDINGS

Cytologic examination of a smear taken from the base of a herpetic lesion will reveal typical features, including ballooning degeneration of cells, intranuclear inclusion bodies, and multinucleated giant cells. However, cytology is non-specific and less sensitive than viral culture.

Diagnosis usually is made by swabbing an infected secretion or ulcer and isolating the virus by cell culture. The virus is identified by staining the infected cells for HSV antigen using immunofluorescence or immunoperoxidase. Alternatively, polymerase chain reaction and restriction endonuclease patterns can be used.[34] Because genital recurrences are much less frequent for HSV-1 than HSV-2, identification of the infecting strain type has prognostic importance and may

be useful for counseling purposes. Serologic detection of antibodies to HSV-2/HSV-1 also can be helpful to make these determinations.

MEDICAL MANAGEMENT

Management of patients with a first clinical episode of genital herpes includes antiviral therapy and counseling regarding the natural history of genital herpes, sexual and perinatal transmission, and how to reduce transmission. The CDC[18] has updated guidelines for the use of antiviral agents. Current recommendations recommend the use of either acyclovir (Zovirax), famciclovir (Famvir) or valacyclovir (Valtrex). All three are nucleoside analogue drugs that act as DNA chain terminators during virus replication in infected cells.

Some of these agents are available in oral, topical, and intravenous formulations. Topical acyclovir therapy is substantially less effective than systemic drug administration. Proper use of the systemic drugs results in decreased duration of lesions and symptoms, and offers the potential to reduce risk of transmission. They do not eliminate the virus from the latent state nor affect subsequent risk, frequency, or severity of recurrences after administration of drugs is discontinued. Antiviral drugs are most effective when given within 1 day of the appearance of symptoms, whether for primary or recurrent disease. The current treatment recommendations[18] found in Box 12-1 are for primary, recurrent and suppressive genital herpes therapy. These protocols, however, also may be used for oral infections.

Daily suppressive antiviral therapy can be implemented for patients with frequent recurrences (more than 5 recurrences per year). Suppressive therapy reduces the frequency of recurrence in 50% to 75% of persons who have 6 or more recurrence per year and reduces asymptomatic viral shedding between outbreaks.[18,2] Safety and efficacy have been documented among patients receiving daily therapy with acyclovir for as long as 6 years, and with valacyclovir and famciclovir for 1 year. Suppressive therapy has not been associated with emergence of clinically significant acyclovir resistance among immunocompetent patients. Nevertheless, current recommendations are to consider stopping suppressive therapy after 1 year to reassess the frequency of recurrence, as the frequency of recurrences often diminishes over time when long-term suppressive therapy is instituted. Intravenous antiviral agents (cidofovir [Vistide] and foscarnet [Foscavir]) are reserved for severe or complicated infections.

CDC-Recommended Regimens for the Treatment of Genital Herpes

Primary episode of genital herpes*
Acyclovir 400 mg orally 3 times a day for 7-10 days, or
Acyclovir 200 mg orally 5 times a day for 7-10 days, or
Famciclovir 250 mg orally 3 times a day for 7-10 days, or
Valacyclovir 1 g orally 2 times a day for 7-10 days.
Recurrent infection
Acyclovir 400 mg orally 3 times a day for 5 days, or
Acyclovir 200 mg orally 5 times a day for 5 days, or
Acyclovir 800 mg orally 2 times a day for 5 days, or
Famciclovir 125 mg orally 2 times a day for 5 days,
Valacyclovir 500 mg orally 2 times a day for 5 days.
Daily suppressive therapy
Acyclovir 400 mg 2 times daily, or
Famciclovir 250 mg orally 2 times a day, or
Valacyclovir 250 mg orally 2 times a day, or
Valacyclovir 500 mg or 1,000† mg orally 1 time a day

*NOTE: Treatment may be extended if healing is incomplete after 10 days of therapy. Higher dosages of acyclovir (i.e., 400 mg orally 5 times a day) were used in treatment studies of first-episode herpes oral infection, including stomatitis or pharyngitis. Whether these forms of mucosal infection require higher doses of acyclovir than used for genital herpes is unknown. Valacyclovir and famciclovir probably are effective for acute HSV oral infection, but clinical experience is lacking.[18]
†Higher doses may be required for patients who have more than 10 recurrences per year.

Acyclovir, famciclovir, and valacyclovir have been assigned pregnancy category C, B, and B, respectively, by the Food and Drug Administration. Accordingly, famciclovir and valacyclovir are considered relatively safe to administer to a pregnant woman.[35]

■ INFECTIOUS MONONUCLEOSIS ■

DEFINITION

Although not classically defined as an STD, infectious mononucleosis is discussed in this chapter because transmission is by intimate personal contact. Infectious mononucleosis is an infection caused, in the majority of cases, by the Epstein-Barr virus (EBV), a lympho-

tropic herpesvirus. Other viruses also can cause acute infectious mononucleosis features. Infectious mononucleosis produces the classic clinical triad of fever, pharyngitis, and lymphadenopathy. Transmission of the virus is primarily by way of the oropharyngeal route during close personal contact (i.e., intimate kissing). Children, adolescents and young adults are most commonly affected. Approximately 10% to 20% of asymptomatic, seropositive adults (antibodies to the Epstein-Barr virus) carry the virus in their oropharyngeal region.[36]

INCIDENCE, PREVALENCE, AND ETIOLOGY

More than 90% of the adults worldwide have been infected with EBV.[37] In the United States, approximately 50% of 5-year-old children and 70% of college freshman have evidence of prior EBV infection.[38,39] The peak rate of acquisition is between 15 and 19 years of age. The annual incidence in this adolescent age group is 3.4 to 6.7 cases per 1000 persons.[38] The incidence has been reported to be 30 times higher in whites than in African-Americans in the United States.[38] No gender predilection exists.

PATHOPHYSIOLOGY

EBV is transmitted primarily through exposure to oropharyngeal secretions and infrequently by infected blood products. The incubation time is 30 to 50 days. A prodromal period of 3 to 5 days precedes the clinical phase, which lasts 7 to 20 days. During the prodromal phase, the virus infects oral epithelial cells and spreads to B lymphocytes. Infected B lymphocytes circulate through the reticuloendothelial system, triggering a marked lymphocytic response. In normal blood smears, large reactive lymphocytes represent approximately 1% to 2% of the cells. In infectious mononucleosis, they constitute at least 10% of the cells. The reactive lymphocytes are not the EBV-infected B lymphocytes but T lymphocytes reacting to the infection.[10] The combination of reactive lymphocytes, cytokines they produce, and B-cell-produced (heterophile) antibodies directed against EBV antigens contribute to the clinical manifestation of the acute infection. Hepatosplenomegaly develops in approximately 40% to 50% of patients, and splenic rupture occurs in 0.1% to 0.2% of all cases.[36] After the acute infection, the virus remains latent in B lymphocytes for the life of the host. Some researchers believe chronic EBV infection can cause fatigue and sleepiness; however, the issue remains controversial.

CLINICAL PRESENTATION

SIGNS AND SYMPTOMS

Infectious mononucleosis usually is asymptomatic when found in children; however, when young adults are affected, approximately 50% are symptomatic. Fever, sore throat, lymphadenopathy occur in 70% to 90% of patients.[40] Additional features include malaise, fatigue, an absolute lymphocytosis (more than 10% reactive lymphocytes), and a positive heterophil antibody test.[36] Approximately one third of the patients develop palatal petechiae during the first week of the illness, and 30% of patients develop an exudative pharyngitis.[41] A generalized skin rash and petechiae of the lips are seen in approximately 10% of cases. Symptoms tend to dissipate by 3 weeks of onset.

LABORATORY FINDINGS

EBV-associated infectious mononucleosis is diagnosed in the laboratory using agglutination assays or solid phase immunoassays. Both detect heterophil antibodies—IgM antibodies that bind to erythrocytes from nonhuman species such as sheep or horses (e.g., Monospot [Ortho Diagnostics] test).[42] Patients with a negative heterophil antibody test should be retested in 7 to 10 days. If the second test is negative, tests for viral capsid antigen IgG and IgM antibody and EBV nuclear antigen should be performed.[36] If these tests are positive the patient has heterophil-negative infectious mononucleosis. A few patients with the classic disease description may be heterophil antibody negative and EBV-IgM negative. For these patients, tests for CMV (cytomegalovirus), *Toxoplasma gondii*, human herpesvirus 6, HIV and adenovirus should be performed.[36]

MEDICAL MANAGEMENT

Treatment of infectious mononucleosis is symptomatic and consists of bed rest, acetaminophen or nonsteroidal anti-inflammatory agents for pain control, and gargling and irrigation with saline solution to provide symptomatic relief of pharyngitis and stomatitis. Vigorous activity is to be avoided to reduce the risk of splenic rupture. In some patients with severe toxic exudative pharyngotonsillitis, pharyngeal edema and upper airway obstruction, a short course of prednisone may be given. Approximately 20% of the patients with symptomatic infectious mononucleosis have concurrent beta-hemolytic

streptococcal pharyngotonsillitis and should be treated with penicillin V if they are not allergic to penicillin. Ampicillin should be avoided because 90% or more patients develop a hypersensitivity skin rash when treated with this drug.[22] Currently no antiviral drugs are effective against EBV.

■ HUMAN PAPILLOMAVIRUS ■ INFECTION

DEFINITION

Human papillomaviruses (HPVs) are small, double-stranded, nonenveloped DNA viruses that infect and replicate in epithelial cells. More than 90 genotypes of HPV exist, with 45 types known to affect genital epithelium.[43] Each HPV subtype exhibits preferential anatomic sites of infection and a propensity for altering epithelial growth and replication. The spectrum of disease induced is dependent on the type of HPV infection, location, and immune response. Subtypes of HPV have been classified as either "high-risk" or "low-risk" types. The low-risk HPVs (HPV-6, HPV-11) cause benign proliferative lesions of mucocutaneous structures; high-risk HPV types (HPV-16, HPV-18, HPV-31, HPV-33, HPV-35) are strongly associated with dysplasia and carcinoma of the uterine and anal tract and other mucosal sites[44] (Table 12-2).

TABLE 12-2

HPV-Associated Oral Mucosal Lesions

Lesion	Most Common HPV Type
Condyloma acuminatum	6, 11
Epithelial dysplasia, carcinoma in situ, squamous cell carcinoma	2, 16, 18
Focal epithelial hyperplasia	13, 32
Lichen planus	11, 16
Oral bowenoid papulosis	6, 11, 16
Squamous papilloma	6, 11
Verruca plana	3, 10
Verruca vulgaris	2, 4, 6, 11, 16
Verrucous carcinoma	2, 6, 11, 16/18

INCIDENCE AND PREVALENCE

HPV infections are one of the three most common STDs in the United States, with an estimated 20 million persons having genital HPV infections[1] that can be transmitted by sexual contact.[45] The exact incidence of HPV infection is unknown because it is not a reportable STD and most cases are asymptomatic or subclinical; but approximately 5.5 million new infections occur every year in the United States,[1] and 10% to 33% of sexually active individuals are infected with the virus.[46] Current estimates indicate that 18% of U.S. women and 8% of men carry genital HPV.[1] The infection is more common in African-American women than in white women. The highest rates of infection are found between the ages of 19 and 26 years.[43] The lifetime number of sexual partners is the most important risk factor identified for genital warts.[47]

ETIOLOGY

Genital HPV can be transmitted by direct contact during sexual intercourse, passage of a fetus through an infected birth canal, or by autoinoculation. Genital lesions usually appear after an incubation period of HPV in epithelium for 3 weeks to 8 months. The most common manifestation of HPV replication is the venereal wart or condyloma acuminatum. HPV types 6 and 11 are the subtypes most frequently associated with condyloma acuminatum. HPV types 2 and 6 also have been identified in condylomata but are not considered the primary etiologic agents.

PATHOPHYSIOLOGY

HPV is transmitted through intimate or sexual contact. The virus either replicates in the nuclei of epithelial cells and increases the turnover of infected cells or remains episomally in a latent state. Active replication results in epithelial hyperplasia, dysplasia, or carcinoma. HPV6 and 11 have a strong tendency to induce condyloma whereas HPV-16 and HPV-18 have a strong tendency to induce malignant transformation. HPV types 31, 33, 35, 39, 45, 51, 52, 54, 56, and 58 have intermediate to high risk for inducing carcinoma.

CLINICAL PRESENTATION

SIGNS AND SYMPTOMS

Although many manifestations of HPV infection exist, the condyloma acuminatum is most common and pertinent to the discussion of STDs. These growths are seen in sexually active individuals in warm, moist, intertriginous areas such as the anogenital skin and mouth, where friction and microabrasion allow entrance of the pathogen. Condyloma appear as small, soft, exophytic papillomatous growths (Fig. 12-10). The surface resembles cauliflower or broccoli and the base is sessile. The borders are raised and rounded. The color varies from pink to dusky gray. Lesions often are multiple and recurrent and can coalesce to form large pebbly growths. Most condylomata are asymptomatic; however, patients may complain of itching, irritation, or bleeding as a result of manipulation or trauma. During pregnancy, condylomata may enlarge because of increased vascularity. Condylomata have occurred on the vagina, anus, mouth, pharynx, or larynx.

LABORATORY FINDINGS

HPV does not grow in cell culture and serologic tests are not routinely performed. Therefore a biopsy should be taken of samples of condyloma acuminatum and examined microscopically. The microscopic appearance is a sessile base, raised epithelial borders, thick spinous spinosum layer (acanthosis), and hyperkeratosis. Identification of HPV within the lesion confirms the diagnosis. This is generally achieved using commercial in situ hybridization kits that detect viral DNA specific to HPV genotypes using RNA probes. Viral subtyping can be important for determining risk of carcinogenesis when cervical tissue and an abnormal Papanicolaou smear is involved (see Chapter 21).

MEDICAL MANAGEMENT

The goal of treatment is the removal of all genital warts present and the amelioration of symptoms.

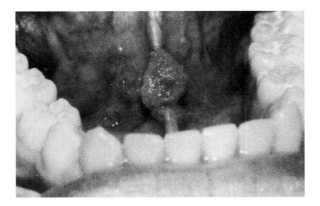

Fig. 12-10 Condyloma acuminatum. (From Miller CS: Seminars in Dermatology 13(2):108-117, 1994. Courtesy Marden Alder.)

Although HPV lesions can be completely removed, eradication of latent HPV is difficult if not impossible. The best response is gained with small warts that have been present for less than 1 year. The medication of first choice by the CDC is[18] podofilox 0.5% (Condylox, Oclassen), which causes necrosis by arresting cells in mitosis. This patient-applied medication should be used twice a day for 3 days, with no treatment for the next 4 days, with a repeat of the cycle up to 4 times.[18] As an alternative, the patient may apply imiquimod (Aldara) 5% cream at bedtime, 3 times per week for up to 16 weeks. Imiquimod is an immune response modifier drug. Most warts dissipate by 8 weeks or less. Other therapies available include surgery (excision, cryotherapy, laser), topical chemical therapy with podophyllum 10% to 25% in tincture of benzoin, trichloroacetic acid 80% to 90% or bichloroacetic acid, or intralesional interferon.[2] Topical and intralesional therapy with 5-fluorouracil, an antimetabolite, has resulted in a greater than 60% response rate.[48] Recurrences are seen in about 10% to 25% of cases (generally within 3 months), even when the entire lesion including the base is removed.[49] Treatment should include the patient's sexual partner to avoid reinfection. Without treatment, lesions may enlarge and spread or regress spontaneously, which occurs in about 20% of patients.[50]

DENTAL MANAGEMENT

MEDICAL CONSIDERATIONS

The dental management of patients with an STD begins with identification. The obvious goal is to identify all individuals who have active disease because many are potentially infectious. Unfortunately, this is not possible in every case because some persons will not provide a history or may not demonstrate significant signs or symptoms suggestive of their disease. The inability to identify potentially infectious patients applies to other diseases, such as HIV infection and viral hepatitis. Therefore all patients must be managed as though they were infectious. The U.S. Public Health Service, through the CDC, has published recommendations for universal precautions to be followed in controlling infection in dentistry that have become the standard for preventing cross-infection[51] (see Appendix A). Strict adherence to these recommendations will, for all practical purposes, eliminate the danger of disease transmission between dentist and patient. Even though these procedures are followed, several significant facts regarding STDs should be remembered (Box 12-2).

BOX 12-2

Dental Management of the Patient with a Sexually Transmitted Disease*

> **Gonorrhea**—little threat of transmission to dentist; oral lesions are possible
> **Syphilis**—untreated primary and secondary lesions infectious; blood also is potentially infectious.
> **Genital herpes**—little threat of transmission to dentist; oral lesions are possible from autoinoculation.
> **HPV infection**—little threat of transmission to dentist; oral lesions are possible.
> Persons with STDs are at risk for HIV infection.
> New cases of syphilis, gonorrhea, and AIDS should be reported to the local/state health department.

*Because many patients with an active STD (as well as with other infectious diseases such as AIDS and hepatitis B) cannot be identified by the dentist, all patients should be considered potentially infectious and managed using universal precautions. Preventive measures should be implemented that include patient education and evaluation, treatment and counseling of sexual partners.

Gonorrhea

The patient with gonorrhea poses little threat of disease transmission to the dentist because of the specific requirements for transmission and the early reversal of infectiousness once antibiotics are administered. Patients in this category can be provided dental care within days of antibiotic treatment.

Syphilis

The lesions of untreated primary and secondary syphilis are infectious as are the patient's blood and saliva. Even after treatment is begun, absolute effectiveness of therapy cannot be determined except by conversion of the positive serologic test to negative; however, early reversal of infectiousness following the institution of antibiotics is to be expected. The time required for this conversion varies from a few months to more than a year. Therefore patients who are being treated or have a positive result on the serologic test for syphilis following treatment should be viewed as potentially infectious. Necessary dental care may be provided unless oral lesions are present. Dental treatment can commence once oral lesions successfully have been treated.

Genital herpes

Localized uncomplicated genital herpes infection poses no problem for the dentist. In the absence of oral lesions,

any necessary dental work may be provided. If oral lesions are present, elective treatment should be delayed until lesions scab over to avoid inadvertent inoculation of adjacent sites. Antiviral agents may be required to prevent oral recurrences after dental treatment.

Infectious Mononucleosis
Patients with infectious mononucleosis may come to the dentist because of oral signs and symptoms. Patients with clinical findings of fever, sore throat, petechiae, and cervical lymphadenopathy must be evaluated to establish a diagnosis of their condition. Screening clinical laboratory tests can be ordered by the dentist (complete blood count, heterophil [Monospot or Monosticon] antibody test, and EBV-antigen testing). The patient also can be referred to a physician for evaluation and treatment.[10,22] Routine dental treatment should be delayed for 3 to 6 weeks until the patient has recovered and the patient's liver is capable of normal metabolism of drugs.

Human Papillomavirus Infection
Although genital condylomata acuminatum do not affect dental management, oral lesions are infectious, and universal precautions apply during oral treatment of patients. The presence of oral lesions necessitates referral to a physician to rule out genital lesions of the patient or the patient's sexual partner. Excisional biopsy is recommended for HPV-associated oral lesions.

PATIENTS WITH A HISTORY OF AN STD

Patients who have had an STD should be approached with a measure of caution because they are in a high-risk group for additional STDs. This can include risk from the inadequate treatment of a previous infection or risk of a new one. Special attention should be given to unexplained lesions of the oral, pharyngeal, and perioral tissues. Also a review of systems may reveal urogenital symptoms. Patients with a history of gonorrhea should give a history of antibiotic therapy. Patients treated for syphilis should receive a periodic STS test for 1 year to monitor conversions from positive to negative. In the absence of medical follow-up care for these disorders, consultation and referral to a physician may be considered.

PATIENTS WITH SIGNS SUGGESTIVE OF AN STD

Patients who have signs or symptoms suggesting an STD or who have unexplained oral or pharyngeal lesions also should be approached with caution. The index of suspicion should be higher if the patient is between 15 and 29 years of age and has risk factors such as being an urban

dweller, single, and from a lower socioeconomic group. Any patient who has these unexplained lesions should be questioned about possible relationships of the lesions with past sexual activity and advised to seek medical care. Herpetic lesions in or around the oral cavity combined with a history of past involvement should be recognized. Patients with acute oral herpes lesions should not receive routine dental care but be given palliative treatment only. For a severe primary oral infection, the patient may require antiviral therapy and referral to a physician.

TREATMENT PLANNING MODIFICATIONS

No modifications in the technical treatment plan are required for a patient with an STD. No adverse interactions exist between the usual antibiotics or drugs used to treat STDs and drugs commonly used in dentistry. Patients with Hutchinson's incisors caused by congenital syphilis may request esthetic repair of their anterior teeth.

REPORTING TO STATE HEALTH OFFICIALS

Dentists should be aware of local statutory requirements regarding reporting STDs to state health officials. Syphilis, gonorrhea, and AIDS are reportable diseases in every state. Local health departments or state STD programs are sources of information regarding this matter.

ORAL COMPLICATIONS AND MANIFESTATIONS

Gonorrhea
The rare presentation of oral gonorrhea is nonspecific and varied and may range from slight erythema to severe ulceration with a pseudomembranous coating. Lesions usually develop within 1 week of contact with an infected person. In the oropharynx, the mucosa becomes fiery red, with tiny pustules and an itching and burning sensation. The patient may be asymptomatic or limited in oral function (eating, drinking, talking). Definitive diagnosis of oral lesions should be attempted.

The initial step in treatment is to ensure that the patient is under the care of a physician and receiving proper antimicrobial therapy. After this, treatment of the oral lesions is symptomatic (see Appendix B). The patient should be assured that oral infection will resolve with the use of appropriate antibiotics.

Syphilis
Syphilitic chancres and mucous patches are usually painless unless they become secondarily infected. Both

lesions are highly infectious. The chancre begins as a papule that erodes into a painless ulcer with a smooth, grayish surface. The size can vary from a few millimeters to 2 to 3 centimeters. A key feature is lymphadenopathy that may be unilateral. The intraoral mucous patch often appears as a slightly raised asymptomatic papule with an ulcerated surface. The lips, tongue, buccal, and labial mucosa may be affected. Both the chancre and mucous patch regress spontaneously regardless of whether antibiotic therapy is used, although chemotherapy is required to eradicate the systemic infection. The gumma is a painless lesion that may become secondarily infected. It is noninfectious and frequently occurs on and destroys the hard palate. Interstitial glossitis, the result of contracture of the tongue musculature after healing of a gumma, is viewed as a premalignant lesion. Oral manifestations of congenital syphilis include peg-shaped permanent central incisors with notching of the incisal edge (Hutchinson's incisors, see Fig. 12-7), defective molars with multiple supernumerary cusps (mulberry molars), atrophic glossitis, a high, narrow palate, and perioral rhagades (skin fissures).

Genital Herpes
Because differentiating between HSV-1 and HSV-2 is impossible clinically, all herpetic lesions of the oral cavity should be treated the same way with antiviral agents (see Appendix B). Oral and perioral herpetic lesions should be considered infectious, regardless of stage (papular, vesicular, or ulcerative), because of (1) the danger of inoculation to a new site on the patient, (2) infection to the dentist (i.e., herpetic paronychia), and (3) aerosol or droplet inoculation of the conjunctivae of either patient or dental personnel. Elective dental treatment should be delayed until the herpetic lesion is completely healed. Once the lesion is crusted, it can be considered as relatively noninfectious.

A problem of particular concern to dentists is herpetic infection of the fingers or nailbeds contracted by dermal contact with a herpetic lesion of the lip or oral cavity of a patient (Fig. 12-11). The infection is called a *herpetic whitlow* or *herpetic paronychia*. It is serious, debilitating, and recurrent. Herpetic whitlow can be triggered to recur as a result of trauma, such as the vibration from operating dental handpieces.

Infectious Mononucleosis
Head, neck, and oral manifestations of infectious mononucleosis include fever, severe sore throat, palatal and lip petechiae, and cervical lymphadenopathy. Lymph nodes in the anterior and posterior cervical chain often are enlarged and tender to palpation.

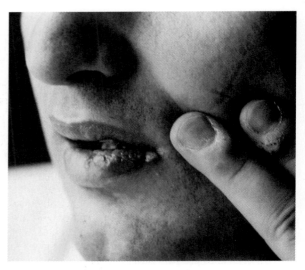

Fig. 12-11 Herpes simplex type 1 infection of the nailbeds (herpetic whitlow, herpetic paronychia) as a result of autoinoculation. (Courtesy R.C. Noble, Lexington, Ky.)

Human Papillomavirus Infections
Condylomata acuminatum commonly occur on the ventral tongue, gingiva, labial mucosa, and palate. Transmission is by direct contact with infected anal, genital, or oral sites, or by self-inoculation. Lesions can be surgically excised, chemically removed with podophyllin, or laser ablated. Caustic chemicals such as podophyllin are to be used with great caution to avoid damage to adjacent uninfected tissue and rinsed several hours after application. In addition, high-speed evacuation should be used during laser eradication to prevent inhalation of the virion-laden plume. Transmission of HPV via inhalation of the plume has been documented to cause laryngeal condylomata.[52]

The dentist also should be cognizant that a condyloma identified in children raises the suspicion of sexual child abuse when autoinoculation by hand to genital contact, nonsexual contact, or maternal fetal transmission have been ruled out. Failure to report signs of child abuse to state health officials is a legal offense in several states.

References

1. Wasserheit J: STD *prevention program*. Milwaukee, Wisc., 2000.
2. Centers for Disease Control: 1993 Sexually transmitted diseases treatment guidelines, MMWR 42(RR-14):1-93, 1993.

3. Gwanzura L et al: Association between human immunodeficiency virus and herpes simplex virus type 2 seropositivity among male factory workers in Zimbabwe, J Infect Dis 177:481-484, 1998.

4. Fox K, Knapp J: Antimicrobial resistance in Neisseria gonorrhoeae, Curr Opin Urol 9:65-70, 1999.

5. Centers for Disease Control: Summary of Notifiable Diseases, United States, 1998, MMWR 47:1-93, 1999.

6. Centers for Disease Control: Summary of notifiable diseases, United States, 1994, MMWR 43:1-80, 1995.

7. Emmert D, Kirchner J: Sexually transmitted diseases in women, Postgrad Med 107:181-184, 189-190, 2000.

8. von Lichtenberg F: Infectious disease: viral, chlamydial, rickettsial, and bacterial diseases. In Cotran R, Kumar V, Robbins S, editors: Robbins' pathologic basis of disease, Philadelphia, 1989, WB Saunders.

9. Escobar V, Farman A, Arm R: Oral gonococcal infection, Int J Oral Surg 13:549-554, 1984.

10. Centers for Disease Control: Summary of notifiable diseases, United States, 1990, MMWR 39:1-65, 1990.

11. Giunta J, Fiuamara N: Facts about gonorrhea and dentistry, Oral Surg 62:529-531, 1986.

12. Jamsky R, Christen A: Oral gonococcal infections: report of two cases, Oral Surg 53:358-362, 1982.

13. Kohn S, Shaffer J, Chomenko A: Primary gonococcal stomatitis, JAMA 219:86, 1972.

14. Merchant H, Schuster G: Oral gonococcal infection, J Am Dent Assoc 95:807-809, 1977.

15. Schmidt H, Hjorting-Hanssen E, Philipsen H: Gonococcal stomatitis, Acta Derm Venereol 41:324-327, 1961.

16. Chue P: Gonorrhea–its natural history, oral manifestations, diagnosis, treatment, and prevention, J Am Dent Assoc 90:1297-1301, 1975.

17. Chue P: Gonococcal arthritis of the temporomandibular joint, Oral Surg 39:572-577, 1975.

18. Centers for Disease Control: 1998 Guidelines for Treatment of Sexually Transmitted Diseases, MMWR 47:1-118, 1998.

19. Noble R: personal communication, 1981.

20. Knapp J et al: Fluoroquinolone resistance in Neisseria gonorrhoeae. Emerg Infect Dis 3:33-39, 1997.

21. Centers for Disease Control: Fluoroquinolone resistance in Neisseria gonorrhoeae–Colorado and Washington, 1995, MMWR 44:761-764, 1995.

22. Rudolph A: Syphilis. In Hoeprich PD, Jordan MC, editors: Infectious disease, ed 4, Philadelphia, 1989, JB Lippincott.

23. Grosskurth H et al: Impact of improved treatment of sexually transmitted diseases on HIV infection in rural Tanzania: randomized controlled trial, Lancet 346:530-536, 1995.

24. Lowhagen G: Syphilis: test procedures and therapeutic strategies, Semin Dermatol 9:152-159, 1990.

25. Thin R: Early syphilis in the adult. In Sexually transmitted diseases, ed 2, New York, 1990, McGraw-Hill.

26. Hook WE 3rd: Acquired syphilis in adults, N Engl J Med 326:1060-1069, 1992.

27. Southwick K et al: An epidemic of congenital syphilis in Jefferson County, Texas, 1994-1995: inadequate prenatal syphilis testing after an outbreak in adults, Am J Public Health 89:557-560, 1999.

28. Zoechling N et al: Molecular detection of Treponema pallidum in secondary and tertiary syphilis, Br J Dermatol 136:683-686, 1997.

29. Fleming D et al: Herpes simplex virus type 2 in the United States, 1976 to 1994, N Engl J Med 337:1105-1111, 1997.

30. Langenberg A et al: A prospective study of new infections with herpes simplex virus type 1 and type 2, N Engl J Med 341:1432-1438, 1999.

31. Nahmias A, Lee F, Bekman-Nahmias S: Sero-epidemiological and sociological patterns of herpes simplex virus infection in the world, Scand J Infect Dis 69:19-36, 1990.

32. Nahmias AJ, Roizman B: Infection with herpes simplex viruses 1 and 2, N Engl J Med 289:781-789, 1973.

33. Goodman J: Infections caused by herpes simplex viruses. In Hoeprich P, Jordan M, editors: Infectious diseases, ed 4, Philadelphia, 1989, JB Lippincott.

34. Fife K: Laboratory diagnosis of herpes simplex virus infections and the realm of rapid diagnostic tests, In Clinical update–herpes simplex: diagnosis and management, Research Triangle Park, NC, 1986, Burroughs Wellcome.

35. Drug information for the health care professional, vols IA and IB, ed 19, Rockville, Md, 1999, United States Pharmacopeial Convention.

36. Godshall S, Kirchner J: Infectious mononucleosis: complexities of a common syndrome, Postgrad Med 107:175-186, 2000.

37. Kaye K, Kieff E: Epstein-Barr virus infection and infectious mononucleosis. In Gorbach S, Bartlett J, Blacklow N, editors: Infectious disease, Philadelphia, 1992, Saunders.

38. Auwaerter P: Infectious mononucleosis in middle age, JAMA 281:454-459, 1999.

39. Schooley R: Epstein-Barr virus (infectious mononucleosis). In Mandell G, Bennett J, Dolin R editors: Mandell, Bouglas, and Bennett's principles and practice of infectious diseases, vol 4, New York, 1995, Churchill Livingstone.

40. Axelrod P, Finestone A: Infectious mononucleosis in older adults, Am Fam Physician 42:1599-1606, 1990.

41. Bailey R: Diagnosis and treatment of infectious mononucleosis, Am Fam Physician 49:879-888, 1994.

42. Linderholm M, Boman J, Juto P, et al: Comparative evaluation of nine kits for rapid diagnosis of infectious mononucleosis and Epstein-Barr virus-specific serology, J Clin Microbiol 32:259-261, 1994.

43. Brown T, Yen-Moore A, Tyring S: An overview of sexually transmitted disease, Part II. J Am Acad Dermatol 41:661-677, 1999.

44. Frisch M et al: Sexually transmitted infection as a cause of anal cancer, N Engl J Med 337:1350-1358, 1997.

45. Koutsky L, Gallowy D, Holmes K: Epidemiology of gential human papillomavirus infection, Epidemiol Rev 10:122-163, 1988.

46. Borg A, Medley G, Garland S: Polymerase chain reaction: a sensitive indicator of the prevalence of human papillomavirus DNA in a population with sexually transmitted disease. Acta Cytologica 39:654-658, 1995.

47. Munk C, Svare E, Poll P, et al: History of genital warts in 10,838 women 20 to 29 years of age from the general population: risk factors and association with Papanicolaou smear history, Sex Transm Dis 24:567-572, 1997.

48. Swinehart J et al: Development of intralesional therapy with fluorouracil/adrenaline injectable gel for management of condyloma acuminata: two phase II clinical studies, *Genitourin Med* 73:481-487, 1997.

49. Edwards L et al: Self-administered topical 5% imiquimod cream for external anogenital warts, *Arch Dermatol* 134:25-30, 1998.

50. Carson D: Common sexually transmitted diseases, *Am Druggist* October:43-49, 1994.

51. Centers for Disease Control: Recommended infection-control practices for dentistry, 1993, MMWR 41(RR-8):1-12, 1993.

52. Hallmo P, Naess O: Laryngeal papillomatosis with human papillomavirus DNA contracted by a laser surgeon, *Eur Arch Otorhinolaryngol* 248:425-427, 1991.

AIDS and Related Conditions

13 CHAPTER

The acquired immune deficiency syndrome (AIDS) is an infectious disease transmitted predominantly by intimate sexual contact and by parenteral means. AIDS first was reported in the United States in 1981. The initial report of the disease came from Los Angeles, where five "healthy" male homosexuals were diagnosed as suffering from an unusual type of pneumonia, caused by the protozoan *Pneumocystis carinii*. These individuals also were found to be immunosuppressed for no obvious reason. From this seemingly innocuous beginning, AIDS has become one of the most significant infectious diseases in history. The Centers for Disease Control (CDC) estimates more than 1.5 million Americans are infected with human immunodeficiency virus (HIV), and that more than 750,000 cases of AIDS exist, with more than 430,000 related deaths reported in the United States.[1,2]

As of the year 2000, a total of 753,907 persons with AIDS, including 8,804 cases in children, had been reported to the CDC.[3] At that time AIDS had resulted in 430,441 deaths, including 5,084 children. The number of cases continues to increase (Table 13-1).[3] However, the number of deaths from AIDS has been decreasing slowly over the past five years (Table 13-2). The disease has been reported with increasing frequency in many European countries and elsewhere in the world. Approximately 30 million people are HIV infected worldwide. The mortality rate for individuals infected with AIDS is virtually 100%.[4]

The AIDS epidemic continues to progress in the United States, although the rate has slowed somewhat in the last few years, according to the CDC.[1,2,4] Still, approximately 4000 new cases per month are reported by the CDC. No vaccine or definitive treatment exists for this nationwide epidemic. The currently approved groups of antiretroviral drugs may help slow the progression of the infection but is far from a cure. The best treatment approach for AIDS is preventive education and counseling for infected patients and their contacts (family, lover, friends, co-workers) and the use of drugs to slow the progress of the disease. Recent changes in the epidemiology of AIDS have been a positive testimony to this approach.[1,3,5]

Because of its frequent association with homosexuality and intravenous (IV) drug abuse, the adverse social implications have caused AIDS to be viewed prejudicially and moralistically by many. However, all segments of society are potentially susceptible to this disease.[1,3,5]

The definition of AIDS by the CDC, as amended in 1993, consists of the cluster of differentiation 4 (CD4) lymphocyte count of less than 200 in a patient who is HIV infected. This revised definition also includes individuals who are HIV infected with pulmonary tuberculosis, recurrent episodes of pneumonia, or invasive cervical carcinoma.[6] Previously, Kaposi's sarcoma or lymphoma, a *Pneumocystis carinii* pneumonia, or other life-threatening opportunistic infection, the wasting syndrome, and/or central nervous system (CNS) syndromes with dementia and associated immunosuppression would fulfill the definition, regardless of the CD4 count.[7,8] That is no longer the case. Because of better pharmacologic management of AIDS patients, some of the opportunistic infections do not occur even with extremely low CD4 counts.[9,10]

From the time of diagnosis, 30% of AIDS patients can be expected to live approximately 2 to 3 years, with most of the others living 10 years or longer. Death usually results from an opportunistic infection and in some cases from complications associated with the various malignancies seen with AIDS. The onset of these complications generally is associated with a low CD4 count. All individuals

TABLE 13-1

AIDS Cases Reported through June 2000, United States

Male Age at Diagnosis (Years)	WHITE, NOT HISPANIC		AFRICAN-AMERICAN, NOT HISPANIC		HISPANIC		ASIAN/ PACIFIC ISLANDER		AMERICAN INDIAN/ ALASKA NATIVE		TOTAL*	
	No.	%	No.	%	No.	%	No.	%	No.	%	No.	%
Under 5	521	(0)	2,110	(1)	766	(1)	16	(0)	12	(1)	3,429	(1)
5-12	340	(0)	458	(0)	280	(0)	9	(0)	6	(0)	1,096	(0)
13-19	850	(0)	863	(0)	501	(0)	25	(1)	22	(1)	2,264	(0)
20-24	7,663	(3)	6,953	(3)	4,178	(4)	170	(4)	80	(4)	19,071	(3)
20-29	37,888	(13)	25,041	(12)	16,175	(14)	606	(12)	326	(18)	80,133	(13)
30-34	68,721	(23)	43,054	(21)	26,650	(24)	1,057	(22)	481	(26)	140,106	(22)
35-39	67,830	(23)	46,981	(23)	24,932	(22)	1,061	(22)	403	(22)	141,414	(23)
40-44	49,471	(17)	37,371	(18)	17,569	(16)	834	(17)	272	(16)	105,887	(17)
45-49	29,899	(10)	21,939	(11)	9,852	(9)	506	(10)	110	(6)	62,395	(10)
50-54	16,198	(5)	11,258	(5)	5,225	(5)	269	(6)	51	(3)	33,052	(5)
55-59	8,740	(3)	6,149	(3)	2,894	(3)	161	(3)	30	(2)	18,002	(3)
60-64	4,816	(2)	3,378	(2)	1,593	(1)	69	(1)	18	(1)	9,886	(2)
65 or older	3,994	(1)	2,834	(1)	1,280	(1)	69	(1)	10	(1)	8,199	(1)
Male subtotal	296,931	(100)	208,389	(100)	111,895	(100)	4,852	(100)	1,821	(100)	624,714	(100)
Female Age at Diagnosis (Years)	No.	%	No.	%	No.	%	No.	%	No.	%	No.	%
Under 5	490	(2)	2,102	(3)	758	(3)	15	(2)	13	(3)	3,383	(3)
5-12	184	(1)	488	(1)	212	(1)	9	(1)	—	—	896	(1)
13-19	258	(1)	1,056	(1)	274	(1)	8	(1)	4	(1)	1,601	(1)
20-24	1,626	(6)	4,256	(6)	1,486	(6)	39	(6)	31	(8)	7,447	(6)
25-29	4,539	(16)	10,701	(14)	4,039	(16)	95	(14)	60	(15)	19,454	(15)
30-34	6,274	(22)	16,188	(22)	5,880	(23)	128	(18)	93	(23)	28,617	(22)
35-39	5,581	(20)	16,236	(22)	5,298	(21)	130	(19)	81	(20)	27,364	(21)
40-44	3,689	(13)	11,403	(15)	3,466	(13)	101	(15)	53	(13)	18,731	(14)
45-49	1,981	(7)	5,702	(8)	1,922	(7)	68	(10)	36	(9)	9,733	(8)
50-54	1,132	(4)	2,832	(4)	1,052	(4)	28	(4)	17	(4)	5,066	(4)
55-59	726	(3)	1,552	(2)	652	(3)	23	(3)	15	(4)	2,969	(2)
60-64	461	(2)	914	(1)	342	(1)	26	(4)	5	(1)	1,750	(1)
65 or older	948	(3)	901	(1)	299	(1)	24	(3)	4	(1)	21,179	(2)
Female subtotal	27,889	(100)	74,331	(100)	25,680	(100)	694	(100)	412	(100)	129,199	(100)
Total†	324,822		282,720		137,575		5,546		2,234		753,907	

*Includes 826 males and 184 females whose race/ethnicity is unknown.
†Includes 3 persons whose gender is unknown.

TABLE 13-2

Estimated U.S. Deaths of Persons with AIDS 1993 Through 1999*

Male Adult/Adolescent Exposure Category	YEAR OF DEATH						
	1993	1994	1995	1996	1997	1998	1999
Men who have sex with men	23,841	25,198	24,740	16,688	8,580	6,741	5,819
Injecting drug use	9,282	10,344	10,779	8,516	5,356	4,439	3,975
Men who have sex with men and inject drugs	3,166	3,475	3,390	2,573	1,427	1,207	1,095
Hemophiliac/coagulation disorder	354	347	328	244	136	112	97
Heterosexual contact	1,591	2,004	2,388	2,106	1,467	1,226	1,187
Receipt of blood transfusion, blood components, or tissue	314	304	261	217	110	80	67
Risk not reported or identified	174	147	103	67	46	28	27
Male subtotal	38,722	41,820	41,989	30,411	17,122	13,833	12,267
Female Adult/Adolescent Exposure Category							
Injecting drug use	3,132	3,687	3,795	3,277	2,144	1,876	1,856
Hemophiliac/coagulation disorder	17	28	29	30	21	16	17
Heterosexual contact	2,655	3,469	3,969	3,434	2,302	1,991	1,929
Receipt of blood transfusion, blood components, or tissue	238	226	233	174	94	75	74
Risk not reported or identified	75	55	56	32	20	15	18
Female subtotal	6,117	7,464	8,081	6,946	4,581	3,972	3,893
Pediatric (<13 years old) Exposure Category	542	585	540	431	219	124	113
Total	45,381	49,869	50,610	37,787	21,923	17,930	16,273

*These numbers do not represent actual deaths of persons with AIDS. Rather, these numbers are estimates adjusted for delays in the reporting of deaths and for redistribution of cases initially reported with no identified risk, but not for incomplete reporting of deaths. Annual estimates are through the most recent year for which reliable estimates are available. See Technical Notes.

infected with HIV-1 eventually will develop AIDS. This will remain true until effective antiviral treatment agents become available. Presently, however, most individuals with AIDS are living longer, including some with CD4 counts that are extremely low (i.e., 10 to 40).[4,9,10]

Several cases of HIV-2 infection have been reported by the CDC and others[11-12] from various countries, including Canada, the United States, South America, and Europe. HIV-2 has been demonstrated to provide some natural immunity to HIV-1 and is much less rapidly de-

veloping. The immunosuppression is not as severe.[12] However, the ultimate mortality from HIV-2 is unknown.[12]

AIDS is the leading cause of death in men 25 to 44 years of age, in the United States, with more than 30 million adults and 1 million children throughout the world infected.[3,13,14] In the last 5 years in the United States a steady increase in the heterosexual transmission of AIDS has occurred, whereas the cases of AIDS associated with blood and blood products is declining. However, over that same time period a 31% decrease was reported in

the incidence of HIV infection in males who have had sex with men. The overall prevalence in that group (over age 13 years) is 15.9 per 100,000.[2,3]

The largest proportionate increase in AIDS cases since 1989 has been among women (blacks, Hispanics, heterosexuals, and those living in the South). More than 80% of these women have a history of IV drug abuse or had sex with a known HIV-infected partner.[2,8,13,14] The impact and importance of AIDS on dentistry has been significant. The CDC has made specific recommendations for dentists managing HIV-infected patients. The American Dental Association has established national guidelines and standards for infection control, identification of potential AIDS patients, and the management of these patients in the dental setting. The Occupational and Safety Administration also has mandated certain standards of practice designed to reduce the likelihood of transmission of blood-borne pathogens to employees in the dental office.

DEFINITION

INCIDENCE AND PREVALENCE

More than 120,000 people had died of AIDS in the United States up to 1992. By 1995 the number had grown to more than 311,000. In 2000 the figure has risen to more than 430,000 (see Table 13-2). More than 1.5 million Americans are believed to have HIV antibodies.[2,3,8] Before 1988 the majority of AIDS cases in the United States were found in four states: California, New York, Florida, and New Jersey. Cities reporting the largest numbers of AIDS cases were New York, San Francisco, Miami, Newark, and Los Angeles.[14] These cities continue to report new cases but not at the rate experienced during 1981 to 1988. By contrast, cities now in the early stages of the epidemic are reporting a doubling of the number of AIDS cases every 6 months to a year. The most dramatic rise in new cases more recently has come from the Southern region of the United States (31%). During that same time, a dramatic increase occurred in the numbers of AIDS cases from small towns and rural areas.[2] In the South, 25% of all new AIDS cases were found in rural areas. Significant numbers of AIDS cases have now occurred in all 50 states (see Table 13-1).

In 1992 approximately 66% of all AIDS cases were reported to involve homosexual or bisexual males. That figure has dropped to 45%, which still represents the largest single group though the general epidemiology has changed significantly.[2] Approximately 7% of these homosexual-bisexual males also are reported to be IV drug users. This 45% figure has decreased from a high of 74%

in late 1988.[13] IV drug users (particularly those who share needles) now constitute some 28% of the AIDS cases, and this figure has increased sharply since 1988. Those with both hemophilia and AIDS represent about 1% of all cases, and transfusion patients about 2%. AIDS found in heterosexuals (not included in the preceding groups) increased from approximately 0.8% in 1985 to 6% in 1992 to the present figure of nearly 10% of all cases of AIDS. AIDS cases in women also have dramatically risen in the past 10 years from 8% to 18%. A group of approximately 4% remains of the reported cases in which the method of transmission is unknown. From 1993 to 1995, the proportion of AIDS cases in whites decreased from 60% to 43%, but the proportion in blacks and Hispanics increased significantly from 25% to 38% and 14% to 18%, respectively[1,2,3,13] (see Table 13-1).

Among the other changes that recently occurred in the epidemiology of AIDS is the increase in the ratio of women to men, particularly in the 30- to 40-year age group in black women (see Table 13-1). A reduction in the number of AIDS cases in the transfusion and hemophiliac groups has occurred because of the testing (started in 1985) of donor blood for HIV antibodies and the heating of factor VIII replacement preparations[2,4] (see Table 13-2).

Generally, the blood supply in the United States is safe from transmission of the HIV virus.[15,16] Nevertheless, a very small risk exists of infection from individuals who become infected and donate blood just before experiencing seroconversion. This risk is estimated to be 1:660,000 for a single unit of blood and 1:222,222 for an average transfusion of 5.4 units of blood.[17,20] The mean time for AIDS to develop after blood transfusion transmission is 7 years.[18,19] The mean incubation period to AIDS for individuals infected with HIV by blood transfusion is 1.97 years for children 1 to 4 years of age, 8.23 years for persons aged 5 to 59, and 5.5 years for individuals over 60 years of age.[19] In a study of persons with hemophilia who had documented data of seroconversion,[20] AIDS was found to develop faster in older patients. Older patients also had an earlier onset of low CD4 cell counts.[20]

Children with AIDS are a true social and emotional concern. In the year 2000, approximately 8700 cases had been reported in the United States[3] (see Table 13-1), 84% of these cases involving mothers with AIDS, mothers who were HIV infected, and mothers who were at increased risk for developing HIV infection. Approximately 9% of the children had received blood transfusions, and 5% had hemophilia. An estimated 1.5 million children are HIV infected worldwide.[17-19] The most common opportunistic infections in children are bacterial; Kaposi's sarcoma is rare.[21-26]

The rate of HIV infection in the general population can only be estimated. The CDC estimated the prevalence in the general U.S. population to be 1 in 4500 in 1989. By 1993 that figure had dropped to 1 in 20,000.[13,14,26] Seroprevalence studies of applicants for U.S. military service during the period between 1985 and 1989 revealed a prevalence of approximately 0.34 per 1000. By 1992 this figure had grown to 1.2 per 1000.[27] The rate was highest for African-Americans and lowest for whites.[1,27] In blind HIV surveillance studies conducted by the CDC in selected hospitals across the United States from 1986 to 1992, the seroprevalence of general admissions was found to be 0.9%.[2] The 65 publicly funded HIV counseling and testing services reporting to the Centers for Disease Control (CDC) have stated that approximately 3% (51,170 of 1,366,537) of the HIV antibody tests were positive during 1990.[6,13] Data from the American Red Cross derived from donated blood indicate that approximately 0.04% of first-time blood donors are HIV infected.[26] Based on CDC estimates, 3,250,000 individuals have been tested since 1985 through public services, and 185,000 (5.7%) were positive for HIV antibodies. Only about half the individuals with negative test results received posttest counseling, compared with approximately 75% of those with positive tests.[28,29] In a follow-up study[14] in 1995, only 10% of individuals tested for HIV were counseled by private clinics compared with more than 60% by public clinics.

In 1991, some 20,000 women had been reported with AIDS. By the end of 1995, that figure was approximately 73,000. In 2000, nearly 130,000 cases of AIDS were in women,[14] 51% of these women IV drug abusers, 34% heterosexual contacts, 8% transfusion recipients, and less than 1% infected from blood products used to treat coagulation disorders. The cause in the remaining women (6%) was undetermined.[2] The highest rate of women diagnosed with AIDS is in the African-American population (see Table 13-1). No gender difference has been found in the rate of progression of HIV infection. A poorer survival rate for women has been found in several studies, but this appears to be related to less access to medical care. Pregnancy in HIV-infected women leads to infection in anywhere from 15% to 50% of the infants, approximately 30% in the United States, although pregnancy itself does not appear to accelerate HIV infection. Women have an increased incidence of *Candida* esophagitis and HIV wasting syndrome over men.[30]

Approximately 10% of the patients with AIDS are over age 50 years. An estimated 1 million homosexual men are over age 65 years. Many of these men engage in regular sexual activity into their 80s. Transfusion of infected blood, use of blood products, sexual activity, and IV drug abuse are the modes of transmission in the older population. Certain problems are unique to older patients with AIDS. HIV-related dementia may be diagnosed as Alzheimer's disease (see Chapter 23). Age changes in the immune system result in an increase in tumors and infections in non-HIV-infected older individuals. Further, the immune suppression found with HIV infection will only enhance the overall degree of immune suppression in older individuals. When dealing with neurologic, neoplastic, and infectious signs and symptoms in older patients, the dentist should consider possible HIV infection and investigate the possibility of the patient being infected.[2,14]

As of the year 2000, more than 30 million cases of HIV infection were estimated worldwide. This figure reflects an increase of 19% in 1 year; 1.5 million children are included in the total figure. AIDS has been reported on 5 continents.[1,3] The majority of cases have been in Africa, Southeast Asia, and the Americas, with the fewest in Central and East Asia. India has nearly the fastest-growing incidence of new AIDS cases in the world, with more than 1.5 million cases.[31]

AIDS also has been reported in more than 30 European countries, with the highest per capita rates appearing in Switzerland and France. The prevalence of HIV infection for various regions of the world is as follows: sub-Saharan Africa (18 million), Southeast Asia (5 million), United States and North America (1.5 million), Latin and South America (2.5 million) and Western Europe (1 million).[3,4,12,23,33]

ETIOLOGY

In 1984 the etiologic agent for AIDS was identified independently by three laboratories. A French team from the Pasteur Institute identified a retrovirus termed the *lymphadenopathy-associated virus* and reported it as the causative agent for AIDS. In the United States, a team from the National Institutes of Health isolated a retrovirus identified as the *human* T *lymphotropic virus* III (HTLV-III) and labeled it as the etiologic agent for AIDS. A team in San Francisco also isolated a retrovirus, AIDS-*related virus* (ARV), and designated it as the causative agent for AIDS. All three viruses were similar retroviruses, with but minor differences in their amino acid sequences.[32] The variations in disease patterns may be accounted for by the slight differences among the AIDS viruses which also makes the production of a vaccine difficult.[32] The three groups essentially were describing the same retrovirus, which can change its antigenicity. Most workers in the field up to 1986 referred to the virus as HTLV-III and considered it to be the causative agent for AIDS. In 1986 the World Health

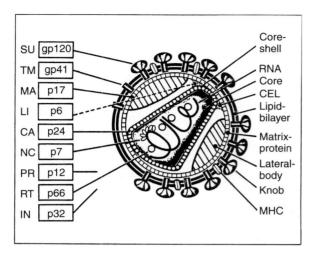

SU	gp120
TM	gp41
MA	p17
LI	p6
CA	p24
NC	p7
PR	p12
RT	p66
IN	p32

Core-shell
RNA
Core
CEL
Lipid-bilayer
Matrix-protein
Lateral-body
Knob
MHC

Fig. 13-1 HIV-1. (From Gelderblom H: *AIDS* 5:620, 1991.)

Organization recommended the AIDS virus be termed the *human immunodeficiency virus* (Fig. 13-1).[32]

What first appeared to be a single virus is now actually known to be a complex family of lentiviruses composed of two subtypes (HIV-1 and HIV-2) with many different strains.[33,34] HIV can infect most human cells; however, the cells most commonly infected are those with CD4 receptors including T-helper lymphocytes (CD4 cells) and macrophages and hence are the cells most involved with HIV infection.[33] Research[34,35] has suggested other receptors are active in allowing HIV to infect human cells. Evidence has surfaced that HIV-antibody complexes interact with Fc or a complement receptor, which facilitates the entry of the virus into the cell. Other cell surface receptors include galactosylcerebroside glycolipids, LFA-1 adhesion receptor, and certain proteases.[34,35]

A small portion of the carboxy-terminal half of the viral envelope (gp120), which represents less than 5% of the total genome, is associated with the most virulent features of HIV infection (see Fig. 13-1). This segment of the gp120 has been referred to as the V_3 loop and may represent the best site for vaccine development.[33,34] Studies[36,37] have indicated that a strong antiviral agent may be produced by suppressor lymphocytes (CD8+ cells). Long-term survivors of HIV infection have been found to have less virulent HIV strains, without the enhancing antibodies to HIV and with strong CD8m T-cell cell antiviral activity.[36,37,38,39]

HIV-1 gene expression is divided into two temporal phases: an early regulatory phase and a later structural phase. In the early phase, a set of small messenger ribonucleic acids (mRNAs) is produced that encode the regulatory proteins: *tat*, *rev*, and *nef*. These are powerful

viral regulators and activators necessary for viral replication. Efforts toward the development of a vaccine have revolved around these regulatory proteins.[36,37] When the viral regions responsible for neutralization enhancement are defined, the development of *nef* proteins to block HIV replication may be possible. (For an in-depth discussion of the function of these viral genes and their products, the reader is referred to the *Textbook of* AIDS *Medicine* by Broder et al.[36])

Recent research also has shown that other factors are involved in cytotoxic T lymphocyte (CTL) activity that may affect viral replication in patients infected with HIV-1.[38] These studies suggest that HIV-1 specific CTL activity is a major component in the host immune response associated with the control of viral replication. This may have important implications in the development of a vaccine.[36-39]

The current attempts to develop a vaccine are directed toward (1) preventing HIV infection and (2) interfering with viral replication, to render the HIV infection less severe. The major efforts to develop a vaccine thus far center around the most virulent portion of HIV, to identify and produce the antiviral agent produced by CD8+ cells, or to develop *nef* (or other) proteins to block HIV replication.[36-39]

PATHOPHYSIOLOGY AND COMPLICATIONS

In addition to its transfer by sexual means and the parenteral transfer of infected blood, AIDS may be transmitted vertically, probably at birth or transplacentally to infants born of infected mothers).[38-40]

The most common method of sexual transmission in the United States is homosexual anal intercourse; however, heterosexual transmission has been documented from infected males to noninfected females. Transmission from infected females to noninfected males also has been reported. Heterosexual transmission of HIV can occur through sexual contact of carriers who are heterosexual IV drug users, bisexual males, or blood recipients of either gender. HIV has been found in saliva, but transmission via saliva has not been demonstrated. HIV also has been isolated from tears, breast milk, cerebrospinal fluid, amniotic fluid, and urine. Blood, semen, breast milk and vaginal secretions are the only fluids that have been demonstrated to be associated with transmission of the virus, however.[7] Casual contact has not been demonstrated as a means of transmission.[36]

More than 1.5 million Americans are estimated to have been exposed to the AIDS virus by the year 2000.[2,3] Current data would suggest that most if not all of these individuals will develop AIDS as defined by the CDC. Antibody positivity to HIV means that the person has been infected with the virus and can be viremic. Individuals who appear to be most susceptible to devel-

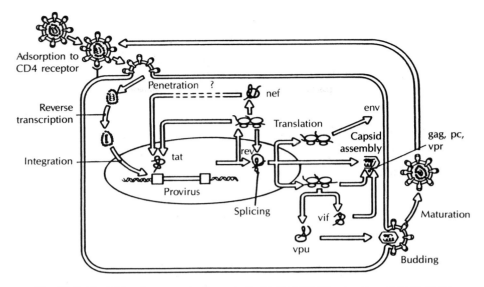

Fig. 13-2 The HIV replication cycle. (From Coffin JM: *AIDS 1990 Year Rev* 4(suppl):S1-S9, 1990.)

oping AIDS are those with repeated exposure to the virus who also have an immune system that has been challenged by repeated exposure to various antigens (semen, hepatitis B, or blood products).

Individuals infected with the virus will develop antibodies usually within 6 to 12 weeks. Most infected individuals will develop a viremia within 2 to 6 weeks. A few may take up to 6 months to achieve seroconversion. In rare cases, as long as 35 months may be required for seroconversion to occur.[7,8] The incubation period for AIDS appears to be lengthy for most individuals (mean 10 to 12 years). Only about 30% percent of individuals with AIDS are dead within 3 years of the diagnosis, whereas approximately 50% live beyond 10 years.[7,8]

Once having gained access to the bloodstream, HIV selectively seeks out T lymphocytes (specifically T4 or T-helper lymphocytes) (Fig. 13-2). The virus binds to the CD4 lymphocyte cell surface specifically by the highly glycosylated outer surface envelope (gp120) proteins. Upon infection, reverse transcriptase catalyzes the synthesis of a haploid, double-stranded DNA provirus, which becomes incorporated into the chromosomal DNA of the host cell. Thus integrated, the provirus genetic material may remain latent in an unexpressed form until events occur that activate it, at which time DNA transcription rapidly occurs and new virons are produced. The virus is lymphotropic; hence the cells it selects for replication are soon destroyed. Once the virus has taken hold, it soon leads to a reduction in the total number of T-helper cells,

and a marked shift in the ratio of T4 to T8 lymphocytes occurs. The normal ratio of T-helper to T-suppressor lymphocytes is about 2:1 (60% T-helper, 30% T-suppressor). In AIDS, the T4/T8 ratio is reversed. The marked reduction in T-helper lymphocytes, to a great degree, explains the lack of immune response seen in AIDS patients and most likely is related to the increase in malignant disease found associated with AIDS: Kaposi's sarcoma, lymphoma, carcinoma of the cervix, and carcinoma of the rectum.[36-40]

The majority (more than 50%) of individuals exposed to the virus at first develop an acute, brief viremia (seroconversion sickness) within 2 to 6 weeks of HIV exposure. A concomitant, temporary fall occurs in CD4 cells (lymphopenia, along with high titers of plasma HIV), but the patients do not develop evidence of immune suppression. Various flu-like symptoms occur in this acute seroconversion sickness that usually last about 2 to 4 weeks. Only an estimated 20% of these individuals will seek medical attention.[36-40] These individuals respond by producing antibodies to HIV (i.e., anti-gp120 and anti-p24) and the cytotoxic T lymphocyte levels increase. The immune abnormalities in HIV disease consist of progressive depletion of CD4+ T lymphocytes with ultimate pancytopenia, impaired lymphocyte proliferative, and cytokine responses to mitogens and antigens; impaired cytotoxic lymphocyte function and natural killer cell activity, anergy to skin testing, and diminished antibody responses to new antigens.[36-40]

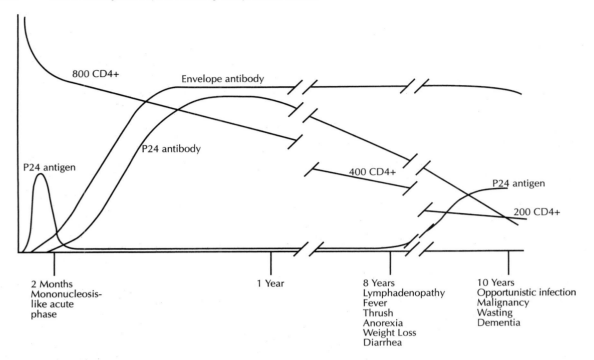

Fig. 13-3 The natural history of HIV infection. (From Brookmeyer R, Gail MH: *AIDS epidemiology: a quantitative approach*, New York, 1994, Oxford University Press, pp 1-18.)

The virus also may infect neurons or macrophages in the central nervous system, allowing the virus to be present within the body in latent form. These individuals may demonstrate a viremia on occasion and hence are considered carriers of the virus who have the potential to infect others. Of special concern is the fact that circulating antibodies fail to neutralize the virus because it has the capacity to alter its antigenicity[36-40] (Fig. 13-3). An alarming characteristic of these patients, in addition to having the potential to be infectious and to develop AIDS, is that approximately 50% of them develop signs of dementia that can be rapidly progressive.[36-40] After a long asymptomatic period, in most cases, while the CD4 count continues to drop and HIV continues to proliferate, the infected individual may develop signs and symptoms such as lymphadenopathy, fever, weight loss, diarrhea, night sweats, pharyngitis, rashes, myalgia and arthralgia, headache, neuropathy and malaise, and eventually AIDS (see Fig. 13-3).[36-40]

Generally, when the CD4 count drops below 200, the patient is susceptible to several opportunistic infections, including *Pneumocytosis carinii* pneumonia, toxoplasmosis, influenza, histoplasmosis, cytomegalovirus (CMV) infec-

tion, and mucocutaneous diseases such as candidiasis. The previously mentioned neoplasms also may appear during AIDS.[40,41]

Tuberculosis (TB) cases in HIV-infected patients have risen dramatically during the past 5 years. The CDC reports that the coincident cases of HIV/AIDS and TB increased from 8% to 17% during that time. The number of cases of TB in the United States during that time increased from approximately 21,000 to 26,000 per year. Most of these cases are in the HIV-infected populations as are the increasing number of multi-drug resistant strains of TB[2,3,13] (see Chapter 8).

CLINICAL PRESENTATION

SIGNS AND SYMPTOMS

In the period 2 to 6 weeks after the initial infection with HIV, more than 50% of patients develop an acute flulike viremia that may last 10 to 14 days.[4,41] Others may not manifest this symptom complex. The patients have the HIV but are antibody negative. They usually will experience seroconversion within 6 weeks to 6 months and

BOX 13-1

Categorization of HIV Exposures

Group I	HIV antibody positive-asymptomatic
Group 2	CD4 <400

Constitutional symptoms (i.e., fever, malaise, lymphadenopathy, diarrhea); opportunistic infections

Group 3	AIDS; CD4 <200

Kaposi's sarcoma, lymphoma, pneumonia, cervical carcinoma, etc.

BOX 13-2

Signs and Symptoms of HIV Infection

Initial exposure or infection (seroconversion syndrome)
Flulike symptoms-fever, weakness, 10 to 14 days
Asymptomatic stage
Serologic evidence of infection
No signs or symptoms
Symptomatic stage
Serologic evidence of infection
T4/T8 ratio reduced to about 1
Persistent lymphadenopathy
Oral candidiasis
Constitutional symptoms-night sweats, diarrhea, weight loss, fever, malaise, weakness
Advanced symptomatic stage
Serologic evidence of infection
T4/T8 ratio suppressed to less than 0.5
HIV encephalopathy
HIV wasting syndrome
Major opportunistic infections
Neoplasms-Kaposi's sarcoma, lymphoma, carcinoma of rectum

Group 1. Immediate post-HIV exposure. After a brief post-seroconversion sickness syndrome, these individuals are antibody positive to HIV but are asymptomatic and show no other laboratory abnormalities.

Group 2. Progressive immunosuppression, HIV-symptomatic stage. Individuals who have various laboratory changes (i.e., lymphopenia: T-helper/T-suppressor ratio; usually less than 1) in addition to being HIV antibody positive, also can show some clinical signs or symptoms, such as enlarged lymph nodes, night sweats, weight loss, oral candidiasis, fever, malaise, and diarrhea.

Group 3. Individuals who have AIDS, including Kaposi's sarcoma, wasting syndrome, lymphoma, cervical or rectal carcinoma, CNS symptoms with dementia, and a life-threatening opportunistic infection (i.e., tuberculosis, pneumonia), a CD-4 count of less than 200 and an altered T-helper/T-suppressor ratio of 0.5 or less; they are HIV antibody positive and can demonstrate generalized lymphadenopathy with severe weight loss, fatigue, chronic diarrhea, chronic fever, and night sweats (see Box 13-2). HIV can infect the CNS and often leads to a progressive form of dementia.

Patients may become confused and disoriented or experience short-term memory deficits. Others can develop severe depression or paranoia and show suicidal tendencies.

LABORATORY FINDINGS

HIV can be isolated from the blood, semen, breast milk, tears, and saliva of many patients with AIDS. Most patients exposed to the virus, with or without clinical evidence of disease, show antibodies to the virus. Patients with advanced HIV infection or AIDS have an altered ratio of T4/T8 lymphocytes, a decrease in total number of lymphocytes, thrombocytopenia, anemia, a slight alteration in the humoral antibody system, and a decreased ability to show delayed allergic reactions to skin testing (cutaneous anergy).

In 1985 several screening tests became available for identification of antibodies to HIV. The enzyme-linked immunosorbent assay (ELISA) is sensitive but has a high rate of false-positive results. Current practice is to screen first with ELISA. If the first results are positive, a second ELISA is performed. All positive results are then rescreened with a second test, the Western blot analysis. This combination of screening tests is accurate more than 99% of the time. Positive ELISA and Western blot test results indicate only that the individual has been exposed to the AIDS virus. If results of the Western blot are indeterminate, HIV infection is rarely, if ever, positive.[37,43] These tests, however, do not indicate the status of the HIV infection or whether AIDS is present.

then will demonstrate antibodies. The severity of the initial acute infection with HIV is predictive of the course the infection will follow. In one study,[42] 78% of the individuals with a long-lasting acute illness developed AIDS within 3 years; by contrast, only 10% of those individuals with no acute illness at seroconversion developed AIDS within 3 years. Once exposure to HIV and seroconversion has occurred, 3 groups of patients may be identified (Boxes 13-1, 13-2; see Fig. 13-3).

BOX 13-3

Drugs of Significance to the Dentist Treating HIV/AIDS Patients*

Antibiotics	Fluconazole
Erythromycin	Amphoterin B
Clarithromycin	Clotrimazole
Streptomycin	**Antivirals**
Clindamycin	Acyclovir
Azithromycin	Ganciclovir
Rifabutin	Valacyclovir
Sulfa drugs (TMP-SMX: Septra, Bactrim)	Zidovudine
Metronidazole	Dideoxyinosine
Pentamidine	Dideoxycytidine
Ethambutol	Foscarnet
Atovaquone	
	Corticosteroids
Antifungals	Dapsone
Nystatin	Vinblastine
Ketoconazole	

*HIV/AIDS patients may be placed on these drugs for management or prophylaxis.

Neither do they show if the patient is viremic, because a special test, the DNA polymerase chain reaction (PCR) for direct detection of the virus would need to be performed. This is considerably more expensive. However, patients with positive results from the ELISA and Western blot tests are considered potentially infectious. An ELISA test developed by Wellcome is 98% sensitive in detecting antibodies to HIV in saliva.[44] A test to detect salivary secretory immunoglobulin A antibodies of nonmaternal origin in newborns of women at risk for HIV infection has been found accurate in detecting infected infants.[45]

Since 1989 HIV-DNA sequences may be readily detected by the DNA PCR assay, which was found to be an equivalent method to culturing the virus itself. Direct detection of HIV by PCR is superior to testing for HIV antigen in serum.[43-45]

Viral load (degree of viremia in blood plasma) is determined using a PCR-based test such as Roche Molecular Systems Inc. Range of detection is 50 copies/ml to over 750,000 copies per ml. The highest viral load is found during the first three months after initial infection and during the late stages of the disease.

MEDICAL MANAGEMENT

No effective treatment or cure for AIDS exists. Antiviral agents have been unsuccessful in killing the HIV virus. However, zidovudine (AZT or Retrovir) has been shown[46,47] to exert significant inhibitory effects on in vitro replication cytopathogenicity of HIV. AZT has been found to prolong life in both asymptomatic and symptomatic HIV-infected individuals,[46,47] although no evidence exists that AZT is effective in preventing infection once exposure to the virus has occurred[46,47] (Box 13-3).

ANTIRETROVIRAL AGENTS

The most effective management of the progression of HIV/AIDS has been with several types of antiretroviral medications. These medications are grouped into three categories (Box 13-4): (1) nucleoside analogs, including zidovudine (Retrovir, formerly known as "Azidothymidine" [AZT]), dideoxyinosine (Videx [ddI]), zalcitabine (HIVID [ddC]), stavudine (Zerit [d4T]), lamivudine (Epivir [3TC]), and abacavir (Ziagen [ABC]); (2) protease inhibitors, including saquinavir (Fortovase), indinavir (Crixivan), ritonavir (Norvir), nelfinavir (Viracept), and amprenavir (Agenerase); and (3) nonnucleoside reverse transcriptase inhibitors, including delavirdine (Rescriptor) and efavirenz (Sustiva). These drugs inhibit HIV replication.[46-48]

One of these medications is started for most HIV-infected patients when immunosuppression becomes pronounced (CD4 is less than 500) and, because of the chronic nature of the infection, continues indefinitely. The current popular therapy is with the so-called "triple therapy" in which two of the nucleoside analogs are combined with a protease inhibitor. See Box 13-4 for the suggested antiretroviral regimens.

Antiretroviral Therapy

Nucleoside analogs: zidovudine (Retrovir) {formerly known as azidothymidine (AZT)}, dideoxyinosine (Videx) (ddI), zalcitabine (HIVID) (ddC), stavudine (Zerit) (d4T) lamivudine (Epivir) (3TC) and abacavir (Ziagen) (ABC);

Protease inhibitors: saquinavir (Fortovase), indinavir (Crixivan), ritonavir (Norvir), nelfinavir (Viracept) and amprenavir (Agenerase);

Non-nucleoside reverse transcriptase inhibitors: delaviridine (Resciptor) and efavirenz (Sustiva).

Common Immunosuppression-Related Diseases Based on T-Helper Cell Level*

T-Helper Cell Count	Disease
400	Most patients have no signs of immunosuppression-associated disease
301 to 400	Bacterial skin infections = staphylococcal
201 to 300	Herpes zoster
	Candidiasis
	Tinea pedia
	Oral hairy leukoplakia
101 to 200	Tuberculosis
	Pneumocystitis carinii pneumonia
	Histoplasmosis
	Coccidioidomycosis
	Cryptococcal meningitis
	Toxoplasmosis
	Herpes simplex
	Cryptosporidiosis
	Kaposi's sarcoma
0 to 100	Wasting syndrome
	Cytomegalovirus
	Lymphoma
	Mycobacterium avium complex

*The T-helper cell range is the common range for the onset of the disease. The disease could first appear at a higher or lower T-cell level.[53]

Usually in the United States antiretroviral therapy will begin as the CD-4 count drops below 500.[48] In many cases, long-term use (more than 6 months) of these medications will result in resistant HIV strains, requiring use of alternative drugs (or combinations of these or other antivirals such as acyclovir), including those to prevent opportunistic infections. The side effects of these medications are numerous and significant to the dental clinician. Anemia is a major side effect as the drugs are toxic to the bone marrow and blood cells. Blood transfusions may be necessary in severe cases. Leukopenia and granulocytopenia occur and predispose the patient to infections, fatigue, muscle pain, rashes, nausea, diarrhea, and headaches. Other side effects may include hepatotoxicity, peripheral neuropathy, and pancreatitis.[48]

Another major directive for management of the HIV/AIDS patient, particularly as the CD4 lymphocyte count drops (to less than 200), is to prevent opportunistic infections such as pneumonia, influenza, TB, and hepatitis B, among others. Effective vaccines and other drugs are available for immunoprophylaxis for many of these infections. Aerosol pentamidine and oral trimethoprim-sulfamethoxazole are effective prophylactic agents for P*neumocystis carinii* pneumonia. Ganciclovir, foscarnet, and acyclovir are used to treat opportunistic viral infections found in AIDS patients. Acyclovir also has been used as a prophylactic treatment for certain viral infections. Attempts to improve the suppressed immune system are being investigated. Ditiocarb (Immuthiol) improves immune competence by modulating T-cell function.[48]

In addition, medical management consists of protecting the patient from exposure to infectious agents and treating infections when they occur with isolation and high doses of antibiotics.[48] Kaposi's sarcoma (epidemic form) associated with AIDS is a much more aggressive lesion than the classic form. Kaposi's sarcoma in cases other than AIDS presents as a vascular tumor that usually is found in older men and may be difficult to manage using surgery or radiation techniques. General treatment of the AIDS patient must be considered to be symptomatic.[48]

OPPORTUNISTIC INFECTIONS

Opportunistic infections are the leading cause of death in HIV/AIDS patients. The dental practitioner must identify the signs and symptoms of these opportunistic infections and realize the special management considerations for those patients who contract these infections or are being treated with prophylactic medications (Table 13-3).[31,41,56]

One of the most common and most serious opportunistic infections in the HIV/AIDS patient is *Pneumocystis carinii* pneumonia, which is caused by a protozoan parasite that invades the lungs (and rarely the lymph nodes). The symptoms are fever, cough, difficulty breathing, weight loss, night sweats, and fatigue. Patients may receive prophylaxis with pentamidine, trimethoprim and sulfamethoxazole (TMP-SMX) (Bactrim, Septra) which are potent medications with substantial side effects. Dapsone also may be used for prophylaxis of *Pneumocystis carinii*, and corticosteroids also may be administered (see Box 13-3). With any of these medications the patient is subject to serious adverse drug effects, including allergic reactions, toxic drug reactions, hepatotoxicity, immunosuppression, anemia, serious drug interactions, and other potential problems. The clinician must have a thorough understanding of all medications and their actions, side effects, warnings, interactions with other drugs, and contraindications before definitive treatment begins. Most often, consultation with the patient's physician is mandatory.[37,41]

Toxoplasmosis is caused by a protozoan parasite and manifests as a latent infection of the central nervous system. Symptoms are generally neurologic and include headaches, dizziness, and seizures. Crytosporidiosis is caused by a protozoan parasite and affects the gastrointestinal tract, resulting in nausea, vomiting, diarrhea, malaise, fever, and weight loss.[41,47]

Candidiasis is a common oral infection but also may be systemic. This fungus may infect the mucous membranes of the mouth, vagina, esophagus, gastrointestinal tract, and skin. A wide range of symptoms exists. Systemic treatment is performed with fluconazole (Diflucan) or ketoconazole (Nizoral). These drugs have a number of significant side effects and drug interactions of which the clinician must be aware.[41,49,50]

Cryptococcus and *Histoplasma* are yeastlike fungi that may infect the lungs, brain, and other tissues, and can be life threatening. Symptoms include fever, weight loss, neurologic symptoms, difficulty breathing, mucosal lesions, headache, nausea, vomiting, and malaise. Treatment is with fluconazole, ketoconazole, or amphotericin B.[50,56]

Because HIV-infected individuals are extremely susceptible to contracting TB, dental practitioners should be aware of its signs and symptoms, such as lymphadenopathy, cough, fever, weight loss, diarrhea, night sweats, and malaise. These manifestations must be evaluated with the potential for *Mycobacterium tuberculosis* infection in mind. Mantoux skin testing (purified protein derivative PPD) of HIV-infected patients is indicated. These patients may be treated or receive prophylaxis with isoniazid (INH). Rifampin, ethambutol, or streptomycin also may be used. An important concern is the multiantibiotic-resistant form of TB (see Chapter 8). Other *Mycobacterium* infectons also may occur such as MAC

(*Mycobacterium avium* and *Mycobacterium intracellulare*). Treatment is with ciprofloxacin (Cipro), amikacin sulfate (Amikin), ethambutol HCl.[50,56]

Viral infections with viruses other than HIV also are common in these patients. Some of these viral infections[57-66] as follows:

Cytomegalovirus
Approximately 90% of all HIV patients become infected with cytomegalovirus (CMV).[56,59] CMV can infect and manifest in most any tissue of the body including the oral cavity (deep, nonhealing ulcerations). Retinitis, esophagitis, and colitis frequently will occur. Ganciclovir (Cytovene) is the usual drug for treatment of CMV infection.[56,59]

Herpes Simplex/Herpes Zoster
Herpes simplex virus (HSV: HSV-1 and HSV-2) and herpes zoster (varicella-zoster virus: VZV) commonly infect individuals who are in an immunocompromised condition. These pathogens infect epithelial tissues and nerve endings. The symptoms are painful inflammatory blisters that follow a sensory nerve tract. These infections usually are treated with acyclovir, which may be used as prophylaxis.[41,56,59]

Epstein-Barr Virus
Epstein-Barr virus is associated with oral hairy leukoplakia in the HIV/AIDS patient. Acyclovir or ganciclovir can reduce or eliminate the lesions if necessary.[60-66]

Human Papillomavirus
Human papillomavirus (HPV) also may infect the oral cavity in HIV/AIDS patients and clinically present as oral warts. These lesions can be excised with lasers.[65,66]

HIV Risk Management
Individuals at risk for HIV infection are advised to reduce their risk of exposure to HIV by practicing safe sex through (1) reducing the number of sexual partners, (2) avoiding anonymous sexual partners, (3) modifying sexual practices to reduce the exchange of bodily secretions (including the use of condoms), (4) reducing the use of drugs such as volatile nitrites and alcohol, and (5) adopting cleanliness procedures before and after the sex act. Suggestions for IV drug users include the following: (1) stop using IV drugs, which would be very difficult for most; (2) avoid sharing needles; (3) clean all apparatus with bleach after each use; (4) seek provision of free needles. HIV-infected mothers should refrain from breastfeeding their infants.[67,68]

The emotional and psychological problems associated with AIDS are numerous and stressful. Psychosocial counseling intervention before testing, at the time of diagnosis, and during the course of the disease is extremely important. The emotional impact on a young

adult faced with the trauma of a fatal disease can be severe. Patients must be helped to deal successfully with the fear of death, the liability of transmitting the disease, and the need to protect themselves from opportunistic infections. They should be encouraged to communicate openly and honestly with lovers, friends, and family who serve as their support group. Psychosocial counseling intervention also can help to resolve problems such as how the patients will support themselves, how medical bills will be paid, and how group therapy may be obtained. Psychosocial counseling can help the patient obtain access to one of the support groups for AIDS patients, provide education and literature about the infections and diseases, and serve as a liaison with community resources such as services agencies for homosexuals, cancer counseling, and civil rights agencies.[40]

DENTAL MANAGEMENT

MEDICAL CONSIDERATIONS

The major considerations for dentists providing care to AIDS patients are to recognize their level of immunosuppression, drug therapies, and potential for opportunistic infections and minimize the possibility of transmission of HIV from an infected patient to dentists, their staff, and other patients. Although saliva has not been demonstrated to have transmitted the virus in a dental situation, the potential for it to do so exists.[67,69] Infected blood can transmit HIV. Dental procedures that result in soft tissue injury allow various amounts of blood to become mixed with saliva. Latex gloves protect the hands of the operator from the mixture of blood and saliva in the mouth of an infected patient, but particles of blood and saliva could be splashed in the eye during various procedures. In addition, if an HIV-infected dentist cuts a finger through a glove, the potential to infect the patient also exists. Blood from the infected dentist could infect the patient through surgical wounds, ulcerations, or active periodontal disease. HIV can be transmitted by needlestick or an instrument wound. However, the frequency of such transfer is low especially with small gauge needles (e.g., 25, 27), such as those for the administration of local anesthesia in dentistry. Needlestick surveillance studies performed by the CDC[15] have noted that 1948 healthcare workers (HCWs) with 2042 percutaneous exposures to blood from HIV-infected patients had a seroconversion rate of 0.29%, and that 668 HCWs with 1051 mucous membrane exposures had no seroconversions.[6,15] Thus the likelihood of mucocutaneous transmission is very low.[70,71]

The CDC has reported 56 known occupational transmissions in HCWs and an additional possible 138 cases.[15] In another study of 710 HCWs who were percutaneously exposed to HIV, the risk of acquiring HIV was directly related to three factors: (1) deep tissue penetration into an artery or vein (odds ratio of 16:1), (2) visible blood contamination on the instrument that caused the percutaneous exposure (odds ratio of 5:2), and (3) the source patient being in the terminal stages of AIDS (odds ratio of 5:1).[72] Additionally, the dentist can do little to prevent accidental percutaneous exposure other than being careful to avoid accidental injury. Needles with a hollow lumen should be handled particularly carefully.[15]

The possibility of developing hepatitis B from a single needlestick injury in a hepatitis B carrier is 6% to 30%, whereas the possibility of developing HIV infection is 0.29%.[7,72] In two studies involving 5150 dental professionals, three dentists were found to be HIV infected; two had risk factors for HIV infection.[15] No risk factors could be identified in the third infected dentist.

An observation study of 1307 general surgical procedures[72] showed a 1.7% rate of parenteral exposure to blood. The risk of exposure increased for procedures lasting longer than 3 hours and when patient blood loss was greater than 300 ml. Awareness of the surgical team to the patient's high-risk or HIV infection status made no difference in the frequency of accidental wounds. Double gloving was found to prevent perforation of the inner glove. This study concluded that preoperative HIV testing would have had no beneficial effect on the frequency of accidental wounding in surgery.[72] According to the CDC, some 6800 AIDS cases had been reported in HCWs, and three of these cases were determined to likely been infected from occupational exposure.[15,70] Included in this study were 46 surgeons and 190 DHCWs.

In summary, while the risk of exposure to HIV and probability of transmission to HCWs is extremely low, the added risks of hepatitis, herpes simplex, and syphilis justify the use of barrier techniques and universal precautions for all patients.

The risk of transmitting HIV from an infected HCW to a patient has been demonstrated in only one instance. This was with the case of a Florida dentist who was found to have infected six of his patients. In look-back studies evaluating the patients treated by 60 HIV-infected HCWs, more than 9000 cases have been studied. The only HCW found to have most likely transmitted infection to his patients was this one dentist,[70,] who eventually died of AIDS. Little risk is involved for the patient being treated by an HIV-infected surgeon or dentist. The possible risk of HIV infection resulting from such treatment is far smaller than the risk of an anesthesia-related death (100 per 1,000,000) or the risk of death from penicillin anaphylaxis (10 to 20 per 1,000,000). The risk in Minnesota for HIV transmission occurring during a surgical procedure has been

estimated[73] to be between 1 per 2,100,000 and 1 per 21,000,000. This risk would be greater in urban areas in other parts of the United States. However, in any case it is very remote.

The available data clearly show little risk for patients to contract HIV from HCWs. A far greater risk exists for infection of HCWs by HIV-infected patients than vice versa. Patients with severe immunosuppression associated with AIDS may be at risk for local or distant postoperative infections after invasive dental procedures that injure tissues and produce transient bacteremias. These patients also may be potential bleeders because of severe thrombocytopenia.[71,74,75]

PREVENTION OF MEDICAL COMPLICATIONS

Patients identified as being carriers of HIV can be managed in the dental office using the protocol first developed for treating hepatitis B carriers but now recommended for all patients.[10,19,69] The use of laboratory screening tests for patients with a history of jaundice, hepatitis, and liver disease will pick up only 20% of the heptatitis B carriers.[19] The other 80% are asymptomatic or have had nonspecific symptoms not identified with hepatitis and hence not picked up by history. The same is true of HIV-exposed individuals; most are asymptomatic and not aware of their exposure. Hence, the history cannot be relied on for identification of infected individuals.[19,41,71] In addition, pretreatment laboratory screening of all patients for HIV exposure is costly, impractical, and contrary to civil rights practices. Screening of all high-risk patients for HIV exposure is possible if these people are identified by history and clinical findings and will consent to screening. However, experience has shown that many individuals in the high-risk groups, homosexual males and IV drug users, are not willing to share that information and when identified are resistant to screening. The American Dental Association[68] and the CDC[70] have recommended that all dental patients be considered as potentially infectious and universal precautions be used. These guidelines have been available since 1985. The federal government, through OSHA, has set standards that describe how to prevent blood-borne pathogen transmission in the workplace. These standards apply to dental offices with one or more employees. The OSHA standard and the infection control procedures recommended by the American Dental Association and the CDC are covered in detail in Appendix A. These recommendations should be used for all patients. If they are followed HIV-infected patients, other patients and dental staff will be best protected from transmission of infectious agents.[70]

PATIENT EVALUATION

The dentist should obtain a health history from the patient with AIDS or a related condition. A head and neck examination, an intraoral soft tissue examination, and a complete periodontal and dental examination on all new patients should be performed. History and clinical findings may indicate the patient who has AIDS or a related condition. Patients with AIDS and those at high risk for it realize their lack of true privacy on questionnaires; in addition, an AIDS phobia or homophobia may exist among members of the dental staff. Thus answers to certain questions may be less than factual. As a result, a patient's history should be obtained whenever possible via caring, understanding, verbal communication with a sharing of knowledge and facts through honesty, the avoidance of direct personal questions, and an openness with the patient. Because of the sensitive social and legal issues involved with AIDS, direct questions are not recommended for inclusion in the health history questionnaire, but certain questions suggestive of a high risk for AIDS or related conditions can be included on the health questionnaire then followed up verbally.

Patients who based on history or clinical findings are found to be at high risk for AIDS or related conditions should be referred for HIV testing, medical evaluation, other appropriate diagnostic procedures, and psychosocial intervention. The dentist should not undertake diagnostic laboratory screening but rather refer the patient to an appropriate medical facility. This should follow a discussion concerning the clinical findings and the possibility that AIDS or a related condition is present. At this time, sexual preference, IV drug use, and so on may be discussed and often will be mentioned by the patient. The patient should be strongly encouraged to seek diagnostic and supportive medical services. The dental health care professional also should encourage the use of professional support services including those offered by social workers, gay rights groups, legal services, economic assistance, and civil rights groups for counseling and support of the patient, and the patient's own support group. The patient must be encouraged to allow the preceding types of activities to take place.

High-risk AIDS patients who, for whatever reasons, fail to receive additional diagnostic testing and evaluation must be considered to have been exposed to the AIDS virus and to be potentially infectious. High-risk AIDS patients and diagnosed AIDS or HIV patients should be treated identically to any other patient that is, with universal precautions. Attention should be directed to the handling of prosthetic procedures and fabrication of prostheses.[67,68,76,77] Biopsy specimens taken from patients also require special attention in processing[19] (see Appendix A). All patients, re-

gardless of their hepatitis or AIDS status, must be treated using universal precautions and barrier techniques (see Appendix A). This is strongly recommended because most HIV carriers and more than 80% of the hepatitis B surface antigen (HBsAg) carriers cannot be identified on the basis of recommended clinical screening procedures.[19]

Several guidelines have emerged regarding the rights of dentists and a patient with AIDS, including:

1. Dental treatment may not be withheld because the patient refuses testing for HIV exposure. The dentist should assume that this type of patient is a potential carrier of HIV and treat that person using barrier techniques just as the dentist would for any other patient.

2. An AIDS patient needing emergency dental treatment may not be refused care because the dentist does not want to treat AIDS patients.

3. No medical or scientific reason exists why AIDS patients seeking routine dental care may be declined treatment by the dentist, regardless of the dentist's reason. However, if the dentist and the patient agree, the dentist may refer this patient to someone who would be more willing to give treatment.

4. A patient who has been under the care of a dentist then develops AIDS or a related condition must be managed by that dentist or by a referral who is satisfactory to the patient and agreed to by the patient. The CDC and the American Dental Association recommend that infected dentists should either inform the patient of the HIV status and receive consent or not perform invasive procedures.

TREATMENT PLANNING CONSIDERATIONS

A major consideration for the dental management of the patient with HIV/AIDS is determining the current CD4 lymphocyte count and level of immunosuppression of the patient. Other points of emphasis in dental treatment planning are the level of viral load, which may be related to both the susceptibility of opportunistic infections and the rate of progression of AIDS. The dentist should be knowledgeable about the presence and status of opportunistic infections and the medications that the patient may be taking for therapy or prophylaxis for these opportunistic infections. Patients who have been exposed to the AIDS virus, and are HIV seropositive but are asymptomatic, may receive all indicated dental treatment. Generally, this is true for those patients having a CD4 count of more than 400. Patients who are symptomatic for the early stages of AIDS (i.e., CD4 less than 200) will have increased susceptibility to opportunistic infections and may be effectively medicated with prophylactic drugs.[59,61]

The patient with AIDS can receive most any dental care needed and desired once the possibility of signifi-

cant immunosuppression, neutropenia, and thrombocytopenia has been ruled out. Complex treatment plans should not be undertaken before an honest and open discussion concerning the long-term prognosis of the patient's medical condition.

Dental management of the HIV-infected patient without symptoms is no different from that for any other patient in the practice. Universal precautions must be used for *all* patients. Any oral lesions found should be diagnosed then managed by appropriate local and systemic treatment or referred for treatment. Lesions that are atypical or require special diagnostic procedures can be managed by the dentist who has experience with those procedures, or the patient can be referred for diagnosis and treatment.[37] Patients with lesions suggestive of HIV infection need to be evaluated for possible HIV infection. Patients with a history of IV drug abuse and infective endocarditis will require antibiotic prophylaxis for invasive dental procedures (see Chapter 2).

Patients may be medicated with drugs that are prophylactic for *Pneumocystis carinii* pneumonia, candidiasis, HSV or CMV, or other opportunistic disease, and these medications must be carefully considered in dental treatment planning. Care in prescribing other medications must be exercised with these, or any, medications for which the patient may experience adverse drug effects, including allergic reactions, toxic drug reactions, hepatotoxicity, immunosuppresion, anemia, serious drug interactions, and other potential problems. The clinician must have a thorough understanding of all medications and their actions, side effects, warnings, interactions with other drugs, and contraindications before definitive treatment begins (see Box 13-3). Most often, consultation with the patient's physician is mandatory.[56,59,61,71]

Patients with severe thrombocytopenia may require special measures before any surgical procedures (including scaling and curettage) are performed. Patients with advanced[57,59] immunosuppression and neutropenia may require prophylaxis for invasive procedures (Box 13-5). Acetaminophen should be used with caution in patients treated with zidovudine (Retrovir), because studies have suggested that granulocytopenia and anemia, associated with zidovudine, may be intensified; also, aspirin should not be given to patients with thrombocytopenia. Antacids, phenytoin, cimetidine, and rifampin should not be given to patients being treated with ketoconazole because of the possibility of altered absorption and metabolism.[51,52,56,58]

Medical consultation is necessary for symptomatic HIV-infected patients before surgical procedures are performed. Current bleeding time and white blood cell count should be available. Patients with abnormal test results may require special management. All these matters need to be discussed in detail with the patient's

Dental Management of the Patient with AIDS or a Related Condition: General Procedures

Consult whenever possible with patient's physician to establish current status; if severe thrombocytopenia is present, platelet replacement may be needed before surgical procedures are performed

Determine if prophylactic antibiotics are needed to protect patient with severe immune neutropenia (<500 cells/mm) from postoperative infection

Render only more immediate treatment needs for patient with advanced AIDS

Provide dental procedures in most cases based on patient's wants and needs

Inform all personnel working with AIDS patient of relative risks involved and how they can be minimized

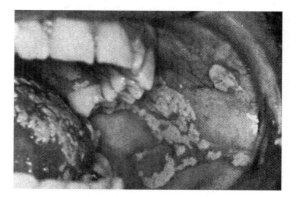

Fig. 13-5 Multiple, large white lesions in a patient with AIDS. The lesions could be removed with a tongue blade. The underlying mucosa was erythematous. Clinical and cytologic findings supported the diagnosis of pseudomembranous candidiasis. (Courtesy Eric Haus, Chicago, Ill.)

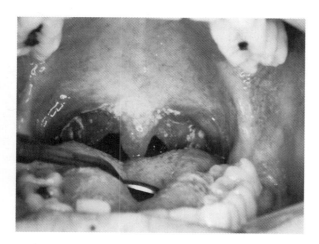

Fig. 13-4 Note the white lesions on the mucosa of the anterior and posterior tonsillar pillars. Cytologic study and culture established the diagnosis of pseudomembranous candidiasis. The patient was found to have AIDS. (Courtesy Sol Silverman, San Francisco, Calif.)

physician.[56,58] Any source of oral or dental infection should be eliminated in HIV-infected patients. They often require more frequent recall appointments for maintenance of periodontal health. Daily use of chlorohexidine mouth rinse may be helpful.

In patients with periodontal disease whose general health status is not clear, periodontal scaling can be done for several teeth to evaluate tissue response and bleeding. If no problems are noted, the rest of the mouth can be treated. Root canal therapy may carry a slightly increased risk for postoperative infection in patients with advanced HIV disease. Infection can be treated with local and systemic measures. Antibiotic prophylaxis is likely not necessary unless severe neutropenia is present[56,58] (less than 500 neutrophils per mm^3).

Individuals with severe symptoms of AIDS may be best managed by treatment of their more urgent dental needs to prevent pain and infection, with deferment of extensive restorative procedures. The main objectives of care are to prevent infection and to keep the patient free of dental or oral pain. Attention must be given to the prevention of infection and excessive bleeding in patients with severe immunosuppression, neutropenia, and thrombocytopenia when planning invasive dental procedures.[67,68] This may involve the use of prophylactic antibiotics in patients with less than 500 cells/mm^3 neutrophiles. White blood cell and differential counts and a platelet count or bleeding time should be ordered before any surgical procedure. If significant thrombocytopenia is present, platelet replacement may be needed. If severe neutropenia is present, antibiotic prophylaxis may be necessary. Medical consultation should precede any dental treatment (see Box 13-5).

ORAL COMPLICATIONS AND MANIFESTATIONS

Clinical findings that suggest a high risk for AIDS or related conditions include candidiasis of the oral mucosa (Figs. 13-4 to 13-7), bluish purple or red lesion or lesions

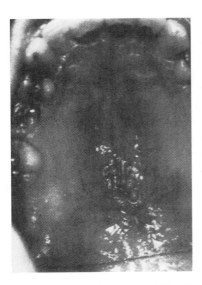

Fig. 13-6 Erythematous palatal lesion in an HIV antibody-positive patient. Smears taken from the lesion showed hyphae and spores consistent with *Candida*. The lesion healed following a 2-week course of antifungal medications. A diagnosis of erythematous candidiasis was made based on clinical laboratory findings. (Courtesy Eric Haus, Chicago, Ill.)

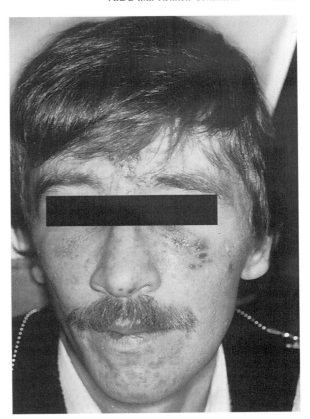

Fig. 13-8 Multiple erythematous lesions on the face of an AIDS patient. The lesions were established by biopsy as Kaposi's sarcoma. (Courtesy Sol Silverman, San Francisco, Calif.)

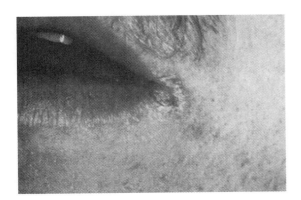

Fig. 13-7 AIDS patient with angular cheilitis. The lesion responded to antifungal medication. (Courtesy Eric Haus, Chicago, Ill.)

that with biopsy are identified as Kaposi's sarcoma (Figs. 13-8 to 13-11), hairy leukoplakia of the lateral borders of the tongue (Figs. 13-12 and 13-13), and other oral lesions associated with HIV infection, some of which have been discussed previously, including herpes simplex, herpes zoster, recurrent aphthous ulcerations, linear gingival erythema (Fig. 13-14), necrotizing ulcerative periodontitis (Fig. 13-15), and necrotizing stomatitis. Other oral conditions found in association with HIV infection are shown

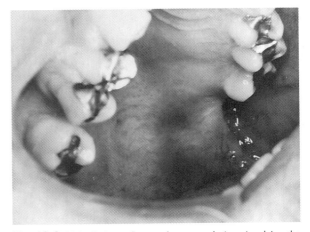

Fig. 13-9 Multiple large, flat, erythematous lesions involving the palatal mucosa. Biopsy revealed the lesions to be Kaposi's sarcoma, and the patient was eventually diagnosed as having AIDS. (Courtesy Sol Silverman, San Francisco, Calif.)

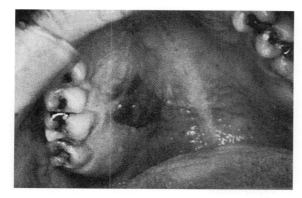

Fig. 13-10 A homosexual man with AIDS. Biopsy of the palatal lesion revealed Kaposi's sarcoma. (Courtesy Sol Silverman, San Francisco, Calif.)

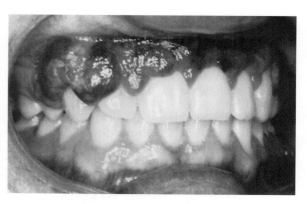

Fig. 13-11 Diffuse, elevated, erythematous lesion on the gingiva that biopsy revealed to be Kaposi's sarcoma. The patient was later diagnosed as having AIDS. (Courtesy Sol Silverman, San Francisco, Calif.)

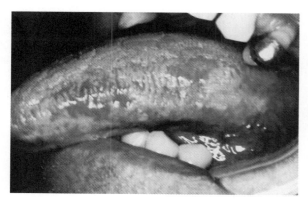

Fig. 13-12 Diffuse white lesion involving the tongue of a male homosexual. Biopsy supported the diagnosis of hairy leukoplakia. (Courtesy Sol Silverman, San Francisco, Calif.)

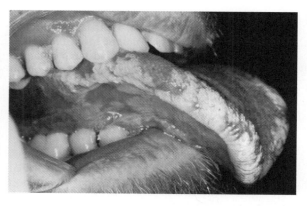

Fig. 13-13 Diffuse white lesion involving the tongue of a male homosexual. Biopsy supported the diagnosis of hairy leukoplakia. (Courtesy Sol Silverman, San Francisco, Calif.)

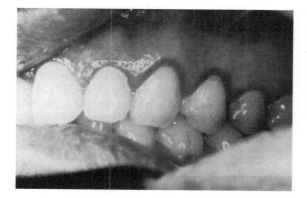

Fig. 13-14 Linear gingival erythema in an HIV-infected patient that extends vestibularly from the gingival margin of the posterior teeth. (Courtesy Sol Silverman, San Francisco, Calif.)

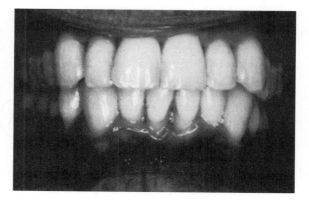

Fig. 13-15 Necrotizing ulcerative periodontitis in an HIV-infected patient. The diagnosis was established after referral of the patient for medical evaluation. (Courtesy Sol Silverman, San Francisco, Calif.)

BOX 13-6

Oral Manifestations of HIV Infections

Fungal infection
Candidiasis*
Pseudomembranous
Erythematous
Hyperplastic
Angular cheilitis
Histoplasmosis
Cryptococcosis
Geotrichosis
Bacterial infections
Linear gingivial erythema*
Necrotizing ulcerative periodontitis*
Necrotizing stomatitis
Mycobacterium avium intracellular
Actinomycosis
Viral infections
Herpes simplex*
Herpes zoster (varicella-zoster)
Cytomegalovirus

Human papillomavirus
Oral warts
Condyloma acuminatum
Focal epithelial hyperplasia
Epstein-Barr virus
Hairy leukoplakia*
Neoplasms
Kaposi's sarcoma*
Non-Hodgkin's lymphoma
Facial palsy
Trigeminal neuropathy
Recurrent aphthous ulceration*
Minor
Major
Herpetiform
Immune thrombocytopenic purpura
Salivary gland enlargement
Xerostomia
Melanotic pigmentation

*More common oral lesions.
Based on Lemp GF et al: N *Engl J Med* 321:1141-1148, 1989; Melnick SL: *Oral Surg* 68:37-43, 1989; Silverman S: *Dent Clin North Am* 35:259-267, 1991; Van Der Waal I, Schulten EA, Pindberg JJ: *Int Dent J* 41:3-8, 1991.

TABLE 13-4

Oral Lesions in HIV-Infected and High-Risk Homosexual and Bisexual Men

Lesion	HIV-positive (n = 2235) (%)	HIV-negative (n = 2962) (%)
Hairy leukoplakia	18.7	0.3
Candidiasis	13.0	1.2
Pseudo- membranous	6.6	0.1
Erythematous	2.1	0.0
Angular cheilitis	0.7	0.2
Kaposi's sarcoma	1.6	0.0
Oral ulcers	2.6	0.9

From Feigal DW et al: AIDS 5:519-525, 1991.

in Box 13-6.[78-89] The prevalence of 6 oral lesions reported to be associated with HIV infection was studied in a large number of homosexual and bisexual men (Tables 13-4 and 13-5).[54] The lesions investigated were hairy leukoplakia, pseudomembranous candidiasis, erythematous candidiasis, angular cheilitis, Kaposi's sarcoma, and oral ulcers. All were much more common in men with HIV infection. Of the men with hairy leukoplakia, 78% had a CD4 cell count below 500 per ml. Hairy leukoplakia, pseudomembranous candidiasis, Kaposi's sarcoma, and angular cheilitis were much more common in HIV-infected men with lower CD4 cell counts. Hairy leukoplakia was found in 20.4% of the HIV infected men, and pseudomembranous candidiasis in 5.8%. The authors concluded that oral lesions can be used as an indirect marker for immune suppresion.[78-89] In one study,[78] a strong relationship was found between an elevation of CD8 lymphocytes before an oral examination and the appearance of oral lesions at the examination. This study involved HIV-infected individuals without symptoms, suggesting that both the CD8 count (increased) and the

TABLE 13-5

Prevalence of Oral Lesions by CD4 Lymphocyte Count on Baseline Examination of 737 HIV-Infected Subjects

		CD4 COUNT ($\times 10^6$/L)		
Lesion	(n = 737) (%)	Less Than 200 (n = 126) (%)	200 to 499 (n = 335) (%)	Greater Than 500 (n = 276) (%)
Hairy leukoplakia	150 (20.4)	43 (34.1)	74 (22.1)	33 (12)
Candidiasis				
Pseudomembranous	43 (5.8)	18 (14.3)	21 (6.3)	4 (1.5)
Erythematous	8 (1.1)	3 (2.4)	3 (0.9)	2 (0.7)
Angular cheilitis	9 (1.2)	5 (4)	2 (0.6)	2 (0.7)
Kaposi's sarcoma	11 (1.5)	8 (6.4)	2 (0.6)	1 (0.4)
Oral ulcers	14 (1.9)	0 (0)	10 (3)	4 (1.5)

From Feigal DW, et al: AIDS 5:519-525, 1991.

TABLE 13-6

Specific Oral Lesions Related to Stage of HIV Infection: Percent of Patients with Lesions

Lesion	Seronegative High-Risk (%)	Seropositive, but Data not Separated into Clinical Stages (%)	Asympto & PGL (%)	ARC (%)	AIDS (%)
Hairy leukoplakia	0.3 to 3	19	8 to 21	9 to 44	4 to 23
Candidiasis	0.8 to 10	11 to 31	5 to 17	11 to 85	29 to 87
Kaposi's sarcoma	0	0.3 to 3	1 to 2	0	35 to 38
Herpes simplex	0 to 0.5	0 to 1	0 to 5	11 to 29	0 to 9
Aphthous ulcerations	0 to 2	0 to 1	2 to 8	11 to 14	2 to 7
Venereal warts	0 to 0.7	0 to 1	0 to 1	0	0 to 1
ANUG	0 to 0.2		1 to 5	0	0 to 7
HIV gingivitis	0		0 to 1	0	51
HIV periodontitis	0		0 to 2	0 to 21	19

ANUG, acute necrotizing ulcerative gingivitis; AIDS, acquired immunodeficiency syndrome; ARC, AIDS-related complex; PGL, persistent generalized lymphadenopathy.
Based on Barone R, et al: *Oral Surg* 69:169-173, 1990; Barr C, et al: IADR 1443:289, 1990; Feigal DW, et al: IADR 65:190, 1989; Little JW, Melnick SL, Rhame FS: *Gen Dent* 42(9):446-450, 1994; Melnick SL, et al: *Oral Surg* 68:37-43, 1989; Roberts MW, Brahim JS, Rinne NF: *J Am Dent Assoc* 116:863-866, 1988; Silverman S Jr, et al: *J Am Dent Assoc* 112:187-192, 1986.

CD4 count (decreased) can be used in the management and evaluation of oral manifestations of HIV infection.[78] In another study of 100 HIV-infected patients, which included 44 with AIDS, 80% were found to have one or more of the HIV-associated oral lesions.[82] In this study, candidiasis was the most commonly found lesion noted in 80.7% of the 44 AIDS patients and in 38% of the 56 HIV-infected individuals. In 6% of all the patients, an oral lesion was the first clinical manifestation of HIV infection.[82] Tables 13-6 and 13-7 summarize the frequency of oral lesions in high-risk and HIV-infected individuals. Seronegative high-risk patients had fewer lesions than did HIV-infected patients, and asymptomatic HIV-infected individuals had an increased frequency of lesions though fewer than in the patients with symptomatic HIV infection or AIDS. In a

TABLE 13-7

Association of Oral Lesions and Stage of HIV Infection: Percent of Patients with Lesions

	PATIENT HIV STATUS		
		HIV Infected	
Seronegative, High Risk (%)	Asymptomatic PGL (%)	ARC (%)	AIDS (%)
I to 9	25 to 30	56 to 85	57 to 92

PGL, Persistent generalized lymphadenopathy 1; ARC, AIDS-related complex; AIDS, acquired immunodeficiency syndrome. Based on Barone R, et al: *Oral Surg* 69:169-173, 1990; Barr C, et al: IADR 1443:289, 1990; Feigal DW, et al: IADR 65:190, 1989; Little JW, Melnick SL, Rhome FS: *Gen Dent* 42(9):446-450, 1994; Roberts MW, Brahim JS, Rinne NF: *J Am Dent Assoc* 116:863-866, 1988; Silverman S Jr, et al: *J Am Dent Assoc* 112:187-192, 1986.

TABLE 13-8

Oral Lesions Found in 106 HIV-Infected Patients

Types/Lesion	Number (%)
Patients with at least one intraoral lesion	30 (28)
Candidiasis	5 (5)
Recurrent herpes	6 (6)
Herpes zoster	0
Kaposi's sarcoma	0
HIV gingivitis	0
HIV periodontitis	2 (2)
Acute necrotizing ulcerative gingivitis	5 (5)
Oral warts	I (I)
Ulcerations	8 (8)
Hairy leukoplakia	10 (9)

From Little JW, Melnick SL, Rhame FS: *Gen Dent* 42(9):446-450, 1994.

TABLE 13-9

Summary of Statistics Related to Oral Candidiasis in HIV-Infected Individuals Taken from 17 Published Reports in the United States

Disease State	PREVALENCE FREQUENCIES			
	Papers	Range	*Weighted Mean (%)	Mean
Oral candidiasis	17	II to 96	30.0	45.2
Erythematous	7	10 to 96	40.5	33.0
Pseudomembranous	6	6 to 69	22.2	25.6
Hyperplastic	6	2 to 20	3.8	3.8
Angular cheilitis	4	I to 23	12.5	16.0

*Weighted by overall number of patients with oral candidiasis in each study.
From Samaranayake LP, Holmstrup P: *J Oral Pathol Med* 18:554-564, 1989.

study of 106 patients with early HIV infection,[26] 28% had a lesion reported to be associated with HIV infection (Table 13-8).

In 1993 a consensus was reached on the classification of oral manifestations of HIV infection and their diagnostic criteria.[49] Candidiasis, hairy leukoplakia, specific forms of periodontal disease (i.e., linear gingival erythema and necrotizing ulcerative periodontitis), Kaposi's sarcoma, and non-Hodgkin's lymphoma are considered to be strongly associated with HIV infection.[49]

Candidiasis

Worldwide, candidiasis is the most common oral manifestation of HIV infection.[51-53] Oral candidiasis, mentioned in the first report on AIDS in the United States,[52] occurs in approximately 45% of AIDS patients in the United States (Table 13-9). Its treatment is mandatory, to stop any spread to the esophagus. Oral candidiasis often occurs in multiple sites within the mouth. Some evidence[53] suggests that erythematous candidiasis precedes pseudomembranous candidiasis. Oral lesions suspected

TABLE 13-10

Antifungal Medications Used for Oral Candidiasis in HIV-Infected Individuals

Medication	Type	Dose	Frequency of Dose	Duration* (Days)
Clotrimazole (topical)				
Mycelex	Oral troche	10 mg	5 times daily	7 to 14
Mycelex-G	Vaginal troche	100 or 500 mg	1 time daily	7 to 14
Nystatin (topical)				
Mycostatin	Vaginal tablets	100,000 units	1 tablet every 6 hours	10 to 14
Milstat	Vaginal tablets	100,000 units	1 tablet every 6 hours	10 to 14
Mycostatin (systemic)	Oral Pastilles	200,000 units	1 tablet every 6 hours	10 to 14
Ketoconazole (systemic)				
Nizoral	Oral tablets	200 mg	1 to 2 tablets daily	10 to 14
Fluconazole (systemic)				
Diflucan	Oral tablets	100 mg	1 tablet daily	10 to 14

*Duration varies based on clinical response. Recurrence is common. Maintenance therapy can be considered using lower dose than treatment dose or every other day dosing with the systemic drugs.

of being candidiasis should be examined using cell study, culture, and biopsy techniques to confirm the clinical diagnosis. These are often white lesions (pseudomembranous candidiasis) that can be scraped off, leaving small points of bleeding; however, many lesions are red (erythematous candidiasis). If the more common causes of oral candidiasis are not found, such as extended antibiotic usage, steroid therapy, radiation therapy, immunosuppressive therapy (i.e., organ transplants), or diabetes mellitus, the dentist should suspect possible immunosuppression secondary to HIV infection.[51-53] The laboratory diagnosis, when used, should involve both Sabouraud and Pagano-Levin plates for primary isolation. The use of these culture media will allow identification of the various strains of *Candida*.[53]

Table 13-10 summarizes the topical and systemic antifungal medications used to treat oral candidiasis of HIV-infected individuals. Studies comparing the efficacies of ketoconazole and fluconazole in treating AIDS patients with oral candidiasis[53] have shown fluconazole to be superior. The yeasts may be developing resistance to the new systemic antifungals. Peridex, Listerine, and hydrogen peroxide are mouth rinses that can be used for patients with candidiasis and other oral lesions associated with HIV infection.

Oral candidiasis found in HIV-infected patients with persistent generalized lymphadenopathy may be of predictive value for the subsequent development of AIDS. In a study of 22 patients with PGL and oral candidiasis,[53] 59% developed AIDS within a median time of 3 months. By contrast, 20 patients with persistent generalized lymphadenopathy without oral candidiasis were followed for a median time of 22 months, and none of these patients developed AIDS.

The appearance of pseudomembranous candidiasis in HIV-infected individuals has been shown to be a strong indicator for the progression of infection to AIDS. The erythematous form of candidiasis also indicates progression toward AIDS. In one study, 169 HIV-infected patients with oral candidiasis were investigated,[53] and 92 had pseudomembranous candidiasis, 37 had erythematous candidiasis, and 40 had both forms. Individuals in all three groups showed a rapid progression to AIDS (mean 25 months) and death (mean 43.8 months).[53]

Kaposi's Sarcoma

The classic lesion of Kaposi's sarcoma is a vascular neoplasm found in older men (over 50) of Jewish and Italian heritage. It usually is confined to the lower extremities and usually runs an indolent clinical course, with 10- to 15-year survivals occurring in more than 37% of the cases. The variant of Kaposi's sarcoma associated with AIDS has been termed *epidemic*. Epidemic Kaposi's sarcoma most often is disseminated throughout the body and runs a fulminant clinical course, with less than 20% survival rate at 2 years if associated with opportunistic infections.[32,80] In a study reported by Silverman,[56] Kaposi's sarcoma was found in the mouth as the first sign of AIDS in 22% of patients with HIV infection. Kaposi's sarcoma was found on the skin and in the mouth at the same time in another 45% of patients.

In the early stages of the AIDS epidemic, Kaposi's sarcoma was found in about 21% of all AIDS patients. From 1984 to 1991, only 13% of reported AIDS patients had Kaposi's sarcoma. Since 1992, this figure has fallen to approximately 9% of all AIDS patients.[59,79] Kaposi's sarcoma is rare in children with AIDS and much less common in IV drug abusers, women, and hemophiliacs with AIDS than in homosexual men with AIDS.[54,59,79] Kaposi's sarcoma in patients with AIDS may be related to the release of HIV-induced growth factors by lymphocytes and macrophages. The growth factors stimulate angiogenesis and proliferation of fibroblasts and vascular (lymphatic) endothelium. In male homosexuals, a sexually transmitted agent plays an important role in the development of this cancer.[57] This also provides an explanation for Kaposi's sarcoma being an uncommon finding in women and children with AIDS. Recent data indicates that Human Herpes Virus 8 (HHV-8) is associated with Kaposi's sarcoma as determined by DNA-PCR.[57]

Hairy Leukoplakia

Hairy leukoplakia is a virus-associated epithelial hyperplasia seen as a corrugated white lesion on the mucosal surface of the mouth, usually involving the lateral borders of the tongue.[64,82,88] It has been reported[88] in HIV-negative renal, liver, and heart transplant patients and in a few HIV antibody-negative homosexual men. Lesions on the ventral surface of the tongue tend to consist of flat, white plaques, whereas lesions on the lateral margins and dorsum of the tongue tend to be more corrugated.[88] Hairy leukoplakia often is infected with *Candida* organisms, which makes the differential diagnosis from oral candidiasis important. Recent studies[55,60,64,82] have demonstrated that EBV replicates within the epithelial cells from hairy leukoplakia. The literature suggests that EBV is not associated with any other oral white lesions that must be differentiated from hairy leukoplakia. Thus hairy leukoplakia may be caused by a reactivation of EBV in the oral mucosa in association with HIV-induced immune deficiency. The diagnosis of hairy leukoplakia is based on the clinical appearance of the lesion, its lack of response to antifungal therapy, and histologic findings.[60,64,82] Confirmation of the diagnosis can be done by immunocytochemistry, in situ hybridization, or electron microscopy. Techniques for the demonstration of EBV in lesions diagnosed by clinical and histologic findings are not available or practical for use by the general dentist, oral surgeon, or oral pathology services. Patients with lesions diagnosed as hairy leukoplakia should be referred to a physician for evaluation of their immune system and HIV antibody testing. Hairy leukoplakia is

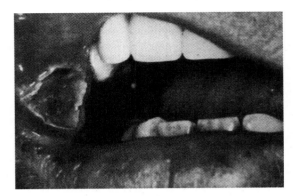

Fig. 13-16 Large aphthous ulcer (major type) found in a patient with AIDS. (Courtesy Eric Haus, Chicago, Ill.)

included in the CDC classification of HIV disease. The finding of hairy leukoplakia is also a predictive value for the subsequent development of AIDS. The probability of AIDS developing in an HIV-infected patient with hairy leukoplakia is 4% by 16 months and 83% by 30 months after the diagnosis of hairy leukoplakia.[60,61] The median time to death following the diagnosis of hairy leukoplakia is 41 months.[60,61]

Aphthous Lesions

In patients with recurrent aphthous ulcers, 3 types of lesions are found. In non-HIV-infected subjects, minor aphthous ulcers are the most common lesions. In HIV-infected patients, herpetiform and major-type (Fig. 13-16) lesions appear to be most common. (Increased numbers of CD8+ cells are found at the base of ulcers in seronegative individuals.) The relative increase in CD8+ cells occurring in symptomatic HIV-infected individuals may, in part, explain the increased prevalence of herpetiform and major-type lesions seen in these people. Most HIV-infected patients with such lesions deny having had them as children.[56,80]

HIV Periodontal Disease

Linear gingival erythema and necrotizing ulcerative periodontitis have been reported to be associated with HIV infection (see Figs. 13-14 and 13-15). Most studies include these conditions in patients with advanced HIV infection. The lesions appear to be related to alterations in the oral bacterial flora, to dysimmunoregulation, and decreased activity of polymorphonuclear leukocytes.[79,81,87] In a study of 97 individuals with early HIV infection (asymptomatic stage),[81] these lesions were rare. The overall periodontal health of these HIV-infected individuals was very good. In recent studies[87] individuals with

TABLE 13-11

Treatment of the Oral Manifestations of HIV Infection

Condition	Regimen
Candidiasis	Topical and systemic antifungal agents
Hair leukoplakia	Usually no treatment: acyclovir, 2.4 to 3 g orally per day for 2 weeks
Herpes simplex	Usually no treatment: acyclovir, 1 to 1.4 g, orally per day for 7 to 10 days
Herpes zoster	Treat promptly to prevent scarring: acyclovir, 800 mg, orally, 5 times per day for 7 to 10 days
Recurrent aphthous ulceration	A small isolated lesion may not need treatment; other lesions can be treated by topical fluocinonide ointment, 0.05%, mixed with Orabase; apply 6 times per day
	Dexamethasone elixir, 0.5 mg/5 ml; rinse and expectorate 2 to 3 times per day
	A large atypical ulcer may require biopsy to rule out lymphoma or rare fungal infections
	Topical fluocinonide
	Metronidazole, orally, 250 mg, four times per day
Xerostomia	Sugarless gum, artificial saliva, topical fluorides; improve oral hygiene
Oral warts	CO_2 laser, surgical excision, cryosurgery, electrosurgery
Periodontal disease	
Linear gingival erythema	Debridement, povidone-iodine, irrigation (Betadine 10%), Peridex (0.12% chlorhexidine gluconate mouth rinse, two times per day)
Necrotizing ulcerative periodontitis	Above plus scaling, root planning; for bone involvement, metronidazole, 230 mg, four times per day, for 4 to 5 days
	Home irrigation with povidone-iodine; use of interproximal brushes
Kaposi's sarcoma	Debridement, dental prophylaxis, and scaling; intralesional vinblastine, CO_2 laser, surgical debulking, radiation
Oral lymphoma	Debridement, scaling, prophylaxis before treatment: radiation, chemotherapy

From Finberg J, Mills J: *Curr Sci* 63:S209-S215, 1990; Fotos PG, Hellstein JW, Vincent SD: *Gen Dent* 39:422-433, 1991; Glick M: *Gen Dent* 38:418-424, 1990; Samaranayake LP, Holmstrup P: *J Oral Pathol Med* 18:554-564, 1989; Scully C, Porter SR, Luker J: *Br Dent J* 170:149-150, 1991; Silverman S: *Dent Clin North Am* 35:259-267, 1991; Stewart JS: AIDS 4(suppl):S217-S221, 1990; Workshop on oral healthcare in HIV disease, *Oral Surg* 73:138-142, 151-155, 1992; Zeitlen S, Shaha A: *J Surg Oncol* 47:230-232, 1991.

HIV have been found to exhibit no more periodontal attachment loss than controls.

Salivary Gland Disease

Several studies[69,84,85] have reported salivary gland enlargement in children and adults with HIV infection. The salivary gland enlargement may involve all the major salivary glands. These patients may have xerostomia. The HIV-associated salivary gland disease (HIV-sgd) is similar histologically to Sjögren's syndrome (see Chapter 24). However, autoantibodies are found in Sjögren's syndrome but are absent in HIV-sgd. Of the patients seen at the Oral AIDS Center at the University of California San Francisco, 6% had HIV-sgd.[86] No evidence has been found of direct invasion of the salivary glands by HIV-1.[85,87] Non-Hodgkin's lymphoma, Kaposi's sarcoma, benign lymphoepithelial cysts, and benign lymphoepithelial lesions have been reported in the major salivary glands of HIV-infected individuals. Human salivary gland secretions have been found to contain a substance that inhibits HIV infection of human lymphocytes. Saliva from healthy women, men, and children was tested[69] and found to contain this factor that, evidence suggests, may be a macromolecule (protein). In a study by Barr et al,[90] only 1% of 218 cultured whole saliva samples from HIV-infected homosexual or bisexual men contained cell-free HIV-1. These data support other studies showing that saliva is not important in the transmission of HIV-1. Saliva has been shown to directly inhibit HIV-1.[45-69] An ELISA test developed by Burroughs-Wellcome, Inc. has been found to be 98% sensitive in detecting antibodies to HIV in saliva. This test may have application for population screening in the future. A test to detect salivary secretory immunoglobulin A antibodies of nonmaternal origin in newborns of women at risk for HIV infection has been found[91] to be accurate in detecting infected infants. One study[45] has shown that saliva might be an appropriate specimen for monitoring drug therapy in HIV-infected individuals.

Lymphadenopathy

Lymphadenopathy, including cervical and submandibular locations, often is an early finding in patients infected with HIV. The lymphadenopathy is persistent and may be found in the absence of any current infection or medications known to cause lymph node enlargement. The nodes tend to be larger than 1 cm in diameter, and multiple sites of enlargement are found.[41,6]

The dentist should perform head and neck and intraoral soft tissue examinations on all patients. White lesions in the mouth must be found and the patient managed in such a way that a diagnosis is established. This may involve cell study, culture, and biopsy by the dentist or referral to an oral surgeon. If red or purple lesions are found and cannot be explained by history (trauma burn, chemical, physical) or proven by clinical observation (healing within 7 to 10 days), a biopsy of them must be performed.[83] Persistent lymphadenopathy must be investigated by referral for medical evaluation, diagnosis, and treatment. Patients with AIDS or a related condition who have developed oral candidiasis can be treated as shown in Table 13-10. Treatment regimens for the various oral lesions associated with HIV infection are shown in Table 13-11 and can be found in Appendix B.

References

1. Brookmeyer R, Gail MH: AIDS *epidemiology: a quantitative approach*, New York, 1994, Oxford Press.
2. Centers for Disease Control: Update: U.S. AIDS Surveillance report, MMWR 49(47):401-402, 2000.
3. Centers for Disease Control: Update: HIV-related knowledge, MMWR 49(47):403-404, 2000.
4. World Health Organization: *The current global situation in the HIV/AIDS pandemic*, Geneva, 1999, World Health Organization.
5. Phillipson TJ, Posner RA: *Private choices and public health. The AIDS epidemic*, Cambridge, Mass, 1993, Harvard University Press.
6. Centers for Disease Control: Update: 1993 revised classification system for HIV infection and expanded surveillance case definition for AIDS, MMWR 41(17):443-445, 1992.
7. Centers for Disease Control: Surveillance for HIV-2 infection in blood donors-United States, MMWR 39:829-831, 1990.
8. Centers for Disease Control: The HIV/AIDS epidemic: the first 10 years, MMWR 40(22):357-363, 1991.
9. Jackson JB et al: Human immunodeficiency virus type 1 detected in all seropositive symptomatic and asymptomatic individuals, J Clin Microbiol 28(1):16-22, 1990.
10. Proceedings of the national symposium on hepatitis B and the dental profession, J Am Dent Assoc 110:614-650, 1985.
11. Centers for Disease Control: Update: AIDS in Europe, MMWR 35:2, 1986.
12. Travers K et al: Natural protection against HIV-1 provided by HIV-2, Science 268:1612-1615, 1995.
13. Centers for Disease Control: Update: trends in AIDS among men who have sex with men U.S. 1989-1994, MMWR 44(4):401-404, 1995.
14. Centers for Disease Control: Update: the first 500,000 AIDS cases, MMWR 44(46):849-852, 1995.
15. Centers for Disease Control: Updated United States Public Health Service Guildelines for the management of occupational exposures to HBV, HCV, and HIV and recommendations for postexposure prophylaxis, MMWR 50(RRII)1-42, 2001.
16. Scully C, Porter SR, Luker J: An ABC of oral health care in patients with HIV infection, Br Dent J 170:149-150, 1991.
17. Weiss SH et al: HTLV-III infection among health care workers; association with needle-stick injuries, JAMA 254:2089-2093, 1985.
18. Proceedings of the national symposium on hepatitis B and the dental profession, J Am Dent Assoc 110:614-650, 1985.
19. American Association of Public Health Dentistry: The control of transmissible diseases in dental practice (position paper), J Public Health Dent 46(1):13-22, 1986.
20. Ward JW, Bush TJ, Perkins HA, et al: The natural history of transfusion-associated infection with human immunodeficiency virus, N Engl J Med 321:947-952, 1989.
21. Tsamtsouris A, Shein B, Rovero J: The pediatric patient HIV infection: an overview for the pedodontist, J Mass Dent Soc 38(1):11-13, 1991.
22. Barr C et al: HIV-associated oral lesions: immunologic and salivary parameters, J Dent Res 69(1443):289, 1990 (abstract).
23. Silverman S Jr et al: Oral findings in people with or at high risk for AIDS: a study of 375 homosexual males, J AM Dent Assoc 112(2):187-192, 1986.
24. Crofts N et al: Testing of saliva for antibodies to HIV-1, AIDS 5:561-563, 1991.
25. Fotos PG, Hellstein JW, Vincent SD: Oral candidiasis revisited, Gen Dent 39:422-433, 1991.
26. Melnick SL et al: Oral mucosal lesions: associations with the presence of antibodies to the human immunodeficiency virus, Oral Surg 68:37-43, 1989.
27. Burke DS et al: Human immunodeficiency virus infections in teenagers: seroprevalence among applicants for US military service, JAMA 263:2074-2077, 1990.
28. Elford J, Bor R, Summers P: Research into HIV and AIDS between 1981 and 1990: the epidemic curve, AIDS 5:1515-1519, 1991.
29. Centers for Disease Control: Publicly funded HIV counseling and testing United States, 1990, MMWR 40(39):666-675, 1991.
30. Barone R et al: Prevalence of oral lesions among HIV-infected intravenous drug abusers and other risk groups, Oral Surg 69:169-173, 1990.
31. Bollinger R: The HIV epidemic in India: magnitude and future projections, Medicine 74(2):97-106, 1995.
32. Curran JW, Morgan WM: AIDS-the beginning, the present, and the future. In Cole HM, Lundberg GD, editors: AIDS *from the beginning*, Chicago, 1986, American Medical Association.
33. Weiss R: The virus and its target cells. In Broder S, Merigan T, Bolognesis D, editors: *Textbook of AIDS medicine*, Baltimore, 1994, Williams & Wilkins.

34. Hahn B: Viral genes and their products. In Broder S, Merigan T, Bolognesis D, editors: *Textbook of AIDS medicine*, Baltimore, 1994, Williams & Wilkins.

35. Cumming PD et al: Exposure of patients to human immunodeficiency virus through the transfusion of blood components that test antibody-negative, N Engl J Med 321:941-946, 1989.

36. Saag M: Natural history of HIV-1 infection. In Broder S, Merigan T, Bolognesis D, editors: *Textbook of AIDS medicine*, Baltimore, 1994, Williams & and Wilkins.

37. Isselbaucher KJ: AIDS and related conditions. In Wilson JD, Braunwald E, Isselbacher KJ, editors: *Harrison's principles of internal medicine*, ed 13, New York, 1994, McGraw-Hill.

38. Pahwa S et al: Spectrum of human T-cell lymphotropic virus type III infection in children, JAMA 255:2299-2305, 1986.

39. Levy JA: Changing concepts in HIV infection: challenges for the 1990s, AIDS 4:1051-1058, 1990.

40. Lederman MM: Acquired immunodeficiency syndrome and related conditions. In Greene HL et al, editors: *Clinical medicine*, ed 2, St Louis, 1993, Mosby.

41. Garfunkel AA, Glick ML: HIV disease: therapy, related and oral conditions-an update, Compend Contin Edu Dent 13(4): 284-290, 1995.

42. Volberding PA et al: Zidovudine in asymptomatic human immunodeficiency virus infection: a controlled trial in persons with fewer than 500 CD4 positive cells per cubic millimeter, N Engl J Med 322:941-949, 1990.

43. Jackson JB et al: Absence of HIV infection in blood donors with indeterminate Western blot tests for antibody to HIV-1, N Engl J Med 322:217-222, 1990.

44. Archibald DW et al: Detection of salivary immunoglobulin A antibodies to HIV-1 in infants and children, AIDS 4:417-420, 1990.

45. Rolinski B et al: Evaluation of saliva as a specimen for monitoring zidovudine therapy in HIV-infected patients, AIDS 5:885-888, 1991.

46. Deeks SG, Volberding PA: Antiretroviral therapy. In Deeks SG, Volberding PA, editors: Treatment of HIV infection, ed 3, San Francisco, 1999, University of San Francisco Press.

47. Fischl MA et al: The safety and efficacy of zidovudine (AZT) in the treatment of subjects with mildly symptomatic human immunodeficiency virus type 1 (HIV) infection, Ann Intern Med 112:727- 737, 1990.

48. Carpenter CC et al: Antiretroviral therapy for HIV infection in 1998: updated recommendations of the International AIDS Society-USA panel, JAMA 280:78, 1998.

49. Clearinghouse on Oral Problems Related to HIV Infection and WHO Collaborating Center on Oral Manifestations of the Immunodeficiency Virus: Classification and diagnostic criteria for oral lesions in HIV infection, J Oral Pathol Med 22(7):289-291, 1993.

50. Van Der Waal I, Schulten EA, Pindborg JJ: Oral manifestations of AIDS: an overview, Int Dent J 41:3-8, 1991.

51. Finberg J, Mills J: Treatment of opportunistic infections, AIDS 1990 Year Rev 4(suppl):S209-S216, 1990.

52. Klein RS et al: Oral candidiasis in high-risk patients as the initial manifestation of the acquired immunodeficiency syndrome, N Engl J Med 311:354-358, 1984.

53. Dodd CL et al: Oral candidiasis in HIV infection: pseudomembranous and erythematous candidiasis show similar rates of progression to AIDS, AIDS 5:1339-1343, 1991.

54. Feigal DW et al: The prevalence of oral lesions in HIV-infected homosexual and bisexual men: three San Francisco epidemiological cohorts, AIDS 5:519-525, 1991.

55. Samaranayake LP, Holmstrup P: Oral candidiasis and human immunodeficiency virus infection, J Oral Pathol Med 18:554-564, 1989.

56. Silverman S: AIDS update: oral manifestations and management, Dent Clin North Am 35:259-267, 1991.

57. Stewart JS: Current approaches to the treatment of HIV-related Kaposi's sarcoma and lymphoma by chemotherapy, AIDS 4(suppl 1):S217-S221, 1990.

58. Statistics from the Centers for Disease Control, AIDS 6:343-345, 1992.

59. Little JW et al: Prevalence of oral lesions among individuals with asymptomatic human immunodeficiency virus infection and early AIDS-related complex, Gen Dent 42(9):446-450, 1994.

60. Greenspan D et al: Oral "hairy" leukoplakia in male homosexuals: evidence of association with both papillomavirus and a herpes-group virus, Lancet 2:831-883, 1984.

61. Greenspan D, Greenspan JS: Management of the oral lesions of HIV infection, J Am Dent Assoc 122(9):26-32, 1991.

62. Greenspan D et al: Relation of oral hairy leukoplakia to infections with the human immunodeficiency virus and the risk of developing AIDS, J Infect Dis 155:475-481, 1987.

63. Greenspan JS et al: Diagnosis and investigation of hairy leukoplakia using noninvasive techniques, J Dent Res 66:184, 1987 (abstract 618).

64. Greenspan JS, Greenspan D: Oral hairy leukoplakia: diagnosis and management, Oral Surg 67:396-403, 1989.

65. Eversole LR et al: Oral condyloma planus (hairy leukoplakia) among homosexual men: a clinical pathologic study of thirty-six cases, Oral Surg 61:249-255, 1986.

66. Greenspan D et al, editors: AIDS and the dental team, Copenhagen, 1986, Munksgaard.

67. Cottone JA, Molinari JA: State-of-the-art infection control in dentistry, J Am Dent Assoc 122(9):33-40, 1991.

68. Council on Dental Therapeutics, American Dental Association: Facts about AIDS for dental professionals, Chicago, 1986, American Dental Association.

69. Fox PC et al: Salivary inhibition of HIV-1 infectivity: functional properties and distribution in men, J AM Dent Assoc 118(6):709-711, 1989.

70. Centers for Disease Control: Update: transmission of HIV infection during an invasive dental procedure in Florida, MMWR 40:21-27, 1991.

71. Ciesielski C et al: Dentists, allied professionals with AIDS, J AM Dent Assoc 122(9):42-44, 1991.

72. Garland FC, Lilienfeld AM, Garland CF: Incidence of human immunodeficiency virus seroconversion in US Navy and Marine Corps personnel, 1986 through 1988, JAMA 262:3161-3165, 1989.

73. Simpson ML: Counseling and testing for human immunodeficiency virus, Minn Med 70:93-94, 1987.

74. Neidle EA: A matter of policy: health groups face the AIDS crisis, J AM *Dent Assoc* 122(9):45-48, 1991.

75. Gerberding JL et al: Risk of exposure of surgical personnel to patients' blood during surgery at San Francisco General Hospital, N *Engl* J 322:1788-1793, 1990.

76. Jacobsen P: Dental treament planning considerations for the HIV/AIDS patient, Personal communication, University of the Pacific, 1995.

77. Schaefer ME: Infection control in dental laboratory procedures, *Can Dent Assoc* J 13(10):81-84, 1985.

78. Melnick SL et al: Increasing CD8;vbm+ T lymphocytes predict subsequent development of intraoral lesions among individuals in the early stages of infection by the human immunodeficiency virus, J *Acquir Immune Defic Syndr* 4:1199-1207, 1991.

79. Beral V et al: Kaposi's sarcoma among persons with AIDS: a sexually transmitted infection? *Lancet* 335:123-127, 1990.

80. MacPhail LA et al: Recurrent aphthous ulcers in association with HIV infection: description of ulcer types and analysis of T-lymphocyte subsets, *Oral Surg* 71:678-683, 1991.

81. Drinkard CR et al: Periodontal status of individuals in early stages of human immunodeficiency virus infection, *Community Dent Oral Epidemiol* 19:281-285, 1991.

82. Greenspan JS et al: Replication of Epstein-Barr virus within the epithelial cells of oral "hairy" leukoplakia, an AIDS-associated lesion, N *Engl* J *Med* 313:1564-1571, 1985.

83. Little JW: Differential diagnosis of white and red/purple lesions in HIV-infected individuals, *Compendium* 11(7):430-438, 1990.

84. Smith FB: Benign lymphoepithelial lesion and lymphoepithelial cyst of the parotid gland in HIV infection, *Arch Pathol Lab Med* 112:742-745, 1988.

85. Zeitlen S, Shaha A: Parotid manifestations of HIV infection, J *Surg Oncol* 47:230-232, 1991.

86. Schiodt M et al: Does HIV cause salivary gland disease? AIDS 3:819-822, 1989.

87. Robinson PG et al: A controlled study of relative periodontal attachment loss in people with HIV infection, J *Clin Periodontol* 27:273-276, 2000.

88. Itin P et al: Oral hairy leukoplakia in a HIV-negative renal transplant patient: a marker for immunosuppression? *Dermatologica* 177:126-128, 1988.

89. Winkler JR et al: Diagnosis and management of HIV-associated periodontal lesions, J Am *Dent Assoc* 119(suppl):25S-34S, 1989.

90. Barr CE et al: Recovery of infectious HIV-1 from whole saliva, J AM *Dent Assoc* 123(2):36-48, 1992.

91. Cowan MJ et al: Maternal transmission of acquired immunodeficiency syndrome, *Pediatrics* 73:382-386, 1984.

Diabetes

14

CHAPTER

*I*n January 2001 the Centers for Disease Control and Prevention (CDC) reported a 6% increase in the incidence of diabetes mellitus in the United States in only 1 year.[1] The major reason for this dramatic increase in cases of diabetes is obesity. The same CDC report estimates that 20% of Americans are classified as obese, which is a 57% increase in the past 10 years. Although the problem extends across all age groups, the largest group of individuals in this category is ages 30 to 39 years.[1]

Diabetes mellitus is a disease complex with metabolic and vascular components. This chronic disease is characterized by hyperglycemia and complications that include microvascular disease of the kidney and eye, and a variety of clinical neuropathies.[2] Diabetes is associated with chronic, premature macrovascular pathology and serious microvascular pathology. The metabolic component involves the elevation of blood glucose associated with alterations in a lipid protein metabolism, resulting from a relative or absolute lack of insulin. Maintenance of good glycemic control can prevent or retard the development of microvascular complications of diabetes.[3] The vascular component includes an accelerated onset of nonspecific atherosclerosis and a more specific microangiopathy that particularly affects the eyes and kidneys. Retinopathy and nephropathy are eventual complications, given sufficient duration, in nearly every individual with diabetes. These complications result in serious morbidity and are so characteristic of diabetes that the classification of diabetic type is dependent on their presence.[4]

In recent years, the classification of diabetes has been reevaluated. In 1975 the American Diabetes Association (ADA) proposed a classification of diabetes that had some problems.[5] In 1979 the National Diabetes Data Group[6] proposed a new classification for diabetes mellitus and related conditions based on dependence on insulin. That terminology basically still holds true; however, the consensus has been to move away from a classification system based on pharmacologic management (Box 14-1). In 1980 the World Health Organization endorsed the substantive recommendations of the National Diabetes Data Group with a few revisions regarding etiologic factors. In 1997 the ADA again changed the classification based on disease etiology.[7] Some of the most recent changes include elimination of the terms *insulin-dependent diabetes mellitus* (IDDM) and *non–insulin-dependent diabetes mellitus* (NIDDM); the terms *type* 1 and *type* 2 *diabetes* are retained but with Arabic instead of Roman numerals. Type 1 diabetes is an absolute insulin deficiency, and type 2 diabetes is the result of insulin resistance with an insulin secretory defect. Also, a new category of malnutrition-related diabetes exists, and the term *impaired glucose tolerance* (IGT) has been retained with a subgrouping of *impaired fasting glucose* added. The term *gestational diabetes mellitus* (GDM) has been retained, and the degree of hyperglycemia has been added.[7] The 1997 ADA classification of diabetes is summarized in Box 14-2.

Diabetes mellitus is of great importance to dentists because they are in a position as members of a health care team to detect new cases of diabetes. They also must be able to render dental care to patients who are already being treated for diabetes without endangering their well-being. A crucial aspect of the identification of the dental patient with diabetes is the ability of the dentist to recognize the level of severity and glycemic control, and the presence of complications from diabetes to consequently manage the patient accordingly. Essential to this determination is knowledge of the patient's blood glucose level at the time of dental treatment.

DEFINITION

INCIDENCE AND PREVALENCE

More than 200 million persons worldwide have diabetes mellitus, and health officials estimate this figure will dou-

BOX 14-1

Prior Classification of Diabetes (1979)

1. Diabetes mellitus
   a. Type I-insulin-dependent diabetes mellitus
   b. Type II-noninsulin-dependent diabetes mellitus
   c. Type III-other types of diabetes
      (1) Pancreatic disease
      (2) Hormonal disease
      (3) Drugs-thiazide, diuretics lithium salts
      (4) Others
2. Impaired glucose tolerance (IGT)
   a. Nonobese IGT
   b. Obese IGT
   c. IGT associated with other conditions
      (1) Pancreatic disease
      (2) Hormonal disease
      (3) Drugs
3. Gestational diabetes mellitus (GDM)
4. Previous abnormality of glucose tolerance (pre-AGT)
5. Potential abnormalities of glucose tolerance (pot-AGT)

From National Diabetes Data Group: *Diabetes* 28:1039-1057, 1979. Reproduced with permission of the American Diabetes Association Inc.

BOX 14-2

Current Classification of Diabetes, American Diabetes Association Inc. (1997)

Type 1	Beta-cell destruction or defect in beta-cell function, usually leading to absolute insulin deficiency
Immune mediated	Presence of islet cell or insulin antibodies that identify the autoimmune process leading to beta-cell destruction
Idiopathic	No evidence of autoimmunity
Type 2	Insulin resistance with relative insulin deficiency
Other specific types	Genetic defects of beta-cell function or insulin action, pancreatic diseases, endocrinopathies, malnutrition, or drug or chemical-induced diabetes
	Impaired fasting glucose (impaired glucose tolerance)
	Abnormalities of fasting glucose (abnormal glucose tolerance)
Gestational diabetes	Any degree of abnormal glucose tolerance during pregnancy

ble or triple within the next 10 years.[1,8] The prevalence of diabetes mellitus has increased more than six-fold in the United States in the last 40 years.[1,9] The CDC estimates that 15.7 million persons in United States have diabetes, representing 5.9% of the population. Approximately 800,000 new cases emerge each year, and about half of these individuals are unaware of their condition. An estimated 11.2% of the general population in the United States has impaired glucose tolerance.[10] The cumulative incidence from birth to age 70 years in a study of individuals in Rochester, Minn.,[5] was 10.5 per 1000 for type 1 and 100.3 per 1000 for type 2. Of the patients with diabetes in the United States, 90% to 95% have type 2.[11] Thus the prevalence of type 2 diabetes is approximately 10 times that of type 1. The vast majority of the undiagnosed cases of diabetes are type 2.[12,13]

The incidence of type 1 diabetes has increased several-fold in children and teenagers during the past 30 years.[5] The distribution of type 2 diabetes increases from 8 per 100,000 at age 15 to 163 per 100,000 at age 65. This rise in the distribution of type 2 diabetes shows the significant association of age and diabetes.

Diabetes mellitus is the third-leading cause of death in the United States and accounts for about 40,000 deaths per year.[5] Kannell and McGee[4] reported the relative risk of morbidity associated with all types of diabetes in the United States. The relative risk for individuals with diabetes acquiring end-stage renal disease is 25 times that of individuals without diabetes. Additionally, 25% of all new cases of end-stage renal disease result from diabetes mellitus.[4] The relative risk for patients with diabetes requiring the amputation of an extremity caused by diabetic complications is more than 40 times that of normal, and more than 20,000 amputations per year are performed on patients with diabetes mellitus, which represents nearly 50% of all nontraumatic amputations.[14,15] Retinopathy occurs in all forms of diabetes.[2-5] As with other complications of diabetes, the development of retinopathy (and blindness) depends on the duration and control of the disease.[16,17] The relative risk of an individual with diabetes becoming blind is 20 times greater than that of other individuals.[14] Increased susceptibility to both myocardial infarction and stroke in patients with diabetes is 2 to 5 times greater than in those without the disease. The severity of these (and other) complications of diabetes is largely dependent on the level and control of hyperglycemia.[18]

The most significant risk factors for type 2 diabetes are family history and obesity. About 60% to 70% of type 2 diabetes patients are obese at the time of diagnosis.[9]

The number of cases of diabetes in the United States will continue to rise because (1) the population is increasing, (2) the life expectancy is increasing, (3) the number of people with obesity is increasing, and (4) persons with diabetes are living longer because of better medical management and are having children who will pass on the disease.

A dental practice serving an adult population of 2000 can expect to encounter about 120 persons with diabetes, about half of whom will be unaware of their condition. Thus it is pertinent that the competent dental practitioner recognizes and properly manages the patient with diabetes.

ETIOLOGY

Diabetes mellitus may be the result of any of the following[7]: (1) a genetic disorder; (2) the primary destruction of islet cells by inflammation, cancer, or surgery; (3) an endocrine condition such as hyperpituitarism or hyperthyroidism; or (4) an iatrogenic disease following the administration of steroids. In this chapter, the discussion is limited to the genetic type of diabetes, the most common type, which also has been called *primary, hereditary,* or *essential* diabetes (see Box 14-2).

The two types of genetic diabetes are type 1 and type 2 diabetes. Both appear to have a genetic component involved in their origin; however, the genetic role in type 2 diabetes is much greater than in type 1 diabetes. In addition to a weak genetic role in type 1 diabetes, environmental factors such as viral infections and autoimmune reactions appear to play important roles in its cause. Studies of identical twins[14,19,20] have shown that if one twin develops type 1 diabetes, the other twin has about a 50% chance of getting the disease. Additionally, if one identical twin develops type 2 diabetes, the other has a 100% chance of also developing it. Obesity plays an important but not well-understood part in the cause of type 2 diabetes.[17,20]

Diabetes mellitus appears to have multiple causes and several mechanisms of pathophysiology. It can be thought of as a combination of diseases that share the cardinal clinical feature of glucose intolerance.[9,21] Each year approximately 1% to 5% of individuals with IGT will develop clinical diabetes.[17] Individuals with IGT have an increased risk for death secondary to atherosclerosis; however, they do not develop microvascular lesions in the retina or kidney as do individuals with overt diabetes mellitus.[17]

GDM is the onset of IGT or clinical diabetes during pregnancy. These patients usually return to normal after the birth of the child but have an increased risk of developing diabetes within 5 to 10 years. In addition, GDM carries an increased risk for loss of the fetus, as well as an increased size of surviving fetuses. Several groups of patients fit into the classification previous abnormality of glucose tolerance (pre-AGT), including patients who have had gestational diabetes, formerly obese individuals who have lost weight, patients with hyperglycemia following myocardial infarction, and patients with posttraumatic hyperglycemia.

Patients who have never had an abnormal glucose tolerance test but are by genetic background at increased risk of developing diabetes mellitus fit into the potential abnormalities of glucose tolerance (post-AGT) classification. Fig. 14-1 illustrates the various types of glycemic abnormalities, their classification, and requirements for insulin.

Patients with clinical signs and symptoms of diabetes mellitus may have type 1, type 2, or another type of diabetes. These individuals show an elevation of the fasting blood glucose, abnormal glucose tolerance test, and microangiopathy.[9]

Type 1 diabetes usually has a sudden onset of clinical symptoms and often is found in individuals under age 40 years; it may, however, occur at any age. Type 2 diabetes generally occurs after age 40 in obese individuals. The incidence of type 2 diabetes increases with age, and insulin secretion may be low, normal, or high. Although most persons with type 2 diabetes are able to secrete insulin for some time, they have decreased numbers of insulin receptors in target cells and decreased postreceptor activity.[20]

The onset of diabetes mellitus in children usually is preceded by a sudden growth spurt. These children have advanced height, bone age, and dental age at the time of onset of the disease compared with siblings without diabetes. Puberty also appears earlier. In approximately 30% of patients with type 2 diabetes, a short period of remission may occur but rarely exceeds 1 year.[9,17,20,21,22]

The etiology of type 1 diabetes has a weak genetic component. Studies[23,24] have shown that a person's susceptibility to type 1 diabetes is linked to the presence of certain genetically determined cell surface antigens found on lymphocytes. The human lymphocyte antigen-D (HLA-D) region is somehow involved in the susceptibility to type 1 diabetes.[23,24]

In persons susceptible to type 1 diabetes, the disease may be triggered to begin developing by an environmental event such as a viral infection. One established relationship in which a viral infection triggers type 1 diabetes is congenital rubella. Another is cytomegalovirus, which has been found in the beta cells of 20% of patients with type 1 diabetes. Other viral infections that have been implicated include mumps, hepatitis, and coxsackievirus.

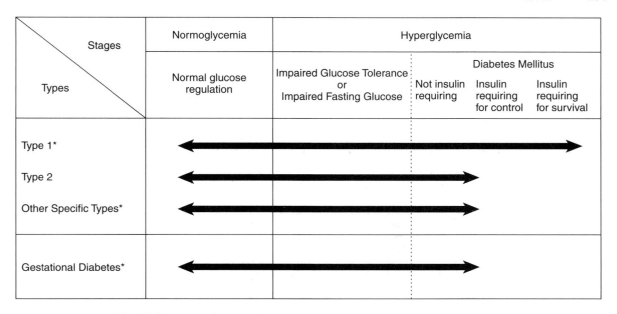

Stages Types	Normoglycemia	Hyperglycemia			
	Normal glucose regulation	Impaired Glucose Tolerance or Impaired Fasting Glucose	Diabetes Mellitus		
			Not insulin requiring	Insulin requiring for control	Insulin requiring for survival
Type 1*	←――――――――――――――――――――――――――――→				
Type 2	←――――――――――――――――――――――→				
Other Specific Types*	←――――――――――――――――――――――→				
Gestational Diabetes*	←――――――――――――――――――――――→				

Fig. 14-1   Diagram of disorders of glycemia; classification and requirements for insulin.

As a result of viral infection or some other event, the susceptible individual appears to develop insulitis with lymphocytic infiltration of the pancreas. An alteration to the surface of the beta cells occurs in some way, and they are converted from "self" to "nonself." An autoimmune destruction of the cells follows. As a result, the pancreatic islet cells do not produce the normal amount of insulin (Fig. 14-2). Islet cell antibodies and insulin antibodies are found in circulation during this stage. However, overt diabetes may not develop for several years.[25,26]

Although little progress has been made in understanding the pathogenesis of type 2 diabetes, researchers know of a strong genetic influence in its etiology (Table 14-1). The modes of inheritance remain unknown except for one variant, maturity-onset diabetes of the young, which is transmitted as an autosomal dominant trait. Type 2 diabetes has no HLA association. Underlying the development of type 2 diabetes are two processes: increased insulin resistance and decreased insulin secretion. A report by Pimenta et al[27] indicated that the primary genetic lesion in type 2 diabetes is pancreatic beta cell dysfunction. Defects in insulin secretion, rather than insulin sensitivity, are most likely the major genetic predisposing factor to the development of type 2 diabetes.[27] Obesity plays a major role in the onset of the disease, as between 60% and 70% of individuals with type 2 diabetes are obese.[5,23,24]

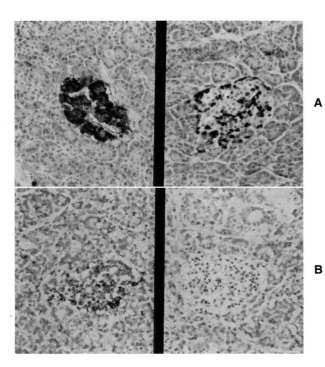

Fig. 14-2   Beta-islet cells in the pancreas of **A,** a normal patient and **B,** a patient with diabetes. Note the staining for insulin production in the normal cells compared with the lack of insulin in the diabetic cells. (Courtesy Richard Estensen, Minneapolis, Minn.)

TABLE 14-1

Hereditary Probability of Developing Type 2 Diabetes in Members of Families

Family Member A	Family Member B	Chance of Developing Diabetes Mellitus (%)
Parent	Parent	85
Parent	Grandparent, aunt, uncle	60
Parent	First cousin	40
I Parent		20
I grandparent		14
I first cousin		2

From Saadoun AP: *Periodont Abstr* 28:116-137, 1980.

Most all individuals with type 2 diabetes have some initial elevation of basal insulin levels. A loss of the first-phase insulin release to a glucose load or meal often occurs. Most patients develop a glucose intolerance even with increased insulin levels. Insulin resistance may occur because of decreased receptors and decreased postreceptor activity. Decreased postreceptor activity accounts for the bulk of insulin resistance.[5,24] Insulin resistance precedes the loss of insulin secretion.[5,24,28]

PATHOPHYSIOLOGY AND COMPLICATIONS

Glucose is the most important stimulus for insulin secretion. Insulin remains in circulation for only several minutes (half-life $[T\frac{1}{2}] = 4$ to 8 minutes), then interacts with target tissues and binds with cell surface insulin receptors. Secondary intracellular messengers are activated and interact with cellular effector systems, including enzymes and glucose transport proteins. Lack of insulin or insulin action allows glucose to accumulate in the tissue fluids and blood.[5]

The mechanisms by which hyperglycemia may lead to microvascular complications include the increased accumulation of polyols through the aldose reductase pathway and of advanced glycolysation end products. Aldose reductase catalyzes the reduction of glucose to sorbitol. An increase in intracellular glucose leads to an increase in sorbitol, which in turn affects glomerular and neural tissue functions.[8] Drugs that inhibit aldose reductase help to prevent diabetic complications such as neuropathy, retinopathy, and nephropathy.[5,13,14,18]

A good correlation exists between the status of the beta cells and the clinical severity of the diabetes.[3,9,18-20,29]

In the early stage of type 1 diabetes, the islets of Langerhans may be enlarged, and a lymphocytic infiltrate exists, which suggests the possibility of an autoimmune response. Later, the islets become smaller, and essentially no insulin is produced. By contrast, most individuals with type 2 diabetes are able to produce some insulin.[9,21,22,29,30] However, the primary defect in type 2 diabetes appears to be a defect in insulin secretion.[27]

The patient with uncontrolled diabetes is deprived of insulin or its action but will continue to use carbohydrates at the usual rates in the brain and nervous system because insulin is not required by these tissues. However, other tissues in the body are unable to take glucose into the cells or use it at a normal rate. Increased production of glucose may occur from glycogen, fat, and protein; thus the rise in blood glucose in diabetic persons results from a combination of underutilization and overproduction from glycogenolysis and fat metabolism.

Hyperglycemia leads to glucose excretion in the urine, which results in an increase in urinary volume. The increased fluid lost through urine may lead to dehydration and loss of electrolytes. With type 2 diabetes, a prolonged hyperglycemia can lead to significant losses of fluid in the urine. When this type of severe dehydration occurs, the urinary output will drop, and a hyperosmolar nonketotic coma can result. This condition is seen most often in elderly patients with type 2 diabeties.[24]

The lack of glucose utilization by many of the cells of the body leads to cellular starvation. The patient often increases intake of food but in many cases still loses weight.

Cortisol secretion often is increased in individuals with type 1 diabetes in response to the stress of the disease, leading to protein breakdown and difficulty incorporating amino acids into proteins. The result is conversion of amino acids to glucose and a loss of body nitrogen in the urine.

As the inability to use glucose progresses in the individuals with type 1 diabetes, the body processes shift to fat metabolism. Body fat stores are mobilized, and the glycerol portion of the triglyceride is separated and converted to glucose. The fatty acids are metabolized through the Krebs cycle; but if excessive fat breakdown continues, the ability of the breakdown product, acetyl-coenzyme A (acetyl-CoA), to be processed through the Krebs cycle fails. An excess of acetone and beta-hydroxybutyric acid (ketones) occurs, which build up in concentration in body fluids and are excreted in the urine.[9,17,21,22]

If these events continue to progress, the person with type 1 diabetes develops metabolic acidosis. For a time, the body may be able to maintain the pH near normal levels; but as the buffer system and respiratory and renal regulators fail to compensate, the body fluids become

TABLE 14-2

Expected Years of Additional Life in Individuals with and Without Diabetes Compared with Given-Age Cohorts

Attained Age of Individual with Diabetes	Expected Years Additional Life of Individual Without Diabetes	Expected Years Additional Life of Individual With Diabetes	Years Lost Because of Diabetes
10	61.5	44.3	17.2
20	51.9	36.1	13.8
30	42.5	30.1	12.4
40	33.3	23.7	9.6

more acidic (i.e., pH falls). Severe acidosis will lead to coma and death if it is not identified and treated. The primary manifestations of diabetes-hyperglycemia, ketoacidosis, and vascular wall disease-contribute to the inability of patients with uncontrolled diabetes to manage infections and heal wounds.[9,17,21] Hyperglycemia may reduce the phagocytic function of granulocytes and facilitate the growth of certain microorganisms. Ketoacidosis delays the migration of granulocytes in the area of injury and decreases phagocytic activity. The vascular wall changes lead to vascular insufficiency, which can result in decreased blood flow to an area of injury and could hamper granulocytic mobilization, as well as reduce oxygen tension. The end results of these effects, and others yet to be identified, are to render the patient with uncontrolled diabetes much more susceptible to infection, reduce the ability to deal with an infection once it is established, and delay the healing of traumatic and surgical wounds.

A study of patients with type 1 diabetes conducted from 1939 to 1981[5] showed the significant effect of the disease on long-term survival. Few deaths occurred among these patients before the age of 30 years. By age 55, only 48% of the women and 34% of the men were still alive. When compared with the general population, women with diabetes lived 22 years less than women without the disease, and men with diabetes lived 24 years less than those without the disease. In another study,[20] diabetes mellitus diagnosed at the age of 10 years was estimated to cause a loss of 17.2 years of life expectancy (Table 14-2). In addition to decreasing life expectancy, the complications of diabetes mellitus lead to significant signs and symptoms that affect the quality of life. The prevalence of diabetic complications are seen in Table 14-3.

TABLE 14-3

Prevalence of Complications in Patients with Insulin-Dependent Diabetes (IDDM)

Complication	Cumulative Prevalence
Visual impairment	14%
Blindness	16%
Renal failure	22%
Stroke	10%
Amputation	12%
Myocardial infarction	21%
Median years of survival after diagnosis of type 1 diabetes	39
Median age at death (years)	49

The complications of diabetes are related to the level of hyperglycemia and pathologic changes within the vascular system and peripheral nervous system (Box 14-3). The vascular complications result from microangiopathy and atherosclerosis. Some evidence[9,17,21] suggests that the microangiopathies seen in persons with diabetes may be a basic part of the disease process and not a later complication. Therefore the case is strong for appropriate glycemic control to prevent or reduce progression of complications. In any case, the vessel changes seen include thickening of the intima, endothelial proliferation, lipid deposition, and accumulation of paraaminosalicylic acid positive material. These changes can be seen throughout the body but have particular

BOX 14-3

Complications of Diabetes Mellitus

Ketoacidosis (type 2 diabetes)
Hyperosmolar nonketotic coma (type 2 diabetes)
Diabetic retinopathy-blindness
Cataracts
Diabetic nephropathy-renal failure
Accelerated atherosclerosis (coronary heart disease [stroke])
Ulceration and gangrene of feet
Diabetic neuropathy (dysphagia; gastric distention; diarrhea; impotence; muscle weakness, cramps; numbness, tingling, deep burning pain)
Early death

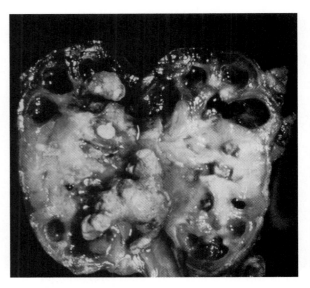

Fig. 14-3   Diabetic nephropathy (cross section of kidney). (Courtesy Richard Estensen, Minneapolis, Minn.)

clinical importance when they occur in the retina and small vessels of the kidney.[9,17,21]

Diabetic retinopathy consists of nonproliferative changes (microaneurysms, retinal hemorrhages, retinal edema, retinal exudates) and proliferative changes (neovascularization, glial proliferation, vitreoretinal traction). Diabetic retinopathy is the leading cause of blindness in the United States. The incidence of blindness in all persons with diabetes is 0.2% per year and 0.6% per year for diabetic individuals with retinopathy. Proliferative retinopathy is most common in type 1 diabetes, with a much lower incidence in type 2 diabetes.[17,21] Cataracts occur at an earlier age and with greater frequency.[4] The typical cataract, senile cataract, is found in 59% of individuals with diabetes ages 35 to 55 years but in only 12% of those without the disease. Young persons with diabetes are more prone to develop metabolic cataracts.[21]

Diabetic nephropathy leads to end-stage renal disease in 30% to 40% of individuals with type 1 diabetes (Fig. 14-3). Renal failure occurs in only 5% of individuals with type 2 diabetes. However, because type 2 diabetes is much more common, the number of persons with renal failure is equal for the two types of diabetes.[25] Renal failure is the leading cause of death in patients with type 1 diabetes. Of all patients using dialysis, 25% have diabetes. The microangiopathy in the kidney usually involves the capillaries of the glomerulus.[17]

Macrovascular disease (atherosclerosis) occurs earlier and is more widespread and more severe in persons with diabetes. With type 1 diabetes, atherosclerosis seems to develop independent of microvascular disease (microangiopathy). Hyperglycemia plays a role in the evolution of atherosclerotic plaques. Individuals with uncontrolled diabeties have increased levels of low-density lipoprotein (LDL) cholesterol and reduced levels of high-density lipoprotein (HDL) cholesterol. Attainment of normal glycemia often will improve the LDL/HDL ratio.

Atherosclerosis increases the risk of ulceration and gangrene of the feet (Fig. 14-4), hypertension, renal failure, coronary insufficiency, myocardial infarction, and stroke.[21]

The most common cause of death in patients with type 2 diabetes is myocardial infarction. By age 55, a third of all individuals with diabetes die of complications from coronary heart disease (CHD). Death rate from CHD in the general population up to age 55 is approximately 8% for men and 4% for women. Women with diabetes treated with insulin have greater risks for CHD than do non–insulin-treated women. This is not true for insulin-treated men. A person with diabetes also has less chance of surviving a myocardial infarction than does a nondiabetic person.[28]

From a clinical standpoint, individuals with diabetes have more complaints concerning nerve disease than any other chronic complication, and growing evidence exists that hyperglycemia is a major factor in the onset and progression of diabetic neuropathy.[14,25] Increased uptake of glucose by Schwann cells leads to the production of intracellular sorbitol, which attracts water into the cell and may cause cellular injury and nerve dysfunction. In the extremities, diabetic neuropathy may lead to muscle weakness, muscle cramps, a deep burning pain, tingling sensations, and numbness. In addition, tendon reflexes, two-point discrimination, and position sense may be

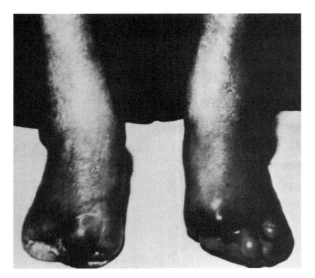

Fig. 14-4 Diabetic gangrene of the feet. (From Falace DA: In Wood NK, editor: *Treatment planning: a pragmatic approach,* St Louis, 1978, Mosby.)

TABLE 14-4

Clinical Pictures of Type 1 and Type 2 Diabetes

	Type 1	Type 2
Frequency (% of person with diabetes)	5-10	90-95
Age at onset (years)	15	40 and over
Body build	Normal or thin	Obese
Severity	Extreme	Mild
Insulin	Almost all	25% to 30%
Plasma glucagon	High, suppressible	High, resistant
Oral hypoglycemic agents	Few respond	50% respond
Ketoacidosis	Common	Uncommon
Complications	90% in 20 years	Less common
Rate of clinical onset	Rapid	Slow
Stability	Unstable	Stable
Family history	Common	More common
Genetic locus	Chromosome 6	Chromosome 11(?)
HLA and abnormal autoimmune reactions	Present	Not present
Insulin receptor defects	Usually not found	Often found

lost.[17,21] Some cases of oral paresthesia and burning tongue are caused by this complication.

Diabetic neuropathy also may involve the autonomic nervous system. Esophageal dysfunction may cause dysphagia, stomach involvement may cause a loss of motility with massive gastric distention, and involvement of the small intestine may result in nocturnal diabetic diarrhea. Sexual impotence and bladder dysfunction also may occur. Diabetic neuropathy is common with both type 1 and type 2 diabetes and may exist in more than 50% of patients.[17,21] Neuropathy progresses over time in type 2 diabetes, and the increase may be greater in patients with hypoinsulinemia.[30]

Other complications found include decubitus ulcerations, gangrenous extremities, cataracts, skin rashes, and deposits of fat in the skin (xanthoma diabeticorum). In individuals who were diagnosed early and are now well controlled, these complications may not develop as quickly or to as great an extent as in those in whom the disease was detected late or was poorly managed.[30]

CLINICAL PRESENTATION

SIGNS AND SYMPTOMS

With type 1 diabetes, the onset of symptoms is sudden. The symptoms include polydipsia, polyuria, polyphagia, loss of weight, loss of strength, marked irritability,

recurrence of bed wetting, drowsiness, and malaise. Patients with severe ketoacidosis may complain of vomiting, abdominal pain, nausea, tachypnea, paralysis, and loss of consciousness.[23,30] The onset of symptoms in type 2 diabetes usually is slow, and the cardinal signs (polydipsia, polyuria, polyphagia, weight loss, and loss of strength) are less commonly seen. The signs and symptoms of type 1 and type 2 diabetes are summarized in Table 14-4 and Box 14-4.

Other signs and symptoms relating to the complications of diabetes are skin lesions, cataracts, blindness, hypertension, chest pain, and anemia. The rapid onset of myopia in an adult is highly suggestive of diabetes mellitus.

Symptoms of Diabetes

Type 1
Cardinal symptoms (common): polydipsia, polyuria, polyphagia, weight loss, loss of strength
Other symptoms: recurrence of bed wetting, repeated skin infections, marked irritability, headache, drowsiness, malaise, dry mouth

Type 2
Cardinal symptoms (much less common):
Usual symptoms: slight weight loss or gain; urination at night, vulvar pruritus, blurred vision, decreased vision, paresthesias, loss of sensation, impotence, postural hypotension

LABORATORY FINDINGS

Two groups of patients should be screened for diabetes mellitus[9,11,17,21,22]: (1) those individuals with signs and symptoms of diabetes or its complications and (2) high-risk ethnic groups (i.e., African-Americans, Hispanics, Native Americans), those with HDL cholesterol levels than 35 mg/100 ml or triglyceride levels greater than 250 mg/100 ml, those who have relatives with diabetes, are obese, are over age 45 years, have had GDM, have delivered large babies, or have had spontaneous abortions or stillbirths should be screened at periodic intervals. For individuals over age 45 the screening should occur routinely at 3-year intervals. Most of the screening for diabetes involves those individuals with undiagnosed type 2 diabetes.[12] Obese individuals, high-risk ethnic groups, those with low HDL cholesterol levels or high triglyceride levels should be screened earlier and more frequently.[9]

The diagnosis of diabetes is established by the presence of a symptom complex consisting of the following[12]:

- Cardinal symptoms of polydipsia, polyphagia, polyuria, loss of strength and unexplained weight loss
- Microangiopathy involving the retina
- Abnormal glucose metabolism by clinical laboratory tests that show glucose and acetone in the urine
- A fasting blood glucose level at or above 126 mg/100 ml
- A 2-hour postprandial (after a 75-g glucose load) blood glucose level at or above 200 mg/100 ml
- A lowered oral glucose tolerance level.

The use of laboratory tests for the diagnosis of diabetes mellitus has changed since 1997. Before then, the glucose tolerance test was considered to be the diagnostic laboratory test. Since then, the fasting glucose level has become the standard laboratory test.[25]

Additionally, the levels of glycohemoglobin (Hb A1c), also known as *glycosylated hemoglobin*, in red blood cells is used for the general assessment of the long-term level (and control) of hyperglycemia in diabetic patients.[31] The use and interpretation of various clinical laboratory tests for evaluating and diagnosing diabetes are described here in general terms.

Blood Glucose Determination

When interpreting the blood glucose level, the dentist should keep in mind that the source of blood, age of the patient, nature of the diet, and physical activity of the patient often will affect the results. Also of great importance is the method used to measure the amount of sugar present in the blood sample.

Most clinical laboratories collect venous blood from the arm for analysis of blood glucose level. Venous glucose levels are lower than arterial glucose levels, with the greatest difference occurring about 1 hour after the ingestion of carbohydrates. After an overnight fast the arterial glucose levels are usually only 2 or 3 mg/100 ml higher than the venous glucose levels.

The capillary blood glucose values are closer to the arterial values than are the venous levels. However, methods that use capillary blood are subject to a greater variation in results because of the dilution of the blood sample with lymph. Normal fasting blood glucose levels range from 60 to 100 mg/100 ml of venous blood.

If the diet has been poor in carbohydrate for several days, and the person is given 75 or 100 mg of glucose just before the blood glucose level is measured, a condition called *starvation hyperglycemia* possible may be produced, which could be misdiagnosed as diabetes mellitus. To prevent this from occurring, the diet should contain at least 250 to 300 g of carbohydrate on each of the 3 days before testing.

Physical activity tends to lower the blood glucose level. Patients who are going to be tested for their blood glucose level should not participate in excessive physical activity.

The most accurate technique for determining blood glucose levels is one that measures only glucose. The Folin and Wu method gives higher results because it also measures other blood sugars (e.g., fructose and lactose). Methods that use glucose oxides give the lowest blood sugar value because they are specific for glucose. Most autoanalyzers use a ferricyanide method, which gives values a little higher than methods that use glucose oxides.

TABLE 14-5

1997 ADA Criteria for the Diagnosis of Diabetes Mellitus

Normal	Impaired Glucose Metabolism	Diabetes Mellitus
Fasting blood glucose <110 mg/dl	Fasting blood glucose 110 mg/dl or greater and <126	Fasting blood glucose 126 mg/dl or greater
2-hr. post-prandial* blood glucose <140 mg/dl	2-hr. post-prandial blood glucose 140 mg/dl or greater <126	2-hr. post-prandial* blood glucose 200 mg/dl or greater

*If the first test performed is the 2-hr. post-prandial test and the value is 200 mg/dl or greater, the physician should order a fasting blood glucose test.

Fasting Venous Blood Glucose. The 1997 ADA criteria for the diagnosis of diabetes mellitus[7] defines diabetes as being present if the fasting blood glucose level is 126 mg/100 ml or greater on two or more occasions.

Two-Hour Postprandial Glucose. For the 2-hour postprandial glucose test, the patient is given a 75- or 100-g glucose load after a night of fasting. Blood glucose levels taken at 2 hours that are 200 mg/100 ml or higher on two or more occasions are diagnostic of diabetes mellitus (Table 14-5).[17,20]

Oral Glucose Tolerance Test

Glucose taken orally is absorbed from the small intestine, the maximum normal rate of absorption being 0.8 g/kg of body weight per hour. The glucose tolerance test reflects the rate of absorption, uptake by tissues, and excretion in the urine of glucose. The glucose load can be given as Glucola, which contains 75 g of glucose in each 7–fl oz bottle. Some laboratories use a 75-g glucose load; others use a 100-g glucose load following a night of fasting. Venous blood samples are drawn from the arm just before and 1, 2, and 3 hours after the ingestion of glucose. Urine samples also are collected at each interval.

The most characteristic alterations seen in diabetes are an increased fasting blood glucose (126 mg/100 ml or higher), an increased peak value (200 mg/100 ml or higher), and a delayed return to normal at the 2- and 3-hour samples. Hypoglycemia may occur in the person with early, mild diabetes 3 to 5 hours after ingestion of glucose. For this reason, some physicians will extend the glucose tolerance test to 5 hours for certain patients. The urine samples should not contain glucose at any point during the test.

As previously mentioned, the glucose tolerance test is no longer the standard for diagnosing diabetes mellitus. This test is used to identify patients with impaired glucose

TABLE 14-6

Glycohemoglobin Measurement as a Laboratory Test for Evaluation of the Patient with Diabetes

Glycohemoglobin Level (% of Total Hemoglobin)	Clinical Interpretation
4 to 8	Normal range in adults
Less than 7.5	Good control of diabetes
7.6 to 8.9	Fair control of diabetes
9 to 20	Poor control of diabetes

absorption and gestational diabetes. Special tests can be performed to measure the release of insulin at various intravenous (IV) glucose infusion levels. However, they are basically for detection of special problems and not part of the routine tests used to diagnose diabetes mellitus.[23,24]

Glycohemoglobin

The extent of glycosylation of hemoglobin A (a nonenzymatic addition of glucose) resulting in the formation of Hb A1c in red blood cells is used for the general assessment of the long-term level (and control) of hyperglycemia in patients with diabetes.[31] The measurement of Hb A1c levels is of value in the detection and evaluation of patients (Table 14-6). Hb A1c is an electrophoretically fast-moving hemoglobin component found in normal persons but increases in the presence of hyperglycemia. It can reflect glucose levels in the blood over the 6 to 12 weeks preceding the test. Normally, patients should have 6% to 8% of Hb A1c. In well-controlled diabetes cases, the level should stay below 7%. The level of hyperglycemia as indicated by the Hb A1c may reach as high as 20% in some uncontrolled cases. Patients

do not have to fast before the test. It can be useful in monitoring the progress of the disease. Normal values must be established for each laboratory. It is now standard practice to measure the Hb A1c levels at least quarterly in patients taking insulin for diabetes mellitus.[29,32] The complications from diabetes are more accelerated in individuals with elevated Hb A1c.[12] Therefore this monitoring is particularly important for those patients who are not monitoring their blood glucose on a regular basis at home.

Urinary Glucose and Acetone

The determination of urinary glucose and acetone is of limited value in detecting overt diabetes. Additionally, finding glucose in the urine is not diagnostic of diabetes. A few people have a low renal threshold for glucose and may "spill" sugar into the urine on that basis. Other conditions may lead to glucose in the urine such as renal disease and the administration of steroids. More important is the fact that failure to find glucose, acetone, or both, in the urine of a patient suspected of having diabetes does not rule out diabetes. Many studies have demonstrated that some persons with overt diabetes at times may not "spill" glucose into the urine, and others may not show any evidence of acetone in the urine. Cases have been reported with blood glucose levels of 300 to 400 mg/100 ml without any evidence of urinary glucose. Except possibly for the patient who has the classic symptoms of diabetes with glucose and acetone in the urine, most physicians depend on blood chemistry values to establish the diagnosis of diabetes.

MEDICAL MANAGEMENT

Diabetes mellitus is not a curable disease. Current evidence supports no precise relationship between hyperglycemia and the vascular complications of diabetes. However, the bulk of evidence weighs in favor of such a relationship; hence, good control of glucose levels is a must. A key observation supporting the concept that good hyperglycemic control prevents complications in individuals with diabetes is to note what happens in transplanted kidneys. When a kidney is transplanted from a healthy person to one with the disease, it develops nephropathy within 3 to 5 years. However, if pancreatic transplantation also is performed, no nephropathy appears to develop.[24] Another example of how proper hyperglycemic control can prevent diabetic complications from occurring is found in the eye. The rate of developing proliferative retinopathy is reduced with good diabetic control[5,18,33] (Box 14-5 and Table 14-7).

BOX 14-5

Treatment of Diabetes Mellitus

Type 1 Diabetes
Diet and physical activity
Insulin
 Conventional
 Multiple injections
 Continuous infusion
 Pancreatic transplantation (Chapter 25)

Type 2 Diabetes
Diet and physical activity
Oral hypoglycemic agents
Insulin plus oral hypoglycemic agents
Insulin

Therapy must be a highly individual process and usually must continue for the rest of the patient's life. This need for lifelong compliance is a problem for many patients. The therapy and test results need to be reevaluated on a continuous basis, and patient education concerning the disease, its complications, and its management also is an ongoing process. The therapeutic goals for most patients are to (1) maintain as close to normal blood glucose levels as possible without repeated episodes of hypoglycemia, (2) strive to maintain normal body weight, and (3) control hypertension and hyperlipidemia, and (4) have a flexible treatment plan that does not dominate the patient's life any more than necessary.[20]

The patient with diabetes may be treated by control of diet and physical activity and the administration of oral hypoglycemic agents and insulin (see Box 14-5). In many cases of type 2 diabetes, the disease can be controlled by weight loss, diet, and physical activity. Total calories must be balanced with physical activity and body weight, and a balanced diet is indicated (with rigid control of the total caloric content). Some physicians will start a patient with diabetes on a diet that has a certain balance of carbohydrate, protein, and fat; others will allow the patient more freedom and will control only the total caloric content.[9,17,21,22]

The Diabetes Control and Complications Trial (DCCT)[34] showed that the most effective strategies for the prevention and treatment of complications from diabetes revolved around intensive treatment of the hyperglycemia. Aldose reductase inhibitors and aminoguanidine may be effective therapeutic agents.[3,11] Antihyper-

tensive drugs (angiotensin-converting enzyme [ACE] inhibitors such as captopril [Capoten]) may be effective in treating the nephropathy.[4,35] Dietary protein restriction also may be effective.[26] Control of the hyperglycemia also will be beneficial in reduction of diabetic neuropathy[23,34] (see Table 14-7).

If control of the diet and physical activity fails to affect the blood glucose level, hypoglycemic agents are used. Many patients with type 2 diabetes can be managed with oral hypoglycemic agents. Four classes of oral hypoglycemia agents exist (Table 14-8). The largest class is sulfonylurea drugs, followed by the biguanides. The third class of drugs is the gamma-glucosidase inhibitors. The final group of drugs is the recently approved thiazolidinediones.[36]

Certain oral hypoglycemics, specifically tolbutamide and related sulfonylurea drugs, were indicted in a report from the University Group Diabetes Program as being ineffective and tending to increase the risk of cardiovascular disease. Since that report, no further studies would seem to support those conclusions.[9,17,21,22] The intensive treatment of hyperglycemia in the Diabetes Control and Complications Trial (DCCT) consisted of the following:

- Hospitalization for the initiation of therapy
- Intensive patient education about diet and diabetes
- Monthly visits and monitoring, patient self-monitoring of blood glucose levels 4 times per day
- Multiple daily insulin injections or use of an insulin-infusion device
- Frequent adjustment of the insulin dosage relative to the blood glucose level, diet, and exercise regimen of the patient

Predefined goals to be attained in the DCCT were fasting blood glucose level 70 to 120 mg/100 ml; post-meal blood glucose level 180 mg/100 ml; and Hb A1c-2 standard deviations above the mean value in normal subjects. The results of the DCCT indicated significant improvement in diabetic status and reduction of diabetic complications across the board. Once complications have started, they progress without intensive therapy for controlling the hyperglycemia. The DCCT supported early intensive therapy, which had a significant effect on limiting the complications of diabetes.[23]

ACE inhibitors can delay the onset and progression of diabetic nephropathy. In one study, patients with type 1 diabetes were treated with captopril and experienced a 50% decrease in renal complications.[35] Another study demonstrated the positive effect of blood pressure control on the progression of complications from type 1 diabetes.[37] This study concluded that control of blood pressure using ramipril (an ACE inhibitor) improved diabetic

TABLE 14-7

Effective Strategies for the Prevention and Treatment of the Complications from Diabetes

Complication/ Strategy	EFFECT IN REDUCTION OF COMPLICATIONS	
	Prevention	Therapy
Retinopathy		
Intensive therapy of hyperglycemia	Yes	Yes
Photocoagulation	Yes	—
Vitrectomy	Yes	—
Aldose reductase inhibitors	Experimental	—
Aminoguanidine	Experimental	—
Antiplatelet therapy	Experimental	—
Nephropathy		
Intensive therapy of hyperglycemia	Yes	Yes
Antihypertensive drugs	Yes	Yes
Dietary protein restriction	Possibly	Possibly
Aldose reductase inhibitors	Experimental	—
Aminoguanidine	Experimental	—
Neuropathic Syndromes		
Intensive therapy of hyperglycemia	Yes	Yes
Aldose reductase inhibitors	Experimental	—
Peripheral Neuropathy		
Amitriptyline	Yes	—
Antidepressant drugs	Yes	—
Capsaicin	Yes	—
Phenytoin	Possibly	—
Carbamazepine	Possibly	—
Gastroparesis		
Erythromycin	Yes	—
Metoclopramide	Yes	—
Cisapride	Yes	—
Domperidone	Possible	—
Aminoguanidine	Experimental	—

nephropathy with respect to slowing the decline of overall renal function, slowing the rate of progression to end-stage renal disease, slowing the clinical course of proteinuria, and improving morbidity and mortality from diabetes.[37] Antihypertensive therapy also is beneficial in slowing the progression of diabetic complications, especially diabetic nephropathy.[38]

Thiazide diuretics are not recommended for use in patients with diabetes because they cause hyperglycemia, hypokalemia, and hypercholesterolemia. Their use has been associated with increased mortality due to cardiovascular disease.[39]

Although the fear of accelerated coronary heart disease has now been discounted, the oral hypoglycemics are still being used less for treatment of type 2 diabetes. The reason for this is that the emphasis is on better hyperglycemia control. Thus a higher percentage of patients with type 2 diabetes are being treated with insulin to prevent or slow the late complications of diabetes.[23] Recently, techniques have improved in transplanting a pancreas or even the islet cells to treat diabetes and its complications.[38,40] Transplantation of a pancreas or implants of islet cells are effective in treating diabetes[41] (see Chapter 25).

In 1984 the second generation of oral hypoglycemic agents became available for use in the United States. The dosage of these new agents is about one hundredth that required for the first-generation oral hypoglycemics. The oral hypoglycemic agents available for treating type 2 diabetes are shown in Tables 14-8 and 14-9. Their mode of action is not completely understood; endogenous insulin must be present for these agents (sulfonylureas) to be effective. In some manner, they appear to stimulate the secretion of insulin, increase the number of cell membrane insulin receptors, and improve insulin postreceptor activity. Some more severe type 2 diabetes cases will require medication with insulin to control complications. A number of patients with type 2 diabetes are being treated with a combination of oral hypoglycemic agents and oral hypoglycemic agents in combination with insulin.[20,23,42]

Patients with type 1 diabetes, patients with type 2 diabetes who are pregnant, and patients who have renal disease or an acute illness should not be treated with oral hypoglycemic agents. If good patient selection is applied, about 80% of the patients with type 2 diabetes will respond to sulfonylurea therapy for a variable time period. Between 5% and 10% per year of those treated

TABLE 14-8

Oral Antidiabetic (Hypoglycemic) Drugs

Class Drug	Daily Dose	Doses/Day
Sulfonylureas (enhance insulin secretion)		
First generation		
Chlorpropamide	100-500 mg	1
Acetohexamide	1500 mg	1
Tolazamide	100-1000 mg	1-2
Tolabutamide	500-3000 mg	2-3
Biguanides (reduce hepatic glucose production)		
Metformin	1500-2500 mg	1-2
Glucovance	?	
Gamma-glucosidase Inhibitors (delay carbohydrate digestion)		
Acarbose	75-300 mg	3
Thiazolidinediones (enhance insulin sensitivity)		
Troglitizone*	400-600 mg	1
Rosiglitazone	4-16 mg	2
Pioglitazone†	15-45 mg	1

*Recent reports of severe drug-related hepatotoxicity. This drug has been removed from the market.
†Recent approval as a drug for the treatment of type 2 diabetes.

TABLE 14-9

Metabolism, Potency, and Activity of Oral Hypoglycemic Agents Used for Type 2 Diabetes

Agent	Maximum Daily Dose (mg/day)	Rate of Metabolism	Duration Activity Known (hr)
Tolazamide	1000	Rapid	24
Acetohexamide	1500	Intermediate	12 to 18
Glyburide	2220	Intermediate	24
Glipizide	2245	Intermediate	24

with sulfonylureas will become nonresponsive to the medication; 3% to 5% of the patients treated with sulfonylureas will experience adverse reactions, including nausea, vomiting, cholestasis, granulomatous hepatitis, blood dyscrasias, rashes, photosensitivity, water retention, and hypoglycemia.

Drug interactions with the sulfonylureas have been reported.[20,24,43] Sulfonylureas actions may be increased by numerous other drugs causing hypoglycemia. Drugs that influence hepatic function and renal clearance must be considered. Barbiturates speed up the liver metabolism of sulfonylureas and can cause hyperglycemia. Sulfonamides compete with the sulfonylureas for metabolic pathways in the liver and can cause hypoglycemia. Warfarin, phenylbutazone, and aspirin also can affect the actions of oral hypoglycemic agents. Patients with type 1 diabetes require insulin to control their blood glucose level, although the amount of insulin needed can be reduced through diet control and adequate exercise.

In the treatment of diabetes mellitus, three types of insulin are available: human (recombinant deoxyribonucleic acid [DNA]), pork, and beef. Pork insulin differs from human insulin in one amino acid and from beef insulin in three. The older animal insulin extracts contained a number of contaminants that caused significant adverse reactions. Allergic reactions at the site of injection were common; on occasion, serious systemic reactions occurred, including hives, angioedema, and anaphylaxis. Another adverse reaction noted with the older animal insulin preparations was lipoatrophy, which consisted of a loss of subcutaneous fat at the injection site. Purified animal extracts of insulin are now available and have greatly reduced the frequency of these reactions in humans. Little difference is noted clinically between the uses of human insulin and purified pork insulin.[6,24]

Another form of synthetic insulin is available that is derived by two processes. Semisynthetic insulin is produced by substituting alanine for threonine in pork insulin. Biosynthetic insulin (lispro insulin) is produced by recombinant DNA methodology in *Escherichia coli* (subtype K-12).[9] Lispro insulin (Humilin) is made by inversion of amino acids in the 28 and 29 positions of the B-chain (proline and lysine). The need for a rapidly acting insulin arose because the absorption of regular insulin from a subcutaneous injection site is too slow to accommodate for the rapid rise in blood glucose after a meal. The slower absorption of regular insulin is because of this form of insulin to self-aggregate, forming hexamers.[9] Lispro insulin has significant advantages over regular insulin when used to control hyperglycemia following the ingestion of a meal. Lispro insulin starts acting within 15 minutes and reaches peak plasma concentrations

within 60 to 90 minutes, and its action lasts for about 4 to 5 hours. Lispro insulin is the short-acting insulin of choice in most patients with diabetes who require insulin therapy.[9]

In April 2000 the Food and Drug Administration approved a new from of synthetic insulin for the treatment of type 1 diabetes. Insulin glargine, which is made from recombinant DNA, is indicated for adults and children and is injected subcutaneously once daily. Another rapidly absorbed insulin, insulin aspart, is undergoing clinical trials for clinical use as a rapidly acting insulin therapeutic agent.

Insulin therapy can be administered by using one of three methods: conventional therapy, multiple subcutaneous injections, and continuous subcutaneous infusion. Conventional therapy is used most often and consists of one or two daily injections of insulin. The multiple injection method consists of injecting short-acting insulin before each meal then a long-acting insulin injection in the evening. In continuous subcutaneous insulin infusion therapy, a small battery-driven pump provides infusion pressure. Sensors are used to detect the need for insulin, or the pump can be programmed to deliver insulin at certain times. The insulin is contained in a syringe or cartridge in the pump, which is worn on a belt. Basal insulin delivery is continuous; however, infusion rates can be adjusted, and larger boluses can be infused at mealtime or with unexpected hyperglycemia. This type of therapy is now standard for intensive insulin therapy and hyperglycemic control in individuals with severe type 1 diabetes.[6,24]

Only one implantable insulin pump is available in the United States. The Minimed implantable insulin pump is implanted directly into the abdominal subcutaneous tissues with a catheter inserted directly into the peritoneal cavity. Insulin secretion is regulated form a handset by the patient, which signals the catheter to deliver insulin on demand.[45] Pancreas transplantation is used in selected patients with diabetes to eliminate the need for exogenous insulin therapy[27] (see Chapter 25).

Insulin is available in short-acting (lispro [1 to 1.5 hr]), regular (4 to 6 hr), neutral protamine Hagedorn (NPH) (intermediate-acting [8 to 12 hr]), and protamine zinc (long-acting [24 to 36 hr]) preparations. Lispro or regular insulin is given first before meals. NPH and lente are intermediate-acting preparations and usually are given once a day in conventional therapy if less than total replacement is needed[35,50] (Table 14-10).

In conventional therapy, regular or lispro insulin can be mixed with either NPH or lente. By using a morning and an early evening injection of regular and NPH insulin, peak insulin levels will be available for breakfast,

TABLE 14-10

Types of Insulin Commonly Used in the United States

Type of Insulin	Action	Buffer Peak (hr)	Duration (hr)
Lispro	Short-acting	None	1 to 1.5
Regular	Rapid	None	4 to 6
Neutral protamine Hagedorn (NPH)	Intermediate	Phosphate	6 to 12
Lente	Intermediate	Acetone	6 to 12
Protamine zinc	Long	Phosphate	14 to 24

lunch, and dinner. A few patients may require a separate injection of long-acting insulin to prevent the dawn phenomenon (a rebound hypoglycemia that occurs in some patients).[17,39]

Patients receiving conventional insulin therapy often use self-glucose monitoring to establish the effectiveness of their hyperglycemia control. These patients can alter their insulin dosage based on the results of the tests. The best results are obtained with a spring-driven lancet holder and an instrument to read the reagent strips that are used to measure the blood glucose levels (Glucometer [Baker, Inc.]). Another method accepted by the Food and Drug Administration is the Glucowatch made by Cygnus Inc., which can monitor blood glucose levels. Using conventional therapy allows two levels of control. *Acceptable control* is defined as maintaining the following blood glucose levels[7,11]: 60 to 130 mg/100 ml fasting and preprandial, less than 200 mg/100 ml postprandial, and greater than 65 mg/100 ml. *Ideal control* is defined as maintaining the following blood glucose levels: 70 to 100 mg/100 ml fasting and preprandial, less than 160 mg/100 ml postprandial, but greater than 65 mg/100 ml.[7,11]

Infection, emotional or physical stress, pregnancy, and surgical procedures usually will disturb the control of a patient's diabetes. This is particularly true in patients taking insulin, and additional control measures must be used during these periods. This often involves increasing the dosage of insulin or administering insulin for a short period to type 2 patients not being managed with insulin.

Diet should be a consideration in the medical management of the patient with diabetes. Naturally, the significance of controlling sugar intake with respect to controlling the hyperglycemia is extremely important. In short-term studies, dietary protein restriction stabilized creatinine clearance, decreased albuminuria, decreased systolic blood pressure, and increased serum albumin concentrations.[26]

BOX 14-6

Signs and Symptoms of Insulin Reaction

Mild Stage
Hunger
Weakness
Tachycardia
Pallor
Sweating
Paresthesias

Moderate Stage
Incoherence
Uncooperativeness
Belligerence
Lack of judgment
Poor orientation

Severe Stage
Unconsciousness
Tonic or clonic movements
Hypotension
Hypothermia
Rapid thready pulse

INSULIN SHOCK

Patients being treated with insulin must follow their diet closely. If they fail to eat in a normal pattern but continue to take their regular insulin injection, they may experience a hypoglycemic reaction caused by an excess of insulin (insulin shock). A hypoglycemic reaction also can be due to an overdose of insulin or an oral hypoglycemic agent. Reaction or shock caused by excessive insulin usually occurs in three well-defined stages, each more severe and dangerous than the preceding (Box 14-6).

Mild Stage

The mild stage is the most common and is characterized by hunger, weakness, trembling, tachycardia, pallor, and sweating; paresthesias may be noted on occasion. It occurs before meals, during exercise, or when food has been omitted or delayed (see Box 14-6).

Moderate Stage

In the moderate stage, as the blood glucose substantially drops, the patient becomes incoherent, uncooperative, and sometimes belligerent or resistive; judgment and orientation are defective. The chief danger during this stage is that patients may injure himself or herself, or someone else (e.g., if the patient is driving) (see Box 14-6).

Severe Stage

Complete unconsciousness with or without tonic or clonic muscular movements occurs during the severe stage. Most of these reactions take place during sleep, after the first two stages have gone unrecognized. This stage also may occur after exercise or the ingestion of alcohol if earlier signs have been ignored. Sweating, pallor, rapid and thready pulse, hypotension, and hypothermia may be present (see Box 14-6).

The reaction to excessive insulin can be corrected by giving the patient sweetened fruit juice or anything with sugar in it. Patients in the severe stage (unconsciousness) are best treated by giving a glucose solution IV; glucagon or epinephrine may be used for transient relief.

DENTAL MANAGEMENT

MEDICAL CONSIDERATIONS

Any undiagnosed dental patient who has the cardinal symptoms of diabetes (i.e., polydipsia, polyuria, polyphagia, weight loss, weakness) should be referred to a physician for diagnosis and treatment. Patients with findings that may suggest diabetes (headache, dry mouth, marked irritability, repeated skin infection, blurred vision, paresthesias, progressive periodontal disease, multiple periodontal abscesses, loss of sensation) should be referred to a clinical laboratory or physician for screening tests.

More recently, patients may be able to readily monitor their blood glucose level using a personal blood glucose monitoring device (e.g., Glucometer). The Glucowatch (Cygnus Inc.) can also be used to monitor blood glucose levels. A patient with an estimated fasting blood glucose level of 126 mg/100 ml or higher should be referred to a physician for medical evaluation and treatment if indicated. A patient with a 2-hour postprandial blood glucose level of 200 mg/100 ml or higher also should be referred.

In a recent study[49] of patients with diabetes entering a dental clinic, a total of 97 patients (mean age of 57.7 years) had their fasting blood glucose determined as a part of their initial dental examination; 28 patients (28.9%) were found to be hyperglycemic (greater than 130 mg/100 ml) (mean = 174.8 ± 40.8 mg/100 ml), whereas 2 patients were found to be hypoglycemic (less than 70 mg/100 ml). This illustrates for dental practitioners how patients with diabetes commonly may not be under good glycemic control.[46-49]

Patients who are obese, are over 45 years of age, or have close relatives who have diabetes should be screened once a year for any indication of hyperglycemia that may reveal the onset of diabetes. Women who have given birth to large babies (greater than 10 lb) or who have had multiple spontaneous abortions or stillbirths also should be screened once a year for diabetes. The use of oral contraceptive agents is not contraindicated in patients with diabetes; however, findings exist of adverse effects of oral contraceptive agents on the progression of complications from diabetes. The above patients are best screened by their physician.

All patients with diagnosed diabetes must be identified by history, and the type of medical treatment they are receiving must be established. The type of diabetes (type 1, type 2, or other types of diabetes) should be determined and the presence of complications noted. Patients being treated with insulin should be asked how much insulin they use and how often they inject themselves each day. They should also be asked whether they monitor their own blood glucose, by which method, how often, and the value of the most recent level. The frequency of insulin reactions and when the last one occurred should be determined. The frequency of visits to the physician should be established, as should when the last Hb A1c test was performed and its result. Whether the patient checks his or her blood for glucose also should be determined. This provides the dentist with information concerning the severity and control of the diabetes (Box 14-7).

Patients with type 2 diabetes who have no evidence of complications and whose disease is under good medical control, as determined by consultation with the patient's physician, will require little or no special attention when receiving dental treatment, unless they develop a significant dental or oral infection possibly accompanied by swelling or fever. By contrast, patients with complications such as renal disease or cardiovascular disease may need to be managed in special ways. Patients being treated with insulin or who are not under good medical management also will require special attention (Box 14-8). This typically may involve consultation with the patient's physician.

BOX 14-7

Detection of the Patient with Diabetes

Known Diabetic Person
1. Detection by history:
   a. Are you diabetic?
   b. What medications are you taking?
   c. Are you being treated by a physician?
2. Establishment of severity of disease and degree of "control"
   a. When were you first diagnosed as diabetic?
   b. What was the level of the last measurement of your blood glucose?
   c. What is the usual level of blood glucose for you?
   d. How are you being treated for your diabetes?
   e. How often do you have insulin reactions?
   f. How much insulin do you take with each injection and how often do you receive injections?

   g. Do you test your urine for glucose?
   h. When did you last visit your physician?
   i. Do you have any symptoms of diabetes at the present time?

Undiagnosed Diabetic Person
1. History of signs or symptoms of diabetes or its complications
2. High risk for developing diabetes
   a. Parents who are diabetic
   b. Gave birth to one or more large babies
   c. History of spontaneous abortions or stillbirths
   d. Obese
   e. Over 40 years of age
3. Referral or screening test for diabetes

Patients who have not seen their physician for a long time, have had frequent episodes of insulin shock, or report signs and symptoms of diabetes may have disease that is unstable. These patients should be referred to their physician for evaluation, or the physician should be consulted to establish the patient's current status.

Some patients with type 1 diabetes who are being treated with large doses of insulin will have periods of extreme hyperglycemia and hypoglycemia (brittle diabetes), even with the best of medical management. These patients require close consultation with the physician before any dental treatment is started.

A major goal in the dental management of patients with diabetes who is being treated with insulin is to prevent insulin shock from occurring during the dental appointment. These patients should be told to take their usual insulin dosage and to eat their normal meals before the dental appointment, which is usually best scheduled in the morning. When such a patient comes for the appointment, the dentist should confirm that the patient has taken insulin and eaten breakfast. In addition, patients should be instructed to tell the dentist if at any time during the appointment they feel symptoms of an insulin reaction occurring. A source of sugar, such as orange juice, cake icing, soda, or Glucola must be available in the dental office to give to the patient if symptoms of an insulin reaction occur (see Box 14-8) (see *Medical Emergencies*).

Any patient with diabetes who is going to receive extensive periodontal or oral surgery procedures other than single simple extractions should be given special dietary instructions after surgery. It is important that the total caloric content and the protein/carbohydrate/fat ratio of the diet remain the same so that control of the disease and proper blood glucose balance are maintained. The patient's physician should be consulted about diet recommendations for the postoperative period. One suggestion is to have the patient use a blender to prepare his or her usual diet so that it can be ingested with minimum discomfort, or special food supplements in a liquid form may be used. The physician also may alter the patient's insulin regimen based on his or her ability to eat properly, as well as the extent of the surgery.

Patients who have brittle diabetes or require a high dosage of insulin (type 1 diabetes) may be at increased risk for postoperative infection. However, prophylactic antibiotics usually are not indicated. If the patient develops an infection the appropriate systemic antibiotics can be given. A protocol for IV sedation often involves fasting before the appointment (i.e., nothing by mouth after midnight); using only half the usual insulin dose; and then supplementing with IV glucose during the procedure. Patients with well-controlled diabetes can be given general anesthesia, if necessary; however, in a dental office, management with local anesthetics is preferable.

BOX 14-8

Dental Management of the Patient with Diabetes*

1. Non–insulin-dependent patient
   All dental procedures can be performed without special precautions, unless complications of diabetes is present
2. Insulin-controlled patient
   a. Usually all dental procedures can be performed
   b. Morning appointments are usually best
   c. Patient advised to take usual insulin dosage and normal meals on day of dental appointment; information confirmed when patient comes for appointment
   d. Patient advised to inform dentist or staff if symptoms of insulin reaction occur during dental visit
   e. Source of glucose (orange juice, soda, Glucola) available and given to patient if symptoms of insulin reaction occur
3. If extensive surgery needed
   a. Consultation with physician concerning dietary needs during postoperative period
   b. Antibiotic prophylaxis can be considered for patients with brittle diabetes and those taking high doses of insulin who also have chronic states of oral infection

*Special precautions may be needed for patient with complications of diabetes, renal disease, heart disease, etc.

BOX 14-9

Dental Management of the Patient with Diabetes and an Acute Oral Infection

1. Non–insulin-controlled patients may require insulin; consultation with physician required
2. Insulin-controlled patients usually will require increased dosage of insulin; consultation with physician required
3. Patient with brittle diabetes or patient receiving high insulin dosage should have culture(s) taken from infected area for antibiotic sensitivity testing
   a. Culture sent for testing
   b. Antibiotic therapy initiated
   c. In cases of poor clinical responses to first antibiotic, a more effective antibiotic selected based on sensitivity test results
4. Infection should be treated using standard methods
   a. Warm intraoral rinses
   b. Incision and drainage
   c. Pulpotomy, pulpectomy, extractions, etc.
   d. Antibiotics

Any patient with diabetes and an acute dental or oral infection presents a significant management problem (Box 14-9). This problem will be even more difficult for patients who take a high insulin dosage and for those who have type 1 diabetes. Infections often cause loss of control over the diabetic condition; as a result, the infection is not handled by the body's defenses as well as it would be in the normal patient. Patients with brittle diabetes (i.e., difficult to control, requires a high dosage of insulin) may require hospitalization during the management of an infection. The patient's physician should be consulted and become a partner during this period.

In a recent study,[48] the risk for infections in patients with diabetes was directly related to their fasting blood glucose levels. If the fasting blood glucose level was below 206 mg/100 ml, no increased risk was present; however, if the fasting blood glucose level was between 207 and 229 mg/100 ml, the risk increased by 20%. Additionally, if the fasting blood glucose level rose above 230 mg/100 ml, an 80% increase occurred in the risk of infection. Therefore dentists must be aware of the level of glycemic control in patients undergoing complex oral surgical procedures because of their increased risk of infection. Judicious monitoring and appropriate use of antibiotics must be considered in the management of these patients.

The basic aim of treatment is to simultaneously cure the oral infection and respond to the need to regain con-

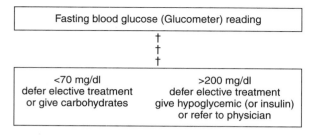

Fig. 14-5 Decision-making diagram for the dental treatment of patients with diabetes depending on blood glucose (Glucometer) reading.

trol of the diabetic condition. Patients receiving insulin usually require additional insulin, which should be prescribed by their physician; noninsulin-controlled patients may need more aggressive medical management of their diabetes, which may include insulin during this period. The dentist must treat the infection very aggressively by incision and drainage, extraction, pulpotomy, warm rinses, and antibiotics. Antibiotic sensitivity testing is recommended for patients with brittle diabetes or who require a high insulin dosage for control. For these patients, penicillin therapy can be initiated, then, if the clinical response is poor, a more effective antibiotic can be selected based on the results of the antibiotic sensitivity testing. Attention also must be paid to the patient's electrolyte balance and fluid and dietary needs.

TREATMENT PLANNING MODIFICATIONS

The patient with diabetes who is receiving good medical management and is under good glycemic control without serious complications such as renal disease, hypertension, or coronary atherosclerotic heart disease can receive any indicated dental treatment. Actually, if the diabetes is under good control, even cardiac transplantation can be safely performed.[12,46] However, patients with diabetes who have serious medical complications may need to have an altered plan of dental treatment (see Chapters 4, 5, 6, 7, and 9). Studies[48,49] have indicated that many dental patients with diabetes are not under good glycemic control, and elevated fasting blood glucose levels render the dental patient more susceptible to complications (Fig. 14-5).

ORAL COMPLICATIONS AND MANIFESTATIONS

The oral complications of poorly controlled diabetes mellitus may include xerostomia; bacterial viral and fungal infections (including candidiasis); poor wound healing;

increased incidence and severity of caries; gingivitis and periodontal disease; periapical abcesses; and burning mouth syndrome. The oral findings in patients with uncontrolled diabetes most likely relate to the excessive loss of fluids through urination, the altered response to infection, the microvascular changes, and possibly the increased glucose concentrations in saliva.[7,19,41,48,50]

The effects of hyperglycemia lead to increased amounts of urine, which deplete the extracellular fluids and reduce the secretion of saliva, thus resulting in the complaint of dry mouth. A high percentage of patients with diabetes present with xerostomia.[15] The complications resulting from xerostomia itself can be devastating. Normally, in a healthy mouth, saliva containing essential electrolytes, glycoproteins, antimicrobial enzymes, and a number of other important constituents continually lubricates and protects the oral mucosa. Saliva in normal quantities and composition serves to cleanse the mouth, clear potentially toxic substances, regulate acidity, neutralize bacterial toxins and enzymes, destroy microorganisms, and maintain the integrity of the teeth and oral soft tissues. When the normal environment of the oral cavity is altered because of a decrease in salivary flow or alterations in salivary composition, a healthy mouth can become susceptible to painful decay and mucosal deterioration. Dry, atrophic, and cracking oral mucosa is the eventual result of xerostomia. Accompanying mucositis, ulcers, and desquamation, and opportunistic bacterial, viral, or fungal infections and an inflamed, depapillated, painful tongue also are common problems. Difficulty in lubricating, masticating, tasting, and swallowing are among the most devastating complications of xerostomia and may contribute to impaired nutritional intake. An increase in the rate of dental caries has been reported in young patients with diabetes and would appear to be related to the reduced salivary flow.[15]

The parotid saliva of persons with uncontrolled diabetes has been reported[50] to contain a slight increase in the amount of glucose. The glucose concentration in parotid saliva from individuals without diabetes varies from 0.22 to 1.69 mg/100 ml, whereas the glucose concentration in parotid saliva from persons with uncontrolled diabetes has been reported to range from 0.22 to 6.33 mg/100 ml. The effect of this slight increase (if any) on the incidence of dental caries and other oral conditions in patients with diabetes remains to be established.

Parotid saliva also has been shown to contain immunoreactive insulin.[50] Precisely from where the insulin is derived and its function in saliva remains to be determined. Several studies[42,50-54] have reported an increased incidence and severity of gingival inflammation, periodontal abscesses, and chronic periodontal disease in

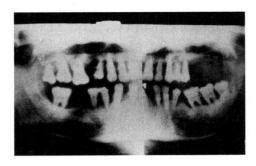

Fig. 14-6   Panoramic radiograph of a young adult with severe, progressive periodontitis. After positive screening for diabetes, the patient was referred to a physician, and the diagnosis of diabetes mellitus was established. The patient required insulin treatment.

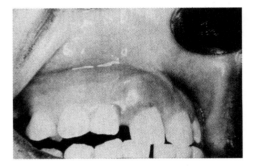

Fig. 14-7   Periodontal abscess in a patient with multiple abscesses. After evaluation by a physician, the diagnosis of diabetes was established.

diabetic patients (Figs. 14-6 and 14-7). On the other hand, a well-controlled study[51] failed to demonstrate any difference in the amount or severity of periodontal disease in young individuals with or without diabetes.

The most impressive study showing an association of periodontal disease and diabetes[20] involved the Pima Indians in the southwestern United States. This tribe has the highest incidence and prevalence of type 2 diabetes in the world. In the study (of 3219 Pima Indians), 736, or 23%, were found to have type 2 diabetes.[20] Among the adults over 35 years of age, 50% had diabetes. The dental status of 2878 of these persons in the study was determined. Periodontal disease was established by loss of epithelial attachment, and loss of crestal alveolar bone was estimated by clinical and radiographic techniques.[20] The prevalence of periodontal disease was significantly greater in those individuals with type 2 diabetes than in the individuals without diabetes. Further, periodontal

disease was found to occur at an earlier age in individuals with diabetes.

Saadoun[42] reported small blood vessel changes in the gingival tissues of patients with diabetes, consisting of flattening of the endothelial cells, accumulation of periodic acid Schiff-positive material in the basement membrane, and a narrowing of the lumina. He also described an increase in the glucose level of the gingival fluids. The neutrophils appeared to be affected secondary to the hypoglycemia, showing decreased phagocytosis, diapedesis, impaired adherence, and impaired chemotaxis.

Saadoun[42] also reported that adults with uncontrolled diabetes who are prone to periodontal disease will have more severe manifestations of the periodontal disease than will individuals without diabetes who are prone to periodontal disease. This relationship is not clear in the patient with controlled diabetes. As a group, patients with diabetes appear to have more severe periodontal disease than those without it, but the differences are not great. Saadoun[42] also concluded that glucose tolerance test results are not a reliable predictor of a patient's periodontal status. The time relationship between the diabetic state and periodontal disease is yet to be established. Cianciola et al[52] evaluated the periodontal status of 263 patients with type 1 diabetes, 59 nondiabetic siblings, and 149 nonrelated nondiabetic patients and concluded that periodontal disease is a complication of type 1 diabetes. The increased periodontal disease found in type 1 diabetes patients could not be explained by increased supragingival plaque accumulations. The periodontal disease found in these young patients (all greater than 30 years of age) usually was asymptomatic and undetected.[52] Kinane and Chestnutt[53] concluded in a comprehensive review of periodontal studies that patients with diabetes have an increased risk of periodontal disease, particularly when hyperglycemia is poorly controlled.

In 1999, the American Academy of Periodontology pointed out in the context of the refined standards for the classification of diabetes that uncontrolled or poorly controlled diabetes is indeed associated with increased risk for periodontitis. Based on the results from multiple studies, the academy determined that periodontal disease is more severe and frequent in poorly controlled diabetics.[54]

A recent study by Lin et al[55] has shown that patients with diabetes did not have a higher coronal or root-surface caries rate than nondiabetic persons, regardless of glycemic control. However an association existed in older adults with diabetes and active caries and tooth loss. This observation was even more significant in patients with diabetes with poor glycemic control.[55] A study performed in Sweden involving children of women with

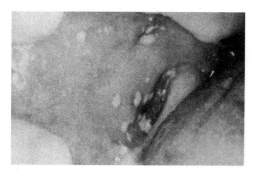

Fig. 14-8 Oral moniliasis in a patient with diabetes. Note the multiple small white lesions on the buccal mucosa. The lesions could be scraped off. Cytologic study and cultures confirmed the clinical impression of infection by Candida albicans.

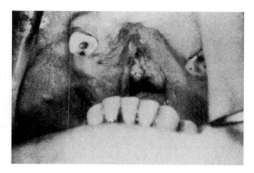

Fig. 14-9 Lesion involving the palate in a patient with diabetes. Cultures established the diagnosis of mucormycosis, a serious fungal infection that may occur in patients with systemic diseases such as diabetes or cancer. Treatment usually includes control of the diabetes, surgical excisions of the lesion, and antibiotics and fungicides.

diabetes[56] showed a much higher frequency of enamel hypoplasia (28%) than in children of mothers who did not have diabetes (3%). The cause of this difference is not known but may be caused by the effects of hyperglycemia on the formation and calcification of the enamel matrix.

Oral fungal infections may be found in the patient with uncontrolled diabetes,[15] including candidiasis and the more rare mucormycosis (Figs. 14-8 and 14-9) (see Appendix B). General agreement exists that healing is delayed in individuals with uncontrolled diabetes and that they are more prone to various oral infections after surgical procedures. Oral lesions are more common in patients with diabetes. A recent report by Guggenheimer et al[58] indicated a significantly higher percentage of oral lesions, especially candidiasis, traumatic ulcers, and de-

layed healing in individuals with type 1 diabetes, as compared with a control population. A report by Bagan-Sebasti et al[58] suggested an association between diabetes mellitus and the atrophic-erosive form of lichen planus. This association was not noticed for the reticular form of lichen planus. Conversely, a study by Van Dis[59] reported no relationship between lichen planus and diabetes. However, in a 1998 report,[60] a higher prevalence of oral lichen planus was found (5.76%) in type 1 diabetes and somewhat higher (2.83%) in type 2 diabetes, compared with a control population. The authors of the study concluded that alterations in the immune system may be responsible for the appearance of lichen planus in diabetes.[60]

Diabetic neuropathy may lead to oral symptoms of paresthesias and tingling, numbness, burning, or pain caused by pathologic changes involving nerves in the oral region. Diabetes has been associated with oral burning symptoms.[61,62] Early diagnosis and treatment of the diabetic state may allow for regression of these symptoms, but in long-standing cases the changes may be nonreversible.

Several studies have suggested that the status of patients thought to be "prediabetic" can be confirmed by gingival biopsy findings of thickened and hyalinized small vessels. However, this technique remains to be proven accurate and beneficial.

References

1. Centers for Disease Control and Prevention: The status of diabetes mellitus in the U.S.: Surveillence report, MMWR 50(3):101-102, 2001.
2. Little JW: Recent advances in diabetes mellitus of interest to dentistry, *Spec Care Dent* 20(2):46-51, 2000.
3. Gray H, Rahilly SO: Toward improved glycemic control in diabetes. What's on the horizon? *Arch Intern Med* 155:1137-1142, 1994.
4. Kannell WB, McGee D: Diabetes and cardiovascular disease: the Framingham study, *JAMA* 241:2035-2038, 1979.
5. Krolewski AS et al: Risk of proliferative diabetic retinopathy in juvenile onset-type I diabetes: a 40-year follow-up study, *Diabetes Care* 9:443-452, 1986.
6. National Diabetes Data Group: Classfication and diagnosis of diabetes mellitus and other categories of glucose intolerance, *Diabetes* 28:1039-1057, 1979.
7. Report of the expert committee on the diagnosis and classification of diabetes mellitus. *Diabetes care,* 20:1181-1194, 1997.
8. Amos AF, McCarty DJ, Zimmet P: The rising global burden of diabetes and its complications: estimates and projections to the year 2010, *Diabet Med* 14:S1-S85, 1997.
9. Burrows W: Diabetes mellitus. In Freeman BA, editor: *Textbook of microbiology,* ed 21, Philadelphia, 1979, WB Saunders.

10. Carter DA et al: Immunoreactive insulin in rat salivary glands and its dependence on age and serum insulin levels, *Proc Soc Exp Biol Med* 209:245-249, 1995.

11. Blackshear PJ: Diabetes mellitus. In Kelly WA, editor: *Textbook of internal medicine*, Philadelphia, 1997, JB Lippincott.

12. Foster DW: Diabetes mellitus. In Fauci AS et al, editors: *Harrison's principles of internal medicine*, ed 14, New York, 1998, McGraw-Hill.

13. DeFronzo RA: Diabetic nephropathy. In Becker KL, editor: *Principles and practice of endocrinology and metabolism*, Philadelphia, 1990, JB Lippincott.

14. Nathan DM: Long-term complications of diabetes mellitus, *N Engl J Med* 328(23):1676-1684, 1995.

15. Rhodus NL: Detection and management of the diabetic patient, *Comp Cont Edu Dent* 8(1):73-80, 1986.

16. Napier JA: Field methods and response rates in Tecumseh community health study, *Am J Pub Health* 52:208-216, 1962.

17. Evanoff GV et al: The effect of dietary protein restriction on the progression of diabetic nephropathy: a 12 month follow-up, *Arch Intern Med* 147:492-495, 1987.

18. Olefsky JM: Diabetes mellitus. In Wyngaarden JB, Smith LH, editors: *Cecil textbook of medicine*, ed 17, Philadelphia, 1997, WB Saunders.

19. Foster DW: Diabetes mellitus. In Wilson JD, Foster DW, Kroneberg HM, editors: *Williams textbook of endocrinology*, ed 9, Philadelphia, 1998, WB Saunders.

20. Shlossman M et al: Type 2 diabetes mellitus and periodontal disease, *J Am Dent Assoc* 121(4):532-536, 1990.

21. Warram JH et al: Excess mortality associated with diuretic therapy in diabetes mellitus, *Arch Intern Med* 10:862-865, 1991.

22. Bartolucci EG, Parkes RB: Accelerated periodontal breakdown in uncontrolled diabetes: pathogenesis and treatment, *Oral Surg* 52:387-390, 1981.

23. Eisenbath GS, Kahn CR: Etiology and pathogenesis of diabetes mellitus. In Becker KL, editor: *Principles and practice of endocrinology and metabolism*, Philadelphia, 1990, JB Lippincott.

24. Faulconbridge AR et al: The dental status of a group of diabetic children, *Br Dent J* 151:253-255, 1981.

25. Clark CM, Lee DA: Prevention of complications of diabetes mellitus, *N Engl J Med* 332(18):1210-1217, 1995.

26. Ekoe JM: Recent trends in prevalence and incidence of diabetes mellitus syndrome in the world, *Diabetes Res Clin Pract* 1:249-264, 1986.

27. Pimenta W et al: Pancreatic beta-cell dysfunction as the primary genetic defect in NIDDM, *JAMA* 273(23):1855-1861, 1995.

28. Kohner M et al: Ponalrestat in early diabetic retinopathy, *Diabetes* 39(suppl 1):61a, 1990.

29. Ganda OP, Weir GC: Oral hypoglycemic agents. In Becker KL, editor: *Principles and practice of endocrinology and metabolism*, Philadelphia, 1990, JB Lippincott.

30. Partanen J, Niskaneb L: Natural history of peripheral neuropathy in patients with non–insulin-dependent diabetes mellitus, *N Engl J Med* 333(2):89-94, 1995.

31. Orchard TJ et al: Factors associated with avoidance of severe complications after 25 years of insulin-dependent diabetes mellitus: Pittsburgh epidemiology of diabetes complications study (I), *Diabetes Care* 13:741-777, 1998.

32. Goteiner DJ: Glycohemoglobin (GHb): a new test for the evaluation of the diabetic patient and its clinical importance, *J Am Dent Assoc* 102(1):57-58, 1981.

33. Krolewski AJ, Warram JH: Natural history of diabetes mellitus. In Becker KL, editor: *Principles and practice of endocrinology and metabolism*, Philadelphia, 1990, JB Lippincott.

34. Diabetes Control and Complications Trial Research Group: The effect of intensive treatment of diabetes on the development and progression of long-term complications from insulin dependent diabetes mellitus, *N Engl J Med* 329:977-986, 1993.

35. Lewis EJ et al: The effect of angiotensin-converting enzyme inhibition on diabetic nephropathy, *N Engl J Med* 329:1456-1460, 1993.

36. Unger RH, Foster DW: Diabetes mellitus. In Wilson JD, Foster DW, Kroneberg HM, editors: *Williams textbook of endocrinology*, ed 9, Philadelphia, 1998, WB Saunders.

37. Rodby RA et al: The study of the intensity of blood pressure management on the progression of type 1 diabetic nephropathy; study design and baseline patient characteristics, *J Am Soc Nephrol* 5(10):1775-1781, 1995.

38. Livi U et al: Mid-term results of heart transplantation in diabetic patients, *J Cardiovac Surg* 35(suppl 1):115-118, 1994.

39. Skillman TG: Diabetes mellitus. In Massaferri EL, editor: *Endocrinology*, ed 3, New York, 1986, Medical Examination Publishing.

40. Sutherland DER: Pancreas transplantation as a treatment for diabetes: indications and outcome. In Bardin CW, editor: *Current therapy in endocrinology and metabolism*, St Louis, 1995, Mosby.

41. Lacy PE: Treating diabetes with transplanted cells, *Sci Am* 50:58-66, 1995.

42. Saadoun AP: Diabetes and periodontal disease: a review and update, *Periodont Abstr* 28:116-139, 1980.

43. Riley WJ et al: A prospective study of the development of diabetes in relatives of patients with insulin-dependent diabetes, *N Engl J Med* 327:1167-1172, 1990.

44. Scheen AJ, Lefebvre PJ: Antihyperglycemia agents. Drug interactions of clinical importance, *Drug Safety* 12(1):32-45, 1995.

45. Duckworth WC: Diabetes mellitus. In Fauci AS et al, editors: *Harrison's principles of internal medicine*, ed 14, New York, 1998, McGraw-Hill.

46. Melchior WR, Bindlish V, Jaber LA: Angiotensin-converting-enzyme inhibitors in diabetic nephropathy, *Ann Pharmacother* 27:344-350, 1993.

47. Brownlee M: Glycation and diabetic complications, *Diabetes* 43:836-841, 1994.

48. Golden EA: Preventing complications of diabetes by controlling hyperglycemia, *Diabetes Care* 22:1408-1418, 1999.

49. Rhodus NL, Vibeto B: Level of glycemic control in diabetic dental patients. *J Am Dent Assoc* 2001. Accepted for publication.

50. Campbell MJ: Glucose in the saliva of the non-diabetic and the diabetic patient, *Arch Oral Biol* 10:197-205, 1965.

51. Shannon IL et al: Glucose tolerance responses in young adults of sharply contrasting periodontal status, SAM-TR-66-9, *US Air Force Sch Aerospace Med* 26:1-6, 1966.

52. Cianciola MJ et al: Prevalence of periodontal disease in IDOM (juvenile diabetes), J Am Dent Assoc 104:653-660, 1982.
53. Kinane DF, Chestnutt IG: Relationship of diabetes to periodontal disease, Curr Opin Periodontol, 4:29-34, 1997.
54. Mealy B: American Academy of Periodontology: position paper diabetes and periodontal diseases, J Periodontol 70:935-949, 1999.
55. Lin, BPJ et al: Dental caries in older adults with diabetes mellitus, Spec Care Dent 19:8-14, 1999.
56. Grahnen H, Edund K: Maternal diabetes and changes in the hard tissues of the primary teeth, Ordontol Rev 18:157,1967.
57. Guggeneheimer J et al: Insulin-dependent diabetes mellitus and oral soft tissue pathologies, Oral Surg Oral Med Oral Pathol 89(5):563-569, 2000.
58. Bagan-Sebastian JV et al: A clinical study of 205 patients with oral lichen planus, J Oral Maxiollofac Surg 50(2):116-118, 1992.
59. Van Dis ML, Parks ET: Prevalence of oral lichen planus in patients with diabetes mellitus, J Oral Surg Oral Med Oral Pathol 79(6):696-701, 1995.
60. Petrou-Amerikanous C et al: Prevalence of oral lichen planus in diabetes according to the type of diabetes, Oral Dis 4: 37-40, 1998.
61. Carlson C, Miller C, Reid K: Psychosocial profiles of patients 2000.
62. Rhodus NL et al: Diagnosis and management of burning mouth syndrome, J Northwest Dent 39:29-41, 2000.

Adrenal Insufficiency

15

CHAPTER

BACKGROUND

The adrenal glands are small (3 to 6 g) endocrine glands located bilaterally at the superior pole of each kidney. Each gland contains an outer cortex and inner medulla. The adrenal medulla functions as a sympathetic ganglion and secretes primarily epinephrine, whereas the adrenal cortex secretes a variety of hormones with multiple actions (Box 15-1). The primary focus of this chapter is on normal adrenal cortical function and hypofunction (i.e., insufficiency).

The adrenal cortex comprises about 90% of the gland and consists of three zones. The outer zone is the zona glomerulosa. The middle zone is the zona fasciculata, and the innermost zone is zona reticularis. The cortex manufactures three classes of adrenal steroids: glucocorticoids, mineralocorticoids, and androgens. All are derived from cholesterol and share a common molecular nucleus. The predominant hormone of the zona glomerulosa is aldosterone, a mineralocorticoid. Aldosterone regulates physiologic levels of sodium and potassium and is relatively independent of pituitary gland feedback. The zona fasciculata secretes glucocorticoids, and the zona reticularis secrete androgens, or sex hormones.

Cortisol, the primary glucocorticoid, is responsible for a wide variety of functions and effects. Some of the more important ones include regulation of carbohydrate, fat, and protein metabolism, maintenance of vascular reactivity, inhibition of inflammation, and maintenance of homeostasis during periods of physical or emotional stress.[1] Cortisol acts as an insulin antagonist (Fig. 15-1), increasing blood levels and peripheral use of glucose; increasing liver glucose output; and initiating lipolysis, proteolysis, and gluconeogenic mechanisms. The anti-inflammatory action of cortisol is modulated by its in-

hibitory action on (1) lysosome release, (2) prostaglandin production, (3) eicosanoid and cytokine release, (4) endothelial cell expression of intracellular and extracellular adhesion molecules (ICAM and ECAM, respectively, that attract neutrophils, and (5) the function of leukocytes.

Regulation of cortisol secretion occurs via the hypothalamic-pituitary-adrenal (HPA) axis (Fig. 15-2). Central nervous system afferents mediating circadian rhythm and responses to stress stimulate the hypothalamus to release corticotropin-releasing hormone (CRH), which stimulates the production and secretion of adrenocorticotropic hormone (ACTH) by the anterior pituitary. ACTH then stimulates the adrenal cortex to produce and secrete cortisol. Plasma cortisol levels are increased within a few minutes after stimulation. Circulating levels

---

BOX 15-1

Secretory Products of the Adrenal Glands

Adrenal Cortex	Adrenal Medulla
Glucocorticoids	Epinephrine*
Cortisol*	Norepinephrine
Corticosterone	Dopamine
Mineralocorticoids	
Aldosterone*	
Deoxycorticosterone	
Sex hormones	
Dehydroepiandrosterone*	
Androstenedione	

*Principal secretory products.

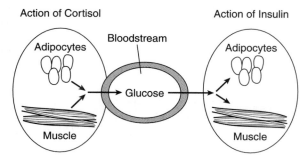

Fig. 15-1 Effect of cortisol and insulin on glucose in the bloodstream.

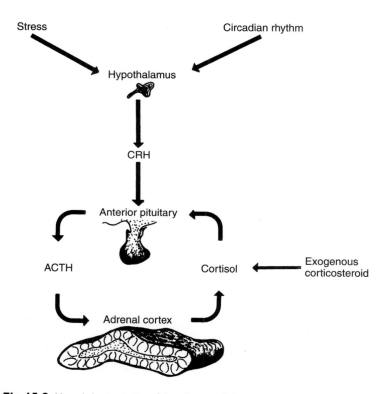

Fig. 15-2 Hypothalamic-pituitary-adrenal axis and the regulation of cortisol secretion.

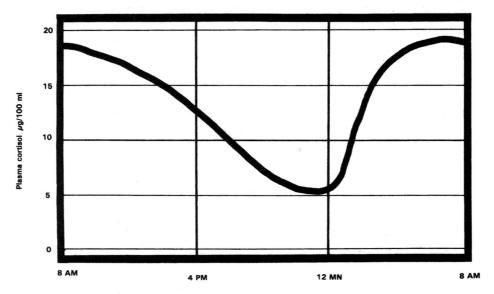

Fig. 15-3 Normal pattern of cortisol secretion over a 24-hour period.

of cortisol inhibit the production of CRH and ACTH, thus completing a negative feedback loop.[2]

Cortisol secretion normally follows a diurnal pattern. Peak levels of plasma cortisol occur about the time of awakening in the morning and are lowest in the afternoon and evening[3] (Fig. 15-3). This pattern is reversed in an individual who habitually works nights and sleeps during the day. The normal secretion rate of cortisol over a 24-hour period is approximately 20 mg.[2,4] During periods of stress, the HPA axis is stimulated, resulting in an increased secretion of cortisol. Anticipation of surgery or an athletic event usually is accompanied by only minimal increases in cortisol secretion. However, surgery itself is one of the most potent activators of the HPA axis.[3] A variety of stressors such as trauma, illness, burns, fever, hypoglycemia, and emotional upset can trigger this effect. The greatest response is found in the immediate postoperative period. However, this can be reduced by morphinelike analgesics or by local anesthesia,[5,6] suggesting that a pain response mechanism increases the requirement for cortisol.

Synthetic glucocorticoids (cortisol-like drugs) are used in the treatment of many diseases, including rheumatoid arthritis, systemic lupus erythematosus, asthma, hepatitis, inflammatory bowel disease, dermatoses, and mucositis. Glucocorticoids are used long-term in patients during immunosuppressive therapy for organ transplantation and joint replacement. In dentistry, corticosteroids are used during perioperative periods for reduction of pain, edema, and trismus following oral surgical and endodontic procedures.[7,8] Many synthetic glucocorticoids are available and differ in potency relative to cortisol and in their duration of action (Table 15-1).

MINERALOCORTICOIDS

Aldosterone is the primary mineralocorticoid secreted by the adrenal cortex and is essential to sodium and potassium balance and to the maintenance of extracellular fluid (i.e., intravascular volume). Its actions are primarily on the distal tubule and collecting duct of the kidney, where it promotes sodium retention, potassium excretion, and fluid retention. Aldosterone secretion is regulated by the renin-angiotensin system, ACTH, and plasma sodium and potassium levels. It is stimulated by a fall in renal blood pressure, resulting from a decrease in intravascular volume or a sodium imbalance.[4] The result is a release of renin, which activates angiotensin. Angiotensin causes aldosterone to be secreted. When blood pressure rises, renin-angiotensin release diminishes, serving as a negative feedback loop that inhibits additional production of aldosterone (Fig. 15-4).

ANDROGENS

Dehydroepiandrosterone is the principal androgen secreted by the adrenal cortex. The effects of adrenal androgens are the same as those of testicular androgens

TABLE 15-1

Glucocorticoids and Their Relative Potency

Compound	Antiinflammatory Potency	Mineralocorticoid Potency	Approximate Equivalent Dose (mg)
Short-acting (<12 hours)			
Cortisol	1	2	20
Cortisone	0.8	2	25
Intermediate-acting (12 to 36 hours)			
Prednisone	4	1	5
Prednisolone	4	1	5
Methylprednisolone	5	0	4
Triamcinolone	5	0	4
Long-acting (>36 hours)			
Paramethasone	10	0	2
Betamethasone	25	0	0.75
Dexamethasone	25	0	0.75

Adapted from Haynes RC: In Gilman AG, Rall TW, Nils AS et al, editors: *Goodman and Gilman's the pharmacological basis of therapeutics*, ed 8, New York, 1990, Pergamon Press; pp 1431-1462.

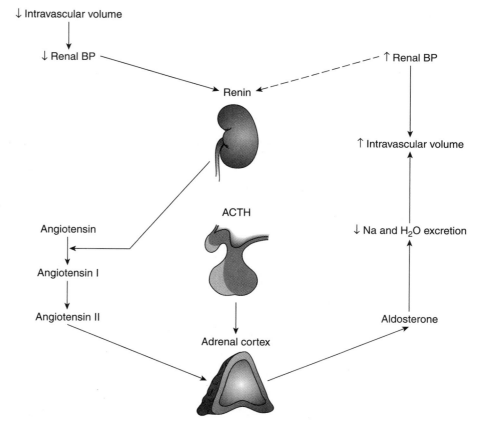

Fig. 15-4 Regulation of aldosterone secretion.

(i.e., masculinization and the promotion of protein anabolism and growth). The activity of the adrenal androgens, however, is only about 20% that of the testicular androgens and is of relatively minor importance.[4]

DEFINITION

Disorders affecting the adrenal glands result in excess or insufficient production of adrenal products. Excess production of the adrenal glands caused by pathophysiologic processes is known as *Cushing's disease.* Insufficient adrenocortical function may occur primarily or secondarily. Primary adrenocortical insufficiency is uncommon and known as *Addison's disease.* Secondary adrenocortical insufficiency results from hypothalamic or pituitary disease or the administration of exogenous corticosteroids, which down regulates adrenal production of cortisol. Long-term use of glucocorticoids can result in clinical features mimicking Cushing's disease. Under these circumstances, the collection of features is known as *Cushing's syndrome.*

EPIDEMIOLOGY: INCIDENCE AND PREVALENCE

Secondary adrenocortical insufficiency is a far more common problem than primary adrenocortical insufficiency. Approximately 5% of the adults in the United States chronically use corticosteroids and thus are at risk for secondary adrenocortical insufficiency. Addison's disease occurs at a rate of approximately 8 cases per 1 million people per year. The estimated prevalence of adrenal insufficiency is 40 to 60 cases per 1 million adults. A dental practice serving 2000 adults can expect to encounter 50 patients who use steroids or have potential adrenal abnormalities.

PATHOPHYSIOLOGY AND COMPLICATIONS

Primary adrenocortical insufficiency is caused by a progressive destruction of the adrenal cortex, usually of an idiopathic nature (most commonly autoimmune) but also resulting from hemorrhage, sepsis, infectious diseases (tuberculosis, human immunodeficiency virus [HIV], cytomegalovirus, and fungal infection), malignancy, adrenalectomy, or drugs.[9] The signs and symptoms of the disease are the result of deficiencies of adrenocortical hormones. Clinical evidence of the deficiency generally arises only after 90% of the adrenal cortices have been destroyed.

The major hormones of the adrenal cortex are cortisol and aldosterone. The presentation of Addison's disease is caused by the lack of these compounds. Lack of cortisol results in impaired glucose, fat, and protein metabolism, hypotension, increased ACTH secretion, impaired fluid excretion, excessive pigmentation, and an inability to tolerate stress. The relationship between corticosteroids and the response to stress is not well understood but probably involves the maintenance of vascular reactivity to vasoactive agents and the maintenance of normal blood pressure and cardiac output. Aldosterone deficiency results in an inability to conserve sodium and eliminate potassium and hydrogen ions, leading to hypovolemia, hyperkalemia, and acidosis.[3]

Secondary adrenocortical insufficiency is a far more common problem and results from hypothalamic or pituitary disease, or the administration of exogenous corticosteroids. The secretion of cortisol is directly dependent on the level of circulating ACTH. As the plasma cortisol level increases, the production of ACTH decreases by virtue of negative feedback to the pituitary and hypothalamus. With the administration of corticosteroids, the feedback system senses the elevated plasma steroid levels and inhibits ACTH production, which in turn suppresses the adrenal production of cortisol (see Fig. 15-2). The result is a partial adrenal insufficiency. The production of aldosterone, being ACTH independent, is not appreciably affected.

Determination of the degree of adrenocortical suppression for a given patient is controversial and generally has been thought to depend on the dosage, and timing and duration of administration. Thus suppression was presumably more likely with supraphysiologic doses taken daily over an extended period. Prediction of suppression, however, based on the history of dosage or length of administration has been unreliable.[10] Assessment of suppression is best accomplished by laboratory evaluation using stimulation tests for functional cortisol production.

A common treatment modification of steroid therapy that attempts to minimize adrenal suppression is the alternate-day regimen. This consists of giving steroids in the morning of every other day instead of daily but at a higher dose to maintain an elevated serum level. Because the cortisol level normally is higher in the morning, a single, large dose given at that time has less suppressant effect on ACTH, and on the off day, the HPA axis is allowed to function normally and produce endogenous steroids. The result is less adrenal suppression than is seen with twice-a-day therapy. Unfortunately, this approach often is not adequate to control symptoms, and many patients must return to daily therapy.

Topically applied and inhaled corticosteroids are rare inducers of adrenal suppression by absorption through the skin, mucous membrane, or pulmonary alveoli. Although the amount of topical steroid required to treat small, noninflamed areas probably does not cause significant suppression, prolonged treatment of large

inflamed areas may be a cause for concern, especially if occlusive dressings are used.[11,13,14] Similar comments can be made concerning the use of inhaled corticosteroids if given in frequent and high doses.[15,16] Daily doses above 1000 to 1500 mg/day (in four divided doses) of beclomethasone dipropionate or budesonide in adults (depending on body mass) generally are considered to be the cutoff point, indicating adrenal suppression is probable.[4,17]

Once corticosteroid administration ceases, the HPA axis regains its responsiveness, and normal ACTH and cortisol secretion resumes eventually. The time required to regain normal adrenal responsiveness is thought to vary from days to months. However, studies from a large review[18] demonstrated a return to stress stimulation of HPA function within 14 days or sooner, in spite of supraphysiologic doses for a month or longer.

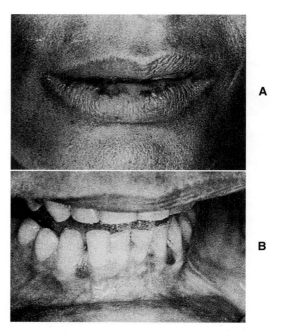

Fig. 15-5 Patient with Addison's disease. Note the bronzing of the skin with pigmentation of **A,** the lip and **B,** the oral mucosa.

CLINICAL PRESENTATION

SIGNS AND SYMPTOMS

Hypoadrenalism

Primary adrenal insufficiency (Addison's disease) has signs and symptoms that relate to a deficiency of aldosterone and cortisol. The most common complaints are weakness, fatigue, and abnormal pigmentation of the skin and mucous membranes (Fig. 15-5). Hypotension, anorexia, and weight loss are additional common findings. If a patient with Addison's disease is challenged by stress (e.g., illness, infection, or surgery), an adrenal crisis can be precipitated. This is a medical emergency manifested by a severe exacerbation of the patient's condition, including sunken eyes, profuse sweating, hypotension, weak pulse, cyanosis, nausea, vomiting, weakness, headache, dehydration, fever, dyspnea, myalgias, arthralgia, hyponatremia, and eosinophilia. If not treated rapidly, the patient may develop hypothermia, severe hypotension, hypoglycemia, and circulatory collapse that can result in death.[19]

Secondary adrenal insufficiency resulting from chronic corticosteroid administration can cause a partial insufficiency limited to glucocorticoids and usually does not produce any symptoms unless the patient is significantly stressed and does not have adequate circulating cortisol to cope with the stress. In that event, an adrenal crisis is possible. An adrenal crisis in a patient with secondary adrenal suppression is rare and tends not to be as severe as that seen with primary adrenal insufficiency since aldosterone secretion is

normal. Thus hypotension, dehydration, and shock seldom are encountered.[3]

Hyperadrenalism

A patient who has been receiving long-term, high-dose corticosteroid therapy can develop signs and symptoms of hyperadrenalism or Cushing's syndrome. A "Cushingoid" person displays weight gain, round or moon-shaped facies (Fig. 15-6), a "buffalo hump" on the back, abdominal striae, and acne. Other findings can include hypertension, heart failure, osteoporosis and bone fractures, diabetes mellitus, impaired healing, mental depression, and psychosis.[19] Chronic steroid use also can increase the risk for insomnia, peptic ulceration, cataract formation, glaucoma, growth suppression, and delayed wound healing.

LABORATORY FINDINGS

Because cortisol deficiency is of most concern from a dental management perspective, remarks in this chapter are limited to tests for the determination of cortisol secretion. These tests include basal plasma ACTH and cortisol, 24-hour urine excretion of 17-hydroxycorticosteroids (17-OHCS), and various stimulation tests.

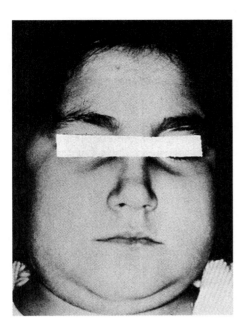

Fig. 15-6 Acquired Cushing's disease. (From Falace DA: Medical considerations: renal, endocrine, infectious, bone, joint, and hemologic disease. In Wood NK, editor: *Treatment planning: a pragmatic approach*, St Louis, 1978, Mosby.)

The usefulness of basal plasma testing and 24-hour urine testing is limited in that they measure cortisol production only at a given point or over a given period of time. These values can be altered by a variety of factors, including ones such as circadian rhythm, diet, and stress.

Normal plasma cortisol concentrations reflect a circadian rhythmicity. Values in the early morning range from 10 to 20 μg/dl, whereas late afternoon values typically range from 3 to 10 μg/dl. Urinary excretion of 17-OHCS ranges from 3 to 8 mg per 24 hours.[3] These plasma and urinary values may be normal in adrenocortical hypofunction, and an abnormality may become evident only with stimulation tests.

Stimulation tests of the HPA axis are a sensitive measure of suppressed endogenous cortisol production. Tests include synthetic ACTH (cosyntropin) stimulation test, insulin-induced hypoglycemia, metyrapone, and CRH tests. The insulin hypoglycemia, metyrapone, and CRH tests evaluate for the hypothalamic-pituitary suppression. The ACTH test directly evaluates the level of adrenal reserve. A positive response (increase in plasma cortisol level) is indicative of adrenal function. However, a subnormal test response, although suggestive of adrenal insufficiency,

has limited correlation with the patient's clinical ability to respond to stress.[20]

MEDICAL MANAGEMENT

PRIMARY ADRENAL INSUFFICIENCY

The primary medical needs of the Addisonian patient are (1) management of the adrenal disease (e.g., elimination of the infectious agent or malignant disease) and (2) hormonal replacement therapy. Glucocorticoid replacement is accomplished at levels that correspond to normal physiologic output of the adrenal cortex, usually being about 25 to 30 mg cortisol per day, with a range of 12.5 to 50 mg daily. Cortisol, 30 mg daily, or prednisone, 7.5 mg daily, provides adequate substitution therapy. Current practice recommends giving two thirds of the dose in the morning and one third in the later afternoon to reflect the normal diurnal cycle. Mineralocorticoid replacement is accomplished by the daily administration of fludrocortisone (0.05 to 0.1 mg). Patients are also encouraged to ingest adequate sodium.[19] Although patients with Addison's disease can lead essentially normal lives with appropriate treatment, the need for supplemental glucocorticoids during periods of illness, trauma, or "stress" remains indefinitely.

SECONDARY ADRENAL INSUFFICIENCY

Secondary adrenal insufficiency can result from hypothalamic-pituitary disorders or chronic steroid use. In the former, treatment involves correcting the ACTH-dependent disorder and replacing the missing glucocorticoid. In the latter, the clinician may be challenged by trying to balance the beneficial effects of steroids with the unwanted adverse effects. Steroids are prescribed in the management of nonendocrine disorders for their anti-inflammatory and immunosuppressive properties. Selection is based on potency, route of administration, duration of action and expected adverse effects. The goal is to achieve resolution of disease symptoms while minimizing adverse effects. Depending on the condition, dosages are generally targeted to be equal to or less than the daily replacement dose of the preparation used. For example, hydrocortisone is usually dispensed at about 20 mg/day, prednisone or prednisolone at 5 mg/day, or dexamethasone at 0.5 mg/day. Such regimens given as a morning dose are less suppressive. Higher and divided daily doses are more suppressive and usually take at least 3 weeks to result in clinical manifestation of glucocortiocoid deficiency. A method for minimizing the

adverse effects of long-term systemic steroid therapy is the alternate-day regimen. This method allows the adrenal gland to function normally during the off day and thus does not tend to cause axis suppression. A tapered dosage schedule is often implemented to discontinue steroid usage, but this may not be necessary in many cases.[21]

Patients who take steroids for the potential of low adrenal reserve and adrenal crisis during and following surgery have been of concern ever since Fraser et al[22] reported in 1952 that a patient experienced refractory hypotension at the end or a routine surgical procedure and died 3 hours later. A similar case was reported a year later.[23] The general consensus has been that these patients should be provided supplemental steroids during periods of stress, trauma, or illness.[9,19] However, this philosophy has been examined over the past decade, and a new approach has emerged. The basis for this change comes from knowledge of adrenal cortical response to physical stressors that has been refined over the past 20 years,[24] which is evidence that few well-documented cases of adrenal crisis exist in the literature.[25,26] Salem and colleagues[26] suggest that clinicians replace glucocorticoids only in an amount equivalent to the normal physiologic response to surgical stress and that the risk of an adverse outcome is dependent on the duration and severity of the surgery, and the overall health of the patient who takes daily steroids.

The factors that influence the need to provide supplemental glucocorticoids are discussed below. Surgery is known to cause increased plasma corticosteroid levels during and after operations. Plasma cortisol levels peak two- to 10-fold above baseline between 4 and 10 hours after the operation.[27,28] The level of the response is based on the magnitude of the surgery and whether general anesthesia is used. Postoperative pain is also contributory, and urine levels of 17-OHCS have been shown to remain increased for 3 to 6 days after the surgery.[28] Kehlet estimates that adults secrete 75 to 150 mg a day in response to major surgery and 50 mg a day during minor procedures.[25] Cortisol secretion in the first 24 hours after surgery rarely exceeds 200 mg.[26,29]

Under conditions of general anesthesia, corticosteroid-treated patients have a significantly lower plasma cortisol response to surgery than patients who have not received corticosteroid drugs.[30,31] This may be an effect of steroid-induced adrenal insufficiency or the use of barbiturate anesthetic drugs that can lower cortisol production.[32,33] Nevertheless, several studies have shown that the vast majority of patients who take chronic daily equivalent or less doses of steroid (e.g., mean dose 5 to 10 mg prednisone daily) for renal transplant or rheumatoid arthritis maintain adrenal function and do not require

supplementation for minor surgical procedures.[21,30,34,35] For minor surgery, the risk of adrenal crisis appears to be low. A significant proportion of patients taking 5 to 50 mg prednisone daily for between 6 days and 10 years who stopped therapy before surgery produced plasma cortisol levels similar to normal subjects for up to 7 days after minor or major surgery and also followed a normal postoperative course.[31,34,36]

If doubt exists as to the adrenal cortical status of a patient scheduled for surgery, a stimulation test of the HPA axis (e.g., CRH stimulation test) is recommended as a preoperative screening evaluation of adrenal function. If biochemical evaluation demonstrates inadequate HPA axis function or insufficient adrenal reserve, or if preoperative testing is not performed, perioperative glucocorticoid coverage should be provided according to the recommendations below.

The current recommendations by Salem et al[26] are as follows:

- For minor surgical stress, the glucocorticoid target is about 25 mg of hydrocortisone equivalent on the day of surgery. For example, an asthmatic patient who takes 5 mg of prednisone every other day should receive 5 mg of prednisone preoperatively.
- For moderate surgical stress, the glucocorticoid target is about 50 to 75 mg per day of hydrocortisone equivalent for up to 1 to 2 days. For example, a systemic lupus erythematosus patient who takes 10 mg prednisone daily should receive 10 mg of prednisone (or parenteral equivalent) preoperatively and 50 mg of hydrocortisone intravenously intraoperatively. On the first postoperative day, 20 mg of hydrocortisone is administered intravenously every 8 hrs (i.e., 60 mg per day). The patient returns to the preoperative glucocorticoid dose on postoperative day 2.
- For major surgical stress, the glucocorticoid target is about 100 to 150 mg per day of hydrocortisone equivalent for 2 to 3 days. For example, a patient with Crohn's disease who takes 40 mg prednisone daily for several years should receive 40 mg prednisone (or the parenteral equivalent) preoperatively and 50 mg hydrocortisone intravenously every 8 hours after the initial dose for the first 48 to 72 hrs after surgery. In comparison, a patient who takes 5 mg prednisone daily who is undergoing a similar major surgery is recommended to receive 5 mg prednisone (or the parenteral equivalent) as a preoperative dose, with 25 mg of hydrocortisone given intraoperatively and 25 mg administered in the 8 hours after surgery. Hydrocortisone 25 mg is prescribed every 8 hours for the subsequent 48 hours.

The above protocol recommends that the steroid be taken within 2 hours of the surgery and the surgeon,

anesthetist and nurses be advised of the possible complications. If the postoperative course is uneventful, the patient is returned to the usual glucocorticoid dosage upon completion of the regimen.

Factors that can complicate the postoperative course and exacerbate adrenal insufficiency include liver dysfunction, sepsis, and certain drugs.[37] Drugs that can lower plasma cortisol levels include aminoglutethimide (an adrenolytic); etomidate (an anesthtic agent); ketoconazole; and inducers of hepatic cytochrome P450 oxygenases (i.e., phenytoin, barbiturates or rifampin) that accelerate degradation of cortisol. In addition, the action of oral anticoagulants can be potentiated by intravenous (IV) high-dose methylprednisolone.[38]

ADRENAL CRISIS

A rare but potentially life-threatening outcome in spite of steroid supplementation is acute adrenal insufficiency (adrenal crisis). This condition requires immediate treatment, including IV injection of a glucocorticoid, usually 100 mg hydrocortisone bolus, and fluid and electrolyte replacement. Intramuscular (IM) injection results in slow absorption and is less desirable for emergency treatment. Over the next 24 hours, 100 mg IV is administered slowly every 6 to 8 hours and if needed, fluid replacement and correction of hypoglycemia. Resolution of the event or condition that precipitated the crisis is also required.

DENTAL MANAGEMENT

In developing recommendations for dental patients with adrenal disease, the dentist must consider the type and degree of adrenal dysfunction and the dental procedure planned. Patients with hyperadrenalism have increased likelihood of hypertension, osteoporosis, and risk of peptic ulcer disease. To minimize risk of adverse outcome, blood pressure should be taken at baseline and monitored during dental appointments. Osteoporosis has a relationship with periodontal bone loss and bone fractures. Treatment planning should address risk for periodontal bone loss and institute measures that promote bone mineralization and avoid extensive neck manipulation if osteoporosis is severe. Because of the risk of peptic ulceration, selection of postoperative analgesics should not include aspirin and nonsteroidal antiinflammatory drugs for long-term steroid users.

Evidence indicates that the vast majority of patients with adrenal insufficiency can receive routine dental treatment without the need for supplemental glucocorticoids.[25,34,35,39] Individuals at risk for adrenal crisis are those who undergo stressful surgical procedures and

have no or extremely low adrenal function because of primary or secondary adrenal insufficiency.

To determine who is risk for adrenal insufficiency or crisis, a thorough medical history must be taken. Past or present history of tuberculosis or HIV increases the risk for adrenal disease and insufficiency, since opportunistic infectious agents can attack the adrenal glands. In addition, adrenal crisis is possible when adrenal insufficient patients discontinue or simply do not take their glucocorticoid before a stressful surgery.

Other than major surgical procedures (e.g., extraction of bony impactions, osteomy, bone resections, cancer surgery), few dental procedures appear to warrant the use of supplemental steroids before, during, or after the operative period. Patients currently taking corticosteroids generally have enough exogenous and endogenous cortisol to handle routine dental procedures, if their usual steroid dose is taken within 2 hours of the surgery. Furthermore, routine dental procedures do not stimulate cortisol production at levels comparable to surgery.[39]

Studies[3,27,36,40] investigating the stress response to minor general and oral surgical procedures have concluded that significant cortisol increases are not generally seen before or during the operation but are increased in the postoperative period approximately 1 to 5 hours after initiating the procedure. The postoperative increase in plasma cortisol levels is likely a response to pain, since postoperative cortisol increases correlate with the loss of local anesthesia[40] and are blunted by the use of analgesics.[27] Consistent with this, Ziccardia and colleagues have reported that supplementation is not required for patients who take corticosteroids when uncomplicated minor surgical procedures of the orofacial complex are performed using local anesthesia with or without conscious sedation.[41-43]

To identify who needs supplementation for moderate to severe surgical procedures, the ACTH stimulation test can be performed. A low biochemical test result demonstrating inadequate adrenal cortical function indicates that supplemental steroids should be provided at a level sufficient for the stress response. However, even if a patient has adrenocortical suppression as diagnosed by an abnormal stimulation test, this does not necessarily reflect how he or she will react clinically or whether an adverse reaction will even occur.[17,18,24] Patients who have their glucocorticoid medication discontinued within a week before surgery have withstood general surgical procedures without the development of adrenal crisis.[17,29,34,36]

Based on the above mentioned studies and the limited number of purported adrenal crisis cases associated with dental procedures,[42,44-46] four factors appear to contribute to risk of adrenal crisis during the perioperative period of oral surgery. These include the severity of surgery, drugs administered, overall health of the patient, and amount of

pain control. Additional factors (e.g., amount of blood loss and a fasting state) can contribute to hypotension and hypoglycemia that can be confused with adrenal crisis but do not require glucocorticoids to resolve.

At present, for minor oral and periodontal surgery, adrenal insufficiency is prevented when circulating levels of glucocorticoids are about 25 mg of hydrocortisone equivalent per day. This is equivalent to a dose of about 6 mg of prednisone. To gain the benefit of the corticosteroid, the drug should be taken within 2 hours of the surgical procedure. Preferably, surgery is scheduled in the morning and stress reduction measures are implemented.

For major oral surgical stress involving use of general anesthesia, procedures lasting more than 1 hour, or significant blood loss, the glucocorticoid target is about 50 to 100 mg per day of hydrocortisone equivalent for the day of surgery and at least 1 postoperative day. Patients should take their normal dose and be provided supplemental hydrocortisone intraoperatively to achieve 100 mg. Hospitalization should be considered for these patients, since blood pressure can be more closely monitored postoperatively in this setting.[47] Hydrocortisone 25 mg is usually prescribed every 8 hours subsequent to surgery for 24 to 48 hours, depending on the procedure and anticipated level of postoperative pain. Box 15-2

BOX 15-2

Dental Management of the Patient with Possible Adrenal Insufficiency

1. Patient past history of systemic corticosteroid use
   a. Evaluate patient
   b. Determine whether systemic corticosteroid taken within last two weeks and reason for discontinuing usage
   c. Determine type, dose and duration of systemic corticosteroid used
   d. Identify signs and symptoms of possible adrenal insufficiency
   e. If major invasive oral procedure is planned and corticosteroid taken within last two weeks consult with physician regarding status and stability (ACTH or CRH test performed). If adrenal insufficient, implement steroid supplementation protocol.*

2. Patient currently taking systemic corticosteroids
   a. Evaluate patient
   b. Determine dose and duration of systemic corticosteroid use
   c. Identify signs and symptoms of possible adrenal insufficiency
   d. For diagnostic and minimally invasive procedures, have patient take usual daily dose and perform oral procedure in morning shortly after corticosteroid taken. Stress reduction measures implemented, blood pressure recorded during procedure.
   e. For major invasive oral procedure, consult with physician regarding status and stability (ACTH or CRH test performed). Implement steroid supplementation protocol.[a]

3. Patient not taking systemic corticosteroids, but may have adrenal insufficiency
   a. Evaluate patient for historical findings associated with risk for adrenal insufficiency
   b. Identify signs and symptoms of adrenal insufficiency
   c. Refer to physician for ACTH testing
   d. If patient found to be adrenal insufficient, defer dental treatment until stabilized with corticosteroid treatment. Then, followed steroid supplementation protocol[a] as defined in 2d and 2e.

*Steroid supplementation protocol for major surgical procedure
- Discontinue drugs that decrease cortisol levels (i.e., ketoconazole) at least 24 hours before surgery with the consent of the patient's physician.
- Have patient take usual morning dose (or the parenteral equivalent as a preoperative dose) and provide supplemental hydrocortisone pre- and intraoperatively to achieve 100 mg within first hour of surgery. Hydrocortisone 25 mg every 8 hours subsequent to surgery for 24 to 48 hours. Perform in hospital environment.
- Provide adequate operative and post-operative analgesia.
- Use barbiturates with caution and knowledge of the potential for adverse effect on plasma cortisol levels.
- Monitor blood pressure (BP) and blood loss throughout procedure. IF BP drops below 100/60 mm Hg, and patient is unresponsive to fluid replacement and vasopressive measures, administer supplemental steroids.
- Communicate with the patient at end of appointment and within 4 hrs post-operatively to determine whether features of weak pulse, hypotension, dyspnea, myalgias, arthralgias, ileus, and fever are present. Signs and symptoms of adrenal crisis dictate transport to a hospital for emergency care.

shows the recommendations for supplementation when orofacial surgical procedures are planned.

Several measures are recommended to minimize the risk of adrenal crisis associated with surgical stress. Surgery should be scheduled in the morning when cortisol levels are highest. Proper stress reduction should be provided as anxiety increases cortisol demand. Use of nitrous oxide-oxygen or benzodiazepine IV sedation[48] is helpful since plasma cortisol levels are not reduced by these agents.[28] In contrast, the reversal of and recovery from general anesthesia and extubation and not the trauma of surgery itself are major determinants of secretion of ACTH, cortisol, and epinephrine.[48,49] Thus general anesthesia increases glucocorticoid demand for these patients. Barbiturates also should be used cautiously since these drugs increase the metabolism of cortisol and reduce blood levels of cortisol.[12,33,50] In addition, drugs that decrease cortisol levels (e.g., ketoconazole) should be discontinued at least 24 hours before surgery with the consent of the patient's physician.

Surgeries lasting more than 1 hour are more stressful than shorter surgeries and should be performed with the consideration for the need of steroid supplementation. Blood and fluid volume loss exacerbate hypotension and increase the risk of adrenal insufficiency–like symptoms. Thus methods to reduce blood loss should be employed. Patients who take anticoagulants are also at greater risk of postsurgical bleeding and hypotension. In addition, inadequate pain control in the postoperative period increases the risk of adrenal crisis. Clinicians should provide good postoperative pain control by using long-acting local anesthetics (e.g., bupivacaine) at the end of the procedure.

Monitoring blood pressure throughout the procedure is critical for recognizing the development of an adrenal crisis. During surgery, blood pressure should be evaluated at 5-minute intervals and before the patient leaves the office. A systolic blood pressure below 100 mm Hg or diastolic at or below 60 mm Hg represents hypotension. The diagnosis of hypotension dictates that the clinician take corrective action. This would include proper patient positioning (i.e., head lower than feet); provision of fluid replacement; vasopressors; and evaluation for signs of adrenal dysfunction versus hypoglycemia. Immediate treatment of an adrenal crisis consists of the administration of 100 mg of hydrocortisone or 4 mg dexamethasone IV and immediate transportation to a medical facility.[3]

TREATMENT PLANNING MODIFICATIONS

Dental treatment of a patient with undiagnosed and untreated adrenal insufficiency should be delayed until the patient is medically stabilized. Otherwise, treatment modifications are not required for patients with medically stable adrenal disorders.

ORAL COMPLICATIONS AND MANIFESTATIONS

In primary adrenal insufficiency, pigmentation of the oral mucous membranes is a common finding (see Fig. 15-5). Patients with secondary adrenal insufficiency may be prone to delayed healing and have increased susceptibility to infection.

References

1. Haynes RC: Adrenocorticotropic hormone; adrenocortical steroids and their synthetic analogs; inhibitors of the synthesis and actions of adrenocortical hormones. In Gilman AG et al, editors: *Goodman and Gilman's the pharmacologic basis of therapeutics*, ed 8, New York, 1990, Pergamon Press.
2. Guyton, AC: *Textbook of medical physiology*, ed 8, Philadelphia, 1991, WB Saunders.
3. Orth DN, Kovacs WJ, Debold CR: The adrenal cortex. In Wilson JD, Foster DW, editors: *Williams textbook of endocrinology*, ed 8, Philadelphia, 1992, WB Saunders.
4. Ganong WF: *Review of medical physiology*, ed 15, 1991, Norwalk, Conn, Appleton & Lange.
5. George JM et al: Morphine anesthesia blocks cortisol and growth hormone response to surgical stress in humans, *J Clin Endocrinol Metab* 38:736-741, 1974.
6. Raff H et al: Inhibition of the adrenocorticotropin response to surgery in humans: interactions between dexamethasone and fentanyl, *J Clin Endocrinol Metab* 65:295-298, 1987.
7. Gersema L, Baker K: Use of corticosteroids in oral surgery, *J Oral Maxillofac Surg* 50:270-277, 1992.
8. Kaufman E et al: Intraligamentary injection of slow-release methylprednisolone for the prevention of pain after endodontic treatment, *Oral Surg Oral Med Oral Pathol* 77:651-654, 1994.
9. Loriaux DL, McDonald WJ: Adrenal insufficiency. In Degroot LJ, editor: *Endocrinology*, vol 2, ed 3, Philadelphia, 1995, WB Saunders.
10. Schlaghecke R et al: The effect of long-term glucocorticoid therapy on pituitary-adrenal responses to exogenous corticotropin-releasing hormone, *N Engl J Med* 326:226-230, 1992.
11. Coskey RJ: Adverse effects of corticosteroids. I. Topical and intralesional, *Clin Dermatol* 4:155-160, 1986.
12. Parnell AG: Adrenal crisis and the dental surgeon, *Br Dent J* 116:294-298, 1964.
13. Patel L et al: Adrenal function following topical steroid treatment in children with atopic dermatitis, *Br J Dermatol* 132:950-955, 1995.
14. Plemons JM, Rees TD, Zachariah NY: Absorption of a topical steroid and evaluation of adrenal suppression in patients with erosive lichen planus, *Oral Surg* 69:688-693, 1990.
15. Hanania NA, Chapman KR, Kesten S: Adverse effects of inhaled corticosteroids, *Am J Med* 98:196-208, 1995.
16. Maxwell DL: Adverse effects of inhaled corticosteroids, *Biomed Pharmacother* 44:421-427, 1990.

17. Toogood JH et al: Personal observations on the use of inhaled corticosteroid drugs for chronic asthma, *Eur J Respir Dis* 65:321-338, 1984.

18. Glick M: Glucocorticosteroid replacement therapy: a literature review and suggested replacement therapy, *Oral Surg* 67:614-620, 1989.

19. Williams GH, Dluky RG: Diseases of the adrenal cortex. In Wilson, JD et al, editors: *Harrison's principles of internal medicine*, ed 2, New York, 1992, McGraw-Hill.

20. Bethune JE: The diagnosis and treatment of adrenal insufficiency. In Degroot LJ et al, editors: *Endocrinology*, vol 2, ed 2, Philadelphia, 1989, WB Saunders.

21. Shapiro R et al: Adrenal reserve in renal transplant recipients with cyclosporine, azathioprine, and prednisone immunosuppression. *Transplantation* 49:1011-1013, 1990.

22. Fraser CG, Preuss FS, Bigford WD: Adrenal atrophy and irreversible shock associated with cortisone therapy, *JAMA* 149:1542-1543, 1952.

23. Lewis L et al: Fatal adrenal cortical insufficiency precipitated by surgery during prolonged continuous cortisone treatment, *Ann Intern Med* 39:116-126, 1953.

24. Chernow B et al: Hormonal responses to graded surgical stress, *Arch Intern Med* 147:1273-1278, 1987.

25. Kehlet H: *Clinical course and hypothalamic-pituitary-adrenocortical function in glucocorticoid-treated surgical patients*, Copenhagen, 1976, FADL's Forlag.

26. Salem M et al: Perioperative glucocorticoid coverage: a reassessment 42 years after emergence of a problem, *Ann Surg* 4:416-425, 1994.

27. Banks P: The adreno-cortical response to oral surgery, *Br J Oral Surg* 8:32-44, 1970.

28. Thomasson B: *Studies on the content of 17-hydroxycorticosteroids and its diurnal rhythm in the plasma of surgical patients*, Turku, Finland, 1959, Mercators Tryckeri Helsingfors.

29. Kehlet H, Binder C: Adrenocortical function and clinical course during and after surgery in unsupplemented glucocorticoid-treated patients, *Br J Anaesth* 45:1043-1048, 1973.

30. Jasani MK et al: Cardiovascular and plasma cortisol responses to surgery in corticosteroid-treated R.A. patients, *Acta Rheum Scand* 14:65-70, 1968.

31. Jasani MK et al: Studies of the rise in plasma 11-hydroxycorticosteroids (11-OHCS) in corticosteroid-treated patients with rheumatoid arthritis during surgery: correlations with the functional integrity of the hypothalmo-pituitary-adrenal axis, *Q J Med* 1968;37:407.

32. Lehtinen A-M, Hovorka J, Widholm O: Modification of aspects of the endocrine response to tracheal intubation by lignocaine, halothane and thiopentone, *Br J Anaesth* 56:239-245, 1984.

33. Oyama T et al: Adrenocortical function related to thiopental-nitrous oxide-oxygen anesthesia and surgery in man, *Anesth Analges Curr Res* 50:727-731, 1971.

34. Bromberg JS et al: Stress steroids are not required for patients receiving a renal allograft and undergoing operation, *J Am Coll Surg* 180:532-536, 1995.

35. Friedman RJ, Schiff CF, Bromberg JS: Use of supplemental steroids in patients having orthopaedic operations, *J Bone Joint Surg* 77:1801-1806, 1995.

36. Plumpton FS, Besser GM, Cole PV: Corticosteroid treatment and surgery. 2. The management of steroid cover, *Anesthesia* 24:12-18, 1969.

37. Singh N et al: Acute adrenal insufficiency in critically ill liver transplant recipients, *Transplant* 59:1744-1745, 1995.

38. Costedoat-Chalumeau N et al: Potentiation of vitamin K antagonists by high-dose intravenous methylprednisolone, *Ann Intern Med* 132:631-635, 2000.

39. Miller CS et al: Salivary cortisol response to dental treatment of varying stress, *Oral Surg Oral Med Oral Pathol Oral Radiol Endod* 79:436-441, 1995.

40. Shannon IL et al: Stress in dental patients. II. The serum free 17-hydroxycorticosteroid response in routinely appointed patients undergoing simple exodontias, *Oral Surg Oral Med Oral Pathol* 15:1142-1146, 1970.

41. Ziccardia VB et al: Maxillofacial considerations in orthotopic liver transplantation, *Oral Surg Oral Med Oral Pathol* 71:21-26, 1991.

42. Ziccardia VB et al: Precipitation of an Addisonian crisis during dental surgery: recognition and management, *Compendium* 13:518, 520, 522-524, 1992.

43. Ziccardia VB: *Personal communication*, 2000.

44. Broutsas MG, Seldin R: Adrenal crisis after tooth extractions in an adrenalectomized patient: report of case. *J Oral Surg* 30:301-302, 1972.

45. Cawson RA, James J: Adrenal crisis in a dental patient having systemic corticosteroids. *Br J Oral Surg* 10:305-309, 1973.

46. Schietler LE, Tucker WM, Christian DG: Adrenal insufficiency: report of a case. *Spec Care Dent* 4:22-24, 1984.

47. Glowniak JV and Loriaux DL: A double-blind study of perioperative steroid requirements in secondary adrenal insufficiency, *Surgery* 121:123-129, 1997.

48. Hempenstall PD et al: Cardiovascular, biochemical, and hormonal responses to intravenous sedation with local analgesia versus general anesthesia in patients undergoing oral surgery, *J Oral Maxillofac Surg* 44:441-446, 1986.

49. Udelsman R et al: Responses of the hypothalamic-pituitary-adrenal and renin-angiotensin axes and the sympathetic system during controlled surgical and anesthetic stress, *J Clin Endocrinol Metab* 64:986-994, 1987.

50. Siker SE, Lipschitz E, Klein R: The effect of preanesthetic medications on the blood level of 17-hydroxycorticosteroids, *Ann Surg* 143:88, 1956.

Thyroid Disease

16
CHAPTER

*T*he patient with thyroid disease is of concern to the dentist from several aspects. The dentist may detect early signs and symptoms of thyroid disease and refer the patient for medical evaluation and treatment. In some cases, this may be lifesaving, whereas in others the quality of life can be improved and complications of certain thyroid disorders avoided.

Patients with untreated thyrotoxicosis may be in danger if the dentist performs surgical or operative procedures. Although uncommon, an acute medical emergency (thyrotoxic crisis or thyroid storm) may be precipitated by dental treatment. Acute infections and trauma also may precipitate a thyrotoxic crisis in the untreated or inadequately treated patient.[1,2]

Patients with thyroid cancer will benefit from the early detection and treatment of their tumors. The role of the dentist is to examine for lesions in the thyroid and surrounding tissues by inspection and palpation. Patients found to have neck lesions that may be related to the thyroid are referred for diagnosis and treatment as indicated. Early detection can lead to cure or prolongation of life. Most thyroid cancers are solitary thyroid nodules.[3,4]

In this chapter, emphasis is placed on disorders involving hyperfunction of the gland (hyperthyroidism or thyrotoxicosis), hypofunction of the gland (hypothyroidism or myxedema or cretinism), thyroiditis, and the detection of lesions that may be cancerous. The standard abbreviations used for thyroid gland function and terminology are shown in Box 16-1.

DEFINITION

The thyroid gland, located in the anterior portion of the neck just below and bilateral to the thyroid cartilage, develops from the thyroglossal duct and portions of the ultimobranchial body. It consists of two lateral lobes connected by an isthmus. The right lobe is normally larger than the left,[5] and in some individuals a superior portion of glandular tissue, or pyramidal lobe, can be identified. Thyroid tissue may be found anywhere along the path of the thyroglossal duct, from its origin (midline posterior portion of the tongue) to its termination (thyroid gland, in the neck). In rare cases the entire thyroid is found in the anterior mediastinal compartment; however, in most individuals the remnants of the duct atrophy and disappear. The thyroglossal duct, passes through the region of the developing hyoid bone, and remnants of the duct can become enclosed or surrounded by the bone.[5] Ectopic thyroid tissue may secrete thyroid hormones or become cystic or neoplastic. In a few individuals, the only functional thyroid tissue is in these ectopic locations.

Enlargements of the thyroid gland, termed a *goiter*, can be diffuse, nodular, singular, functional, or nonfunctional. On a functional basis, thyroid enlargement can be divided into the three types listed in Table 16-1. Simple goiter accounts for about 75% of all thyroid swellings. Most of these goiters are nonfunctional and thus do not cause hyperthyroidism. The goiter of Graves' disease is associated with hyperthyroidism. Hashimoto's thyroiditis leads to hypothyroidism. In contrast, patients with subacute thyroiditis develop a transient period of hyperthyroidism. Hypothyroidism can occur as a congenital or acquired condition. Thyroid cancer often presents as a single nodule but can present as multiple lesions or in rare cases occur within a benign goiter.[1,2,4]

EPIDEMIOLOGY

Incidence and Prevalence

Worldwide, the most common thyroid disorder is iodine deficiency (diet-related) goiter. In many of these cases, hypothyroidism develops, and in some, hyperthyroidism

results. This type of goiter is called *endemic* if more than 10% of a local population is affected.[1,2,6,7]

In the United States, where current levels of iodine intake are adequate, the prevalence of goiter ranges from 0.5% to 7%. The incidence of new single nodules is about 0.1% per year. The incidence of nodular thyroid disease is about 0.1% to 1.5% per year.[4,6]

BOX 16-1

Standard Abbreviations Used for Thyroid Gland Function and Terminology

T_4	Thyroxine
T_3	Triiodothyronine
rT_3	Reverse triiodothyronine
TSH	Thyroid-stimulating hormone
TRH	Thyrotropin-releasing hormone
TT_4	Total thyroxine
TT_3	Total triiodothyronine
FTI	Free triiodothyronine
FT_4	Free thyroxine
T_3U	Triiodothyronine uptake
FT_4I	Free thyroxine index
FT_3I	Free triiodothyronine index
TTG	Thyroid globulin
TBG	Thyroid-binding globulin
TTR	Transthyretin
TBA	Thyroid-binding albumin

A recent study[8] examined thyroid size and function in genetically similar populations from a region of low iodine intake (Jutland, Denmark) and a region of high iodine intake (Iceland). Women from the low iodine intake region in Jutland had a high prevalence of goiter (12.2%) compared with women from Iceland (1.9%). The rate of goiter in men from both regions was similar. Thyroid dysfunction was common in both areas. In the high iodine region of Iceland, hypothyroidism was more common. In contrast, goiter and thyrotoxicosis were more common in the low iodine region of Jutland. This and two other studies[9,10] show the importance of avoiding very high and very low iodine diets.

Few good studies demonstrate the prevalence of thyroid disorders.[11,12] Among patients with hyperthyroidism, 60% to 80% have Graves' disease. The annual incidence of Graves' disease in women over a 20-year period is about 0.5 cases per 1000, with the highest risk of onset between 40 and 60 years.[11] Studies in Great Britain have shown about 25 to 30 cases of hyperthyroidism per 10,000 women. The mean age at the time of diagnosis was 48 years. Some 2% of the women had established cases. The incidence of new cases was 3 per 1000 women per year. These studies showed that hyperthyroidism was 10 times more common in women than in men. The incidence of the disease in the United States has been reported to be 3 cases per 10,000 women per year.[12] The prevalence of Graves' disease is similar among whites and Asians, and it is lower among African-Americans.[11]

Hypothyroidism in Great Britain occurs at a rate of 3 cases per 1000 women per year. The number of estab-

---

TABLE 16-1

Causes of Goiter in Regions with Normal Iodine Intake

Type of Goiter	Relative Frequency	Thyroid Function
Primary Goiter		
Simple goiter	Very Common	Usually normal
Thyroid cancer	Infrequent	Usually normal
Secondary Goiter: Thyrostimulatory		
Graves' disease	Infrequent	Increased
Hashimoto's thyroiditis	Common	Decreased
Congenital hereditary goiter	Rare	Decreased
Secondary Goiter: Thyroinvasive		
Hashimoto's thyroiditis	Common	Usually decreased
Subacute thyroiditis	Infrequent	Transient increase
Riedel's thyroiditis	Rare	Transient increase
Metastatic tumors to the thyroid	Rare	May be decreased

From Emerson CH: Thyroid nodules and goiter. Greene HL, editor: *Clinical medicine*, ed 2, St Louis, 1996, Mosby.

lished cases was reported to be 14 per 1000 women. The number of established cases in men was 1 per 1000. The mean age at diagnosis was 57 years. About one third of all cases resulted from surgical or radiation treatment for hyperthyroidism.[12]

In the United States, hypothyroidism occurs in 3% to 4% of ill older patients admitted to the hospital. It is five to six times more common than hyperthyroidism. It is estimated that 10% of the women over the age of 40 years have a thyroid hormone deficiency caused by autoimmune thyroid disease.[7] Both hypothyroidism and hyperthyroidism are about four to five times more common in women than in men in the United States.[12,13]

Subclinical hypothyroidism and hyperthyroidism are common, well-defined conditions that often progress to overt disease. In addition, concerns are evident that the subclinical states may contribute to hyperlipidemia, cardiac dysfunction, and osteoporosis.[1,2,14]

Thyroid nodules were found in 4.2% of the Framingham population, with an increased prevalence in women and older individuals. The frequency of cancer in solitary thyroid nodules has been reported to be about 1% to 5%. Thyroid cancer is found in 8% to 20% of surgically removed thyroid nodules. In autopsy studies of thyroid nodules, about 3% are cancerous.[3,4] The estimated number of cases

of thyroid cancer in the United States in the year 2000 was 18,400, with 75% of cases occurring in women.[15]

PATHOPHYSIOLOGY AND ETIOLOGY

The thyroid gland secretes three hormones: thyroxine (T_4), triiodothyronine (T_3), and calcitonin. The tissue developing from the ultimobranchial bodies is thought to give rise to the parafollicular cells, which produce calcitonin. Calcitonin is involved, with parathyroid hormone and vitamin D, in regulating serum calcium and phosphorous levels and skeletal remodeling. This hormone and its actions also are considered in Chapter 9. T_4 and T_3 are hormones that affect metabolic processes throughout the body and are involved with oxygen use.

An adequate supply of iodine is needed for the synthesis of thyroid hormone. This requires the daily uptake of sufficient iodide to allow the synthesis of approximately 100 μg of T_4, which is 65% iodine by weight. Box 16-2 shows the various factors that can influence the 24-hour uptake of iodine.

Blood levels of T_4 and T_3 are controlled through a servofeedback mechanism mediated by the hypothalamic-pituitary-thyroid axis. Increased or decreased metabolic demand appears to be the main modifier of the system.

BOX 16-2

Factors that Influence 24-hour Thyroid Iodine Uptake

Factors That Increase Uptake

Increased Hormone Synthesis

Hyperthyroidism

Response to glandular hormone depletion
Recovery from thyroid suppression
Recovery from subacute thyroiditis
Antithyroid agents

Excessive hormone losses
Nephrotic syndrome
Chronic diarrheal states
Soybean ingestion

Normal Hormone Synthesis

Iodine deficiency
Dietary insufficiency
Excessive loss (dehalogenase defect, pregnancy)

Hormone biosynthetic defects

Factors That Decrease Uptake

Decrease Hormone Synthesis

Primary hypofunction
Primary hypothyroidism
Antithyroid agents
Hormone biosynthetic defects
Hashimoto's disease
Subacute thyroiditis

Secondary hypofunction

Exogenous thyroid hormone

Not Reflecting Decreased Hormone Synthesis

Increased availability of iodine
Diet or drugs
Cardiac or renal insufficiency

Increased hormone release
Very severe hyperthyroidism (rare)

From Larsen PR, Davies TF, Hay JD: The thyroid gland. In Wilson JD et al, editors: *Williams textbook of endocrinology*, ed 9, Philadelphia, 1999, WB Saunders.

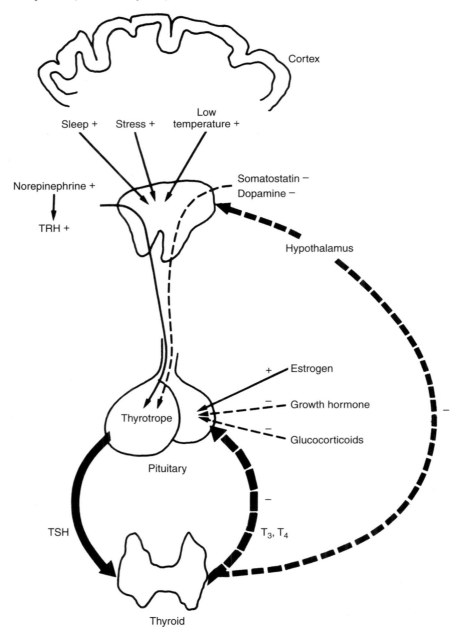

Fig. 16-1 Hypothalamic-pituitary-thyroid axis involved in the control of thyroid secretion. The secretion of thyrotropin (thyroid-stimulating hormone [TSH]) is regulated by interaction of a releasing factor (thyroid-releasing hormone [TRH]) and an inhibitory factor (somatostatin). Thyroid hormones (T_3 and T_4) act directly on the pituitary to inhibit TSH secretion. Thyroid hormones also act at the hypothalamic level to stimulate somatostatin release. T_4 is converted to T_3 in the liver, kidney, and heart and in the pituitary and hypothalamus. T_3 is more potent than T_4 at all sites. (From Mazzaferri EL: The thyroid. In Mazzaferri EL, editor: *Endocrinology*, ed 3, New York, 1986, Medical Examination Publishing.)

Drugs, illness, thyroid disease, and pituitary disorders can affect the control of this balance. Recent findings[13,16,17] also show that age has some effect on the system (Fig. 16-1).

Under normal conditions, thyrotropin-releasing hormone is released by the hypothalamus in response to external stimuli (stress, illness, metabolic demand, low levels of T_3, and to a lesser degree, T_4). Thyrotropin-releasing hormone stimulates the pituitary to release thyroid-stimulating hormone (TSH), which causes the thyroid gland to secrete T_4 and T_3.[1,2,13]

T_4 and T_3 also have a direct influence on the pituitary. High levels turn off the release of TSH, and low levels turn it on. The effect of T_3 on the pituitary is greater than that of T_4.[1,2,13] T4 is the main hormone secreted by the thyroid. The level of T_4 in the peripheral blood is 60 times that of T_3. T_4 is converted to T_3 peripherally by deiodination. T_3 is the more active hormone and is the main effector principle.[1,2,13] A small amount of an inactive form of T_3, called *reverse* T_3 (rT_3), is found in circulation.[2]

Goitrins are antithyroid agents that inhibit thyroid hormone synthesis. Foods such as cabbages, turnips, and rutabagas contain them. Thiocyanate, perchlorate, thiourea, methimazole, and propylthiouracil are goitrins. Methimazole and propylthiouracil block both the iodination of tyrosine and the coupling of monoiodotyrosine and diiodotyrosine to form iodotyrosine.[1,2,16]

The thyroid gland is the only source of T_4 and produces about 20% of T_3. Thus under normal conditions, 20% of the circulating pool of T_3 comes from the thyroid gland and the rest (80%) comes from the peripheral monodeiodination of T_4. In cases of hyperthyroidism, 30% to 40% of circulating T_3 comes from the thyroid.[2,5]

The conversion of T_4 to T_3 can be inhibited by fasting, illness, steroids, and certain drugs (e.g., propylthiouracil). Iodine must be available for the synthesis of T_4 and T_3. The inorganic form of iodine as used by the gland comes from the peripheral degradation and deodination of thyroid hormone and the diet. A minimum of 60 μg of iodine per day is required for thyroid hormone synthesis, and at least 100 μg per day is needed to eliminate all signs of iodine deficiency from the population. In the United States the daily intake of iodine is in the range of 500 μg. Much of this is supplied by the use of iodized salt. A gradual increase in the dietary intake of iodine in the United States has occurred in recent years. Iodine, which is stored in the thyroid gland, appears to be oxidized to a higher valence by a preoxidase and then combines with thyrosyl to form either monoiodotyrosine or diiodotyrosine. These compounds, by an oxidative coupling reaction, form either T_4 or T_3.[1,2]

The thyroid hormones are stored in the colloid of the thyroid gland. A 3- to 4-month reserve is maintained. Of the organic iodine content of the thyroid gland, 35% is stored as T_4, with about 5% to 8% as T_3. Phagocytosis of colloid droplets starts the secretion process. The colloid droplets are digested by proteases; once freed, thyroid globulin (TG), T_4, T_3, and small amounts of rT_3 are secreted into the blood.[1,16]

In the blood, T_4 and T_3 are almost entirely bound to plasma proteins. The binding plasma proteins are thyroxine-binding globulin (TBG), transthyretin, and thyroid-binding albumin. A small amount of T_3 and T_4 are bound to high-density lipoproteins. The most important thyroid hormone-binding serum protein is TBG. TBG binds about 70% of T_4 and 75% to 80% of T_3. The remaining T_4 and T_3 is bound by transthyretin and thyroid-binding albumin. Only 0.02% to 0.03% of FT_4 and about 0.3% of FT_3 are found in plasma.[1,2]

Low T_4 and T_3 plasma levels often are found in ill and medicated older persons. Protein abnormalities can affect total T_4 and T_3 levels. Illness can reduce the conversion of T_4 to T_3 and increase rT_3. Drugs and illness also can affect the free levels of T_4 and T_3. The main age-related change seen in much older individuals is a fall in T_3 because of the reduced peripheral conversion of T_4 to T_3.[1,2,13]

Thyroid hormone influences the growth and maturation of tissues, cell respiration and total energy expenditure. The hormone is involved in the turnover of essentially all substances, vitamins, and hormones. Some of the thyroid hormone actions take place at the level of the mitochondria to influence oxidative metabolism or at the level of the plasma membrane and endoplasmic reticulum to influence the activity of Ca^{2+}-ATPase, and the transcellular flux of substrates and cations. The primary action of thyroid hormone is expressed by binding to one or more intracellular receptor complexes, which, in turn, bind to specific regulatory sites in the chromosomes to influence genomic expression.[2]

Antibodies to various structures within the thyroid are associated with autoimmune diseases of the thyroid. Graves' disease and Hashimoto's thyroiditis have such an association. Three autoantibodies are most often involved with autoimmune thyroid disease. These are TSH receptor antibodies (TSHRAb), thyroid preoxidase antibodies (TPOAb), and thyroglobulin antibodies (TgAb).[1]

TSHRAb are not found in the general population but are found in 80% to 95% of patients with Graves' disease and in 10% to 20% of patients with autoimmune thyroiditis. Most TSHRAb in Graves' disease are stimulating antibodies, which stimulate the release of thyroid hormone. However, blocking antibodies to the TSH receptor (TSHR-blocking Ab) also are found, blocking the release of thyroid hormone. The ratio of these TSH receptor antibodies determines the clinical status of the patient in regards to function of the thyroid gland.[1,2,11]

Thyroid Function Tests in Hyperthyroidism and Hypothyroidism

Test*	Hyperthyroidism	Normal Range	Hypothyroidism
T_4	Elevated	60-150 nmol/L	Decreased
T_3	Elevated	70-190 nmol/L	Decreased
TSH	None or very decreased	0.3-5.0 mμ/L	Elevated
TBG	Elevated	12-30 mg/L	Decreased
rT_3	Elevated	10-40 nmol/L	Decreased
FT_4	Elevated	1.3-3.8 ng/L	Decreased
FT_3	Elevated	260-480 png/L	Decreased
RAIU	Elevated	10% to 30% per 24 hr	Decreased

*Most frequently used tests: T_4, T_3, TSH, TBG
Modified from Nickolai TF: *Thyroid*. In Rose LF, Kay D, editors: *Internal medicine for dentistry*, ed 2, St Louis, 1990, Mosby; Smaliridge RC: *Thyroid disease*. In Becker K-L, editor: *Principles and practice of endocrinology and metabolism*, Philadelphia, 1990, JB Lippincott; Wartofsky L: Diseases of the thyroid. In Wilson JD et al, editors: *Harrison's principles of internal medicine*, ed 14, New York, 1998, McGraw-Hill.

TgAb are found in about 10% to 20% of the general population. These antibodies are found in 50% to 70% of patients with Graves' disease. TgAb are found in 80% to 90% of patients with autoimmune thyroiditis.[1]

TPOAb are found in 8% to 27% of the general population. In Graves' disease, about 50% to 80% of the patients have these antibodies. TPOAb are found in 90% to 100% of patients with autoimmune thyroiditis.[1]

LABORATORY TESTS

Direct tests of thyroid function involve the administration of radioactive iodine. Measurement of the thyroid radioactive iodine uptake (RAIU) is the most common of these tests. [131]I has been used for this test, but ^{123}I is preferred because it exposes the patient to a lower radiation dose. The RAIU is measured 24 hours after the administration of the isotope (Table 16-2). The RAIU varies inversely with the plasma iodide concentration and directly with the functional state of the thyroid. In the United States the normal 24-hour RAIU is 10% to 30%. The RAIU discriminates poorly between normal and hypothyroid states. Values above the normal range usually indicate thyroid hyperfunction.[2]

Several tests are available that measure the thyroid hormone concentration and binding in blood. Highly specific and sensitive radioimmunoassays are used to measure serum T_4 and T_3 concentrations and rarely to measure rT_3 concentration (Table 16-2). Elevated levels usually indicate hyperthyroidism, and lower levels usu-

ally indicate hypothyroidism. The free hormone levels usually correlate better with the metabolic state than do total hormone levels. Indirect assays are used to estimate the free T_4 level.[2]

The measurement of the basal serum TSH concentration is useful in the diagnosis hyperthyroidism and hypothyroidism. Very sensitive methods are now available, such as immunoradiometric or chemiluminescent, to measure serum TSH. In cases of hyperthyroidism the TSH level is almost always low or nondetectable (see Table 16-2). Higher levels indicate hypothyroidism, and lower levels signify hyperthyroidism.[2]

Other tests used in selected cases include TSH stimulation test, T_3 suppression test, and radioassay techniques for measuring TSHRAb, TSHR-blocking Ab, TPOAb, and TgAb.[1,2,13,16,18]

A thyroid scan is a common test used to localize thyroid nodules and to locate functional ectopic thyroid tissue. [123]I or ^{99}Tc is injected, and a scanner localizes areas of radioactive concentration. This technique allows for the identification of nodules 1 cm or larger. When a pinhole thyroid scan is used, 2- to 3-mm lesions can be detected.[1,2,16]

Ultrasonography also is used to detect thyroid lesions. Nodules 1 to 2 mm in size can be identified. The technique also is used to distinguish solid from cystic lesions, measure the size of the gland, and guide needles for aspiration of cysts or biopsy of thyroid masses. Computed tomography (CT) and magnetic resonance imaging (MRI) are expensive procedures helpful mainly

BOX 16-3

Disorders of Thyrotoxicosis

Thyrotoxicosis Caused by Primary Thyroid Hyperfunction Graves' disease Toxic multinodular goiter Toxic adenoma **Thyrotoxicosis Caused by Secondary Thyroid Hyperfunction** Pituitary adenoma—TSH secretion Nonadenomatous inappropriate TSH secretion Trophoblastic hCG-secretion tumors	**Thyrotoxicosis without Thyroid Hyperfunction** Hormonal leakage • Subacute thyroiditis • Chronic thyroiditis with transient thyrotoxicosis Thyrotoxicosis factitia (thyroid hormone use) Hamburger thyrotoxicosis (bovine thyroid in ground beef) Ectopic thyroid tissue • Struma ovarii • Metastatic thyroid cancer Iatrogenic thyrotoxicosis (overdosage of thyroid hormone)

From Burth HB: Thyroid disease. In Bardin CW. editor: *Current therapy in endocrinology and metabolism*, ed 5, St Louis, 1996, Mosby.

in the postoperative management of patients with thyroid cancer. They are used for the preoperative evaluation of larger lesions of the thyroid, greater than 3 cm that extend beyond the gland into adjacent tissues.[1,2,16,19]

THYROTOXICOSIS (HYPERTHYROIDISM)

ETIOLOGY, PATHOPHYSIOLOGY, AND COMPLICATIONS

The term *thyrotoxicosis* refers to an excess of T_4 and T_3 in the bloodstream. This excess may be caused by ectopic thyroid tissue, Graves' disease, multinodular goiter, thyroid adenoma, subacute thyroiditis, ingestion of thyroid hormone (thyrotoxicosis factitia), food-containing thyroid hormone, or pituitary disease involving the anterior portion of the gland (Box 16-3). In this section the signs and symptoms, laboratory tests, treatment, and dental considerations for the patient with Graves' disease are considered in detail and serve as the model for other conditions that can result in similar clinical manifestations. It should be emphasized that multinodular goiter, ectopic thyroid tissue, and neoplastic causes of hyperthyroidism are rare compared with toxic goiter (Graves' disease).[1,2,20]

The basic cause of Graves' disease is not understood, but an immunoglobulin or family of immunoglobulins directed against the TSH receptor mediates the thyroid stimulation. These include TSHRAb and TSHR-blocking Ab, which inhibit the binding of TSH to its receptors. Graves' disease is now considered to be an autoimmune disease.[1,2,11]

Patients with Graves' disease often have in their serum high titers of TSHRAb and low titers of TSHR-blocking Ab. The level of TSHRAb in serum does not correlate with the severity of symptoms of the disease. In addition, infants whose mothers have Graves' disease will show a transient period of goiter, ophthalmopathy, and clinical manifestations of Graves' disease. As the disease disappears, the level of serum TSHRAb diminishes.[1,2,11,21]

In contrast to the preceding data, a familial tendency has been noted for the transmission of this disorder, with an increased incidence of about 20% reported in monozygotic twins compared with a much lower rate in dizygotic twins. No single gene is known to cause Graves' disease or be necessary for its development. A well-established association with certain human lymphocyte antigen (HLA) alleles varies among racial groups. In whites, HLA-DR3 and HLA-DQA*0501 are associated with Graves' disease. The risk of Graves' disease in the HLA-identical siblings of an affected patient is much lower than the risk in a monozygotic twin, suggesting the involvement of non-HLA genes. Graves' disease also is associated with polymorphisms of the cytotoxic T-lymphocyte antigen 4 (CTLA-4) gene in several racial groups.[11]

In addition, ^{131}I uptake tests have been shown to be increased in about 20% of the immediate relatives of patients with Graves' disease, particularly in sisters and daughters.[22]

The chief risk factor for Graves' disease is female gender. This may be in part due to the modulation of the autoimmune response by estrogen. This disorder is much more common in women (7:1) and may manifest itself at

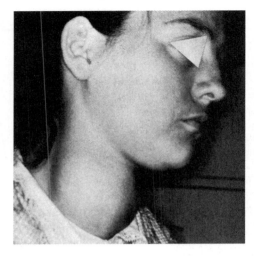

Fig. 16-2 Woman with toxic goiter (Graves' disease).

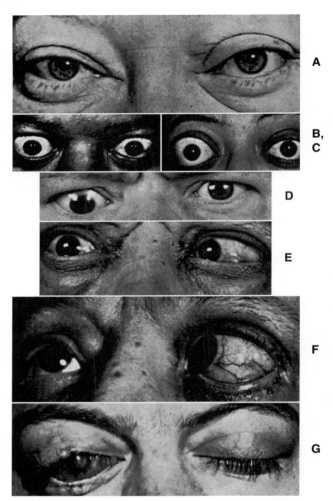

A

B,
C

D

E

F

G

Fig. 16-3 Graves' orbitopathy. **A,** Palpebral edema. This patient's eyes protruded anteriorly 1 cm more than normal, but no "pop-eye" appearance is present, owing to edema of the surrounding structures. **B,** Marked widening of palpebral fissures and slight palpebral swelling. **C,** Unequal degrees of ophthalmopathy. **D,** Unilateral lid retraction. **E,** Palpebral swelling, presumably because of fat pads and edema; paralysis of right external rectus muscle. **F,** Marked conjunctival injection and chemosis, together with ophthalmoplegia. **G,** Failure to close lids on right because of marked exophthalmos, corneal scarring, and panophthalmitis; the eye had to be enucleated. (From Larsen PR, Davies TF, Hay ID: The thyroid gland. In Wilson JD et al, editors: *Williams textbook of endocrinology*, ed 9, Philadelphia, WB Saunders, 1999.)

puberty, pregnancy, or menopause (Fig. 16-2). Emotional stress such as severe fright or separation from loved ones has been reported to be associated with its onset. The disease may occur in a cyclic pattern and then "burn itself out" or continue in an active state.[11]

CLINICAL PRESENTATION

Signs and Symptoms

The clinical picture in Graves' disease is caused by direct and indirect effects of the excessive thyroid hormones. The most common symptoms are nervousness, fatigue, a rapid heartbeat or palpitations, heat intolerance, and weight loss. These symptoms are present in more than 50% of all patients who have the disease. With increasing age, weight loss and decreased appetite become more common, and irritability and heat intolerance are less common. Atrial fibrillation is rare in patients younger than 50 years old but is found in approximately 20% of older patients. The patient's skin is warm and moist, the complexion rosy, and the patient may blush readily. Palmar erythema may be present, profuse sweating is common, and excessive melanin pigmentation of the skin occurs in many patients; however, pigmentation of the oral mucosa has not been reported. In addition, the patient's hair becomes fine and friable, and the nails soften.[1,2,11,16]

Graves' ophthalmopathy, found in approximately 50% of the patients, is characterized by edema and inflammation of the extraocular muscles, and an increase in orbital connective tissue and fat. The ophthalmopathy is an organ-specific autoimmune process strongly linked to Graves' hyperthyroidism. Although the hyperthyroidism can be suc-

cessfully treated, the ophthalmopathy often produces the greatest long-term disability for patients with this disease. Figs. 16-3 and 16-4 demonstrate the signs associated with ophthalmopathy (eyelid retraction, proptosis, periorbital edema, chemosis, and bilateral exophthalamos). The dis-

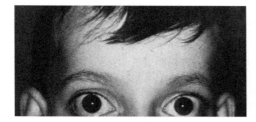

Fig. 16-4 Exophthalmos in a child with Graves' disease.

ease may progress to visual loss by exposure keratopathy or compressive optic neuropathy.[2,11,23]

Most thyrotoxic patients show eye signs not related to the ophthalmopathy of Graves' disease. These signs (stare with widened palpebral fissures, infrequent blinking, lid lag, jerky movements of the lids, and failure to wrinkle the brow on upward glaze) result from sympathetic overstimulation and usually clear when the thyrotoxicosis is corrected.[2,11]

Another complication, found in about 1% to 2% of the patients with Graves' disease, is dermopathy (Fig. 16-5). In focal areas of the skin, the hyaluronic acid and chondroitin sulfate concentrations in the dermis are increased. This may occur from lymphokine activation of fibroblasts. The accumulation causes compression of the dermal lymphatics and nonpitting edema. Early lesions contain a lymphocytic infiltrate. Nodular and plaque formation may occur in chronic lesions. The lesions are most common over the anterolateral aspects of the shin. Patients with dermopathy almost always will have severe ophthalmopathy.[1,2,11]

The increased metabolic activity caused by excessive hormone secretion increases circulatory demands, and an increased stroke volume and heart rate often develop in addition to widened pulse pressure, resulting in the patient complaining of palpitations. Supraventricular cardiac dysrhythmias develop in many patients. Congestive heart failure may occur and often is somewhat resistant to the effects of digitalis. Patients with untreated or incompletely treated thyrotoxicosis are highly sensitive to the actions of epinephrine or other pressor amines, and these agents must not be administered to them; however, once the patient is well managed from a medical standpoint, these agents can be resumed.

Dyspnea not related to the effects of congestive heart failure may occur in some patients. The respiratory effect is caused by reduction in the vital capacity secondary to weakness of the respiratory muscles.

Weight loss even with an increased appetite is a common finding in younger patients. Stools are poorly

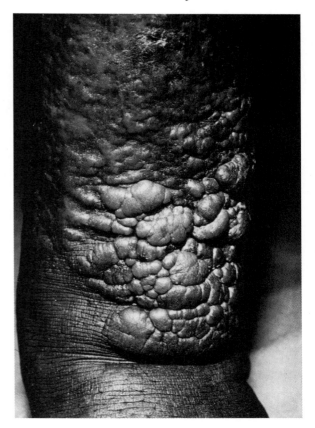

Fig. 16-5 Chronic pretibal myxedema in a patient with Graves' disease and orbitopathy. The lesions are firm and nonpitting with a clear edge to feel. (From Larsen PR, Davies TF, Hay ID: The thyroid gland. In Wilson JD et al, editors: *Williams textbook of endocrinology,* ed 9, Philadelphia, WB Saunders, 1999.)

formed, and the frequency of bowel movements is increased. Anorexia, nausea, and vomiting are rare but, when they occur, may be the forerunners of thyroid storm. Gastric ulcers are rare in patients with thyrotoxicosis. Many of these patients have achlorhydria, and about 3% develop pernicious anemia.

Thyrotoxic patients tend to be nervous and often show a great deal of emotional lability, losing their tempers easily and crying often; severe psychic reactions may occur. These patients cannot sit still and are always moving. A tremor of the hands and tongue, along with lightly closed eyelids, is often present; in addition, a generalized muscle weakness may lead to the patient complaining of easy fatigability (Box 16-4 and Table 16-3).

The effect of the excessive thyroid hormone on mineral metabolism is complex and not well understood. In

BOX 16-4

Clinical Findings in the Patient with Thyrotoxicosis

Skeletal System
Increased bone turnover
Rate of resorption exceeds that of formation
Osteoporosis (common in elderly)

Cardiovascular System
Palpitations
Tachycardia
Arrhythmias (10% to 15% atrial fibrillation)
Cardiomegaly, congestive heart failure
Angina, myocardial infarction

Gastrointestinal System
Weight loss—may have increased appetite
Decreased absorption of vitamin A
Pernicious anemia (3%)

Central Nervous System
Anxiety, restlessness, sleep disturbances
Emotional lability

Impaired concentration
Weakness
Tremors (hands, fingers, tongue)

Skin
Erythema
Hyperpigmentation
Thin fine hair, areas of alopecia
Soft nails—may lift from distal bed

Eyes
Retraction of upper lid, exophthalmos corneal ulceration, ocular muscle weakness

Other
Increased risk for diabetes mellitus
Decreased serum cholesterol level
Increased risk for thrombocytopenia

TABLE 16-3

Frequency of Signs and Symptoms in 332 Thyrotoxic Patients

Symptom	Young and Adult Patients (%)	Elderly Patients (%)
Nervousness	99	10
Heat intolerance	89	63
Palpitations	89	63
Tachycardia	82	58
Weight loss	85	75
Increased appetite	64	11
Angina	0	20
Tremor	0	55
Signs		
Tachycardia	100	58
Goiter	100	63
Tremor	97	89
Eye signs	71	57
Atrial fibrillation	10	39
Muscle weakness	0	39

From Mazzaferri EL: The thyroid. In Mazzaferri EL, editors: *Endocrinology*, ed 3, New York, 1986, Medical Examination Publishing.

addition, the role of calcitonin only complicates the problem; however, thyrotoxic patients have an increased excretion of calcium and phosphorus in their urine and stools, and radiographs demonstrate increased bone loss. Hypercalcemia occurs sometimes, but the serum levels of alkaline phosphatase usually are normal.[1,2,11] The bone age of young individuals is advanced (see Chapter 9). Kenny et al[24] showed that postmenopausal women with hyperparathyroidism have more fractures and height loss than controls.

Glucose intolerance and rarely diabetes mellitus may accompany hyperthyroidism. Those with diabetes who are treated with insulin require an increased dose of insulin if they develop Graves' disease.[11]

The individual red blood cells (RBCs) in patients with thyrotoxicosis are usually normal; however, the RBC mass is enlarged to carry the additional oxygen needed for the increased metabolic activities. In addition to the increase in total numbers of circulating RBCs, the bone marrow reveals an erythroid hyperplasia, and requirements for vitamin B_{12} and folic acid are increased. The white blood cell (WBC) count may be decreased because of a reduction in the number of neutrophils, whereas the absolute number of eosinophils may be increased. Enlargement of the spleen and lymph nodes occurs in some patients. The platelets and clotting mechanism usually are normal, but thrombocytopenia has been reported.[24]

From Larsen PR, Davies TF, Hay JD: The thyroid gland. In Wilson JD et al, editors: *Williams textbook of endocrinology*, ed 9, Philadelphia, 1999, WB Saunders.

TABLE 16-4

Antithyroid Treatment Methods Used to Manage the Patient with Thyrotoxicosis

Acute Stage of Treatment

Propylthiouracil	100 to 150 mg every 8 hr
Methimazole (Tapazole)	10 to 20 mg every 8 hr
Propranolol	20 to 40 mg every 6 hr
Dexamethasone	2 mg every 6 hr
Lithium (used with propylithiouracil)	800 to 1200 mg/day

Second Stage of Treatment

Propylthiouracil	50 to 100 mg every 8 hr
Surgery	
Radioiodine[131]	

The increased metabolic activities associated with thyrotoxicosis lead to increased secretion and breakdown of cortisol; however, serum levels remain within normal limits.

Laboratory Findings

The T_4, T_3, TBG, and TSH tests can be used to screen for hyperthyroidism. The normal values for these tests and the results found in hyperthyroidism are shown in Table 16-2. However, current practice is to screen patients suspected of being hyperthyroid with the TSH serum level and measure or estimate the free T_4 concentration. A low TSH level and a high free T_4 concentration are classic for hyperthyroidism. Some patients are hyperthyroid with a low TSH level and normal free T_4 concentration, but they have an elevated free T_3 level. A few patients have a normal or elevated TSH and a high free T_4. These patients either have a TSH-secreting pituitary adenoma or have thyroid hormone-resistance syndrome.[11]

No general agreement exists on whether serum TSH receptor antibodies should be measured in the differential diagnosis of Graves' disease. The newer assays have a high degree of sensitivity—up to 99%. A positive assay may indicate the presence of either TSHRAb or TSHR-blocking Ab. A positive test in a clinically hyperthyroid patient would indicate the presence of TSHRAb.[11]

MEDICAL MANAGEMENT

Treatment of patients with thyrotoxicosis may involve antithyroid agents that block hormone synthesis, iodides, radioactive iodine, or subtotal thyroidectomy (Table 16-4). The most common antithyroid agents used are propylthiouracil, carbimazole, and methimazole, all of which inhibit thyroid preoxidase and thus the synthesis of thyroid hormone. Propylthiouracil also blocks the extrathyroidal deiodination of T_4 to T_3. Carbimazole is the drug of choice in the United Kingdom and propylthiouracil is the drug of choice in North America. The usual length of treatment is up to 18 months. When the "block-replace" regimen is used, no added benefit occurs after 6 months of treatment. In the block-replace regimen, an antithyroid agent is given along with T_4. Antithyroid agents may cause a mild leukopenia, but drug therapy is not stopped unless the WBC count is more severely depressed. In rare cases, agranulocytosis may occur. If sore throat, fever, and/or mouth ulcers develop, most physicians advise the patient to stop the antithyroid medication and have a WBC count performed.[1,2,11]

Radioactive iodine is the preferred initial treatment for Graves' disease in North America. It is contraindicated in pregnant women and those who are breast-feeding. Radioactive iodine can induce or worsen ophthalmopathy, particularly in smokers. Weetman[11] recommends antithyroid drug treatment for patients younger than 50 years of age with their first episode of Graves' disease and radioactive iodine for those over 50 years of age. The main side effect of radioactive iodine treatment is hypothyroidism. The incidence of cancer is unchanged or slightly reduced in patients treated with radioactive iodine, but the risk of death from thyroid cancer and possibly other cancers is slightly increased. Patients with severe hyperthyroidism should be treated with an antithyroid drug for 4 to 8 weeks before radioactive iodine therapy is initiated. This approach reduces the slight risk of thyrotoxic crisis if radioactive iodine was given initially.[11]

Subtotal thyroidectomy is preferred by some patients with a large goiter and is indicated in patients with a coexistent thyroid nodule whose nature is unclear. The patient is first treated with an antithyroid drug until euthyroidism is achieved. Then inorganic iodide is administered for 7 days before surgery. In major centers, hyperthyroidism is cured in more than 98% of the cases, with low rates of operative complications. Postoperative hypothyroidism is a complication of the surgical treatment becoming more common as near-total thyroidectomy is approached.[11]

If exophthalmos is present, it follows a course independent of the therapeutic metabolic response to antithyroid treatment modalities and usually is irreversible. The adrenergic component in thyrotoxicosis can be managed by using beta-adrenergic antagonists such as propranolol. Propranolol alleviates adrenergic manifestations such as sweating, tremor, and tachycardia.[1,2,11]

A delay in the recovery of the hypothalamus-pituitary-thyroid axis occurs in the majority of patients with

Graves' disease treated with ^{131}I and is manifested by a transient central hypothyroid phase.[25]

The clinical presentations of thyroid disorders often are subtle in older adults and may be confused with "normal" aging. To avoid delay in diagnosis, some authors recommend routine TSH screening of all patients age 60 and older in the primary care practice. When hyperthyroidism is caused by Graves' disease, symptomatic therapy with a beta-blocker or antithyroid drugs is initiated, followed by definitive thyroid ablation with radioiodine.[26]

Management of Thyrotoxic Crisis

Patients with thyrotoxicosis who are untreated or incompletely treated may develop thyrotoxic crisis, a serious but fortunately rare complication that may occur at any age and has an abrupt onset. Thyrotoxic crisis occurs in less than 1% of the patients hospitalized for thyrotoxicosis.[13] Most patients who develop thyrotoxic crisis have a goiter, wide pulse pressure, eye signs, and long history of thyrotoxicosis.[5] Precipitating factors are infections, trauma, surgical emergencies, and operations. Early symptoms are extreme restlessness, nausea, vomiting, and abdominal pain; fever, profuse sweating, marked tachycardia, cardiac arrhythmias, pulmonary edema, and congestive heart failure soon develop. The patient appears to be in a stupor, and coma may follow. Severe hypotension develops, and death may occur. These reactions appear to be associated, at least in part, with adrenocortical insufficiency.[1,2]

Immediate treatment for the patient in a thyrotoxic crisis consists of large doses of antithyroid drugs (200 mg of propylthiouracil); potassium iodide; propranolol (to antagonize the adrenergic component); hydrocortisone (100 to 300 mg); dexamethasone (2 mg orally every 6 hours, to inhibit release of hormone form the gland and the peripheral conversion of T_4 to T_3); intravenous (IV) glucose solution; vitamin B complex; wet packs; fans; and ice packs. Cardiopulmonary resuscitation is sometimes needed.[1,2]

Thyrotoxicosis Factitia

Thyrotoxicosis that results from the ingestion, usually chronic, of excessive quantities of thyroid hormone is referred to as *thyrotoxicosis factitia*. This condition usually occurs in patients with underlying psychiatric disease, or in individuals such as nurses and physicians with access to the medication. In other cases patients may not be aware that they are taking the hormone or some other thyroid active agent (iodocasein), but it is part of a weight reduction program.[1]

Other causes of Thyrotoxicosis

Thyrotoxicosis has been reported to occur in patients who ate ground beef containing large quantities of bovine thy-

roid. Functional ectopic thyroid tissue can result in thyrotoxicosis. Thyroid tissue can be found in ovarian teratomas (*struma ovarii*). In rare cases, hyperfunctioning metastases of follicular carcinoma can cause thyrotoxicosis.[1]

■ THYROIDITIS ■

DEFINITION

Thyroiditis includes disorders of various causes including Hashimoto's thyroiditis; subacute thyroiditis; pyogenic thyroiditis; chronic fibrosing (Riedel's) thyroiditis; and chronic thyroiditis with transient thyrotoxicosis (Table 16-5). The most common type, Hashimoto's thyroiditis, will be discussed.[1,2]

ETIOLOGY, PATHOPHYSIOLOGY, AND COMPLICATIONS

Hashimoto's thyroiditis is a common inflammatory disease of the thyroid in which autoimmune factors play an important role. It occurs most often in middle-age women and is the most common cause of sporadic goiter in children. The prevalence of Hashimoto's thyroiditis is increasing, and the disorder is more common in the United States than in Europe. Lymphocytic infiltration of the gland and presence in the serum of increased concentrations of immunoglobulins and antibodies against several components of the thyroid gland support an autoimmune cause. The most important of these are antithyroglobulin antibody (TgAb) and antithyroid preoxidase antibody (anti-TPOAb). In most cases, destruction of the epithelial cells and degeneration of the follicular basement membrane occurs. Hormone synthesis is impaired by the destruction of epithelial cells and a defect in the organic binding of thyroid iodine. Hashimoto's thyroiditis may coexist with other diseases of an autoimmune nature such as type 1 diabetes mellitus, pernicious anemia, and Sjögren's syndrome.[1,2]

CLINICAL PRESENTATION

SIGNS AND SYMPTOMS

Goiter is the hallmark of Hashimoto's thyroiditis. The goiter is usually moderate in size, rubbery firm in consistency, and moves freely with swallowing. In cases of sudden onset, the clinical picture suggests subacute thyroiditis with pain present. Patients may be euthyroid during the early phases of the disease. Over time, most patients develop hypothyroidism as lymphocytes replace functioning

TABLE 16-5

Thyroiditis

Type	Cause	Clinical Findings	Thyroid Function	Treatment
Hashimoto's thyroiditis	Autoimmune related	Goiter is moderate in size, rubbery firm	Euthyroid early Few with transient hyperfunction Most develop hypothyroidism	Thyroid hormone In rare cases with compression of vital tissues surgery is indicated
Subacute thyroiditis	Viral infection	Enlarged, firm, tender, gland with pain that may radiate to ear, jaw, or occipital region	Hyperthyroidism with return to euthyroid state	Aspirin Prednisone Propranolol for symptoms of thyrotoxicosis
Pyogenic thyroiditis	Bacterial infection	Pain and tenderness in gland, fever, malaise, skin over the gland warm and red	Euthyroid	Incision and drainage, appropriate antibiotics
Chronic fibrosing thyroiditis (Riedel's)	Unknown	Enlarged gland that is stony hard and fixed to surrounding tissues	Usually remain euthyroid but in some cases hypothyroidism may occur	Usually none, if vital structures are compressed surgery is indicated Thyroid hormone
Chronic thyroiditis with transient thyrotoxicosis	Not established	Enlarged gland that is firm and nontender	Hyperthyroidism for 5 to 6 months then return to euthyroid state	Propranolol for symptoms of thyrotoxicosis

tissue. In a few cases the patient develops transient hyperthyroidism, later to be followed by hypothyroidism.[1,2]

LABORATORY FINDINGS

Early in the course of Hashimoto's disease the patient is euthyroid, but the TSH level is often slightly increased and the RAIU is increased. Increasing titers of autoantibodies are found early in the disease; anti-TPOAb and anti-TgAb are the most important from a clinical standpoint. Fine needle biopsy of the thyroid gland at this stage helps to confirm the diagnosis. Later in the disease the serum levels of T_4 and T_3 start to fall, and the TSH level continues to increase. At this stage the patient is hypothyroid and requires treatment with hormone replacement.[1,2]

MEDICAL MANAGEMENT

Early in the course of the disease, patients with Hashimoto's disease have small goiters, are asympto-matic, and do not require treatment. Patients with larger goiters and/or mild hypothyroidism are treated with thyroid hormone replacement. More recent goiters usually respond by decreasing in size. Long-standing goiters often do not respond to hormone treatment. In these cases, unsightly goiters or those compressing adjacent structures can be treated by surgery after an attempt to decrease their size using hormone therapy. Patients with full-blown hypothyroidism require hormone replacement treatment.[1,2]

■ HYPOTHYROIDISM ■

DEFINITION

The causes of hypothyroidism (Box 16-5) can be divided into three main categories: (1) primary, or permanent loss or atrophy of thyroid tissue; (2) goitrous hypothyroidism (hypothyroidism with compensatory thyroid enlargement due to impairment of hormone synthesis); and (3) insufficient stimulation of a normal gland (hy-

---

BOX 16-5

Causes of Hypothyroidism

Primary Atrophic Hypothyroidism
Primary idiopathic hypothyroidism (probably end-stage Hashimoto's disease)
Postablative (iatrogenic)
- ^{131}I
- Surgery
- Radiation for nonthyroid malignancy

Sporadic athyreotic hypothyroidism (agenesis or dysplasia)
Endemic cretinism (less common, agoitrous form)
Unresponsiveness to TSH

Goitrous Hypothyroidism
Hashimoto's thyroiditis
Riedel's struma
Endemic iodine deficiency
Iodine-induced hypothyroidism
Antithyroid agents
- Thionamides, Thiouylenes, Thiocyanate
- Perchlorate
- Lithium, Resorcinol

Inherited defects of hormone synthesis
Amyloidosis, sarcoidosis, hemochromatosis, scleroderma

Transient
Withdrawal of thyroid hormone treatment in patients with an intact thyroid
Removal of toxic adenoma or subtotal thyroidectomy for Graves' disease
Following postpartum lymphocytic thyroiditis
Following ^{131}I treatment of Graves' disease

Central Hypothyroidism
Secondary (pituitary) hypothyroidism
Panhypopituitarism (tumors, infiltrative disorders, Sheehan's syndrome)
Isolated TSH deficiency
TSH synthesis defect
Defect in TSH receptor
Tertiary (hypothalamic) hypothyroidism (idiopathic, traumatic, tumors)

Resistance to Thyroid Hormone Action

From Larsen PR, Davies TF, Hay JD: The thyroid gland. In Wilson JD et al, editors: *Williams textbook of endocrinology,* ed 9, Philadelphia, 1999, WB Saunders.

---

pothalamic or pituitary disease or defects in the TSH molecule). Primary and goitrous hypothyroidism account for 95% of all cases. Acquired impairment of thyroid function affects about 2% of adult women and about 0.1% to 0.2% of adult men in North America. Neonatal screening programs in many areas of the world show that hypothyroidism is present in one of every 4000 newborns.[1]

Hypothyroidism can be congenital or acquired. Permanent hypothyroidism occurs about once in every 3500 to 4000 live births in the United States. Transient hypothyroidism occurs in 1% to 2% of newborns. Most infants with permanent congenital hypothyroidism have thyroid dysgenesis: ectopic, hypoplastic, or thyroid agenesis. The acquired form may follow thyroid gland or pituitary gland failure. Radiation of the thyroid gland (radioactive iodine); surgical removal; and excessive antithyroid drug therapy are responsible for the majority of these cases of hypothyroidism; however, some cases appear with no identifiable cause.[5]

CLINICAL PRESENTATION

Signs and Symptoms
Neonatal cretinism is characterized by dwarfism; being overweight; a broad, flat nose; wide-set eyes; thick lips; a large, protruding tongue; poor muscle tone; pale skin; stubby hands; retarded bone age; delayed eruption of teeth; malocclusions; a hoarse cry; an umbilical hernia; and mental retardation. All of these characteristics can be avoided with early detection and treatment (Fig. 16-6).

The onset of hypothyroidism in older children and adults is characterized by a dull expression; puffy eyelids; alopecia of the outer third of the eyebrows; palmar yellowing; dry, rough skin; dry, brittle, and coarse hair; increased size of the tongue; slowing of physical and mental activity; slurred, hoarse speech; anemia; constipation; increased sensitivity to cold; increased capillary fragility; weight gain; muscle weakness; and deafness (Table 16-6).

The accumulation of subcutaneous fluid (intra- and extracellularly) is usually not as pronounced in patients with pituitary myxedema as it is in those with primary (thyroid) myxedema. The serum cholesterol levels are el-

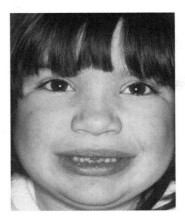

Fig. 16-6 Cretinism. (From Neville, Damm, Allen, et al: Oral and Maxillofacial Pathology, ed 2, Philadelphia, WB Saunders, 2002.)

TABLE 16-6

Signs and Symptoms of Myxedema in 400 Patients

Clinical Findings	Patients (%)
General	
Dry thick skin and/or dry hair	89
Fatigue	70
Edema; puffy hand, face, eyes	67
Cold intolerance	58
Hoarseness	48
Weight gain (15 lb or greater)	48
Central Nervous System	
Mental and physical slowness	57
Sleepiness	25
Headache	22
Gastrointestinal System	
Constipation	37
Anorexia	14
Nausea or vomiting	13
Musculoskeletal System	
Arthritis	15
Muscle cramps	10
Cardiovascular system	
Shortness of breath	19
Hypertension	18
Slow pulse	14
Genitourinary System	
Menstrual disturbances	17
Special Senses	
Blurred vision	7
Tinnitus	7

From Mazzaferri EL: The thyroid. In Mazzaferri EL, editor: *Endocrinology*, ed 3, New York, 1986, Medical Examination Publishing.

evated in thyroid myxedema and are closer to normal values in the patients with pituitary myxedema. Untreated patients with severe myxedema may develop hypothermic coma that usually is fatal. The T_4, T_3, TBG, and TSH tests are used to screen for hypothyroidism. The normal values for those tests and results found in hypothyroidism are shown in Table 16-2.

MEDICAL MANAGEMENT

Patients with hypothyroidism are treated with synthetic preparations containing sodium levothyroxin (Synthyroid) (LT_4) (Table 16-7) or sodium liothyronine (Leotrix) (LT_3).[5] The usual prescription for ideal body weight for LT_4 is 75 μg to 112 μg per day for women and 125 μg to 200 μg per day for men. Hypothyroid patients receiving warfarin or other related oral anticoagulants when treated with T_4 may have further prolonging of the prothrombin time and could be at risk for hemorrhage. In addition, hypothyroid patients with diabetes have a decreased need for insulin or sulfonylureas may become hyperglycemic when treated with T_4.[26] Patients with untreated hypothyroidism are sensitive to the actions of narcotics, barbiturates, and tranquilizers, so these drugs must be used with caution. Smoking can worsen the disease.[27] Stressful situations such as cold, operations, infections, or trauma may precipitate a hypothyroid (myxedema) coma in untreated hypothyroid patients. The external manifestations of severe myxedema, bradycardia, and severe hypotension are just about always present. Myxedematous coma occurs most often in severely hypothyroid elderly patients. It is more common during the winter months, and has a high mortality rate. Hypothyroid coma is treated by parenteral levothyroxin (T_4), steroids, and artificial respiration. Hypertonic saline and glucose

may be required to alleviate dilutional hyponatremia and the occasional hypoglycemia.[1,2]

■ THYROID CANCER ■

DEFINITION

Most cases of thyroid cancer have a good prognosis and are responsive to therapy. Thyroid cancers account for 0.4% of all cancer deaths. Most of the thyroid cancers are

TABLE 16-7

Recommended Replacement Dosage of Sodium Levothyroxine (Synthetic Sodium LT₄) in Childhood and Adult Hypothyroidism

Age (yr)	Dose of sodium Levothyroxine (Synthyroid) (µg/kg/day)
0 to 1	9
1 to 5	6
6 to 10	4
11 to 20	3
21 to 65	2.2
Over 65	1.8

From Mazzaferri EL: The thyroid. In Mazzaferri EL, editor: *Endocrinology*, ed 3, New York, 1986, Medical Examination Publishing.

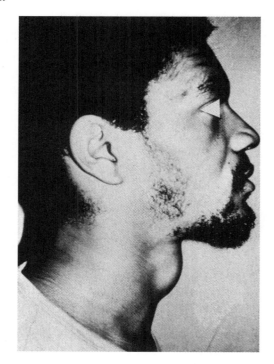

Fig. 16-7 Man with a thyroglossal duct cyst.

derived from follicular cells. Thyroid carcinomas are present as enlarging thyroid nodules or masses, which may be painful or fixed. They may be associated with vocal cord paralysis or enlarged cervical lymph nodes. Surgery is the primary treatment for thyroid carcinoma. It often is combined with RAI treatment.[1]

Patients found to have solitary thyroid nodules must be evaluated by use of thyroid function tests, thyroid scanning, and fine-needle aspiration biopsy. These tests must be considered for patients with a history of head and neck radiation, a family history of thyroid cancer, dysphagia, hemoptysis, or shortness of breath. Other indications for the use of these tests are firm, fixed nodules; ipsilateral lymphadenopathy; and high patient concern toward cancer. Patients with a negative history and minimal clinical findings can be followed to observe for increased size of the lesion. If this occurs, the above tests should be used.[3,7]

DENTAL MANAGEMENT

CLINICAL EXAMINATION

Examination of the thyroid gland should be part of a head and neck examination performed by the dentist. The anterior neck region can be scanned for indications of old surgical scars; the posterior dorsal region of the tongue should be examined for a nodule that could represent lingual thyroid tissue; and the area just superior and lateral to the thyroid cartilage should be palpated for the presence of a pyramidal lobe. Although difficult to detect, the normal thyroid gland can be palpated in many patients.[1,2] It may feel rubbery and may be more easily identified by having the patient swallow during the examination. As the patient swallows, the thyroid rises; lumps in the neck that may be associated with it also rise (move superiorly). Nodules in the midline area of the thyroglossal duct move upward with protrusion of the patient's tongue (Fig. 16-7).

An enlarged thyroid gland caused by hyperplasia (goiter) feels softer than the normal gland. Adenomas and carcinomas involving the gland are firmer on palpation and are usually seen as isolated swellings. Patients with Hashimoto's disease or Riedel's thyroiditis have a much firmer gland on palpation than the normal gland.

If a diffuse enlargement of the thyroid is detected, auscultation should be employed to examine for a systolic or continuous bruit that can be heard over the hyperactive gland of thyrotoxicosis or Graves' disease as a result of engorgement of the gland's vascular system.

Dental Management of the Thyrotoxic Patient

Detection of undiagnosed disease
- Symptoms
- Signs
- Referral for medical diagnosis and treatment

Patient with diagnosed disease
- Determination of original diagnosis
- Past therapy
- Present medication
- Assessment of clinical status (symptoms, signs, thyroid tests)
- Referral for reevaluation if signs and symptoms found
- Consultation before starting dental treatment

Avoidance of following in untreated or poorly treated patient
- Surgical procedures

- Acute infection
- Epinephrine and other pressor amines (in local anesthetics, gingival retraction cords)

Recognition and management of initial therapy for thyrotoxic crisis
- Seeking of medical aid
- Wet packs, ice packs
- Hydrocortisone (100 to 300 mg)
- Intravenous glucose solution
- Cardiopulmonary resuscitation

Patient under good medical treatment
- Avoidance of acute oral infections
- Treatment of all chronic oral infections
- Implementation of normal procedures and management

MEDICAL CONSIDERATIONS

THYROTOXICOSIS

The dentist should be aware of the clinical manifestations of thyrotoxicosis so that undiagnosed or poorly treated disease can be detected and the patient referred for medical evaluation and treatment (Box 16-6). By doing this, dentists may be able to help reduce the morbidity and mortality rates associated with thyrotoxicosis.

Patients with untreated or poorly treated thyrotoxicosis are susceptible to developing an acute medical emergency called *thyrotoxic crisis*, which is another important reason for detection and referral. Symptoms include restlessness, fever, tachycardia, pulmonary edema, tremor, sweating, stupor, and finally coma and death if treatment is not provided. If a surgical procedure is performed on these patients, a crisis may then be precipitated. In addition, an acute oral infection could precipitate a crisis. If a crisis occurs, the dentist should be able to recognize what is happening, begin emergency treatment, and seek immediate medical assistance. The patient can be cooled with cold towels, given an injection of hydrocortisone (100 to 300 mg), and started on an IV infusion of hypertonic glucose (if equipment is available). Vital signs must be monitored, and cardiopulmonary resuscitation initiated if necessary. Immediate medical assistance should

be sought, and when available, other measures such as antithyroid drugs and potassium iodide can be started.

Although the role of chronic infection and thyrotoxicosis is unclear, these sources should be treated as in any other patient. Once the patient has been identified and referred for medical management, the treatment of oral foci of infection can be accomplished. Patients with extensive dental caries or periodontal disease, or both, can be treated after medical management of the thyroid problem has been effected.

The use of epinephrine or other pressor amines (in local anesthetics or gingival retraction cords, or to control bleeding) must be avoided in the untreated or poorly treated thyrotoxic patient. However, the well-managed or euthyroid thyrotoxic patient presents no problem in this regard and may be given normal concentrations of these vasoconstrictors.

Once the thyrotoxic patient is under good medical management, the dental treatment plan is unaffected. If acute oral infection occurs, however, consultation with the patient's physician is recommended as part of the management program.

HYPOTHYROIDISM

In general, the patient with mild symptoms of untreated hypothyroidism is not in danger when receiving dental

BOX 16-7

Dental Management of the Hypothyroid Patient

Detection of undiagnosed disease
- Symptoms
- Signs
- Referral for medical diagnosis and treatment

Patient with diagnosed disease
- Determination of original diagnosis
- Past therapy
- Present medication
- Assessment of clinical status (symptoms, signs, thyroid tests)
- Referral for reevaluation if signs and symptoms of hyperthyroidism or hypothyroidism are found

Avoidance of following in untreated or poorly treated patient
- Surgical procedures
- Oral infection
- Central nervous system depressants (narcotics, barbiturates, etc)

Recognition and management of initial stages of myxedematous coma
- Seeking of medical aid
- Hydrocortisone (100 to 300 mg)
- Artificial respiration

Patient under good medical treatment
- Avoidance of acute oral infections
- Implementation of normal procedures and management

therapy. Central nervous system (CNS) depressants, sedatives, or narcotic analgesics may cause an exaggerated response in patients with mild to severe hypothyroidism. These drugs must be avoided in all patients with severe hypothyroidism and used with care (reduced dosage) in patients with mild hypothyroidism; however, a few patients with untreated severe symptoms of hypothyroidism may be in danger if dental treatment is rendered. This is particularly true of elderly patients with myxedema. A myxedematous coma can be precipitated by CNS depressants, surgical procedures, and infections; thus once again, the major goal of the dentist is to detect these patients and refer them for medical management before any dental treatment is rendered (Boxes 16-7 and 16-8).

Patients with less severe forms of hypothyroidism also should be identified when possible, because the quality of their life can be greatly improved with medical treatment. In young individuals, permanent mental retardation can be avoided with early medical management. In addition, oral complications of delayed eruption of teeth, malocclusion, enlargement of the tongue, and skeletal retardation can be prevented with early detection and medical treatment.

Once the hypothyroid patient is under good medical care, no special problems are presented in terms of dental management, except for dealing with the malocclusion and enlarged tongue if present.

THYROID CANCER

Palpation and inspection of the thyroid gland should be part of the routine head and neck examination performed by the dentist. If a thyroid enlargement is noted, even though the patient appears euthyroid (normal thyroid function), a referral should be made for evaluation before dental treatment is rendered. A diffuse enlargement may be simple goiter, subacute thyroiditis, or chronic thyroiditis. The patient may be hyperthyroid, hypothyroid, or euthyroid. Isolated nodules may turn out to be an adenoma or carcinoma. Growing nodules in diffusely enlarged glands or in glands with multinodular involvement may represent thyroid carcinoma and need to be evaluated by a physician.

ORAL COMPLICATIONS AND MANIFESTATIONS

THYROTOXICOSIS

Osteoporosis may be found involving the alveolar bone. Dental caries and periodontal disease appear more rapidly in these patients. The teeth and jaws develop more rapidly, and premature loss of the deciduous teeth with early eruption of the permanent teeth is common. Euthyroid infants of hyperthyroid mothers have been reported with erupted teeth at birth. A few patients with thyrotoxicosis have been found to have a lingual "thyroid," consisting of thyroid tissue below the area of the foramen cecum.

If the dentist detects a lingual tumor in a euthyroid patient, the patient should be evaluated by a physician

BOX 16-8

Medical Problems of Concern to the Dentist in a Patient with Undiagnosed or Poorly Controlled Thyroid Disease

Hyperthyroidism
Adverse interaction with catecholamines (epinephrine)
Life-threatening cardiac arrhythmias
Congestive heart failure
Complications of underlying cardiovascular pathologic conditions
Thyrotoxic crisis can be precipitated by
• Infection
• Surgical procedures

Hypothyroidism
Exaggerated response to central nervous system depressants
• Sedatives
• Narcotic analgesics
Myxedematous coma can be precipitated by central nervous system depressants
Infection
Surgical procedures

for the presence of a normal thyroid gland before the mass is surgically removed. This usually is done with radioactive iodine scanning.[1,2]

The pain associated with subacute thyroiditis may radiate to the ear, jaw, or occipital region. Hoarseness and dysphagia may be present. Patients may complain of palpitations, nervousness, and lassitude. On palpation the thyroid is enlarged, firm, often nodular, and usually very tender.[1,2]

HYPOTHYROIDISM

Infants with cretinism may demonstrate thick lips, enlarged tongue, delayed eruption of teeth, and resulting malocclusion. The only specific oral change manifested by adults with acquired hypothyroidism is an enlarged tongue.

References

1. Reed Larson P, Davies TF, Hay ID: The thyroid gland. In Wilson JD et al, editors: *Williams textbook of endocrinology*, ed 9, Philadelphia, 1998, WB Saunders.
2. Wartofsky L: Diseases of the thyroid. In Fauci AS et al, editors: *Harrison's principles of internal medicine*, ed 14, New York, 1998, McGraw-Hill.
3. Cooper DS: Solitary thyroid nodule. In Bardin CW, editor: *Current therapy in endocrinology and metabolism*, ed 5, St Louis, 1994, Mosby.
4. Emerson CH: Thyroid nodules and goiter. In Greene H et al, editors: *Clinical medicine*, ed 2, St Louis, 1996, Mosby.
5. Mazzaferri EL: The thyroid. In Mazzaferri EL, editor: *Endocrinology*, ed 3, New York, 1986, Medical Examination Publishing.
6. Gharib H: Diffuse nontoxic and multinodular goiter. In Bardin CW, editor: *Current therapy in endocrinology and metabolism*, ed 5, St Louis, 1994, Mosby.
7. Carnell NE, Wilber JF: Primary hypothyroidism. In Bardin CW, editor: *Current therapy in endocrinology and metabolism*, ed 5, St Louis, 1994, Mosby.
8. Laurberg P: Iodine intake and the pattern of thyroid disorders: a comparative epidemiological study of thyroid abnormalities in the elderly in Iceland and in Jutland, Denmark, J Clin Endocrinol Metab 83:765-772, 1998.
9. Martino E: Environmental iodine intake and thyroid dysfunction during chronic amiodarone therapy, Ann Intern Med 101:28-34, 1994.
10. Laurberg P: High incidence of multinodular toxic goiter in the elderly population in a low iodine intake area versus high incidence of Graves' disease in the young in a high iodine intake area: comparative surveys of thyrotoxicosis epidemiology in East-Jutland Denmark and Iceland, J Intern Med 229:415-420, 1991.
11. Weetman AP: Graves' disease, N Engl J Med 343(17):1236-1248, 2000.
12. Tunbridge WMG, Caldwell G: The epidemiology of thyroid diseases. In Braverman LE, Utiger RD, editors: *Werner and Ingbar's the thyroid*, ed 6, Philadelphia, 1991, JB Lippincott.
13. Green MF: The endocrine system. In Pathy MSJ, editor: *Principles and practice of geriatric medicine*, ed 2, New York, 1991 John Wiley & Sons.
14. Hart IR: Management decisions in subclinical thyroid disease, Hosp Pract 30(1):43-50, 1995.
15. Greenlee R et al: Cancer statistics: 2000, CA Cancer J Clin 50:7-33, 2000.
16. Nickolai TF: The thyroid gland. In Rose LF, Kaye D, editors: *Internal medicine for dentistry*, ed 2, St Louis, 1990, Mosby.
17. Wartofsky L: Introduction of thyroid disease. In Becker KL, editor: *Principles and practice of endocrinology and metabolism*, Philadelphia, 1990, JB Lippincott.
18. Smallridge RC: Evaluation of thyroid function: blood tests. In Becker K, editor: *Principles and practice of endocrinology and metabolism*, Philadelphia, 1990, JB Lippincott.
19. Weber AL, Randolph G, Aksoy FG: The thyroid and parathyroid glands. CT and MR imaging and correlation with pathology and clinical findings, Radiol Clin North Am 38(5):1105-1129, 2000.
20. Bogazzi F et al: The age of patients with thyrotoxicosis factitia in Italy from 1973 to 1996, J Endocrinol Invest 22(2):128-133, 1999.
21. Safran MS: Testing of thyroid function. In Greene H et al, editors: *Clinical medicine*, ed 2, St Louis, 1996, Mosby.

22. Ingbar SH, Woeber KA: The thyroid gland. In Williams RH, editor: *Textbook of endocrinology*, ed 5, Philadelphia, 1974, WB Saunders.

23. Yeatts RP: Graves' ophthalmopathy, *Med Clin North Am* 79(1): 195-209, 1995.

24. Kenny AM: Fracture incidence in postmenopausal women with primary hyperparathyroidism, *Surgery* 118(1):109-114, 1995.

25. Uy HL, Reasner CA, Samuels MH: Pattern of recovery of the hypothalamic-pituitary-thyroid axis following radioactive iodine therapy in patients with Graves' disease, *Am J Med* 99(2):173-179, 1995.

26. Hurley DL, Gharib H: Detection and treatment of hypothyroidism and Graves' disease, *Geriatrics* 50(4):41-44, 1995.

27. Muller B et al: Impaired action of thyroid hormone associated with smoking in women with hypothyroidism, *N Engl J Med* 333(15):964-969, 1995.

Pregnancy and Breast-Feeding

17

CHAPTER

A pregnant patient, while not considered medically compromised, poses a unique set of management considerations for the dentist. Dental care must be rendered to the mother without adversely affecting the developing fetus. Although providing routine dental care to pregnant patients is generally safe, the delivery of dental care involves some potentially harmful elements, including ionizing radiation and drug administration. Thus the prudent practitioner minimizes exposure of the patient to potentially harmful procedures or avoids them altogether when possible.

Additional considerations arise during the postpartum period if the mother elects to breast-feed her infant. Although most drugs are only minimally transmitted from the maternal serum to the breast milk and the infant's exposure is not significant, the dentist should avoid using any drug known to be harmful to the infant.

DEFINITION

PHYSIOLOGY AND COMPLICATIONS

To define rational management guidelines, a review of the normal processes of pregnancy and fetal development is first necessary. Endocrine changes are the most significant basic alterations that occur with pregnancy. They result as the production of maternal and placental hormones increase and activity of target end organs are modified.

Fatigue is a common physiologic finding in the first trimester that has psychologic impact. A tendency also exists for syncope and postural hypotension. During the second trimester, patients typically have a sense of well being and relatively few symptoms. During the third trimester, increasing fatigue, discomfort, and mild depression may be seen.

Several cardiovascular changes occur. Blood volume increases 40%, cardiac output increases 30% to 40%, whereas the red blood cell volume increases only about 15% to 20%.[1] In spite of the increase in cardiac output, blood pressure falls (usually to 100/70 mm Hg or lower) during the second trimester, with a modest increase in the last month of pregnancy. Corresponding to the increase in blood volume are additional cardiovascular changes, including high flow/low resistance circulation, tachycardia, and heart murmurs. A benign systolic murmur develops in 90% of pregnant women but disappears shortly after delivery.[2] A murmur of this type would be considered physiologic or functional. However, a murmur that preceded pregnancy or persisted after delivery would need further evaluation to determine its significance.

During late pregnancy, a phenomenon known as *supine hypotensive syndrome* may occur that manifests by an abrupt fall in blood pressure, bradycardia, sweating, nausea, weakness, and air hunger when the patient is in a supine position.[3] These symptoms are caused by impaired venous return to the heart resulting from compression of the inferior vena cava by the gravid uterus. This leads to decreased blood pressure, decreased cardiac output, and impairment or loss of consciousness. The remedy for the problem is to roll the patient over onto her left side, which lifts the uterus off the vena cava. Blood pressure should return rapidly to normal.

Blood changes in pregnancy include anemia and a decreased hematocrit value.[1] Anemia occurs because blood volume increases more than red blood cell mass does. As a result, a fall in hemoglobin and a marked need for additional folate and iron occurs. Approximately 20% of pregnant women have iron deficiency, a problem exaggerated with significant blood loss. White blood cell count also increases because of a neutrophilia. This increased level of neutrophils can complicate interpretation of the complete blood count during infection.

Although changes in platelets are usually insignificant, several blood clotting factors (especially fibrinogen; factors VII, VIII, IX, and X, and fibrin-split products) are increased. This hypercoagulation state increases the risk of thrombosis.[1]

Changes in respiratory function during pregnancy include reduced expiratory reserve volume due to enlargement of the uterus in the cephalad direction and increased demand on the lungs for oxygen. These ventilatory changes cause increased rate of respiration (tachypnea) and dyspnea that is aggravated by the supine position.

Pregnancy predisposes the expectant mother to an increased appetite and often a craving for unusual foods. As a result, the diet may be imbalanced, high in sugars, or nonnutritious. This can adversely affect the mother's dentition and contribute to significant weight gain. Taste alterations and an increased gag response are also common; the latter may make up to 90% of pregnant women vulnerable to nausea and vomiting. Symptoms of nausea and vomiting are worse during the first trimester.

The general pattern of fetal development should be understood when dental management plans are being formulated. Normal pregnancy lasts approximately 40 weeks. During the first trimester, formation of organs and systems occurs. Thus the fetus is most susceptible to malformation during this period. After the first trimester, the majority of formation is complete, and the remainder of fetal development is devoted primarily to growth and maturation. Thus the chances of malformation are markedly diminished after the first trimester. A notable exception to this is the fetal dentition, which is susceptible to dental staining caused by the administration of tetracycline during later pregnancy.

Complications of pregnancy are infrequent when prenatal care is provided and the mother is healthy. Unfortunately, complications occur more often in expectant mothers who harbor pathogens and in nonwhites over whites in the United States.[4] Common complications include infections, glucose abnormalities (gestational diabetes in 1% to 3%), and hypertension. Each increases the risk for perinatal mortality and congenital anomalies. Hypertension is of particular interest because it can lead to end organ damage or preeclampsia, a clinical condition manifest by hypertension, proteinuria, edema, and blurred vision. Preeclampsia progresses to eclampsia if seizures and coma develop. The cause of eclampsia is unknown but may involve the renin-angiotensin system. Complications of pregnancy that are unresponsive to diet modification and palliative care ultimately require drugs for adequate control.

Another consideration relating to fetal growth is spontaneous abortion (miscarriage). Spontaneous abortion, the natural termination of pregnancy before the 20th week of gestation, occurs in more than 15% of all pregnancies, the majority of which are caused by intrinsic fetal abnormalities.[5] Therefore it is most unlikely that any dental procedure would be implicated in spontaneous abortion. Febrile illnesses and sepsis, however, can precipitate a miscarriage; therefore prompt treatment of odontogenic infection and periodontitis is advised.

The fetus has a limited ability to metabolize drugs because of its immature liver and enzyme systems. Pharmacologic challenge of the fetus is to be avoided when possible.

During the postpartum period, the mother may suffer from lack of sleep and postpartum depression. In 5% to 10% of women, postpartum thyroiditis with transient thyrotoxicosis occurs.

DENTAL MANAGEMENT

MEDICAL CONSIDERATIONS

Management recommendations during pregnancy should be viewed as general guidelines, not immutable rules. The dentist should determine the general health of the patient through a thorough medical history. Inquiries regarding current physician, history of gestational diabetes, miscarriage, hypertension, and morning sickness should be made. If possible, contacting the patient's obstetrician or physician to discuss her medical status, dental needs, and proposed dental treatment is helpful. This is beneficial from the standpoint of planning treatment and also demonstrates to the patient a caring concern about her and her baby. In a 1992 survey of obstetricians,[6] 91% of respondents indicated that they preferred not to be contacted in regard to "routine" dental care. However, 88% wanted to be consulted before the dentist prescribed antibiotics and 54% wanted a consultation before the dentist prescribed analgesics.

Pregnancy is a special event in a woman's life and hence is an emotionally charged one. Therefore establishing a good patient-dentist relationship that encourages openness, honesty, and trust is an integral part of successful management. This kind of relationship greatly decreases stress and anxiety for both patient and dentist.

As with all patients, monitoring vital signs is important to identify undiagnosed abnormalities and the need for corrective action. At a minimum, blood pressure, pulse, and respirations should be taken. Systolic pressure values at or above 140 mm Hg and diastolic pressure at or above 90 mm Hg are signs of hypertension (see Chapter 4). Confirmed hypertensive values

dictate that the patient be referred to a physician to ensure that preeclampsia is properly diagnosed and managed.

Preventive Program

An important objective in planning dental treatment for a pregnant patient is to establish a healthy oral environment and an optimum level of oral hygiene. This essentially consists of a plaque-control program that minimizes the exaggerated inflammatory response of gingival tissues to local irritants that commonly accompany the hormonal changes of pregnancy. The relationship of plaque and other local irritants, hormonal alterations, and periodontal disease is well known and can be clearly explained to the patient.[7] Studies performed during the past 25 years have demonstrated that the reduction of oral streptococcal levels in the pregnant mother reduces the risk of the infant being infected and developing caries.[8-10] In addition, maternal periodontal disease increases the infant's risk for low birth weight.[11]

Accordingly, acceptable oral hygiene techniques should be taught, reinforced, and monitored. Diet counseling, with emphasis on limiting the intake of refined carbohydrates, should be provided. Coronal scaling and polishing or root curettage may be performed whenever necessary. Preventive plaque-control measures should be provided and emphasized throughout pregnancy, including the first trimester.

Several studies have shown the benefits of prenatal fluoride. Glenn[12] and Glenn et al[13] have shown that when a daily 2.2-mg tablet of sodium fluoride was administered to mothers during the second and third trimester in combination with fluoridated water, 97% of the offspring remained virtually free of caries for up to 10 years. Not only was medical or dental defects, including fluorosis, absent in these children, but also an association with decreased premature delivery and increased birth weight was seen in the fluoride treatment group. The conclusion was that fluoride tablet supplementation from the third through ninth month of pregnancy was safe and effective. In another study sponsored by the National Institute of Dental Research, more than 1200 women and their offspring were studied. Half of the women received prenatal fluoride and the other half received placebo.[14] After 5 years, offspring from the prenatal fluoride group had 45% fewer caries than the placebo group offspring, and 96% were free of caries. Similarly, in a study of 65 pregnant women, salivary streptococcal levels were significantly reduced in mothers and their offspring from a regimen that included diet counseling, prophylaxis, systemic fluoride, daily fluoride, and chlorhexidine mouth rins-

TABLE 17-1

Treatment Timing During Pregnancy

First Trimester	Second Trimester	Third Trimester
Plaque control	Plaque control	Plaque control
Oral hygiene instruction	Oral hygiene instruction	Oral hygiene instruction
Scaling, polishing, curettage	Scaling, polishing, curettage	Scaling, polishing, curettage
Avoid elective treatment; urgent care only	Routine dental care	Routine dental care

ing.[10] These findings indicate that the use of prenatal fluoride and oral hygiene measures benefit the mother and newborn without risk and should be discussed with the patient and obstetrician.

TREATMENT TIMING

Other than as part of a good plaque-control program, elective dental care is best avoided during the first trimester because of potential vulnerability of the fetus (Table 17-1). The second trimester is the safest period in which to provide routine dental care. Emphasis should be placed on controlling active disease and eliminating potential problems that could occur later in pregnancy or in the immediate postpartum period, since providing dental care during these periods is often difficult. Extensive reconstruction or significant surgical procedures are best postponed until after delivery because pregnancy is a temporary condition.

The early part of the third trimester is still a good time to provide routine dental care; but after the middle of the third trimester, elective dental care is best postponed. This is because of the increasing feeling of discomfort that the expectant mother may have and is not necessarily applicable to all patients. Prolonged time in the dental chair should be avoided to prevent the complication of supine hypotension. If supine hypotension develops, rolling the patient onto her left side affords return circulation to the heart. Problems can be minimized by scheduling short appointments, allowing the patient to assume a semireclined position, and encouraging frequent changes of position.

TABLE 17-2

Comparative Radiation Exposures to Fetal or Embryonic Tissues

Source of Radiation	Absorbed Exposure (cGy)
Upper gastrointestinal series	0.330
Chest radiograph	0.008
Skull radiograph	0.004
Daily (cosmic) background radiation	0.0004
Full mouth dental series (18 intraoral radiographs, D film, lead apron)	0.00001

Adapted from DiSaia PJ. In Scott JR et al, editors: *Danforth's obstetrics and gynecology*, ed 6, Philadelphia, 1990, JB Lippincott, p 1127.[23]

DENTAL RADIOGRAPHS

Dental radiography is one of the more controversial areas in the management of a pregnant patient. Irradiation should be avoided during pregnancy, especially during the first trimester, because the developing fetus is particularly susceptible to radiation damage.[15] However, should dental treatment become necessary, radiographs may be required to accurately diagnose and treat the patient. Therefore the dentist must be aware of how to proceed safely in this situation.

The safety of dental radiography has been well established, provided features such as fast exposure techniques (e.g., high-speed film or digital imaging), filtration, collimation, and lead aprons are used. Of all aids, the most important for the pregnant patient is the protective lead apron. Studies have shown that when an apron is used during contemporary dental radiography, gonadal and fetal radiation is less than 0.01 microSieverts (μSv).[16-18]

The dentist must keep in perspective the facts of radiation biology. Animal and human data[19-24] clearly support the conclusion that no increase in gross congenital anomalies or intrauterine growth retardation occurs as a result of exposures during pregnancy totaling less than 5 to 10 centiGray (cGy).[25]* For comparison, the following can be considered[23,24] (Table 17-2):

- A medical chest radiograph results in an estimated fetal or embryonic dose of 0.008 cGy

- A skull radiograph results in 0.004 cGy
- Natural background radiation is approximately 0.0008 cGy daily
- A full mouth series of dental radiographs with a lead apron results in 0.00001 cGy

When further assessing risks of dental radiography during pregnancy, three reports should be kept in mind. The first states that the maximum risk attributable to 1 cGy (which is more than 1000 full mouth series with E-speed film and rectangular collimation or 10% to 20% of the threshold dose) of in utero radiation exposure has been estimated[20] to be approximately 0.1%. This is a quantity thousands of times less than the normal anticipated risks of spontaneous abortion, malformation, or genetic disease. The second report calculates the risk of a first-generation fetal defect from a dental radiographic examination to be 9 in 1 billion.[26] The third report found that the gonadal dose to women, after full mouth radiographs, is less than 0.01 μSv, which is at least 1000-fold below the threshold shown to cause congenital damage to newborns.[18] These figures indicate that with use of the lead apron, rectangular collimation, and E-speed film or faster techniques, one or two intraoral films are truly of minute significance in terms of radiation effects to the developing fetus. In terms that can be explained to a patient, consider the following: the gonadal/fetal dose of 2 periapical dental films (when a lead apron is used) is 700 times less than 1 day of average exposure to natural background radiation in the United States.[27,28]

Despite the negligible risks of dental radiography, the dentist should not be cavalier regarding its use during pregnancy (or at any other time, for that matter). Radiographs should be used selectively and only when necessary and appropriate to aid in diagnosis and treatment. Bite-wing, panoramic, or selected periapical films are recommended for minimizing patient dose. To further reduce the radiation dose, the following measures should be employed: rectangular collimation, E-speed film or faster techniques, lead apron, high kilovoltage (kV) or constant beams, and a quality assurance program.

An additional consideration is the pregnant dental auxiliary or dentist. The maximum permissible radiation dose for whole-body exposure of the pregnant dental care worker is 0.005 Gy or 5 millisieverts (mSv) per year. This is equivalent to the maximum permissible radiation dose of the nonoccupationally exposed public and ten-fold less than the level of occupationally exposed nonpregnant workers (50 mSv).[25] The National Commission of Radiation Protection and Measurements reports that production of congenital defects is negligible from fetal exposures of 50 mSv.[25,29] To further ensure

---

*1 cGy (0.01 Gy) = 1 rad (roentgen, R) (e.g., 1R = 0.01 Gy = 0.01 Sievert (Sv) = 10 mSv

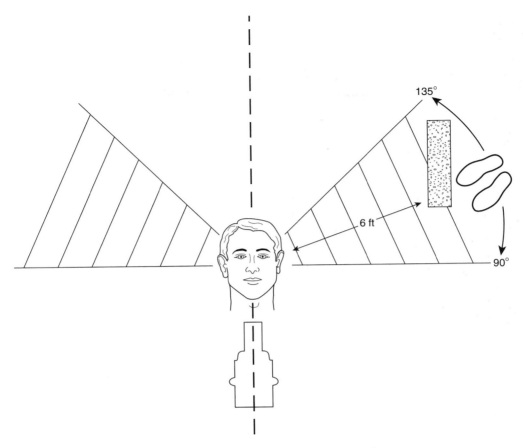

Fig. 17-1 Proper operator position during exposure of x-rays.

safety, the pregnant operator should wear a film badge, stand more than 6 feet from the tube head, and position herself between 90 and 130 degrees of the beam, preferably behind a protective wall (Fig. 17-1). When these guidelines are followed, no contraindication to pregnant women operating the x-ray machine occurs. However, dentists should familiarize themselves with federal (Code of Federal Regulations, Code 10, Part 20, Section 20.201) and state regulations that would supercede these guidelines.

DRUG ADMINISTRATION

During Pregnancy

Another controversial area in treating the pregnant dental patient is drug administration. The principal concern is that a drug may cross the placenta and be toxic or teratogenic to the fetus. Additionally, any drug that is a res-

piratory depressant can cause maternal hypoxia, resulting in fetal hypoxia, injury, or death.

Ideally, no drug should be administered during pregnancy, especially the first trimester. However, adhering to this rule is sometimes impossible. Most of the commonly used drugs in dental practice can be given during pregnancy with relative safety, although a few exceptions occur. Table 17-3 is a suggested approach to drug usage for pregnant patients.

Before prescribing or administering a drug to a pregnant patient, the dentist should be familiar with the Food and Drug Administration[33] categorization of prescription drugs for pregnancy based on their potential risk of fetal injury. These categories, although not without limitations,[34] are meant to aid clinicians and patients with decisions about drug therapy. Counseling should be provided to make sure that women who are pregnant clearly understand the nature and magnitude of risk associated with a drug.

TABLE 17-3

Drug Administration During Pregnancy and Breast-Feeding

Drug	FDA Catagory (prescription drug)	Use During Pregnancy	Risk	Use During Breast-feeding
Local Anesthetics				
Lidocaine	B	Yes		Yes
Prilocaine	B	Yes		Yes
Etidocaine	B	Yes		Yes
Mepivacaine	C	Use with caution; consult physician	Fetal bradycardia	Yes
Bupivacaine	C	Use with caution; consult physician	Fetal bradycardia	Yes
Articaine	Not assigned			
Analgesics				
Aspirin	C/D[3]	Caution; avoid in third trimester	Postpartum hemorrhage Constriction ductus arteriosus	Avoid
Acetaminophen	B	Yes		Yes
Ibuprofen, flurbiprofen	B	Caution; avoid in second half of pregnancy	Delayed labor	Yes
Diflunisal, etodolac, mefenamic acid	C/D[3]	Use with caution; consult physician	Delayed labor	No
Naproxen	B/D[3]	Caution; avoid in second half of pregnancy	Delayed labor	Yes
Codeine	C/D*	Use with caution; consult physician	Neonatal respiratory depression	Yes
Hydrocodone	C/D[3]	Use with caution; consult physician	Neonatal respiratory depression	—
Oxycodone	C/D[3]	Use with caution; consult physician	Neonatal respiratory depression	—
Propoxyphene	C	Use with caution; consult physician	Neonatal respiratory depression	Yes
Pentazocine	C	Use with caution; consult physician	Neonatal respiratory depression	Yes

Adapted from Drug information for the health care professional, vols IA and IB, ed 19, Rockville, Md., 1999, United States Pharmacopeial Convention; Moore PA. Selecting drugs for the pregnant dental patient, JADA 129:1281-1286, 1998; and Briggs GG, Freeman RK, Yaffe SJ. Drugs in Pregnancy and Lactation. A reference guide to fetal and neonatal risk. ed 5, Baltimore, 1998, Williams & Wilkins.
D* = Risk Category D if used for prolonged period or high dose; D[3] = Risk Category D if administered in third trimester.

TABLE 17-3

Drug Administration During Pregnancy and Breast-Feeding—cont'd

Drug	FDA Catagory (prescription drug)	Use During Pregnancy	Risk	Use During Breast-feeding
Antibiotics				
Penicillins	B	Yes		Yes
Erythromycin	B	Yes; avoid estolate form		Yes
Cephalosporins	B	Yes		Yes
Tetracycline	D	Avoid	Tooth discoloration, inhibits bone formation	Avoid
Metronidazole	B	Yes		Yes
Clindamycin	B	Yes		Yes
Sedative/Hypnotics				
Barbiturates	D	Avoid	Neonatal respiratory depression	Avoid
Benzodiazepines	D/X	Avoid	Possible risk for oral clefts with prolonged exposure	Avoid
Nitrous oxide	Not assigned		Best used in second and third trimesters and for <30 minutes; consult physician	Yes
Corticosteroids				
Prednisone	B	Yes		Yes

Adapted from Drug information for the health care professional, vols IA and IB, ed 19, Rockville, Md., 1999, United States Pharmacopeial Convention.; Moore PA. Selecting drugs for the pregnant dental patient, JADA 129:1281-1286, 1998; and Briggs GG, Freeman RK, Yaffe SJ. Drugs in Pregnancy and Lactation. A reference guide to fetal and neonatal risk. ed 5, Baltimore, 1998, Williams & Wilkins.
D* = Risk Category D if used for prolonged period or high dose; D³ = Risk Category D if administered in third trimester.

The current pregnancy labeling categories are as follows:

A. Controlled studies in humans have failed to demonstrate a risk to the fetus, and the possibility of fetal harm appears remote.

B. Animal studies have not indicated fetal risk, and human studies have not been conducted; *or* animal studies have shown a risk, but controlled human studies have not.

C. Animal studies have shown a risk, but controlled human studies have not been conducted, or studies are not available in humans or animals.

D. Positive evidence of human fetal risk exists, but in certain situations the drug may be used despite its risk.

E. Evidence of fetal abnormalities and fetal risk exists based on human experience, and the risk outweighs any possible benefit of use during pregnancy.

Obviously, drugs in category A or B are preferable for prescribing. However, many drugs that fall into category C are administered during pregnancy, and therefore these drugs present the most difficulty for the dentist and physician in terms of therapeutic and medicolegal decisions.

Physicians may advise against the use of some of the approved drugs or conversely may suggest the use of a questionable drug. The listed guidelines are general ones. An example of the occasional use of a questionable drug would be a narcotic for a pregnant patient in severe pain.

Anesthetics

Local anesthetics administered with epinephrine are considered relatively safe for use during pregnancy. Both the local anesthetic and the vasoconstrictor cross the placenta; however, subtoxic threshold doses have not been shown to cause fetal abnormalities. It is advisable to limit the dose to the amount required.

Analgesics

The analgesic of choice during pregnancy is acetaminophen. Aspirin and nonsteroidal antiinflammatory drugs have risks for constriction of the ductus arteriosus, as well as postpartum hemorrhage and delayed labor (see Table 17-3). The risk of these adverse events increases when administered in the third trimester. Prolonged or high doses of opioids are associated with congenital abnormalities and respiratory depression.[30,35]

Antibiotics

Penicillins, erythromycin (except in estolate form), and cephalosporins (first and second generation) are considered safe to the mother and developing child. However, these antibiotics have lower maternal blood levels compared with controls because of a shorter half-life and increased volume of distribution. For example, in one study, 2 of 10 pregnant mothers failed to have detectable drug blood levels of erythromycin up to 4 hours after antibiotic administration.[36] An increased dose or more frequent administration may be required if an infection is not readily brought under control with antibiotic use. Tetracycline's use is contraindicated during pregnancy. They bind to hydroxyapatite, causing brown discoloration of teeth, hypoplastic enamel, inhibition of bone growth, and other skeletal abnormalities.[37]

Anxiolytics

Few anxiolytics are considered safe during pregnancy. However, a single exposure of nitrous oxide oxygen (N_2O-O_2) for less than 35 minutes has not been associated with any human fetal anomalies, including low birth rate.[38] In contrast, chronic N_2O-O_2 inhalation analgesia can cause cellular abnormalities in animals (e.g., inactivation of methionine synthetase and vitamin B_{12}, altered DNA metabolism) and birth defects. Accordingly, the following guidelines are recommended if N_2O-O_2 is used during pregnancy:

- Use of N_2O-O_2 inhalation should be minimized to 30 minutes.
- At least 50% oxygen should be delivered to ensure adequate oxygenation at all times.
- Appropriate oxygenation should be provided to avoid diffusion hypoxia at the termination of administration.
- Repeated and prolonged exposures to nitrous oxide are to be prevented.
- The second or third trimester are safer periods of treatment because organogenesis occurs during the first trimester.[1]

An additional consideration is for the female dentist or dental auxiliary who is pregnant. They should not be exposed to persistent trace levels of nitrous oxide in the operatory. Female dental health care workers who are chronically exposed to nitrous oxide for more than 3 hours per week, when scavenging equipment is not used, have decreased fertility and increased spontaneous abortions.[39] Implementation of National Institute for Occupational Safety and Health recommendations can reduce occupational exposure to nitrous oxide (Box 17-1).[40]

DRUG ADMINISTRATION

During Breast-feeding

A potential problem arises when a nursing mother requires the administration of a drug in the course of dental treatment. The concern is that the administered drug can enter the breast milk and be transferred to the nursing infant, in whom exposure may result in adverse effects.

The data on which to draw definitive conclusions about drug dosage and effects via breast milk are limited. However, retrospective clinical studies and empiric observations, coupled with known pharmacologic pathways, allow recommendations to be made. A significant fact is that the amount of drug excreted in the breast milk usually is not more than 1% to 2% of the maternal dose. Therefore most drugs are of little pharmacologic significance to the infant.[30,41]

Agreement exists that a few drugs, or categories of drugs, are definitely contraindicated for nursing mothers. These include lithium, anticancer drugs, radioactive pharmaceuticals, and phenindione.[30,42,43] Table 17-3 contains recommendations adapted from the American Academy of Pediatrics regarding the administration of commonly used dental drugs during breast-feeding.[42] As with drug use during pregnancy, individual physicians may wish to modify these recommendations, which should be viewed only as general guidelines for treatment.

In addition to careful drug selection for the nursing mother, authorities suggest she take the drug just after

Control of Nitrous Oxide in the Dental Office During Pregnancy

1. Inspect nitrous oxide equipment and replace defective tubing and parts.
2. Check pressure connections for leaks and fix leaks.
3. Ensure mask fits well and is secure. Observe reservoir bag is not over or underinflated.
4. Provide operatory ventilation of 10 or more room air exchanges per hour.
5. Use scavenging system and appropriate mask sizes. Vacuum should provide up to 45 L/min.
6. Connect and turn on vacuum pump of scavenging system before nitrous oxide.
7. Conduct air sampling regularly. Maintain low exposure limits (e.g., 25 ppm*) when pregnant dental health care workers are involved.

Adapted from McGlothlin JD, Crouch KG, Mickelsen RL: Control of nitrous oxide in dental operatories. Cincinnati: U.S. Department of Health and Human Services, Public Health Service, Centers for Disease Control and Prevention, National Institute for Occupational Safety and Health, Division of Physical Sciences and Engineering, Engineering Control Technology Branch, 1994; DHHS publication no. (NIOSH) 94-129. (ETTB report no. 166-04).
*This limit is a NIOSH recommendation. In contrast, Yagiela suggests a time-weighted average (TWA) lower limit of 100 ppm for an 8 hour workday. Yagiela JA. Health hazards and nitrous oxide: a time for reappraisal. Anesth Prog 38:1-11, 1991.

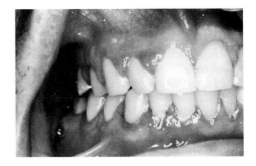

Fig. 17-2 Generalized gingivitis, "pregnancy gingivitis," in a woman in the sixth month of pregnancy.

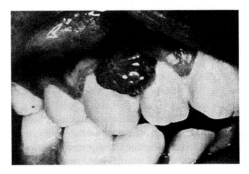

Fig. 17-3 Pyogenic granuloma, "pregnancy tumor," occurring during pregnancy.

breast-feeding and avoid nursing for 4 hours or more if possible. This should result in decreased drug concentration in the breast milk.[44]

TREATMENT PLANNING MODIFICATIONS

No technical modifications are required for the pregnant patient. However, full mouth radiographs, reconstruction, crown and bridge procedures, and significant surgery are best delayed until after pregnancy. A prominent gag reflex also may dictate a delay in certain dental procedures. Although dental amalgam has not been shown to be hazardous to pregnant women or the developing fetus,[41] several European countries and Canada have national recommendations advising to limit or avoid the placement and replacement of amalgams during pregnancy.[42]

ORAL COMPLICATIONS AND MANIFESTATIONS

The most common oral complication of pregnancy is pregnancy gingivitis (Fig. 17-2). This condition results from an exaggerated inflammatory response to local irritants and less than meticulous oral hygiene during periods of increased secretion of estrogen and progesterone and altered fibrinolysis.[7] The gingival inflammation of pregnancy gingivitis begins at the marginal and interdental gingiva usually in the second month of pregnancy. Progression of the condition leads to fiery red and edematous interproximal papillae that are tender to palpation. In approximately 1% of gravid women, the hyperplastic response may exacerbate in a localized area, resulting in a pyogenic granuloma or "pregnancy tumor" (Fig. 17-3). The most common location of a pyogenic granuloma is the labial aspect of the interdental papilla. The lesion is generally asymptomatic; however, toothbrushing may traumatize the lesion and cause bleeding.

These hyperplastic gingival changes become apparent around the second month and continue until after parturition, at which time the gingival tissues usually regress and return to normal, provided proper oral hygiene measures are implemented and any calculus present is removed.[7] Surgical or laser excision is occasionally required if symptoms, bleeding, or interference with mastication dictate. Pregnancy does not cause periodontal disease but can modify and worsen what is already present.

A relationship between dental caries and the physiologic processes of pregnancy has not been demonstrated. Caries activity is attributed to the presence of cariogenic bacteria in the mouth, a diet containing fermentable carbohydrates, and poor oral hygiene. Control of the carious process through fluoride and chlorhexidine is important because maternal saliva is the primary vehicle for the transfer of cariogenic streptococci to the infant.[47,48]

Many women are convinced that pregnancy causes tooth loss (i.e., "a tooth for every pregnancy") or that calcium is withdrawn from the maternal dentition to supply fetal requirements (i.e., "soft teeth"). Calcium is present in the teeth in a stable crystalline form and hence is not available to the systemic circulation to supply a calcium demand. However, calcium is readily mobilized from bone to supply these demands. Therefore although calcium supplementation for the purpose of preventing tooth loss or soft teeth is unwarranted, the physician may prescribe calcium for general nutritional requirements of mother and infant.

Tooth mobility, localized or generalized, is an uncommon finding during pregnancy. Mobility is a sign of gingival disease, disturbance of the attachment apparatus, and mineral changes in the lamina dura. Since vitamin deficiencies can contribute to this and other congenital problems (e.g., folate deficiency and spina bifida), when discussing oral hygiene, the dentist should take this opportunity to educate the patient about the benefits of the use of multivitamins. Daily removal of local irritants, adequate levels of vitamin C, and delivery of the newborn should result in the reversal of tooth mobility.

Pregnant women often have a hypersensitive gag reflex. This, in combination with morning sickness, may contribute to episodes of regurgitation and lead to halitosis and enamel erosion.

References

1. Hume RF, Killam AP: Maternal physiology. In Scott JR et al, editors: *Danforth's obstetrics and gynecology*, ed 6, Philadelphia, 1990, JB Lippincott.

2. Cunningham FG, MacDonald PC, Gant NF: *Williams obstetrics*, ed 18, Norwalk, Conn, 1989, Appleton and Lange.

3. Bottoms SF, Scott JR: Transfusions and shock. In Scott JR et al, editors: *Danforth's obstetrics and gynecology*, ed 6, Philadelphia, 1990, JB Lippincott.

4. Ventura SJ et al: Births: final data for 1998, *Natl Vital Stat Rep* 48:1-100, 2000.

5. Scott JR: Spontaneous abortion. In Scott JR et al, editors: *Danforth's obstetrics and gynecology*, ed 6, Philadelphia, 1990, JB Lippincott.

6. Shrout MK et al: Treating the pregnant dental patient: four basic rules addressed, J Am Dent Assoc 123:75-80, 1992.

7. Löe H: Periodontal changes in pregnancy, J Periodontol 36:209-217, 1965.

8. Kohler B, Bratthall D, Krasse B: Preventive measures in mothers influence the establishment of the bacterium *Streptococcus mutans* in their infants, Arch Oral Biol 28:225-231, 1983.

9. Kohler B, Andréen I: Influence of caries-preventive measures in mothers on cariogenic bacteria and caries experience in their children, Arch Oral Biol 39:907-911, 1994.

10. Brambilla E et al: Caries prevention during pregnancy: results of a 30-month study, JADA 129:871-877, 1998.

11. Dasanayake AP: Poor periodontal health of the pregnant woman as a risk factor for low birth weight, Ann Periodontl 3:206-212, 1998.

12. Glenn FB: Immunity conveyed by a fluoride supplement during pregnancy, J Dent Child 44:391-395, 1977.

13. Glenn FB, Glenn WD III, Duncan RC: Fluoride tablet supplementation during pregnancy for caries immunity: a study of the offspring produced, Am J Obstet Gynecol 143:560-564, 1982.

14. Leverett DH: Clinical trial of the effect of prenatal fluoride supplements in preventing dental caries, *Final Report (7/83-6/91)*:1-54, Bethesda, Md, National Institute of Dental Research, April 1992.

15. Serman NJ, Singer S: Exposure of the pregnant patient to ionizing radiation, Ann Dent 53:13-15, 1994.

16. Bean LR Jr, Devore WD: The effects of protective aprons in dental roentgenography, Oral Surg 28:505-508, 1969.

17. Laws PW: *The x-ray information book. A consumer's guide to avoiding unnecessary medical and dental x-rays*, New York, 1983, Farrar, Straus, and Giroux.

18. White SC: 1992 assessment of radiation risk from dental radiography, Dentomaxillofac Radiol 21:118-126, 1992.

19. Brent RL: Environmental factors: radiation. In Brent RL, Harris MI, editors: *Prevention of embryonic, fetal and perinatal disease*, Fogarty International Center Series on Preventive Medicine, vol 3, Department of Health, Education, and Welfare Publication No. 76-853:1799-1807, 1976.

20. Brent RL: The effects of embryonic and fetal exposure to x-ray, microwaves, and ultrasound, Clin Obstet Gynecol 26:484-510, 1983.

21. Brent RL: Ionizing radiation, Contemp Obstet Gynecol 30:20-29, 1987.

22. Brent RL, Gorson RO: Radiation exposure in pregnancy, Curr Probl Radiol 2:1-48, 1972.

23. DiSaia PJ: Radiation therapy in gynecology. In Scott JR et al, editors: *Danforth's obstetrics and gynecology*, ed 6, Philadelphia, 1990, JB Lippincott.

24. Mole RH: Radiation effects on pre-natal development and their radiological significance, Br J Radiol 52:89-101, 1979.

25. National Council on Radiation Protection and Measurements: Recommendations on limits for exposure to ionizing radiation, NCRP Report, No 91, 1987.

26. Danforth RA, Gibbs SJ: Diagnostic dental radiation. What's the risk, J Calif Dent Assoc 28:28-35, 1980.

27. Gonad doses and genetically significant dose from diagnostic radiology: United States, 1964 and 1970, DHEW (FDA) Pub No 76-8034, 1976.

28. Freeman JP, Brand JW: Radiation doses of commonly used dental radiographic surveys, Oral Surg Oral Med Oral Pathol 77:285-289, 1994.

29. National Council on Radiation Protection and Measurements: Ionizing radiation exposure of the population of the United States, NCRP Report, No 93, 1987.

30. Briggs GG, Freeman RK, Yaffe SJ: Drugs in pregnancy and lactation: a reference guide to fetal and neonatal risk, ed 5, Baltimore, 1998, Williams and Wilkins.

31. Moore PA: Selecting drugs for the pregnant dental patient, JADA 129:1281-1286, 1998.

32. United States Pharmacopeial Convention: Drug information for the health care professional, vols IA and IB, ed 19, Rockville, Md, 1999, The Convention.

33. Pregnancy categories for prescription drugs, FDA Drug Bull 12:24-25, 1982.

34. Food and Drug Administration: Content and format of labeling for human prescription drugs; pregnancy labeling; public hearing—FDA. Notice of public hearing; request for comments, Fed Regist 62:41061-41063, 1997.

35. Heinonen OP, Slone D, Shapiro S: Birth defects and drugs in pregnancy, Littleton, Mass, 1977, Publishing Sciences Group.

36. Larsen B, Glover DD: Serum erythromycin levels in pregnancy, Clin Therap 20:971-977, 1998.

37. Cohlan SW, Bevelander G, Tiamsic T: Growth inhibition of prematures receiving tetracycline, Am J Dis Child 105:453-461, 1963.

38. Crawford JS, Lewis M: Nitrous oxide in early human pregnancy, Anaesthesia 41:900-905, 1986.

39. Rowland AS et al: Nitrous oxide and spontaneous abortion in female dental assistants, Am J Epidemiol 141:531-538, 1995.

40. McGlothlin JD et al: Control of anesthetic gases in dental operatories, Scand J Work Environ Health 18(Suppl 2):103-105, 1992.

41. Wilson JT et al: Drug excretion in human breast milk: principles, pharmacokinetics and projected consequences, Clin Pharmacokinet 5:1-66, 1980.

42. American Academy of Pediatrics Committee on Drugs: The transfer of drugs and other chemicals into human milk, Pediatrics 93:137-150, 1994.

43. Niebyl JR: Teratology and drugs in pregnancy and lactation. In Scott JR et al, editors: Danforth's obstetrics and gynecology, ed 6, Philadelphia, 1990, JB Lippincott.

44. Berlin CM: Pharmacologic considerations of drug use in the lactating mother, Obstet Gynecol 58(Suppl 5):17S-23S, 1981.

45. Larrson K: Teratological aspects of dental amalgam, Adv Dent Res 6:114-119, 1992.

46. Minister of Supply and Services, Canada: Health Canada: the safety of dental amalgam, Montréal, 1996, The Minister.

47. Berkowitz RJ, Hones P: Mouth to mouth transmission of the bacterium Streptococcus mutans between mother and child, Arch Oral Biol 4:377-379, 1985.

48. Caufield PW: The fidelity of initial acquisition of mutans streptococci by infants from their mothers, J Dent Res 74:681-685, 1995.

*A*llergic diseases are increasing in prevalence and are contributing significantly to health care costs.[1] For example, the number of children with allergies has recently doubled in certain areas.[1]

One of the most common medical emergencies that can occur in the dental office is that of an acute allergic reaction. The following four reasons signify why the dentist must know about allergy: (1) to identify patients with a true allergic history so acute medical emergencies that might occur in the dental office because of an allergic reaction can be prevented; (2) to recognize oral soft tissue changes that might be caused by an allergic reaction; (3) to identify and plan appropriate dental care for patients who have severe alterations of their immune system because of radiation, drug therapy, or immune deficiency disorders; and (4) to recognize signs and symptoms of acute allergic reactions and manage these problems appropriately. To accomplish these goals, the dentist first must have a basic understanding of allergy.

DEFINITION

EPIDEMIOLOGY: INCIDENCE AND PREVALENCE

Researchers estimate[1,2] that 15% to 25% of all Americans are allergic to some substance, including about 4.5% who have asthma, 4% who are allergic to insect stings, and 5% who are allergic to one or more drugs. Allergic reactions account for about 6% to 10% of all adverse drug reactions.[2-6] Of these, 46% consist of erythema and rash, 23% urticaria, 10% fixed drug reactions, 5% erythema multiforme, and 1% anaphylaxis.[2,3] About a 1% to 3% risk for an allergic reaction is possible when using a drug. Fatal drug reactions occur in about 0.01% of surgical inpatients and 0.1% of medical inpatients.[1,2]

Drugs are the most common cause of urticarial reactions in adults, and food and infections are the most common cause of these lesions in children. Urticaria occurs in 15% to 20% of young adults. In approximately 70% of the patients with chronic urticaria, no etiologic agent can be identified.[1,7]

Iodinated organic compounds used as radiographic contrast media result in about 1 death for every 1,400 to 60,000 diagnostic procedures.[8] Animal insulin used to treat type 1 diabetic patients causes an allergic reaction in about 10% to 56% of these individuals, and reports[8] have stated that some 25% of patients with diabetes who are allergic to insulin react to penicillin.

About 5% to 10% of the individuals given penicillin develop an allergic reaction, and 0.04% to 0.20% of these experience an anaphylactic reaction to the drug. Death occurs in about 10% of those individuals who had an anaphylactic reaction.[3,7,8]

A report of 151 deaths worldwide from anaphylactic reactions to penicillin[7] found that in 85% of the cases, death occurred within 15 minutes after administration of the drug; in 50% of the cases the allergic reaction started immediately after the administration. A history of having been given penicillin[7] (Box 18-1) occurred in 70% of the individuals. The most common causes of anaphylactic death are penicillin, bee stings, and wasp stings; individuals with an atopic history are more susceptible to anaphylactic death than are patients with no history of allergy.[1,3,8] Common causes of anaphylaxis of significance to the dentist are listed in Box 18-2.

In rare cases, antihistamines have been reported[8] to cause urticaria from an allergic response to the colored coating material of the capsule. In addition, azo and non-azo dyes used in toothpaste have been reported to cause anaphylacticlike reactions. Additionally, analine dyes used to coat certain steroid tablets have caused serious allergic reactions.[8]

Parabens (used as preservatives in local anesthetics) have caused anaphylactoid reactions.[3,4] Seng[10] reported that the sulfites (sodium metabisulfite or acetone sodium bisulfite) used in local anesthetic solutions to prevent oxidation of the vasoconstrictors can cause serious allergic reactions. The group of patients most susceptible to allergic reactions from sulfites are the 9-11 million persons with asthma in the United States.

ETIOLOGY

Allergic diseases are conditions resulting from an immunologic reaction to a noninfectious foreign substance (antigen). They are actually a series of repeat reactions to a foreign substance. The reactions involve different types of immunologic hypersensitivity (Box 18-3) and elements of the nonspecific and specific branches of the immune system (Box 18-4). The three

---

BOX 18-1

Summary of 151 Cases of Penicillin-Related Anaphylactic Deaths

21 (14%)	Had history of allergies
106 (70%)	Had received penicillin before; 25% had experienced sudden allergic reaction
128 (85%)	Died within 15 minutes of administration
75 (50%)	Experienced symptoms right after first administration of drug
3 (2%)	Were related to oral penicillin

From Idsoe O et al: *Bull WHO* 38:159-188, 1968.

BOX 18-2

Causes of Anaphylactic Reactions in Humans of Importance to the Dentist

Causative Agent
Antibiotics
Penicillins
Sulfonamides
Vancomycin
Amphotericin B
Cephalosporins
Nitrofurantoin
Ciprofloxacin
Tetracyclines
Streptomycin
Chloramphenicol

Miscellaneous Drugs/Therapeutic Agents
Acetylsalicylic acid
Succinylcholine
d-Tubocurarine
Antitoxins
Progesterone
Thiopental
Vaccines
Protamine sulfate
Nonsteroidal antiinflammatory drugs (NSAIDs)
Opiates
Mechlorethamine

Diagnostic Agents
Sodium dehydrocholate
Radiographic contrast media
Sulfobromophthalein
Benzylpenicilloyl polylysine (Pre-Pen)

Hormones
Insulin
Parathormone
Corticotropin
Synthetic adrenocorticotropic hormone (ACTH)

Enzymes
Streptokinase
Penicillinase
Chymotrypsin
Asparaginase
Trypsin
Chymopapain

Blood Products
Whole blood
Plasma
Gamma globulin
Cryoprecipitate
Immunoglobulin A (IgA)

Latex

Adapted from Patterson R: In Patterson R, editor: *Allergies*, ed 5, Philadelphia, 1997, JB Lippincott, pp 593-596.

branches of the immune system are humoral, cellular, and nonspecific. The functions of the humoral and cellular branches of the immune system are shown in Table 18-1.[1,2,9,10]

The foreign substances that trigger hypersensitivity reactions are termed *allergens* or *antigens*.[1] Box 18-5 shows some of the characteristics of antigens. Playing central roles in the two branches of the specific immune system are two types of lymphocytes. B lymphocytes are key in the humoral branch, and T lymphocytes are key in the cellular branch. The three branches of the immune system do not operate independently. T lymphocytes play an important role in the regulation of B lymphocytes. The initial function of humoral and cellular branches of the immune system is the recognition of antigens; however, for the eradication of antigens, cells and chemicals from the nonspecific branch of the immune system are necessary.

Under some circumstances the repeated contact or exposure to an antigen may cause an inappropriate response (hypersensitivity) that can be harmful or destructive to the host's tissues; thus hypersensitivity reactions can involve either the cellular or humoral components of the immune system.[1,3,11]

Reactions that involve the humoral system most often occur soon after contact with the antigen;[1] three types of hypersensitivity reaction involve elements of the humoral immune system (types I, II, and III).[1,12,13] Type IV hypersensitivity reactions involve the cellular immune system. Allergic reactions that involve the cellular immune system often have delayed onset. Examples include contact dermatitis, graft rejection, graft-versus-host disease, some drug reactions, and some types of autoimmune disease.[1,13]

PATHOPHYSIOLOGY AND COMPLICATIONS

Humoral Immune System

B lymphocytes recognize specific foreign chemical configurations via receptors on their cell membranes. For the antigen to be recognized by specific B lymphocytes,

---

BOX 18-3

Coombs and Gell Classification of Immunologic Hypersensitivity Reactions

Type I = Anaphylactic or IgE-mediated
Type II = Cytotoxic
Type III = Immune complex-mediated
Type IV = Cell-mediated or delayed

BOX 18-4

The Immune System

1. **Nonspecific**
   a. Mechanical reflexes
      (1) Coughing, sneezing
      (2) Action of cilia
      (3) Sphincter control of bladder
   b. Secretion of bactericidal substances
      (1) Stomach acid
      (2) Earwax (cerumen)
      (3) Enzymes in tears or saliva
   c. Phagocytic cells
      (1) Neutrophils
      (2) Monocytes
      (3) Marcophages
   d. Circulating chemicals
      (1) Complement
      (2) Interferon

2. **Specific**
   a. Humoral immunity
      (1) Protection against bacterial infection
      (2) Clones of B lymphocytes
      (3) Recognition of chemical configuration
      (4) Plasma cells produce antibodies
      (5) Eradication of antigen
   b. Cellular immunity
      (1) Protection against viral infection, tuberculosis, leprosy
      (2) Transplant rejection
      (3) T lymphocytes produce cytokines
      (4) Eradication of antigen

Adapted from Thomson NC, Kirkwood EM, Lever RS: In Thomson NC et al, editors: *Handbook of clinical allergy*, Oxford, 1990, Blackwell Scientific, pp 1-36.

it must first be processed by T lymphocytes and macrophages. Each clone (family) of B lymphocytes recognizes its own specific chemical structure. Once recognition has taken place, the B lymphocytes differentiate and multiply, forming plasma cells and memory B lymphocytes. The memory B lymphocytes remain inactive until contact with the same type of antigen occurs. This contact transforms the memory cell into a plasma cell to produce immunoglobulins (antibodies) specific for the antigen involved.[1] Box 18-6 lists the functions for the five classes of immunoglobulins. Note that immunoglobulin E (IgE) is the key antibody involved in the pathogenesis of type I hypersensitivity reactions.[1,14] The normal functions of the humoral immune system are shown in Box 18-7.

Type I, type II, and type III hypersensitivities involve elements of the humoral immune system. Type I hypersensitivity is summarized in Box 18-8. These are immunoglobulin E (IgE)-mediated reactions leading to the release of chemical mediators from mast cells and basophils in various target tissues. The role of IgE is clear in these reactions, but that of the other sensitizing antibody IgG4 is not well understood.[1]

Type I Hypersensitivity Reactions. Type I hypersensitivity reactions are related to the humoral immune system. They usually occur soon after the second contact with an antigen; however, it also is common to find individuals who have had repeated contacts with a drug or material before finally becoming allergic to it (Fig. 18-1).[1,15] *Anaphylaxis* is an acute reaction involving the smooth muscle of the bronchi in which the antigen-antibody complex formed causes histamine release from

BOX 18-5

Antigens

Materials considered foreign by body
Large molecular size
Certain degree of molecular complexity
Polysaccharides rarely induced cell-mediated immune response rarely induced by polysaccharides (T-independent antigens)
Have multiple antigenic determinants or antibody bindings sites (epitopes)
Do not produce same reaction in all humans

Adapted from Thomson NC, Kirkwood EM, Lever RS: In Thomson NC et al, editors: *Handbook of clinical allergy*, Oxford, 1990, Blackwell Scientific, pp 1-36.

TABLE 18-1

Functions of the Immune System

Function	Humoral	Cellular
Processing of antigen	T-helper cells and macrophages	Macrophages plus antigens of major histocompatibility complex (MHC)
Cellular recognition of antigen	Receptors on B lymphocytes sensitive to specific chemical configurations	T lymphocytes with receptors to specific subsets of MHC antigens
Cellular response to presentation of antigen	Specific clones of B lymphocytes multiply and produce plasma cells and memory cells	Specific clones of T lymphocytes multiply and produce effector T cells and memory T cells
Cellular action against antigen	Plasma cells produce specific immunoglobulins (antibodies); memory cells become plasma cells, with later antigen contact	Effector T cells produce cytokines Memory T cells become effector T cells, with later antigen contact
Eradication of antigen	Reaction with specific antibody facilitated by nonspecific branch of immune system; removed by cells of nonspecific branch	Destruction of antigen by cytokines and elements of nonspecific branch of immune system

Adapted from Thomson NC, Kirkwood EM, Lever RS: In Thomson NC et al, editors: *Handbook of clinical allergy*, Oxford, 1990, Blackwell Scientific, pp 1-36.

BOX 18-6

Functions of Immunoglobulins

1. **IgG**
   a. Most abundant immunoglobulin
   b. Small size allows diffusion into tissue spaces
   c. Can cross placenta
   d. Opsonizing antibody—facilitates phagocytosis of microorganisms by neutrophils
   e. Four subclasses: IgG1, IgG2, IgG3, IgG4 (IgG can bind to mast cells)

2. **IgA**
   a. Two types
      (1) Secretory (dimer, secretory components) found in saliva, tears, nasal mucus; secretory component protects from proteolysis
      (2) Serum (monomer)
   b. Does not cross placenta
   c. Last immunoglobulin to appear in childhood

3. **IgM**
   a. Large molecule
   b. Confined to intravascular space
   c. First immunoglobulin produced
   d. Activates complement
   e. Good agglutinating antibody

4. **IgE**
   a. Very low concentration in serum (0.004%)
   b. Increased in parasitic and atopic diseases
   c. Binds to mast cells and basophils
   d. Key antibody in pathogenesis of type I hypersensitivity reactions

5. **IgD**
   a. Low concentration in serum
   b. Little importance

Adapted from Thomson NC, Kirkwood EM, Lever RS: In Thomson NC et al, editors: *Handbook of clinical allergy,* Oxford, 1990, Blackwell Scientific, pp 1-36

the mast cells. The smooth muscle contracts, and this may lead to acute respiratory distress or failure.[1,3] *Atopy* is a hypersensitivity state influenced by hereditary factors. Hay fever, asthma, urticaria, and angioneurotic edema are examples of atopic reactions. The most common lesions associated with atopic reactions are urticaria, which is a superficial lesion of the skin, and angioneurotic edema, which is a lesion occurring in the deeper layer of the skin or in other tissues such as the larynx or tongue. In true allergic reactions, these lesions result from the effect of antigens and their antibodies (IgE) on mast cells in various locations in the body. The antigen-antibody complex causes the release of mediators (histamine) from the mast cells; these mediators then produce an increase in the permeability of adjacent vascular structures, resulting in a loss of intravascular fluid into the surrounding tissue spaces. This reaction accounts for the edematous lesions of urticaria, angioneurotic edema, and the secretions associated with hay fever.[1]

Common agents that can cause acute urticaria include shellfish, nuts, eggs, milk, antibiotic drugs and insect bites (bee stings). The humoral antibodies involved in anaphylaxis and atopy are IgE antibodies that are fixed to and sensitize mast cells so that when they encounter the antigen, they release histamine.[1,13,14]

Type II Hypersensitivity Reactions. The key elements involved in type II hypersensitivity are shown in Box 18-9. These reactions are IgG- or IgM-mediated. The classic example of type II (cytotoxic) hypersensitivity is transfusion reaction resulting from mismatched blood.[1,2]

Type III Hypersensitivity Reactions. Type III hypersensitivity is summarized in Box 18-10. These reactions take place in blood vessels and involve soluble immune complexes. They constitute what is referred to as *immune complex–mediated hypersensitivity.* Their key feature is vasculitis. Clinical examples are systemic lupus erythematosus and streptococcal glomerulonephritis.[1,2]

Cellular Immune System
The cellular or delayed immune system has T lymphocytes playing the central role. The primary function of this system is to recognize and eradicate antigens that are fixed in tissues or within cells. This system is involved in protection against viruses, tuberculosis, and leprosy. Antibodies are not operative in the cell-mediated immune system. Effector T lymphocytes produce various cytokines that serve as the active agents of this system.

Type IV Hypersensitivity Reactions. Type IV hypersensitivity reactions involve the cellular immune system. They include infectious contact dermatitis,

BOX 18-7

Functions of the Humoral Immune System

1. **First encounter with antigen (primary response)**
   a. Latent period
      (1) Antigen is processed
      (2) B lymphocyte clone selected
      (3) Differentiation and proliferation
      (4) Plasma cells produce specific immunoglobulins
   b. Specific IgM level increases first in serum followed by IgG
   c. IgM levels will later fall to zero
   d. IgG levels will fall; however, some remain

2. **Second encounter with antigen (secondary response)**
   a. Latent period is shorter
      (1) Antigen is processed
      (2) Memory cells selected; become plasma cells
      (3) Plasma cells produce specific immunoglobulins
   b. IgM levels increase first
   c. IgG levels increase to 50 times level found in primary response
   d. IgM levels will later fall
   e. IgG levels will later fall but significant serum level is usually maintained

Adapted from Thomson NC, Kirkwood EM, Lever RS: In Thomson NC et al, editors: *Handbook of clinical allergy*, Oxford, 1990, Blackwell Scientific, pp 1-36

BOX 18-8

Type I Hypersensitivity

1. IgE antibody–mediated
2. Immediate response
3. Usual allergens (antigens)
   a. Dust
   b. Mites
   c. Pollens
   d. Animal danders
   e. Food
   f. Drugs (haptens)
4. Symptoms
   a. Anaphylaxis
   b. Hay fever
   c. Asthma
   d. Urticaria, angioedema
   e. Symptoms on occasion
5. Frequency-affects about 10% of population
6. Inherited tendency

Adapted from Thomson NC, Kirkwood EM, Lever RS: In Thomson NC et al, editors: *Handbook of clinical allergy*, Oxford, 1990, Blackwell Scientific, pp 1-36.

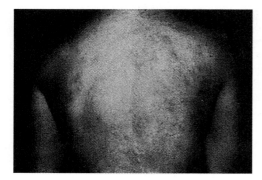

Fig. 18-1 This patient had taken penicillin a number of times without any problem. However, he developed a generalized urticarial reaction following the injection of penicillin for treatment of an acute oral infection.

BOX 18-9

Type II Hypersensitivity

1. Antibody-mediated
2. Cytotoxic hypersensitivity
   a. Antibodies combine with host cells recognized as foreign
   b. Foreign antigens bind to host cell membranes during induced hemolytic anemias or thrombocytopenia
3. Common examples
   a. Transfusion reactions from mismatched bloods
   b. Rhesus incompatibility
   c. Goodpasture's syndrome

Adapted from Thomson NC, Kirkwood EM, Lever RS: In Thomson NC et al, editors: *Handbook of clinical allergy,* Oxford, 1990, Blackwell Scientific, pp 1-36.

BOX 18-10

Type III Hypersensitivity

1. Antibody-mediated via immune complex formation
2. Also known as immune complex–mediated hypersensitivity
3. Local form is Arthus reaction
4. Immune complex formation
   a. Hypersensitivity state-complexes persist and lodge in blood vessel walls, initiating inflammatory reaction
   b. Large complexes
   c. Removed by neutrophils and macrophages
   d. Soluble complexes (more antigen than antibody)
      (1) Most harmful
      (2) Penetrate vessel wall
      (3) Lodge on basement membrane
   e. Complement is activated
      (1) Vascular permeability increased
      (2) Neutrophils attracted
      (3) Neutrophils release enzymes
      (4) Vasculitis results
5. Sensitive sites
   a. Renal glomeruli
   b. Synovial membranes
6. Examples
   a. Systemic lupus erythematosus
   b. Poststreptococcal glomerulonephritis

Adapted from Thomson NC, Kirkwood EM, Lever RS: In Thomson NC et al, editors: *Handbook of clinical allergy,* Oxford, 1990, Blackwell Scientific, pp 1-36.

transplant rejection, and graft-versus-host disease (Box 18-11). The events in type IV hypersensitivity (contact dermatitis) include dendritic cells and Langerhans cells process and present the antigen to undifferentiated T lymphocytes. Some of the more common antigens causing contact dermatitis include metal jewelry, perfumes, rubber products, chemicals such as formaldeahyde, and medicines such as topical anesthetics. Type IV hypersensitivity reactions usually are delayed and appear about 48 to 72 hours after contact with the antigen.[1,2]

Infectious-type allergic reactions are exemplified by the tuberculin skin test, in which a person who has previously been exposed to *Myobacterium tuberculosis* develops, along with a second exposure in the form of an intradermal injection of altered bacteria, a delayed response, usually within 48 to 72 hours. The response is characterized by induration, erythema, swelling, and sometimes ulceration at the site of injection.

Contact allergy occurs when a substance of low molecular weight that is not antigenic by itself comes in contact with a tissue component (primarily a protein) and forms an antigenic complex. This small molecule is called a *hapten* (or one half of an antigen), and the resulting complex causes sensitization of T lymphocytes. Poison ivy is an example of a contact allergy, wherein the reaction is delayed (with response occurring 48 to 72 hours after contact with the allergen).

Graft rejection occurs when organs or tissues from one body are transplanted into another body. A cellular rejection of the transplanted tissue occurs, unless the donor and recipient are genetically identical or the host's immune response has been suppressed.

Graft-versus-host reaction is an unusual phenomenon that occurs in bone marrow transplant patients whose cellular immune system has been rendered deficient by whole-body radiation. Lymphocytes transferred to the host attempt to destroy the host's tissues.[1,2]

Nonallergic Reactions

Other agents may cause mast cells to release their mediators without inciting a true allergic reaction, which is true in cases of chronic urticaria caused by certain drugs, temperature changes, and emotional states and in some reactions to drugs. Most so-called *anaphylactic reactions* to local anesthetics do not involve an antigen-antibody re-

Type IV Hypersensitivity

1. Mediated by T lymphocytes ④⑤
2. Does not involve antibodies
3. Also called delayed-type hypersensitivity (Response not seen until about 2 days following antigenic exposure)
4. Examples include
   a. Contact dermatitis
   b. Graft rejection
   c. Graft-versus-host reaction
   d. Some type of drug hypersensitivity
   e. Some types of autoimmune disease

Adapted from Thomson NC, Kirkwood EM, Lever RS: In Thomson NC et al, editors: *Handbook of clinical allergy*, Oxford, 1990, Blackwell Scientific, pp 1-36.

action but are a result of damage to the mast cells through other mechanisms. These reactions are termed anaphylactoid or *anaphylaxislike*.[8]

Because from the clinical standpoint the management of both anaphylactic and anaphylacticlike reactions is similar, these types of drug reactions are viewed as true allergic reactions. Certain cases of urticaria and angioneurotic edema can occur based on a similar pathogenesis and are not considered true allergic reactions.

The nonallergic cases of urticaria, angioneurotic edema, and anaphylacticlike reactions are caused by the nonspecific release of vasoactive amines from mast cells or the activation of some other form of nonspecific immunologic effector mechanisms.[5,8] The reader is referred to a text on allergic diseases for an in-depth discussion of the origin of these reactions.

MEDICAL MANAGEMENT

Patients with atopy may receive injections to gradually desensitize them so that they are no longer allergic to the antigen. Some individuals with severe asthma may be forced to move to an area of the country that does not contain the antigen (e.g., in the case of allergy to pollen).[1,12] Patients with asthma (see Chapter 8), immune complex injury, or cytotoxic immune reactions may be treated with systemic steroids, whereas patients with hay fever or urticaria are treated with antihistamines.

Signs and Symptoms Suggestive of an Allergic Reaction

Urticaria
Swelling
Skin rash
Chest tightness
Dyspnea, shortness of breath
Rhinorrhea
Conjunctivitis

Patients who have received an organ transplant often take steroids and immunosuppressive drugs. A variety of treatments have been used for patients with contact dermatitis, including topical steroids. From a dental standpoint, the patient being treated for an allergic problem has an increased chance of being allergic to another substance, and if this individual is taking steroids, his or her reaction to stress may be impaired (see Chapter 15). Additionally, if the patient has received an organ transplant, he may be susceptible to infection (see Chapter 25).

DENTAL MANAGEMENT

MEDICAL CONSIDERATIONS

The dentist is often confronted with problems related to allergy. One of the most common concerns is the patient who reports an allergy to a local anesthetic, antibiotic, or analgesic. The history then must be expanded, specifically trying to determine exactly what the offending substance was and exactly how the patient reacted to it. If the adverse reaction was of an allergic nature, one or more of the classic signs or symptoms of allergy should have been present (Box 18-12). If these signs or symptoms were not reported, the patient probably did not experience a true allergic reaction. Common examples of mislabeled allergy include syncope after injection of a local anesthetic and nausea or vomiting after the ingestion of codeine. Adverse drug reactions are listed in Box 18-13.

Local Anesthetics

The most common reaction associated with local anesthetics is a toxic reaction, resulting usually from an

Adverse Drug Reactions

Predictable
  Dose-related
  No immunologic basis
  Account for about 80% of all adverse reactions to drugs
  Direct toxicity
  Overdoses
  Drug interactions
  Side effects of drugs
Unpredictable
  Not dose-related
  Unrelated to expected pharmacologic effects
  Allergy
  Pseudoallergy (anaphylactoid reactions)
  Idiosyncrasy
  Intolerance
  Paradoxical reactions (cause histamine release but
    not IgE-mediated
  Often underlying genetic defect present

Adapted from Weiler JM, Maves KK: In Lichtenstein LM, Fauci AS, editors: *Current therapy in allergy, immunology, and rheumatology,* ed 5, St Louis, 1997, Mosby, pp 132-139.

BOX 18-14

Adverse Reactions to Local Anesthetics

Toxic
  Central nervous system stimulation
  Central nervous system depression
Vasoconstrictor
Anxiety
Allergic

BOX 18-15

Signs and Symptoms of a Toxic Reaction to Local Anesthetic

Talkativeness
Slurred speech
Dizziness
Nausea
Depression
Euphoria
Excitement
Convulsions

BOX 18-16

Signs and Symptoms of a Psychomotor Response to the Injection of a Local Anesthetic

Hyperventilation
Vasovagal syncope (Bradycardia, Pallor, Sweating)
Sympathetic stimulation (Anxiety, Tremor, Tachycardia,
  Hypertension)

inadvertent intravenous injection of the anesthetic solution (Box 18-14). Excessive amounts of an anesthetic also can cause a toxic reaction or a reaction to the vasoconstrictor. The signs and symptoms associated with toxic reactions to a local anesthetic are shown in Box 18-15. The signs and symptoms of a vasoconstrictor reaction include tachycardia, apprehension, sweating, and hyperactivity. Another common reaction to local anesthetics involves the anxious patient who, because of concern about receiving a "shot," experiences tachycardia, sweating, paleness, and syncope (Box 18-16). True allergic reactions to the local anesthetics (amides) most commonly used in dentistry are rare.[17]

If the patient's history supports a toxic or vasoconstrictor reaction, the dentist should explain the nature of the previous reaction (see Box 18-15) and avoid injecting the local anesthetic solution IV by aspirating before the injection and limiting the amount of solution to the recommended dose. If the patient's history supports an interpretation of fainting and not a toxic or allergic reaction, the dentist's primary task will be to work with the patient to reduce anxiety during dental visits. If the history supports a true allergic reaction to a local anesthetic, the dentist should try to identify the type of local anesthetic that was used. Once this has been done, a new anesthetic with a different basic chemical structure can be used. The two main groups of local anesthetics in dentistry[18] are (1) paraaminobenzoic acid (PABA) esters (procaine [Novocain] and tetracaine [Pontocaine]) and (2) amides (lidocaine [Xylocaine], mepivacaine [Carbocaine], and prilocaine [Citanest]). The benzoic acid ester anesthetics may cross-react with each other, whereas the amide anesthetics usually do not cross-react. Cross-reaction does not occur between ester and amide local anesthetics.[5]

BOX 18-17

Referral of Patient with a History of Anesthetic Allergy to an Allergist

1. History shows reaction consistent with allergic response
   a. Allergic to anesthetic that is identified
   b. Allergic to anesthetic that cannot be identified
   c. Allergic to several anesthetics involving both amides and esters
2. Skin testing not indicated because of variable results
3. Provocative dose testing (PDT)
4. Selection and recommendation of alternative local anesthetic based on results of PDT

Procaine is the local anesthetic with the highest incidence of allergic reactions. Its antigenic component appears to be PABA, one of the metabolic breakdown products of procaine. Cross-reactivity has been reported[19,20] between lidocaine and procaine; however, this could be traced to the presence of a germicide, methylparaben, which has been used in small amounts as a preservative and is chemically similar to PABA. Thus a patient who is allergic to procaine may react to lidocaine solution if it contains methylparaben. Lidocaine that does not contain methylparaben can now be readily obtained and should be used when dealing with a patient who has an allergic history to procaine.[19,20]

Patients with a history of being allergic to local anesthetics and who cannot identify the specific agent used present more of a problem. The nature of the reaction must be established, and if it is consistent with an allergic reaction the next step should be to attempt to identify the anesthetic used. When the patient is unable to provide this information, the dentist can attempt to contact the previous dentist involved. If this fails, the following two options are available: (1) an antihistamine (diphenhydramine [Benadryl]) can be used as the local anesthetic or (2) the patient can be referred to an allergist for provocative dose testing (PDT) (Box 18-17). The use of diphenhydramine is often the more practical option. A 1% solution of diphenhydramine that contains 1:100,000 epinephrine can be easily compounded by a pharmacist, but it must be confirmed that methylparaben is not used as a preservative. This solution induces anesthesia of about 30 minutes average duration and can be used for infiltration or block injection. When it is used for a mandibular block, 1 to 4 ml of solution is needed. Some

patients have reported a burning sensation, swelling or erythema after a mandibular block with 1% diphenhydramine, but these effects were not serious and cleared within 1 or 2 days. No more than 50 mg of diphenhydramine should be given during a single appointment. Diphenhydramine also can be used in the patient who gives a history of being allergic to both ester and amide local anesthetics.[21,22]

The dentist also may elect to refer the patient to an allergist for evaluation and testing, which usually includes both skin testing and PDT. Most investigators agree that skin testing alone for allergy to local anesthetics is of little benefit because false-positive results are common; therefore the allergist also should perform PDT. Having samples of one's usual anesthetic agents without vasoconstrictors sent along for specific testing is a great help.

Based on the patient's history, the allergist selects a local anesthetic for testing that is least likely to cause an allergic reaction, which is usually an anesthetic from the amide group because they do not usually cross-react with each other.[5] At 15-minute intervals, 0.1 ml of test solution is injected subcutaneously, with concentrations increasing from 1:10,000 to 1:1000 to 1:100 to 1:10, followed by undiluted; next, 0.5 ml of undiluted test solution is tried; and finally 1 ml of undiluted solution. During PDT, the allergist should be prepared to deal with any adverse reaction that might occur and report to the dentist on the drug selected, the final dose given, and the absence of any adverse reaction. Under these conditions, a local anesthetic with no reaction can be used in the tested patient, and the risk of an allergic reaction is then no greater than in the general population.[19] Schatz and Greenberger[24] report that they have not dealt with a single patient for whom a safe local anesthetic could not be found using the PDT procedure.

When administering an alternative anesthetic to a patient with a history of a local anesthetic allergy, the dentist should follow these steps:
1. Inject slowly, aspirating first to make sure that a vessel is not being injected.
2. Place one drop of the solution into the tissues.
3. Withdraw the needle and wait 5 minutes to see what reaction, if any, occurs. If no allergic reaction occurs, as much anesthetic as needed for the procedure should be deposited. Be sure to aspirate before making the second injection (Box 18-18).

Penicillin
The use of penicillin has been increasing tremendously throughout the world during the last 30 years, particularly in the United States. Approximately 2.5 million persons in the United States are allergic to penicillin,

BOX 18-18

Dental Management of a Local Anesthetic Allergy

1. Establish history of previous reaction following use of local anesthetic
2. Establish history of previous reaction and type of anesthetic used
   a. Syncopal
   b. Allergic
      (1) Soft-tissue swelling
      (2) Skin rash
      (3) Rhinitis
      (4) Difficulty breathing
3. If reaction was consistent with allergic reaction
   a. Select anesthetic from different chemical group
      (1) Paraaminobenzoic acid (procaine)
      (2) Amide (lidocaine, mepivacaine)
   b. Aspirate, inject one drop of alternate anesthetic, and wait 5 minutes; if no reaction occurs, inject after aspirating rest of anesthetic needed (be prepared to deal with allergic reaction if one should occur)
   c. In cases of allergic reaction to several local anesthetic agents or if anesthetic used previously cannot be identified, consider using diphenhydramine
4. If history of multiple allergies is present or if type of local anesthetic used previously cannot be identified, refer patient to allergist for PDT

BOX 18-19

Penicillin Reactions

Anaphylaxis
In 0.04% to 0.2% of patients
Fatal reaction in 1 per 100,000 treated individuals
Atopic predisposition not risk factor for anaphylaxis, but is for fatal reaction

Risk of Reaction Dependent on
History of prior reaction
Time interval since prior reaction
Persistence of specific IgE antibodies
History of multiple drug sensitivities

Most Useful Parameter to Assess Risk in Patients with History of Penicillin Reaction is Skin Testing with Major and Minor Determinants
Negative result—Very little risk
Positive result—High risk for serious reaction to penicillin-Risk for cross-reaction with cephalosporin

Adapted from Kaplan MS: In Lichtenstein LM, Fauci AS, editors: *Current therapy in allergy, immunology, and rheumatology*, ed 5, St Louis, 1997, Mosby, pp 126-132.

and allergic reactions occur in 5% to 10% of patients who receive penicillin and related drugs. About 0.04% to 0.2% of the patients treated with penicillin develop an anaphylactic reaction, and about 10% of those individuals die, accounting for some 400 to 800 deaths per year. Box 18-19 shows the risk assessment of penicillin reactions.[1-3,8,9,25,26]

The possibility of sensitizing a patient to penicillin increases according to the route of administration as follows[2,3,23,27]: oral administration results in sensitization of only about 0.1% of patients, intramuscular (IM) injection in about 1% to 2%, and topical application in about 5% to 12%. Based on these data, the use of penicillin in a topical ointment is contraindicated. Additionally, if the dentist has a choice, the oral route is preferable for administration whenever possible. Several authors[1,38] report that less serious reactions occur if oral administration of penicillin is used instead of parenteral. However, Idsoe

et al[23] suggest that the early data on penicillin reactions involved primarily parenteral administration and thus are biased. They suggest the risk is equally great for a serious allergic reaction with both routes. Antibodies produced against penicillin cross-react with the semisynthetic penicillins and can cause severe reactions in patients allergic to penicillin.[1,3,23] Nevertheless, the synthetic penicillins do seem to cause fewer new sensitizations in patients who are not allergic to penicillin at the time of administration.[23] Patients with a history of penicillin allergy should be given erythromycin or clindamycin for the treatment of oral infections or clindamycin for prophylaxis against infective endocarditis.

Skin testing for allergy to penicillin is much more reliable than skin testing for allergy to a local anesthetic; however, some risk is involved, and the allergist must be prepared for adverse reactions. Several points should be considered in the use of skin testing for pencillin sensitivity. To be cost-effective, the test should be conducted only on patients with a history of penicillin reaction who need penicillin for a serious infection. An important fact to remember is that penicillin reactivity declines with time; hence, a patient may have reacted to the drug years ago but is now no longer sensitive (negative skin test).

The length of time for retaining sensitivity is variable and is dependent on IgE levels.[21,23] Most anaphylactic reactions to penicillin occur in patients who have been treated in the past with penicillin but reported no adverse reactions.[8,9]

When skin testing for penicillin sensitivity is performed, both metabolic breakdown products of penicillin (the major derivative, penicilloyl polylysine, and the minor derivative mixture must be tested; 95% of penicillin is metabolized to the major determinant and 5% to the minor determinants.[8,9] If skin tests are negative to both breakdown products, the patient is considered not allergic to penicillin; however, if positive tests are obtained for one or both of the breakdown products, the patient is considered to be allergic to penicillin and the drug should not be used.[23] When penicillin must be used, the patient with a positive skin test can be desensitized to it.[8,9] Patients with a positive skin test to minor derivative mixture have a higher incidence of anaphylactic reactions than do patients with a positive test to the major derivative.[23,24]

In dentistry, wherein alternative antibiotics can be selected, reactions to penicillin are preventable by merely not using penicillin in patients who have a history of penicillin allergy. Additionally, drugs that may cross-react including ampicillin, carbenicillin, and methicillin should be avoided in these patients.[19]

Cephalosporins cross-react in 5% to 10% of penicillin-sensitive patients. The risk is greatest with first- or second-generation drugs. Cephalosporins are metabolized to their major determinant, cephaloyl, which can cross-react with the major determinant of penicillin. Cephalosporins usually can be used in patients with a history of distant, nonserious reaction to penicillin.[25] However, skin testing is recommended by some authors for these patients. If the patient's skin test to penicillin is negative, then either penicillin or a cephalosporin may be used. If the penicillin skin test is positive, a skin test for the specific cephalosporin selected should be performed. If this skin test is negative, the cephalosporin that was tested can be used. Box 18-20 summarizes the use of cephalosporins in patients with a history of penicillin hypersensitivity.[9]

Patients with a negative history of allergy to penicillin can be treated with the drug when indicated, and it should be given by the oral route. The patient is observed for 30 minutes after the first dose, if possible and is advised to seek immediate care if any of the signs or symptoms of an allergic reaction occur after he or she has left the dental office (Box 18-21).

Analgesics

Aspirin may cause gastrointestinal upset, but this can be avoided if it is taken with food or a glass of milk. The dis-

---

BOX 18-20

Use of Cephalosporins for Patients with a History of Penicillin Hypersensitivity

1. Cephalosporins metabolized to major determinant, cephaloyl
2. Cephaloyl can cross-react with major determinant of penicillin (penicilloyl polylysine)
3. Risk of adverse reaction to cephalosporin is controversial
   a. Greatest with first- or second-generation drugs
      (1) Cephaloridin, 16.5%
      (2) Cephalothin, 5%
      (3) Cephalexin, 5.4%
   b. Anaphylaxis
      (1) Positive history of penicillin reaction, 0.1%
      (2) Negative history of penicillin reaction, 0.4%
   c. Urticaria
      (1) Positive history of penicillin reaction, 1.3%
      (2) Negative history of penicillin reaction, 0.4%
4. Patient with history of penicillin reaction, first skin test for penicillin sensitivity
   a. Negative—use either penicillin or cephalosporin
   b. Positive
      (1) Avoid penicillin
      (2) Skin test specific cephalosporin; use if result is negative

Adapted from Kaplan MS: In Lichtenstein LM, Fauci AS, editors: *Current therapy in allergy, immunology, and rheumatology*, ed 5, St Louis, 1997, Mosby, pp 126-132.

---

comfort may include "heartburn," nausea, vomiting, or gastrointestinal bleeding. Aspirin should not be used by patients with an ulcer, gastritis, or a hiatal hernia and should be used with care by patients whose condition predisposes them to nausea, vomiting, dyspepsia, or gastric ulceration. Aspirin also is known to prolong the prothrombin time and to inhibit platelet function, which is usually of little clinical importance except in patients with a hemorrhagic disease or a peptic ulcer. In these patients aspirin must be avoided. Many individuals, estimated at 2 per 1000, are allergic to salicylates.[7,25] Allergic reactions to aspirin can be serious, and deaths have been reported.[24,25]

Aspirin provokes a severe reaction in some patients with asthma. They may react in the same way to other nonsteroidal antiinflammatory drugs (NSAIDs) that inhibit cyclooxygenase, which is the key enzyme in generating prostaglandin from arachidonic acid. The typical re-

Procedures for Prevention of a Penicillin Reaction

1. Have emergency kit for treatment
2. Take medical history on all patients, including
   a. Previous contact with penicillin
   b. Reactions to penicillin
   c. Allergic reactions to other agents
3. Do not use penicillin in patient with history of reactions to drugs
4. Tell patient when you are going to give penicillin
5. Do not use penicillin in topical preparations
6. Do not use penicillinase-resistant penicillins unless infection is caused by penicillinase-producing staphylococci
7. Use oral penicillin whenever possible
8. Use disposable syringes for injection of penicillin
9. Have patient wait in office for 30 minutes after first dose of penicillin
10. Inform patient about signs and symptoms of allergic reaction to penicillin, and if these occur to seek immediate medical assistance

action consists of acute bronchospasm, rhinorrhea, and urticaria. Most individuals with asthma who react to NSAIDs also have nasal polyps and lack IgE-mediated allergy to airborne allergens. The mechanism for this reaction does not appear to be allergic but is still undefined.[1-4]

The dentist should be aware of the many multiple-entity analgesic preparations that include aspirin or other salicylates. These agents must not be given to the patient who may be endangered by an adverse reaction associated with aspirin or other salicylates.[28]

Many NSAIDs are now available, and most can cause some degree of gastrointestinal irritation. NSAIDs also are inhibitors of prostaglandin formation, platelet aggregation, and prothrombin synthesis. Most have the potential for cross-sensitivity with patients who exhibit an asthma-like reaction to aspirin. NSAIDs should not be given to certain patients with asthma, patients with an ulcer or hemorrhagic disease, and patients who are pregnant or nursing.[25] The new COX-2 inhibitors (celecoxib and rofecoxib) are now available, effective, and cause much less gastrointestinal disturbance.

Codeine is a commonly used narcotic analgesic in dentistry. Emesis, nausea, and constipation may occur with analgesic doses of codeine. Miosis and adverse renal, hepatic, cardiovascular, and bronchial effects are not likely to occur with therapeutic doses, however.[28]

Most of the reported reactions to codeine consist of non-allergic gastrointestinal manifestations; nevertheless, these may be severe enough to preclude the use of codeine in certain patients. Alternate drug selections can be made by referring to a current pharmacology text, the *Physicians' Desk Reference,* or *Accepted Dental Therapeutics.*

Rubber Products

A number of reports have demonstrated that certain health care workers and patients are at risk for hypersensitivity reactions to latex or agents used in the production of rubber gloves or related materials (e.g., rubber dam, blood pressure cuff, catheters). An obstetrics and gynecology physician developed latex anaphylaxis from surgical gloves.[29] Intraoperative cardiovascular collapse was reported in five patients because of latex gloves.[29] Sussman et al[13] reported that latex caused hypersensitivity reactions in 14 persons, including health care workers. All 14 cases had positive latex skin tests. Warpinski et al[6] found allergic reactions to latex, including anaphylaxis, in 4 atopic patients. Gonzalez,[32] in a review of allergy to latex products, found that about 3% of hospital physicians and nurses were affected. However, most of these reactions were type IV, resulting from agents used in the production of rubber products. Type I allergic reactions to latex are rare. Based on these findings, it can be concluded that serious type I hypersensitivity reactions may occur in physicians, dentists, other health care workers, and patients from contact with latex products such as gloves, rubber dam, balloons, or catheters.

Dentists should be aware that latex allergy can present as anaphylaxis during dental work when the patient or dentist has been sensitized to latex. Anaphylaxis may result in the sensitized individual after contact with rubber gloves, rubber dam material, blood pressure cuffs, or any other product containing latex. Studies[34] have shown that latex-allergic individuals have IgE antibodies for specific latex proteins. Latex skin tests are a satisfactory method to identify individuals who may be sensitized to latex.[34,35]

Dental Materials and Products

Type I, type III, and type IV hypersensitivity reactions have been reported to result from various dental materials and products.[36-40] Topical anesthetic agents have been reported to cause type I reactions consisting of urticarial swelling. Mouth rinses and toothpastes containing phenolic compounds, antiseptics, astringents, or flavoring agents have been known to cause type I, type III, and type IV hypersensitivity reactions involving the oral mucosa or lips. Hand soaps used by dental care workers also have been reported as a cause of type IV reactions. Some of the dental agents that can lead

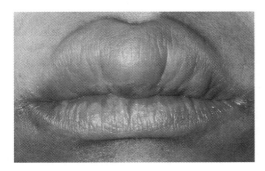

Fig. 18-2 Angioneurotic edema of the upper lip that occurred soon after the injection of a local anesthetic. (From Neville, Damm, Allen, et al: Oral and Maxillofacial Pathology, ed 2, Philadelphia, WB Saunders, 2002.)

to type IV hypersensitivity (contact stomatitis) include dental amalgam, acrylic, composite resin, nickel, eugenol, rubber products, talcum powder, mouthwashes, and toothpastes.[30-40]

Other Conditions

Allergic patients being treated with steroids should be managed as described in Chapter 15. Patients who have had an organ transplant should be managed as described in Chapter 25. The dental management of patients with asthma primarily is concerned with preventing severe asthma attacks from occurring in the dental office and dealing with an attack if one happens. In addition, certain important drug considerations must be taken for these patients[1,2] (see Chapter 8).

TREATMENT PLANNING MODIFICATIONS

The dentist should obtain a history of any allergic reactions from each patient. If a patient has a history of allergy to drugs or materials that may be used in dentistry, a clear entry should be made in the dental record, and any further contact or use of the antigen(s) should be avoided in that patient. Most allergic patients can receive any indicated dental treatment as long as the antigen is avoided and special preparations are made for those patients receiving steroids.

ORAL COMPLICATIONS AND MANIFESTATIONS

Hypersensitivity

Type I Hypersensitivity. Oral lesions may be produced by type I hypersensitivity reactions. An atopic reaction to various foods, drugs, or anesthetic agents may occur within or around the oral cavity and is usually char-

---

BOX 18-22

Oral or Paraoral Type I Hypersensitivity Reactions

1. Urticarial swelling (or anginoeurotic edema)
   a. Reaciton occurs soon after contact with antigen
   b. Reaction consists of painless swelling
   c. Itching and burning may occur
   d. Lesion may remain for 1 to 3 days
2. Treatment
   a. Reaction not involving tongue, pharynx, or larynx and no respiratory distress present requires 50 mg of diphenhydramine four times a day until swelling diminishes
   b. Reaction involving tongue, pharynx, or larynx with respiratory distress present requires
      (1) 0.5 ml of 1:1000 epinephrine, IM or SC
      (2) Oxygen
      (3) Once immediate danger over, 50 mg of diphenhydramine four times a day until swelling diminishes

---

acterized by urticarial swelling or angioneurotic edema (Fig. 18-2).[1] This reaction is generally rapid, with the lesion developing within a short time after contact with the antigen. It is a painless, with soft tissue swelling produced by transudate from the surrounding vessels that may lead to itching and burning. The lesion is usually present for 1 to 3 days and then begins to resolve spontaneously. Oral antihistamines should be given; diphenhydramine, 50 mg every 4 hours, orally, is the recommended regimen, Treatment is given for 1 to 3 days. Further contact with the antigen must be avoided (Box 18-22).

Type III Hypersensitivity. Foods, drugs, or agents that are placed within the oral cavity can cause white, erythematous, or ulcerative lesions based on type III hypersensitivity or immune complex reactions. The lesions develop rather quickly, usually within a 24-hour period, after contact with the offending antigen. Some cases of aphthous stomatitis (Fig. 18-3) may be caused by type III hypersensitivity, although most are related to lymphocyte dysfunction. Fig. 18-4 demonstrates an allergic dermatitis that occured after orthodontic brackets and archwires (containing nickel) were placed. Erythema multiforme represents an immune complex reaction.[36]

About half the patients with erythema multiforme (Figure 18-5) are found to have a predisposing factor such

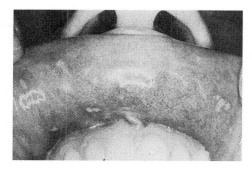

Fig. 18-3 Aphthous stomatitis that occurred in a man found to be allergic to the toothpaste he was using.

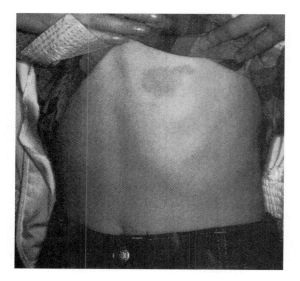

Fig. 18-4 Allergic rash on the abdomen of a patient whom had just had orthodontic brackets and archwires placed. The patient was tested and found to be allergic to the nickel in the wires.

as a drug allergy or herpes simplex infection involved in the onset of their disease.[10,36]

Sulfa antibiotics are the most common drug associated with the onset of erythema multiforme, and sulfonyl urea hypoglycemic agents (e.g., tolbutamide, tolazamide, glyburide, glipizide), used to treat some individuals with diabetes, have been found to be associated with the onset of erythema multiforme. Many patients with erythema multiforme can be managed by symptomatic therapy including a bland mouth rinse, syrup of diphenhydramine, and triamcinolone acetonide (Kenalog) in Orabase. A few patients with more severe involvement may require systemic steroids. (See Appendix B for treatment regimens.) If a drug appears to be associated with the onset of the disease, any further contact with it should be avoided. Box 18-23 summarizes oral type III hypersensitivity reactions.

Type IV Hypersensitivity. Contact stomatitis is a delayed allergic reaction associated with the cellular immune response in most cases. Because of the delayed nature of the reaction after contact with the allergen in cases of contact stomatitis, the dentist must inquire about contacts with materials that may have occurred 2 to 3 days before the lesions appeared.[36] The antigen may be found in dental materials, toothpaste, mouth rinses, lipsticks, face powders, and so on.[36-38] In many cases no further treatment is necessary once the source of the antigen has been identified and removed from further contact with the patient; however, if the tissue reaction is severe or persistent, topical corticosteroids should be used. A good preparation to use topically is triamcinolone acetonide in Orabase (see Appendix B for treatment regimens).

Various dental materials have been reported as a cause of allergic reactions in patients. Impression materials containing an aromatic sulfonate catalyst have been reported to cause a delayed allergic reaction in post-

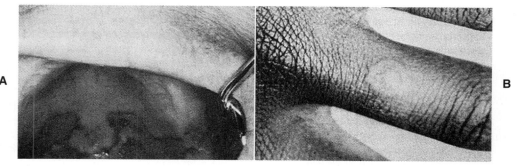

Fig. 18-5 Erythema multiforme that developed following oral administration of a drug used to treat an oral infection. **A,** Ulceration of the palatal mucosa. **B,** Target lesion of the finger.

menopausal women. The reaction consisted of tissue ulceration and necrosis that became progressively worse with each exposure.[36-38]

Some papers[36-37] have reported oral lesions found in close association with amalgam restorations. These (mucosal) lesions were described as whitish, reddish, ulcerative, or lichenoid and were thought to be caused by toxic irritation or a hypersensitivity reaction to the silver amalgam restoration. When these restorations were removed, the lesions most often cleared. In some of the studies, skin testing for mercury sensitivity was performed. All the reports suggested that some of the oral lesions were a result of toxic injury to the mucosa and others were a result of type IV hypersensitivity reaction to mercury in the amalgams.[36-37]

No well-done studies exist that relate nonspecific symptoms such as depression, fatigue, and headaches to the effects of mercury in amalgam restorations. The practice of avoiding use of amalgam restorations in patients with nonspecific symptoms has, at present, no scientific basis.[37] However, to remove any amalgam restorations in contact with oral mucosa that shows lesions consistent with a toxic or hypersensitivity reaction to mercury is rational.

On rare occasions, dental composite materials have been reported[30] to cause allergic reactions. The acrylic monomer used in denture construction has caused an allergic reaction[38]; however, the vast majority of tissue changes under dentures are from trauma and secondary infection with bacteria or fungi.[38] Gold, nickel, and mercury have been reported[40] to cause allergic reactions resulting in tissue erythema and ulceration.

The dentist may want to test certain agents that are thought to be possible antigens causing oral lesions.

Type III Hypersensitivity Reactions

1. Usually occur within 24 hours following contact with antigen
2. Consist of
   a. Erythema
   b. Rash
   c. Ulceration
3. Treatment requires
   a. Topical steroids
   b. Systemic steroids (in severe cases)
   c. Identification of antigen
   d. Avoidance of any further contact with antigen

Oral epimucous testing for contact stomatitis consists of placing the suspected antigen in contact with the oral mucosa and observing over a period of several days for any reaction (e.g., erythema, sloughing, ulceration) that might indicate an allergy to the test material. In most cases, a reaction is not expected to develop for at least 48 to 72 hours. Various techniques have been used to conduct epimucous testing for suspected allergens. One of these is placing the suspected allergen in a rubber suction cup, placing the cup on the buccal mucosa, and observing at intervals for erythema or ulceration under the cup. Another technique is to place a sample of the suspected antigen in a depression on the palatal aspect of an overlay denture. The denture is inserted and holds the allergen in contact with the palatal mucosa.

Another technique consists of incorporating the allergen into Orabase, applying the Orabase in the mucobuccal fold, and periodically observing for a reaction. Alternately, the antigen can be incorporated into an oral adhesive spray. Skin testing and oral epimucous testing for potential antigens are not foolproof, by any means; in certain patients, they give unreliable tissue responses. The response in some cases may be caused by trauma, and in others in which no tissue reaction occurs, the patient may still be allergic to the substance.

The basic management of contact stomatitis is to remove common sources of antigens known to cause hypersensitivity reactions to see if the lesions clear. Skin or mucosal testing for sensitivity also can be performed. Once the offending agent or antigen has been identified, the patient should be told to avoid any future contact with the antigen. Again, if the lesions persist, topical steroids can be applied (see Appendix B).

Lichenoid Drug Eruptions

Some patients with skin and/or oral lesions identical to those of lichen planus will be found to have taken certain drugs before the onset of their lesions.[34,35] If these drugs are withdrawn, the lesions clear within several days (in most patients) or within a few weeks. The agents most commonly associated with the onset of the lichenoid lesions are levamisole (Levantine) and the quinidine drugs. Other agents found to be associated are the thiazide drugs, methyldopa, and photographic dyes (e.g., paraphenylenediamine).[34,35] Biopsy of a lichenoid lesion shows the same microscopic picture as seen in lichen planus, with the additional finding of eosinophils in the subepithelial infiltrate. These lesions are related to the cellular immune system and therefore could be placed under the heading of contact stomatitis; however, the true nature of the reactions is not clear.[34,35]

MANAGEMENT OF SEVERE TYPE I HYPERSENSITIVITY REACTIONS

Even when the dentist has taken appropriate precautions, an allergic reaction may occur in the patient. Most of these are mild and of a nonemergency nature; however, some may be severe and life threatening (anaphylactic). The dentist must be ready to deal with either type. In handling the anaphylactic reaction, the dentist should remember that it has an allergic etiology. In other words, the reaction should occur soon after (i.e., minutes) the injection, ingestion, or application of a topical anesthetic, medication, drug, local anesthetic, or dental product. The dentist must take the following actions immediately: (see *Management of Common Medical Emergencies in the Dental Office*).

1. Place the patient in a head-down or supine position.
2. Make certain that the airway is patent.
3. Administer oxygen.
4. Be prepared to send for help and to support respiration and circulation. The rate and depth of respiration should be noted, as should the patient's other vital signs. Most reactions in dental patients consist of simple fainting, which can be managed well by the preceding actions. In addition, the dentist may administer aromatic spirits of ammonia by inhalation, which will encourage breathing through reflex stimulation.

If the initial steps have not solved the emergency problem, and it is of an allergic cause, the dentist is faced with either an edematous-type reaction or an anaphylactic reaction.

Angioneurotic Edema

If the immediate type I hypersensitivity reaction has resulted in edema of the tongue, pharyngeal tissues, or larynx, the dentist must take additional emergency steps to prevent death from respiratory failure. At this point, if the patient has not responded to the initial procedures and is in acute respiratory distress, the dentist should do the following:

1. Inject 0.3-0.5 ml of 1:1000 epinephrine IM (into the tongue) or subcutaneous (SC).
2. Support respiration, if indicated, by mouth-to-mouth breathing or bag and mask; be sure the chest moves when either of these methods is used.
3. Check the carotid or femoral pulse; if a pulse cannot be detected, closed chest cardiac massage should be initiated. By this time, someone in the office should have called a nearby physician or hospital.

Anaphylaxis

An anaphylactic reaction usually takes place within minutes. The signs and symptoms associated with anaphylactic reactions are listed in Box 18-24. In contrast to the severe edematous reaction, in which respiratory distress occurs first, both respiratory and circulatory depression occur early in the anaphylactic reaction. Anaphylaxis

---

BOX 18-24

Signs and Symptoms of Anaphylaxis

Itching of soft palate
Nausea, vomiting
Substernal pressure
Shortness of breath
Hypotension
Pruritus
Urticaria
Laryngeal edema
Bronchospasm
Cardiac arrhythmias

BOX 18-25

Anaphylaxis

Basis
1. First contact with antigen results in formation of antibodies by plasma cells
2. Antibodies circulate in bloodstream (IgE antibodies)
3. Antibodies attach to target tissues (mast cells near smooth muscle of bronchi)
4. Next contact with antigen may result in combining of antigen and antibody
5. Antigen-antibody complex causes degranulation of mast cell(s) with release of histamine
6. Smoth muscle contracts and vessels lose fluid, etc.
7. Acute respiratory distress and cardiovascular collapse may occur within minutes

Management
1. Call for medical help
2. Place patient in supine position
3. Check for open airway
4. Administer oxygen
5. Check pulse, blood pressure, respiration
   a. If depressed or absent, inject 0.3 to 0.5 ml 1:1000 epinephrine IM in tongue
   b. Provide cardiopulmonary resuscitation if needed
   c. Repeat injection of 0.5 ml 1:1000 epinephrine if no response

often is fatal unless vigorous, immediate action is taken. Because it occurs within minutes after contact with the antigen, the dentist should take the following steps[18] (Box 18-25):

1. Have someone in the office call for medical aid at a nearby physician or hospital.
2. Place the patient in a supine position.
3. Make certain the airway is patent.
4. Administer oxygen.
5. Check the carotid or femoral pulse and respiration; if no pulse is present and the respiration is depressed
6. Inject 0.3-0.5 ml of 1:1000 epinephrine IM (into the tongue) or SC. Support circulation by closed chest cardiac massage. Support respiration by mouth-to-mouth breathing. Repeat the injection of epinephrine if no response occurs.

References

1. Kay AB: Allergies and allergic diseases, *New Eng J Med*, 344(1):30-37, 2001.
2. Hagner BF, Fauci AS: Disorders of the immune system. In Harrison et al, editors: *The principles of internal medicine*, ed 14, New York, 1998, McGraw-Hill.
3. Patterson R: Anaphylaxis. In Patterson R, editor: *Allergic diseases*, ed 5, Philadelphia, 1997, JB Lippincott.
4. *Physicians' desk reference*, ed 55, Montvale NJ, 1999, Medical Economics.
5. Incaudo G et al: Administration of local anesthetics to patients with a history of prior adverse reaction, *J Allergy Clin Immunol* 61:339-345, 1978.
6. Warpinski JR et al: Allergic reaction to latex: a risk factor for unsuspected anaphylaxis, *Allergy Proc* 12(2):95-102, 1991.
7. Idsoe O et al: Nature and extent of penicillin side-reactions, with particular reference to fatalities from anaphylactic shock, *Bull WHO* 38:159-188, 1968.
8. Czarnetzki BM: *Urticaria*, New York, 1986, Springer-Verlag.
9. James J et al: Oral lichenoid reactions related to mercury sensitivity, *Br J Oral Maxillofac Surg* 25(6):474-480, 1987.
10. Seng GF, Gay BJ: Dangers of sulfites in dental local anesthetic solutions: warning and recommendations, *J Am Dent Assoc* 113:769-770, 1986.
11. Norman PS, Lichtenstein LM: Immune responses in man. In Harvey A et al, editors: *The principles and practice of medicine*, ed 21, New York, 1997, Appleton-Century-Crofts.
12. Aaronson DW, Rosenberg M: Asthma, general concepts. In Patterson R, editor: *Allergic diseases*, ed 5, Philadelphia, 1997, JB Lippincott.
13. Sussman GL, Tarlo S, Dolvich J: The spectrum of IgE-mediated responses to latex, *JAMA* 265(21):2844-2847, 1991.
14. Thomson NC, Kirkwood EM, Lever RS: Basic immunological mechanisms. In Thomson NC et al, editors: *Handbook of clinical allergy*, Oxford, 1990, Blackwell Scientific.
15. Austen, KF: Diseases of immediate type hypersensitivity. In Wilson JD et al, editors: *Harrison's principles of internal medicine*, ed 12, New York, 1991, McGraw-Hill.
16. Nguyen DH et al: Intraoperative cardiovascular collapse secondary to latex allergy, *J Urol* 146:571-574, 1991.
17. Malamed SF: Diphenhydramine hydrochloride, its uses as a local anesthetic in dentistry, *Anesth Prog* 20:76-82, 1973.
18. American Dental Association: *Accepted dental therapeutics*, Chicago, 1998, The American Dental Association.
19. Giovannitti JA, Bennett CR: Assessment of allergy to local anesthetics, *J Am Dent Assoc* 98(5):701-706, 1979.
20. Kaplan MS: Penicillin allergy. In Lichtenstein LM, Fauci AS, editors: *Current therapy in allergy, immunology, and rheumatology*, ed 5, St Louis, 1997, Mosby.
21. Reed CE: Drug allergy. In Wyngaardin JB, Smith LH, editors: *Cecil textbook of medicine*, ed 17, Philadelphia, 1985, JB Lippincott.
22. Larson CE: Methylparaben, an overlooked cause of local anesthetic hypersensitivity, *Anesth Prog* 24:72-74, 1977.
23. Idsoe O et al: Nature and extent of penicillin side-reactions, with particular reference to fatalities from anaphylactic shock, *Bull WHO* 38:159-188, 1968.
24. Schatz M, Greenberger PA: Drug allergy. In Patterson R, editor: *Allergic diseases*, ed 5, Philadelphia, 1997, JB Lippincott.
25. Holroyd SV, Wynn RL: *Clinical pharmacology in dental practice*, ed 4, St Louis, 1987, Mosby.
26. Weiler JM, Maves KK: Drug reactions. In Lichtenstein LM, Fauci AS, editors: *Current therapy in allergy, immunology, and rheumatology*, ed 5, St Louis, 1997, Mosby.
27. Williams BG: Oral drug reaction to methyldopa, *Oral Surg* 56:375-377, 1983.
28. Greenberg MS: Dental correlations: immunological and allergic disorders. In Rose LF, Kaye D, editors: *Internal medicine for dentistry*, ed 2, St Louis, 1990, Mosby.
29. Chen MD, Greenspoon JS, Long TL: Latex anaphylaxis in an obstetrics and gynecology physician, *Am J Obstet Gynecol* 166:968-969, 1992.
30. Nathanson D: Delayed extra-oral hypersensitivity to dental composite materials, *Oral Surg* 47:329-333, 1979.
31. Shafer WG, Hine MK, Levy BM: *A textbook of oral pathology*, ed 4, Philadelphia, 1983, WB Saunders.
32. Gonzalez E: Latex hypersensitivity: a new and unexpected problem, *Hosp Pract* 27(2):145-148, 1992.
33. Thomson NC, Kirkwood EM, Lever RS: Contact dermatitis. In Thomson NC et al, editors: *Handbook of clinical allergy*, Oxford, 1990, Blackwell Scientific.
34. Stenman E, Bergman M: Hypersensitivity reactions to dental materials in a referred group of patients, *Scand J Dent Res* 97(1):76-83, 1989.
35. Eversole LR: Allergic stomatitis, *J Oral Med* 34:93-102, 1979.
36. Dahl BL: Tissue hypersensitivity to dental materials, *J Oral Rehabil* 5:117-120, 1978.
37. Holmstrup P: Reactions of the oral mucosa related to silver amalgam: a review, *J Oral Pathol Med* 20(1):1-17, 1991.
38. Fernstrom AL: Location of the allergenic monomer in warm-polymerized acrylic dentures. I. *Swed Dent J* 4:253-260, 1980.
39. Weinstein L: Chemotherapy of microbial diseases. In Goodman LS, Gilman A, editors: *The pharmacological basis of therapeutics*, ed 7, New York, 1985, Macmillan.
40. Wiesenfeld D et al: Allergy to dental gold, *Oral Surg* 57:158-160, 1984.

Bleeding Disorders

19

CHAPTER

A number of procedures performed in dentistry may cause bleeding. Under normal circumstances, these procedures can be performed with little risk to the patient; however, the patient whose ability to control bleeding has been altered by drugs or disease may be in grave danger unless the dentist identifies the problem before performing any dental procedure. In most cases, once the patient with a bleeding problem has been identified, steps can be taken to greatly reduce the risks associated with dental procedures.

DEFINITION

Bleeding disorders are conditions that alter the ability of blood vessels, platelets, and coagulation factors to maintain hemostasis. Inherited bleeding disorders are genetically transmitted. Acquired bleeding disorders occur secondary to diseases affecting vascular wall integrity, platelets, coagulation factors, drugs, radiation, or chemotherapy for cancer.

Most bleeding disorders are iatrogenic. Every patient who receives coumarin to prevent recurrent thrombosis has a potential bleeding problem. Most of these patients are receiving anticoagulant medication because they have had a recent myocardial infarction, a cerebrovascular accident, or thrombophlebitis. Patients who have atrial fibrillation or had open-heart surgery to correct a congenital defect, replace diseased arteries, repair or replace damaged heart valves, or have had recent total hip or knee replacement also may be receiving long-term anticoagulation therapy. In addition, some individuals treated with aspirin for cardiovascular disorders or chronic illnesses, such as rheumatoid arthritis have potential bleeding problems.

EPIDEMIOLOGY: INCIDENCE AND PREVALENCE

Patients on low-intensity warfarin therapy (international normalized ratio [INR] 2.0 to 3.0) for prophylaxis of venous thromboembolism have a risk of major bleeding of less than 1% and about an 8% risk for minor bleeding. Patients on high-intensity warfarin therapy (INR 2.5 to 3.5) have up to a five-fold greater risk for bleeding.[1]

The most common inherited bleeding disorder is von Willebrand's disease (vWD). It affects about 1% of the population in the United States. The disease usually is inherited as an autosomal dominant trait. Hemophilia A, factor VIII deficiency, is the most common of the inherited coagulation disorders. The overall prevalence of hemophilia A in the United States is about 1 case for every 20,000 people; however, because of its genetic mode of transfer, certain areas of the United States, such as North Carolina, are found to contain many more persons with hemophilia than other areas. About 80% of all genetic coagulation disorders are hemophilia A, 13% are hemophilia B (Christmas disease, factor IX deficiency), and 6% are factor XI deficiency.[2-4]

Patients with acute or chronic leukemia may have clinical bleeding tendencies because of thrombocytopenia, which may result from overgrowth of malignant cells in the bone marrow that leaves no room for red blood cells or platelet precursors. In addition, leukemic patients may develop thrombocytopenia from the toxic effects of the various chemotherapeutic agents used to treat the disease. The incidence of leukemia is discussed in Chapter 20.

Obtaining accurate information is difficult about the incidence of other systemic conditions, such as liver disease, renal failure, thrombocytopenia, and drug-induced vascular wall defects that may render the patient susceptible to prolonged bleeding after injury or surgery. However, when considering the prevalence of the drug-

influenced or disease-produced defects in the normal control of blood loss, a busy dental practice will contain a large number of patients who may be potential "bleeders."

ETIOLOGY

A pathologic alteration of blood vessel walls, a significant reduction in the number of platelets, defective platelets or platelet function, a deficiency of one or more coagulation factors, the administration of anticoagulant drugs, a disorder of platelet release, or the inability to destroy free plasmin can result in significant abnormal clinical bleeding. This can occur even after minor injuries and may lead to death in some patients if immediate action is not taken.

The classification given in Box 19-1 is based on bleeding problems in patients with normal numbers of platelets (nonthrombocytopenic purpuras), decreased numbers of platelets (thrombocytopenic purpuras), and disorders of coagulation.

Infections, chemicals, collagen disorders, or certain types of allergy can alter the structure and function of the vascular wall to the point at which the patient may have a clinical bleeding problem. A patient may have normal numbers of platelets, but they may be defective or unable to perform their proper function in the control of blood loss from damaged tissues. If the total number of circulating platelets is reduced below 50,000/mm^3 of blood, the patient may be a bleeder. In some cases the total platelet count is reduced by unknown mechanisms; this is called *primary* or *idiopathic thrombocytopenia*. Chemicals, radiation, and various systemic diseases (e.g., leukemia) may have a direct effect on the bone marrow and may result in secondary thrombocytopenia.[5-7]

BOX 19-1

Classification of Bleeding Disorders

1. Nonthrombocytopenic purpuras
   a. Vascular wall alteration
      (1) Scurvy
      (2) Infections
      (3) Chemicals
      (4) Allergy
   b. Disorders of platelet function
      (1) Genetic defects (Bernard-Soulier disease)
      (2) Drugs
         (a) Aspirin
         (b) NSAIDs
         (c) Alcohol
         (d) Beta-lactam antibiotics
         (e) Penicillin
         (f) Cephalothins
      (3) Allergy
      (4) Autoimmune disease
      (5) von Willebrand's disease (secondary factor VIII deficiency)
      (6) Uremia
2. Thrombocytopenic purpuras
   a. Primary—idiopathic
   b. Secondary
      (1) Chemicals
      (2) Physical agents (radiation)
      (3) Systemic disease (leukemia)
      (4) Metastatic cancer to bone
      (5) Splenomegaly
      (6) Drugs
         (a) Alcohol
         (b) Thiazide diuretics
         (c) Estrogens
         (d) Gold salts
      (7) Vasculitis
      (8) Mechanical prosthetic heart valves
      (9) Viral or bacterial infections
3. Disorders of coagulation
   a. Inherited
      (1) Hemophilia A (deficiency of factor VIII)
      (2) Hemophilia B (deficiency of factor IX)
      (3) Others
   b. Acquired
      (1) Liver disease
      (2) Vitamin deficiency
         (a) Biliary tract obstruction
         (b) Malabsorption
         (c) Excessive use of broad-spectrum antibiotics
      (3) Anticoagulation drugs
         (a) Heparin
         (b) Coumarin
         (c) Aspirin and NSAIDs
      (4) DIC
      (5) Primary fibrinogenolysis

NSAIDs, nonsteroidal antiinflammatory drugs; DIC, disseminated intravascular coagulation.

Patients may be born with a deficiency of one of the factors needed for blood coagulation. For example, factor VIII deficiency (hemophilia A) or factor IX deficiency (hemophilia B or Christmas disease). Congenital deficiencies of the other coagulation factors have been reported but are rare. When congenital deficiency of a coagulation factor occurs only a single factor is affected.

Acquired coagulation disorders are the most common cause of prolonged bleeding. Liver disease and disseminated intravascular coagulation (DIC) can lead to severe bleeding problems. Many of the other acquired coagulation disorders may become apparent in patients only after trauma or surgical procedures. In contrast to the congenital coagulation disorders where only one factor is affected, the acquired coagulation disorders usually have multiple factor deficiencies.[4,8]

The liver produces all the protein coagulation factors; thus any patient with significant liver disease may have a bleeding problem. In addition to a possible disorder in coagulation, the patient with liver disease who develops portal hypertension and hypersplenism may be thrombocytopenic as a result of splenic over activity, which leads to increased sequestration platelets in the spleen.[9]

Any condition that so disrupts the intestinal flora that vitamin K is not produced in sufficient amounts will result in a decreased plasma level of the vitamin K dependent coagulation factors. Vitamin K is needed by the liver to produce prothrombin (factor II) and factors VII, IX, and X. Biliary tract obstruction, malabsorption syndrome, and excessive use of broad-spectrum antibiotics can lead to low levels of prothrombin and factors VII, IX and X on this basis.[8]

Drugs, such as heparin and coumarin derivatives, can cause a bleeding disorder because of disruption of the coagulation process. Aspirin, other nonsteroidal antiinflammatory drugs (NSAIDs), penicillin, cephalosporins, and alcohol also can interfere with platelet function.

PATHOPHYSIOLOGY

The three phases of hemostasis for controlling bleeding are vascular, platelet, and coagulation. The coagulation phase is followed by the fibrinolytic phase that dissolves the clot (Box 19-2).

Vascular Phase
The vascular phase begins immediately after injury and involves vasoconstriction of arteries and veins in the area of injury, retraction of arteries that have been cut, and buildup of extravascular pressure by blood loss from cut vessels. This pressure aids in collapsing the adjacent capillaries and veins in the area of injury. Vascular wall in-

---

BOX 19-2

Normal Control of Bleeding

1. Vascular phase
   a. Vasoconstriction in area of injury
   b. Begins immediately after injury
2. Platelet phase
   a. Platelets and vessel wall will become "sticky"
   b. Mechanical plug of platelets seals off openings of cut vessels
   c. Begins seconds after injury
3. Coagulation phase
   a. Blood lost into surrounding area coagulates through extrinsic and common pathways
   b. Blood in vessels in area of injury coagulates through intrinsic and common pathways
   c. Takes place more slowly than other phases
4. Metabolic (fibrinolytic) phase
   a. Release of antithrombotic agents
   b. Spleen and liver destroy the antithrombotic agents

---

tegrity is important to maintain the fluidity of blood. The smooth endothelial lining consists of a nonwettable surface that under normal conditions will not activate platelet adhesion or coagulation. In fact, the endothelial cells synthesize and secrete three potent antiplatelet agents: prostacyclin, nitric oxide, and certain adenine nucleotides.[10,11]

Vascular endothelial cells also are involved with both antithrombotic and prothrombotic activities. The major antithrombotic activity consists of the secretion of heparin-like glycosaminoglycans (heparin sulfate) that catalyze inactivation of serine proteases such as thrombin and factor Xa by antithrombin III. Endothelial cells also produce thrombomodulin, which will combine with thrombin to form a complex that activates protein C. The activated protein C (APC) then binds to endothelial-released protein S causing proteolysis of factor Va and factor VIIIa that inhibits coagulation. Tissue-type plasminogen activator (tPA) is released by injured endothelial cells to initiate fibrinolysis.

The vessel wall components contribute prothrombotic activities. The exposure of vessel wall subendothelial tissues, collagen and basement membrane, by chemical or traumatic injury serves as a tissue factor (old term was tissue thromboplastin) and initiates coagulation via the extrinsic pathway. The endothelial cell synthesis of factor V promotes thrombin formation. In addition, an in-

ducible endothelial cell prothrombin activator may directly generate thrombin. Injured endothelial cells release adenosine diphosphate (ADP), which induces platelet adhesion. Vessel wall injury also promotes platelet adhesion and thrombus formation by exposure of subendothelial von Willebrand Factor (vWF). Endothelial cells also contribute to normal homeostasis and vascular integrity by synthesis of type IV collagen, fibronectin, and vWF.[10,11]

Platelet Phase

Platelets are cellular fragments from the cytoplasm of megakaryocytes that last 8 to 12 days in the circulation. About 30% of the platelets are sequestered in the microvasculature or spleen and serve as a functional reserve. Platelets do not have a nucleus thus they are unable to repair inhibited enzyme systems by drugs such as aspirin. Aged or nonviable platelets are removed and destroyed by the spleen and liver. Platelet structure consists of three areas: a peripheral zone, a sol-gel zone (cytoskeleton), and an organelle zone.[10,12] Box 19-3 outlines the component parts and function of these structures.

The functions of platelets include maintenance of vascular integrity, formation of a platelet plug to aid the initial control of bleeding, and stabilization of the platelet plug by involvement in the coagulation process. About 10% of the platelets are used to nurture endothelial cells, allowing for endothelial and smooth muscle regeneration.

Subendothelial tissues at the site of injury are exposed and, through contact activation, cause the platelets to become sticky and adhere to the subendothelial tissues (vWF/glycoprotein Ib). ADP released by damaged endothelial cells initiates aggregation of platelets (primary wave); and when the platelets release their secretions, a second wave of aggregation results. Binding with fibrinogen (glycoprotein IIb) that is converted to fibrin stabilizes the platelet plug. The result of the preceding processes is a clot of platelets and fibrin attached to the subendothelial tissue.[6,10,12] Box 19-4 summarizes the function of platelets.

A product of platelets, thromboxane, is needed to induce platelet aggregation. The enzyme cyclooxygenase is key in the process for generation of thromboxane. Endothelial cells, through a similar process (also dependent on cyclooxygenase), generate prostacyclin, which inhibits platelet aggregation. Aspirin acts as an inhibitor of cyclooxygenase, and this causes irreversible damage in the platelets. However, endothelial cells can, after a short period, recover and synthesize cyclooxygenase; thus aspirin has only a short effect on the availability of prostacyclin from these cells. The net result of aspirin therapy is to inhibit platelet aggregation. This effect can last for up to 9

BOX 19-3

Platelet Structure and Function

1. Peripheral zone (stimulus receptor-transmitter region)
   a. Exterior coat (glycocalyx, blood groups, HLA)
   b. Plasma membrane (receptors)
      (1) Glycoprotein Ib (von Willebrand's factor)—adhesion to subendothelium
      (2) Glycoproteins IIb and IIIa (fibrinogen, fibronectin)
      (3) ADP, thrombin, epinephrine, serotonin
   c. Phospholipid portion of plasma membrane
      (1) Factor V
      (2) Factor VIII
      (3) Platelet factors III and IV
   d. Open canalicular system—allows pathway for granules to exterior
2. Sole-gel zone (cytoskeleton)
   a. Submembranous filaments
   b. Microtubules—contraction facilitates secretion
      (1) Actin
      (2) Myosin
3. Organelle zone (metabolic and secretory)
   a. Dense granules (ADP)
   b. Alpha granules (platelet factor IV, growth factor)
   c. Lysosomes (acid hydrolases)
   d. Dense tubular system
      (1) Prostaglandin synthesis
      (2) Calcium secretion
   e. Mitochondria (ATP generation for energy)

HLA, human lymphocyte antigen; ADP, adenosine diphosphate; ATP, adenosine triphosphate.
Modified from Harmening DM: *Clinical hematology and fundamentals of hemostatsis*, ed 2, Philadelphia, 1992, FA Davis.

---

days (time needed for all old platelets to be cleared from the blood).[10]

Coagulation Phase

The process of the fibrin-forming (coagulation) system is shown in Fig. 19-1. The overall time involved from injury to a fibrin-stabilized clot is about 9 to 18 minutes. Platelets, blood proteins, lipids, and ions are involved in the process. Thrombin is generated on the surface of the platelets, and bound fibrinogen is converted to fibrin.[10,13,14]

Coagulation of blood involves the factors shown in Table 19-1 and Box 19-5. Many of the coagulation factors are proenzymes that become activated in a "waterfall" or

Platelet Functions and Activation

1. Maintain vascular integrity
   a. Nurturing endothelial cells
   b. Endothelial and smooth muscle regeneration
2. Initial control of bleeding (platelet plug)
   a. Contact activation (subendothelial)
   b. Stickiness
   c. Adhesion
   d. Aggregation (ADP initiated)
      (1) Platelet changes shape (spherical)
      (2) Calcium and fibrinogen (glycoprotein-IIb and glycoprotein-IIIa) form bridges between platelets
   e. Secretion release (second-wave aggregation)
      (1) ADP, serotonin, calcium (dense granules)
      (2) Irreversible changes in platelets
3. Stabilization of platelet plug—contributes to coagulation process
   a. Binding of fibrinogen
   b. Exposure of platelet factor III on surface
   c. Factor V and factor VIII complexes on surface
   d. Thrombin generated on surface as result of intrinsic and extrinsic pathways
   e. Conversion of fibrinogen to fibrin

Blood Coagulation Factors

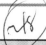

Factor	Name
I	Fibrinogen
II	Prothrombin
III	Thromboplastin
IV	Calcium
V	Labile factor, proaccelerin, accelerator (Ac) globulin
(VI)	Not assigned
VII	Proconvertin, serum prothrombin conversion accelerator (SPCA), cothromboplastin, autoprothrombin I
VIII	Antihemophilic factor (AHF), antihemophilic globulin (AHG), von Willebrand's factor (vWF)
IX	Plasma thromboplastin component (PTC) (Christmas factor)
X	Stuart-Prower factor
XI	Plasma thromboplastin antecedent (PTA)
XII	Hageman factor
XIII	Fibrin-stabilizing factor
Fitzgerald factor	High-molecular-weight kininogen (HMWK)
Fletcher factor	Prekallikrein

Modified from Harmening DM: *Clinical hematology and fundamentals of hemostasis*, ed 2, Philadelphia, 1992, FA Davis.

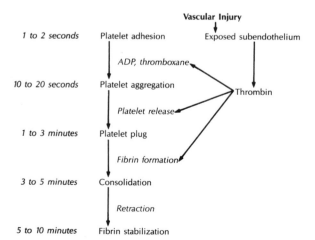

Fig. 19-1 Fibrin-forming (coagulation) system. (From Harmening DM: *Clinical hematology and fundamentals of hemostasis*, ed 2, Philadelphia, 1992, FA Davis.)

cascade manner—that is, one factor becomes activated and it, in turn, activates another, and so on in an ordered sequence. For example, the proenzyme factor XI is activated to the enzyme factor XIa by contact with injury exposed subendothelial tissues in vivo to start the intrinsic pathway. In vitro, the intrinsic pathway is initiated by contact activation of factor XII. Coagulation proceeds through two pathways, the intrinsic and the extrinsic. Both utilize a common pathway to form the end product, fibrin.[10,13,14] Fig. 19-2 shows these coagulation pathways.

The (faster) extrinsic pathway is initiated through tissue factor (an integral membrane protein), released or exposed by injury to tissues, which activates factor VII (VIIa). In the past the trigger for initiating the extrinsic pathway was referred to as a tissue *thromboplastin*. It has since been shown that the real activator is the tissue fac-

BOX 19-5

Classification of the Coagulation Factors

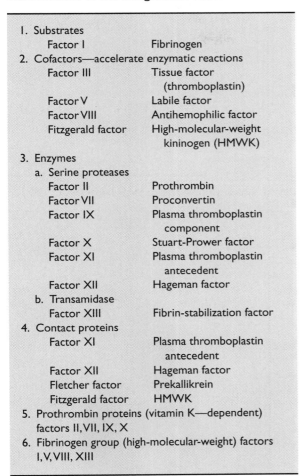

1. Substrates
   Factor I   Fibrinogen
2. Cofactors—accelerate enzymatic reactions
   Factor III   Tissue factor
                     (thromboplastin)
   Factor V   Labile factor
   Factor VIII   Antihemophilic factor
   Fitzgerald factor High-molecular-weight
                     kininogen (HMWK)
3. Enzymes
   a. Serine proteases
      Factor II   Prothrombin
      Factor VII   Proconvertin
      Factor IX   Plasma thromboplastin
                     component
      Factor X   Stuart-Prower factor
      Factor XI   Plasma thromboplastin
                     antecedent
      Factor XII   Hageman factor
   b. Transamidase
      Factor XIII   Fibrin-stabilization factor
4. Contact proteins
   Factor XI   Plasma thromboplastin
                     antecedent
   Factor XII   Hageman factor
   Fletcher factor   Prekallikrein
   Fitzgerald factor HMWK
5. Prothrombin proteins (vitamin K—dependent)
   factors II, VII, IX, X
6. Fibrinogen group (high-molecular-weight) factors
   I, V, VIII, XIII

Modified from Harmening DM: *Clinical hematology and fundamentals of hemostasis*, ed 2, Philadelphia, 1992, FA Davis.

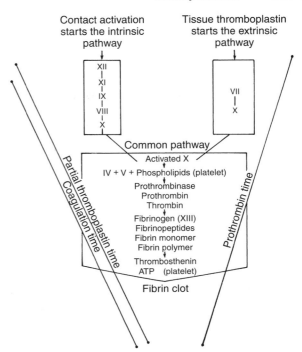

Fig. 19-2 Pathways for the coagulation of blood.

tor (TF). The nomenclature, extrinsic pathway, continues to be used today, despite being somewhat outdated. This is because TF is not always extrinsic to the circulatory system. TF is expressed on the surface of vascular endothelial cells and leukocytes.[14]

Thrombin generated by the faster extrinsic and common pathway is used to accelerate the slower intrinsic and common pathway. The activation of factor XII acts as a common link between the component parts of the homeostatic mechanism: coagulation, fibrinolytic, kinin, and complement systems. As a result thrombin is generated, which in turn converts fibrinogen to fibrin, activates factor XIII, enhances factor V and factor VIII activity, and stimulates aggregation of more platelets.[10,14]

Fibrinolytic Phase

The fibrin-lysing (fibrinolytic) system is needed to prevent coagulation of intravascular blood away from the site of injury and to dissolve the clot once it has served its function in homeostasis (Fig. 19-3). This system involves plasminogen, a proenzyme for the enzyme plasmin produced in the liver, and various plasminogen activators and inhibitors of plasmin. The prime endogenous plasminogen activator is tissue-type plasminogen activator (t-PA), which is released by endothelial cells at the site of injury. Two other endogenous plasminogen activators are prourokinase (scu-PA) and urokinase (u-PA). Streptokinase (SK) acts as an exogenous plasminogen activator. Alpha-2 antiplasmin and three plasminogen activator inhibitors, PAI-1, PAI-2, and PAI-3, are present in plasma to inhibit the plasminogen activators. The actions of plasmin are to destroy fibrin and fibrinogen producing fibrin degradation products, destroy factors V and VIII,

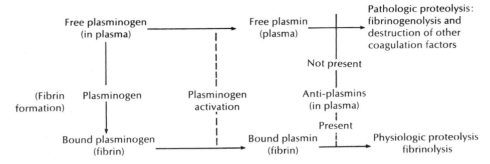

Fig. 19-3 Plasminogen system.

Fibrin-Lysing (Fibrinolytic) System

1. Activation of coagulation also activates fibrinolysis
2. Active enzyme: plasmin
3. Plasminogen activated to plasmin
   a. Tissue-type plasminogen activator (t-PA)
   b. Prourokinase (scu-PA)
   c. Urokinase (u-PA), streptokinase
4. Tissue plasminogen activator (TPA)
   a. Produced by endothelial cells
   b. Released by injury
   c. Activates plasminogen bound to fibrin
   d. Circulating plasminogen not activated
   e. TPA will dissolve clot, not cause systemic fibrinolysis
5. Action of plasmin
   a. Splits large pieces of alpha and beta polypeptides from fibrin
   b. Splits small pieces of gamma chains
   c. First product is X monomer
   d. Each X monomer splits into one E fragment and two D fragments
   e. Split products are called fibrin-split products (FSPs) and fibrin-degradation products (FDPs)
6. Action of fibrin-degradation products
   a. Increase vascular permeability
   b. Interfere with thrombin-induced fibrin formation

Modified from Harmening DM: *Clinical hematology and fundamentals of hemostasis,* ed 2, Philadelphia, 1992, FA Davis.

enhance conversion of factor XII into XIIa, amplify conversion of prekallikrein to kallikrein, and cleave complement (C3) into fragments. The fibrin-forming and fibrinlysing systems are intimately related; activation of the fibrin-forming (coagulation) system also activates the fibrinolytic system. The t-PA released by injured endothelial cells binds to fibrin as it activates the conversion of fibrin-bound plasminogen to plasmin. Circulating plasminogen (i.e., not fibrin-bound) is not activated by t-PA. Thus t-PA is efficient in dissolving a clot without causing systemic fibrinolysis.[10,14]

The action of plasmin on fibrin and fibrinogen is to split off large pieces that are broken up into smaller and smaller segments. The final smaller pieces are called *split products.* The split products also are referred to as fibrindegradation products (FDPs). These can be important clinically if they are allowed to accumulate. FDPs increase vascular permeability and interfere with thrombin-induced fibrin formation and can be the basis for clinical bleeding problems.[10,14] Box 19-6 summarizes the fibrinlysing system.

The antiplasmin factors present in circulating blood rapidly destroy free plasmin but are relatively ineffective against plasmin that is bound to fibrin (Box 19-7). Thus under normal conditions, once an injury has occurred, coagulation will proceed to the formation of fibrin. At the same time, both bound plasminogen and free plasminogen become activated to plasmin. The free plasmin is rapidly destroyed, and it does not interfere with the formation of a clot. The bound plasmin is not inactivated, and it is free to dispose of the fibrin clot after its function in homeostasis has been fulfilled. In a sense, the clot is "programmed" to self-destruct at the time of its formation.[10,14]

Timing of Clinical Bleeding
A significant disorder in either the vascular or the platelet phase leads to an immediate clinical bleeding problem

following injury or surgery. These phases are concerned with controlling blood loss immediately after an injury and if defective, will lead to an early problem. However, if the vascular and platelet phases are normal and the coagulation phase is abnormal, the bleeding problem will

BOX 19-7

Protease Inhibitors

1. Plasmin and kallikrein in circulation eliminated by
   a. Liver
   b. Lymphoid system
   c. Serine protease inhibitors in blood
2. Plasma protease inhibitors
   a. Antithrombin III (AT-III)
   b. Alpha$_2$-macroglobulin
   c. Alpha$_2$-antiplasmin
   d. Alpha$_2$-antitrypsin
   e. C-I esterase inhibitor
   f. Protein C and S inhibitors*
3. Antithrombin III (AT)
   a. Also called heparin cofactor or factor Xa inhibitor
   b. Major physiologic inhibitor of thrombin and factor Xa
   c. In natural state a slow inhibitor
   d. Activity increased 100 times with heparin
   e. Deficiency causes thrombosis
4. Protein C (serine protease)
   a. Cleaves factors V and VIII
   b. Increases release of t-PA
   c. Acts as cofactor with protein S*
   d. Deficiency causes thrombosis

*Protein S (a vitamin K–dependent fibrinolytic agent manufactured in the liver) is needed, along with protein C (another fibrinolytic agent from the liver), for the destruction of factors V and VIII.

Modified from Harmening DM: *Clinical hematology and fundamentals of hemostasis*, ed 2, Philadelphia, 1992, FA Davis.

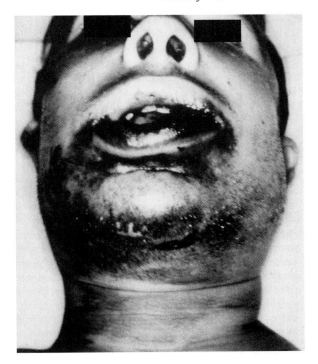

Fig. 19-4 Patient with hemophilia who has massive areas of ecchymoses secondary to trauma.

not be detected until several hours after the injury or surgical procedure. In the case of small cuts, for example, little bleeding would occur until several hours after the injury, and then a slow trickle of bleeding would start. If the coagulation defect were severe, this slow loss of blood could continue for days. Even with this "trivial" rate, a significant loss of blood might occur: 0.5 ml per minute or about 3 units per day.[14-16]

CLINICAL PRESENTATION

SIGNS AND SYMPTOMS

Signs of bleeding may appear in the skin or mucous membranes or after trauma or invasive procedures. Jaundice, spider angiomas, and ecchymoses may be seen in the person with liver disease. A fine tremor of the hands when held out also may be observed in these patients. In about 50% of persons with liver disease, a reduction of platelets occurs secondary to hypersplenism that results from the effects of portal hypertension, and these individuals may show petechiae on the skin and mucosa.[15,17-20]

The most common objective findings in patients with genetic coagulation disorders are ecchymoses, hemarthrosis, and dissecting hematomas (Fig. 19-4). The signs seen most commonly in patients with abnormal platelets or thrombocytopenia are petechiae and ecchymoses (Fig. 19-5).

Patients with acute or chronic leukemia may reveal one or more of the following signs: ulceration of the oral mucosa, hyperplasia of the gingivae, petechiae of the skin or mucous membranes, ecchymoses of skin or mucous membranes, and lymphadenopathy (Figs. 19-6   19-7). Chapter 20 discusses these findings in greater detail.

A number of patients with bleeding disorders may show no objective signs that suggest their underlying problem. Severe or chronic bleeding can lead to anemia with features of pallor, fatigue, and so on. Anemia is discussed in detail in Chapter 20.

A
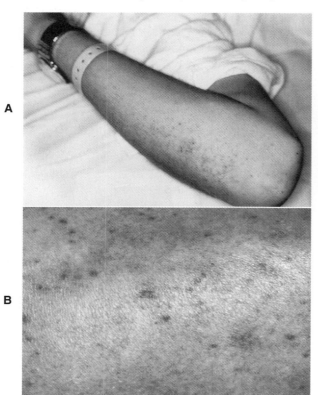

B

Fig. 19-5 A, Arm of a patient with thrombocytopenia, shows numerous petechiae. **B,** Close-up view of the petechiae.

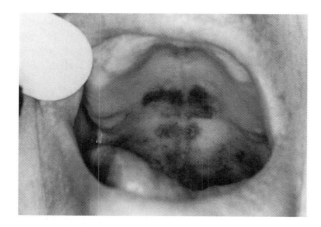

Fig. 19-6 Areas of ecchymoses on the mucosa of the hard and soft palate in a patient with chronic lymphocytic leukemia.

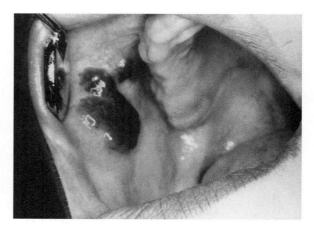

Fig. 19-7 Cheek lesion that might appear to be an area of ecchymoses. However, the lesion blanched with pressure and was determined to be a capillary hemangioma.

LABORATORY TESTS

Several tests are available to screen patients for bleeding disorders and to help pinpoint the specific deficiency. In general, screening is done in dentistry when the patient gives a history of a bleeding problem, a family member with a history of a bleeding problem, and/or when signs of bleeding disorders are found in the clinical examination. The dentist can order the screening tests or the patient can be referred to a hematologist for screening. In medicine, routine screening is done for patients before major surgical procedures such as open-heart surgery.

When screening for possible bleeding disorders, three tests are recommended by Rodgers[16] to be used in the initial screen. These tests are the partial thromboplastin time (PTT); the prothrombin time (PT); and the platelet count. If no clues are evident as to the cause of the bleeding problem and the dentist is ordering the tests from a commercial laboratory, two additional tests can be added to the initial screen: platelet function analyzer (PFA-100) if available (if not, then the Ivy bleeding time [BT]) and the thrombin time.

Patients with positive screening tests need to be evaluated further to identify the specific deficiency and to rule out the presence of inhibitors. A hematologist orders these tests. The hematologist establishes a diagnosis based on the additional testing and makes recommendations for the management of the patient found to have a significant bleeding problem.

Screening Tests
Partial Thromboplastin Time. PTT is used to check the intrinsic system (factors VIII, IX, XI, and XII) and the

common pathways (factors V and X, prothrombin, and fibrinogen). It also is the best single screening test for co-agulation disorders. Phospholipid platelet substitute is added to the patient's blood to initiate the coagulation process. This material acts, as a partial thromboplastin and cannot trigger the extrinsic pathway. For the PTT test, activation is accomplished by the glass wall of the test tube or by adding a contact activator such as kaolin. When a contact activator is added, the test is referred to as the *activated* PTT (*aPTT*). A control must be run with the test sample, and the results can be interpreted only if the control value falls within the normal range of results for the laboratory performing the test.

The aPTT varies from laboratory to laboratory; hence, the dentist must be aware of the normal range for the laboratory being used. In general the aPTT ranges from 25 to 35 seconds and results in excess of 35 seconds are considered abnormal or prolonged.

The aPTT screens for the following intrinsic pathway deficiencies: prekallikrein; HMW kiningen; and factors VIII, IX, XI, and XII. Deficiencies of factor XII, prekallikrein, and HMW kiningen result in a prolonged aPTT test, but these deficiencies do not cause clinical bleeding problems. The aPTT is prolonged in cases of mild to severe deficiency of factors VIII, IX, or XI. The aPTT is more sensitive to deficiencies of factors VIII and IX. The test is abnormal when a given factor is 15% to 30% below its normal value. In the unusual cases higher levels than normal result with one of the intrinsic pathway coagulation factors, the aPTT is shortened (less than 25 seconds).[16]

Prothrombin Time. PT is used to check the extrinsic pathway (factor VII) and the common pathway (factors V and X, prothrombin, and fibrinogen). Three of these are vitamin K–dependent (factors VII and X and prothrombin) and are depressed by coumarin-like drugs. Thus the PT is used to evaluate the effect of the coumarin-like drugs. For this test, tissue thromboplastin is added to the test sample to serve as the activating agent. Again, a control must be run and results vary from one laboratory to another. In general the normal range is 11 to 15 seconds, and results in excess of 15 seconds are considered abnormal or prolonged. The PT is prolonged if the plasma level of any factor is below 10% of its normal value. When the test is used to evaluate the level of anticoagulation with coumarin-like drugs the INR format is recommended. The INR is a method that standardizes PT assays.

Platelet Count. The platelet count is used to screen for possible bleeding problems because of thrombocytopenia. The normal platelet count is 140,000 to 400,000/mm³ of blood; however, clinical bleeding problems usually are associated with platelet counts of less than 50,000/mm.³ A peripheral blood smear also is used to examine for the presence of platelets.[5,16,21]

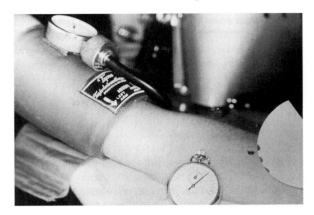

Fig. 19-8 Ivy bleeding time. Midway through the test, blood can still be blotted onto the filter paper.

Ivy Bleeding Time. The Ivy BT is used to screen for inherited disorders of platelet function. It is a crude screen and is performed by measuring how long it takes for bleeding to stop from a fresh cut of defined size. A blood pressure cuff is placed on the arm, and the pressure is raised to 30 mm Hg. A wound is made on the inner surface of the forearm with a sterile lancet, and every 15 seconds, it is blotted with a piece of sterile filter paper. The test is finished when no blood can be absorbed by the filter paper (Fig. 19-8). The normal range for the BT is 1 to 6 minutes, with a time greater than 6 minutes considered abnormal or prolonged. The bleeding time is prolonged in many cases of vWD; Bernard-Soulier disease; Glanzmann's disease (thrombasthenia); by drugs such as aspirin and NSAIDs; and renal failure (uremia).[16]

In the past the Ivy BT was used to screen for thrombocytopenia, functional platelet disorders, and vascular disorders. However, the BT does not discriminate among vessel defects, thrombocytopenia, or platelet quality defects. The test does not reproduce well because no two wounds are the same. In cases of vessel defects, the test is inconsistently abnormal. The BT tends to decrease with advancing age. Test results depend on platelet numbers, quality of the platelets, hematocrit, skin quality, certain components of coagulation, and technique. No correlation is evident between preoperative BT and blood loss and need for transfusion.

The BT can best be used to screen for inherited disorders of platelet function in the patient with a clinical history of mucocutaneous bleeding with normal screening results using the aPTT, PT, and platelet count. In patients with vWD, repeating the screening tests is common including the BT to demonstrate the problem.[16]

Platelet Function Analyzer 100. An in vitro system for the detection of platelet dysfunction, PFA-100 is available in some laboratories. It provides a quantitative measure of platelet function in anticoagulated whole blood. The system consists of a microprocessor-controlled instrument and a disposable test cartridge containing a biologically active membrane. The types of cartridges available are a standard cartridge containing collagen-ADP and a collagen-epinephrine cartridge. The instrument aspirates a blood sample under constant vacuum from the sample reservoir through a capillary and a microscopic aperture cut into the membrane. The presence of either ADP or epinephrine and the high shear rates generated under the standardized flow conditions result in platelet attachment, activation, and aggregation, which slowly builds to a stable platelet plug of the aperture. The time required to obtain full occlusion of the aperture is reported as the "closure time." The collagen epinephrine cartridge is used to screen for aspirin effect. The instrument has been reported to be highly accurate in discriminating normal from abnormal platelet function. The PFA-100 may soon be added to the screening protocol for bleeding disorders.[22-29]

Thrombin Time. In this test, thrombin is added to the patient's blood sample as the activating agent. It converts fibrinogen in the blood to insoluble fibrin, which constitutes the essential portion of a blood clot. Again, a control must be run, and results vary from laboratory to laboratory. This test bypasses the intrinsic, extrinsic and most of the common pathway. For example, patients with hemophilia A or factor V deficiency have a normal TT. Generally, the normal range for the TT test is 9 to 13 seconds, and results in excess of 16 to 18 seconds are considered abnormal or prolonged.

Diagnostic Tests

When one or more of the screening tests are found to be abnormal, the hematologist runs additional tests to pinpoint the bleeding disorder's specific defect.

Platelet Disorders. The platelet count is very effective in identifying patients with thrombocytopenia. It is not effective in identifying patients with disorders of platelet function such as vWD, Bernard-Soulier disease, Glanzmann's disease, uremia, or drug-induced platelet release defects. The BT may be prolonged in these patients but the test results are inconsistent. Platelet aggregation tests, ristocetin-induced agglutination, platelet release reaction, and other tests may have to be performed to demonstrate the nature of the clinical bleeding problem.[16,23]

Additional laboratory tests are needed to establish the diagnosis and type of vWD. These consist of a ristocetin cofactor activity, ristocetin-induced platelet aggregation, immunoassay of vWF, multimeric analysis of vWF, and specific assays for factor VIII.

Disorders of the Intrinsic Pathway. The screening tests show a prolonged aPTT, normal PT, and normal platelet count (except in some cases of vWD). The specific missing factor is identified by specific assays. Mixing studies also are done to exclude factor inhibitors (antibodies to the factor). Some acquired coagulation disorders can produce a prolonged aPTT with a normal PT. These include the Lupus inhibitor, antibodies to factor VIII and heparin therapy.[16,23]

Disorders of the Extrinsic Pathway. A normal aPTT and a prolonged PT suggest a factor VII deficiency, which is very rare, or inhibitors to factor VII. Factor VII deficiency is confirmed by specific assay. Mixing studies are used to rule out factor VII inhibitors.[16]

Disorders of the Common Pathway. A prolonged aPTT and a prolonged PT in a patient with a history of a congenital bleeding disorder indicate a common pathway factor deficiency. A congenital deficiency of factors V and X, prothrombin, or fibrinogen is rare. When both of these tests are prolonged it usually indicates an acquired common pathway factor deficiency. Often multiple factors are found to be deficient. Conditions that can cause both tests to be abnormal are vitamin K deficiency, liver disease, and DIC. A prolonged PT alone usually indicates a common pathway factor deficiency, with the rare exception an inherited factor VII deficiency. When both tests are prolonged in a patient with a history suggestive of a congenital bleeding problem, the next step in the laboratory is to exclude or identify an abnormality of fibrinogen. This involves measuring the plasma fibrinogen level and performing tests for D-dimer of fibrin degradation products. Once a problem involving fibrinogen has been ruled out, the next step is to perform specific assays for deficiency of factors V or X or prothrombin.[16]

Inhibitors of Coagulation. Once a congenital deficiency of a coagulation factor has been demonstrated by laboratory testing, the patient's blood is tested for the presence of antibodies (inhibitor) to the deficient factor. These tests are called *mixing studies* or *inhibitor screens*. A small amount of the patient's blood is added to a normal blood sample. If an inhibitor is present, it will not allow the blood sample to coagulate.[16]

Degradation Products of Fibrin or Fibrinogen. In patients with prolonged aPTT, PT, and TT, the defect involves the last stage of the common pathway, which is the activation of fibrinogen to form fibrin to stabilize the clot. The plasma level of fibrinogen is determined, and if it is within normal limits, then tests for fibrinolysis are performed. These tests examine for the presence of fibrinogen and/or fibrin degradation products. The tests used are the staphylococcal-clumping assay, agglutina-

tion of latex particles coated with antifibrinogen antibody, and the euglobulin clot lysis time.[16]

Disorders with Normal Primary Screening Results. Patients with vascular abnormalities that can cause clinical bleeding may not be identified using the recommended screening tests. The BT is the only test that might be abnormal in these patients. However, it has clearly been shown that the BT is inconsistent in these patients. Thus this test is not reliable for identifying these patients. In most cases the diagnosis is based on history and clinical findings.[16]

A small group of patients give a history of significant bleeding problems and when screened using current recommended methods, will have negative test results. It appears that current methods are unable to demonstrate whatever disorder these patients may have. A clear-cut history of prolonged bleeding after trauma or surgical procedures is always more significant than negative laboratory data.[16]

MEDICAL MANAGEMENT

In this section, conditions that may cause clinical bleeding are considered. The emphasis is placed on the detection of patients with a potential bleeding problem and the management of these patients if surgical procedures are needed.

Disorders affecting the vascular, platelet, coagulation and fibrinolytic phases are discussed. Hemophilia, vWD, Bernard-Soulier disease, DIC, disorders of platelet release, and primary fibrinogenolysis are described in some detail to demonstrate the nature of certain genetic and acquired bleeding disorders. These diseases show the role of various factors involved in the control of excessive bleeding following injury and what happens when these factors are defective. Table 19-2 summarizes the nature of the defects and the medical treatment for excessive bleeding in patients with the disorders covered in this section. Table 19-3 lists the commercial products available to treat bleeding problems in these disorders.

VASCULAR DEFECTS

Bleeding disorders caused by vascular abnormalities may be caused by structural malformation of vessels, hereditary disorders of connective tissue, and acquired connective tissue disorders.

Hereditary hemorrhagic telangiectasia (Osler-Weber-Rendu syndrome) is an autosomal dominant disorder characterized by multiple telangiectatic lesions involving the skin and mucous membranes. These lesions are associated with epistaxis and other bleeding complications.

The bleeding results because of an inherent mechanical fragility of vessels. Lesions usually appear in affected individuals by the age of 40, and increase in number with age.[30]

Ehlers-Danlos disease, osteogensis imperfecta, pseudoxanthoma elasticum, and Marfan syndrome are hereditary disorders of connective tissue that can have associated bleeding problems. In some patients with Ehlers-Danlos disease, an abnormal type III collagen is produced, which leads to vessel wall weakness. These patients are prone to arterial aneurysms and bleeding from spontaneous rupture of vessels. Surgery in these patients should be avoided if at all possible. If surgery must be done, extreme care needs to be taken in manipulation of vascular tissues. In pseudoxanthoma elasticum, a genetic defect leads to calcification of elastic fibers. Bleeding can result when the calcified vessels rupture. Bruising; epistaxis; and bladder, joint, and gastrointestinal bleeding are common.[30]

Acquired connective tissue disorders that can be complicated by bleeding include scurvy, small vessel vasculitis, paraproteins, and skin disorders. In scurvy the deficiency of vitamin C leads to the lack of peptidyl hydroxylation of procollagen, resulting in weakened collagen fibers. The abnormal collagen results in defective perivascular supportive tissues, which can lead to capillary fragility and delayed wound healing. Patients on chronic steroids develop thinning of the connective tissues that can result in bleeding after minor trauma.[30]

Small vessel vasculitis can be caused by a variety of conditions that cause inflammation of small vessels including arterioles, venules, and capillaries. Serum sickness can lead to purpura by immune-complex deposits into vessel walls. Drugs such as penicillin, hydralazine, sulfonamides, and thiazides diuretics and hepatitis have been associated with serum sickness-like reactions.[30]

Various paraproteins, when deposited in the vessel wall, can lead to purpura. Patients with multiple myeloma or systemic amyloidosis may have light chain deposits in the cutaneous blood vessels. The vessels become fragile and lead to purpura after minor trauma.[30]

Hypergammaglobulinemic purpura is a disorder characterized by polyclonal hypergammaglobulinemia associated with recurrent attacks of purpura. Cryoglobulins are immunoglobulins that can be deposited in dermal vessels. These vessels tend to be fragile and purpura often results. Cryoglobulins can be formed in lymphoproliferative, autoimmune or inflammatory disease. Cryofibrinogens are associated with malignancies or inflammatory processes. These patients usually have an elevated total fibrinogen level. Cutaneous purpura is common and is thought to be the result of fibrin thrombi obstructing small dermal vessels.[30]

TABLE 19-2

Medical Treatment of Bleeding Disorders

Condition	Defect	Medical Treatment
von Willebrand's disease	Deficiency or defect in vWF causing poor platelet adhesion and in some cases deficiency of F-VIII	DDAVP EACA F-VIII replacement that retains vWF
Hemophilia A	Deficiency or defect in F-VIII.	DDAVP EACA F-VIII
	Some patients develop antibodies (inhibitors) to F-VIII	Porcine F-VIII, PCC, APCC, F-VIIa, and/or steroids for patients with inhibitors
Hemophilia B	Deficiency or defect in F-IX	F-IX
Primary thrombocytopenia (idiopathic thrombocytopenia)	Platelets destroyed by autoimmune processes	Prednisone IV gamma globulin Platelet transfusion
Secondary thrombocytopenia	Deficiency of platelets because of accelerated destruction or consumption, deficient production, or abnormal pooling	Platelet transfusion
Bernard-Soulier disease	Genetic defect in platelet membrane, absence of Glycoprotein Ib causes disorder in platelet adhesion	Platelet transfusion
Liver disease	Multiple coagulation factor defects Patients with portal hypertension may be thrombocytopenic	Vitamin K Replacement therapy only for serious bleeding or before surgical procedures. DDAVP provides some benefit.
DIC	Multiple coagulation factor defects due to triggered consumption Formation of fibrin and fibrinogen degradation products due to fibrinolysis Thrombocytopenia	Treatment of primary disorder Heparin Cryoprecipitate for replacement of fibrinogen Platelet transfusion Other blood product replacements lead to mixed results

*v*WF, von Willebrand factor; F-VIII, factor VIII; DDAVP (1-desamino-8-D-arginine vasopressin); EACA, epsilon-aminocaproic acid; PCC, prothrombin complex concentrates; APCC, activated prothrombin complex concentrates; F-VIIa, activated factor VII; F-IX, factor IX; DIC, disseminated intravascular coagulation.

Purpura can be associated with the following six skin diseases: Schamberg's progressive pigmentary dermatosis, Majocchi's purpura annularis, eczematoid-like purpura, pigmented purpura lichenoid dermatitis, itching purpura, and lichen aureus.[30] These are commonly classified as pigmented purpura. The pigmented purpuric eruptions consist of red-brown skin pigmentations (caused by hemosiderin deposits) associated with purpura or petechiae. The lesions tend to develop on the lower extremities in middle-age people and are usually chronic.

PLATELET DISORDERS

von Willebrand's Disease

The most common inherited bleeding disorder is vWD, which is caused by an inherited defect involving platelet adhesion. Platelet adhesion is affected be-

TABLE 19-3

Antihemophilic Factor (F-VIII), Factor IX, and Factor VIIa (Recombinant) Concentrates Available in the United States

Factor	Product	Source of Factor	Risk of Infection with HIV and Hepatitis Viruses
Factor VIII (AHF) Concentrates	Alphanate	Human plasma	No
	Hemofil M	Human plasma	No
	Humate-P	Human plasma	Yes (HBV, HCV)
	Koate-HP	Human plasma	No
	Monarc-M	Human plasma	No
	Monoclate-P	Human plasma	No
	Bioclate	Recombinant	No
	Helixate	Recombinant	No
	Kogenate	Recombinant	No
	Recombinate	Recombinant	No
	Hyate: C	Porcine plasma	No
	Antihemophilic Factor	Porcine plasma	No
Factor IX Concentrates	AlphaNine SD	Human plasma	No
	Mononine	Human plasma	No
	BeneFix	Recombinant	No
Factor IX Complex	Konyne-80 factor IX Complex	Human plasma	Yes (low risk)
	Proplex T factor IX Complex	Human plasma	Yes (low risk)
	Profinine SD	Human plasma	Yes (low risk)
	Bebulin VH	Human plasma	Yes (Hepatitis) Yes (low risk for HIV)
Activated Factor IX Complex	Autoplex T	Human plasma	Yes (low risk)
	Feiba VH	Human plasma	Yes (low risk)
Factor VIIa Concentrates	NovoSeven	Recombinant	No

AHF, antihemophilia factor; HIV, human immunodeficiency virus; HBV, hepatitis B virus; HCV, hepatitis C virus.
Modified from Rodgers GM, Greenberg CS: Inherited coagulation disorders. In Lee et al, editors: Wintrobe's clinical hematology, ed 10, Lippincott-Williams and Wilkins, 1999 Philadelphia; Shord SS, Lindley CM: Coagulation products and their uses, Am J Health-Syst Pharm 57(15):1403-1417, 2000.

cause of a deficiency in vWF or a qualitative defect in the factor. The disease has several variants, depending on the severity of genetic expression. Most of the variants are transmitted as autosomal dominant traits (types 1 and 2). These variants of the disease tend to result in mild to moderate clinical bleeding problems. Type 1 disease has a partial deficiency of vWF. The type 2 variants (2A, 2B, 2M, and 2N) have various qualitative defects in vWF. In type 2N the vWF variants have a decreased affinity for factor VIII. Type 3 is transmitted as an autosomal recessive trait that leads to a severe deficiency of vWF.[4]

vWF binds factor VIII in circulating blood. Unbound factor VIII is destroyed in circulation. Thus variants of vWD with a significant reduction in vWF or with a vWF that is unable to bind factor VIII can show signs and symptoms of hemophilia A in addition to those associated with defective platelet adhesion. This is found in all cases of type 3 diseases, in many of the cases with type 2N disease, and in some cases of type 1 disease. Reduction of factor VIII may occur in the other variants of vWD, but when it occurs, it usually is not severe.[4]

Type 1 is the most common form of the vWD. It accounts for about 70% to 80% of the cases of vWD. The

greater the deficiency of vWF in type 1 disease, the more likely are the signs and symptoms of hemophilia A that are found. Type 2A accounts for 15% to 20% of the cases. The other variants of the disease are uncommon. In mild cases, bleeding occurs only after surgery or trauma. The more severe cases, type 2N and type 3, can have spontaneous epistaxis or oral mucosal bleeding.[4,31]

The cause of the platelet dysfunction in vWD is a deficiency or qualitative defect of vWF, which is made from a group of glycoproteins. Megakaryocytes and endothelial cells produce these glycoproteins. They form into a single monomer that polymerizes into huge complexes, which are needed to carry factor VIII and to allow platelets to adhere to surfaces. As stated above, nonbound factor VIII does not survive long in blood. Thus a deficiency of vWF results in a similar decrease in plasma factor VIII levels. The complex of vWF and factor VIII attaches to the surface of circulating platelets, and it is from this location that the factors contribute to hemostasis.[4,31]

The mild variants of vWD are characterized by a history of cutaneous and mucosal bleeding because of a lack of platelet adhesion. In the more severe forms of the disease where factor VIII levels are low, hemarthroses and dissecting intramuscular hematomas are part of the clinical picture. Petechiae are rare in these patients. However, gastrointestinal bleeding, epistaxis, and menorrhagia are very common. Serious bleeding can occur in these patients after trauma or surgical procedures. Patients with the more severe forms of vWD may give a family history of bleeding and also may report having had problems with bleeding after injury or surgery. Patients with mild forms of the disease may have a negative history for bleeding problems. Laboratory investigation is needed to make the diagnosis. Screening laboratory tests may show a prolonged BT, a prolonged aPTT, normal platelet count, normal PT, and normal TT. The PFA-100 has been reported to be very sensitive screening test to identify patients with mild forms of the disease.[23,32] Additional laboratory tests are needed to establish the diagnosis and type of vWD. These consist of a ristocetin cofactor activity, ristocetin-induced platelet aggregation, immunoassay of vWF, multimeric analysis of vWF, and specific assays for factor VIII.[4]

Treatment depends on the clinical condition of the patient and the type of vWD involved. Treatment options that are available include cryoprecipitate, factor VIII concentrates that retain high-molecular-weight vWF multimers (Humate-P, Koate HS) or desmopressin (1-desamino-8-D-arginine vasopressin [DDAVP]). DDAVP can be given parenterally or by nasal spray one hour before surgery. Parenterally, the dose of DDAVP is 0.3 micrograms per kg of body weight, with a maximum dose of 20 to 24 micrograms. The nasal spray, Stimate, contains 1.5 mg

of DDAVP per ml and is given in a dose of 300 mg/kg. Usually one dose is sufficient. If a second dose is needed it is given 8 to 24 hours after the first dose. DDAVP should be used with caution in older patients with cardiovascular disease because of the potential risk of drug-induced thrombosis.[4,33,34]

Patients with type 1 vWD are the best candidates for DDAVP therapy. DDAVP treatment must not be started without prior testing for which variant form of vWD is involved. It is not effective for type 3 vWD and most variants of type 2 vWD. These patients are treated with factor VIII replacement that retains the high-molecular-weight vWF multimers (Humate-P or Koate HS). In patients with type 2 variants with qualitative defects in vWF, Humate-P or Koate HS supplies functional high-molecular-weight vWF and factor VIII for those with decreased levels. In patients with type 3 vWD, these replacement agents supply deficient materials, vWF, and factor VIII. Women are often given oral contraceptive agents to suppress menses and avoid excessive physiologic loss of blood.[4,33,34]

Bernard-Soulier Disease

Bernard-Soulier disease also represents a disorder of platelet adhesion; however, in this disease the platelets are defective and unable to interact with vWF. The basic defect is the absence of a glycoprotein-Ib from the membrane of the platelet. Glycoprotein-Ib appears to function as a receptor for vWF. Laboratory tests show a low platelet count, large platelets, faulty platelet adhesion, and poor aggregation with ristocetin. The only effective therapy for bleeding problems in patients with Bernard-Soulier disease is transfusion with normal platelets.[33,35,36]

Glanzmann's Thrombasthenia

Glanzmann's thrombasthenia is a disorder of platelet aggregation because of genetic quantitative or qualitative abnormality of the platelet membrane complex glycoprotein IIb-IIIa. These platelets can adhere to the subendothelium but cannot bind to fibrinogen, thus a total lack of platelet-to-platelet interaction is evident. Bleeding in this condition is very unpredictable. Treatment consists of platelet transfusions.[35]

Disorders of Platelet Release

Platelets participate directly in the clotting cascade by serving as constituents of factor X and prothrombin-converting complexes through the release of PF3. The potency of this release effect is increased the more often platelets participate in the clotting process. In certain cases, the platelets can fail to complete the release reaction of PF3. Sometimes this is caused by a defective production of thromboxane, other times to a deficiency in the production of dense granule ADP.

Defective thromboxane production almost always results from the administration of antiinflammatory drugs. The best example is aspirin, which inactivates cyclooxygenase, the first enzyme of the prostaglandin-thromboxane synthetic pathway. Other drugs that interfere with thromboxane formation include NSAIDs (indomethacin, phenylbutazone, ibuprofen, sulfinpyrazone); beta-lactam antibiotics; calcium channel blocking drugs (verapamil, diltiazem, and nifedipine); phenytoin; nitrates; phenothiazines; and tricyclic antidepressants. All platelet-release defects produce about the same clinical picture.

In otherwise healthy individuals the impairment of platelet function produced by drugs usually is of no clinical significance. However, in patients with coagulation disorders, uremic or thrombocytopenic patients, and patients receiving heparin or coumarin anticoagulants, drug-induced platelet dysfunction can result in serious bleeding. BT may be normal or prolonged, and platelet function studies often show an absence of secondary-wave aggregation. Patients can be screened with the standard screening tests; if these are normal, surgical procedures can be performed. Surgery can still be performed in patients with a BT that is moderately prolonged (6 to 20 minutes) if no other bleeding disorders are present.[33,35]

Uremia may interfere with platelet function. This effect can be severe with prolonged BTs and grossly abnormal platelet function tests. These patients are in danger of bleeding to death if injury occurs or surgery is performed. They respond to dialysis, cryoprecipitate, or kidney transplant but not to platelet replacement. Although beta-lactam antibiotics (penicillin and cephalothins) can cause platelet dysfunction, usually no treatment is required. Alcohol can, in some undetermined way, impair platelet function, which may be severe enough to contraindicate surgery unless corrective measures are taken.[33,35]

COAGULATION DISORDERS

Hemophilia A

The hemostatic abnormality in hemophilia A is caused by a deficiency or defect of factor VIII. Factor VIII circulates in the plasma bound to vWF. Unbound factor VIII is destroyed. Until recently, factor VIII was thought to be produced by endothelial cells and not by the liver as most coagulation factors. However, when several liver transplant patients with hemophilia had their disease corrected by the transplant, it became clear that liver parenchymal cells also produce factor VIII.[31]

Hemophilia A is an X-linked recessive trait. The defective gene is located on the X chromosome. An affected man will not transmit the disease to his sons; however

all of his daughters will be carriers of the trait because they inherit his X chromosome. A female carrier will transmit the disorder to half of her sons and the carrier state to half of her daughters. The severity of bleeding varies from kindred to kindred. Within a given kindred the clinical severity of the disorder is constant; for example, relatives of severe hemophiliacs are likely to be affected severely. The mutation rate for the responsible gene is unusually high, which explains why a rare condition such as hemophilia A would not die out after several generations. Because of the high mutation rate of the responsible gene, a negative family history is of little value in excluding the possibility of hemophilia A.[4]

The assay of factor VIII activity can be used to identify female carriers of the trait. About 35% of the carriers will show a decrease in factor VIII (about 50% of normal factor VIII levels). The other carriers may have normal levels of factor VIII. Immunoassays for vWF can greatly improve the detection rate of carriers of hemophilia A. Polymorphic DNA probes are now available that are capable of detecting 90% of affected families and 96% or more of carriers.[4]

Hemophilia A can manifest in women. This occurs in a mating between an affected male and a female carrier. One half of the daughters of such a mating would inherit two abnormal X chromosomes, one from the affected father and one from the carrier mother. These daughters would have homozygous hemophilia. In addition, hemophilia may occur in a minority of heterozygous carriers. Rare cases of hemophilia in females have been reported because of a newly mutant gene.[4]

Normal homeostasis requires at least 30% factor VIII activity. Symptomatic patients usually will have factor VIII levels below 5%. Severe forms of the disease occur when the level is less than 1% of normal. Patients with levels between 1% and 5% have moderate disease. Those with factor VIII levels between 5% and 30% have a mild form of the disease. The majority of patients with hemophilia A have factor VIII levels below 5%.[31]

Patients with severe hemophilia A bleed extensively from trivial injuries. However, the most characteristic bleeding manifestations associated with hemophilia A, such as hemarthrosis, often develop without significant trauma. The frequency and severity of bleeding problems in hemophiliacs are generally related to the blood level of factor VIII. Patients with severe hemophilia (less than 1% of factor VIII) experience severe, spontaneous bleeding. Hemarthrosis and soft-tissue hematomas are common. Gastrointestinal and genitourinary bleeding also is common in severe hemophiliacs. Intracranial hemorrhage accounts for about 25% of deaths associated with hemophilia. Spontaneous bleeding may occur in these patients from the mouth, gingiva, lips, tongue, and nose. Those

with moderate hemophilia (1% to 5% of factor VIII) have moderate bleeding with minimal trauma or surgery. Hemarthrosis and soft-tissue hematomas occur less often. Individuals with mild hemophilia (5% to 30% of factor VIII) may develop mild bleeding with major trauma or surgery. Hemarthroses and soft-tissue hematomas are seldom found in these patients.[4,34]

Hemophiliacs usually do not bleed abnormally from small cuts such as razor nicks. However, after larger injuries, bleeding out of proportion to the extent of the injury is common. The bleeding may be massive and life threatening, or it may persist as a slow continuous oozing for days, weeks or months. The onset of excessive bleeding is usually delayed. At the time of surgery or injury hemostasis appears to be normal. Bleeding of sudden onset and serious proportions may develop several hours or even several days later. Venipuncture, if skillfully performed, is of no danger to the hemophiliac because of the elasticity of the venous walls.[4]

A complication that poses great difficulties in the management of patients with hemophilia is the appearance of factor VIII inhibitors. These inhibitors are usually immunoglobulin G (IgG) antibodies. Factor VIII inhibitors develop in patients who have received multiple factor VIII replacement therapy. About 10% to 20% of individuals with hemophilia have factor VIII inhibitors. Half of these patients have inhibitors that remain at low, stable levels (remaining constant over time). The other half have inducible inhibitors whose level increases in response to factor VIII replacement therapy. Patients with inducible inhibitors should not receive human factor VIII replacement for the treatment of bleeding.[4,31,34]

In an emergency, control of bleeding in patients with inducible inhibitors may require high doses of porcine factor VIII (Hyate: C); prothrombin complex concentrates (PCC); activated PCC products (anti-inhibitor coagulant complex [Autoplex]); plasmapheresis; and/or steroids. In some patients, large doses of factor VIII for periods of months or years have been reported to produce immune tolerance to factor VIII.[37]

Recently, the Food and Drug Administration approved recombinant factor VIIa for commercial use in managing acute bleeding in hemophiliacs with inducible inhibitors. Elective surgery in general is avoided in these patients. In contrast, patients with stable low-titer antibodies may respond to higher than normal doses of factor VIII.[4,31,34]

All types of general surgical procedures can now be performed in individuals without inducible inhibitors of factor VIII. The expected rate of postoperative bleeding problems is 6% to 23%; with orthopedic surgery on the knee, it increases up to 40%. Patients with mild deficiency of factor VIII often can undergo surgical procedures when DDAVP is used alone or in combination with epsilon-aminocaproic acid (EACA). DDAVP transiently increases the factor VIII level. DDAVP can be given parenterally, 0.3 mg/kg or an intranasal dose of 300 mg/kg. A second dose can be given if needed 8 to 24 hours after the first dose.[4,8,33,34]

EACA is a potent antifibrinolytic agent that can inhibit plasminogen activators present in oral secretions and stabilize clot formation in oral tissue. Patients with more severe antihemophilic factor (AHF) deficiency require factor VIII replacement. EACA also is given to patients receiving factor replacement. Aspirin, aspirin-containing drugs, and NSAIDs, which impair platelet function and may cause severe bleeding, must not be used. Factor VIIa, a new recombinant product, is now being used for some cases of severe hemophilia A with inducible inhibitors.[4,8,33,34]

Development of gene therapy for hemophilia (factor VIII) and hemophilia B (factor IX, also known as Christmas disease,) is proceeding at a fast pace. Success with both molecules has been demonstrated in mouse and canine models of hemophilia A and B. Clinical approaches to gene therapy for hemophilia in humans include ex vivo gene therapy, in vivo gene therapy, and nonautologous gene therapy.[39] Ex vivo gene therapy involves taking cells from the intended recipients, which are then explanted, genetically modified to secrete factor VIII or IX, and reimplanted into the donor. In vivo gene therapy consists of injecting factor VIII or IX encoding vectors directly into the recipients. In nonautologous gene therapy universal cell lines engineered to secrete factor VIII or IX are enclosed in immunoprotective devices before being implanted into recipients. These techniques have not reached human clinical trials.

Hemophilia B

In hemophilia B (Christmas disease), factor IX is deficient or defective. Hemophilia B is inherited as an X-linked recessive trait. Factor IX levels below 10% have been reported in a few women. Like hemophilia A, the disease primarily manifests in males. Severely affected patients (those with less than 1% of factor IX) are less common than in hemophilia A. The clinical manifestations of the two disorders are identical. Screening laboratory tests results are similar for both diseases. Specific factor assays for factor IX establish the diagnosis. Purified factor IX products (see Table 19-3) are recommended for the treatment of minor and major bleeding. Recombinant factor IX is now available for clinical use.

Disseminated Intravascular Coagulation

DIC has been reported to occur in about 1 in 1000 hospital admissions. The syndrome is associated with a number of disorders such as infection, obstetric complica-

tions, cancer, and snakebites. In fact, worldwide, the most common cause of DIC is snakebites. DIC is a condition that results when the clotting system is activated in all or a major part of the vascular system. Despite widespread fibrin production, the major clinical problem is bleeding, not thrombosis. DIC is caused when large quantities of thromboplastic substances are introduced into the vascular system and "trip" the clotting cascade. Acute DIC can be caused by obstetric complications (abruptio placentae, missed abortion, amniotic fluid embolism); infection; injuries and burns; antigen-antibody complexes; shock; and acidosis.

Symptoms of acute DIC include severe bleeding from small wounds; purpura; and spontaneous bleeding from the nose, gums, gastrointestinal tract, or urinary tract. Traumatic hemolytic anemia can occur because the red blood cells are "sliced" by fibrin strands. On rare occasions, bilateral necrosis of the renal cortex has developed. Chronic DIC may occur in association with certain types of cancer. Malignant cells can release thromboplastic material as they die within the tumor mass. Antigen-antibody complexes associated with systemic lupus erythematosus may cause chronic DIC. In the chronic form of the disease, thrombosis is more common than bleeding.[8,31]

Thromboplastic substances (e.g., antithrombin III, protein C, and phagocytes) can be aided by tissue acidosis and circulatory stasis and when released in large quantities, may swamp the body's defenses. The thromboplastic substances act on factors XII and VII and platelets; the result is triggering every component of the coagulation system. Plasmin is generated by factor XIIa, thrombin, and plasminogen activators released by monocytes and endothelial cells.[8,31]

The excessively generated plasmin splits both fibrinogen and newly generated fibrin, releasing fibrin-split products, which have strong anticoagulation properties of their own. Thrombin, exposed collagen, and tissue factor activate platelets. This activation releases platelet factor-3, which feeds back to accelerate the clotting cascade; in addition, the activated platelets are consumed as they aggregate and adhere to damaged tissue.

The net effect in acute DIC is to reduce the levels of fibrinogen, factors V, VIII, and XIII; decrease the platelet count; and cause numerous fibrin-split products to appear in the blood. The end result is a complex bleeding disorder caused by clotting factors and platelet deficiencies and is complicated by the anticoagulant effects of fibrin-split products. The classic laboratory findings with DIC are prolonged PT, aPTT, TT, Ivy BT; decreased platelet count and serum fibrinogen; and a marked increase in fibrin-split products.[8,31]

The treatment of DIC includes an attempt to reverse the cause; control of the major symptom (either bleeding or thrombosis); and a prophylactic regimen to prevent recurrence in cases of chronic DIC. The consumed coagulation factors need to be replaced along with the missing platelets. Fibrinogen levels must be restored. Cryoprecipitate is used if bleeding is the major problem. Fresh frozen plasma also can be used. If thrombosis is the major problem (early in the process), IV heparin is used. Long-term heparin infusion is used for prophylaxis in cases of chronic DIC.[8,31]

FIBRINOLYTIC DISORDERS

Fibrinolysis and Fibrinogenolysis

Primary fibrinogenolysis may develop if active plasmin is generated in the circulation at a time when the clotting cascade is not in operation. It can occur in patients with liver disease, cancer of the lung, cancer of the prostate, or heatstroke. Severe bleeding results from the depletion of fibrinogen (split by plasmin) and the formation of fibrin-split products (with their anticoagulant properties) from the fibrinogen.[31]

Laboratory test results are similar to those in DIC, with the following important exceptions:
1. Platelet count is normal.
2. Euglobulin lysis time is shortened in primary fibrinogenolysis and is normal in DIC (the euglobulin lysis test is a crude measurement of circulating plasmin).
3. The fibrin-split products of primary fibrinogenolysis clump with the staphylococcal clumping assay (same for DIC), but no fibrin monomers can be released by paracoagulation with ethanol (in DIC, a loose complex of fibrin monomers is released from fibrin-split products and then polymerizes to form a gel).[31]

Fibrinogenolysis can be treated with EACA or tranexamic acid, which inhibits both plasmin and plasmin activators; however, these drugs can be dangerous if used in DIC because diffuse thromboses may result. Thus excluding the diagnosis of DIC before starting antifibrinolytic agents is very important. Using a specific test such as D-dimer measurement can do this.[8,31]

RISK OF INFECTION WITH REPLACEMENT PRODUCTS

The use of cryoprecipitates, factor VIII concentrates, and fresh frozen plasma carries several important risks. For example, transmission of hepatitis B virus (HBV); hepatitis C virus (HCV); and the human immunodeficiency virus (HIV) can occur.[4]

In the 1980s, more than 90% of multiply transfused hemophiliacs became HIV positive and ultimately developed AIDS. Many of these patients have died from the

disease. The advent of sterile concentrates, together with rigid donor testing started in 1985, and the availability of recombinant products have greatly reduced the risk of HIV infection with blood product administration. AIDS cases in association with hemophilia B have been less common, probably because rarity of the condition. A look at hemophilia mortality from 1900 to 1990 demonstrates the terrible impact of HIV infection. Survival increased in 1970 when factor VIII replacement first became available to 1980 with a median life expectancy of 68 years. From 1980 to 1990 this decreased to 49 years. Most of this effect was caused by infection with HIV from contaminated blood products.

The identification of an etiologic agent for AIDS, the development of a screening test to determine exposure to the AIDS virus, and the heating of blood concentrates all have enabled the blood pool in the United States to become "safe" (current risk for HIV infection from transfusion is less than 1:660,000).[40] However, because of the risk to individuals needing repeated replacement of blood products, alternate sources and substitutes for therapeutic blood components are used.[41-43] Porcine factor VIII concentrate is used for patients with lower levels of inhibitor to factor VIII. Ultrapure preparations of AHF are now available (see Table 19-3), produced by recombinant DNA or monoclonal antibody techniques.[31,42]

THROMBOSIS AND ANTITHROMBOTIC THERAPY

Thrombosis is the formation, from the components of blood, of an abnormal mass within the vascular system. It involves the interaction of vascular, cellular, and humoral factors within a flowing stream of blood. Thrombosis and the complicating emboli that can result are one of the most important causes of sickness and death in developed countries. Thrombosis is of greater overall clinical importance in terms of morbidity and mortality than all of the hemorrhagic disorders combined. Excessive activation of coagulation or inhibition of anticoagulant mechanisms may result in hypercoagulability and thrombosis. Injury to the vessel wall, alterations in blood flow, and changes in the composition of blood are major factors leading to thrombosis.[1]

Inherited thrombotic disorders can be caused by deficiency of antithrombin III; heparin cofactor II; protein C; protein S; thrombomodulin; plasminogen; t-PA; an activated protein C resistance (factor V Leiden); dysfibrinogenemia; and homocysteinemia. Acquired deficiencies of most of the above also have been reported. Patients should be considered for laboratory evaluation for inherited thrombotic disorders if they are less than 45 years of age with recurrent thrombosis. In addition, patients who have had a single thrombotic event and have a family history of thrombosis should be tested.[1]

The pathologic basis for arterial thrombosis involves atherosclerotic vascular disease associated with platelet thrombi. Thrombin is a major mediator in this type of thrombosis. Drug therapy for arterial thrombi involves agents with antithrombin and antiplatelet activity. Venous thrombi usually occur in normal vessel wall, with stasis or hypercoagulability being the major predisposing factors. Drugs that prevent thrombin formation or lyse fibrin clots are the major agents used to treat venous thrombi.[1]

Heparin is used in high-dose to treat thromboembolism (intravenous [IV] bolus of 5000 units and IV infusion over a 5- to 10-day period) and in low-dose form as a prophylaxis of thromboembolism. Heparin itself is not an anticoagulant. Plasma antithrombin III (ATIII) is the actual anticoagulant with heparin serving as a catalyst. Patients over the age of 40 years who are going to have major surgery should receive prophylaxis with graded compression elastic stockings, low-dose heparin therapy, or intermittent pneumatic compression. If heparin prophylaxis is used, 5000 units are given subcutaneously (SQ) 2 hours before surgery and every 8 to 12 hours until the patient is ambulatory. Low-molecular weight heparin can be used instead of regular heparin and is rapidly becoming the treatment of choice. Patients undergoing total hip or knee replacement should receive postoperative low-molecular weight heparin.[1]

Standard heparin consists of an unfractionated heterogeneous mixture of polysaccharide chains with a mean molecular weight of 12,000 to 16,000 Daltons. It inhibits factor Xa and thrombin equally. Treatment with standard heparin usually consists of IV infusion in a hospital setting and requires monitoring with aPPT. Standard heparin has a half-life of 1 to 2 hours. Low-molecular weight heparin (LMWH) is prepared by depolymerization of unfractionated heparin chains yielding heparin fragments with a mean molecular weight of 4000 to 6000 Da. LMWH preparations have greater activity against factor Xa than thrombin. LMWHs exhibit less binding to plasma proteins, endothelial cells, and macrophages than standard heparin. Thus they have better bioavailability when administered SQ, longer half-lives, and more predictable anticoagulant effects. The LMWHs are administered SQ in the abdomen. The dosage is based on body weight and no laboratory monitoring is needed. The half-life of the LMWHs is about 2 to 4 hours. Treatment with the LMWHs can occur on an outpatient basis.[41-46]

Six LMWH preparations have been approved for the treatment of deep-vein thrombi and asymptomatic pul-

monary embolism: *ardeparin* (Normiflo); *dalteparin* (Fragmin); *enoxaparin* (Lovenox); *nadroparin* (Fraxiparine); *reviparin* (Clivarin); and *tinzaparin* (Innohep). Their mean molecular weight ranges from 4200 Da for enoxaparin to 6000 Da for ardeparin and dalteparin. Their anti-Xa:thrombin ratio varies from 1.9 for ardeparin and tinzaparin to 3.8 for enoxaparin.[45]

Patients with deep vein thrombosis or pulmonary embolism are usually treated with IV heparin in dosages sufficient to prolong the aPTT to a range corresponding to a heparin level of 0.2 to 0.4 micro/ml (1.5 to 2.5 times control value). The heparin therapy is continued for at least 5 days or longer. Oral anticoagulation with warfarin is started early and should overlap the heparin treatment for 4 to 5 days. The heparin treatment is stopped after 5 to 10 days and the warfarin treatment is continued for at least 3 months. Complications with heparin treatment include thrombocytopenia or thrombosis. Starting warfarin therapy early after heparin is first started minimizes these complications. Overdose of heparin can cause significant clinical bleeding.[1]

Warfarin and Coumadin are oral anticoagulants that inhibit the biosynthesis of the vitamin K–dependent coagulation proteins (factors VII, IX, and X and prothrombin). These drugs are bound to albumin, metabolized by hydroxylation by the liver, and excreted in the urine. The PT is used to monitor warfarin therapy because it measures three of the vitamin K–dependent coagulation proteins: factors VII and X, and prothrombin. The PT is particularly sensitive to factor VII deficiency. Therapeutic anticoagulation with warfarin takes 4 to 5 days.[1]

The PT has been shown to be imprecise and variable. Little comparability of PT values taken in different laboratories is seen. These differences are caused by the source of thromboplastin (human brain, rabbit brain); the brand of thromboplastin; and the type of instrumentation used. This has caused problems with bleeding as a result of a high degree of anticoagulation based on an artificially low PT.[47]

In 1985 the International Committee on Thrombosis and Homeostasis requested that all the lots of thromboplastin have their international sensitivity index (ISI) indicated. The ISI establishes the reference standard of 1.0 to human brain-derived thromboplastin. An ISI greater than 1.0 designates a less sensitive thromboplastin, whereas a value less than 1.0 indicates a more sensitive thromboplastin. This allowed uniformity of the results by the introduction of the INR calculated by the formula, $INR = (PTR)^{ISI}$, the prothrombin time ratio (PTR) corresponding to the patients' PT divided by that of reference control plasma. The INR index allows for the interpretation of PT with respect to other laboratories.[47,48]

The consequences of the absence of uniformity in the control of anticoagulant therapy are important and serious. The principal complication of oral anticoagulants is bleeding and stroke. Moreover, the global mortality caused by hemorrhagic complications is about 0.1% to 0.5% for treatments of short duration and much higher in prolonged therapy. The uncertainty concerning the degree of anticoagulation inherent in the use of a single PTR may be the source of many of these bleeding or thromboembolic complications.[47,48]

A study reported by Andrews[49] demonstrated the advantage of the INR system. The rate of bleeding in anticoagulated patients monitored using the PTR was 6.7% (1.2% major and 5.5% minor), and with INR, it was 2.9% (0.00% major and 2.9% minor).

The INR system has slowly been accepted and adapted by clinicians and laboratories but still has minor problems with use of thromboplastins with high ISI values, incorrect ISI values assigned by manufactures, and laboratories using a different reagent-instrument combinations than used by the manufacture.[1,50-54]

The recommended INR goal for a patient on low-intensity warfarin therapy is 2.5 with a range of 2.0 to 3.0. With a patient on high-intensity anticoagulation therapy, the INR goal is 3.0 with a range of 2.5 to 3.5.[1,46,55] Table 19-4 shows the conditions recommended for low-intensity and high-intensity warfarin therapy and the recommended INR and PTR values.

Scardi[56] reported on new strategies being developed for managing care of patients taking warfarin for anticoagulation therapy. One promising modality has the patients performing their PT measurements at home. This model is possible because of point-of-care instrumentation for prothrombin testing. One instrument now available is the CoaguChek (Hoffman La Roche).[57] These portable monitors can measure a PT from a finger-stick sample of whole blood and provide results within seconds. Whether this may turn out to be a management strategy that will maximize the benefit-risk ratio of anticoagulant therapy has not yet been determined.

ANTIPLATELET DRUGS

Platelets are an important contributor to arterial thrombi. Antiplatelet treatment has been reported to reduce overall mortality form vascular disease by 15% and reduce nonfatal vascular complications by 30%. Aspirin is the prototypical antiplatelet drug. Aspirin exerts its antithrombotic action by irreversibly inhibiting platelet cyclooxygenase, preventing synthesis of thromboxane A_2, and impairing platelet secretion and aggregation. Aspirin is the least expensive, most widely used, and most widely studied antiplatelet drug. NSAIDs such as ibuprofen and

TABLE 19-4

Recommended Therapeutic Range for Warfarin Therapy

Indication	INR	PROTHROMBIN TIME RATIO		
		ISI = 1.0	ISI = 1.8	ISI = 2.8
Low-Intensity	2.0 to 3.0	2.0 to 3.0	1.5 to 1.8	1.3 to 1.5
Prophylaxis of venous thrombosis (high-risk surgery)				
Treatment of venous thrombosis				
Treatment of pulmonary embolism				
Prevention of systemic embolism				
Tissue heart valves				
Acute MI				
Atrial fibrillation				
Valvular heart disease				
High-Intensity	2.5 to 3.5	2.5 to 3.5	1.7 to 2.0	1.4 to 1.6
Mechanical Prosthetic heart valves				
Prevention of recurrent myocardial infarction				
Treatment of thrombosis associated with antiphospholipid antibodies				

INR, International normalized ratio; ISI, international sensitivity index.
From Hirsh J, Fuster V: AHA medical/scientific statement: guide to anticoagulant therapy, part 2: oral coagulants. *Circulation* 89(3):1469-1480, 1994; Rodgers GM: Thrombosis and antithrombotic therapy. In Lee et al, editors: Wintrobe's clinical hematology, ed 10, Philadelphia, 1999, Williams and Wilkins.

indobufen act as reversible inhibitors of cyclooxygenase and are used clinically to some extent. Dipyridamole, which increases cyclicademosine monophosphate; Ticlopidine and Clopidogrel, which inhibit the fibrinogen receptor glycoprotein IIb-IIIa; Abciximab, a monoclonal antibody (C7E3-Fab); and Integrelin, Tyrafiban, and Lamifiban, which are peptide disintegrin inhibitors (platelet fibrinogen receptor inhibitors) are all used as antiplatelet agents. However, dipyridamole alone has been reported to be ineffective and now when used is given with aspirin.[1]

PREOPERATIVE HEMOSTASIS EVALUATION

Rodgers[16] does not recommend routine preoperative screening for potential bleeding disorders in patients with a negative history and clinical findings scheduled for minor surgery such as dental extractions, biopsy procedures, and others. He recommends that patients with a negative history for excessive bleeding scheduled for major surgery should be screened using the platelet count and aPTT. Patients with an equivocal bleeding history scheduled for major surgery involving hemostatic impairment (heart bypass machine) should be screened using PT, aPTT, platelet count, BT, factor XIII assay and euglobulin clot lysis time. All patients with a positive bleeding history scheduled for minor or major surgery should be screened using PT, aPTT, platelet count, BT, factor XIII assay, and euglobulin clot lysis time.[16] If these tests are negative, Rodgers[16] suggests the following tests be performed before the surgery, factors VIII and IX assays, TT, alpha-2-antiplasmin assay, post-aspirin BT, and factor XI assay.

Our suggestions for dentistry are in large part based on the recommendations of Rodgers.[16] Patients with a significant history of a bleeding disorder should be referred to a hematologist for all screening and diagnostic testing. Patients with a history suggestive of a possible bleeding disorder can be screened by the dentist using a commercial laboratory or referred to a hematologist for

screening. If the dentist orders the screening tests we recommend that the aPTT, PT, TT, platelet count, and PFA-100 (if available) be used. If the PFA-100 is not available, then the Ivy BT is suggested.

DENTAL MANAGEMENT

PATIENT IDENTIFICATION

The four methods by which the dentist can detect the patient who may have a bleeding problem are listed below. The skill developed with these methods determines how well dentists can protect certain patients from the danger of excessive bleeding following dental surgical treatment. The four methods are (1) a good history, (2) physical examination, (3) screening clinical laboratory tests, and (4) observation of excessive bleeding following a surgical procedure (Box 19-8).

HISTORY AND SYMPTOMS

A good history is the best single screening procedure to identify the patient with a possible bleeding disorder. The history should include questions concerning the following six topics:
1. Presence of bleeding problems in relatives
2. Excessive bleeding following operations, surgical procedures and tooth extractions
3. Excessive bleeding following trauma
4. Use of drugs for prevention of coagulation or chronic pain
5. Past and present illness
6. Occurrence of spontaneous bleeding

BLEEDING PROBLEMS IN RELATIVES

The male offspring of parents with a family history of hemophilia are at risk for the disease. Children of a parent with vWD, type 1, are at risk, with about 33% of the children affected. Children of parents with a hereditary disorder of connective tissue or hereditary hemorrhagic telangiectasia are at risk for a bleeding disorder. In the rare cases of a family history of disorders of platelet function, such as Bernard-Soulier syndrome or Glanzmann's thrombasthenia, the bleeding disorder can be passed to offspring.

Bleeding Problems after Operations and Tooth Extraction
Each new patient should be questioned concerning excessive bleeding after major or minor operations. The number of individuals who have had an appendectomy, tonsillectomy, or tooth extraction is large. Persons who

---

BOX 19-8

Detection of the Patient Who Is a "Bleeder"

1. History
   a. Bleeding problems in relatives
   b. Bleeding problems after operations and tooth extractions
   c. Bleeding problems after trauma (cuts, and so on)
   d. Medications that may cause bleeding problems
      (1) Aspirin
      (2) Anticoagulants
      (3) Long-term antibiotic therapy
   e. Presence of illnesses that may have associated bleeding problems
      (1) Leukemia
      (2) Liver disease
      (3) Hemophilia
      (4) Congenital heart disease
      (5) Renal disease—uremia
   f. Spontaneous bleeding from nose, mouth, ears, and so on
2. Examination findings
   a. Jaundice, pallor
   b. Spider angiomas
   c. Ecchymoses
   d. Petechiae
   e. Oral ulcers
   f. Hyperplastic gingival tissues
   g. Hemarthrosis
3. Screening laboratory tests
   a. PT
   b. aPTT
   c. TT
   d. PFA-100 or BT
   e. Platelet count
4. Surgical procedure—excessive bleeding following surgery may be first clue to underlying bleeding problem

PT, Prothrombin time; aPTT, activated partial thromboplastin time; TT, thrombin time; BT, bleeding time (Ivy); PFA-100, platelet function analyzer.

---

have had such procedures without a bleeding problem do not have a significant inherited coagulation disorder. However, although they did not have a significant acquired bleeding problem at the time the operative procedure was performed, this does not mean that they are free of such a problem that could have been acquired since the last surgery. Establishing the length of prolonged

bleeding and the amount of blood that was lost is important. For example, normally a small amount of blood may ooze from an extraction site for several hours or so. Blood oozing from an extraction site for several days is abnormal unless a local infection was present. Some blood may be found on a pillow the next day after an extraction, but to find the pillow soaked with blood would be abnormal. Another area to ask about is the need for blood replacement after surgery; this would be most important if it was required during the postoperative period. The patient should be asked if the excessive bleeding started soon after minor surgical procedures or was it delayed in its onset. When excessive bleeding has been reported after minor surgery, the patient should be asked if he or she sought medical attention and treatment. If treatment was rendered, the dentist should attempt to establish what type of treatment was given.

Bleeding Problems After Trauma

All new dental patients should be asked if they have experienced any recent trauma, and, if so, whether excessive bleeding followed it. The more severe the trauma, the more likely the presence of an underlying bleeding disorder. Small cuts in patients with coagulation disorders may not cause excessive bleeding initially because the vascular and platelet phases may be sufficient to control blood loss, even if a defect in coagulation is found. However, small cuts in patients with platelet or vascular deficiencies usually result in excessive bleeding, and in patients with severe coagulation disorders, it may lead to bleeding several hours after the injury.

When excessive bleeding occurs after trauma in patients with coagulation disorders, it usually is delayed because the immediate control of blood loss by vasoconstriction, extravascular pressure, and platelet plugging proceeds normally. However, when these effects begin to lessen, they are not replaced by the formation of a good clot of fibrin as happens in normal coagulation. This is when the bleeding occurs in the patient who has a coagulation defect.

Medications That May Cause Bleeding

All new and recall dental patients should be asked if they are taking an anticoagulant drug such as heparin (IV); low-molecular weight heparin (SQ); dipyridamole; or a coumarin derivative. If the patient is receiving one of these drugs, the dentist should contact the patient's physician to determine the degree of anticoagulation being maintained and the purpose for which the drug is being used. All patients should be asked if they have been taking aspirin or drugs that contain aspirin. Patients also should be asked if they have had recent treatment with a broad-spectrum antibiotic and about excessive use of alcohol.

Presence of Illnesses with Associated Bleeding Problems

The past and current medical status of patients needs to be reviewed. They should be questioned concerning a history of liver disease, biliary tract obstruction, malabsorption problems, infectious diseases, genetic coagulation disorders, chronic inflammatory diseases, chronic renal disease, or leukemia or other types of cancer and whether they have received radiation therapy or been exposed to large amounts of radiation. It must be determined if patients with cancer are being treated with chemotherapy, since this can cause significant suppression of platelet production.

Spontaneous Bleeding

Each patient should be asked about a history of spontaneous bleeding, including gingival, nasal, urinary, rectal, gastrointestinal, oral, pulmonary, and vaginal sources of bleeding. If spontaneous bleeding has occurred, the frequency, amount of blood lost, appearance of the blood, and steps that were necessary to stop it should be determined.

SCREENING LABORATORY TESTS

The dentist can use five clinical laboratory tests to screen patients for bleeding disorders (Box 19-9). These tests are the platelet count, PFA-100, APTT, PT, and TT. If the PFA-100 is not available, then the Ivy BT can be used.

The platelet count is ordered to screen for thrombocytopenia. The PFA-100 is used to screen for functional defects of platelets. The BT is used to screen for functional platelet disorders and vascular disorders but the results tend to be inconsistent. The BT is most helpful in cases of congenital bleeding disorders with mucocutaneous sign and symptoms. The aPTT test is used to measure the status of the intrinsic and common pathways of coagulation. This test reflects the ability of blood still within vessels in the area of injury to coagulate. It will be prolonged in coagulation disorders affecting the intrinsic and common pathways (hemophilia, liver disease) and also in cases of excessive fibrinolysis.

The PT test is used to measure the status of the extrinsic and common pathways of coagulation. This test reflects the ability of blood lost from vessels in the area of injury to coagulate. It will be prolonged in cases of factor VII deficiency and disorders affecting the common pathway and fibrinolysis. This test usually is normal in patients with intrinsic pathway defects (hemophilia).[58,59]

The TT test uses thrombin as the test-activating agent; hence, it measures only the ability of fibrinogen to form an initial clot. Since fibrin-degradation products tend to prolong the TT, this test becomes reasonably sensitive for fibrinolysis disorders. When done with the PT and aPTT tests, it allows for the identification of coagulation dis-

Screening Laboratory Tests for the Detection of a Potential "Bleeder"

1. PT—activated by tissue thromboplastin
   a. Tests extrinsic and common pathways
   b. Control should be run
   c. Normal (11 to 15 seconds, depending on laboratory)
   d. Control msut be in normal range
2. aPTT—Initiated by phospholipid platelet substitute and activated by addition of contact activator (kaolin)
   a. Tests intrinsic and common pathways
   b. Control should be run
   c. Normal (25 to 35 seconds, depending on laboratory)
   d. Control must be in normal range
3. TT—activated by thrombin
   a. Tests ability to form initial clot from fibrinogen
   b. Controls should be run
   c. Normal (9 to 13 seconds)
4. PFA-100*
   a. Tests platelet function
   b. Normal if adequate number of platelets of good quality present
   c. Normal (60 to 120 seconds)
5. Platelet count
   a. Tests platelet phase for adequate number of platelets
   b. Normal (140,000 to 400,000/mm^3).
   c. Clinical bleeding problem can occur if less than 50,000/mm^3

*If the platelet function analyzer 100 (PFA-100) is not available, use by the Ivy BT, which tests platelet function and vascular phase (often inconsistent results) as normal 1 to 6 minutes.

Selection of Screening Laboratory Tests for Detecting the Patient with a Potential Bleeding Problem Based on History and Examination Findings

1. No clinical or historical clues to bleeding problem; excessive bleeding occurs after surgery
2. History or clinical findings or both suggest possible bleeding problem but no clues to cause the following:
   PT
   aPTT
   TT
   PFA-100 or BT
   Platelet count
3. Aspirin therapy: PFA-100 or BT
4. Coumarin therapy: PT
   Low-molecular weight heparin: aPTT
5. Possible liver disease: Platelet count, PT
6. Chronic leukemia: Platelet count
7. Malabsorption syndrome or long-term antibiotic therapy: PT
8. Renal dialysis (heparin): aPTT
9. Vascular wall alteration: BT (results often inconsistent)
10. Primary fibrinogenolysis (active plasmin in circulation), cancers (lung, prostate): TT

orders involving the last "stage" of the sequence. For example, if the PT, aPTT, and TT were all prolonged, the problem in the coagulation system would be at the point of conversion of fibrinogen to the initial clot.

If positive, the results of these screening tests direct the hematologist to the possible source of a bleeding disorder and allow for the selection of more specific tests to identify the nature of the defect.[4,8,14,16]

MEDICAL CONSIDERATIONS

No surgical procedures should be performed on a patient suspected of having a bleeding problem based on history and examination findings. Such a patient should be screened by the dentist ordering the appropriate clinical laboratory tests or referred to a hematologist for screening. Patients screened by the dentist with abnormal test results should be referred to a hematologist for diagnosis, treatment and management recommendations. Patients under medical care who may have a bleeding problem should not receive dental treatment until consultation with the patient's physician has taken place and appropriate preparations have been made to avoid excessive bleeding after dental procedures.

Ten clinical situations often present the dentist with the problem of whether a given patient has a bleeding problem. Each of these situations is discussed in detail (Box 19-10).

No Clinical or Historical Clues to Bleeding Problem

A person with a potential bleeding problem may have no subjective or objective findings that suggest the condition. The first indication may be prolonged bleeding after a dental surgical procedure. For this, local measures should be taken to control the bleeding; if these fail, a

hematologist may have to be consulted. Once the problem is under control, the patient should be screened with the appropriate laboratory tests (PT, aPTT, BT, platelet count, and TT) by the dentist through a commercial clinical laboratory or by a hematologist.

History or Clinical Findings, or Both, Suggest a Possible Bleeding Problem But Not Clues to Its Cause

When no clues are evident regarding the cause of a potential bleeding problem in a patient, all five screening laboratory tests should be performed. The stronger the history of excessive bleeding, the more advantageous it is to refer the patient to a hematologist for screening and diagnosis. In other cases the patient's physician can order these tests, or the dentist can order them from a clinical laboratory facility (see Box 19-9).

Aspirin Therapy

Patients receiving aspirin therapy may have a bleeding problem based on the drug's effect on platelets. Some of these patients have been receiving high doses (20 g or more, or four or more tablets) of aspirin each day for a prolonged period (more than a week). Others are taking one tablet a day or one every other day to prevent coronary thrombosis. Even this low dosage of aspirin is enough to inhibit platelet thromboxane production and platelet aggregation. Although these are nonreversible effects, they may or may not be clinically significant.[8,60] If the BT is moderately prolonged in these patients, they will not experience excessive bleeding with minor surgery unless some other bleeding disorder is present.

The best screening test for aspirin effect is the PFA-100, if this is not available then the Ivy BT can be used. Although aspirin affects platelets and the coagulation process through its effect on platelet release, it does not usually lead to a significant bleeding problem unless the BT is greater than 20 minutes. If surgery must be performed under emergency conditions, and the BT is in excess of 20 minutes, DDAVP can be used to shorten the BT. This should be done in consultation with the patient's physician or hematologist.[8,36,61] On a less urgent basis, with approval from the physician, the aspirin can be discontinued for three days, which allows for a sufficient number of new platelets to arrive into the circulation.

NSAIDs can also inhibit platelet cyclooxygenase, thereby blocking the formation of thromboxane A_2. These drugs produce a systemic bleeding tendency by impairing thromboxane-dependent platelet aggregation and thus prolonging the BT. However, these drugs inhibit cyclooxygenase reversibly, and the duration of their action depends on the specific drug dose, serum level, and half-life. Generally if the clinician waits three half-lives of the drug, levels will be sufficiently elimi-

nated to allow for normal platelet function to return. It should be remembered that the clinical risks of bleeding with aspirin or nonaspirin NSAIDs are enhanced by the use of alcohol or anticoagulants and associated conditions such as advanced age, liver disease, and other co-existing coagulopathies.[60]

Coumarin Therapy

Box 19-11 summarizes the dental management of the patient taking warfarin or Coumadin. If the history establishes that a patient is receiving one of the coumarin drugs, the dentist should consult the patient's physician concerning the reason for taking the drug and the level of anticoagulation reported in terms of the PT or INR. Most patients are held at a PT ratio of about 1.5 to 2 times normal or an INR of about 2.0 to 3.0, whereas patients with mechanical prosthetic heart valves are held at a PT ratio of 2.0 to 3.0 or a INR of 2.5 to 3.5. Most physicians are aware of the recommendations of the American Medical Association and the American Dental Association suggesting that the patient be at a level of anticoagulation of about 1.5 to 2 times the normal PT before a surgical procedure is attempted. If bleeding occurs, local measures can be used to control it.[58]

In patients with a PT greater than 2.0 or a INR greater than 3.0 the dentist needs to consult with the patient's physician regarding possible reduction of the anticoagulant dosage before surgery. Minor surgery can be safely performed in patients with PT of up to 2.5 and INR up to 3.5. In general, treating these patients without reducing the dose of the anticoagulant is safer. If the physician wants the dose reduced, he or she will give directions to the patient to reduce the dosage of anticoagulant. Current information does not support stopping the drug, which increases the risk for thrombotic events. At least 3 to 4 days must pass for the effect of the reduced dosage to be reflected in a decrease in the PT or INR.[8]

On the day of surgery, the physician or dentist should order a PT or INR before the procedure to be certain that the desired reduction of anticoagulation effect has occurred.

A review by Wahl[62] found little to no risk of significant bleeding after dental surgical procedures in patients with a PT of 1.5 to 2 times normal. Wahl also reported that data showed little risk, even if the PT is up to 2.5 times normal. A study by Benoliel[63] also suggested that dental surgery could be performed without major bleeding complications in patients receiving anticoagulation therapy at higher than two times the normal PT. Devani[64] reported no differences in clinical bleeding problems in patients whose anticoagulant was discontinued (mean INR = 1.6) and those who remained on their medication (mean INR = 2.7). The authors concluded that there was no justification to alter

BOX 19-11

Dental Management of the Patient Taking Warfarin or Coumadin for Whom Invasive Procedures Are Planned

Preoperative

Consult
Confirm diagnosis
Status of medical condition
Confirm PTR or INR level
Type of surgery or invasive procedures planned
Need for dosage reduction
• Based on level of anticoagulation
• Based on the amount of expected bleeding

Dental
Free of acute injection; if infection present treat prior to performing elective dental care
Good oral hygiene

Level of anticoagulation and need for altering dosage to avoid excessive bleeding
PTR (1.5 to 2.0) or INR (2.0 to 3.0): Dosage does not need to be altered
PTR (2.0 to 2.5) or INR (2.5 to 3.5): Dosage may be altered
PTR (2.5 or >) or INR (3.5 or >): Delay invasive procedure until dosage decreased

Decision is made to alter dosage of anticoagulation medication
Physician will reduce patient's dosage
Affect of reduced dosage takes 3 to 5 days
Dental appointment needs to be scheduled within 2 days once desired reduction in PTR or INR has been confirmed

Operative
Confirm status of PTR or INR on day of surgery
Use good surgical technique
Control bleeding by local means
• Pressure packs
• Gelfoam/thrombin
• Oxycel
• Surgicel
• Microfibrillar collagen
• Tranexamic acid
• Fibrin glue (not available in United States)

Postoperative
Avoid aspirin and NSAIDs (Celecoxib and Rofecoxib can be used in reduced dosage)
Acetaminophen can be used with reduced dosage and can be combined with codeine
Tell patient to call if bleeding occurs during first 24 to 48 hours
See patient in 48 to 72 hours and observe for the following:
• Healing
• Infection: Treat if present
• Bleeding: Use local means to control is present
Patients whose anticoagulant dosage was reduced
• If free of complications (if not treat and once controlled)
• Call patient's physician and have patient returned to normal anticoagulation dosage

PTR, Prothrombin time ratio (patient's PT/control PT); INR, international normalized ratio [INR = (PTR)^{ISI}]; ISI, international sensitivity index, based on sensitivity of thromboplastin used in PT; NSAIDs, nonsteroidal antiinflammatory drugs.

coumadin dosage if an INR of 4 or less is found. Giglio[65] has suggested the following guidelines: single tooth extraction or minimally invasive procedures, indicated if INR is less than 4; for cases where moderate bleeding is expected, reduce the INR, depending on risk to patient; adjust coumadin to an INR less than 3 if significant bleeding is expected; and avoid any surgery if the INR is greater than 5. Based on this information, our suggestion is to obtain medical consultation to reduce the level of anticoagulation before surgery is performed on patients with PT values higher than 2.5 or INR values higher than 3.5.

If infection is present, surgery should be avoided until the infection has been treated. When the patient is free of acute infection and the PT is 2.5 times normal or less or the INR is less than 3.5 or less, surgery can be performed. The procedure should be done with as little trauma as possible. If excessive postoperative bleeding occurs, Gelfoam with thrombin can be used to control it. In some patients, it may be helpful to construct a splint before surgery to cover the surgical area, which will protect the clot, and Gelfoam with thrombin can be packed beneath the splint. In addition, primary closure over the sockets is desirable.

Oxycel, Surgicel, or microfibrillar collagen may be used in place of Gelfoam. However, thrombin should not be used in combination with these agents because it is inactivated

as a result of pH factors, thus representing an additional cost with no real benefits. Local application of an inhibitor of fibrinolysis also can be used (tranexamic acid).[66]

The dentist must be aware that certain drugs will affect the action of warfarin (Coumadin). Drugs the dentist may use that potentiate the anticoagulant action of warfarin are acetaminophen, metronidazole, salicylates, broad-spectrum antibiotics, erythromycin and the new COX-2-specific inhibitors (Celecoxib and Rofecoxib). Other drugs that have the same effect are cimetidine, chloral hydrate, phenytoin, propranolol, and thyroid drugs. Drugs the dentist may use that will antagonize the anticoagulant action of warfarin are barbiturates, steroids, and nafcillin. Other drugs that have the same effect are carbamazepine, cholestyramine, griseofulvin, rifampin, and trazodone.[1,67]

Postoperative pain control can be obtained by using minimal dosage of acetaminophen with or without codeine. Aspirin and NSAIDs must be avoided. Although when used in the indicated dosage, the COX-2-specific inhibitors (Celecoxib and Rofecoxib) do not affect platelet count, PT, and PPT and do not inhibit platelet aggregation. However, they can increase the PT and INR in patients taking warfarin and if used, the dosage should be reduced.

Heparin Therapy

Most patients treated with standard heparin are hospitalized and will be on warfarin once discharged. Dental emergencies in these patients during hospitalization should be treated as conservatively as possible, avoiding invasive procedures. Patients receiving hemodialysis are treated with heparin. The half-life of heparin is only 1 to 2 hours, thus by waiting until the day after dialysis these patients can receive invasive dental treatment. The dental management of these patients is presented in Chapter 9.

The dentist may see patients being treated on an outpatient basis with a LMWH. These would include patients with recent total hip or knee replacement and those being treated on an outpatient basis for deep-vein thrombi or asymptomatic pulmonary embolism. No clear guidelines are yet available for managing these patients for invasive dental procedures. Elective surgical procedures can be delayed until the patient is off the LMWH, which in most cases will be in 3 to 6 months. If an invasive procedure most be performed, the dentist has several options. First, the dentist should consult with the patient's physician regarding the need for and type of surgery. The half-life of the LMWHs is much less than one day. Thus the physician could suggest that the drug be stopped and the surgery be performed within 1 to 2 days. The other option is to go ahead with the surgery and deal with any bleeding complications on a local basis.

Possible Liver Disease

A patient with a history of jaundice or heavy alcohol use may have significant liver disease. Most of the coagulation factors are produced in the liver; therefore if enough liver damage has occurred, the patient could have a serious bleeding problem because of a defect in the coagulation phase. In addition, about 50% of patients with significant liver disease (portal hypertension present) will be thrombocytopenic as a result of platelets being sequestered in the spleen. Alcohol also can have a direct effect on homeostasis by interfering with platelet function. The PT test can be used to screen for a defect in the coagulation phase in patients with a history that indicates liver disease (see Chapter 10 for blood tests indicative of alcoholism). A platelet count should be obtained to see if the platelet phase has been affected. The amount of liver damage may not be great enough to affect the coagulation phase, but the effect on the platelet phase could be severe enough to lead to a serious bleeding problem. If both the PT and the platelet count are normal, surgery can be performed on these patients with little risk of a postoperative bleeding problem. If both tests are abnormal, then the dentist should consult with the patients physician regarding management of the patient prior to the surgery. This may involve vitamin K administration, platelet replacement, or other special physician-directed procedures.

Chronic Leukemia

Chapter 20 describes the management of patients with leukemia.

Malabsorption Syndrome or Long-term Antibiotic Therapy

In patients with malabsorption syndrome or patients receiving long-term antibiotic therapy, the bacteria in the intestine that produce vitamin K may be adversely affected. The liver needs vitamin K for the production and function of prothrombin (factor II) and related coagulation factors (factors VII, IX, and X). The PT test can be ordered to screen for a possible bleeding problem; and if it is normal, surgery can be performed on these patients without risk of a bleeding problem. The patient's physician should be consulted regarding the patient's health status before surgery, because complicating factors can occur, in addition to the possible bleeding problem that would contraindicate surgery. Parenteral vitamin K may have to be administered in some of these cases.

End-stage Renal Disease and Renal Dialysis

The management of the patient end-stage renal disease (ESRD) and those on renal dialysis is covered in Chapter 9.

Vascular Wall Alteration

Patients with autoimmune disease, infectious disease, structural malformations of vessels, hereditary disorders of connective tissue, scurvy, steroid therapy, small vessel vasculitis, or with deposits of paraproteins may have alterations of the vessel wall that can result in excessive bleeding after surgical procedures. No reliable screening tests can detect those patients that will be bleeders. The Ivy BT test can be used to identify the potential bleeders, but as stated before, the Ivy BT is inconsistent and will not detect many of the bleeders. The dentist must rely on the medical history (questions related to excessive bleeding problems); clinical findings; and consultation with the patient's physician to detect these patients.

MANAGEMENT OF THE PATIENT WITH A SERIOUS BLEEDING DISORDER

The dental treatment of patients with thrombocytopenia, hemophilia A, and vWD is used here to demonstrate how patients with serious bleeding disorders can be managed to avoid significant bleeding complications.

Before any dental treatment is performed for a patient with a bleeding disorder, the dentist must consult with the patient's physician to determine the severity of the disorder and the need for special preparations for dental treatment. Patients with significant bleeding disorders are at increased risk for spontaneous gingival bleeding or excessive bleeding following minor trauma to the oral tissues. They can be at even greater risk if surgical procedures are performed without special preparations. Good oral hygiene is a must for these patients. Care should be taken in the placement of intraoral radiographic films to avoid trauma to the oral tissues. In general, block anesthesia and intramuscular injections must be avoided unless appropriate replacement factors have been used in patients with a factor deficiency.[50,58,68]

Infiltration anesthesia usually can be given without replacement therapy. Simple restorative procedures often can be performed without replacement therapy or endodontic treatment of nonvital teeth. However, overinstrumentation and overfilling must be avoided. When performed, complex restorative procedures usually require replacement therapy. However, care must be taken with the placement of wedges; bands (restorative or orthodontic); and archwires.[58,68]

Conservative periodontal procedures including polishing with a prophy cup and supragingival calculus removal often can be done without replacement therapy. In children, primary teeth should be removed soon after they become loose. Local bleeding control usually can be obtained by use of pressure, thrombin, or microfibrillar collagen. If bleeding continues, topical AHF (factor VIII) can be applied to the "wounds."[50,58,68]

Thrombocytopenia

Patients found to have severe thrombocytopenia or a severe coagulation disorder most often require hospitalization and special preparation for surgery. A hematologist should be involved with the diagnosis, presurgical evaluation, preparation, and postsurgical management of these patients.

Surgical treatment including extractions requires special preparation. For patients with thrombocytopenia, the platelet count should be at least 50,000/mm^3 before surgery is attempted. Continuous transfusion of platelets may be required, or a single preoperative platelet transfusion can be given 30 minutes before the dental surgery. All bleeding sites should be packed with microfibrillar collagen and EACA (100 mg/kg orally), which is given just before surgery and then continued for 8 days (50 mg/kg every 6 hours, orally).[68-70]

In children with acute idiopathic thrombocytopenia (ITP) with platelet counts less than 20,000/mm^3, prednisone or IV gamma globulin increases the platelet count to more than 50,000/mm^3 within 48 hours in about 90% of the cases. Once the platelet count is over 50,000/mm^3, the needed surgical procedures can be performed. Adults with chronic ITP are usually followed without treatment. The incidence of bleeding problems is correlated with the platelet count. Patients with platelet counts greater than 60,000/mm^3 rarely have spontaneous bleeding and may only require treatment if extensive surgical procedures are planned. Adults with chronic ITP with platelet counts less than 20,000/mm^3 or with significant mucosal membrane bleeding with platelet counts less than 50,000/mm^3 must have their platelet count corrected before any surgery. Treatment may include glucocorticoids, IV immunoglobulins, followed by platelet transfusions.[7,9,71]

Hemophilia

The patient with hemophilia A (factor VIII deficiency) can be used to illustrate some of the management problems involved in dealing with a serious coagulation disorder. Consultation with a hematologist is necessary. The hematologist first establishes the diagnosis and determines the degree of factor VIII deficiency, whether any factor VIII inhibitors are present, and the need for hospitalization. The type of replacement material is selected (Box 19-12; see Table 19-3), and the hematologist determines the dosage of the replacement material.[8,16]

Extractions have been performed for patients with a mild deficiency of factor VIII using only DDAVP and EACA, and postoperative bleeding problems have been minimal.[72] Additionally, tranexamic acid (a long-acting

BOX 19-12

Dental Management of the Patient with Hemophilia

Preoperative

Hematology consult
Confirm diagnosis and severity of disease
Presence of inhibitors (antibodies to factor VIII)
• No inhibitors
• Stable inhibitors
• Inducible inhibitors
Determine treatment location
• Patients with mild to moderate hemophilia are usu-
  ally treated in the dental setting
• Patients with severe hemophilia or those with
  inhibitors are usually treated in hopsital
• Also influenced by type of dental treatment: sur-
  gery, extractions or operative
• The more invasive the procedure the more likely
  the patient will be treated in hospital
Management recommendations
• DDAVP: 0.3 μg/kg (maximal dose, 20 to 24 μg),
  parenterally, I hour (hr) before procedure
• EACA: 6 g every 6 hrs, orally, for 3 to 4 days
• Factor VIII replacement: Loading (0 or 30-40 U/kg,
  IV), maintenance (10-40 U/kg, IV q 12 hrs)
• Porcine factor: VIII, PCC, APCC, or F-VII, and
  steroids
Dental
• Treat any acute oral infection
• Establish good oral hygiene
• Construct splints for patients with moderate to
  severe hemophilia who are having multiple extrac-
  tions

Operative
Use good surgical technique
Use microfibrillar collagen, tranexamic acid, fibrin
  glue, or gelfoam with thrombin to control
  bleeding
Use pressure packs (mild cases)
Place splints (moderate and severe cases)
Hematologist will monitor treatment of hospitalized
  patients)

Postoperative
Patients treated in the dental office may require second
  dose of DDAVP or replacement factor
Hospitalized patients will require additional doses of
  DDAVP, factor VIII, or other agents
Patients given factor VIII replacement need to be exam-
  ined for signs of allergy
• Hospitalized patients: Hematologist will do this
• Dental office: Dentist needs to do this, any questions
  about findings consult with hematologist
Examine patient 24 to 48 hours after surgery for the
  following:
• Signs of infection: Treat if present
• Bleeding: Use local measures to control, if not effec-
  tive other systemic measures as indicated
• Healing
Avoid aspirin, aspirin containing compounds, and
  NSAIDs (the new COX-2-specific inhibitors,
  Celecoxib and Rofecoxib, can be used).
  Acetaminophen with or without codeine is suggested
  for most patients.

DDAVP, I-desamino-8-D-arginine vasopressin; EACA, epsilon-aminocaproic acid; PCC, prothrombin complex concentrates; APCC,
activated prothrombin complex concentrations; NSAIDs, nonsteroidal antiinflammatory drugs.

antifibrinolytic) has been used.[73] In patients with mild hemophilia without inhibitors, DDAVP can be given I hour
before the procedure by nasal spray (300 mg/kg) or parenterally (0.3 micrograms/kg, up to a maximal dose of 20
to 24 micrograms). EACA also can be given orally to prevent fibrinolysis (6 g every 6 hours to adults and 100
mg/kg every 6 hours for children) for 3 to 4 days following
tooth extraction.[4] Patients with moderate factor VIII deficiency and no inhibitors can be given a single dose of factor VIII concentrate 10 to 30 minutes before the procedure. Factor VIII has a half-life of 8 to 12 hours. EACA also
is given orally every 6 hours for 3 to 5 days. If bleeding

occurs after the first 8 to 12 hours, additional infusions of
factor VIII will be needed.[4,31,34,70]

A 1993[74] study demonstrated the use of a fibrin glue to
treat patients with various bleeding disorders including
hemophilia prior to extraction. Eighty patients with various bleeding disorders underwent 135 extractions without preventive replacement hematologic therapy. For
local homeostatic control, Beriplast (aprotinin as the active component),[74,75] a fibrin glue, was used for homeostatic control. The concentration of the aprotinin (an antifibrinolytic agent) in the fibrin glue had to be increased
by the investigators to 10,000 kabivitrium international

units/ml from 1,000 to prevent secondary bleeding in severe hemophiliacs. The results were as follows: in 12 severe hemophiliacs receiving 1000 KIU/ml of aprotinin, 9 of 12 had secondary bleeding, 3 of 25 severe hemophiliacs receiving 10,000 KIU/ml of aprotinin had secondary bleeding, and none of the 43 patients with coagulopathies other than severe hemophilia had secondary bleeding. Swish and swallow rinses of tranexamic acid were used before and after extractions in the severe hemophiliacs on the high dose of aprotinin.[74]

Patients with more severe deficiencies of factor VIII without factor VIII inhibitors can receive most oral surgical procedures if proper factor VIII replacement is effectively achieved. Even patients with stable levels of factor VIII inhibitors can have oral surgery performed if large doses of factor VIII replacement are used. However, patients with inducible factor VIII inhibitors still present great problems and are at high risk for serious bleeding if surgery is attempted.[4] Elective surgery is not recommended for these patients. Periodontal surgery is not suggested, and extractions are performed only when no alternate treatment is available. Both nonactivated and activated prothrombin complex concentrates with EACA have been tried in patients with high titers of factor VIII inhibitors, but success has been limited. Porcine factor VIII concentrate has been used with some success. Cortisone also has been tried in patients with inducible inhibitors to interfere with their action. Plasmapheresis may clear the blood of inhibitors for a short time.[4,31,34,42]

The dentist before surgery can make splints so mechanical displacement of the clot in wounds healing by secondary intention is prevented. Care should be taken in the construction of the splints so that pressure does not occur on soft tissues, which could lead to tissue necrosis. All extraction sites should be packed with microfibrillar collagen, and the wound should be closed with absorbable sutures for primary healing whenever possible. Endodontic procedures should be done rather than extractions whenever possible because the risk for serious bleeding is less.[18,19,41,50,58]

The administration of local anesthetics is a major concern in dental treatment for the patient with hemophilia. Hematomas, airway obstruction, and death have occurred as complications of block anesthesia in these individuals. In general, block injections or intramuscular injections should not be given unless the patient has a plasma factor VIII level of 50% or greater. Patients with severe hemophilia (1% or less of factor VIII) should be given replacement therapy before any local anesthetic is administered.[68]

In many cases, the patient must be hospitalized for surgical procedures. This decision should be made based on the dental procedure and in consultation with the patient's hematologist. Patients with a mild-to-moderate form of hemophilia without inhibitors can be managed on an outpatient basis using DDAVP and EACA or tranexamic acid or using replacement therapy plus EACA. When replacement therapy is used, the dentist and hematologist must observe the patient for any signs of allergic reaction and be prepared to take appropriate action. Box 19-12 reviews the role and function of the hematologist and dentist in managing the hemophiliac. Postoperative pain control can usually be obtained using acetaminophen with or without codeine or the new COX-2-specific inhibitors, Rofecoxib and Celecoxib (see Box 19-12).

von Willebrand's Disease

Surgical procedures can be performed in patients with mild vWD (type I and some type II variants) by using DDAVP and EACA. Patients with more severe types of vWD will require cryoprecipitate or factor VIII concentrates such as Humate-P that retain vWF multimers to replace the missing vWF and factor VIII. A recent study[76] reported the results of bleeding complications in 63 consecutive patients with vWD. Of the cases, 31 had type 1 vWD, 22 had type 2 variants of vWD, and 10 had type 3 vWD. All patients had extractions or periodontal surgery performed. All cases received tranexamic acid before and for 7 days after surgery. Fibrin glue (not available in the United States) was used as local therapy in several patients during surgery. Desmopressin or factor VIII concentrates with vWF were given systemically as indicated. Of the patients, 29 were treated with tranexamic acid and local measures and did not experience excessive bleeding. Desmopressin was given to 24 patients, and six received factor VIII with vWF. Excessive bleeding after surgery occurred in only two patients. The authors[76] concluded that tranexamic acid, fibrin glue, and desmopressin can prevent bleeding complications in the vast majority of patients with vWD (84%). Box 19-13 reviews the role and function of the hematologist and dentist in the management of patients with vWD.

TREATMENT PLANNING MODIFICATIONS

With proper preparation, most indicated dental treatment could be provided for patients with various bleeding problems. Patients with congenital coagulation defects must be encouraged to improve and maintain good oral health, because most dental treatment for these patients at present is complicated by the need for replacement of the missing factor. Dental treatment often requires hospitalization for patients with severe defects. Patients with bleeding problems secondary to diseases that may be in the terminal phase should, in general, be offered only conservative dental treatment. Aspirin and

BOX 19-13

Dental Management of the Patient with von Willebrand's Disease

Preoperative

Hematology consult

Confirm diagnosis; establish variant and treatment modality

- Type 1: partial deficiency of vWF; DDAVP usually effective, F-VIII with vWF in a few cases
- Type 2: qualitative defects in vWF; DDAVP usually effective, F-VIII with vWF in some cases
- Type 3: severe deficiency of vWF; F-VIII with vWF in all cases

Test for DDAVP response if use is planned (most type 1 and many type 2 patients)

Establish dosage for F-VIII replacement and need for EACA

Location: most patients can be treated in dental office; those with type 3 may be hospitalized

Dental

- Treat any acute oral infection
- Good oral hygiene
- Construct splints for multiple extractions in patients with type 3 and type 2 N variants

Operative

Hematologist/Dentist

Treatment with DDAVP before procedure

Treatment with EACA before procedure

Factor VIII replacement before procedure: Humate-P or Koate-HP

Dental

Use good surgical technique

Control bleeding using local measures

- Pressure packs
- Microfibrillar collagen
- Gelfoam with thrombin
- Fibrin glue (not available in the United States)
- Tranexamic acid

Place splint

Postoperative

Hematologist/Dentist

Examine for signs of bleeding within 24 to 48 hours

Type 1 and type 2 patients: additional dose of DDAVP and EACA as indicated

Type 3 and some type 2 patients: additional doses of factor VIII and EACA as needed

Examine for signs of allergy to factor VIII

Dental

Examine for signs of infection or delayed healing within 24 to 48 hours

If infection occurs treated by local and systemic means

Bleeding can be managed using local means if these fail additional systemic therapy may be needed

Avoid aspirin and NSAIDs; can use acetaminophen with or without codeine. Also, the new

Cox-2-specific inhibitors, Celecoxib and Rofecoxib, can be used.

vWF, von Willebrand factor: *F-VIII*, factor VIII; *DDAVP*, 1-desamino-8-D-arginine vasopressin (desmopressin acetate); *EACA*, epsilon-aminocaproic acid; *Humate-P*, factor VIII that retains vWF; *Koate-HP*, factor VIII that retains vWF; *NSAIDs*, nonsteroidal antiinflammatory drugs.

other NSAIDs should not be used for pain relief in patients who have known bleeding disorders or who are receiving anticoagulant medication. This includes the various compounds that contain aspirin, such as Anacin, Synalgos-DC, Fiorinal, Bufferin, Alka-Seltzer, Empirin with Codeine, and Excedrin.

ORAL COMPLICATIONS AND MANIFESTATIONS

Patients with bleeding disorders may experience spontaneous gingival bleeding. Oral tissues (e.g., soft palate, tongue, buccal mucosa) may show petechiae, ecchy-moses, jaundice, pallor, and ulcers. Spontaneous gingival bleeding and petechiae usually are found in patients with thrombocytopenia.

Hemarthrosis of the temporomandibular joint (TMJ) is a rare finding in patients with coagulation disorders and is not found in patients with thrombocytopenia. Individuals with leukemia may reveal a generalized hyperplasia of the gingiva. Patients with neoplastic disease may show osseous lesions on radiographs, oral ulcers, or tumors. These patients also may have drifting and loosening of teeth and may complain of paresthesias (e.g., burning of the tongue, numbness of the lip) (see Chapter 21).[17,18,58]

References

1. Rodgers GM: Thrombosis and antithrombotic therapy. In Lee GR et al, editors: *Wintrobe's clinical hematology*, ed 10, Philadelphia, 1999, Lippincott Williams & Wilkins.
2. Kasper CK et al: Hematologic management of hemophilia A for surgery, JAMA 253:1279-1283, 1985.
3. Kitchens CS: Surgery in hemophilia and related disorders, J Med 65:34-45, 1986.
4. Rodgers GM, Greenberg CS: Inherited coagulation disorders. In Lee GR et al, editors: *Wintrobe's clinical hematology*, ed 10, Philadelphia, 1999, Lippincott Williams & Wilkins.
5. Handin RI: Disorders of the platelet and vessel wall. In Fauci AS et al, editors: *Harrison's principles of internal medicine*, ed 14, New York, 1998, McGraw-Hill.
6. Parise LV et al: Platelets in hemostasis and thrombosis. In Lee GR et al, editors: *Wintrobe's clinical hematology*, ed 10, Philadelphia, 1999, Lippincott Williams & Wilkins.
7. Levine SP: Thrombocytopenia: pathophysiology and classification In Lee GR et al, editors: *Wintrobe's clinical hematology*, ed 10, Philadelphia, 1999, Lippincott Williams & Wilkins.
8. Grosset ABM, Rodgers GM: Acquired coagulation disorders. In Lee GR et al, editors: *Wintrobe's clinical hematology*, ed 10, Philadelphia, 1999, Lippincott Williams & Wilkins.
9. Levine SP: Miscellaneous causes of thrombocytopenia. In Lee GR et al, editors: *Wintrobe's clinical hematology*, ed 10, Philadelphia, 1999, Lippincott Williams & Wilkins.
10. Harmening DM: Introduction to hemostasis—an overview of hemostatic mechanism, platelet structure and function, and extrinsic and intrinsic systems. In Harmening DM, editor: *Clinical hematology and fundamentals of hemostasis*, ed 2, Philadelphia, 1992, FA Davis.
11. Rodgers GM: Endothelium and the regulation of hemostasis. In Lee GR et al, editors: *Wintrobe's clinical hematology*, ed 10, Philadelphia, 1999, Lippincott Williams & Wilkins.
12. Stenberg PE, Hill RJ: Platelets and megakaryocytes. In Lee GR et al, editors: *Wintrobe's clinical hematology*, ed 10, Philadelphia, 1999, Lippincott Williams & Wilkins.
13. Handin RI: Disorders of coagulation and thrombosis. In Fauci AS et al, editors: *Harrison's principles of internal medicine*, ed 14, New York, 1998, McGraw-Hill.
14. Greenberg CS, Orthner CL: Blood coagulation and fibrinolysis. In Lee GR et al, editors: *Wintrobe's clinical hematology*, ed 10, Philadelphia, 1999, Lippincott Williams & Wilkins.
15. Barber A et al: The bleeding time as a preoperative screening test, Am J Med 78:761-765, 1985.
16. Rodgers GM, Bithell TC: The diagnostic approach to the bleeding disorders. In Lee GR et al, editors: *Wintrobe's clinical hematology*, ed 10, Philadelphia, 1999, Lippincott Williams & Wilkins.
17. Rodeghiero F et al: Hyper-responsiveness to DDAVP for patients with type I von Willebrand's disease and normal intraplatelet von Willebrand factor, Eur J Haematol 40(2):163-167, 1988.
18. Stajcic Z: Primary wound closure in hemophiliacs undergoing dental extractions, Int J Oral Maxillofac Surg 18(1):14-16, 1989.
19. Wintrobe MM et al: Clinical hematology. In Wintrobe MM, editor: *Clinical hematology*, ed 8, Philadelphia, 1981, Lea & Febiger.
20. Zieve PD: Bleeding disorders. In Harvey A et al, editors: *The principles and practice of medicine*, ed 19, New York, 1976, Appleton-Century-Crofts.
21. Rodgers GM: Overview of platelet physiology and laboratory evaluation of platelet function, Clin Obstet Gynecol 42(2):349-359, 1999.
22. Von Pape K, Aland E, Bohner J: Platelet function analysis with PFA-100(R) in patients medicated with acetylsalicylic acid strongly depends on concentration of sodium citrate used for anticoagulation of blood sample, Thromb Res 98(4):295-299, 2000.
23. Kundu SK et al: Description of an in vitro platelet function analyzer–PFA-100, Semin Thromb Hemost 21(Suppl 2):106-112, 1995.
24. Mammen EF, Alshameeri RS, Comp PC: Preliminary data from a field trial of the PFA-100 system, Semin Thromb Hemost 21(Suppl 2):113-121, 1995.
25. Rand ML, Carcao MD, Blanchette VS: Use of the PFA-100 in the assessment of primary, platelet-related hemostasis in a pediatric setting, Semin Thromb Hemost 24(6):523-529, 1998.
26. Mammen EF et al: PFA-100 system: a new method for assessment of platelet dysfunction, Semin Thromb Hemost 24(2):195-202, 1998.
27. Escolar G et al: Evaluation of acquired platelet dysfunctions in uremic and cirrhotic patients using the platelet function analyzer (PFA-100): influence of hematocrit elevation, Haematologica 84(7):614-619, 1999.
28. Hezard N et al: Use of the PFA-100 apparatus to assess platelet function in patients undergoing PTCA during and after infusion of cE3 Fab in the presence of other antiplatelet agents, Thromb Haemost 83(4):540-544, 2000.
29. Homoncik M et al: Monitoring of aspirin (ASA) pharmacodynamics with the platelet function analyzer PFA-100, Thromb Haemost 83(2):316-321, 2000.
30. Rees MM, Rodgers GM: Bleeding disorders caused by vascular abnormalities. In Lee GR et al, editors: *Wintrobe's clinical hematology*, ed 10, Philadelphia, 1999, Lippincott Williams & Wilkins.
31. Handin RI: Disorders of coagulation and thrombosis. In Isselbacher KJ et al, editors: *Harrison's principles of internal medicine*, ed 13, New York, 1994, McGraw-Hill.
32. Fressinaud E et al: Screening for von Willebrand disease with a new analyzer using high shear stress: a study of 60 cases, Blood 91(4):1325-1331, 1998.
33. Handin RI: Disorders of platelet and vessel wall. In Isselbacher KJ et al, editors: *Harrison's principles of internal medicine*, ed 13, New York, 1994, McGraw-Hill.
34. Shord SS, Lindley CM: Coagulation products and their uses, Am J Health-Syst Pharm 57(15):1403-1418, 2000.
35. Levine SP: Qualitative disorders of platelet function. In Lee GR et al, editors: *Wintrobe's clinical hematology*, ed 10, Philadelphia, 1999, Lippincott Williams & Wilkins.
36. Handin RI: Anticoagulant, fibrinolytic, and antiplatelet therapy. In Isselbacher KJ et al, editors: *Harrison's principles of internal medicine*, ed 13, New York, 1994, McGraw-Hill.

37. Brackmann HH et al: German recommendations for immune tolerance therapy in type A haemophiliacs with antibodies, *Haemophilia* 5(3):203-206, 1999.

38. Kaufman RJ: Advances toward gene therapy for hemophilia at the millennium, *Hum Gene Ther* 10(13):2091-2107, 1999.

39. Hortelano G, Chang PL: Gene therapy for hemophilia, *Artif Cells Blood Substit Immobil Biotechnol* 28(1):1-24, 2000.

40. Schroeder ML: Principles and practice of transfusion medicine. In Lee GR et al, editors: *Wintrobe's clinical hematology*, ed 10, Philadelphia, 1999, Lippincott Williams & Wilkins.

41. Handin RI: Clotting disorders. In Wilson JD et al, editors: *Harrison's principles of internal medicine*, 12 ed, New York, 1991, McGraw-Hill.

42. McGlasson DL: Defects of plasma clotting factors. In Harmening DM, editor: *Clinical hematology and fundamentals of hemostasis*, ed 2, Philadelphia, 1992, FA Davis.

43. Kahn RA, Allen R, Baldassare J: Alternate sources and substitutes for therapeutic blood components, *Blood* 66:1-12, 1985.

44. Gould MK: Concise Review: Efficacy and cost-effectiveness of low-molecular-weight heparins in acuted deep venous thrombosis. In Fauci AS et al, editors: *Harrison's principles of internal medicine*, ed 14, New York, 2000, McGraw-Hill.

45. Elliott G: Concise review: low-molecular-weight heparin in the treatment of acute pulmonary embolism. In Fauci AS et al, editors: *Harrison's principles of internal medicine*, ed 14, New York, 2000, McGraw-Hill.

46. Dalen JE et al: Update on the Fifth ACCP Consensus Conference on Antithrombotic Therapy, 1999; Tucson, Arizona.

47. Steinberg MJ, Moores JF: Use of INR to assess degree of anticoagulation in patients who have dental procedures, *J Oral Surg Oral Med Oral Path* 80:175-177, 1995.

48. Helft G, Vacheron A, Samama MM: Current biological surveillance of oral anticoagulant treatment, *Arch Mal Coeur Vaiss* 88(1):85-89, 1995.

49. Andrews TC et al: Complications of warfarin therapy monitored by the international normalized ratio versus the prothrombin time ratio, *Clin Cardiol* 18(2)80-82, 1995.

50. Ublansky JH: Comprehensive dental care for children with bleeding disorders–a dentist's perspective, *J Can Den Assoc* 58(2):111-114, 1992.

51. Hirsh J, Poller L: The international normalized ratio. A guide to understanding and correcting its problems, *Arch Intern Med* 154(3)282-288, 1994.

52. Lassen JF, Brandslund I, Antonsen S: International normalized ratio for prothrombin times in patients taking oral anticoagulants: critical difference and probability of significant change in consecutive measurements, *Clin Chem* 41(3):444-447, 1995.

53. Lassen JF et al: Interpretation of serial measurements of international normalized ratio for prothrombin times in monitoring oral anticoagulant therapy, *Clin Chem* 41(8 Pt 1):1171-1176, 1995.

54. Hobbs FD et al: Is the international normalized ratio reliable? A trial of comparative measurements in hospital laboratory and primary care settings, *J Clin Pathol* 52:494-497, 1999.

55. Hirsh J, Fuster V: AHA medical/scientific statement: guide to anticoagulant therapy, part 2: oral anticoagulants, *Circulation* 89(3):1469-1480, 1994.

56. Scardi S, Mazzone C: Anticoagulant prophylaxis: from clinical trials to clinical practice, *G Ital Cardiol* 28(2):178-186, 1998.

57. Schardt-Sacco D: Update on coagulopathies, *Oral Surg Oral Med Oral Pathol Oral Radiol Endod* 90:559-563, 2000.

58. Lynch MA: Hematologic diseases and related problems. In Lynch MA, editor: *Burket's oral medicine diagnosis and treatment*, ed 7, Philadelphia, 1977, JB Lippincott.

59. Kelly MA: Common laboratory tests: their use in the detection and management of patients with bleeding disorders, *Gen Dent* 38(4):282-285, 1990.

60. Schafer AI: Effects of nonsteroidal antiinflammatory drugs on platelet function and systemic hemostasis, *J Clin Pharmacol* 35(3):209-219, 1995.

61. Beck KH: Desmopressin effect on acetylsalicylic acid impaired platelet function, *Semin Thromb Hemost* 21(Suppl 2):32-39, 1995.

62. Wahl MJ: Myths of dental treatment in anticoagulated patients, *J Am Den Assoc* 131(1):77-81, 2000.

63. Benoliel R: Dental treatment for the patient on anticoagulant therapy: prothrombin time–what difference does it make? *Oral Surg* 62:149-151, 1986.

64. Devani P, Lavery K, Howell C: Dental extractions in patients on warfarin: is alteration of anticoagulant regime necessary? *Br J Oral Maxillofacial Surg* 35:107-111, 1998.

65. Giglio J: Complications of dentoalveolar surgery. In Kwon P, Laskin D, editors: *Clinician's manual of oral and maxillofacial surgery*. (Ill): London, 1997, Quintessence.

66. Lippert S, Gutschik E: Views of cardiac-valve prosthesis patients and their dentists on anticoagulation therapy, *Scan J Den Res* 102(3):168-171, 1994.

67. Hylek EM: Acetaminophen and other risk factors for excessive warfarin anticoagulation, *JAMA* 279(9):657-662, 1998.

68. Cohen SG, Glick M: Dental correlations, factor deficiencies. In Rose LF, Kaye D, editors: *Internal medicine for dentistry*, ed 2, St Louis, 1990, Mosby.

69. Sindet-Pedersen S: Haemostasis in oral surgery, *Dan Med Bull* 38(6):427-443, 1991.

70. Speirs RL: Haemostasis, *Dent Update* 18(4):166-171, 1991.

71. Levine SP: Thrombocytopenia caused by immunologic platelet destruction. In Lee GR et al, editors: *Wintrobe's clinical hematology*, ed 10, Philadelphia, 1999, Lippincott Williams & Wilkins.

72. Ghirardini A et al: Clinical evaluation of subcutaneously administered DDAVP, *Thromb Res* 49(3):363-372, 1988.

73. US Food and Drug Administration: Recent drug approvals. Tranexamic acid, *FDA Drug Bull* 17(1):9, 1987.

74. Radocz M et al: Dental extractions in patients with bleeding disorders. The use of fibrin glue. *Oral Surg Oral Med Oral Path* 75(3):280-282, 1993.

75. O'Brien JG: Effects of tranexamic acid and aprotinin, two antifibrinolytic drugs, on PAF-induced plasma extravasation in unanesthetized rats. *Inflammation* 24(5):411-429, 2000.

76. Federici AB et al: Optimising local therapy during oral surgery in patients with von Willebrand disease: effective results from a retrospective analysis of 63 cases, *Haemophilia* 6(2):71-77, 2000.

Disorders of Red and White Blood Cells

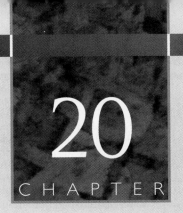

20
CHAPTER

Disorders of the red and white blood cells (RBCs and WBCs) can influence dental treatment (Box 20-1). The dentist should be able to detect patients with these abnormalities by history, clinical examination, and screening laboratory tests. Patients with disorders of the WBCs or RBCs may be susceptible to abnormal bleeding, delayed healing, infection, or mucosal ulceration. Some of these diseases can be fatal. Thus these disorders must be detected early and affected patients referred promptly to a physician for diagnosis and treatment before invasive dental procedures are performed. Patients with known life-threatening disorders who are under medical care should not receive dental care until after consulting with the patient's physician.

■ ANEMIA ■

DEFINITION

About 1% of the circulating erythrocyte mass is generated by the bone marrow each day. Precursors of erythrocytes are reticulocyte, and they comprise 1% of the total red cell count. The normal red cell is about 33% hemoglobin by volume. Hemoglobin (Hb), the oxygen-carrying molecule of erythrocytes, consists of two pair of globin chains (i.e., α plus β, δ, or γ) that form a shell around four oxygen-binding heme groups. Healthy adults have about 95% Hb A ($\alpha2\beta2$) and small amounts of Hb A2 ($\alpha2\delta2$) and Hb F ($\alpha2\gamma2$). Genes on chromosome 16 encode the alpha globin chains; the beta chains are encoded on chromosome 11.[1] Oxygen demand serves as the stimulus for erythropoiesis. This occurs mainly in the kidney, which releases erythropoietin, a hormone that stimulates the bone marrow to release RBCs. About 95% of erythropoietin is produced by cortical cells in the kidney. The other

5% is produced by the liver. Hypoxia is the main stimulant of erythropoietin.[2]

Anemia is defined as a reduction in the oxygen-carrying capacity of the blood and usually is related to a decrease in number of circulating RBCs or to an abnormality in the Hb contained within the RBCs. Anemia is not a disease but rather a symptom complex that may result from decreased production of RBCs (iron deficiency, pernicious anemia, folate deficiency), blood loss, or increased rate of destruction of circulating RBCs. In the latter case, defectively constructed RBCs cause hemolytic anemia. Hemolytic anemias are divided into extracorpuscular or intracorpuscular defects. The two diseases caused by intracorpuscular defects—glucose-6-phosphate deficiency and sickle cell anemia—are discussed here to demonstrate the problems presented by the hemolytic anemias.[3] All the various causes of anemia are not covered in detail in this chapter. Examples have been selected to demonstrate the clinical problems involved in the management of patients with anemia.

IRON-DEFICIENCY ANEMIA

Iron-deficiency anemia is a microcytic anemia caused by excessive blood loss. The blood loss can be caused by menses or bleeding from the gastrointestinal tract, gastrectomy, or a malabsorption syndrome that reduces absorption of iron from the gastrointestinal tract. It is common in children with poor dietary intake and women who are menstruating or pregnant. The repeated loss of blood associated with menses can lead to depletion of iron and result in a mild state of anemia. On occasion, when taking a history from a woman, the dentist may want to ask of the onset, nature, and regularity of the patient's menstruation cycle. Women with a history of regular periods but with heavy flow may be anemic and should receive medical advice and treatment. A patient with a change in

BOX 20-1

Classification and Features of Blood Dyscrasias

1. Red blood cell (RBC) disorders
   a. Anemia—low oxygen-carrying capacity of blood, often caused by decreased number of circulating RBCs
   b. Polycythemia—increased number of circulating RBCs
2. White blood cell (WBC) disorders
   a. Leukocytosis—increased number of circulating WBCs
   b. Leukopenia—decreased number of circulating WBCs
   c. Myeloproliferative disorders
      (1) Acute myeloid leukemia—immature neoplastic malignancy of myeloid cells
      (2) Chronic myeloid leukemia—mature neoplastic malignancy of myeloid cells
   d. Lymphoproliferative disorders
      (1) Acute lymphoblastic leukemia—immature neoplastic malignancy of lymphoid cells
      (2) Chronic lymphocytic leukemia—mature neoplastic malignancy of lymphoid cells
      (3) Lymphomas
         (a) Hodgkin's disease—malignant growth of lymphocytes primarily in lymph nodes
         (b) Non-Hodgkin's disease—B or T cell malignant neoplasms, many types and locations
         (c) Burkitt's lymphoma—B cell malignancy involving bone and lymph nodes
      (4) Multiple myeloma—overproduction of malignant plasma cells involving bone

the pattern, onset, length, or rate of menstrual flow should be encouraged to seek medical evaluation. Patients who have stopped having periods long before expected should be referred for medical evaluation, as should those who have had bleeding in between regular periods.

During pregnancy, the expectant mother experiences an increased demand for additional iron and vitamins to support the growth of her fetus, and unless sufficient amounts of these nutrients have been provided in some form, she may become anemic. Approximately 20% of pregnant women have iron deficiency anemia. In obtaining the health history, the dentist should establish if the patient has other children and when they were born, because the closer together the pregnancies were, the greater is the risk for the patient to develop iron-deficiency anemia. Once the baby is born, the mother may lose additional iron during delivery and breast-feeding

By contrast, mild anemia in men usually indicates the presence of a serious underlying medical problem (e.g., gastrointestinal bleeding or malignancy). Under normal physiologic conditions, men lose little iron, and iron-deficiency anemia is rare. Therefore any man found to be anemic should be referred for medical evaluation.

FOLATE-DEFICIENCY ANEMIA AND PERNICIOUS ANEMIA

Vitamin B_{12} (cobalamin) and folic acid are needed for the maturation of RBCs in bone marrow. Vitamin B_{12} is a cofactor in methionine-associated enzymatic reactions required of protein synthesis, and thus the maturation of RBCs. Folate is needed for enzymatic reactions related to synthesis of deoxyribonucleic acid (DNA), ribonucleic acid (RNA), and proteins. A deficiency in the daily intake or absorption (because of celiac disease or tropical sprue) of these vitamins can result in anemia. Folate is found in fruits and leafy vegetables. Its absorption and metabolism is interfered with by alcohol consumption and certain drugs (methotrexate). Pernicious anemia is caused by a deficiency of intrinsic factor, a substance secreted by the stomach parietal cells that is necessary for the absorption of vitamin B_{12}.

Pernicious anemia is usually a disease of late adult life. It most often occurs in 40-year-old to 70-year-old northern Europeans of fair complexion, with one notable exception. An early onset in black American women, 21% of whom were under the age of 40, has been observed.[2] Most patients with pernicious anemia have chronic atrophic gastritis with decreased intrinsic factor and hydrochloric acid secretion. Antibodies against intrinsic factor also are found in the serum of 50% to 70% of the patients. This finding suggests that the disease may be an autoimmune process.

Patients with pernicious anemia are at increased risk for gastric carcinoma, myxedema, rheumatoid arthritis, neuropsychiatric and neuromuscular abnormalities, the latter due to a defect in myelin synthesis.[2] Early symptoms include weakness; fatigue; palpitations; syncope; tingling of the fingers and toes (paresthesias); numbness; uncoordination; and muscular weakness. Competitive binding assays for serum cobalamin and folate are used for initial screening of the deficiency.[4] Use of the Schilling test with radioactive cyanocobalamin and the intrinsic factor antibody test

help establish the diagnosis of pernicious anemia.[2,4] Early detection is important, so treatment, which involves vitamin B_{12} injections, can be started before neurologic symptoms progress beyond correction. Folic acid will correct the anemia but will not stop the progression of neurologic symptoms. The vitamin B_{12} deficiency still will exist but may be undetected, which is why federal regulations require that vitamins sold over the counter cannot contain a significant amount of folic acid. A form of megaloblastic anemia similar to pernicious anemia has been reported[5] as a consequence of gastric bypass surgery.

GLUCOSE-6-PHOSPHATE DEHYDROGENASE DEFICIENCY

The search during World War II for a substitute quinine led to the discovery of glucose-6-phosphate dehydrogenase (G-6-PD) deficiency. Since then, glucose metabolism in the RBC has been established. Glucose enters the RBC by a carrier mechanism independent of insulin. About 90% of the glucose is metabolized by the glycolytic pathway. The remaining glucose is metabolized by the hexose monophosphate shunt pathway. The byproduct of the glycolytic pathway is adenosine triphosphate, which provides the energy for the cell. The byproduct of the hexose monophosphate shunt pathway is nicotinamide adenine dinucleotide phosphate (NADPH), which is used to reduce various cellular oxidants.[3]

G-6-PD is an enzyme needed for the hexose monophosphate shunt pathway. This enzyme is deficient in more than 400 million persons worldwide, making this disorder the most common enzymopathy of humans.[6] At present, more than 350 G-6-PD variants exist. They are grouped into five classes (I-V), with class I being severely deficient, based on the level of enzyme deficiency.[7] The G-6-PD gene is located on the X chromosome; thus the disease inheritance is gender-linked. G-6-PD A, the most common variant associated with hemolysis, is found in 11% of African-Americans. G-6-PD MED, the second-most common variant associated with hemolysis, occurs in ethnic groups of Mediterranean origin.[3] Not surprisingly, G-6-PD deficiency has an association with sickle cell anemia.[8]

Blockage of the hexose monophosphate shunt pathway in individuals with G-6-PD deficiency allows the accumulation of oxidants in the RBCs. These substances, which produce methemoglobin and denatured Hb, precipitate to form Heinz bodies; the Heinz bodies attach to cell membranes. Alteration of the cell membranes leads to hemolysis of the cell.[5]

The clinical features of G-6-PD deficiency involve acute intravascular hemolysis, which can be severe.

Jaundice, palpitations, dyspnea, and dizziness may result. Infection is the most common event that triggers hemolysis in G-6-PD A deficiency. Drugs are the most common trigger for hemolysis in G-6-PD MED deficiency.[6] Of more than 40 drugs that can induce hemolysis, those having dental significance include acetylsalicyclic acid, acetophenetidin (phenacetin), dapsone, ascorbic acid, and vitamin K.[3] Fava bean ingestion is the most common dietary cause of hemolytic anemia in persons with G-6-PD deficiency.

Screening tests for NADPH can be used to detect individuals with G-6-PD deficiency. More sensitive tests use direct spectrophotometric measurement of NADPH. Other tests used to detect this deficiency include the cyanide-ascorbate assay and the cytochemical estimation.[3]

SICKLE CELL ANEMIA

Sickle cell hemoglobin (Hb S) was the first Hb variant to be recognized of the more than 600 inherited human Hb variants (hemoglobinopathies) that exist. Of these, more than 90% have single amino acid substitutions in the Hb chain. Hb S is the result of substitution of a single amino acid, valine for glutamic acid, at the sixth residue of the β chain. In contrast, the thalassemias, another type of hemoglobinopathy, are caused by deletion or mutations of the α or β globin gene that result in reduced (or absent) synthesis of one or more globin chain.[9] The hemoglobinopathies are more commonly found in regions of malarial endemicity and in populations who have migrated from these regions, as the mutated gene(s) confer advantage against infection by *Plasmodium falciparum* (i.e., malaria). Hemoglobinopathies including sickle cell anemia are inherited as autosomal recessive traits.[10,11]

Sickle cell disorders are distinguished by the number of globin genes affected. The two most common types are sickle cell trait and sickle cell (disease) anemia. Sickle cell trait is the heterozygous state in which the affected individual carries one gene for Hb S. Approximately 8% to 10% of African-Americans carry the trait. In central Africa, up to 25% of the population may be carriers. Sickle cell anemia is the homozygous state. A gene from each parent contributes to formation of the Hb S molecule responsible for the disease. The RBC in sickle cell anemia becomes sickle-shaped when blood experiences lowered oxygen tension or decreased pH, or when the patient becomes dehydrated.[11-13] About 50,000 African-Americans (about 0.003% to 0.15%, or 1 in 600, have sickle cell anemia.[10,13-16]

Distortion of the RBC into a sickled shape is the result of deoxygenation or decreased blood pH, causing

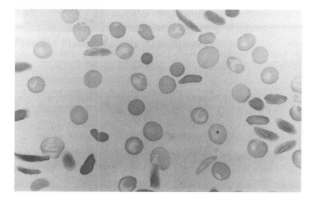

Fig. 20-1 Sickle cell anemia. Peripheral blood smear showing abnormal sickle-shaped red blood cells (RBCs) in sickle cell anemia. (Courtesy R. Estensen, Minneapolis, Minn.)

partial crystallization of Hb S, polymerization, and re-alignment of the defective Hb molecule (Fig. 20-1). Cellular rigidity and membrane damage occur, with irreversible sickling the final result. The net effect of these changes is erythrostasis, increased blood viscosity, reduced blood flow, hypoxia, increased adhesion of RBCs, vascular occlusion, and further sickling.[10,13] Sickling crises are rare in individuals with the sickle cell trait.[10]

In patients with sickle cell anemia, more than 80% of the Hb is Hb S. Diagnosis requires use of red cell indices, electrophoresis, and chromatography (usually high performance liquid chromatography).[1,17] Management is based on routine prophylactic penicillin for infants and early antibiotic use to prevent severe infections.[8] The clinical signs and symptoms of sickle cell anemia are the result of chronic anemia and small blood vessel occlusion. They include jaundice, pallor, dactylitis (hand and foot warmth and tenderness), leg ulcers, organomegaly, cardiac failure, stroke, and attacks of abdominal and bone pain (aseptic necrosis). Aplastic crises, where the patient becomes acutely ill, the production of red cells stops, and severe anemia occurs, may develop from infection, hypersensitivity reactions, hypoxia, systemic disease, acidosis, dehydration, or trauma.

Without the provision of contemporary health care, 50% of persons with sickle cell anemia will die before the age of 30 years. Because folic acid deficiency may play a role in the cause of the crises, folic acid dietary supplements are given daily to most patients with sickle cell anemia. In addition, penicillin prophylaxis is used at least for the first 5 years of life. Therapeutic strategies include the use of hydroxyurea (with or without erythropoietin), which induces the production of Hb F and thus prevents the formation of Hb S polymers.[10,18,19] Once a

crisis develops, high doses of folic acid, analgesics for pain, hydration, and blood transfusions are used to treat the patient.[8,10] Bone marrow transplantation (BMT) has been used in children with sickle cell anemia and has met with moderate success (25% to 30% cure rate) but is associated with mortality.[20]

Individuals with the sickle cell trait generally have no symptoms unless they are placed in situations in which abnormally low concentrations of oxygen are present (e.g., in an unpressurized airplane or through the injudicious administration of general anesthesia). Patients with sickle cell trait are much more resistant to sickling stimuli because only 20% to 45% of their Hb is Hb S. Patients with sickle cell trait are not at risk during dental treatment unless severe hypoxia, severe infection, or dehydration occurs.[10,13,14,16]

RENAL DISEASE

The kidney produces the hormone erythropoietin, which stimulates RBC production by the bone marrow. If significant renal damage occurs, the lack of production of this hormone results in anemia (see Chapter 9).

CLINICAL PRESENTATION

SIGNS AND SYMPTOMS

Symptoms of anemia include fatigue, palpitations, shortness of breath, abdominal pain, bone pain, tingling of fingers and toes, and muscular weakness. Signs of anemia may include jaundice, pallor, cracking, splitting and spooning of the fingernails, increased size of the liver and spleen, lymphadenopathy, and blood in the stool. Patients with anemia may complain of a sore or painful tongue, smooth tongue, or redness of the tongue. Some patients may complain of a loss of taste sensation.

SCREENING LABORATORY TESTS

If the dentist identifies a patient with signs or symptoms that suggest anemia, this patient should be sent to a commercial laboratory for a complete blood count and differential, or referred to a physician for evaluation. The Hb level, hematocrit, and RBC indices (mean corpuscular Hb and volume) are the tests used to screen the patient. In addition, a total WBC count and platelet count should be obtained (see Chapter 1).

All African-American patients should be questioned about the presence of sickle cell disease in their family histories. If no history of an individual having been screened for sickle cell disease exists, the dentist should

arrange for the patient to be tested. This can be done in the dental office using the Sickledex Test (Hb solubility test, distributed by Johnson & Johnson), in a commercial clinical laboratory, or by a physician.

■ WHITE BLOOD CELL DISORDERS ■

DEFINITION

Three groups of WBCs are found in the peripheral circulation: granulocytes, lymphocytes, and monocytes. Of the granulocyte population, 90% is composed of neutrophils; the remainder is composed of eosinophils and basophils. The circulating lymphocytes are of three types: T lymphocytes (thymus mediated); B lymphocytes (bursa-derived); and natural killer cells. Lymphocytes are subdivided by the surface markers they exhibit and the cytokines they produce.[21]

The primary function of neutrophils is to defend the body against certain infectious agents by phagocytosis and enzymatic destruction. The eosinophils and basophils are involved with inflammatory allergic reactions. The T lymphocytes (T cells) are involved with the delayed, or cellular, immune reaction, whereas the B lymphocytes (B cells) play an important role in the immediate, or humoral, immune system involving the production of plasma cells and immunoglobulins. The monocytes serve as phagocytes and mediate the immune and inflammatory response through the production of more than 100 substances, such as cytokines and growth factors (see Chapter 18). Monocytes also serve as antigen-presenting cells.

The majority of WBCs are produced primarily in the bone marrow (granulocytes and monocytes; Chapter 1), and these cells form several "pools" in the marrow: (1) the mitotic pool, which consists of immature precursor cells; (2) a maturing pool, which consists of cells undergoing maturation; and (3) a storage pool of functional cells, which can be released as needed.

The WBCs released by the bone marrow that are found circulating in the peripheral blood form two pools of cells, a marginal one and a circulating one. Cells in the marginal pool adhere to vessel walls and are readily available. When infection threatens the body, the storage and marginal pools can be called on to help fight the invading organisms.

Growth-promoting substances called *colony-stimulating factors* (CSFs) are responsible for the growth of committed granulocyte-monocyte stem cells. The major function of CSFs is to amplify leukopoiesis rather than recruit new stem cells into the granulocyte-monocyte differentiation pathway. Thus by the local release of CSFs, the bone marrow can increase the production of granulocytes and monocytes. This process occurs in response to infection.[22]

LEUKOCYTOSIS AND LEUKOPENIA

The number of circulating WBCs normally ranges from 4500 to 11,000/mm³ in adults.[8] The differential WBC count is an estimation of the percentage of each cell type per cubic millimeter of blood. A normal differential count consists of neutrophils, 50% to 60%; eosinophils, 1% to 3%; basophils, less than 1%; lymphocytes, 20% to 30%; and monocytes, 3% to 7%. The term *leukocytosis* is defined[8] as an increase in the number of circulating WBCs to more than 11,000/mm³, and *leukopenia* as a reduction in the number of circulating WBCs (usually to less than 4500/mm³).

Many causes of leukocytosis are known. Exercise, pregnancy, and emotional stress can lead to increased numbers of WBCs in the peripheral circulation. Leukocytosis resulting from these causes is called *physiologic leukocytosis*. Pathologic leukocytosis can be caused by infections, neoplasia, and necrosis. Pyogenic infections induce a type of leukocytosis characterized by an increased number of neutrophils. If excessive numbers of immature neutrophils (stab cells) are released into the circulation in response to a bacterial infection, a shift to the left is said to have occurred. Tuberculosis, syphilis, and viral infections produce a type of leukocytosis characterized by increased numbers of lymphocytes. Protozoan infections often produce a type of leukocytosis that increases the numbers of monocytes. Allergies and parasitic infections caused by certain helminths increase the number of circulating eosinophils. Cellular necrosis increases the numbers of circulating neutrophils. Leukemia (cancer of the WBCs) is characterized by a great increase in the numbers of circulating immature leukocytes. Carcinomas of glandular tissues may cause an increase in the number of circulating neutrophils. Acute bleeding also can result in a leukocytosis.

Many causes of deficient numbers of leukocytes (less than 4500/mm³) in the blood are also evident. Leukopenia may occur in the early phase of leukemia and lymphoma as a result of bone marrow replacement by excessive proliferation of WBCs. Leukopenia also occurs during agranulocytosis (reduction of granulocytes) and pancytopenia (decrease in WBCs and RBCs) that result from toxic effects of drugs and chemicals. An important form of leukopenia involves the cyclic depression of circulating neutrophils, a disorder called *cyclic neutropenia*, in which patients have a periodic decrease (at least 40% drop) in the number of neutrophils (about every 21 to 28 days). During the period in which few circulating

neutrophils are present, the patient is susceptible to infection and oral manifestation (see Oral Complications and Manifestations in this chapter).[14,24] Familial and chronic idiopathic forms of neutropenia also contribute.[23]

Patients with leukocytosis or leukopenia can have bone marrow abnormalities that can cause thrombocytopenia. Infectious diseases associated with leukocytosis and leukopenia are discussed in Chapters 8, 12, and 13.

LEUKEMIA AND LYMPHOMA

Leukemia is cancer of the WBCs affecting the bone marrow and circulating blood. It involves exponential proliferation of a clonal myeloid or lymphoid cell and occurs in both an acute and chronic forms. This section includes a description of six types of leukemia: (1) acute lymphocytic, (2) acute myeloid, (3) chronic lymphocytic, (4) chronic myeloid, (5) hairy cell, and (6) acute T-cell leukemia.

Lymphoma is cancer of lymphoid organs and tissues. This section includes a discussion of three types of lymphoma (Hodgkin's disease, non-Hodgkin's lymphoma, and Burkitt's lymphoma) and a plasma cell malignancy (multiple myeloma). These diseases are of importance to the dentist because the initial signs often occur in the mouth (e.g., Waldeyer's ring) and in the head and neck region, and precautions must be taken before any dental treatment is provided.

Leukemia and lymphoma account for about 8% of all new malignancies each year in the United States, which amounts to approximately 93,000 cases per year.[25] These patients are usually immunosuppressed because of the disease itself or secondary to the treatment used to control it. Hence, they are prone to develop serious infections and often are bleeders because of thrombocytopenia.

Leukemia

Leukemia occurs in all races, at any age at an incidence of 10.4 per 100,000.[26] Approximately 30,000 new cases per year are diagnosed in the United States.[15,25] The incidence of leukemia has remained somewhat stable in the United States since about 1956. The mortality rate also has remained stable, at about 6.8 deaths per 100,000 population per year, with 50% to 60% of the deaths caused by acute leukemia. All types of leukemia are somewhat more common in men. The male/female ratio for acute leukemia is about 3:2, and for chronic leukemia, it is about 2:1. About 50% of all leukemia is the acute form.

The cause of leukemia remains unknown (Box 20-2). Increased risk is found in association with large doses of ionizing radiation; certain chemicals (benzene); and infection with a few viruses (Epstein Barr virus [EBV] and

---

BOX **20-2**

Etiology of the Leukemias

1. Host factors
   a. Heredity
      (1) Generally not inherited disease
      (2) High concordance among identical twins if one twin develops disease early
      (3) A few leukemic families have been reported
   b. Chromosome abnormalities—increased risk in:
      (1) Down syndrome
      (2) Turner's syndrome
      (3) Klinefelter's syndrome
      (4) Fanconi's anemia
   c. Immunodeficiency syndromes (hereditary types)
   d. Chronic bone marrow dysfunction
2. Environmental factors
   a. Ionizing radiation
      (1) Radiation therapy
      (2) Occupational exposure
      (3) Atomic bomb survivors
   b. Chemical and drugs
      (1) Benzene (organic solvents)
      (2) Chloramphenicol
      (3) Phenylbutazone
      (4) Arsenic pesticides
      (5) Alkylating chemotherapeutic agents
   c. Viruses
      (1) HTLV-I (adult T cell leukemia)
      (2) HTLV-II (atypical hairy cell leukemia)

Adapted from Champlin R, Golde DW: In Wilson JD et al, editors: *Harrison's principles of internal medicine,* ed 12, New York, 1991, McGraw-Hill, pp 1552-1561; List AF, Spier CM, Dalton US: In Hiddeman W et al, editors: *Haematology and blood transfusion: acute leukemias,* ed 34, New York, 1992, Springer-Verlag, pp 3-10; O'Mura GA: In Rose LF, Kaye D, editors: *Internal medicine for dentistry,* ed 2, St Louis, 1990, Mosby, pp 317-324; Perkins ML: In Harmening DM, editor: *Clinical hematology and fundamentals of hemostasis,* ed 2, Philadelphia, 1992, FA Davis, pp 266-292.

human lymphotropic virus [HTLV]-1).[15,36] Cigarette smoking and exposure to electromagnetic fields also have been proposed to be causative. Box 20-2 lists the various factors that have been implicated in the etiology of human leukemias. Acute and chronic forms of leukemia are based on the degree of maturation of cells and survival time of the patient. The diagnosis of leukemia is made by examination of peripheral blood and bone mar-

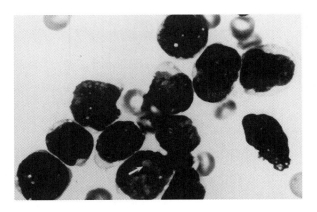

Fig. 20-2 Acute lymphoblastic leukemia. Peripheral blood smear showing many lymphoblasts with large nuclei and large nucleoli (*arrow*), representative of acute lymphoblastic leukemia. (Courtesy R. Estensen, Minneapolis.)

row stained with Wright-Giemsa. Cytochemical staining, immunophenotyping, and cytogenetic analyses are used to characterize the type and subtype, allow for specific treatment approaches, and detect residual disease following therapy. Hemorrhage and infection, often complications of chemotherapy, are the chief causes of death.

Acute Leukemia. Acute leukemia has a sudden onset and leads to death in 1 to 3 months if untreated.[27] It consists of increased numbers of immature WBCs in the bone marrow and peripheral circulation (Fig. 20-2). The two types of acute leukemia are acute myeloid (AML) and acute lymphoblastic (ALL). Both types make patients susceptible to excessive bleeding, poor healing, and infection after surgical procedures.[28]

AML is characterized by cytogenetic abnormalities (e.g., translocation and rearrangement of chromosomes) that affect transcriptional cascades of myeloid precursor cells. It arises either *de novo* in younger adults or secondarily in elderly because of myelodysplasia. An age-related increase in incidence occurs from 3.5 per 100,000 persons younger than 45 years to 35 per 100,000 by age 90. The mean age of AML in the United States is 63 years.[29] AML produces a leukemic infiltration of marrow and organs that causes cytopenia and diverse nonspecific signs and symptoms including bone pain. The anemia and thrombocytopenia usually manifest as fatigue, weakness, dyspnea on exertion, pallor, bleeding and small hemorrhages (petechiae, ecchymoses) of the skin and mucous membranes.[30] Because of granulocytopenia at least one third of patients have recurrent infections, oral ulcerations, and fever. Enlargement of the tonsils, lymph nodes, spleen, and gingiva occurs as a result of leukemic infiltration of these tissues. Infiltration of

the central nervous system (CNS) and the skin as a raised, nonpruritic rash termed *leukemia cutis* also occurs.

The diagnosis of AML is made by the presence of at least 30% myeloblasts in the bone marrow. According to the French-American-British classification, nine subtypes of AML have been identified that differ by myeloid lineage and morphology (Table 20-1). Little difference is evident in the clinical findings among the subtypes, except that disseminated intravascular coagulation is found associated most often with M3 and M4, whereas M5 is more likely to have extramedullary involvement of the gingiva, skin, and CNS.[31,32]

Treatment involves chemotherapy (Table 20-2 and Box 20-3); BMT; or in specific cases (e.g., M3, acute promyelocytic leukemia), tretinoin (vitamin A analogue) and chemotherapy. The prognosis of AML in adults who are 60 years or older is poor. Chemotherapy can produce remission in 60% to 80% of these older patients, but the duration is short (Table 20-3). Additional adverse prognostic factors include previous chemotherapy for AML, WBC more than 20,000 per mm^3 a patient, elevated serum lactate dehydrogenase, and those who develop preleukemia syndrome.[30,31] In contrast, complete remission is gained in 70% to 80% of adults under age 60 years who undergo intensive treatment and more than 90% in promyelocytic leukemias treated with tretinoin.[33]

ALL typically occurs in children. It accounts for about 50% of all neoplasms in children and 80% of leukemias in children. A remarkable peak of incidence occurs in children who are 2 to 4 years old, with 75% of cases in this age group. Boys are affected slightly more often than girls. The disease is associated with chromosomal anomalies that commonly result in 50 to 65 chromosomes (e.g., hyperdiploidy).[34] The clinical presentation of ALL is similar to AML, but with bone and joint pain that can affect walking, and a higher propensity of central nervous system disease. Laboratory evaluation almost always reveals depressed levels of Hb, hematocrit, and platelets reflecting large replacement of marrow by lymphoblasts.

ALL is classified based on the type, size, and immunophenotype of the neoplastic lymphocytes. The classification system consists of three groups: L-1 (small cells); L-2 (larger cells); and L-3 (Burkitt-type, large, homogeneous B marker cells).[35] More than 90% of the leukemic lymphoblasts in ALL contain a nuclear enzyme, terminal deoxynucleotidyl transferase (Tdt), which serves as a marker for this disease. Tdt can be found in leukemic lymphoblasts of AML, but this is rare.[31] The immature leukemic cells in about 80% of the patients with ALL, in addition to being Tdt$^+$, have a common ALL (B cell) antigen (CD10, originally designated CALLA) and CD19, CD22, and HLA-DR.[31] The leukemic cells in 20% of the patients with ALL are T cell types, Tdt$^+$, and CD10$^-$. In 15%

TABLE 20-1

Classification of Acute Leukemias and Associated Clinical,* Cytologic, Immunologic Abnormalities

FAB Subtype	Common Name (% of Cases)	RESULTS OF STAINING			Cell Surface Markers	Chromosomal Abnormalities
		Myeloperoxidase and Sudan Black	Nonspecific Esterase	PAS		
Acute Myeloid Leukemias (AMLs)						
M0	Acute myeloblastic leukemia with minimal differentiation (3%)	−	−	−	For subtypes M0-M5, about 90% of cases will react with at least one of the anti-myeloid antibodies listed: Anti-CD13	inv and t
M1	Acute myeloblastic leukemia without maturation (15-20%)	+	±|	−		various
M2	Acute myeloblastic leukemia with maturation (25-30%)	+	±|	+	Anti-CD14	t(8;21)
M3	Acute promyelocytic leukemia (5-10%)	+	+	+	Anti-CD33	t(15;17)
M4	Acute promyelocytic leukemia (20%)	+	+++	++	Anti-CD34	inv and t
M4Eo	Acute myelomonocytic leukemia with abnormal eosinophils (5-10%)	+	+++	++		inv and t
M5	Acute myocytic leukemia (2-9%)	−	+++	++		t(9;11)
M6	Erythroleukemia (3-5%)	+	−	++	Antiglycoporin antispectrin	
M7	Acute megakaryocytic leukemia (3-12%)	−	±|	+	CD41, CD61	t
Acute Lymphoblastic Leukemias (ALLs)						
L1, Childhood variant	Small, uniform blasts, nucleoli indistinct	−	−	+++	About 80% react with anti-CD10; 20% with T-Cell phenotype: antiCD1, 2, 3, 5, or 7	t(9;22), t(4;11) and t(1;9)
L2, Adult variant	Larger, more irregular nucleoli present	−	−	++		
L3, Burkitt-like	Large with strong basophilic cytoplasm and vacuoles	−	−	−	Anti-CD19, 20	t(8;14)

***Signs of Leukemia:** Pallor, lymphadenopathy, petechiae, ecchymoses, gingival enlargement, oral ulcerations, loose teeth, pulpal abscess, enlarged tonsils, gingival bleeding.

Symptoms of Leukemia: Dyspnea, palpitations, fever, weakness, recurrent infections, spontaneous gingival bleeding, weight loss, sore throat, bone and organ pain (Modified from Applebaum FR: The Acute Leukemias. In Goldman L, Bennett JC editors: *Cecil textbook of medicine*, ed 21, Philadelphia, 2000, WB Saunders, p 955).

TABLE 20-2

Classes of Drugs Used to Treat Leukemias

Class of Drug	Chemotherapeutic Agent	Mechanism of Action
Alkylating agents	Busulfan, Carmustine, Cyclophosphamide, Dacarbazine, Lomustine Nitrogen Mustard Derivative: Chlorambucil	Produce alkyl radicals causing cross-linking of DNA and inhibition of DNA synthesis in rapidly replicating tumor cells
Antibiotics	Bleomycin, Daunorubicin, Doxorubicin, Idarubicin, Mitomycin C	Disrupt cellular function such as RNA synthesis or inhibit mitosis
Antimetabolites	Folic acid analogs: Methotrexate	Disrupt enzymatic processes or nucleic acid synthesis
	Purine analogs: Cladribine, Fludarabine, Fluorouracill 6-Mercaptopurine, Thioguanine	
	Pyrimidine nucleoside analogs: Arabinosyl cytosine (Ara-C, Cytarabine)	
Biologicals	Interferon alfa	Causes a direct antiproliferative effect on CML progenitor cells
	Monoclonal antibodies eg., Rituximab (Rituxan)	Binds antigen target on malignant lymphocyte
	All-trans retinoic acid (Tretinoin)	Induces differentiation and apoptosis of malignant promyelocytes in APML
Enzymes	Asparaginase	Inhibits synthesis of asparagine which is required for protein synthesis in leukemic lymphoblasts
Mitotic inhibitors	Vincristine, Vinblastine	Act as mitotic spindle inhibitors causing metaphase arrest
	Etoposide	Topoisomerase II inhibitor
Steroid	Prednisone	Hormone that has anti-inflammatory and antilymphocytic properties

BOX 20-3

Chemotherapeutic Protocols Used to Treat Leukemias and Lymphomas

Acute lymphoblastic leukemia (ALL): *Induction:* Vincristine + prednisone + asparaginase + daunorubicin or doxorubicin ± cyclophosphamide. *CNS prophylaxis:* Intrathecal methotrexate (± intrathecal cytarabine ± intrathecal hydrocortisone) ± systemic high-dose methotrexate with leucovorin. *Maintenance:* Mercaptopurine + methotrexate; High-dose chemotherapy + bone marrow infusion.

Acute myeloid leukemia (AML): *Induction:* Cytarabine + either daunorubicin or idarubicin ± etoposide. *For acute promyelocytic leukemia (APL):* tretinoin ± further induction therapy. *CNS prophylaxis:* Intrathecal cytarabine or methotrexate ± intrathecal hydrocortisone. *Post Induction:* High-dose cytarabine ± other drugs; High-dose chemotherapy + bone marrow infusion.

Chronic myeloid leukemia (CML): Interferon alfa ± cytarabine; Chronic phase Hi-dose chemotherapy + bone marrow infusion ± donor lymphocyte infusions. Accelerated: Cytarabine + daunorubicin or idarubicin; Hi-dose chemotherapy + bone marrow infusion. Blast phase: *Lymphoid:* vincristine + prednisone + asparaginase + doxorubicin or daunorubicin ± cytophosphamide + intrathecal methotrexate (± maintenance with mercaptopurine + methotrexate). Myeloid: Cytarabine + daunorubicin or idarubicin.

Chronic lymphocytic leukemia (CLL): Fludarabine ± cyclophosphamide; Chlorambucil or cyclophosphamide ± prednisone.

Hodgkin's and Non-Hodgkins' lymphomas: Doxorubicin + bleomycin + vinblastine + dacarbazine.

Burkitt's lymphomas: Cyclophosphamide + doxorubicin + vincristine + prednisone (CHOP) + high dose methotrexate + intrathecal methotrexate; Cyclophosphamide + doxorubicin + vincristine + etoposide + bleomycin + methotrexate + prednisone.

From Geller RB, Dix SP: Oral chemotherapy agents in the treatment of leukaemia, *Drugs* 58 Suppl 3:109-118, 1999; and Perry MC, Anderson CM, Donehower RC: In Abdeloof MD et al. editors: *Clinical Oncology,* ed 2, New York 2000, Churchill Livingstone; 387-419.

TABLE **20-3**

Clinical Factors in Acute and Chronic Leukemias

Factor	TYPE OF LEUKEMIA			
	ALL	**AML**	**CLL**	**CML**
Age	Children (75%)	Adults (85%)	Over 40 years	30 to 50
Prognosis	Very good	Poor	Good	years
Survival (mean)	—	2 years	Stage I (19 months)	Poor
			Stage IV (12 years)	3 to 4 years
Remissions	90%	60% to 80%	—	—
Duration	Usually long term	9 to 24 months	—	—
Cures	50% to 70%	10% to 30%	—	—
	ALL	**AML**	**CLL**	**CML**
Age	Adults (25%)	Children (15%)	Children (rare)	Children (rare)
Prognosis	Poor	Poor	—	—
Survival (mean)	26 months	—	—	—
Remissions	50% to 70%	56% to 66%	—	—
Duration	10 to 19 months	8 to 12 months	—	—
Cures	20%	20% to 40%	—	—

ALL, Acute lymphocytic leukemia; AML, acute myelogenous leukemia; CLL, chronic lymphocytic leukemia; CML chronic myelogenous leukemia.

Adapted from Canellos GP: In Petersdorf RG et al, editors: *Principles of internal medicine*, ed 10, New York, 1983, McGraw-Hill; Champlin R, Golde DW: In Wilson JD et al, editors: *Harrison's principles of internal medicine*, ed 12, New York, 1991, McGraw-Hill, pp 1552-1561; Clarkson B: In Petersdorf RG et al, editors: *Harrison's principles of internal medicine*, ed 10, New York, 1983, McGraw-Hill; O'Mura GA. In Rose LF, Kaye D, Editors: *Internal medicine for dentistry*, ed 2, St Louis, 1990, Mosby; pp 317-324; Perkins ML: In Harmening DM, editor: *Clinical hematology and fundamentals of hemostasis*, ed 2 , Philadelphia, 1992, FA Davis, pp 266-292.

of the patients, leukemic lymphocytes are the null cell type and lack Tdt, CD10, and T-cell and B-cell antigens. A mature B-cell phenotype is detected in less than 5% of the patients with ALL.[31,36]

The prognosis for children with ALL is very good, with cures now being obtained in more than 70% of cases. The prognosis is worse in those more than 30 years of age, with blast count greater than 50,000 per mm³, with mature B-cell ALL phenotype, with multiorgan involvement and chromosomal translocations t (;22) or t (4;11). Remission can be achieved with chemotherapy; however the duration of remission is short. The overall long-term survival (cure) rate for adults is less than 20%.[31,36] Relapse can result in second remission in 75% but less than 30% of these are cured.

Treatment of Acute Leukemia. The ability to cure a patient of acute leukemia is related to tumor burden and the rapid elimination of malignant WBCs. The normal bone marrow consists of 0.3% to 5% blast cells. Patients with acute leukemia have 100-fold more (about a trillion) blast cells. Once effective chemotherapy has been given, the number of blast cells is reduced from tril-

lions to billions, leukemic cells can no longer be detected, and the patient is said to be in *remission*. With a 5-day generation time for the remaining undetectable leukemic cell mass, 10 doublings in 50 days could restore the leukemic cell mass to a trillion cells, and the patient would again show signs and symptoms of leukemia. This would constitute a short remission with a relapse.[37]

Three phases are administered in chemotherapy of acute leukemias. The purpose of the first phase (induction) is to hit hard and induce a state of remission by killing tumor cells with cytotoxic agents. Agents used to treat the acute leukemias are shown in Table 20-2 and Box 20-3. The second phase (consolidation or intensification) is to consolidate the kill of remaining leukemic cells. The third phase (remission) is to provide maintenance treatment to prevent any remaining leukemic cell mass from expanding. During induction and consolidation, myeloid growth factors (granulocyte colony stimulating factor [G-CSF] and granulocyte monocyte colony stimulating factor [GM-CSF]) are administered at some institutes to shorten the duration

of neutropenia and reduce the incidence of severe infections.

Patients are cured of leukemia when no leukemic cells remain. Long-term survival occurs when the leukemic cell mass is greatly reduced and kept from increasing over a long period. In general, once a patient relapses, a second remission is more difficult to induce and, if it occurs, will be of a shorter duration.[31,36] BMT is generally reserved for those under the age of 45 years and children and young adults who relapse when a suitable sibling match is available (allogeneic).[31,36] The marrow transplant, or more recently, peripheral blood stem cell transplant, is preceded by high-dose chemotherapy (including busulfan) and radiation therapy.

Another concern of treatment of patients with acute leukemia is that leukemic cells can migrate to areas in the body where chemotherapeutic agents cannot reach them. These areas are called *sanctuaries*, and they require special treatment. The most important sanctuary in patients with ALL is the CNS. Thus patients with ALL will be treated by cranial irradiation plus intrathecal methotrexate in addition to the usual antileukemic agents. Another important sanctuary (in males) is the testes.[31,36]

Chronic Leukemia. Chronic myeloid and chronic lymphocytic (CLL) are the two types of chronic leukemia. The more common form in the United States is CLL. The chronic leukemias have a slower onset of symptoms, a better prognosis, and more mature WBCs than acute leukemias. About 25% of the patients are identified during routine examinations.[31,37]

Chronic myeloid leukemia (CML) has an incidence of 1 to 2 cases per 100,000 population.[25] The majority of patients with CML are 45 to 55 years of age at the onset. Their WBC count is usually around 200,000/mm³ at the time of diagnosis, and the symptoms include an enlarged and painful spleen, abdominal fullness, pallor, weight loss, fever, anemia, leukocytosis, bleeding problems and purpura, and increased serum vitamin B_{12} levels.[38] Lymphadenopathy is rare in the early phase of the disease. At least 20% of the patients with CML are asymptomatic at the time of diagnosis. They are identified by the marked elevation of their white cell count during routine examinations (Fig. 20-3).

Of the leukemic cells in CML, 95% have the Philadelphia (Ph) chromosome, a shortened chromosome 22 resulting from reciprocal translocation between the long arms of chromosomes 9 and 22, which can be found in the metaphase and contributes abnormal tyrosine kinase activity and myeloid proliferation.[39] The Ph chromosome revealed by cytogenetic analysis is part of the standard diagnostic workup. This abnormal chromosome and its hybrid BCR-ABL gene product are used to monitor patient response to therapy.

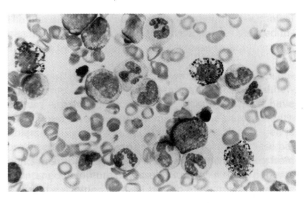

Fig. 20-3 Chronic myeloid leukemia. Peripheral blood smear showing granulocytes in all stages of maturation typical of this type of leukemia. (Courtesy R. Estensen, Minneapolis, Minn.)

CML progresses from a chronic phase (3 to 5 years) to an accelerated phase and then a blast phase (or crisis). During the indolent phase of CML, the leukemic cells are functional; thus infection is not a major problem. However, once transformation to the blastic stage has occurred, the leukemic cells are immature and nonfunctional; infection then becomes a major problem. About 25% of CML patients per year undergo a transformation to the blast phase of the disease after 6 to 12 months following diagnosis. The blast phase consists of 30% or more leukemic cells in peripheral blood or marrow.[40] More than 85% of the patients with CML die in the blast phase, and patients without the Philadelphia chromosome have worse prognosis. The overall prognosis for CML is poor, with survival from time of diagnosis being about 3.5 years.[11,18,41]

CML is treated in the chronic phase with hydroxyurea, hydroxycarbamide or busulfan which results in good symptom and blood count control. Use of other alkylating agents, cytarabine, whole-body radiation therapy plus BMT, stem-cell transplantation, and interferon alfa (see Table 20-2 and Box 20-3) have yielded remission in 50% at 5 years. BMT is a poor option once transformation to the blastic stage has occurred.[31,41]

Chronic lymphocytic leukemia is the most common type of leukemia in adults.[15] Patients with CLL are older than those with CML (mean age 60 years). Both CML and CLL are rare in children.

Of the patients with CLL, 95% have neoplastic B cells.[42] A trisomy 12 chromosomal abnormality is present in the leukemic cells of 40% of patients. In most cases, monoclonal immunoglobulin can be demonstrated on the cell surface. Less than 5% of the patients with CLL have leukemic cells of T-cell origin. The diagnosis of CLL is made when lymphocytosis (more than 50,000 per mm³)

exists for more than 1 month. CLL patients have an enlarged spleen, lymphadenopathy, and decreased serum immunoglobulin levels that contributes to susceptibility to infections. Less frequently, CLL patients develop associated anemia and thrombocytopenia.

CLL is classified using an international staging system. Three stages are identified: stage A (two or fewer lymph node groups, no anemia or thrombocytopenia); stage B (three or more lymph node groups, no anemia or thrombocytopenia); and stage C (anemia and thrombocytopenia, any number of lymph node groups). The lymph node groups include cervical, axillary, inguinal, liver, and spleen. The mean survival time for patients with stage A disease is more than 10 years; with stage B, about 5 years; and with stage C, only about 2 years. Treatment of CLL has had little effect on survival times. Patients in the asymptomatic phase usually are not treated. Only moderate effectiveness has been reported for some treatments in the reduction of lymphocyte counts and palliation of symptoms. Chlorambucil, prednisone, fludarabine or cladribine, and ionizing radiation have been used in the treatment of CLL with some benefit.[31,33-37]

A form of chronic lymphocytic leukemia called *hairy cell leukemia* has been described. These patients have leukemic B cells with hairlike cytoplasmic projections. This form of chronic leukemia is usually found in men over the age of 40. The patient may have an enlarged spleen, a hemocytopenia, and an associated vasculitis-like disorder (e.g., erythema nodosum or polyarteritis nodosa). More than 50% of affected patients will survive longer than 8 years from the time of diagnosis. Patients with atypical hairy cell leukemia appear to have a viral cause for their disease (HTLV-II). Other human leukemias caused by virus infection are African Burkitt's (EBV) and acute T cell (HTLV-I).[31,37,41]

Complications of Chronic Leukemia. In general, patients with a chronic leukemia have anemia and bleeding problems associated with thrombocytopenia. These can be caused by the leukemia itself and the effects of chemotherapy. Infection is less of a problem in patients with a chronic leukemia than in those with an acute leukemia because the cells are more mature and functional in chronic leukemias. However, in the later stages of both CML and CLL, infection can become a serious complication.[38] Splenectomy because of massive splenomegaly can also increase the risk of infection. Table 20-4 lists parameters in comparison of acute and chronic leukemias.

Lymphomas

Lymphomas represent the seventh-most common malignancy worldwide. They are grouped as B-cell and T-cell neoplasms and into low-, intermediate- and high-

TABLE 20-4

Comparison of Acute and Chronic Leukemias

Parameter	Acute	Chronic
Clinical onset	Sudden	Insidious
Course (untreated)	Less than 6 months	2 to 6 years
Leukemic cells	Immature	Mature
Anemia	Mild to severe	Mild
Thrombocytopenia	Mild to severe	Mild
WBC	Variable	Increased
Organomegaly	Mild	Prominent
Age	Adults and children	Adults

Adapted from Perkins ML: *Clinical hematology and fundamentals of hemostasis*, Philadelphia, 1992, FA Davis, pp 266-292.

grade categories. Of 14 types, three lymphoma are considered in this section: Hodgkin's disease, non-Hodgkin's lymphoma, and Burkitt's lymphoma. In addition, multiple myeloma is described because it represents a lymphoproliferative disorder of clinical importance to the dentist.

Hodgkin's Disease. Hodgkin's disease results from uncontrolled growth of lymphocytes. The cause remains unknown, but two peaks of incidence occur, one in early adulthood and the other peak around the fifth decade of life.[32] Hodgkin's disease affects about 7500 Americans per year.[25,32] The initial presentation is a mass or group of firm, nontender, enlarged lymph nodes, often (i.e., more than 50% of cases) affecting the mediastinal nodes or neck nodes.[32] Later, fever, weight loss, sweating, pruritus, and fatigue develop. Enlarging tumorous nodes can cause lung or vascular obstruction or can eventually spread to the liver or spleen. Diagnosis of lymphoma is made from nodal biopsy or bone marrow aspirate. Microscopically, Hodgkin's disease typically shows large multinucleated Reed-Sternberg reticulum (monoclonal B) cells (Fig. 20-4). Survival time varies from short- to long-term and relates to the stage of the disease and symptoms.[43] Staging is determined from biopsies, history, physical examination, and computed tomography scans. Radiation (therapeutic dose of 4000 centigrays [cGy]) and chemotherapy (e.g., alkylating agents, MOPP [nitrogen mustard, vincristine, procarbazine, prednisone]) are used for treatment. An increased risk for developing acute leukemia occurs in 3% to 10% of patients who receive alkylating agents as part of therapy.[43]

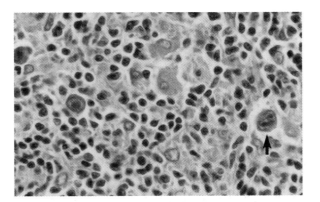

Fig. 20-4 Hodgkin's disease. Photomicrograph showing the involved tissue with a characteristic Reed-Sternberg cell *(arrow)* containing an "owls-eye" nucleus. (Courtesy M. Cibull; Lexington, Ky.)

TABLE 20-5

Comparison of Non-Hodgkin's and Hodgkin's Lymphomas

Parameter	Non-Hodgkin's	Hodgkin's
Cellular derivation	90% B cell 10% T cell	Unresolved
Site		
Localized	Uncommon	Common
Nodal	Discontiguous	Contiguous
Extranodal	Common	Uncommon
Abdominal	Common	Uncommon
Mediastinal	Uncommon	Common
Bone marrow	Common	Uncommon
Symptoms (fever, night sweats, weight loss)	Uncommon	Common
Curability	Less than 25%	Greater than 75%

From Nadler LM: In Wilson JD et al, editors: H*arrison's principles of internal medicine*, ed 12, New York, 1991, McGraw-Hill, pp 1599-1612.

Patients with Hodgkin's disease are also prone to infections and inflammation.

Non-Hodgkin's Lymphoma. Non-Hodgkin's lymphoma (NHL) is a lymphoproliferative disorder, primarily (90%) of B-cell origin.[32] Although the cause of NHL is not completely understood, the disease is related to persistent inflammation, immunodeficiency states, EBV infection, and in cases of gastric lymphoma, to *Helicobacter pylori* infection of the stomach. Each year about 50,000 new cases are reported, and all races and age groups are affected. NHL results in 25,000 deaths per year and is the seventh leading cause of death in the United States.[25,26] The condition has been reported[32] in association with acquired immunodeficiency syndrome (AIDS) (about 10% of AIDS cases) and in these cases, appears to be EBV-associated. NHL is also a potential complication of Sjögren's syndrome.[32]

More than 20 variations of NHL occur, and classification is based on pattern of distribution (diffuse or nodular); cell type (lymphocytic, histiocytic, mixed); and degree of differentiation of the cells (well, moderate, poor). Unlike Hodgkin's disease, which often begins with a single focus of tumor, NHL is usually multifocal when first detected.[32,44] The most prominent sign of NHL is nontender, lymph node swelling of greater than 2 weeks duration.[32,44] Additional signs and symptoms include persistent fever of unknown cause, weight loss, malaise, sweating, painful lymphadenopathy, abdominal or chest pain, and on occasion extranodal tumors.[44,45,46] Head, neck, and intraabdominal manifestations occur fairly often.[45,46] Less frequently, an oral presentation (e.g., a firm swelling arising from the posterior hard palate) may be seen.

NHLs are radiosensitive and the typical total dose is 4000 to 5000 cGy. More advanced stage disease (e.g., widespread lymphoid and organ involvement) requires the addition of chemotherapy. Cure rates exceed 50% in cases of localized disease. Patients who have advanced disease and undergo radiotherapy and chemotherapy have a median survival of about 2 years.[44] Bone marrow transplants and monoclonal antibodies against antigens expressed by malignant lymphocytes (e.g., Rituxan) combined with chemotherapy also have helped patients who poorly respond to traditional therapies. Extranodal lymphomas in the oral-pharyngeal region have a poor prognosis. Table 20-5 compares the findings of Hodgkin's disease and NHL.

Burkitt's Lymphoma. Burkitt's lymphoma is a malignant, monomorphic B lymphocyte proliferation associated in the majority of cases with EBV and translocation of the *c-myc* gene from chromosome 8 to the immunoglobulin gene on chromosome 14 [t(8;14)] or 2 [t(2;8)]. It affects children and young adults at a rate of 0.05 cases per 100,000 and has been reported as a development in AIDS.[37] Burkitt's lymphoma is found most often in Central Africa, where it usually is seen as a tumor of the jaws. In the United States the disease initially involves lymph nodes of the abdomen and bone marrow. The American form has a worse prognosis. Diagnosis is based on the radiographic features and histologic pattern of numerous small, noncleaved atypical

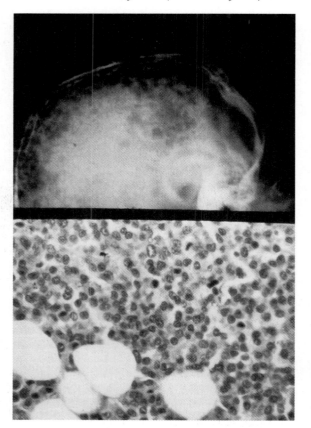

Fig. 20-5 Multiple myeloma. Punched-out lytic lesions in the skull containing malignant plasma cells shown in lower frame. (Courtesy R. Estensen, Minneapolis, Minn.)

CD10[+] lymphocytes interspersed with histiocytes ("starry sky" pattern). Intraoral radiographs demonstrate osteolytic jaw lesions and tooth displacement, usually developing distal to the last mandibular molar. Radiation and chemotherapy are used for treatment of Burkitt's lymphoma. Those that live beyond 2 years often enjoy long-term remission.

Multiple Myeloma. Multiple myeloma is a lymphoproliferative disorder consisting of an overproduction of cloned malignant plasma cells. Its origin remains unknown. Incidence is equal among men and women, and mean survival is only 2 years. Each year, about 10,000 new cases occur.[26,47] Most cases occur in persons older than 65 years. The disease consists of plasma and myeloma cell proliferation, immunoglobulin production, and bone marrow replacement (Fig. 20-5). The bone marrow replacement leads to anemia, leukopenia, thrombocytopenia, hypercalcemia, and eventually a decrease in plasma immunoglobulins. During the early to middle stages of disease, increased plasma viscosity contributes to altered platelet function, excessive bleeding, and renal impairment. Additional signs and symptoms include weakness, weight loss, recurrent infections, bone pain, anemia, pathologic fractures and Bence-Jones proteins (abnormal immunoglobulin light chains) in the urine.

Dental radiographs may show "punched-out" lesions or mottled areas representing areas of tumor. These osteolytic lesions are more common in the posterior body of the mandible and can be associated with cortical plate expansion. Extramedullary plasma cell tumors can occur in the oral pharynx. An amyloid-like protein is found sometimes in oral soft tissues as a result of multiple myeloma, and these areas may be swollen and painful. Biopsy and special amyloid stains can be used for diagnosis.[47] Treatment of multiple myeloma consists of chemotherapeutic agents (alkylating agents) and localized radiotherapy. Patients undergoing chemo- or radiotherapy are susceptible to infection, bony fracture, and excessive bleeding. Biphosphonates and antibiotics are used to maintain bone strength and treat infections, respectively.

DENTAL MANAGEMENT

MEDICAL CONSIDERATIONS

The dentist should search for signs and symptoms of anemia or WBC disorders in patients who are seen for dental treatment. A patient with the classic signs or symptoms of anemia, leukemia, or lymphoma, for example, should be referred directly to a physician. Patients with signs and symptoms suggestive of these disorders should be screened by appropriate laboratory tests and/or biopsy of soft tissue and osseous lesions. Screening laboratory tests can be obtained by sending the patient to a commercial clinical laboratory or to a physician. Screening tests should include total and differential WBC counts; a smear for cell morphologic study; a Hb or hematocrit count; a Sickledex test (for African-Americans); and a platelet count. If the screening tests are ordered by the dentist and one or more are abnormal, the patient should be referred for medical evaluation and treatment.

Patients with anemia may have a serious underlying disease such as peptic ulcer or carcinoma, in which early detection may be lifesaving. Patients with sickle cell anemia may be in grave danger if the disease is not detected before dental treatment is started. Undetected leukemic patients may develop serious bleeding problems after any surgical procedure, may have problems with healing

of surgical wounds, and are prone to postsurgical infections. Thus it is important for the dentist to attempt to identify these patients through history and clinical examination before starting any treatment.

Anemias

Patients with G-6-PD dehydrogenase deficiency have an increased incidence of drug sensitivity with sulfonamides, aspirin, and chloramphenicol being the prime offenders.[2,20] Penicillin, streptomycin, and isoniazid also have been linked to hemolysis in these patients. Dental infection and drugs that contain phenacetin may accelerate the rate of hemolysis in patients with this type of anemia.[14,48] Thus dental infections should be avoided and, if they occur, must be dealt with effectively. The astute clinician will realize that febrile illness and elevated bilirubin are features of this condition. Drugs containing phenacetin should not be used in these patients.

African-Americans with sickle cell anemia can receive routine dental care during noncrisis periods; however, long and complicated procedures should be avoided. Good dental repair and preventive dental care are important because oral infection can precipitate a crisis. If infection occurs, it must be treated expeditiously using local and systemic measures such as incision and drainage, heat, high doses of appropriate antibiotics, pulpectomy, and/or extraction. If cellulitis develops, the patient's physician must be consulted and hospitalization considered.[13,14] Adequate fluid intake to avoid dehydration is important. Dental management considerations of the patient with sickle cell anemia are summarized in Box 20-4.

For routine dental care, the appointments should be short (to reduce stress) for patients with sickle cell anemia. The use of a local anesthetic is acceptable (avoid general anesthesia); however, inclusion of small amounts of epinephrine in the local anesthetic is controversial in that some authors believe it may impair circulation and cause vascular occlusion. Smith et al[13] suggest that a local anesthetic without a vasoconstrictor be used for routine dental care. When a surgical procedure must be performed, they recommend using a local anesthetic with epinephrine 1:100,000 to obtain hemostasis and profound anesthesia. The use of nitrous oxide-oxygen (N_2O-O_2) also is controversial; however, N_2O-O_2 given with at least 50% oxygen concentration using a high flow rate and proper ventilation, appears to have a good margin of safety.[37]

Intravenous (IV) sedation must be used with extreme caution in patients who have a history of sickle cell anemia. Barbiturates and narcotics should be avoided because suppression of the respiratory center by these agents leads to hypoxia and acidosis, which could pre-

---

BOX 20-4

Dental Management of the Patient with Sickle Cell Anemia

1. Confirm with patient's physician the condition is stable
2. Arrange short appointments
3. Avoid long and complicated procedures
4. Maintain good dental repair
5. Institute aggressive preventive dental care
   a. Oral hygiene instruction
   b. Diet control
   c. Toothbrushing and flossing
   d. Fluoride gel application
6. Avoid oral infection; treat aggressively when present
7. Use local anesthetic without epinephrine for routine dental care; for surgical procedures use 1:100,000 epinephrine in local anesthetic
8. Avoid barbiturates and strong narcotics; sedation with diazepam (Valium) can be used
9. Use prophylactic antibiotics for major surgical procedures
10. Avoid liberal use of salicylates; pain control with acetaminophen and codeine
11. Use nitrous oxide-oxygen with greater than 50% oxygen, high flow rate, good ventilation

---

cipitate an acute crisis. Light sedation with diazepam (Valium) or nalbuphine hydrochloride can be used.[13] Additional oxygen by nasal canula and liberal use of IV fluids during sedation is advised.[49] General anesthesia is not recommended when the Hb level falls below 10 g/100 ml. High doses of salicylates should be avoided because the "acid" effect could cause a crisis. Pain control can be attempted with acetaminophen and small doses of codeine.[13]

Prophylactic antibiotics are recommended for major surgical procedures to prevent wound infection or osteomyelitis. Penicillin is the drug of choice in nonallergic patients. Intramuscular or IV antibiotics should be considered for use in sickle cell anemic patients who have an acute dental infection. Dehydration must be avoided during surgery and the postoperative period. Consultation with the patient's physician is a must before any surgical procedure. The dentist needs to establish the patient's current status and, if blood transfusion is indicated, to correct severe anemia or its complications before surgery.[13]

BOX 20-5

Dental Management of the Leukemic Patient

1. Detection
   a. History
   b. Examination
   c. Screening laboratory tests
      (1) White cell count
      (2) Differential white cell count
      (3) Smear for cell morphologic study
      (4) Hemoglobin or hematocrit level
      (5) Platelet count
2. Referral
   a. Medical diagnosis
   b. Treatment
3. Consultation before any dental care is rendered
   a. Current status
   b. Review of dental treatment needs
   c. Dental management plan
4. Routine dental care
   a. None for patient with acute symptoms
   b. Once disease is under control, patient may receive indicated dental care

   c. Scaling and surgical procedures
      (1) Bleeding time on day of procedure; if normal, proceed; if prolonged, delay or obtain platelet replacement
      (2) Prophylactic antibiotic therapy to prevent postoperative infection (if severe neutropenia is present)
5. Emergency dental care
   a. Treatment of oral ulcers (see Appendix B)
      (1) Antibiotics
      (2) Bland mouth rinse
      (3) Antihistamine solutions
      (4) Orabase
   b. Oral candidiasis—treat with antifungal medication (see Appendix B)
   c. Conservative management of pain and infection
      (1) Antibiotic sensitivity testing
      (2) Antibiotics, heat for infection
      (3) Strong analgesics for pain

White Blood Cell Disorders

New dental patients under medical treatment for leukemia, lymphoma, and multiple myeloma must be identified by health history and their current status established by consultation with the physician. With special considerations, the patient who is in remission can receive most indicated dental treatment (Box 20-5). Patients with acute signs or symptoms of the disease (e.g., oral infections) in general should receive only conservative emergency dental care until the infection has been treated and the patient has returned to a "normal" state.

For the recently diagnosed leukemic patient, the dentist should be involved early during the treatment planning stages of cancer therapy.[22] Guidance from the dentist helps prevent severe oral infections. For example, in addition to providing oral prophylaxis and hygiene instructions, the dentist may recommend root canal therapy or extraction of teeth susceptible to acute exacerbations during chemotherapy. The focus of treatment is on elimination of risks of infection, and assessment for sequelae of radiation and chemotherapy damage. Dental attention is given to oral hygiene procedures including the use of fluoride gels; encouraging a noncariogenic diet, eliminating mucosal and periodontal disease; pro-

tecting salivary glands (with lead lined stents or drugs); and eliminating sources of mucosal injury.[13,51] Extraction should be considered if periodontal pocket depths are greater than 5 mm, periapical inflammation is present, the tooth is nonfunctional or partially erupted (third molar), and the patient is noncompliant with oral hygiene measures and routine dental care.[52]

Guidelines for extraction in patients before chemotherapy include scheduling a minimum of 10 to 14 days (3 weeks preferable) between the time of extraction and onset of chemo- or radiotherapy; obtaining primary closure; avoiding intraalveolar hemostatic packing agents; avoiding invasive procedures if the platelet count is less than 50,000/ mm^3; transfusing if the platelet count is less than 40,000; and using prophylactic antibiotics if the WBC count is less than 2000 or the neutrophil count is less than 500 (or 1000 at some institutions).[52]

The use of prophylactic antibiotics in patients with severe WBC disorders is dependent on the type of medical treatment the patient is receiving, the status of the disease and the dental procedure planned. Patients in remission usually do not require prophylaxis. A neutrophil count above 1000 usually indicates no need for prophylaxis. Antibiotic regimens are empirical. Penicillin VK 2 gram, 1 hour before the procedure and

500 mg four times daily for 1 week is a reasonable selection, when needed.

If scaling or surgical procedures are planned for a patient who has leukemia that is under good medical control, a platelet count should be obtained on the day of the procedure. This is done to ensure that an adequate number of platelets are present. The number of platelets can be depressed in these patients by the leukemic process or by the agents used to treat the process. If the count is low, or the bleeding time abnormal, the procedure should be delayed until the patient's physician is consulted. In patients whose disease is under good control but who are still thrombocytopenic, platelet replacement by the physician can be instituted if a dental procedure must be done. Dental management of the patient receiving radiation or chemotherapy is discussed further in Chapter 21.

TREATMENT PLANNING MODIFICATIONS

Anemia
Elective surgical procedures are best avoided in patients with sickle cell anemia. Routine dental care can be rendered for patients with sickle cell trait and those with disease who are in a noncrisis state. Special emphasis should be placed on oral hygiene procedures to avoid dental caries and gingival inflammation and infection.

White Blood Cell Disorders
Meticulous oral hygiene with frequent dental examination and scaling is important in minimizing the destructive effects of white blood disorders. Patients with leukemia and/or lymphoma that are in a state of remission can receive routine dental care as indicated. Patients with advanced disease and who have limited prognosis, as in many cases of acute leukemia and multiple myeloma, should receive emergency care only; complex restorative procedures, extensive dental restorations, and other procedures usually are not indicated. A platelet count or bleeding time should be obtained before any surgical procedure; if abnormal, platelet replacement may be indicated.

ORAL COMPLICATIONS AND MANIFESTATIONS

Anemia
The oral findings in patients with anemia usually relate to the underlying cause of the anemia. The oral mucosa often will appear pale. Patients with nutritional causes of anemia (e.g., vitamin B_{12} or iron deficiency) may show loss of papillae from the tongue and atrophic changes of the oral mucosa (Fig. 20-6). Angular cheilitis and aphthae

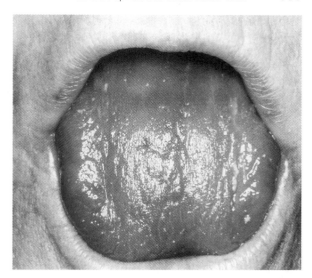

Fig. 20-6 Smooth red tongue in a patient found to have pernicious anemia (vitamin B_{12} deficiency caused by lack of intrinsic factor).

may be found. These patients also may complain of burning or sore tongue. Some patients with iron deficiency anemia develop Plummer-Vinson syndrome, which is characterized by a sore mouth; dysphagia (resulting from muscular degeneration in the esophagus with esophageal stenosis, "webbing"); and an increased frequency of carcinoma of the oral cavity and pharynx. Patients with this syndrome should be followed up closely for any oral or pharyngeal tissue changes that might be early indicators of carcinoma.[14,24]

Patients with hemolytic anemia may show pallor and oral evidence of jaundice caused by hyperbilirubinemia secondary to excessive erythrocyte destruction. The trabecular pattern of the bone on dental radiographs may be affected because of hyperplasia of marrow elements in response to the increased destruction of RBCs. The bone will appear more radiolucent with prominent lamellar striations.[14,24]

Patients with sickle cell anemia also may show pallor and evidence of jaundice in the oral tissues. Erythropoietic activity is increased, and dental radiographic findings associated with the bone marrow hyperplasia include increased widening and decreased numbers of trabeculations and generalized osteoporosis. The trabeculae between teeth may appear as horizontal rows or as a "stepladder" because of compensatory marrow expansion (Fig. 20-7). The lamina dura may appear more dense and distinct. Areas of sclerosis have been reported. Vasoocclusive events can promote ischemic

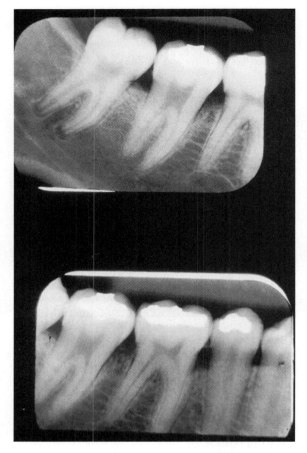

Fig. 20-7 Radiographs of the mandible in a patient with sickle cell anemia. Note the prominent horizontal trabeculations and dense lamina dura.

necrosis within the mandible and peripheral neuropathy. Patients with sickle cell anemia often have delayed eruption of teeth and dental hypoplasia.[13,14,24]

White Blood Cell Disorders

Patients with neutropenia are unable to provide a protective response against oral microbes. Accordingly, these individuals develop gingival inflammation, mucosal ulcerations, and severe destruction of the periodontium with attachment loss when oral hygiene is less than optimal. Periodontal therapy that includes oral hygiene instruction, frequent scaling, and antimicrobial therapy can reduce the adverse effects of this disorder.[23]

Leukemic patients are prone to the development of a variety of oral conditions associated with the malignancy and treatment. A brief list includes gingival enlargement, ulcerations, oral infections, mucositis, graft-versus-host disease, and alterations in growth and development. Fortunately, improved therapy protocols over the past two decades have resulted in a decline in the incidence (to about 30% of patients) of oral complications.[28]

Localized or generalized gingival enlargement is caused by inflammation and infiltrates of atypical and immature WBCs (Figs. 20-8 and 20-9). It occurs in up to 36% of those with acute leukemia and about 10% of those with chronic leukemia.[23] A localized mass of leukemic cells (in the gingival or other sites) is specifically known as a *granulocytic sarcoma* or *chloroma*. Generalized gingival enlargement is more common and is particularly prevalent when oral hygiene is poor and in patients who have AML. The combination of poor oral hygiene and gingival enlargement contribute to gingival bleeding and fetor

B

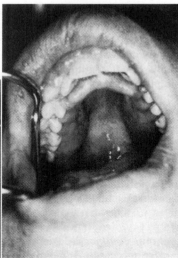

A

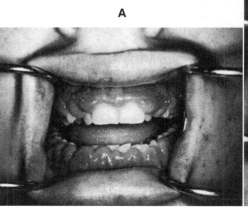

Fig. 20-8 A, Severe gingival hyperplasia in a patient with acute nonlymphoblastic leukemia. Gingival biopsy revealed numerous immature white blood cells (WBCs) in the tissues. **B,** Palatal view of the hyperplasia.

oris. Plaque control measures, chlorhexidine, and chemotherapy promote resolution of the condition.

Active leukemia often is associated with severe gingival bleeding when gingival tissues are edematous and significant thrombocytopenia is present. The dentist should make efforts to improve oral hygiene and use local measures to control the bleeding. A gelatin sponge with thrombin or microfibrillar collagen can be placed over the area, or an oral antifibrinolytic rinse can be used. If local measures fail, medical help will be needed and may involve platelet transfusion.[53]

The mucosa of the mouth and gastrointestinal tract grow rapidly and are likely to be affected by cancer therapy. Thus these patients often develop mucositis. The mucositis usually begins 7 to 10 days after onset of chemotherapy and resolves after the cessation of chemotherapy. Cytotoxic agent treatments affect epithelial cells that have high replication rates.[54] Accordingly, younger persons have greater prevalence of mucositis. Affected mucosa becomes red, raw, and tender. Breakdown of the epithelial barrier produces oral ulcerations that may become secondarily infected and can serve as a source of systemic infection (Fig. 20-10). Oral hygiene should be maintained to minimize infection complications. A bland mouth rinse can be used to clean the surface of the ulcer (commercial mouth rinses are not recommended because they contain alcohol and tend to irritate ulcerated tissues). Following the bland mouth rinse, use of a topical anesthetic and systemic analgesics make the mouth more comfortable. Various solutions of antihistamines that have local anesthetic properties are effective, and a thin layer of Orabase is useful in protecting ulcers from surface irritation. (See Appendix B for suggested regimens.) This protocol can be repeated four to six times a day. In addition, removing sharp edges of teeth and restorations is palliative. Antiseptic and antimicrobial rinses (e.g., Chlorhexidine) are recommended to promote the healing of oral ulcerations and prevent oral infections.[5,14,24,53,55] Additional novel cytoprotective agents (e.g., defensin salivary protein, IL-11, keratinocyte growth factor 1 and 2, lysofiline, misoprostol, PGE1, and TBGB3) are currently being investigated.

Opportunistic infections are common in leukemic patients because (1) of the immaturity of the malignant leukocytes, (2) chemotherapy induces an immunocompromised state, and (3) use of broad-spectrum antibiotics produces selective antimicrobial killing. A common opportunistic infection is acute pseudomembranous candidiasis. When this complication occurs, the patient should be treated with antifungal medications listed in Appendix B. Infrequently, patients develop unusual oral fungal infections (torulopsis, aspergillosis, mucormycosis) or fungal septicemia that may originate from the oral cavity. These patients require potent systemic antifungal agents such as fluconazole or amphotericin B.

Another common infection in patients receiving chemotherapy is recurrent herpes simplex virus (HSV) infection.[56,57] Herpetic lesions tend to be larger and take longer to heal than herpetic lesions found in nonleukemic patients. Generally, antiviral agents (acyclovir, valacyclovir, famciclovir) are prescribed to HSV antibody-positive patients who are undergoing chemotherapy to prevent recurrences. In patients that develop HSV infections, diagnosis can be made rapidly using an enzyme-linked immunoassay.[58] Immunocompromised leukemic patients also are susceptible to varicella-zoster and

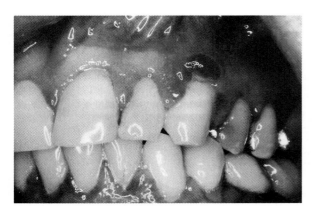

Fig. 20-9 Localized area of gingival inflammation in a patient with only moderately good oral hygiene. The lesion would not clear up following removal of the local irritants. Biopsy revealed immature WBCs compatible with leukemic infiltrate. The patient was referred, and a diagnosis of acute nonlymphoblastic leukemia established.

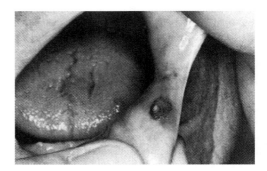

Fig. 20-10 Multiple intraoral ulcers involving the mucosa of the lower lip in a patient with chronic lymphocytic leukemia.

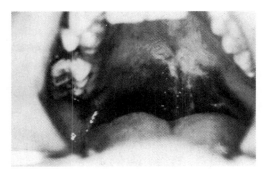

Fig. 20-11 Palatal ecchymoses in a leukemic patient.

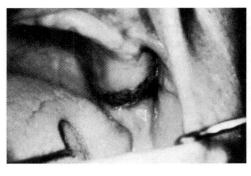

Fig. 20-13 Non-Hodgkin's lymphoma in a patient who came to the dentist complaining of loose maxillary denture.

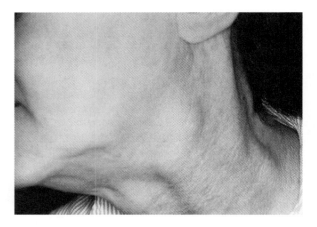

Fig. 20-12 Lymphadenopathy involving the cervical lymph nodes in a patient with Hodgkin's disease.

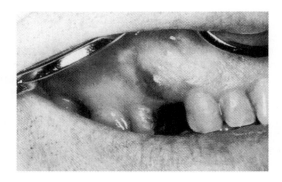

Fig. 20-14 Lesion on the alveolar ridge that was found on radiographs to involve the underlying alveolar bone. The patient had non-Hodgkin's lymphoma.

cytomegalovirus infection. Lesions have been documented in the oral cavity.[54]

Signs of infection often are masked in patients with untreated leukemia, those who were nonresponsive to treatment, or those who have relapsed following treatment. The swelling and erythema usually associated with oral infection often are less marked. In these patients, severe infection can be present with minimal clinical signs. Such infections often develop from invasion by bacteria that do not cause oral infections in most patients seen by the dentist. Unusual infections may be caused by *Pseudomonas*, *Klebsiella*, *Proteus*, *Escherichia coli*, or *Enterobacter*. Often these infections will present as oral ulcerations. When oral infection develops in such patients, a specimen of exudate should be sent for culture, diagnosis, and antibiotic sensitivity testing. If a bacterial infection is suspected, penicillin therapy should be started (if the pa-

tient is not allergic to penicillin). If the clinical course shows little or no improvement in several days, laboratory data should be used to select a more appropriate antimicrobial agent.

Small or large areas of submucosal hemorrhage may be found in the leukemic patient (Fig. 20-11). These lesions result from minor trauma (e.g., tongue biting) and are related to thrombocytopenia. Leukemic patients also may complain of spontaneous gingival hemorrhage that is aggravated by poor oral hygiene, and some will complain of paresthesias resulting from leukemic infiltration of the peripheral nerves.

Graft-versus-host disease (GVHD) is a common sequela of patients who undergo BMT. It occurs when immunologically active donor cells react against histocompatibility antigens of the host. The acute stage develops within the first 100 days (median: 2 to 3

weeks) and is marked by a rash; mucosal ulcerations; elevated liver enzymes; and diarrhea. The chronic stage appears between 3 and 12 months and produces features that mimic Sjögren's syndrome and includes thickening and lichenoid changes of the skin and mucosa, arthritis, xerostomia, xeropthalmia, mucositis, and dysphagia.

A small number of leukemic patients complain of paresthesias resulting from leukemic infiltration of the peripheral nerves or from side effects of chemotherapy (vincristine). An adverse effect of cyclosporin use in BMT patients is gingival overgrowth.

Patients with Hodgkin's disease or non-Hodgkin's lymphoma may present with cervical lymphadenopathy and extranodal or intraoral tumors (Figs. 20-12 to 20-14). This is of particular concern in immunosuppressed patients and individuals with Sjögren's syndrome who are at increased risk for the development of lymphoma. These patients should be periodically monitored for the development of orofacial neoplasia.[59]

Intraoral lymphoma most commonly involves Waldeyer's ring (soft palate and oropharynx)[60]; less often the salivary glands and mandible are affected. Intraoral lymphomas appear as a rapidly expanding (or chronic), unexplained swellings of head and neck lymph nodes, palate, gingival, buccal sulcus or floor of the mouth. The enlargements can be painless or painful. Infrequently, patients have deep "crateriform" oral ulcers and fever.[61] Presence of these orofacial abnormalities requires prompt evaluation either by biopsy via needle, incisional or excisional.

Patients with lymphoma sometimes complain of burning mouth symptoms similar to those noted in patients with leukemia that may be related to drug toxicity, xerostomia, candidiasis, or anemia[28] (see Appendix B for management regimens). Patients who have received more than 3000 rads (cGy) are susceptible to xerostomia and would benefit from salivary substitutes or pilocarpine.[52] Radiation also can damage taste buds, cause trismus of the masticatory muscles, and stunt craniomandibular growth and development. Osteoradionecrosis is a long-term risk associated with radiation doses in excess of 5000 (cGy) to the jaws. The usual dose of irradiation to patients with lymphoma seldom puts them at risk for osteoradionecrosis, but they can develop xerostomia.[47] Protocols to reduce the risk of osteoradionecrosis have included use of prophylactic antibiotics and/or hyperbaric oxygen, and antibiotics during the week of healing (see Chapter 21 and Box 21-10).[62]

Patients with multiple myeloma may have jaw lesions, soft tissue lesions, and soft tissue deposits of amyloid. The bone and soft tissue lesions often are painful.[47]

References

1. Clarke GM, Higgins TN: Laboratory investigation of hemoglobinopathies and thalassemias: review and update, *Clin Chem* 46:1284-1290, 2000.
2. Beck WS: Megaloblastic anemias. I. Cobalamin deficiency. In Beck WS, editor: *Hematology,* ed 5, Cambridge, Mass. 1991, MIT Press.
3. Beck WS, Tepper RI: Hemolytic anemias. IV. Metabolic disorders. In Beck WS, editor: *Hematology,* ed 5, Cambridge, Mass. 1991, MIT Press.
4. Allen RH: Megaloblastic anemias. In Goldman L, Bennett JC editors: *Cecil's textbook of medicine,* ed 21, Philadelphia, 2000, WB Saunders.
5. Dreizen S et al: Malignant gingival and skin "infiltrates" in adult leukemia, *Oral Surg* 55:572-579, 1983.
6. Beutler E: Glucose-6-phosphate dehydrogenase deficiency, *N Engl J Med* 324:169-174, 1991.
7. Ruwende C, Hill A: Glucose-6 phosphate dehydrogenase deficiency and malaria, *J Mol Med* 76:581-588, 1998.
8. Steinberg MH: Management of sickle cell disease, *N Engl J Med* 340:1021-1030, 1999.
9. Olivieri NF: The β-thalassemias, *N Engl J Med* 341:99-109, 1999.
10. Bunn HF: Hemoglobin. II. Sickle cell anemia and other hemoglobinopathies. In Beck WS, editor: *Hematology,* ed 5, Cambridge, Mass. 1991, MIT Press.
11. May DA: Dental management of sickle cell anemia patients, *Gen Dent* 39:182-184, 1991.
12. List AF, Spier CM, Dalton WS: Multidrug resistance and its circumvention in acute leukemia. In Hiddemann W et al, editors: *Haematology and blood transfusion: acute leukemias,* ed 34, New York, 1992, Springer-Verlag.
13. Smith HB, McDonald DK, Miller RI: Dental management of patients with sickle cell disorders, *J Am Dent Assoc* 114:85-87, 1987.
14. Lynch MA: Hematologic diseases and related problems. In Lynch MA, editor: *Burket's oral medicine; diagnosis and treatment,* ed 7, Philadelphia, 1977, JB Lippincott.
15. Perkins ML: Introduction to leukemia and the acute leukemias. In Harmening DM, editor: *Clinical hematology and fundamentals of hemostasis,* ed 2, Philadelphia, 1992, FA Davis.
16. Wintrobe MM, Lee GR, Boggs DR, et al: *Clinical hematology,* ed 8, Philadelphia, 1981, Lea & Febiger.
17. Davies SC et al: Screening for sickle cell disease and thalassaemia: a systematic review with supplementary research, *Health Technol Assess* 4:1-99, 2000.
18. Charache S et al: Effect of hydroxyurea on the frequency of painful crises in sickle cell anemia, *N Engl J Med* 332(20):1317-1322, 1995.
19. Rodgers GP et al: Augmentation by erythropoietin of the fetal-hemoglobin response to hydroxyurea in sickle cell disease, *N Engl J Med* 328(2):73-80, 1993.
20. Davies SC, Roberts IA: Bone marrow transplant for sickle cell disease—an update, *Arch Dis Child* 75:3-6, 1996.
21. Roit I, Brostoff J, Male D: *Immunology,* ed 4, London, Mosby, 1996.

22. Sciubba J et al: National Institutes of Health consensus development conference statement: oral complications of cancer therapies: diagnosis, prevention, and treatment, J Am Dent Assoc 119:179-183, 1989.

23. Kinane D: Blood and lymphoreticular disorders, *Periodontology* 21:84-93, 2000.

24. Shafer WG, Hine MK, Levy BM: *A textbook of oral pathology*, ed 4, Philadelphia, 1983, WB Saunders.

25. Greenlee RT, Murray T, Bolden S, Wingo PA: Cancer statistics, 2000, CA 50:7-33, 2000.

26. http://www-seer.ims.nci.nih.gov/, *Surveillance, epidemiology and end results*, National Cancer Institute, 2000.

27. Clarkson B: The acute leukemias. In Petersdorf RG et al, editors: *Harrison's principles of internal medicine*, ed 10, New York, 1983, McGraw-Hill.

28. Childers NK et al: Oral complications in children with cancer, *Oral Surg Oral Med Oral Pathol* 75:41-47, 1993.

29. Linet MS, Devesa SS: Descriptive epidemiology of the leukemias. In Henderson ES, Lister TA, editors: *Leukemia*, ed 5, Philadelphia, 1990, WB Saunders.

30. Lowenberg B, Downing JR, Burnett A: Acute myeloid leukemia, N Engl J Med 30:1051-1062, 1999.

31. Champlin R, Golde DW: The leukemias. In Wilson JD et al, editors: *Harrison's principles of internal medicine*, ed 12, New York, 1991, McGraw-Hill.

32. Nadler LM: The malignant lymphomas. In Wilson JD et al, editors: *Harrison's principles of internal medicine*, ed 12, New York, 1991, McGraw-Hill.

33. Geller RB, Dix SP: Oral chemotherapy agents in the treatment of leukaemia, *Drugs* 58(Suppl 3):109-118, 1999.

34. Micallef-Eynaud PD et al: Cytogenetic abnormalities in childhood acute lymphoblastic leukemia, *Pediatr Hematol Oncol* 10:25-30, 1993.

35. Bennett JM et al: Proposals for the classification of the acute leukemias: French-American-British cooperative group, Br J Haematol 33:451-458, 1976.

36. Appelbaum FR: The acute leukemias. In Goldman L, Bennett JC editors: *Cecil textbook of medicine*, ed 21, Philadelphia, 2000, WB Saunders.

37. O'Mura GA: The leukemias. In Rose LF, Kaye D, editors: *Internal medicine for dentistry*, ed 2, St Louis, 1990, Mosby.

38. Canellos GP: The chronic leukemias. In Petersdorf RG et al, editors: *Harrison's principles of internal medicine*, ed 10, New York, 1983, McGraw-Hill.

39. Keating, MJ: Chronic leukemias. In Goldman L, Bennett JC editors: *Cecil textbook of medicine*, ed 21, Philadelphia, 2000, WB Saunders.

40. Faderl S et al: The biology of chronic myeloid leukemia, N Engl J Med 341:164-172, 1999.

41. Adamson JW: The myeloproliferative diseases. In Wilson JD et al, editors: *Harrison's principles of internal medicine*, ed 12, New York, 1991, McGraw-Hill.

42. Wierda WG, Kipps TJ: Chronic lymphocytic leukemia, *Curr Opin Hematol* 6:253-261, 1999.

43. Moormeir JA, Williams SF, Golomb HM: The staging of Hodgkin's disease, *Hematol Oncol Clin North Am* 3:237-251, 1989.

44. Shipp MA, Harris NL: Non-Hodgkin's lymphoma. In Goldman L, Bennett JC editors: *Cecil textbook of medicine*, ed 21, Philadelphia, 2000, WB Saunders.

45. Eisenbud L et al: Oral presentations in non-Hodgkin's lymphoma: a review of thirty-one cases. I, *Oral Surg* 56:151-156, 1983.

46. Eisenbud L et al: Oral presentations in non-Hodgkin's lymphoma: a review of thirty-one cases. II, *Oral Surg* 57:272-280, 1984.

47. Silverman S, editor: *Oral cancer*, ed 2, New York, 1985, American Cancer Society.

48. American Dental Association: *Accepted dental therapeutics*, ed 39, Chicago, 1982, American Dental Association.

49. Sansevere JJ, Milles M: Management of the oral and maxillofacial surgery patient with sickle cell disease and related hemoglobinopathies, J Oral Maxillofac Surg 51(8):912-916, 1993.

50. Peterson DE: Prevention of oral complications in cancer patients, Prev Med 23:763-765, 1994.

51. Semba SE, Mealey BL, Hallmon WW: Dentistry and the cancer patient: part 2: oral health management of the chemotherapy patient, *Compendium* 15(11):1378-1388, 1994.

52. Peterson DE: *Personal communication*, 1995.

53. Greenberg MS: Leukemia, dental correlations. In Rose LF, Kaye D, editors: *Internal medicine for dentistry*, ed 2, St Louis, 1990, Mosby.

54. Sonis S: Oral complications of cancer chemotherapy. In Peterson D, Sonis S, editors: *Epidemiology, frequency, distribution, mechanisms and histopathology*, The Hague, 1983, Martinus Nijhoff.

55. Ferretti GA et al: Chlorhexidine for prophylaxis against oral infections and associated complications in patients receiving bone marrow transplants, J Am Dent Assoc 114:461-467, 1987.

56. Barrett AP: A long-term prospective clinical study of orofacial herpes simplex virus infection in acute leukemia, *Oral Surg Oral Med Oral Pathol* 61:149-152, 1986.

57. Redding SW: Role of herpes simplex virus reactivation in chemotherapy-induced oral mucositis, NCI *Monogr* 9:103-105, 1990.

58. Laga EA et al: Evaluation of a rapid enzyme-linked immunoassay for the diagnosis of herpes simplex virus in cancer patients with oral lesions, *Oral Surg Oral Med Oral Pathol* 75:168-172, 1993.

59. Kassan SS et al: Increased risk of lymphoma in sicca syndrome, Ann Intern Med 89:888-892, 1978.

60. Kaugars GE, Burns JC: Non-Hodgkin's lymphoma of the oral cavity associated with AIDS, *Oral Surg Oral Med Oral Pathol* 67:433-436, 1989.

61. Raut A, Huryn J, Pollack A, Zlotolow I: Unusual gingival presentation of post-transplantation lymphoproliferative disorder: a case report and review of the literature, *Oral Surg Oral Med Oral Pathol Oral Radiol Endod* 90:436-441, 2000.

62. Maxymiw WG, Wood RE, Liu FF: Postradiation dental extractions without hyperbaric oxygen, *Oral Surg Oral Med Oral Pathol* 72:270-274, 1991.

Cancer

21
CHAPTER

*I*mprovements in health care and sanitation have contributed to increasing life span of persons worldwide. Concordant with the increased longevity, the incidence of cancer has increased over the past 50 years. At present, the probability of developing cancer from birth to death in the United States in men is 44% and in women 38%.[1]

Because patients diagnosed with cancer are experiencing increased survival as a result of improved diagnostics and advances in antineoplastic therapy, an increased likelihood exists of dentists treating patients in various phases of cancer therapy. For optimum oral health, the dentist should be an integral part of the cancer patient's health care team. Knowledge of cancer progression, treatment modalities, the location of cancer therapy (hospital or outpatient facility), and the likely outcome all affect the dental treatment plan. Maintenance of proper oral hygiene is critical for reducing local and systemic complications associated with chemotherapy, radiation therapy, and marrow and stem cell transplantation. In addition, dentists have the unique opportunity to reduce the risk of cancer by providing advice regarding cancer screening, a healthy diet, counseling regarding smoking cessation and risks associated with alcohol consumption, and by performing cancer screening procedures.

This chapter focuses on common cancers that may affect patients who require dental care. The text does not attempt to include all cancers, but instead provides an overview of cancer, a discussion of common cancers, and the oral considerations of these patients. A discussion of lymphoma and leukemia is found in Chapter 20.

DEFINITION

Cancer is a condition characterized by uncontrolled growth of aberrant neoplastic cells. Cancerous cells kill by destructive invasion of tissues—that is, direct extension and spread to distant sites by metastasis through blood, lymph, or serosal surfaces.[2] Malignant cells arise from genetic and acquired mutations, chromosomal translocations, and over- or underexpression of factors (oncogenes, growth factor receptors, signal transducers, transcription factors) that cause cells to lose their ability to regulate deoxyribonucleic acid (DNA) synthesis and the cell cycle.[2] Cellular abnormalities of malignancy result in three common features: uncontrolled proliferation, ability to recruit blood vessels (i.e., neovascularization), and ability to spread.

EPIDEMIOLOGY: INCIDENCE AND PREVALENCE

Each year about 1.2 million new cases of cancer are diagnosed in the United States and about 560,000 persons die of the disease (Table 21-1).[1] This does not include the 1.3 million cases of basal and squamous cell skin cancers that also occur annually.[1] In 1998, for the first time, the total number of new cancer cases and cancer death rates in the United States declined. However, cancer remains the second-leading cause of death behind heart disease in the United States.

ETIOLOGY AND PREVENTION

Carcinogenesis is a complex multistep process that involves the accumulation of mutations and the loss of regulatory control over cell division, differentiation, apoptosis, and adhesion (Fig. 21-1). The process originates at the level of gene and cell cycle control, either by a hereditary mutation, acquired mutation or inappropriate expression of a transcription factor. At least three to six somatic mutations are needed to transform a normal cell into a malignant cell. Acquired mutations can arise from

TABLE 21-1

Common Cancers and 5-year Survival, United States 2000

Cancer Site	Estimated No. of Cases USA (% of Total)	5-year Survival
Breast	184,200 (15.1%)	86%
Prostate	180,400 (14.7%)	93%
Lung	164,000 (13.4%)	14%
Colon/rectum	130,200 (10.7%)	62%
Lymphoma	62,300 (5.1%)	83%*
Bladder	53,200 (4.6%)	81%
Leukemia	30,800 (2.5%)	43%
Oropharynx	30,200 (2.5%)	53%
Stomach	21,500 (1.8%)	21%
Liver	15,300 (1.3%)	5%
Cervix	12,800 (1.1%)	71%

*Hodgkins lymphoma
Adapted from Greenlee RT, et al: Cancer statistics, 2000, CA *Cancer J Clin* 50:7-33, 2000.

exposure to hazardous chemicals and pathogens that lead to activation of oncogenes, inactivation of tumor suppressor genes (pRb and p53), and chromosomal abnormalities (translocations, deletions, insertions). The accumulation of these abnormalities leads to a cell that becomes functionally independent and aggressive. Natural killer cells provide surveillance for cancerous cells. Reduced numbers or function of natural killer cells, which occur during immunosuppression, increase the risk for cancer.

Research over several decades has focused on agents that will prevent carcinogenesis at the cellular level. National efforts currently focus on the reduction or elimination of factors known to be associated with cancer. Recommendations from the American Cancer Society[2,4] are to minimize exposure to tobacco smoke; environmental and occupational carcinogens (e.g., asbestos fibers, arsenic compounds, chromium compounds, pesticides); decrease intake of fat and exposure to ultraviolet light; moderate the intake of alcohol; obtain an adequate intake of dietary fiber and antioxidants (vitamins C and E, selenium); and perform moderate levels of physical activity.

PATHOPHYSIOLOGY AND COMPLICATIONS

The loss of regulatory control in a cell destined to become a cancer cell results in a series of pathologic changes that include hyperproliferative epithelium, dysplasia, and finally carcinoma. Dysplastic tissue is characterized by atypical cell proliferation, nuclear enlargement, failure of maturation and differentiation short of malignancy. Malignant cells exhibit antigenic, karyotypic, biochemical and membrane changes that cause loss of contact inhibition, changes in chromosomal morphology and increased permeability. Malignant tumors lack cell cycle control and replicate rapidly, becoming clinically detectable after about 30 cell doublings when the mass contains about 10^9 cells (1 g). A three-log increase to 10^{12} cells produces a tumor that weighs 1 kg and is often lethal. After reaching clinically detectable size, tumors slow in growth as they reach anatomic boundaries and begin to outgrow their blood supply. Malignant tumors overcome the limitation of anatomic boundaries by losing cell adherence and by metastasizing. Metastasis is a distinct form of cancerous spread that occurs when malignant cells enter blood or lymphatic vessels and travel to distant sites. Metastasis is related to factors produced by tumors cells that allow individual cells to invade tissues and endothelium. It often results in end-organ failure and death.

CLINICAL PRESENTATION

SIGNS AND SYMPTOMS

Cancers often present as a palpable mass that increase in size over time. Preceding the development of the tumor are subtle changes that are dependent on the anatomic site involved and the cell type of origin. Initial features can include a change in surface color, a lump, enlarged lymph node, or altered organ function. Symptoms include pain and paresthesia. Tumors permitted to increase in size often result in a reddened epithelial surface (due to increased blood vessels) that ulcerates.

STAGING

Most cancers are assigned a stage (I, II, III, or IV) by the medical team based on the size of the tumor and how far it has spread. Generically speaking, Stage I is localized and confined to the organ of origin. Stage II is regional in nearby structures. Stage III is extensive beyond the regional site crossing several tissue planes and Stage IV is widely disseminated. This system often is supplemented by detailed and specific staging systems developed for particular cancers and generally

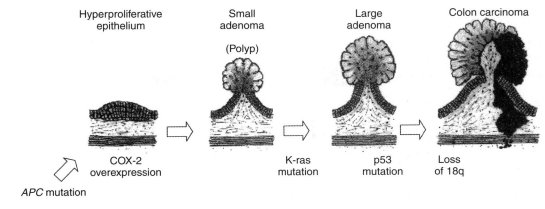

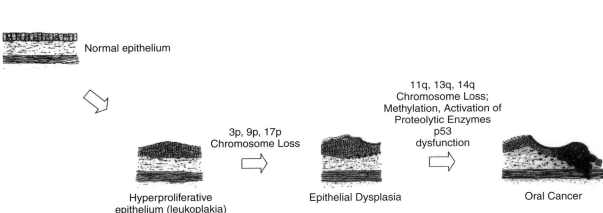

Fig. 21-1 Carcinogenesis: pathologic sequence in gastrointestinal mucosa. Examples in colon and oral mucosa. (Modified from Jänne PA and Mayer RJ: Chemoprevention of colorectal cancer, *N Engl J Med* 342:1960-1968, 2000).

does not apply to leukemia, as leukemia is a disease of the blood cells that does not usually form a solid mass or tumor.[2] The TNM system is frequently employed, where T is tumor size, N is nodal involvement and M is metastases (Box 21-1). The prognosis of patients depends in large part on the stage of disease at the time of diagnosis.

LABORATORY FINDINGS

The diagnosis of cancer is dependent on microscopic examination of an adequate sample of tissue taken from the lesion (Box 21-2). Tissue can be obtained by cytologic smears, needle biopsy, or incisional or excisional biopsy. Cells can also be subjected to flow cytometry, chromosomal analyses, in situ hybridization or other molecular procedures to identify specific cancer markers, ploidy, and DNA analysis. Serum tumor markers such as carcinoembryonic antigen (CEA) for colorectal carcinoma (CA 15-3 or CEA in breast cancer and CA 125 for ovarian cancer) have low sensitivity for the detection of early stage cancers but are useful in monitoring disease progression and response to therapy.

MEDICAL MANAGEMENT

Treatment strategies for cancer are based on eliminating fast multiplying cancer cells without killing the host (see Chapter 20). Therapeutic modalities include surgery; radiation (external beam or implants); cytotoxic, chemotherapeutic, and endocrine drugs; and possibly stem cell or bone marrow transplantation. Surgery often

---

BOX 21-1

International TNM System of Classification and Staging of Oral Carcinomas

T—Size of Tumor
T_{IS}, Carcinoma in situ
T_1, Tumor <2 cm in size
T_2, Tumor >2 cm to <4 cm in size
T_3, Tumor >4 cm in size
T_4, Massive tumor with deep invasion into bone, muscle, skin, etc.

N—Regional Lymph Node Involvement
N_0, No palpable nodes
N_1, Single, homolateral palpable node <3 cm in diameter
N_2, Single, homolateral palpable node, 3 to 6 cm, *or* Multiple, homolateral nodes, none >6 cm
N_3, Single or multiple, homolateral nodes, one >6 cm, *or* Bilateral nodes (stage each side of neck), *or* Contralateral nodes

M—Metastases
M_0, No known distant metastasis
M_1, Distant metastasis—PUL (pulmonary), OSS (osseous), HEP (liver), BRA (brain)

Stage Classification

0 (carcinoma in situ)	T_{is}, N0, M0
I	T_1, N_0, M_0
II	T_2, N_0, M_0
III	T_3, N_0, M_0 or T_1, T_2, or T_3, N_1, M_0
IVA	T_4, N_0, M_0 or T_4, N_1, M_0 or Any T, N_2, M_0
IVB	Any T, N_3, M_0
IVC	Any T, any N, M_1

T, tumor; N, node; M, metastasis.

BOX 21-2

Microscopic Criteria of Malignancy

Cytoplasm:	Scant cytoplasm, increased nucleus to cytoplasm ratio, tight molding of cytoplasmic membrane around nucleus
Nucleus:	Enlargement with variation in size, irregular membrane with sharp angles, hyperchromasia, irregular chromatin distribution with clumping, prominent nucleoli, abundant or abnormal mitotic figures
Relationships:	Variation in cell size and shape, abnormal stratification, decreased cohesiveness

---

is used when anatomy permits to debulk a tumor or if the cancer is limited in size. Radiation (often greater than 50 Gray [Gy]) kills cells by damaging cancer cell DNA and chromosomes needed for cell replication and is used when the tissue cannot be excised and when cells are most susceptible to this form of therapy. Chemotherapeutic agents are most effective against rapidly growing tumors by adversely affecting the DNA synthesis or protein synthesis of cancerous cells. A wide range of cancer chemotherapeutic compounds exist. They are divided into the several categories: alkylating agents,

antimetabolites, hormones, antibiotics, mitotic inhibitors, and miscellaneous drugs (Table 21-2; see Table 20-2). Tumoricidal efficacy is gained from use of the chemotherapeutic drugs in combination. High-dose multidrug protocols are employed in hospital settings to induce myelosuppression for patients with leukemia, lymphoma (see Chapter 20), and more recently, breast cancer who are scheduled to undergo bone marrow transplantation. Opportunistic infections are a major concern during the myelosuppressive period. Patients who receive outpatient chemotherapy are administered a lower-dose regimen on a three to four week schedule and are at lower risk for opportunistic infections.

BREAST CANCER

Breast cancer is the most-common type of cancer in the United States, with 98% of cases occurring in women.[1] In 1997, approximately 181,000 of breast cancer were reported in United States, with more than 44,000 persons dying of the disease that year[7] The incidence increases with age. Risk factors include early menarche, late menopause, and nulliparity (women who do not bear children).[8] All breast cancers are the result of somatic genetic abnormalities. The most important risk factor of breast cancer is family history of the disease with 5-10% of cases arising in high-risk families.[9-12] The most common mutations identified in breast cancer cells are in the BRCA1 and BRCA2 genes.[13] These mutations confer a 50% to 85% lifetime risk of breast cancer. Abnormalities also have been identified in genes (bcl-2, c-myc, c-myb and p53) and gene products (Her2/neu and cyclin D1) that reg-

TABLE 21-2

Chemotherapy Drugs of Choice for Common Cancers

Cancer	Drugs of Choice
Breast	*Risk reduction:* Tamoxifen Adjuvant: Doxorubicin + cyclophosphamide ± fluorouracil followed by paclitaxel; Cyclophosphamide + methotrexate + fluorouracil; Tamoxifen for receptor-positive and hormone-response *Metastatic:* Doxorubicin + cyclophosphamide ± fluorouracil; Cyclophosphamide + methotrexate + fluorouracil Tamoxifen or toremifene for receptor-positive and/or hormone-responsive Paclitaxel + trastuzumab for tumors overexpressing HER2 protein
Cervix	*Locally advanced:* Cisplatin ± fluorouracil Metastatic: Cisplatin; ifosfamide with mesna; Bleomycin + ifosfamide with mesna + cisplatin
Colorectal	Adjuvant: Fluorouracil + leucovorin Metastatic: Fluorouracil + leucovorin + irinotecan
Head and neck	Cisplatin + fluorouracil or paclitaxel
Kaposi's sarcoma	Liposomal doxorubicin or daunorubicin; Doxorubicin + bleomycin + vincristine
Leukemia and lymphoma	See Box 20-3
Liver	Hepatic intra-arterial floxuridine, cisplatin, doxorubicin or mitomycin
Lung	
Nonsmall cell	Paclitaxel + cisplatin or carboplatin; Cisplatin + vinorelbine; Gemcitabine + cisplatin
Small cell	Cisplatin or carboplatin + etoposide (PE)
Melanoma	*Adjuvant:* Interferon alfa *Metastatic:* Dacarbazine
Multiple myeloma	Melphalan or cyclophosphamide + prednisone; Vincristine + doxorubicin + dexamethasone (VAD)
Prostate	Gonadotropin-releasing hormone (GnRH) agonists (leuprolide or goserelin) ± antiandrogen (flutamide, bicalutamide, or nilutamide)
Renal	Interleukin-2

Adapted from Drugs of choice for cancer chemotherapy, *Med Lett Drugs Ther* 42:83-92, 2000.

ulate the cell cycle and DNA replication.[13,14] Gonadal steroid hormones, growth factors, and various chemokines (IL-6) influence the behavior and dissemination of the disease. Cancer in one breast increases the risk for cancer development in the other.

Breast cancer often is detected as a lump in the breast with or without nipple discharge, breast skin changes and breast pain. Mammography detects the mass in only 75% to 85% of patients (Fig. 21-2). In a small percentage of patients the first sign is an axillary mass. Diagnosis is made from a tissue core biopsy of breast tissue.[15] Most breast cancers are infiltrating ductal carcinomas whereas a smaller percentage are infiltrating lobular carcinomas, medullary carcinomas, mucinous carcinoma or tubular carcinoma.[8] Metastasis occurs after the cancer becomes clinically detectable and

is primarily to regional lymph nodes and within the chest wall, bone, lung, and liver.

Treatment of breast cancer depends on the histologic type of cancer and stage. Cellular markers such as the Her2/*neu* molecule (target of drug herceptin) and the sodium/iodide symporter (NIS) aid in the diagnosis and treatment planning.[16] Lumpectomy (when the tumor is less than 5 cm), or lumpectomy plus radiotherapy is preferred to radical mastectomy. Axillary node dissection is performed if the regional sentinel node is positive. Hormone therapy (tamoxifen) and chemotherapy combined with local therapy is recommended when invasive carcinoma exceeding 1 cm in diameter or axillary lymph nodes are positive. The combination of fluorouracil, doxorubicin, and cyclophophamide usually is administered for 4 to 6 months, given at 3- to 4-week intervals. At

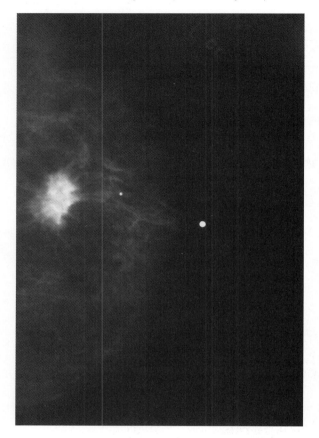

Fig. 21-2 Mammogram showing a radiodense area in the breast suggestive of a malignancy that should be sent for biopsy. (Courtesy A.R. Moore, Lexington, Ky.)

present, metastatic breast cancer is incurable. Accordingly, the American Cancer Society[4] recommends a mammogram and professional clinical examination every year for women 40 years of age and older (Table 21-3). Women 20 to 29 years of age should have a professional breast examination at least every 3 years. Women 20 years of age and older should perform a breast self-examination every month. The American Geriatrics Society[17] recommends mammography every 2 or 3 years for healthy women between the ages of 65 and 85.

CERVICAL CANCER

Cancer of the uterine cervix occurred in 12,800 women in the United States in 1998, and 4,800 women died of the disease.[18] Cervical cancer is relatively uncommon in developed countries because of intensive screening programs being in place. Since the widespread use of screen-ing Papanicolaou (Pap) smears, that detect asympto-matic cancerous precursor lesions at early stages, the in-cidence of cervical cancer has decreased dramatically from 32 cases per 100,000 women in the 1940s to 8.3 cases per 100,000 women in the 1980s. However, approx-imately 30% of these patients die of the disease within 5 years, and the death rate for African-Americans is more than twice the national average.[4]

Human papillomaviruses (HPVs), epitheliotropic sex-ually transmitted DNA viruses, are the major etiologic factor in cervical carcinogenesis.[21] These viruses dysreg-ulate the cell cycle and tumor suppressor genes (p53 and pRb) via overexpression of viral early genes E6 and E7.[20,21] Certain HPV strains (HPV16, 18, 45, 56) are classi-fied as high risk types, as they are associated with the majority of cases (Fig. 21-3).[22] HPV types 30, 31, 33, 35, 39, 51, 52, 58, and 66 are classified as intermediate onco-genic risk. In addition to viral infection, chronic cigarette smoking, multiple sexual partners and immunosuppres-sion increase the risk of cervical cancer.[20,23]

Cervical cancer typically has a long asymptomatic pe-riod before the disease becomes clinically evident. The cancer classically presents in women who are between 40 and 60 years of age. The earliest preinvasive changes are diagnosed by Pap smear.[19] Further evaluation is made by colposcopy and colposcopic-directed biopsy. If neoplas-tic cells penetrate the underlying basement membrane of the uterine cervix, widespread dissemination can occur. Metastases often affect renal tissues resulting in ureteral obstruction and azotemia. Treatment is based on the stage of the disease and involves hysterectomy in the early stages and radiation therapy for disease that ex-tends to or invades local organs.[19] The 5-year survival rate is relatively high (see Table 21-1) but drops below 50% when the cancer extends to and beyond the pelvic wall.[24]

The American Cancer Society[4] recommends that a Pap smear and professional pelvic examination be performed in women at the onset of sexually activity or at 18 years of age. Because immunosuppression is associated with cervical cancer, the Centers for Disease Control and Prevention (CDC) advises all women with human im-munodeficiency virus (HIV) to receive semiannual screen-ing beginning the first year after diagnosis.[25] Health care providers may elect to screen less often when three an-nual examinations in a row are negative.[17]

COLORECTAL CANCER

Cancer of the large bowel (colon and rectum) is the most common malignancy of the gastrointestinal tract and overall the fourth-most-common cancer of persons living in the United States. This cancer was diagnosed in 130,200 persons in the United States in 1998.[1] Colorectal

Screening Recommendations of the American Cancer Society

Breast	Self exam (age 20 years and over)	every month
	Clinical exam (20-40 years; over 40)	every 3 years; every year
	Mammography (40-49; 50 and over)	every 1-2 years; every year
Colon	Sigmoidoscopy (50 and over)	every 3-5 years
	Fecal occult blood test (50 and over)	every year
	Digital rectal exam (40 and over)	every year
Cervical	Papanicolaou test (women 18 and over, and sexually active)	every year*
	Pelvic examination	
Prostate	Prostate examination (men 50 and over)	every year
	Blood tests for prostate specific antigen (PSA)	
Health counseling and cancer checkups† (men and women over 40)		every year

*If 3 or more consecutive satisfactory normal annual examinations, screening may be performed less frequently
†To include examination for cancers of the thyroid, testes, prostate, ovaries, lymph nodes, oral region and skin.
These recommendations are often applied 5 to 10 years earlier for specific cancers in persons with a family history of cancer and when specific racial (e.g., African-American) populations are at increased risk.

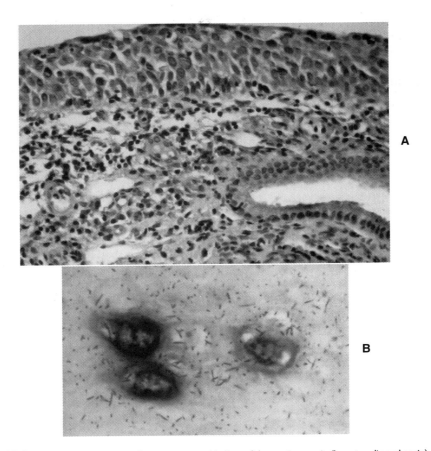

Fig. 21-3 A, Biopsy specimen revealing cancerous epithelium of the uterine cervix (hematoxylin and eosin). **B,** Human papillomavirus DNA detected in cervical epithelium by in situ hybridization. (Courtesy M. Cibull, Lexington, Ky.)

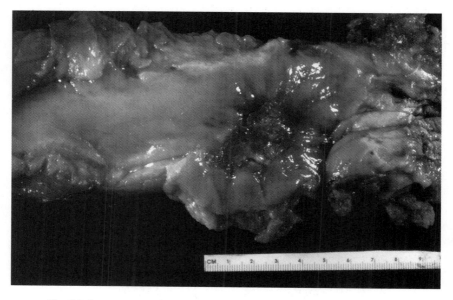

Fig. 21-4 Destructive effects of colon cancer. (Courtesy M. Cibull, Lexington, Ky.)

cancer accounts for about 10% of all cancer in the United States and has a 5-year survival rate of 61%. Over the past two decades, mortality has decreased for white women and men but increased in African-American men and women.

The vast majority of colorectal cancers are adenocarcinomas (Fig. 21-4). Inherited predisposition and environmental factors contribute to their development. Genetic abnormalities in chromosome 5 (in familial adenomatous polyposis); chromosome 17 (p53 gene); and chromosome 18 (DCC gene) are contributory.[26] An initiating and probably obligatory event is the oncogenic activation of the adhesion protein, beta-catenin, resulting from its overexpression, or loss of its negative regulator the adenomatous polyposis cancer protein (APC).[27] These abnormalities result in an upregulation in cell cycle signaling. Patients with chronic inflammation (ulcerative colitis) have approximately 10 to 20 times the risk of colorectal cancer as the general population.[28] The risk also increases with high fat content diet (40% of total calories); low dietary fiber intake,[29] and smoking cigarettes for 20 years or more.[30] By contrast, use of nonsteroid antiinflammatory drugs (NSAIDs) and folate reduces the risk for colorectal cancer.[31,32] Colonic adenomas (polyps) have malignant potential; however, less than 5% develop into carcinomas. The exception to this rule is in Gardner's syndrome, in which virtually all affected patients develop malignant polyposis by age 40 unless treated.

Colorectal cancer is not often seen until age 40 and increases in incidence after age 50. Risk rises sharply by age 60 and doubles every decade until it peaks at age 75 years.[28] Spread is by direct extension through the bowel wall and invasion of adjacent organs by lymphatics and the portal vein to the liver. The major signs and symptoms of colorectal cancer are rectal bleeding, abdominal pain, and change in bowel habits (constipation). Presenting symptoms may include those referable to invasion of adjacent organs (kidney, liver, vagina).[28]

Colonoscopy is the preferred approach for evaluating a patient for colorectal cancer. This approach permits tissue and brush biopsies to be performed. Staging of the patient is aided by endoscopic ultrasonography and computed tomography (CT) scanning. Surgical excision is the treatment of choice with lesions encroaching the distal 5 cm of the colon, resulting in colostomy. Radiation therapy is used for rectal and anal cancer. Chemotherapy (fluorouracil and leucovorin for up to 6 months or more recently, topoisomerase I inhibitors [camptothecins] and oxaliplatin) are used when metastatic spread occurs. Liver metastases have been treated with hepatic arterial therapy with implantable pumps and injection ports that deliver chemotherapeutic agents.[28]

The poor prognosis of advanced colorectal cancer (Stages III or IV) emphasizes the need for annually screening of at-risk adults. Digital rectal examination, fecal occult blood test, stool DNA testing,[33] sigmoidoscopy, colonoscopy, and barium enema with air contrast

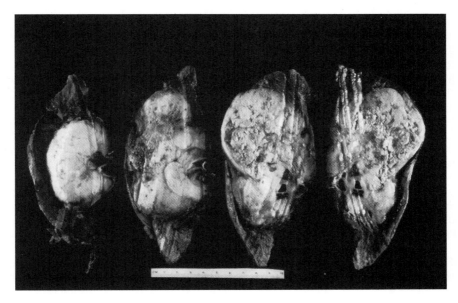

Fig. 21-5 Large cell undifferentiated carcinoma infiltrating the entire lung shown in cross section. (Courtesy M. Cibull, Lexington, Ky.)

are the screening procedures for colorectal cancer. The American Cancer Society[4] recommends that screening start at age 50 for both men and women and even earlier if a family history exists, especially first-degree relatives of colorectal cancer, present inflammatory bowel disease, a personal history of colorectal cancer or adenomatous polyp, or a family history of hereditary colorectal cancer syndromes (e.g., familial adenomatous polyposis, Peutz-Jeghers, Gardner's syndrome). Digital rectal examination and a test for occult blood should be performed once a year. Sigmoidoscopy is recommended every 5 years and colonoscopy every 10 years. A barium enema can be performed in place of the sigmoidoscopy and colonoscopy.

LUNG CANCER

Lung cancer is the cause of 14% of cancer cases and is the leading cause of cancer deaths (almost 157,000 deaths annually) in the United States (see Table 21-1).[1] Although it maintains a similar incidence with breast and prostate cancer, the number of deaths caused by lung cancer exceeds the two combined. The number of new cases has been declining in men since 1984; by contrast, the incidence in women increased in the 1980s and 1990s and only recently declined.[1,34] Lung cancer is more prevalent in industrialized countries, but increased incidence in nonindustrialized countries has resulted from the introduction of cigarettes into these regions. Overall, more than 85% of cases are related to smoking tobacco with a

dose-dependent effect. In 60% of human lung cancers, the p53 tumor suppressor gene is mutated. Current evidence suggests that polycyclic aromatic hydrocarbons (e.g., benzopyrene metabolite) of tobacco smoke form adducts within the p53 gene that contribute to an abnormally functioning p53.[35] Deletions in chromosomes 3p and 9p and overexpression of the *ras* and *myc* oncogenes and growth factor receptor c-erbB-2 appear to be important malignant steps. Risk of lung cancer increases in persons who are exposed to certain inorganic minerals (asbestos and crystalline silica), metals (arsenic, chromium, and nickel), and ionizing radiation (e.g., radon).[36]

Histologically, lung cancers are divided into two groups. About 80% are non–small-cell lung cancers (large cell undifferentiated 10%; squamous cell carcinoma [SCC] 30%; and adenocarcinoma 40%) and 20% are small-cell lung cancers (i.e., oat cell carcinoma) (Fig. 21-5).[37] Small-cell cancers have a rapid growth rate and metastasize early.[38]

Lung cancer is a clinically silent disease until late in its course. Tumors that grow locally can produce a cough or change the nature of a chronic cough. Cancers that invade adjacent structures can produce chest pain and dyspnea, hemoptysis or produce syndromes (e.g. Horner's syndrome) from disruption of nerves in the chest and neck or endocrine, cutaneous or neurologic manifestations.[36] Metastases to the brain, bone, adrenal gland, and liver produce features associated with malfunction of these organs and lymphadenopathy. During advanced

disease, patients present with anorexia, weight loss, weakness, and profound fatigue.

The diagnosis of lung cancer is made by imaging studies, bronchoscopy, bronchial washings, brush and tissue biopsies, and histological examination of the cells and tissue. Stages I and II nonsmall-cell lung cancers are treated by surgical resection. Radiotherapy is used for more advanced nonsmall-cell lung cancers and when patients with Stage I or II disease refuse or are medically unfit for surgery.[38] Chemotherapy using two or three agents (e.g., cisplatin, carboplatin, etoposide, vinblastine, vindesine) is employed in combination with radiotherapy for Stages III and IV non small cell lung cancers. Chemotherapy is the mainstay of treatment for small-cell lung cancer. Adjuvant radiotherapy is used in patients with limited disease. Stage I lung cancer and Stage II squamous cell lung cancers are associated with 5-year survival rates of more than 50%.[39] The 5-year survival rate for all stages of lung cancer, at present, is just 14%.[1] Despite the poor prognosis, national recommendations have not been made in the United States to deploy diagnostic image screening for the detection of lung cancer even in high-risk persons.

PROSTATE CANCER

Prostate cancer is the second most common cancer (approximately 180,000 cases per year) and the most common cancer of men in the United States (see Table 21-1). It is the second-leading cause of cancer deaths among men. Prostate cancer develops in approximately 9% of white and 11% of African-American men.[40] Family history and race (African-Americans) are definitive risk factors for the development of this disease.

At present, the etiologic factors of prostate cancer remain unknown. High dietary fat intake and mutations in chromosome 1 (1q24-25) and X (Xq27-28) appear to increase the risk for prostate cancer.[41-44] Overexpression of the c-*myc* oncogene also is commonly detected in solid tumors such as prostate cancer.[44]

More than 90% of all prostate carcinomas are adenocarcinomas. They typically arise at multiple locations within the gland. Cancer of the prostate produces few signs and symptoms other than problems in urination (hesitancy, decreased force of urination) that, if present, occur late in the course of the disease. Thus screening procedures are paramount to the successful management of this disease. Methods used to screen for prostate cancer include the digital rectal examination (DRE) in combination with blood tests for prostate specific antigen (PSA), and endorectal ultrasound (see Table 21-3). The amount of nonbound or free PSA (expressed as the percent of the total PSA) and PSA velocity (change in the PSA level over time) aid in the diagnosis. The upper nor-

mal level for the PSA is 4 ng/ml. Transrectal ultrasound-guided needle biopsy is recommended when the patient has the following:

- PSA value over 10 ng/ml
- A positive DRE (palpable nodule or abnormality); even if the PSA value is less than 4 ng/ml, a positive DRE represents about 25% of all prostate cancer
- PSA value between 4 ng/ml and 10 ng/ml, a negative DRE, and a free PSA value less than 25%
- PSA value less than 4 ng/ml, a negative DRE, and a PSA value that has increased from 1 year to the next by 0.75 ng/ml (PSA velocity) or more
- PSA value between 2 ng/ml and 4 ng/ml, a negative DRE, and free PSA level of less than 25%

Radionuclide scanning or pelvic magnetic resonance imaging (MRI) is recommended for men diagnosed with prostate cancer with a PSA greater than 10 ng/mL to determine the extent of the disease. Metastasis occurs by lymphatic or hematogenous dissemination. Lymphatic spread is usually to thoracic and pelvic regions. Hematogenous spread is usually to bone. Bony metastasis is often identified in the pelvis, spine, and femur (Fig. 21-6).

Treatment options include radical prostatectomy, external-beam radiation, interstitial seed radiation, and cryosurgery. Androgen deprivation therapy is offered in cases of more advanced disease. Prognosis correlates with the histologic grade and stage of the tumor, with persons who have limited disease (stage I) having the best prognosis.

SKIN CANCER

Of the three primary types of skin cancer, basal cell carcinoma is the most common type, followed by SCC (discussed under oral cancer) and melanoma. Basal cell carcinoma occurs in about 500,000 new persons annually in the United States. They are slow-growing, locally invasive tumors that arise in the basal layer of epithelium generally as a result of chromosomal changes caused by chronic exposure to ultraviolet light (particularly UVB radiation). Evidence suggests that mutation and inactivation of the human "patched" gene located in chromosome 9 (9q22.3) is probably a requirement for the development of basal cell carcinoma.[45]

Basal cell carcinomas are more common in older persons with lighter skin and blond and red hair type. However, diagnosis in the second and third decade is becoming more common.[46] About 85% appear on sun-exposed surfaces of the head and neck (including the lip). Four types of basal cell carcinomas are recognized: nodular, superficial, sclerosing (morpheaform) or pigmented forms. Each type presents as a gradual local growth. Classically, the nodular basal cell carcinoma is a pearly

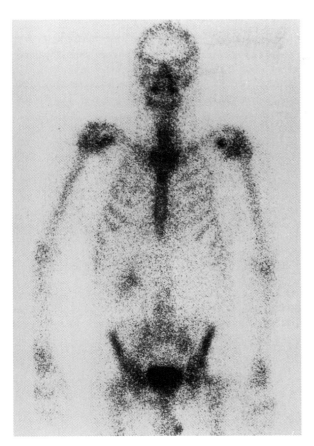

Fig. 21-6 Radionuclide scan showing increased uptake of technetium at sites of bony metastasis from prostate cancer. (Courtesy Dale Miles, Lexington, Ky.)

papule with telangiectasias, a rolled waxy border and a central ulceration ("rodent ulcer") (Fig. 21-7). A history of intermittent encrustation and bleeding is common. The less common types appear reddish, pigmented or scarlike. Basal cell carcinomas are readily removed with cryotherapy and surgical excision. Contemporary therapy results in over 95% cure rate. Because basal cell carcinomas are locally invasive and destructive, preventive measures that include reduced sun exposure and frequent examination of sun-exposed skin by a health care provider is important in preventing recurrences. Inadequate treatment results in spread to deeper structures, but rarely do these tumors metastasize.

Melanoma is a malignant neoplasm arising from melanocytes. This cancer occurs primarily in skin but can occur at any site where melanocytes are found, including the oral cavity. The incidence of melanoma is increasing faster than any other cancer,[47] with approximately 48,000 new cases of melanoma reported in the United States annually.[1] Ultraviolet light sun exposure is the major etiologic factor. Because of increased time spent outdoors and thinning of the atmosphere,[48] the rate of melanoma has increased from 1 in 1500 persons in 1935 to 1 in 75 persons in 2000.[49] Increased risk also is associated with light skin type, severe sunburns as a child, overall nevus count greater 50, light and red hair color, and extensive freckling. Men are more commonly affected, as are persons over age 50. Cytogenetic studies have implicated chromosomes 1p and 9p as possible locations for genetic alterations predisposing for melanoma.[50]

Approximately 30% of melanomas arise from previously existing pigmented lesions, particularly ones with a history of trauma. Clinical features of melanoma are

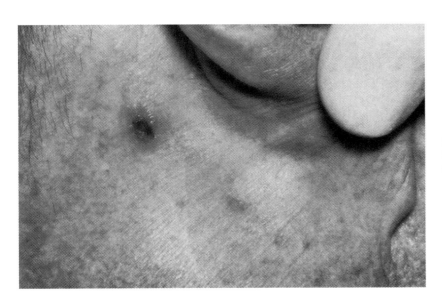

Fig. 21-7 Basal cell carcinoma presenting as a "rodent ulcer" behind the ear of a dental patient.

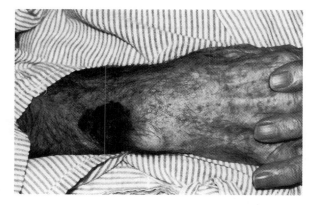

Fig. 21-8 Malignant melanoma of the arm. The arms, face and neck are visible surfaces to be examined by the dentist.

Features of Some Common Cancers that Appear in the Oral Cavity, Head and Neck

Basal cell carcinoma	Slightly raised lesion with rolled waxy border and central ulceration on sun-exposed surface
Squamous cell carcinoma	Nonhealing white, red-white lesion, ulcer or fungating mass of the lateral tongue, floor of the mouth, lip
Kaposi's sarcoma	Purple plaques or nodules of the palate, gingival or face
Melanoma	Brown, black enlarging plaque of skin, palate (+ satellite lesions)
Mucoepidermoid carcinoma	Dome-shaped swelling with central ulceration of palate, retromolar region, or lytic osseous lesion
Leukemia	Gingival enlargement, and bleeding, skin pallor, small hemorrhages of the skin and mucous membranes and bruising
Lymphoma	Enlarged, nonpainful lymph nodes, palatal or pharyngeal swellings, retromolar ulcerations
Advanced breast, prostate and renal cancer	Lytic osseous metastases in the mandible

characterized by A,B,C, D—that is, Asymmetry, irregular Border, Color variegation, and Diameter greater than 6 mm. The color is usually deep and may be brown, gray, blue, or jet black (Fig. 21-8). Multiple colors is a prominent sign. Bleeding, ulceration, firmness and satellite lesions are characteristic of established lesions. Early diagnosis and complete resection are critical to long-term survival, as cure rates approach 100% for those persons having a melanoma with a depth of 0.75 mm or less. In contrast, a depth of 1.6 mm or greater confers only a 20% to 30% 10-year survival.[51] Vaccine therapies for melanoma are currently under clinical trial.[52]

Prevention of skin cancer is achieved from the use of sun protection measures (sunscreens and clothing) and periodic screening. The American Cancer Society[4] recommends self-examination once a month using a full-length mirror and a hand mirror to see the back and other hard to see areas of the body. Professional examination of the skin should be done every 3 years from 20 to 40 years of age, and after 40 years of age, it should be done every year.

ORAL CANCER

Oral cancer includes a variety of malignant neoplasms that occur within the mouth (Box 21-3). More than 90% of cases are attributed to SCC. About 9% are carcinomas that arise from salivary gland tissues and other tissue types such as sarcomas and lymphomas.[53] The remaining 1% or so are metastatic from elsewhere in the body, most commonly from lung, breast, prostate and kidney.[54] In the year 2000, the American Cancer Society reported 30,200 cancers of the oral cavity and pharynx and 7800 deaths because of this disease in the United States.[4]

Oropharyngeal cancer represents about 3% of all cancers in the United States. The vast majority of oral cancers occur in patients over age 45 years, and the incidence increases with each decade over age 40 for men and women until age 65.[53,55] Cancer in African-American men and women is increasing faster than in whites and other racial groups.[1,56] Over the past 20 years, little change has occurred in incidence and 5-year survival rates (see Table 21-1).[1,55,57] The 5-year survival rates for all stages of oral cavity and pharyngeal cancer (53%) remain lower for African-American (34%) than for whites (56%).[1]

The biochemical factors of oral SCC has not been fully elucidated. At least 80% of cases are associated with the multiple cellular abnormalities resulting from chronic

and excessive exposure to carcinogens found in smoking tobacco,[58] and alcohol (including mouthwashes with high alcohol content),[59,60] smokeless tobacco,[61] and betel leaf that contains areca nut.[62] Ultraviolet light exposure and immunodeficiency (e.g., HIV infection, solid-organ transplant recipients)[63,64] are associated with approximately 10% of cases, particularly of the lip. HPV (high-risk types) infection can be detected in about 30% of cases.[65-67] Plummer-Vinson syndrome and a vitamin A deficiency also increase the risk of cancer of the oral cavity and oropharynx.[68] Other factors suggested to play a minor role in the cause of oral cancer include arsenic compounds used in the treatment of syphilis, nutritional deficiencies, heavy exposure to materials such as wood and metal dusts, and *Candida* infection.[53,69]

The cellular changes and contributory processes that result in SCC are shown in Fig. 21-1. At the subcellular level, chronic exposure of mucosal cells to carcinogens results in activation of oncogenes and gene mutations and deletions. The most common deletion in smoking tobacco-related oral SCCs (66% of SCCs of the aerodigestive tract) occurs in chromosome 9 (9p21-22).[70,71] The most frequently detected mutation occurs in p53.[58]

Overexpression of epidermal growth factor receptor (EGFR) and activation of the *ras* and *c-myc* oncogenes play contributory roles.[72] HPV's involvement appears to be the result of its early gene (E6 and E7) products that increase the degradation of the p53 protein and protect cells from p53-induced apoptosis/tumor suppression.[73,74] The result of these processes alter a normal cell into a dysplastic cell that eventually develops increased DNA content, functional independence, and loss of adherence. Eventually these cells also promote angiogenesis (i.e., a malignant cell).

Oral SCC has a variable appearance. It may be a white or red patch, an exophytic mass, an ulceration, a granular raised lesion, or combinations of these (Figs. 21-9 and 21-10). White lesions that cannot be scraped off and are clinically nonspecific, called *leukoplakia*, are potential precursors lesions. About 19% of leukoplakias are dysplastic, and about 4% are considered SCC at initial biopsy. Leukoplakias that are not cancerous when first biopsied have about a 6% chance of developing into cancer over time.[68,75,76] Thus the overall incidence of SCC in oral leukoplakia approximates 10% (see Table 21-4). The malignant transformation rates for homogeneous and mixed leukoplakias is higher (as high as 17.5%).[68] Leukoplakias with areas of erythema have a three- to five-time greater chance of being cancerous at initial biopsy or developing into cancer than do homogeneous leukoplakias.[68,75] Nonspecific red lesions involving the oral mucosa (erythroplakia), although less common than white lesions (Table 21-4) are malignant in more than 60% of cases at initial biopsy.[77-78]

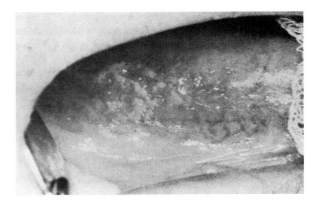

Fig. 21-9 A clinical cause for this tongue lesion could not be identified, and its appearance was not highly suggestive of cancer. Nevertheless, it was diagnosed as early squamous cell carcinoma (SCC) by histopathology. In such cases, it would be appropriate for the dentist to request a biopsy of the lesion.

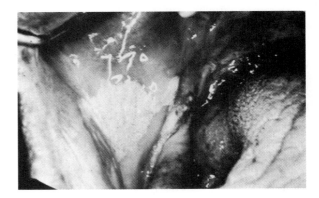

Fig. 21-10 SCC appearing as erythroleukoplakia (a red patch in a diffuse white lesion).

The majority of early carcinomas are asymptomatic and have an erythroplastic component (see Table 21-4).[55,68] Advanced lesions are more often ulcerated with raised margins and induration (Fig. 21-11). Pain is often absent until late in the course of the disease. High-risk sites include the floor of the mouth; lateral (posterior) and ventral (anterior) surfaces of the tongue (Fig. 21-12); soft palate; and surrounding tissues.[55,68,79] These areas are less keratinized and more susceptible to carcinogens. The buccal mucosa and gingivae also are common sites, especially in regions where social oral habits result in carcinogens being placed in close proximity to these tissues.[80] Carcinoma of the upper lip and dorsum of the tongue (e.g., due to use of arsenic compounds) are rare.

Color Characteristics of Oral Squamous Cell Carcinomas (SCCs)*

Color	% of Total SCCs
Only white lesions	24.8
White lesions with erythroplakia	60.0
Only erythroplakia (red) lesions	33.3
Other	1.9

*From 207 asymptomatic intraoral squamous cell carcinomas. Adapted from Mashberg A, Samit A: CA *Cancer J Clin* 46:328-345, 1995.

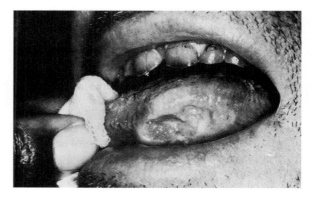

Fig. 21-12 Tongue lesion with a high chance of being cancerous, based on its clinical appearance (size, margins, induration). Direct referral to a cancer treatment center for diagnosis and therapy is indicated. This lesion was diagnosed as SCC.

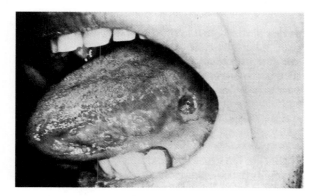

Fig. 21-11 SCC appearing as an ulcerated lesion with induration and raised margins.

Oral SCC spreads by local infiltration into surrounding tissues or metastasis to regional lymph nodes through lymphatic channels. Spread to local structures results in induration, fixation, and lymphadenopathy. Routes of lymph node metastasis are through first-station drainage nodes (buccinator, jugulodigastric, submandibular, and submental) and then second-stage nodes (parotid, jugular, and the upper and lower posterior cervical nodes).[81] Distant metastasis is rare but occurs more commonly to the lung, liver, and bone. Lesions of the floor of the mouth, tongue, and posterior sites tend to metastasize earlier than carcinomas located in anterior oral sites such as the lip. Moreover, about 40% of patients with SCC of the tongue and floor of the mouth lack evidence of metastases at the time of treatment but develop metastatic disease later. Lesions in the maxillary region have a greater tendency to metastasize than do those in the mandibular region. Oral cancer can lead to death by (1) local obstruction of the pathway for food and air; (2) infiltration into major vessels of the head and neck (resulting in significant blood loss); (3) secondary infections; (4) impaired function of other organs through distant metastases; (5) general wasting; or (6) complications of therapy.

In advanced cases of oral carcinoma, the patient may complain of weight loss and difficulty in breathing or nerve involvement that may cause local musculature to become atrophic or result in unilateral paralysis (e.g., loss of the gag reflex when soft palate involved). Other symptoms include hoarseness, dysphagia, intractable ulcers, bleeding, numbness, loosening of teeth, difficulty opening, and a change in the fit of a denture. The diagnosis of oral cancer is made based on microscopic examination of tissue or cells taken from the lesion. Vital staining with toluidine blue can aid in identifying the location from which to biopsy.[68] The international tumor-node-metastases (TNM) system of classification and staging is used to evaluate and classify a tumor's status (see Box 21-1).[4,53,81]

Most early oral SCCs are amenable to surgery, whereas stage III or IV cancers (and those involving bone, vascular structures and multiple lymph nodes) are usually treated with combination therapy (irradiation and surgery). Radiation is by (1) interstitial, (2) implantation, or more commonly, (3) external beam methods,[68] usually within 6 weeks of surgical resection. The tumoricidal dose of external beam radiation ranges from 5000 to 7000 Centigray (cGy), given in separate doses of 150 to 200 cGy over a 6- to 7-week period, with 4 or

5 treatment days followed by 2 or 3 nontreatment days.[81,82] Hyperfractionation employs slightly lower daily doses and is delivered twice a day. "Prophylactic" neck dissection is performed to minimize the development of metastases after treatment of the primary tumor. Radiosensitizers, topical 5-fluorouracil, laser surgery[83] photodynamic therapy (PDT) using a photosensitizing drug, Photofrin II, and 630-nm light from an argon dye laser also have been used as alternative treatment methods.[53,81,84] A combination of radiotherapy and chemotherapy (cisplatin, 5-fluorouracil or taxanes) is reserved for patients when the chance of cure is poor.[53] Selective intraarterial infusion of a chemotherapeutic agent (cisplatin) also has been used successfully in a select group of patients.[85]

The overall 5-year survival rate (53%) of oral SCC is virtually unchanged for 30 years.[1] Higher survival rates are associated with early diagnosis, younger age, early cancers (stages I and II), anterior sites, cancer depth of 5 mm or less, and carcinomas that do not infiltrate bone.[86,87] Recurrences are frequent, especially if patients fail to stop using tobacco and alcohol products.

DENTAL MANAGEMENT

RECOGNITION OF CANCER AND MEDICAL CONSIDERATIONS

The dentist has an important role in the management of the patient with cancer. A primary role is early recognition of the disease. Accordingly, dentists are advised to take a consistent approach for ascertaining pertinent medical, historical, and clinical information from the patient. The dentist should question the patient carefully for signs and symptoms of cancer, particularly those in the head and neck region. Matters involving cancer can be approached by asking the patient questions such as, "Have you experienced any change in your health since your last visit?" or "Are you aware of a lump or bump developing under your arm or in your neck for no apparent reason, a lesion changing color, pain in any body region, or abnormal bleeding from any site, such as blood in the stool?" Such questions allow patients to recall events and situations pertinent to the pathogenesis of disease and may permit them to discuss the condition with you. Questions of the social history regarding overall health, exercise, diet, vitamin intake, tobacco and alcohol use, and cancer in family members are also important and allow the dentist to globally assess the risk of cancer in the patient. The dentist also is in a prime position to discuss the benefits of cancer screening of organ systems (e.g., breast, colon, rectum, cervix, mouth, ovary, prostate,

and skin) and its impact on survival. Certain medical centers and programs offer free cancer screening and patients should be encouraged to take advantage of these services.

After the interview, clinical examination is mandatory to reveal clues of underlying cancer. A head and neck and intraoral soft tissue examination should be performed on each dental patient as he or she enters the practice. This examination, which can be life-saving in the patient with an early cancerous lesion, should be repeated on a regular basis as often as possible, but at least during dental recall visits. It is important to remember that the early stages of cancer are often subtle, and cancer is most amenable to treatment when the lesion is small or asymptomatic and has not spread. The dentist also should remember that the clinical features vary with the type of cancer and location. Lesions clinically suspicious for cancer and those that fail to heal within 14 days despite measures to alleviate it should be biopsied by a skilled clinician. In addition, patients with hard, fixed, and/or matted lymph nodes should be referred directly to a head and neck surgeon or a cancer treatment center. Each patient should be advised of the concern in a frank and open manner. Patients with other signs and symptoms suggestive of cancer should be worked up with laboratory tests and imaging studies. Screening laboratory tests can be obtained by sending the patient to a hospital, a commercial clinical laboratory or a physician. Blood tests should include a total red blood cell (RBC) and white blood cell (WBC) count; a differential white cell count; a smear for cell morphologic study; hemoglobin; hematocrit count; and a platelet count. If the screening tests are ordered by the dentist and one or more are abnormal, the patient should be referred for medical evaluation and treatment.

TREATMENT PLANNING MODIFICATIONS

Dental treatment planning for the patient with cancer begins with the establishment of the diagnosis. Planning involves (1) pretreatment evaluation and preparation of the patient; (2) oral health care during cancer therapy, which includes hospital and out-patient care; and (3) posttreatment management of the patient, including long-term considerations. Cancers that are amenable to surgery and do not affect the oral cavity require few treatment plan modifications. However, certain cancers affect oral health either directly because of surgery or indirectly due to chemotherapy or immunesuppression. The focus of the remainder of this chapter is on those treatments and complications that can affect the oral cavity.

Pretreatment Evaluation and Considerations

The dentist should be aware of the type of treatment selected for the patient and whether the cancer stands a good chance of being controlled. A patient who is to receive palliative therapy may not want replacement of missing teeth; however, this patient must be free of active dental disease that could worsen during cancer therapy. By contrast, a patient who has cancer in stage I or II and no evidence of regional spread can be managed for future dental care as a normal patient. An exception is that the dentist should consider recalling this patient for more frequent examinations for evidence of metastases, recurrence of the lesion, or presence of a new cancer. This is particularly important for patients with oral cancer who are at increased risk for a second primary cancer in the respiratory system, upper digestive tract, or oral cavity. The risk for a second oral cancer in smokers whose habits remained unchanged is about 30%, as compared with 13% for those who quit.[68]

A pretreatment oral evaluation is recommended[88] for all cancer patients before the initiation of cancer therapy to (1) rule out oral disease that may exacerbate during cancer therapy, (2) provide a baseline for comparison and monitoring sequelae of radiation and chemotherapy damage, (3) detect metastatic lesions, and (4) minimize oral discomfort during cancer therapy.[88-90] The evaluation should include a thorough clinical and radiographic examination and review of the blood laboratory findings. Edentulous regions should be surveyed to rule out impacted teeth, retained root tips, and latent osseous disease that could exacerbate during immunosuppressive cancer therapy. A panoramic film is acceptable; however, supplemental bitewing and periapical films may be required to adequately visualize dental and osseous structures.

Pretreatment care should include oral hygiene instructions, the encouragement of a noncariogenic diet, calculus removal, prophylaxis and fluoride treatment, and elimination of all sources of irritation and infection. In children undergoing chemotherapy, mobile primary teeth and those expected to be lost during chemotherapy should be extracted, and gingival opercula should be evaluated for surgical removal to prevent entrapment of food debris. Orthodontic bands should be removed before starting chemotherapy.

If head and neck radiation and immunosuppressive chemotherapy is scheduled, the following recommendations[91] should be considered:

- Reduce radiation exposure to noncancerous tissues (salivary glands) with lead-lined stents, beam sparing procedures, or the use of anticholinergic (biperiden)[92] or parasympathicomimetic (pilocarpine HCl, Salagen) drugs during and after radiotherapy should be discussed with the radiation oncologist and patient.[90,93-97]
- Nonrestorable teeth with poor or hopeless prognosis, acute infection or severe periodontal disease

---

BOX 21-4

Guidelines for Tooth Extraction in Patients Scheduled to Receive Head and Neck Radiation (including the mouth) or Chemotherapy

Indicators of Extraction:

Pocket depths 6 mm or greater, excessive mobility, purulence on probing

Periapical inflammation present

Tooth is broken-down, nonrestorable, non-functional or partially erupted and the patient is non-compliant with oral hygiene measures

Patient has no interest in saving tooth/teeth

Tooth is associated with a inflammatory (e.g., pericoronitis), infectious or malignant osseous disease

Extraction Guidelines:

Extraction performed with minimal trauma at least 2 weeks,* ideally 3 weeks, before initiation of radiation therapy

At least 5 days (in maxilla) before initiation of chemotherapy

At least 7 days (in mandible) before initiation of chemotherapy

Trim bone at wound margins to eliminate sharp edges

Obtain primary closure

Avoid intra-alveolar hemostatic packing agents that can serve as a nidus of microbial growth

Transfuse if the platelet count is less than 50,000/mm³

Delay if the white blood count is less than 2,000/mm³ or the absolute neutrophil is less than 1000/mm³ or expected to be this level within 10 days; alternatively prophylactic antibiotics (cephalosporin) can be used with extractions that are mandatory

---

*In *select* circumstances when healing will not be compromised, a minimum of 10 days can be used.
Biological modifiers that promote healing (e.g., vitamin C) may be useful in these circumstances.
Alternatively, if these time recommendations can not be met before initiation of chemotherapy, a root canal can be performed to reduce the number of viable microbes, then the extraction can be performed after the white blood cell count returns to sufficient levels.
Adapted in part from Rankin KV, Jones DL: *Oral health in cancer therapy,* Texas Cancer Council, 1999.

that may predispose the patient to complications (e.g., sepsis, osteoradionecrosis) should be extracted; sharp, bony edges trimmed and smoothed; and primary closure obtained (Box 21-4).[98,99] Chronic inflammatory lesions in the jaws and potential

Complications of Head and Neck Radiotherapy and Myelosuppressive Chemotherapy

Nausea and vomiting (acute onset)
Mucositis—starts about second week
Ulceration (C)
Taste alteration—starts about second week
Xerostomia (R)—starts about second week
Secondary infections (fungal, bacterial, viral)
Bleeding (C)
Radiation caries (R) (delayed onset)
Hypersensitive teeth (acute and delayed onset)
Muscular dysfunction (R) (delayed onset)
Osteoradionecrosis (R) (delayed onset [More common in mandible, less common in maxilla])
Pulpal pain and necrosis (delayed onset [R]—orthovoltage, not found with cobalt-60)

(C) = limited to, or more prominent with chemotherapy
(R) = limited to, or more prominent with radiotherapy

sources of infection should be examined and treated or eradicated before radiation or chemotherapy.

- Adequate time for wound healing before the induction of radiation therapy or myelosuppressive chemotherapy should be provided for extractions and surgical procedures (see Box 21-4).
- Symptomatic nonvital teeth should be endodontically treated at least 1 week before initiation of head and neck radiation or chemotherapy. However, dental treatment of asymptomatic teeth even with periapical involvement can be delayed.
- Prioritize treatment of infections, extractions, periodontal care and irritations before treatment of carious teeth, root canals therapy, and replacement of faulty restorations. Temporary restorations can be placed and certain treatment (cosmetic, prosthodontic, endodontic) can be delayed when time is limited.
- Tooth scaling and prophylaxis should be provided before initiation of cancer therapy to optimize oral health and reduce the risk of oral complications such as mucositis and infection. Removable prosthodontic appliances should be removed during therapy.
- Patients who will be retaining their teeth and undergoing head and neck radiation therapy must be informed concerning the problems associated with decreased salivary function, which includes xerostomia and increased risk of oral infections, including radiation caries[68,81,95,100] and the risk for osteoradionecrosis (Box 21-5).

Dental preparation of the cancer patient who is going to be treated by surgery is not as critical as for the patient undergoing head and neck radiation and chemotherapy. However, active oral infection should be treated, teeth that are broken down should be removed, and teeth that may be used for the retention of a prosthetic appliance can be restored as needed. The better the dental health of the patient, the lower will be the risk of dental infection complicating the healing process. For the oral cancer patient, the dentist should consider consultation with the maxillofacial prosthodontist so proper coordination of the patient's dental and tooth replacement needs can occur during the presurgical and postsurgical phases.

Oral Care During Cancer Therapy

The oral health of the cancer patient needs to be maintained during cancer therapy, as oral complications develop in a significant portion of patients (more than 400,000) who receive cancer radiation and chemotherapy.[89] Patients undergoing head and neck radiation and in-patient chemotherapy should have oral infections and potential problems eliminated before cancer therapy, with their routine dental care delayed until after cancer therapy is complete. Outpatient chemotherapy requires dental treatment to be provided at appropriate times between cycles. This section discusses oral complications that occur during and after chemotherapy and irradiation of head and neck structures that may require modifications in oral health care management.

Management of Complications of Radiation and Chemotherapy

General management considerations of radiation and chemotherapy are seen in Box 21-6. Acute toxicities reactions are seen during and immediately after radiation and chemotherapy. Acute toxicities are directly proportional to the amount of radiation or cytotoxic drug to which the tissues are exposed, and are more evident in rapidly dividing cells. Delayed toxicities can occur several months to years after radiation therapy.

Radiation therapy induces cell necrosis, microvascular damage, parenchymal and stromal damage. The production of oxygen-free radicals from ionizing radiation is one of the leading causes of cell damage. Cells that have rapid turnover are more susceptible to the damage. For this reason, hypoxic cells and slowly replicative cells are more resistant to radiation than those that are well oxygenated and mitotically active. Box 21-7 lists the effects of radiotherapy on different oral tissues.

Most chemotherapeutic agents will cause alopecia; breakdown of the mucous membranes (mucositis); depression of the bone marrow (infection, bleeding,

---

BOX 21-6

Radiation Effect on Normal Tissues in the Path of the External Beam

Mucosa and Lamina Propria
Epithelial changes (atrophy), mucositis, vascular changes, intimal thickening, luminal stenosis, obliteration, decreased blood flow

Muscle
Fibrosis, vascular changes

Bone
Decreased number of osteocytes, decreased numbers of osteoblasts, decreased blood flow

Salivary Glands
Atrophy of acini, vascular changes, fibrosis

Pulp
Necrosis (orthovoltage)

---

anemia); gastrointestinal changes (diarrhea, malabsorption); and altered nutritional status, and it can also induce cardiac and pulmonary dysfunctions.[5] Bone marrow suppression and mucositis associated with chemotherapy are predictable, dose dependent, and usually manageable. Patients receiving chemotherapy may manifest erythema and ulceration of the oral mucosa, infection of the surrounding tissues, excessive bleeding with minor trauma, xerostomia, anemia, and neurotoxicity.[68,81,89]

Mucositis. Mucositis, inflammation of the oral mucosa, results from the direct cytotoxic effects of radiation or antineoplastic agents on rapidly dividing oral epithelium and the upregulation of proinflammatory cytokine expression (see Appendix B).[101,102] Mucositis occurs in up to 40% of patients undergoing chemotherapy[103] and is often a dose-limiting factor for chemotherapy and a cause of dose interruption of radiation therapy. It develops more often in nonkeratinized mucosa (buccal and labial mucosa, ventral tongue) and adjacent to metallic restorations by the end of the second week of radiation therapy (if the dose is 200 cGy per week; Fig. 21-13). Mucositis develops most often between the seventh and

---

BOX 21-7

Management of the Patient with Oral Complications of Radiotherapy and Chemotherapy

Mucositis
  Eliminate infection, irritations, establish good oral hygiene
  Mouth rinses (3 choices similar in controlling mucositis[108]):
    1. Salt and sodium bicarbonate mouthwash (1 tspn each in pint of water)
    2. Elixir of diphenhydramine (Benadryl) or viscous lidocaine 0.5% in Milk of Magnesia, Kaopectate or sucralfate
    3. Chlorhexidine 0.12% (can be formulated in water by pharmacist)
  Anti-inflammatory: topical steroids, kamillosan liquidim
  Protectants: Orabase
  Avoid tobacco, alcohol, carbonated drinks
  Soft diet, maintain hydration
  Use humidifier, vaporizer
  Consider topical and systemic antimicrobials if severe
  Biological response modifiers (under investigation)
Xerostomia
  Sugarless lemon drops, sorbitol-based chewing gum, buffered solution of glycerine and water, salivary substitutes (see Box 21-9)

Radiation caries
  Educate patient concerning the risks and motivate to maintain optimum oral hygiene
  Custom trays for the daily application of fluoride constructed of soft flexible mouth guard material. Trays hold 5 to 10 drops of a 1% to 2% acidulated fluoride gel, applied 5 minutes each day. If the 1% to 2% acidulated gel is found to be irritating to the tissues; 0.5% neutral sodium fluoride gel can be substituted. Alternative: A single brush-on application of 5000 ppm fluoride (PrevDent) may be more effective for some patients.
  Frequent dental recall
  Patient compliance confirmed by monthly recall during first year.
  Restore early carious lesions
Secondary infection—Culture, cytologic study, antibiotics, antifungal agents, antiviral agents
Sensitivity of teeth—Topical fluorides
Loss of taste—Zinc supplementation
Osteoradionecrosis (see Box 21-10)
Muscular dysfunction—Tongue blades to help retain maximum opening of jaws and access to oral cavity

See Appendix B for medications, dosage, and duration of use.

fourteenth day after chemotherapy (especially VP16, epotoside, methotrexate) when the effects of the drugs produce an extremely low WBC count (*nadir*). It generally subsides one to 2 weeks after the completion of treatment. Young cancer patients with higher division rates have a greater prevalence of chemotherapy-induced mucositis than older cancer patients.[101,104]

Mucositis produces red, raw and tender oral mucosa with epithelial sloughing similar to a severe oral burn. Oral ulcerations can result from breakdown of the epithelial barrier and infection by viral, bacterial or fungal organisms.[105,106] Patients typically complain of ulceration, pain, dysphagia, loss of taste, and difficulty in eating, and it increases the risk for oral and systemic infection. If the major salivary glands have been irradiated, xerostomia (Fig. 21-14) comes after the initial onset of mucositis. The

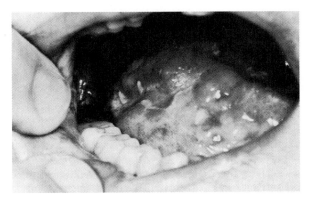

Fig. 21-13 Extensive mucositis that developed from the effects of radiation on the oral mucosa. (Courtesy R. Gorlin, Minneapolis, Minn.)

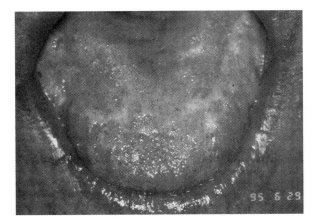

Fig. 21-14 Severe xerostomia that developed from the effects of radiation on the oral mucosa. Note the angular cheilitis.

complications of mucositis and xerostomia make the patient extremely uncomfortable and increases the difficulty of maintaining proper nutritional intake.

During this acute phase, the goal is to maintain the mucosal integrity[107] and oral hygiene. Patients are generally managed by use of the following[108]: (1) a bland mouth rinse (salt and soda water) to keep ulcerated areas as clean as possible; (2) topical anesthetics (viscous lidocaine 0.5%) and/or an antihistamine solution (benzydamine HCl [Tantum rinse], diphenhydramine [Benadryl], promethazine [Phenergan]) can provide pain control or can be combined with milk of magnesia (Maalox), Kaopectate, or sucralfate to serve as a coating agent (for protection of the ulcerated areas); (3) antimicrobial rinses such as chlorhexidine;[105] (4) antiinflammatory agents (kamillosan liquidim or topical steroids [dexamethasone]); (5) adequate hydration; (6) a diet consisting of soft foods, protein, and vitamin supplementation at therapeutic levels; (7) oral lubricants and lip balms containing water base, beeswax base, or vegetable oil base (e.g., Surgi-Lube); (8) humidified air (humidifiers or vaporizers); (9) avoidance of alcohol, tobacco, and irritating foods (e.g., citrus fruits and juices and hot, spicy dishes; Box 21-7, Appendix B).[107] Dentures should not be worn until the acute phase of mucositis resolves. Dentures should be cleaned and soaked with an antimicrobial solution daily to prevent infections.

Secondary Infections. During radiation and chemotherapy, patients are prone to secondary infections. Because of the quantitative decrease in actual salivary flow and compositional alterations in saliva, several organisms (bacterial, fungal, and viral) can opportunistically infect the oral cavity. Moreover, if the patient is immunosuppressed from chemotherapy, and the white blood count falls below 2000 cells/mm,[3] the immune system is less able to manage these infections. Opportunistic infections are also common in patients who receive chemotherapy and broad-spectrum antibiotics.

The most frequent organism opportunistically infecting the oral cavity in individuals undergoing cancer therapy (who have hyposalivation and immunosuppression) is *Candida albicans*. Cytologic study, potassium hydroxide (KOH) staining, microscopic examination, and *Candida*-specific cultures are often performed to provide a definitive diagnosis. Candidal infections can produce pain, burning, taste alterations, and intolerance to certain foods, especially acidic citrus fruits or spicy foods. They present clinically in four different forms ranging from denuded epithelium to hyperplastic lesions. During cancer therapy, the most common type is pseudomembranous candidiasis, which produces white plaques that are easily scraped off, leaving behind tiny petechial hemorrhages

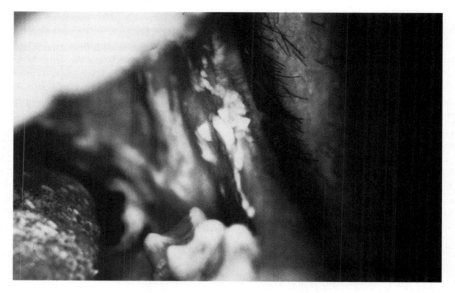

Fig. 21-15 Oral candidiasis (pseudomembranous form) in a patient undergoing chemotherapy. (Courtesy G. Ferretti, Lexington, Ky.)

(see Fig. 21-15). Slightly less prevalent is the erythematous, atrophic form, which manifests as a red patch accompanied by a burning sensation (see Appendix B). The other forms of candidiasis (angular cheilosis and the less common hypertrophic form, which presents as a thick, white plaque that cannot be scraped off) are more commonly detected in patients with chronic hyposalivation.

Candidiasis is best managed by topical oral antifungal agents. These include nystatin (oral suspension 100,000 international units [IU]/ml 4 to 5 times daily); clotrimazole (Mycelex lozenges 10 mg 5 times day); or other preparations (e.g., vaginal topical antifungal agents). Prophylactic use of antifungal agents may be required in patients undergoing chemotherapy who have frequent recurrent infections. Ketoconazole (Nizoral), fluconazole (Diflucan), or itraconazole (Sporanox) may be used if systemic therapy is warranted or if patients develop unusual oral fungal infections (torulopsis, aspergillosis, mucormycosis) or fungal septicemia (possibly from the oral cavity). Alternatively, the physician may place the patient on granulocyte (monocyte) colony stimulating factor (G[M]-CSF) that elevates the neutrophil count to normal levels and can contribute to resolution of the lesions.[109]

Bacteria and viruses may be the cause of other secondary infections. Oral bacterial infections may appear with typical signs of swelling, erythema, and fever. Alternatively, these features can be masked in patients with low WBC counts due to chemotherapy.[94,106] In immunosuppressed patients, a shift occurs in the oral flora

to gram-negative organisms that normally inhabit the gastrointestinal or respiratory tract such as *Pseudomonas, Klebsiella, Proteus, Escherichia coli,* or *Enterobacter.* The most common presentation is an oral ulceration. Thus dentists should culture all nonhealing oral ulcerations in such patients, and these specimens should be sent for diagnosis and antibiotic sensitivity testing. If a bacterial infection is suspected, appropriate antibacterial therapy should be initiated. Antimicrobial sensitivity data are important for the selection of an effective antibiotic when the clinical course shows little or no improvement in several days.

Recurrent herpes simplex virus eruptions develop often during chemotherapy if antivirals are not prophylactically prescribed. They are infrequent during radiation therapy.[110] Herpes recurrences in cancer patients undergoing chemotherapy tend to be larger and take longer to heal than herpetic lesions found in nonimmunocompromised patients (Fig. 21-16).[111,112] Anti-viral agents (acyclovir, famciclovir, or valacyclovir) are recommended prophylactically for HSV-antibody–positive patients who are undergoing chemotherapy to prevent recurrences.[113] A daily dose of at least 1 g acyclovir-equivalent is needed to suppress HSV recurrences. Because these ulcers can mimic the appearance of aphthous and can occur on nonkeratinized mucosa in immunocompromised cancer patients, obtaining a culture or use of an enzyme-linked immunoassay is important for accurate diagnosis. Laboratory tests also help distinguish the infection from

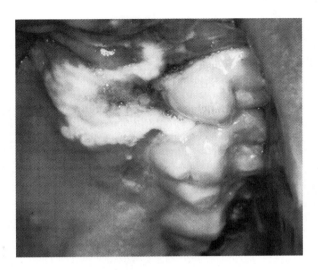

Fig. 21-16 Recurrent herpes simplex virus infection presenting as a large ulcer on the palate of a patient undergoing chemotherapy.

other oral herpes virus infections such as varicella zoster and cytomegalovirus that can occur in these patients.[101] Antiviral sensitivity testing should be considered for patients with unresolving or extensive infections and those in poor general health.

Bleeding. Cancer patients who undergo total body irradiation or high-dose chemotherapy or have bone marrow involvement due to disease are also susceptible to thrombocytopenia. Gingival bleeding and submucosal hemorrhage as a result of minor trauma (e.g., tongue biting or toothbrushing) can occur when the platelet count drops below 50,000 cells/mm.[3] Palatal petechiae, purpura on the lateral margin of the tongue, and gingival bleeding/oozing are common features. Gingival hemorrhage is aggravated by poor oral hygiene. When gingival tissues bleed easily and the platelet count is severely reduced, the patient should avoid vigorous brushing of the teeth and begin using softer devices such as toothettes or gauze wrapped around a finger and dampened in warm water or an antimicrobial solution (chlorhexidine prepared by the pharmacist in water). During this stage, patients should be instructed not to use toothpicks, water-irrigating appliances, or dental floss. To control gingival bleeding, local measures, such as pressure with a gelatin sponge with thrombin or microfibrillar collagen placed over the area or an oral antifibrinolytic rinse (aminocaproic acid [Amicar] syrup 250 mg/mL) placed in a soft vinyl mouthguard can be used to control bleeding. If local measures fail, medical help should be obtained and platelet transfusion considered.

Neural and Chemosensory Changes. Many patients receiving radiation therapy experience diminished sense of taste, probably as a result of damage to the microvilli of the taste cells.[114] Patients receiving chemotherapeutic agents complain of bitter tastes, unpleasant odors, and conditioned aversions to foods.[98] To minimize sensory stimulation, the dentist should avoid wearing colognes or perfume when in contact with patients undergoing radiation/chemotherapy.

In most patients, the ability to taste returns in 3 to 4 months after completion of radiotherapy. In cases of chronic loss of taste, zinc supplementation has been reported to improve taste perceptions. Silverman[68] recommends 220 mg of zinc two times per day for patients with severe chronic loss of taste. However, currently, no effective treatment is available for completely restoring damaged taste.

Neurotoxicity is a side effect of chemotherapeutic agents, particularly vincristine and vinblastine. Although, more commonly, this complication arises in the peripheral nerves, patients can experience odontogenic pain that mimics irreversible pulpitis due to these agents. The pain is more common in the molar region and can be bilateral.[115] Proper diagnosis requires the clinician to be familiar with the chemotherapy drug regimen and is aided by the absence of clinical or radiographic abnormalities.

OTHER CONSIDERATIONS

Many cancer patients have indwelling catheters (Hickman catheters or ports) that are susceptible to infection. The American Heart Association's regimen for endocarditis antibiotic prophylaxis is recommended for these patients before invasive dental procedures.[116] In contrast, prosthetic implants (breast, penile, oral) that have been placed to restore esthetics or function due to cancerous tissue or cancer treatment are not considered at risk for bacterial seeding from oral invasive procedures and do not require antibiotic coverage.[116-119]

Whether a patient is receiving inpatient or outpatient chemotherapy, the dentist should be familiar with the patient's WBC count and platelet status before dental care. In general, routine dental procedures can be performed if the granulocyte count is greater than 2000/mm,[3] the platelet count is greater than 50,000/mm,[3] and the patient feels capable of withstanding dental care.[90] For outpatient care, this is generally 17 days after chemotherapy

If urgent care is needed and the platelet count is below 50,000/mm[3] consultation with the patient's oncologist is required. Platelet replacement may be indicated if invasive or traumatic dental procedure are to be

Recommendations for Invasive Oral Procedures in the Cancer Patient Who is Undergoing Chemotherapy in an Out-Patient Setting

Provide routine care when:
  the patient feels best—generally 17 to 20 days after chemotherapy
  granulocyte count* > 2000 cells/mm³
  platelet count*† > 50,000 cells/mm³
If indwelling catheter (or port) present—
  Amoxicillin 2 g 1 hr before procedure, or if allergic to penicillin
  Clindamycin 600 mg 1 hr before procedure

*Consultation with physician recommended when values lower than indicated in table.
†Platelet values below 50,000 may cause significant bleeding in patients.

performed and topical therapy using pressure, thrombin, microfibrillar collagen, and splints may be required (see Chapter 19).

If urgent dental care is needed and the granulocyte count is less than 2000 cells/mm³, consultation with the physician is recommended and antibiotic prophylaxis should be provided. The dentist should be aware that use of prophylactic antibiotics for these patients is rational but without scientific evidence of effectiveness. The potential adverse effects of antibiotics should be kept in mind when making the decision to use them. No standard antibiotic regimen is recommended for prophylaxis. The drug(s), duration, and dosage to be used for prophylaxis should be established in consultation with the patient's oncologist.[120] Penicillin V, 500 mg, every 6 hours starting at least 1 hour before any invasive procedure that involves bone, pulp, or periodontium and continuing for at least 3 days is a reasonable regimen. Periodontal infections and patients who are allergic to penicillin will require the selection of alternative antibiotics.

Post Cancer Treatment Management

After cancer therapy, consultation with the physician is recommended to determine whether the patient is cured, in remission, or completing palliative care. If cancer therapy is completed and remission or a cure is the outcome, the cancer patient should be placed on an oral recall program. Usually, the patient is seen once every 1 to 3 months during the first 2 years and at least every 3 to 6 months thereafter. After 5 years, the patient should be examined at least once per year. This recall program is important for the following reasons[53,68,81] (1) a patient with cancer tends to develop additional lesions, (2) latent metastases may develop, (3) the initial lesions may recur, and (4) complications related to therapy can be detected and managed. The usual long-term complications associated with the cancer and its therapy include chronic xerostomia, loss of taste, altered bone, and related problems. Recall appointments are also important to ensure that the dentate patient continues to maintain good oral hygiene (including daily brushing, flossing, and the continued use of daily fluoride gel applications), and detection of oral soft tissue and hard tissue disease occurs early, before inflammation and infection involves the underlying bone leading to necrosis. Patients who have completed palliative care should be afforded preventive oral care and dental procedures they desire and can withstand.

Hyposalivation and Its Sequela. Salivary gland tissue is moderately sensitive to radiation damage. Because of this, acinar tissue that is in the field of radiation can be permanently damaged during head and neck radiation therapy, resulting in hyposalivation. The degree of hyposalivation is directly related to the radiation field and dose (i.e., the dose delivered to the major salivary glands), and baseline salivary function. Dosages in excess of 3000 cGy are the most damaging, especially if shielding or medication is not provided to the patient during radiation. Irradiated salivary glands become dysfunctional due to acinar atrophy, vascular alterations, chronic inflammation, and loss of salivary parenchymal tissue.[89] Usually, a 50% to 60% reduction of salivary flow occurs in the first week postirradiation therapy.[121] After radiation therapy, saliva is reduced in volume and altered in consistency, pH, and immunoglobulin concentration. The consistency is mucinous, thick, sticky, and ropy because the serous acini are more sensitive to radiation than mucous acini. Unfortunately, the pathologic changes often progress several months after radiotherapy has ceased, and the radiation-induced salivary gland damage and dysfunction is permanent. In most cases, no recovery of salivary gland function occurs.

The direct effects of hyposalivation include extreme dryness of the oral mucosa. Of major significance is the discomfort, inconvenience, and substantial diminution of quality of life that accompanies oral dryness. Clearly, saliva is an important host defense mechanism against oral disease, serving a variety of important functions in the oral cavity. In a healthy mouth, copious saliva containing essential electrolytes, glycoproteins, immunoglobulins, hydrolytic enzymes (amylase), antimicrobial enzymes, and a number of other important factors continually lubricates and protects the oral mucosa.

Saliva in normal quantities and composition serves to cleanse the mouth, clear potentially toxic substances, regulate acidity, buffer decalcifying acids, neutralize bacterial toxins and enzymes, destroy microorganisms, and remineralize enamel with inorganic elements (e.g., calcium and phosphorus), thus maintaining the integrity of the teeth and soft tissues.[96,100,122,123]

When the normal environment of the oral cavity is altered because of a decrease in or total absence of salivary flow or because of alterations in salivary composition, a healthy mouth becomes susceptible to painful deterioration and decay. Dry, atrophic, and fissured oral mucosa and soft tissues are usual results of the hyposalivary condition along with accompanying ulcers and desquamation, opportunistic bacterial and fungal infections, inflamed and edematous tongue, caries, and periodontal disease. Extreme difficulty in lubricating and masticating food (sticking to the tongue or hard palate) and difficulty swallowing food (dysphagia)[124] are common and among the most devastating and potentially most systemically impacting manifestations of hyposalivation in these individual.[125,126] Additionally, lack of or altered taste perception (hypogeusia or dysgeusia) and tolerance for certain acidic foods (citrus fruits, acetic acid, vinegar, and so on) are substantially altered in these individuals. As a result, nutritional intake in these individual may be impaired.[100,124,126]

The manifestation of salivary hypofunction in patients having undergone irradiation therapy for head and neck cancer include severe xerostomia (less than 0.2 mL/min unstimulated salivary flow); mucositis; cheilitis; glossitis; fissured tongue; glossodynia; dysgeusia; dysphagia; and a severe form of caries called *radiation caries* (Fig. 21-17).[100] Radiation caries is estimated to occur 100 times more often in patients who have received head and neck radiation compared with normal individuals.[100] It can progress within months, advancing towards pulpal tissues and resulting in periapical infection that extends to the surrounding irradiated bone. Extensive infection and necrosis can result. A prescription for concentrated fluoride toothpaste (5000 ppm) should be provided to these patients for use in custom trays or brush on application (see Box 21-7), and an assessment of salivary flow should be made.

After a proper diagnostic assessment that determines the level of unstimulated and stimulated salivary flow, xerostomia is managed according to the three categories delineated in Box 21-9. First is the provision of additional moisture and lubrication to the oral cavity and oropharynx. This may be accomplished by either simulation of oral fluids or stimulation of endogenous saliva. Several artificial salivas are available, some of which provide a

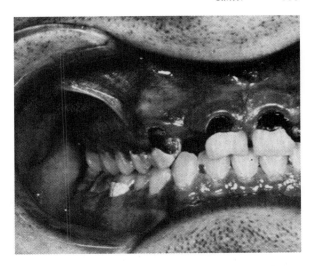

Fig. 21-17 Note the extensive cervical caries in a patient who received radiotherapy. (Courtesy R. Gorlin, Minneapolis, Minn.)

modicum of symptomatic relief from oral dryness. However, synthetic saliva solutions alone do not appear to be satisfactory for relief of the complaints associated with chronic xerostomia. Generally, they are compounded from carboxymethylcellulose or hydroxymethylcellulose. Some contain fluoride and supersaturated calcium and phosphate ions. An artificial saliva that has been particularly effective but is found only in Europe, is Saliva-Orthana, which contains some natural animal mucins. Mouthkote contains a plant glycoprotein that reproduces the lubricating mucosal protection normally provided by saliva. Xero-Lube, Optimoist, Glandosane, and Salivart are other examples of artificial salivas that primarily are compounds of carboxymethylcellulose and may be effective. A gel form of artificial saliva that provides long-lasting relief, especially at night, is Oral Balance. This contains two antimicrobial enzymes (lactoperoxidase and glucose oxidase), which normally are found in saliva.

Patients should be encouraged to drink plenty of water and other fluids with the exception of diuretics such as coffee or tea. Ethanol and tobacco should be avoided or minimized, since these dry the oral mucosa. Also, postradiation cancer patients who sip drinks constantly to keep the oral mucosa moist should avoid sipping drinks that contain a fermentable carbohydrate or carbonic acid, as exposed cementum and dentin breakdown rapidly (in less than 6 months), resulting in radiation caries. Sugarless mints, candies, or chewing gum are beneficial in producing some additional moisture.

BOX 21-9

Management of Salivary Dysfunction*

1. Moisture–Lubrication
General
   a. Drink–sip water, liquids (that lack fermentable carbohydrate and carbonic acid)
   b. Avoid ethanol, tobacco, coffee, tea, hot spicy foods
   c. Use sugarless candy/gum
Products (over the counter [OTC] and prescription)
OTC Oral balance apply ½ tspn 5 to 6 times daily

Rx Pilocarpine HCl 2% (Salagen)† 5 mg, tid or qid
Rx Anethole trithione (Sialor)† 25 mg tid
Rx Bethanechol chloride (Urecholine)† 25 mg tid
Rx Cevimeline (Evoxac)† 30 mg caps tid
Rx Artificial salivas: Glandosane spray, Moi-Stir, Mouthkote, Optimoist, Roxane Saliva Substitute, Salivart spray, Salix lozenges or generic (sodium carboxymethylcellulose 0.5% aqueous solution)

2. Soft Tissue Lesions–Soreness
OTC Oral balance

OTC Biotene mouthwash

Rx Diphenhydramine (Benadryl) + Maalox + nystatin elixir‡ (± Sucralfate) (± 0.5% viscous lidocaine)
Rx Dexamethasone (Decadron Elixir) 0.5 mg/5 ml§
Rx Triamcinolone 0.1% (in hydrocortisone acetate [Orabase] Orabase-HCA)
Rx Clotrimazole (Mycelex) 60-mg troches
Rx Nystatin and triamcinolone ointment (Mycolog II, Tristatin II, Mytrex)

3. Prevention of Caries–Periodontal Disease
   a. Meticulous personal oral hygiene
   b. Avoid acidic drinks
   c. Toothpaste (Biotene)
   d. Regular hygiene recalls and dental prophylaxis
   e. Mechanical brushes, waterpik, NaHCO₄ rinses

Rx Neutral NaF 1.0%–trays (Prevident 5000)
Rx Chlorhexidine gluconate (Peridex, Periguard)

*Salivary gland dysfunction, hyposalivation, or xerostomia should be managed by the diagnosis and according to the signs, symptoms, and severity of its manifestations in the oral cavity. Decreases in the quantity, and alterations in the composition of beneficial constituents of saliva render the patient subject to many problems. The strategies for management will vary from individual to individual as to severity and are divided into the above three major areas.
†Caution in use in patients who have chronic obstructive pulmonary disease (COPD) and patients at risk for myocardial infarction (MI)
‡Rx: Benadryl 25 mg/10 ml + nystatin 100,000 IU/ml + Maalox 4 ml; eq 15 ml.
§Rx: Decadron Elixir 0.5%/5 ml. Dispense 100 ml. Sig: 1 tsp. tid swish-swallow.

Considerable research has been performed with various sialogogue drugs such as pilocarpine HCl (Salagen); anethole trithione (Sialor)[95] and recently, cevimeline (Evoxac).[96,123,127] Pilocarpine is the prototype parasympathomimetic drug derived from the pilocarpus plant. It is an alkaloid, muscarinic-cholinergic agonist and is known to stimulate smooth muscle and exocrine secretions.[128] Pilocarpine has been extensively tested in safety and efficacy trials, and it appears to be very promising as a sialogogue.[96,123,127] These parasympathomimetic drugs appear to be effective for stimulating salivary flow in most patients who have some residual salivary acinar function.[96,127,129] However, certain side effects occur, and patients have to be carefully screened (i.e., cardiovascular disease, diabetes, concomitant medications) before being placed on these drugs. Of particular note is that approximately

50% of the patients who used pilocarpine and experienced increased salivary flow noticed symptomatic improvement in their dry mouth. Therefore although the drug increases salivary flow and provides endogenous beneficial constituents to the oral cavity, patients may still need adjunctive artificial salivas in order to feel more comfortable.

Fungal Infection. Opportunistic infection with *Candida albicans* is very prevalent in the postirradiation patient, with more than 80% of these individuals exhibiting infection with the fungus if proper diagnostic testing is used (see Secondary Infections, above).

Tooth Sensitivity. During and following radiotherapy, the teeth may become hypersensitive, which could be related to the decreased secretion of saliva and the lowered pH of secreted saliva. The topical application of a fluoride gel should be of benefit in reducing these symptoms.

Muscle Trismus. Radiation therapy of the head and neck can cause damage to the vasculature of muscles (obliterative endoarteritis) and thus trismus of the masticatory muscles and joint capsule. To minimize the effects of radiation on the muscles around the face and the muscles of mastication, a mouth block should be placed when the patient is receiving external beam irradiation. The patient also should perform daily stretching exercises to improve trismus, and apply warm moist heat. One exercise is for the patient to place a given number of tongue blades in the mouth at least three times a day for ten minute intervals. By slowly increasing the number of tongue blades, muscle stretching will occur and more normal function will ensue.[53]

Prosthodontics. Patients should avoid wearing their dentures during the first 6 months after completion of the radiotherapy because mild trauma to the altered mucosa can result in ulcerations and possible necrosis of underlying bone (see Osteoradionecrosis below). Once patients start to wear their dentures, they must be told to come to the dentist if any sore spots develop so the dentures can be adjusted. Ill-fitting dentures should be replaced by new ones. In severe cases of chronic xerostomia, a small amount of petrolatum can be applied to the mucosal surface of the denture to help with adhesion.[130] Implants can be placed 12 to 18 months after radiation therapy but require knowledge of tissue irradiation fields, degree of healing and vascularity of the region. For example, implants placed in the maxilla and the anterior mandible are less of a risk for osteoradionecrosis than those placed in the posterior mandible.

Osteoradionecrosis. Osteoradionecrosis (ORN) is a condition characterized by exposed bone that fails to heal (present for 6 months) after high-dose radiation to the jaws.[131] ORN results from radiation-induced changes (hypocellularity, hypovascularity, and ischemia) in the jaws. Most cases result from damage to tissues overlying the bone as opposed to direct damage to the bone.[82] Accordingly, soft tissue necrosis usually precedes ORN and is variably present at the time of diagnosis. Risk is greatest in posterior mandibular sites, for patients whose jaws have received in excess of 6500 cGy, who continue to smoke, and undergo a traumatic (i.e., extraction) procedure.[68,132] Risk is greater for dentate patients than edentulous patients and when periodontal disease is present. Nonsurgical procedures that are traumatic (e.g., curettage) or cause a reduction of blood supply to the region (use of vasoconstrictors) can result in ORN. Spontaneous ORN also occurs. The risk remains throughout a patient's lifetime.[131]

If the dentist is unsure of the amount of radiation received and invasive procedures are planned, the radiation oncologist should be contacted to determine the total dose to the head and neck region before initiating care. Clinicians should be aware that risk of ORN increases with increasing dose to the jaws (e.g., 7500 cGy is a greater risk than 6500 cGy).[68] Patients determined to be at risk should be provided the appropriate preventive measures. Protocols to reduce the risk of osteoradionecrosis include selection of endodontic therapy over extraction, use of nonlidocaine local anesthetics that contain no or low concentration of epinephrine; atraumatic surgical procedures (if surgery is necessary); prophylactic antibiotics plus antibiotics during the week of healing (penicillin VK for seven days); and hyperbaric oxygen before invasive procedures (Box 21-10).[91,133,134] Hyperbaric oxygen involves sequential daily dives under two atmospheres of oxygen pressure in a chamber.

The use of prophylactic antibiotics to prevent infection after surgical procedures in postradiation patients minimizes bacterial invasion of the surgical site. However, the effectiveness of such coverage can be greatly reduced because of altered blood flow to the affected bone. The dentist should be aware that reduction in blood flow after radiotherapy is much greater in the mandible than the maxilla because of the limited source and lack of collateral circulation, which accounts for the greater frequency and severity of osteoradionecrosis in the mandible. The use of hyperbaric oxygen treatment at the time of extraction is gaining more support but is costly and cannot be repeated later with the same effect.[134]

Once necrosis occurs, conservative management usually is indicated. The exposed bone (Fig. 21-18) should be irrigated with a saline or antibiotic solution, and the patient should be directed to use oral irrigating devices to clean the involved area. However, extreme pressures should be avoided when these devices are prescribed.

BOX 21-10

Recommendations to Prevent Osteoradionecrosis in the Head and Neck Irradiated Patient

1. Extract teeth with questionable and hopeless prognosis at least 2 weeks before radiotherapy
2. Avoid extractions during radiotherapy
   Mandible at greater risk than maxilla
   Posterior sites at greater risk than anterior sites
3. Minimize infection
   Prophylactic antibiotic use
      2 gram penicillin VK orally 1 hour before surgical procedure
   After surgery, continue with penicillin VK 500 mg four times a day for 1 week
4. Minimize hypovascularity after radiotherapy
   Use nonlidocaine local anesthetic (e.g., Prilocaine plain or forte) for dental procedures
   Minimize or avoid vasoconstrictor, if must use consider low concentration epinephrine (1:200,000 or less)
   Consider hyperbaric oxygen*

5. Minimize trauma
   Endodontic therapy is preferred over extraction (assuming the tooth is restorable)
   Atraumatic surgical technique
   Avoid periosteal elevations
   Limit extractions to two teeth per quadrant per appointment
   Irrigate with saline, obtain primary closure, eliminate bony edges or spicules
6. Maintain good oral hygiene
   Use oral irrigators
   Use antimicrobial rinses (chlorhexidine)
   Use daily fluoride gels
   Eliminate smoking
   Frequent postoperative recall appointments

*Alternatives include: Referral of patient in need of extractions to oral and maxillofacial surgeon who has experience with these patients or discuss the use hyperbaric oxygen (HBO) with a medical specialist. HBO treatments often consists of 20 pre-extraction dives and 10 postsurgical dives.

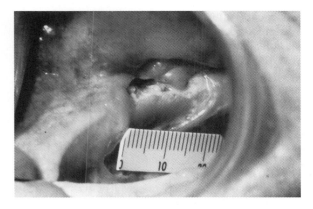

Fig. 21-18 Osteoradionecrosis. Exposed necrotic bone in the posterior mandible edentulous ridge of a patient who previously received radiation therapy to the head and neck region.

Bony sequestrum should be removed to allow for epithelialization. If swelling and suppuration are present, broad-spectrum antibiotics are used. Severe cases benefit from hyperbaric oxygen treatment (60- to 90-minute dives, 5 days per week for a total of 20 to 30 dives).[82,135]

Cases that do not respond to conservative measures may require surgical resection of involved bone.[68,81,134]

Carotid Atheroma. Patients who have received neck irradiation (more than or equivalent to 45 Gy) are more likely to develop carotid artery atheromas (calcified atherosclerotic plaques) after treatment than are risk-matched control patients who have not been irradiated.[136] These lesions (see Fig. 22-7) can be detected by panoramic radiography and are a risk factor for stroke that warrants referral of the patient to their physician for evaluation.

References

1. Greenlee R et al: Cancer statistics, 2000, CA *Cancer J Clin* 50:7-33, 2000.
2. Simone J: Oncology. In Goldman L, Bennett J, editors: *Cecil textbook of medicine*, ed 21, Philadelphia, 2000, WB Saunders.
3. Vogelstein B, Kinzler K: The multistep nature of cancer, *Trends Genet* 9:138-141, 1993.
4. Society AC: Prevention and early detection of cancer. web site: *http://www2.cancer.org/prevention/index.cfm*, 2000.
5. Skeel R, Lachant N: *Handbook of cancer chemotherapy*, ed 4, Boston, 1995, Little, Brown and Co.

6. Armitage J: Bone marrow transplantation, N Engl J Med 330:827-838, 1994.

7. Chu K et al: Recent trends in U.S. breast cancer incidence, survival, and mortality rates, J Natl Cancer Inst 88:1571-1579, 1996.

8. Hortobagyi G: Treatment of breast cancer, N Engl J Med 339:974-984, 1998.

9. Anderson D: Familial versus sporadic breast cancer, Cancer 70:Suppl:1740-1746, 1992.

10. King M, Rowell S, Love S: Inherited breast and ovarian cancer: what are the risks? What are the choices? JAMA 269:1975-1980, 1993.

11. Eng C et al: Familial cancer syndromes, Lancet 343:709-713, 1994.

12. Colditz C et al: Family history, age, and risk of breast cancer: prospective data from the Nurses' Health Study, JAMA 270:338-343, 1993.

13. McKenzie K, Sukemar S: Molecular genetics of human breast cancer, Prog Clin Biol Res 394:183-209, 1997.

14. Brenner A, Aldaz C: The genetics of sporadic breast cancer, Prog Clin Biol Res 396:63-82, 1997.

15. D'Angelo P, Galliano D, Rosemurgy A: Stereotactic excisional breast biopsies utilizing the advanced breast biopsy instrumentation system, Am J Surg 174:297-302, 1997.

16. Tazebay U et al: The mammary gland iodide transporter is expressed during lactation and in breast cancer, Nat Med 6:871-878, 2000.

17. Paist S: Screening and preventive interventions in older patients: which ones are useful? Hospital Med 35:16-21, 1999.

18. Landis S et al: Cancer statistics, 1998, CA Cancer J Clin 48: 6-29, 1998.

19. Canavan T, Doshi N: Cervical cancer, Am Family Phys 61: 1369-1376, 2000.

20. Southern S, Herrington C: Differential cell cycle regulation by low- and high-risk human papillomaviruses in low-grade squamous intraepithelial lesions of the cervix, Cancer Res 58:2941-2945, 1998.

21. zur Hausen H: Papillomaviruses in human cancers, Proc Assoc Amer Physicians 111:581-587, 1999.

22. Lorincz A et al: Human papillomavirus infection of the cervix: relative risk associations of 15 common anogenital types, Obstet Gynecol 79:328-337, 1992.

23. Wigle D, Mao Y, Grace M: Smoking and cancer of the uterine cervix: hypothesis, Am J Epidemiol 111:125-127, 1980.

24. DiSaia P, Creasman W: Clinical gynecologic oncology, ed 5, St. Louis, 1997, Mosby.

25. Centers for Disease Control: 1998 guidelines for treatment of sexually transmitted diseases, MMWR 47:1-111, 1998.

26. Hill M: Molecular and clinical risk markers in colon cancer trials, Eur J Can 36:1288-1291, 2000.

27. Polakis P, Hart M, Rubinfeld B: Defects in the regulation of beta-catenin in colorectal cancer, Adv Exp Med Biol 470:23-32, 1999.

28. Levin B: Neoplasms of the large and small intestines. In Goldman L, Bennett J, editors: Cecil textbook of medicine, 21, Philadelphia, 2000, WB Saunders.

29. Fuchs C et al: Dietary fiber and the risk of colorectal cancer and adenoma in women, N Engl J Med 340:169-176, 1999.

30. Chao A et al: Cigarette smoking and colorectal cancer mortality in the cancer prevention study II, J Natl Cancer Inst 92:1888-1896, 2000.

31. Berkel H et al: Nonsteroidal antiinflammatory drugs and colorectal cancer, Epidemiol Rev 18:205-217, 1996.

32. Janne P, Mayer R: Chemoprevention of colorectal cancer, N Engl J Med 342:1960-1968, 2000.

33. Ahlquist D et al: Colorectal cancer screening by detection of altered human DNA in stool: feasibility of a multitarget assay panel, Gastroenterology 119:1219-1227, 2000.

34. Ries L et al: SEER cancer statistics review, 1973-1996, Bethesda, Md, 1999, National Cancer Institute.

35. Smith L et al: Targeting of lung cancer mutational hotspots by polycyclic aromatic hydrocarbons, J Natl Cancer Inst 92:803-811, 2000.

36. Miller Y: Pulmonary neoplasms. In Goldman L, Bennett J, editors: Cecil textbook of medicine, ed 21, Philadelphia, 2000, WB Saunders.

37. Travis W, Travis L, Devesa S: Lung cancer, Cancer 75:191-202, 1995.

38. Hoffman P, Mauer A, Vokes E: Lung cancer, Lancet 355:479-485, 2000.

39. Park B, Louie O, Altorki N: Staging and the surgical management of lung cancer, Radiologic Clin N Am 38:545-561, 2000.

40. Partin A: Diseases of the Prostate. In Goldman L, Bennett J, editors: Cecil textbook of medicine, ed 21, Philadelphia, 2000, WB Saunders.

41. Jarvik G et al: Confirmation of prostate cancer susceptibility genes using high-risk families. IV. Applications panel, J Nat Cancer Inst 26:81-87, 1999.

42. West D et al: Adult dietary intake and prostate cancer risk in Utah: a case-control study with special emphasis on aggressive tumors, Cancer Causes Control 2:85-94, 1991.

43. Giovannucci E et al: A prospective study of dietary fat and risk of prostate cancer, J Natl Cancer Inst 85:1571-1579, 1993.

44. Ozen M, Pathak S: Genetic alterations in human prostate cancer: a review of current literature, Anticancer Res 20:1905-1912, 2000.

45. Gailani M, Bale A: Developmental genes and cancer: role of patched in basal cell carcinoma of the skin, J Natl Cancer Inst 89:1103-1109, 1997.

46. Cox N: Basal cell carcinoma in young adults, Br J Dermatol 127:26-29, 1992.

47. Grin C, Rigel D, Friedman R: Worldwide incidence of malignant melanoma. In Balch C et al, editors: Cutaneous melanoma, Philadelphia, 1992, JB Lippincott.

48. Green A et al: Sun exposure, skin cancers and related skin conditions, J Epidemiol 9(6 Suppl):S7-13, 1999.

49. Rigel D, Friedman R, Kopf A: The incidence of malignant melanoma in the United States: Issues as we approach the 21st century, J Am Acad Dermatol 34:839-847, 1996.

50. Platz A, Ringborg U, Hansson J: Hereditary cutaneous melanoma, Semin Cancer Biol 10:319-326, 2000.

51. Parker F: Skin diseases of general importance. In Goldman L, Bennett J, editors: Cecil textbook of medicine, ed 21, Philadelphia, 2000, WB Saunders.

52. Haigh P et al: Vaccine therapy for patients with melanoma, *Oncology* 13:1561-1574, 1999.

53. US Department of Health, Education and Welfare: Management guidelines for head and neck cancer, *Public Health Service Publication* No. 80-2037, 1979.

54. Zacharides N: Neoplasms metastatic to the mouth, jaws and surrounding tissues, *J Craniomaxillofac Surg* 17:283-290, 1989.

55. Mashberg A, Feldman L: Clinical criteria for identifying early oral and oropharyngeal carcinoma: erythroplakia revisited, *Am J Surg* 1565:273-275, 1988.

56. Boring C, Squires T, Tong T: Cancer statistics, 1992, CA *Cancer J Clin* 42:19-38, 1992.

57. National Institutes of Health NCI: *Measures of progress against cancer*, 1994.

58. Brennan J et al: Association between cigarette smoking and mutation of the p53 gene in squamous cell carcinoma of the head and neck, *N Engl J Med* 332:712-717, 1995.

59. Mashberg A, Meyers H, Garfinkel L: Alcohol as a primary risk factor in oral cancer, CA *Cancer J Clin* 31:146-155, 1981.

60. Feldman J et al: A case-control investigation of alcohol, tobacco, and diet in head and neck cancer, *Prev Med* 4:444-463, 1975.

61. Winn D: Smokeless tobacco and cancer: the epidemiologic evidence, CA *Cancer J Clin* 38:236-243, 1988.

62. Merchant A et al: Pan without tobacco: an independent risk factor for oral cancer, *Int J Cancer* 86:128-131, 2000.

63. King G et al: Increased prevalence of dysplastic and malignant lip lesions in renal-transplant patients, *N Engl J Med* 332:1052-1057, 1995.

64. Penn I: Occurrence of cancers in immunosuppressed organ transplant recipients. In Terasaki P, editor: *Clinical transplants*, vol 53-62, Los Angeles, 1990, UCLA Tissue Typing Laboratory.

65. Miller C, White D: Human papillomavirus expression in oral mucosa, premalignant conditions, and squamous cell carcinoma: a retrospective review of the literature, *Oral Surg Oral Med Oral Pathol Oral Radiol Endod* 82:57-68, 1996.

66. Smith E et al: Human papillomavirus and risk of oral cancer, *Laryngoscope* 108:1098-1103, 1998.

67. Watts S, Brewer E, Fry T: Human papillomavirus DNA types in squamous cell carcinomas of the head and neck, *Oral Surg* 71:701-707, 1991.

68. Silverman S, Jr: *Oral cancer*, ed 4, Hamilton, 1998, American Cancer Society, BC Decker Inc.

69. Krogh P: The role of yeasts in oral cancer by means of endogenous nitrosation, *Acta Odontol Scand* 48:85-88, 1990.

70. Ahsee K et al: An allelotype of squamous carcioma of the head and neck using microsatellite markers, *Cancer Res* 54:1617-1621, 1994.

71. Nawroz H et al: Allelotype of head and neck squamous cell carcinoma, *Cancer Res* 54:1152-1155, 1994.

72. Wong D et al: Molecular biology of human oral cancer, *Crit Rev Oral Biol Med* 7:319-328, 1996.

73. Hickman E, Bates S, Vousden K: Perturbation of the p53 response by human papillomavirus type 16 E7, *J Virol* 71:3710-8, 1997.

74. Shally M et al: The E6 variant proteins E6I-E6IV of human papillomavirus 16: expression in cell free systems and bacteria and study of their interaction with p53, *Virus Res* 42:81-96, 1996.

75. Silverman S, Rosen R: Observations on the clinical characteristics and the natural history of oral leukoplakia, *J Am Dent Assoc* 76:772-777, 1968.

76. Silverman SJ, Gorsky M, Lozada F: Oral leukoplakia and malignant transformation; a follow-up study of 257 patients, *Cancer* 53:563-568, 1984.

77. Mashberg A: Erythroplasia: the earliest sign of asymptomatic oral cancer, *J Am Dent Assoc* 96:615-620, 1978.

78. Shafer W, Waldron C: Erythroplakia of the oral cavity, *Cancer* 36:1021-1028, 1975.

79. Mashberg A, Samit A: Early diagnosis of asymptomatic oral and oropharyngeal squamous cancers, CA *Cancer J Clin* 46:328-345, 1995.

80. Zain R, Ikeda N, Yaacob H: *Oral mucosal lesions survey of adults in Malaysia*, Selangor, Malaysia, 1995, Interoffice Equipment SDN. BHD., Ministry of Health, University of Malaysia.

81. Million RR, Cassisi MJ: *Management of head and neck cancer*, Philadelphia, 1984, JB Lippincott.

82. Suntharalingam M: Principles and complications of radiation therapy. In Ord R, Blanchaert R, editors: *Oral cancer: the dentist's role in diagnosis, management, rehabilitation, and prevention*, Chicago, 2000, Quintessence Publishing.

83. Maxson B, Scott R, Headington J: Management of oral squamous cell carcinoma in situ with topical 5-fluorouracil and laser surgery, *Oral Surg* 68:44-48, 1989.

84. Nauta J et al: In vivo photo-detection of chemically induced premalignant lesions and squamous cell carcinoma of the rat palatal mucosa, *J Photochem Photobiol B* 39:156-166, 1997.

85. Robbins K et al: Phase I study of highly selective supradose cisplatin infusions for advanced head and neck cancer, *J Clin Oncol* 12:2113-2120, 1994.

86. Jones K et al: Prognostic factors in the recurrence of stage I and II squamous cell cancers of the oral cavity, *Arch Otololaryngol* 118:483-485, 1992.

87. Wallner P et al: Patterns of care study; analysis of outcome survey data anterior two-thirds of tongue and floor of mouth, *Am J Clin Oncol* 9:50-57, 1986.

88. Sciubba J et al: National Institutes of Health consensus development conference statement: oral complications of cancer therapies-diagnosis, prevention, and treatment, *J Am Dent Assoc* 119:179-183, 1989.

89. National Institutes of Health Consensus Development Panel: *Oral complications of cancer therapies: diagnosis, prevention, and treatment*, vol 9, Washington, DC, 1990, US Department of Health and Human Services.

90. Peterson D: Prevention of oral complications in cancer patients, *Prev Med* 23:763-765, 1994.

91. Rankin K, Jones D: *Oral health in cancer therapy*, 1999, Texas Cancer Council.

92. Rode M et al: The effect of pilocarpine and biperiden on salivary secretion during and after radiotherapy in head and neck cancer patients, *Int J Radiat Oncol Biol Phys* 45:373-378, 1999.

93. Zimmerman R, Mark R, Juillar G: Timing of pilocarpine treatment during head and neck radiotherapy: concomitant administration reduces xerostomia better than postradiation pilocarpine, *Int J Rad Oncol* 36:155, 1996.

94. Semba S, Mealey B, Hallmon W: Dentistry and the cancer patient: Part 2, oral health management of the chemotherapy patient, *Compendium* 15:1378-1388, 1994.

95. Epstein J, Schubert M: Synergistic effect of sialogogues in management of xerostomia after radiation therapy. *Oral Surg Oral Med Oral Pathol* 64:1179-1182, 1987.

96. Fox P: Pilocarpine for the treatment of of xerostomia associated with salivary gland dysfunction, *Oral Surg Oral Med Oral Pathol* 61:243-245, 1986.

97. Poole T, Flaxman N: Use of protective prostheses during radiation therapy, *J Am Dent Assoc* 112:485-488, 1986.

98. Naylor G, Terezhalmy G: Oral complications of cancer chemotherapy: prevention and management, *Spec Care Dentist* 8:150-156, 1988.

99. Fattore L, Baer R, Olsen R: The role of the general dentist in the treatment and management of oral complications of chemotherap, *Gen Dent* 35:374-377, 1987.

100. Dreizen S et al: Prevention of xerostomia related dental caries in irradiated cancer patients, *J Dent Res* 56:99-104, 1977.

101. Sonis S: Oral complications of cancer chemotherapy. In Sonis S, Peterson D, editors: *Epidemiology, frequency, distribution, mechanisms and histopathology.* The Hague, 1983, Martinus Nijhoff.

102. Sonis S: Oral complications of cancer therapy. In DeVita V, Hellman S, Rosenberg S, editors: *Cancer: principles and practice of oncology*, ed 5, Philadelphia, 1997, Lippincott-Raven.

103. Scully C, Epstein J: Oral health care for the cancer patients, *Eur J Cancer B Oral Oncol* 32B:281-292, 1996.

104. Childers N et al: Oral complications in children with cancer, *Oral Surg Oral Med Oral Pathol* 75:41-47, 1993.

105. Ferretti G et al: Chlorhexidine for prophylaxis against oral infections and associated complications in patients receiving bone marrow transplants, *J Am Dent Assoc* 114:461-467, 1987.

106. Peterson D, D'Ambrosio J: Nonsurgical management of head and neck cancer patient, *Dent Clin N Amer* 38:425-445, 1994.

107. Epstein J, Schubert M: Oral mucositis in myelosuppressive cancer therapy, *Oral Surg Oral Med Oral Pathol Oral Radiol Endod* 88:273-276, 1999.

108. Dodd M et al: Randomized clinical trial of the effectiveness of 3 commonly used mouthwashes to treat chemotherapy-induced mucositis, *Oral Surg Oral Med Oral Pathol Oral Radiol Endod* 90:39-47, 2000.

109. Luzzi G, Jones B: Treatment of neutropenic oral ulceration in human immunodeficiency virus infection with G-CSF, *Oral Surg Oral Med Oral Pathol Oral Radiol Endod* 81:53-54, 1996.

110. Redding S, Luce E, Boren M: Oral herpes simplex virus infection in patients receiving head and neck radiation, *Oral Surg Oral Med Oral Pathol* 69:578-580, 1990.

111. Redding S: Role of herpes simplex virus reactivation in chemotherapy-induced oral mucositis, *NCI Monogr* (9):103-105, 1990.

112. Miller CS, Redding SW: Diagnosis and management of orofacial herpes simplex virus infections, *Dent Clin North Am* 36:879-895, 1992.

113. Centers for Disease Control and Prevention: 1998 Guidelines for Treatment of Sexually Transmitted Diseases, *MMWR* 47:1-118, 1998.

114. Conger A: Loss and recovery of taste acuity in patients irradiated in the oral cavity, *Radiat Res* 53:338-347, 1973.

115. Robbins M: Oral Care of the Patient Receiving Chemotherapy. In Ord R, Blanchaert R, editors: *Oral cancer: the dentist's role in diagnosis, management, rehabilitation, and prevention*, Chicago, 2000, Quintessence Publishing.

116. Dajani A et al: Prevention of bacterial endocarditis: recommendations by the American Heart Association, *Clin Infect Dis* 25:1448-1458, 1997.

117. Little J: Dent Teamwork. *Preventing bacterial infections.* 7:28-32, 1994.

118. Marx R, Morales M: The use of implants in the reconstruction of oral cancer patients, *Dent Clin North Am* 42:177-202, 1998.

119. Little J, Rhodus N: The need for antibiotic prophylaxis of patients with penile implants during invasive dental procedures: a national survey of urologists, *J Urol* 148:1801-1804, 1992.

120. Peterson D: Pretreatment strategies for infection prevention in chemotherapy patients, *NCI Monogr* 9:61-71, 1990.

121. Makkonen T, Edelman L, Forsten L: Salivary flow and caries prevention in patients receiving radiotherapy, *Proc Finn Dent Soc* 82, 1986.

122. Mandel I: In defense of the oral cavity. In Kleinberg I ES, Mandel I, editors: *Saliva and dental caries*, New York, 1979, Information Retrieval.

123. Mandel I, Katz R: The effect of pilocarpine and a beta-adrenergic blocking agent on human saliva, *Pharmacol Ther Dent* 1:71-82, 1971.

124. Rhodus N, Moller K: Dysphagia in post-irradiation therapy head and neck cancer patients, *J Cancer Res Ther Control* 4:49-55, 1994.

125. Hughes C et al: Oral pharngeal dysphagia: a common sequela of salivary gland dysfunction, *Dysphagia*, 1989.

126. Stuchell R, Mandel I: Salivary gland dysfunction and swallowing disorders, *Otolaryngol Clin North Am* 21:649-661, 1988.

127. Greenspan D, Daniels T: Effectiveness of pilocarpine in postradiation xerostomia, *Cancer* 59:1123-1125, 1987.

128. Dawes C: The composition of human saliva secreted in response to a gustatory stimulus and to pilocarpine, *J Physiol* 183:360-368, 1966.

129. LeVeque F, Montgomery M, Potter D, et al: A multicenter, randomized, double-blind, placebo-controlled, dose-titration study of oral pilocarpine for treatment of radiation-induced xerostomia in head and neck cancer patients, *J Clin Oncol* 1124-31.

130. Vergo T, Kadish S: Dentures as artificial saliva reservoirs in the irradiated edentulous cancer patient with xerostomia, *Oral Surg* 51:229-233, 1981.

131. Epstein J et al: Postradiation osteonecrosis of the mandible: a long-term follow-up study, *Oral Surg Oral Med Oral Pathol Oral Radiol Endod* 83:657-662, 1997.

132. Marciani R, Ownby H: Osteoradionecrosis of the jaw, J *Oral Maxillofac Surg* 46:218-223, 1986.

133. Maxymiw W, Wood R, Liu F: Postradiation dental extractions without hyperbaric oxygen, *Oral Surg Oral Med Oral Pathol* 72:270-274, 1991.

134. Myer R, Marx R: Use of hyperbaric oxygen in postradiation head and neck surgery, NCI *Monogr* 9:151-157, 1990.

135. McKenzie M et al: Hyperbaric oxygen and postradiation osteonecrosis of the mandible, *Eur J Cancer* B *Oral Oncol* 29B:201-207, 1993.

136. Freymiller E, Sung E, Friedlander A: Detection of radiation-induced cervical atheromas by panoramic radiography, *Oral Oncol* 36:175-179, 2000.

Neurological Disorders

22

CHAPTER

Four of the more common and significant neurological diseases are epilepsy, stroke, Parkinson's disease, and multiple sclerosis. Cerebrospinal fluid shunts also are discussed because of the risk for bacterial seeding after an invasive dental procedure. Alzheimer's disease, a closely related disorder, is covered in Chapter 23.

■ EPILEPSY ■

DEFINITION

Epilepsy is a term that describes a group of disorders characterized by chronic, recurrent, paroxysmal changes in neurologic function (seizures) caused by abnormal and spontaneous electrical activity in the brain. Seizures may be convulsive (i.e., accompanied by motor manifestations) or manifested by other changes in neurologic function (i.e., sensory, cognitive, emotional).[1] In the past, much confusion existed about the nature and classification of epilepsy, but recent efforts have increased the understanding of these disorders.

In the 1800s, Hughlings Jackson's discourse on epilepsy concluded that "a convulsion is but a symptom, and implies only that there is an occasional, an excessive, and a disorderly discharge of nerve tissue." This has proven accurate; however, it is too limited because many forms of epilepsy exist besides the tonic-clonic generalized convulsion. Many of them are focal, limited, and nonconvulsive.

Today, epilepsy describes a group of chronic conditions whose major manifestation is the occurrence of epileptic seizures.[1] It is characterized by discrete episodes, which tend to be recurrent and often unprovoked, in which a disturbance of movement, sensation, behavior, perception, and consciousness exists. The symptoms are the result of excessive temporary neuronal discharging, which results from intracranial or extracranial causes.[2]

Although seizures are required for the diagnosis of epilepsy, not all seizures imply epilepsy. Seizures may occur during many medical or neurologic illnesses including stress, sleep deprivation, fever, alcohol or drug withdrawal, and syncope.[1]

The classification of epilepsy currently accepted (Box 22-1) was developed by the International League Against Epilepsy.[3] This classification is based on clinical behavior and electroencephalographic changes. For example, partial seizures are limited in scope and clinical manifestations, and involve motor, sensory, autonomic, or psychic abnormalities. Partial seizures are subdivided as simple when consciousness is preserved and complex when consciousness is impaired. Generalized seizures are more global in scope and manifestation. They involve an altered consciousness state and frequently abnormal motor activity. Discussion in this section is limited to generalized tonic-clonic seizures (idiopathic grand mal) because these represent the most severe expression of epilepsy that the dentist is likely to encounter.

EPIDEMIOLOGY: INCIDENCE AND PREVALENCE

Approximately 10% of the population will have at least one epileptic seizure in a lifetime, and the overall incidence is 0.5%.[1] Seizures are most common during childhood, with as many as 4% of children having at least one seizure during the first 15 years of life. Most children outgrow the disorder.[4] About 4 in 1000 children do not outgrow the disorder and require medical care. Seizures also are common in the elderly, with an estimated annual incidence of 134 per 100,000.[5,6] Cerebrovascular disease is the most common factor underlying seizures in the elderly.

Classification of Epileptic Seizures

I. **Partial (focal, local)**
   Simple partial seizures
   Complex partial seizures
   Partial seizures evolving to secondarily generalized seizures

II. **Generalized (convulsive or nonconvulsive)**
   Absence seizures (petit mal)
   Myoclonic seizures
   Tonic-clonic seizures (grand mal)
   Tonic seizures
   Atonic seizures

III. **Unclassified epileptic seizures**

From Commission on Classification and Terminology of the International League Against Epilepsy: *Epilepsia* 22:489-501, 1981.

ETIOLOGY

The etiology of epilepsy is known in many patients. Common causes include head trauma, developmental abnormalities, intracranial neoplasm, hypoglycemia, cerebrovascular disease, drug withdrawal, and febrile illness (meningitis, encephalitis). Seizures also are found with genetic conditions such as Down syndrome, tuberous sclerosis, and neurofibromatosis. Many patients, however, have epilepsy of unknown cause. This is termed *idiopathic* or *primary epilepsy.*

Although the underlying cause of idiopathic generalized epilepsy is unknown, seizures sometimes can be evoked by specific stimuli. Approximately 1 of 15 patients reports that seizures occurred after exposure to flickering lights, monotonous sounds, music, or a loud noise. Of interest have been reports[7] of epileptic seizures in youngsters exposed to flickering lights and geometric patterns while playing video games. Syncope and diminished oxygen supply to the brain also are known to be associated with seizure.

PATHOPHYSIOLOGY AND COMPLICATIONS

The basic event underlying an epileptic seizure is an excessive focal neuronal discharge that spreads to thalamic and brainstem nuclei. The cause of this abnormal electrical activity is not precisely known, although a number of theories exist.[1,8] These include altered neuronal membrane potentials, altered synaptic transmission, diminution of inhibitory neurons, increased neuronal excitability, and decreased electrical threshold for epileptic activity. During the seizure the blood becomes hypoxic and lactic acidosis occurs.

No specific type of brain lesion is absolutely correlated with epileptic seizures. In other words, a lesion in one location of the brain may be epileptogenic in one patient but not in another. In many cases no identifiable lesion exists, which seems to suggest a biochemical abnormality.[8]

Approximately 60% to 80% of patients with epilepsy achieve complete control over their seizures; the remainder achieve only partial or poor control.[8,9] A significant problem with epileptic patients is one of compliance (i.e., making sure that patients take their medication as directed). This problem is common to many chronic disorders, such as hypertension, because the patients may have to take medication for the rest of their lives even though they remain asymptomatic. Complications of seizures include oral, head and neck trauma, and aspiration pneumonia.

Other problems related to anticonvulsant drugs are adverse effects and toxicity. Adverse effects are discussed under *Medical Management.* Common examples of toxicity are phenytoin-induced ataxia and phenobarbital-induced drowsiness. Also, patients who have frequent and severe seizures may experience altered mental function, dullness, confusion, or argumentativeness.

A serious acute complication of epilepsy (especially tonic-clonic) is the occurrence of repeated seizures over a short time without a recovery period. This is called *status epilepticus* and constitutes a medical emergency. Patients may become seriously hypoxic and acidotic during this event and suffer permanent brain damage or death. Patients with epilepsy also are at increased risk for sudden death and death due to accident.

CLINICAL PRESENTATION

SIGNS AND SYMPTOMS

The clinical manifestations of generalized tonic-clonic convulsions (grand mal seizure) are classic. An aura (a momentary sensory alteration that produces an unusual smell or visual disturbance) precedes the convulsion in one third of patients. Irritability is another premonitory signal. After the aura warning, the patient emits a sudden "epileptic cry" (caused by spasm of the diaphragmatic muscles) and immediately loses consciousness. The tonic phase consists of generalized muscle rigidity, pupil dilation, eyes rolling upward or

TABLE 22-1

Anticonvulsants Used in the Management of Generalized Tonic-Clonic (Grand Mal) Seizures

Generic Name	Trade Name	Usual Daily Adult Dose (mg)	Dental Considerations
Drugs of Choice			
Phenytoin*	Dilantin	300 to 400	Gingival hyperplasia, increased incidence of microbial infections, delayed healing, gingival bleeding (leukopenia), osteoporosis
Carbamazepine*	Tegretol	800 to 1600	Xerostomia, microbial infections, delayed healing, ataxia, gingival bleeding (leukopenia and thrombocytopenia), ataxia, osteoporosis. Drug interactions: Propoxyphene, erythromycin
Valproic acid*	Depakene, Depakote	1000 to 3000	Excessive bleeding and petechiae, decreased platelet aggregation, increased incidence of microbial infections, delayed healing gingival bleeding (leukopenia and thrombocytopenia), drowsiness. Drug interactions: Aspirin and NSAIDs
Lamotrigine*	Lamictal	75 to 200	Ataxia may require help getting into and out of the dental chair, risk for developing Stevens-Johnson syndrome
Alternatives			
Clonazepam*	Klonopin	1 to 2	Drug interactions: CNS depressants
Felbamate	Felbatol	1800-4800	Risk of aplastic anemia, Stevens-Johnson syndrome
Gabapentin	Neurotin	300-3600	
Oxcarbazepine	Trileptal	300-900	Liver enzyme induction but less than carbamazepine
Phenobarbital*	Luminal	60 to 120	Sedation, liver enzyme induction. Drug interaction: Central
Primidone*	Mysoline	750 to 1250	nervous system (CNS) depressants
Vigabatrin	Sabril	500-1000	Drug Interactions: CNS depressants

*Pre-existing liver disease can exacerbate adverse effects associated with anti-epileptics. Drugs of choice for absence (petit mal) seizures: ethosuximide (Zarontin), valproate, lamotrigine, or clonazepam. Drugs of choice for status epilepticus: lorazepam 4 to 8 mg, or diazepam, 10 mg, intravenously.

to the side, and loss of consciousness. Breathing may stop because of spasm of respiratory muscles. This is followed by clonic activity that consists of uncoordinated beating movements of the limbs and head, forcible jaw closing, and head rocking. Incontinence of urine or feces may occur. After a few minutes, movement ceases, muscles relax, and a gradual return to consciousness occurs accompanied by stupor, headache, confusion, and depression. Several hours of rest or sleep may be needed to fully regain cognitive and physical abilities.

LABORATORY FINDINGS

The diagnosis of epilepsy generally is based on the history of seizures and an abnormal electroencephalogram (EEG). Seizures produce characteristic spike and wave patterns on an EEG. Other diagnostic procedures useful to rule out other causes of seizures include computed axial tomography (CAT), magnetic resonance imaging (MRI), single photon emission computed tomography (SPECT), lumbar puncture, serum chemistry profiles, and toxicology screening.[8]

MEDICAL MANAGEMENT

The medical management of epilepsy usually is based on long-term drug therapy. Phenytoin (Dilantin), carbamazepine (Tegretol) and valproic acid are considered first-line treatments. Several other drugs are available for control of generalized tonic-clonic seizures (Table 22-1).[9]

These drugs reduce the frequency of seizures by elevating the seizure threshold of motor cortex neurons, depressing abnormal cerebral electrical discharge, and limiting the spread of excitation from abnormal foci. They are efficient at blocking sodium or calcium channels of the motor neurons. Adverse effects of phenytoin include anemia, ataxia, gingival overgrowth, cosmetic changes (coarsening of facial features, hirsutism, facial acne, gingival overgrowth), lethargy, skin rash and gastrointestinal disturbances. Phenobarbital is considered a second-line drug,[10] and can induce hepatic microsomal enzymes that can increase metabolism of concurrently used drugs. Several antiseizure medications (see Table 22-1) can cause drowsiness, sedation, ataxia, weight gain, cognitive impairment and hypersensitivity reactions.[11] Adverse effects are more common at the start of therapy when drugs are administered rapidly or at high dose. For these reasons, and to facilitate compliance, single-drug therapy and a slow increase in dose is recommended. Unfortunately, the use of combination therapy frequently is necessary. Drug therapy is usually continued in children until a 1- to 2-year seizure-free period is obtained or until around age 16 years. Attempts to taper antiepileptic drug therapy are made thereafter.

Vagus nerve stimulation (VNS) is reserved for patients who have had unsatisfactory seizure control with several medications, and is an option for some before brain surgery. VNS is similar to an implantable cardiac pacemaker, in which a subcutaneous pulse generator is implanted in the left chest wall and delivers electrical signals to the left vagus nerve through a bipolar lead.[12] The stimulated vagus nerve provides direct projection to regions in the brain potentially responsible for the seizure. The device generally is used in combination with antiepileptic medications.

DENTAL MANAGEMENT

MEDICAL CONSIDERATIONS

The first step in the management of an epileptic dental patient is identification. This is best accomplished by the medical history and discussion with the patient or family members. Once a patient with epilepsy is identified, the dental practitioner must learn as much as possible about the seizure history, including type of seizures, age at onset, cause (if known), current and regular use of medications, frequency of physician visits, degree of seizure control, frequency of seizures, date of last seizure, and any known precipitating factors. In addition, a history of previous injuries associated with seizures and their treatment may be helpful (Box 22-2).

Fortunately, most epileptic patients are able to attain good control of their seizures with anticonvulsant drugs and are therefore able to receive normal routine dental care. In some instances, however, the history may reveal a degree of seizure activity that suggests noncompliance or a severe seizure disorder that does not respond to anticonvulsants. For these patients a consultation with the physician is advised before dental treatment is rendered. A patient with poorly controlled disease may require additional anticonvulsant or sedative medication, as directed by the physician.

Patients who are taking anticonvulsants may suffer from the toxic effects of these drugs, and the dentist should be aware of their manifestations. In addition to the more common adverse effects (see Table 22-1), occasionally allergy may be seen as a rash, erythema multiforme, or worse (Stevens-Johnson syndrome). Phenytoin, carbamazepine, and valproic acid can cause bone marrow suppression, leukopenia, and thrombocytopenia, resulting in an increased incidence of microbial infection, delayed healing, and gingival and postoperative bleeding.[13] Valproic acid can decrease platelet aggregation, leading to spontaneous hemorrhage and petechiae.[14]

Propoxyphene and erythromycin should not be administered to patients taking carbamazepine because of interference with metabolism of carbamazepine, which could lead to toxic levels of the anticonvulsant drug. Aspirin and nonsteroidal antiinflammatory drugs (NSAIDs) (see Table 22-1) should not be administered to patients taking valproic acid; they can further decrease platelet aggregation, leading to hemorrhagic episodes.[13] No contraindication is indicated to the use of local anesthetics in proper amounts in these patients. Patients who have a VNS device implanted in their chest do not need antibiotic prophylaxis before invasive dental procedures.

Seizure Management

In spite of appropriate preventive measures taken by the dentist and patient, the possibility always exists that an epileptic patient may have a generalized tonic-clonic convulsion in the dental office. The dentist and staff should anticipate this occurrence and be prepared for it. Preventive measures include knowing the patient's history, scheduling the patient at a time within a few hours of taking the anticonvulsant medication, using a mouth prop, removing dentures, and discussing with the patient the urgency of mentioning an aura as soon as it is sensed. The clinician also should be aware that irritability is often a symptom of

BOX 22-2

Dental Management of the Epileptic Patient

1. Identification of patient by history
   a. Type of seizure
   b. Age at time of onset
   c. Cause of seizures (if known)
   d. Medications
   e. Frequency of physician visits (name and phone number)
   f. Degree of seizure control
   g. Frequency of seizures
   h. Date of last seizure
   i. Known precipitating factors
   j. History of seizure-related injuries
2. Provide normal care—well-controlled seizures pose no management problems
3. If questionable history or poorly controlled seizures, consultation with physician before dental treatment—may require modification of medications
4. Be alert to adverse effects of anticonvulsants
   a. Drowsiness
   b. Slow mentation
   c. Dizziness
   d. Ataxia
   e. Gastrointestinal upset
   f. Allergic signs (rash, erythema multiforme)
5. Patients taking valproic acid (Depakene) or carbamazepine (Tegretol) may have bleeding tendencies because of platelet interference—order pretreatment bleeding time; if grossly abnormal, consultation with physician
6. Be prepared to manage grand mal seizure
   a. Consider placing a ligated mouth prop at beginning of procedure
   b. Chair back in supported supine position
7. Manage the seizure
   a. Clear area
   b. Turn patient to side (to avoid aspiration)
   c. Do not attempt to use padded tongue blade
   d. Passively restrain
8. After the seizure
   a. Examine for traumatic injuries
   b. Discontinue treatment, arrange for patient transport

impending seizure. If sufficient time in the premonitory stage occurs, 0.5 to 2 mg of lorazepam can be given sublingually or 2 to 10 mg diazepam can be given intravenously.[15]

If the patient has a seizure while in the dental chair, the primary task of management is to protect the patient and try to prevent injury. No attempt should be made to move the patient to the floor. Instead, the instruments and instrument tray should be cleared from the area, and the chair should be placed in a supported supine position (Fig. 22-1). The patient's airway should be maintained patent. No attempt should be made to restrain or hold the patient down. Passive restraint should be used only to prevent injury from the patient's hitting nearby objects or falling out of the chair.

If a mouth prop (e.g., a padded tongue blade between the teeth to prevent tongue biting) is used, it should be inserted at the beginning of the dental procedure. Trying to insert a mouth prop is not advised during the procedure, as doing so may damage the patient's teeth or oral soft tissue and may be nearly an impossible task. An exception would be if the patient senses a pending seizure and can cooperate.

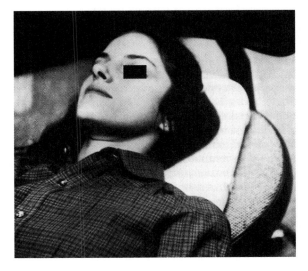

Fig. 22-1 Dental chair in the supine position with the back supported by the operator or the assistant's stool.

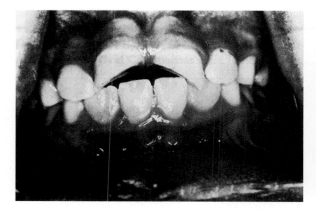

Fig. 22-2 Fractured teeth sustained during a grand mal seizure. (Courtesy G. Ferretti, Lexington, Ky.)

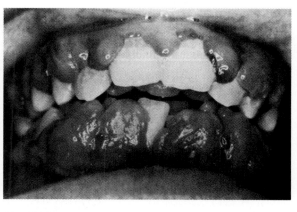

Fig. 22-3 Phenytoin-induced gingival overgrowth. (Courtesy H. Abrams, Lexington, Ky.)

Seizures generally do not last more than a few minutes. Afterward, the patient can fall into a deep sleep and cannot be aroused. Oxygen (100%), maintenance of a patent airway and mouth suction should be provided during this phase. Alternatively, the patient can be turned to the side to control the airway and minimize aspiration of secretions. In a few minutes, the patient will gradually regain consciousness but may be confused, disoriented, and embarrassed. Headache is a prominent feature of this period. If the patient does not respond within a few minutes, the seizure may be associated with low serum glucose and glucose may need to be delivered.

No further treatment should be attempted after generalized tonic-clonic seizures, although an examination for sustained injuries (e.g., lacerations or fractures) should be performed. In the event of avulsed or fractured teeth (Fig. 22-2) or a fractured appliance, an attempt should be made to locate the tooth or fragments to rule out aspiration. A chest radiograph may be required to locate a missing fragment or tooth.

In the event a seizure becomes prolonged (status epilepticus) or is repeated, intravenous lorazepam of 4 to 8 mg, or 10 mg of diazepam is generally effective in controlling it. Lorazepam is more efficacious and longer lasting.[15,16] Oxygen and respiratory support should be provided because respiratory function may be depressed postictally.

TREATMENT PLANNING CONSIDERATIONS

Because gingival overgrowth is associated with phenytoin administration, every effort should be made to maintain a patient at an optimum level of oral hygiene.

This may require frequent visits for monitoring progress. If significant gingival overgrowth exists, surgical reduction will be necessary. However, this must be accompanied with an increased awareness of oral hygiene needs and a positive commitment by the patient to maintain oral cleanliness.

A missing tooth or teeth should be replaced if possible to prevent the tongue from being caught in the edentulous space during a seizure (as commonly happens). Generally, a fixed prosthesis or implant is preferable to a removable one. The removable prosthesis is dislodged more easily. For fixed prostheses, all-metal units should be considered when possible to minimize the chance of fracture. When placing anterior castings, the dentist may wish to consider using three quarter crowns or retentive nonporcelain facings.

Removable prostheses are, nevertheless, sometimes constructed for epileptic patients. Metallic palates and bases are preferable to all acrylic. If acrylic is used, it should be reinforced with wire mesh.

ORAL COMPLICATIONS AND MANIFESTATIONS

The most significant oral complication seen in epileptic patients is gingival overgrowth associated with phenytoin (Fig. 22-3) and rarely with valproic acid[17,18] and vigabatrin.[19] The incidence of phenytoin-induced gingival overgrowth in epileptics ranges from 0% to 100%, with an average of approximately 42%.[20] A greater tendency to develop gingival overgrowth exists in youngsters than adults. The anterior labial surfaces of the maxillary and mandibular gingivae are most commonly and severely affected.

Meticulous oral hygiene is important for preventing and significantly decreasing its severity.[21-23] Good home care must always be combined with the removal of irritants, such as overhanging restorations and calculus. Frequently, enlarged tissues interfere with function or appearance, and surgical reduction will become necessary.

Traumatic injuries such as broken teeth, tongue lacerations, and lip scars also are common in patients who suffer from generalized tonic-clonic seizures. Stomatitis, erythema multiforme and Stevens-Johnson syndrome are rare adverse effects associated with phenytoin, valproic acid, lamotrigine, phenobarbital and carbamazepine use. These complications are more common during the first 8 weeks of treatment.[24]

■ STROKE ■

DEFINITION

Stroke is a generic term used to refer to a cerebrovascular accident, a serious and often fatal neurologic event caused by sudden interruption of oxygenated blood to the brain. This in turn results in focal necrosis of brain tissue and possibly death. Even if a stroke is not fatal, the survivor often is to some degree debilitated in motor function, speech, or mentation. The scope and gravity of stroke are reflected in the fact that stroke is the third most common cause of death in the United States (behind heart disease and cancer) and 5% of the population over age 65 years has had one.[25]

EPIDEMIOLOGY: INCIDENCE AND PREVALENCE

Although the incidence of stroke has declined, it still remains one of the most significant health problems in the United States. Each year in the United States about 600,000 people suffer new or recurrent strokes.[26] This translates to 1 stroke occurring about every minute, with 75% of persons surviving their stroke annually. Approximately 4.5 million persons living in 2001 had survived a stroke.[26] Risk is associated with race, with African-Americans having a 38% greater risk of first stroke than do whites.[27]

Stroke resulted in the death of 158,000 Americans in 1998.[26] African-Americans and racial minorities in the United States have higher stroke mortality than whites. The risk of death from stroke in African-Americans age 35 to 74 years is 2 to 4 times greater than that of non-Hispanic whites. African-American males and persons living in the South and Northwest are at greatest risk.[28] American Indians and Alaska natives are also at increased risk. While risk of stroke increases with age, on average 28% of people who suffer a stroke are under the age of 65 years. The chance of having a stroke before age 70 is 1 in 20 for both genders.[26]

ETIOLOGY

Stroke is caused by the interruption of blood supply to the brain most commonly by thrombosis (60% to 80% of cases) of a cerebral vessel. Other common causes of interruption of cerebral blood flow include cerebral embolism and intracranial hemorrhage. Cerebrovascular disease is the primary factor associated with stroke via atherosclerosis, hypertensive vascular disease, and cardiac pathosis (myocardial infarction, atrial fibrillation), the latter increasing the risk of thrombi and emboli.[29] Approximately 10% of persons who have had a myocardial infarction will have a stroke within 6 years.[26] Additional factors that increase the risk for stroke include the occurrence of transient ischemic attacks, a previous stroke, high dietary fat, obesity and elevated blood lipid levels, physical inactivity, uncontrolled hypertension, cardiac abnormalities, diabetes mellitus, elevated and homocysteine levels, elevated hematocrit, elevated antiphospholipid antibodies, heavy tobacco smoking, increasing age (risk doubles each decade after 65 years) and periodontal disease.[30-32] Increased risk for hemorrhagic stroke also occurs with use of phenylpropanolamine, an alpha-adrenergic agonist.[33] This has led to the Food and Drug Administration ordering the removal of phenylpropanolamine from over-the-counter cold remedies and weight loss aids.[34] Intake of fruits and vegetables and medium levels of exercise have a protective effect against stroke.[35-36]

PATHOPHYSIOLOGY AND COMPLICATIONS

The pathologic changes associated with stroke result from infarction, intracerebral hemorrhage, or subarachnoid hemorrhage. Cerebral infarctions most commonly are caused by atherosclerotic thrombi or emboli of cardiac origin (Fig. 22-4). The extent of an infarction is determined by a number of factors, including site of the occlusion, size of the occluded vessel, duration of the occlusion, and collateral circulation.[37] The production and circulation of proinflammatory cytokines, clotting factors as well as arterial inflammation contribute to platelet aggregation. The neurological abnormalities that present depend on the result of excitotoxicity, free radicals, the inflammatory reaction, and mitochondrial and DNA damage, and apoptosis of the region supplied by the damaged artery.[38]

The most common cause of intracerebral hemorrhage is hypertensive atherosclerosis, which results in

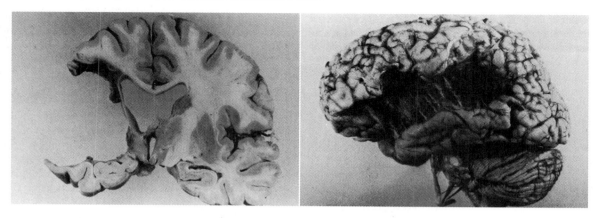

Fig. 22-4 Residual damage many years after a cerebral infarction.

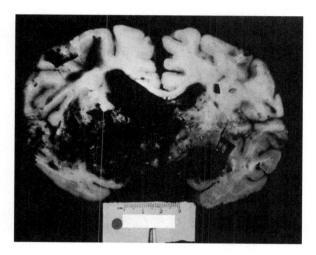

Fig. 22-5 Cerebral hemorrhage caused by hypertensive vascular disease.

microaneurysms of the arterioles. The vessels within the circle of Willis often are affected. Rupture of these micro-aneurysms within brain tissue leads to extravasation of blood, which displaces brain tissue and causes increased intracranial volume until the resulting tissue compression halts bleeding[37] (Fig. 22-5). The most common cause of subarachnoid hemorrhage is rupture of a saccular aneurysm at the bifurcation of a major cerebral artery.

The most serious outcome of stroke is death, occurring in 8% of those experiencing ischemic strokes and 38% to 47% of those with hemorrhagic strokes within a month of the event, and overall in about 23% of patients by one year.[26] Mortality rates are directly related to the type of stroke,[29] with 80% dying after an intracerebral hemorrhage, 50% after a subarachnoid hemorrhage, and 30% after occlusion of a major vessel by a thrombus. Death from a stroke may not be immediate (sudden death) but rather may occur hours, days, or even weeks after the initial stroke episode.

If the victim survives, an excellent chance exists that a neurologic deficit or disability of varying degree and duration will remain. Of those surviving the stroke, 10% recover with no impairment, 50% have a mild residual disability, 15 to 30% are disabled and require special services, and 10% to 20 % require institutionalization.[26,39] Approximately 50% of those who survive the acute period (the first 6 months) are alive 7 years later.[39,40]

The type of deficit residual from a stroke is directly dependent on the size and location of the infarct or hemorrhage. Deficits include unilateral paralysis, numbness, sensory impairment, dysphasia, blindness, diplopia, dizziness, and dysarthria. Return of function is unpredictable and usually takes place slowly, over several months. Even with improvement, patients frequently are left with some permanent residual problem, such as difficulty in walking, using the hands, performing skilled acts, or speaking.

CLINICAL PRESENTATION

SIGNS AND SYMPTOMS

Familiarity with the warning signs and symptoms and phases of stroke can lead to appropriate action that may be lifesaving. Four events associated with stroke are the (1) transient ischemic attack (TIA), (2) reversible ischemic

BOX 22-3

Differences Between Right-Sided Brain Damage and Left-Sided Brain Damage

Right-Side Brain Damage	Left-Side Brain Damage
Paralyzed left side	Paralyzed right side
Spatial-perceptual deficits	Language and speech problems
Thought impaired	Decreased auditory memory (cannot remember long instructions)
Quick impulsive behavior	Slow, cautious, disorganized behavior
Patient cannot use mirrors	Memory deficits—language based
Difficulty performing tasks (toothbrushing)	Patients anxious
Memory deficits	
Neglect of left side	

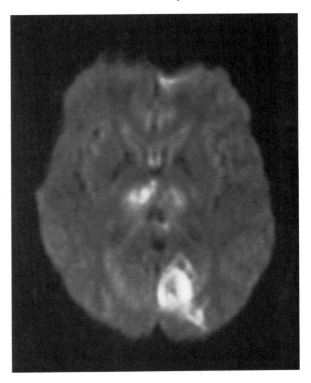

Fig. 22-6 Magnetic resonance perfusion scan of the brain demonstrating edema in the basilar artery region and occipital lobe caused by a cerebrovascular accident. (Courtesy C. Lee, Lexington, Ky.)

neurologic deficit (RIND), 3) stroke-in-evolution, and 4) a completed stroke. These events are defined principally by their duration.

A TIA is a "mini" stroke caused by a temporary disturbance in blood supply to a localized area of the brain. It often causes numbness of the face, arm, or leg on one side of the body (hemiplegia), weakness, tingling, numbness, or speech disturbances that usually last less than 10 minutes. Most commonly, a major stroke is preceded by 1 or 2 TIAs within several days of the first attack.[29] A RIND is a neurologic deficit similar to a TIA that does not clear within 24 hours, but there is eventual recovery.[29]

A *stroke-in-evolution* is a neurologic condition caused by occlusion or hemorrhage of a cerebral artery in which the deficit has been present for several hours and continues to worsen during a period of observation.[29] Signs of stroke include hemiplegia, temporary loss of speech or trouble in speaking or understanding speech; temporary dimness or loss of vision, particularly in one eye (could be confused with migraine); unexplained dizziness, unsteadiness, or a sudden fall.

Residual deficits that remain after a stroke include language disorders, hemiplegia, and paresis, a form of paralysis with loss of sensory function and weakened motor power. Box 22-3 illustrates the different behavioral patterns of right-sided brain damage versus left-sided brain damage. Of note, the majority of stroke patients have their intellect remain intact; however, large, left-sided stroke has been documented to be associated with cognitive decline.[41]

LABORATORY FINDINGS

Patients suspected of having had a stroke usually are submitted to a variety of laboratory and diagnostic imaging tests to rule out conditions that can produce neurologic alterations such as diabetes mellitus, uremia, abscess, tumor, acute alcoholism, drug poisoning, and extradural hemorrhage.[29] Laboratory tests often include urinalysis, blood sugar level, complete blood count, erythrocyte sedimentation rate, serologic tests for syphilis, blood cholesterol and lipid levels, chest radiographs, and electrocardiogram. Various abnormalities may be disclosed by these test results, depending on the type and severity of stroke as well as its causative factors. A lumbar puncture also may be ordered by the physician in an effort to check for blood or protein in the cerebrospinal fluid (CSF) and for altered CSF pressure.[29,42] Doppler blood flow, EEG, CAT scanning, arteriography, and MRI (Fig. 22-6) including diffusion and perfusion studies of

the brain are important for determining the extent and location of arterial injury.

MEDICAL MANAGEMENT

The first aspect of stroke management is prevention. This is accomplished by identifying risk factors in individuals (e.g., hypertension, diabetes, atherosclerosis, cigarette smoking) and attempting to reduce or eliminate as many of these as possible. Antiplatelet therapy (see Chapter 19) and carotid endarterectomy are methods of preventive treatment in some patients who have experienced a TIA.

If a patient has a stroke, treatment is generally three-fold. The immediate task is to sustain life during the period immediately following the stroke. This is done by means of life-support measures and transport to a hospital. The second task is emergency efforts to prevent further thrombosis or hemorrhage, and attempt to lyse the clot in cases of thrombosis or embolism. Thrombolysis and improved neurological outcome have been achieved with intravenous tissue-type plasminogen activator (rt-PA) and intra-arterial prourokinase.[43] Of the two, intravenous administration of rt-PA within 3 hours of ischemic stroke onset is the only approved therapy.[44-46]

After the initial time period, efforts to stabilize the patient continue with anticoagulant medications such as heparin, coumarin, aspirin, and dipyridamole combined with aspirin (Aggrenox) in cases of thrombosis or embolism. Heparin is administered intravenously during acute episodes, whereas coumarin, dipyridamole, aspirin, subcutaneous low molecular weight heparin, or platelet receptor antagonists (clopidogrel, abciximab, ticlopidine) are employed for prolonged periods. Corticosteroids may be used acutely after a stroke to reduce the cerebral edema that accompanies cerebral infarction. This can markedly lessen complications. Surgical intervention may be indicated for removal of a superficial hematoma or management of a vascular obstruction. The latter usually is accomplished by thromboendarterectomy or by bypass grafts in the neck or thorax. Valium, Dilantin or other anticonvulsants are prescribed to manage seizures that may accompany the postoperative course of stroke.

If the patient survives, the third and final task is institution of preventive therapy, administration of medications that reduce the risk of another stroke, and initiation of rehabilitation. Rehabilitation generally is accomplished by intense physical, occupational, and speech therapy (if indicated). Although marked improvement is common, many patients are left with some degree of permanent deficit.

The future holds much promise for the introduction of drugs that reduce the risk for stroke and that are neuroprotective.[47] Of the many drugs being tested, two currently stand out for their ability to reduce risk of recurrent stroke. They include nimodipine (calcium channel blocker) for the prevention of ischemic neurologic deficits after subarachnoid hemorrhage[48] and the use of the lipid-lowering statins drugs for reducing risk of ischemic stroke in patients with history of coronary artery disease.[49,50]

DENTAL MANAGEMENT

MEDICAL CONSIDERATIONS

Some primary tasks of the dentist are stroke prevention and identification of the stroke-prone individual. Patients with a history or clinical evidence of hypertension, diabetes mellitus, coronary atherosclerosis, elevated blood cholesterol or lipid levels, or cigarette smoking are predisposed to stroke as well as to myocardial infarction. The dentist should encourage these individuals to seek medical care and to eliminate or control all possible risk factors (Box 22-4).

A patient who has had a stroke or TIA is at greater risk for having another than a person who has not had one.[29,40] These individuals should be approached with a degree of caution. Deferral of treatment for 6 months is advised because patients are at an increased risk of recurrent strokes during this period. Although a decreased risk exists after 6 months, risk remains, with 14% of those who survive a stroke or TIA having a recurrence within one year.[26] Further, patients suffering a TIA or RIND are unstable and should not receive elective dental care. Medical consultation and referral to a physician are mandatory.

A patient taking coumarin or antiplatelet drugs is at risk for abnormal bleeding (Box 22-4). The status of coumarin anticoagulation is monitored by the prothrombin time or international normalized ratio (INR) status. A prothrombin time level 2.5 times normal or less (normal being 11 to 14 seconds) or an INR level of 3.5 or less is acceptable for performing most invasive and noninvasive dental procedures. If the prothrombin time is greater than 2.5 seconds or the INR greater than 3.5 and oral surgery is planned, significant bleeding could occur, and the physician should be consulted to decrease the dosage of the anticoagulant. In these cases, reducing the dose of anticoagulant is recommended over interruption of anticoagulation therapy as the risk for significant adverse outcome is minimized by the reduction approach[51] (see Chapter 19).

BOX 22-4

Dental Management of the Stroke Patient

1. Identification of risk factors
   a. Hypertension
   b. Diabetes mellitus
   c. Coronary atherosclerosis
   d. Elevated blood cholesterol or lipid levels
   e. Cigarette smoking
   f. TIA or previous stroke
   g. Increasing age
2. Encouragement to control risk factors (referral to physician if appropriate)
3. History of stroke
   a. Having had a stroke places patient at high risk for having another—use caution
   b. Urgent dental care only during first 6 months
   c. Patient with TIAs or RINDs—no elective care
   d. Anticoagulant drugs predispose to bleeding problems
      (1) Aspirin ± dipyridamole (Aggrenox); or Clopidogrel (Plavix), Abciximab (ReoPro), Ticlopidine (Ticlid): pretreatment bleeding time <20 minutes
      (2) Coumarin—pretreatment prothrombin time should be <2.5 seconds or INR <3.5. Higher levels require consultation with physician to reduce dose.
      (3) Heparin (IV)—use palliative emergency dental care only, or discontinue 6 to 12 hours before surgery with physician's approval; restart heparin after clot forms (6 hours later). Heparin (subcutaneous, low molecular weight)—generally no changes required
      (4) Use measures that minimize hemorrhage
      (5) Have non-adrenergic hemostatic agents and devices available
4. Short stress-free, midmorning appointments scheduled
5. Monitoring of blood pressure and oxygen saturation
6. Minimum amount of anesthetic with vasoconstrictor used
7. No epinephrine in retraction cord

The effect of aspirin and dipyridamole on platelet aggregation is monitored by the bleeding time (BT). Any BT greater than 10 minutes has the potential for a slightly increased risk of bleeding during the procedure; however, this risk usually does not become significant until the BT exceeds 20 minutes.[22] Abnormal results should be discussed with the physician. Postoperative pain should be managed with acetaminophen-containing products.

Management of stroke-prone patients or patients with a history of stroke includes the use of short midmorning appointments that are as stress-free as possible. Assisted transfer to the dental chair may be needed. Do not overestimate the patient's abilities, especially since some stroke patients may be able to verbalize but do not realize the extent of paresis present. Dental care providers should move slowly around the patient and speak clearly while facing the patient with the mask off. Effective communication techniques are listed in Box 22-5.

Blood pressure should be monitored to ensure good control. Pain control is important. Nitrous oxide-oxygen may be given if good oxygenation is maintained at all

BOX 22-5

Effective Communication Techniques for the Stroke Patient

Face the patient
Use slower, more deliberate, less complex pattern of speech
Communicate at eye level
Be positive
Ask yes/no questions—simple and brief
Give frequent, accurate, and immediate feedback
Use simple drawings to explain procedures
Do not underestimate or overestimate their abilities
Do not raise voice or use baby talk
Do not wear a mask when talking to the patient
Communicate also with significant other/personal care provider

Data from Henry R: Personal communication, 1995; and Ostuni E: *J Am Dent Assoc* 125:721-727, 1994.

times. A pulse oximeter should be used to ensure oxygenation is adequate. A local anesthetic with 1:100,000 or 1:200,000 epinephrine may be used in judicious amounts (4 ml or less).[52] Gingival retraction cord impregnated with epinephrine should not be used.

A patient who develops signs or symptoms of a stroke in the dental office should be provided oxygen and the EMS should be activated. Transport to a medical facility should not be delayed, as thrombolytic agents should be administered within 3 hours to be most effective in reestablishing arterial flow.[43,53] The dental staff should remember that stroke patients have feelings of grief, loss, and depression, and should treat these patients with compassion.

TREATMENT PLANNING MODIFICATIONS

Technical modifications may be required for patients with residual physical deficits who have difficulty obtaining adequate oral hygiene. For these patients, extensive bridgework is not a good choice. However, fixed prostheses may be more desirable than removable because of difficulty of daily placement and removal. Individualized treatment plans are important. All restorations should be placed with ease of cleansability in mind. Hygiene may be facilitated by an electric toothbrush, a large-handled toothbrush, or a water irrigation device. Flossing aids should be prescribed, and loved ones and personal care providers should be instructed on how and when to provide these services. Frequent professional prophylaxis is advisable.

ORAL COMPLICATIONS AND MANIFESTATIONS

A stroke-in-evolution may be evident by slurred speech, weak palate, or difficulty swallowing. After a stroke, loss or difficulty in speech, unilateral paralysis of the orofacial musculature, and loss of sensory stimuli of oral tissues may occur. The tongue may be flaccid, with multiple folds, and deviate on extrusion. Dysphagia is common. Patients with right-sided brain damage may neglect the left side. Thus food and debris may accumulate around teeth, beneath the tongue, or in alveolar folds. Patients may need to learn to clean teeth or dentures with only one hand, or may require assistance to maintain oral hygiene.

Calcified atherosclerotic plaques have been demonstrated in the carotid arteries of elderly and diabetic patients in panoramic films (Fig. 22-7).[54-56] This feature indicates a risk for stroke[57] and warrants a referral to the patient's physician for evaluation.

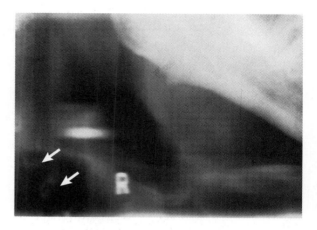

Fig. 22-7 Cervical region of a panoramic film showing two calcifications (arrows) within the carotid artery of an elderly patient.

■ PARKINSON'S DISEASE ■

DEFINITION

Parkinson's disease, first described by James Parkinson[58] in 1817, is a progressive, neurodegenerative disorder of neurons that produce dopamine. The loss of these neurons results in characteristic motor disturbances (tremor, stiffness, shuffling gait, and diminished facial expression). The dopaminergic neurons are found in nigrostriatal pathway of the brain. Approximately 80% of the dopamine in these neurons must be depleted before symptoms of the disease arise.[59,60]

EPIDEMIOLOGY: INCIDENCE AND PREVALENCE

Parkinson's disease is a common disease of the central nervous system (CNS) affecting about 1 million Americans or 100 per 100,000 persons. Each year 50,000 individuals are diagnosed with the disease. About 1% of the population over age 50 years, and 2.5% of the population over age 70 have the disease. With the aging phenomenon of the United States, a three- to fourfold increase in Parkinson disease frequency is predicted in the next 50 years.[61] Parkinson's disease is not limited to seniors, and a particular form of the disease can strike teenagers. Men are affected slightly more often than women; no racial predilection exists.

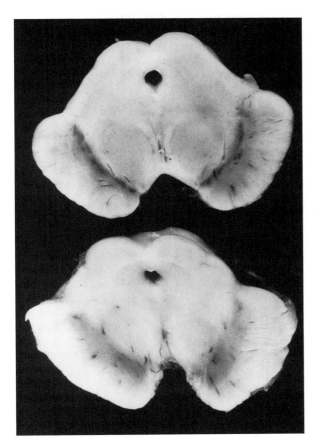

Fig. 22-8 Parkinson's disease. Normal pigmentation of dopaminergic neurons in the substantia nigrans of a healthy patient (top); in contrast with depleted and depigmented dopaminergic neurons of the substantia nigrans in a patient who has Parkinson's disease (bottom).

ETIOLOGY

Parkinson's disease is caused by depletion of the dopaminergic neurons, which are manufactured in the substantia nigra (Fig. 22-8) and released in the caudate nucleus and putamen (the nigrostriatal pathway). Although the cause of Parkinson's disease is unknown, many factors have been identified that are associated with the development of the disease. These include genetic mutation (mutation in chromosome 4),[62] stroke, brain tumor, and head injury (e.g., boxing) that damage the cells of the nigrostriatal pathway. Exposure to manganese (in miners and welders), mercury, carbon disulfide, certain agricultural herbidices, street heroin contaminated with a meperidine analogue (1-methyl-4-phenyl-1,2,3,6-tetrahydropyridine)

can be neurotoxic and give rise to Parkinson's disease symptoms.[59]

PATHOPHYSIOLOGY AND COMPLICATIONS

The neuropathologic findings of Parkinson's disease include degeneration and loss of pigmented neurons primarily of the substantia nigra as well as destructive lesions of the circuitry to the limbic system, motor system, and centers regulating autonomic functions. Damaged neurons display neuronal cytoskeleton changes including eosinophilic intraneuronal inclusion bodies (Lewy bodies)[63] and Lewy neurites in their neuronal processes. At the microscopic level, the inclusion bodies occur in regions of the presynaptic protein alpha-synuclein.[64] Although the exact cause of neuronal cell death is not known, many investigators suggest that the most common causes are the result of metabolic compromise, excitotoxicty and oxidative stress.[65] Degeneration of other regions in the brain such as the cholinergic nucleus basalis can result in depression and impaired neurotransmitter function.

CLINICAL PRESENTATION

SIGNS AND SYMPTOMS

Parkinson's disease results in resting tremor (that is attenuated during activity), muscle rigidity, slow movements (bradykinesia), and facial impassiveness (mask of Parkinson's disease) (Fig. 22-9). The tremor is rhythmic and fine and is best seen in the extremity at rest. The tremor produces a "pill-rolling rest tremor" and handwriting changes. Cogwheel-type rigidity (decreased arm swing with walking), stooped posture, unsteadiness, imbalance (gait instability) and falls also are common features. In addition, pain, (musculoskeletal, sensory [burning, numbness, tingling] or akathisia—subjective feeling of restlessness—restless leg syndrome), orthostatic hypotension and bowel and bladder dysfunction occur in approximately 50% of patients. Cognitive impairment of memory and concentration occurs to varying degrees depending on the destruction of the cortical-basal ganglia-thalamic neural loops. Mood disturbances (depression, dysthymia, apathy, anxiety) occur in approximately 40% of patients; dementia occurs in approximately 25% of patients.[66] Psychosis, related to dopaminergic medications, occurs in approximately 20% of patients.[67]

LABORATORY FINDINGS

Because no diagnostic test for Parkinson's disease exists, the diagnosis requires a thorough history, clinical

PARKINSON'S DISEASE

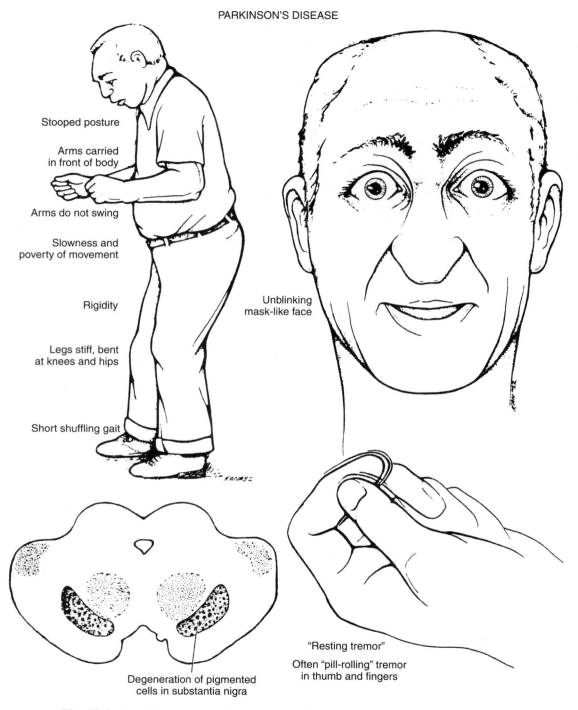

Stooped posture

Arms carried
in front of body

Arms do not swing

Slowness and
poverty of movement

Rigidity

Legs stiff, bent
at knees and hips

Short shuffling gait

Unblinking
mask-like face

"Resting tremor"

Often "pill-rolling" tremor
in thumb and fingers

Degeneration of pigmented
cells in substantia nigra

Fig. 22-9 Clinical features of Parkinson's disease. (From Poritsky R: *Neuroanatomical Pathways,* Philadelphia, 1984, WB Saunders.)

examination, specific tests and images to rule out diseases that can produce similar symptoms such as Wilson's disease, arteriosclerotic pseudoparkinsonism, multiple stem atrophy, and progressive supranuclear palsy.

MEDICAL MANAGEMENT

Between the 1960s and 1990s, the mainstay of treatment for Parkinson's disease was replacement of the neurotransmitter dopamine with levodopa (L-dopa), an immediate precursor of dopamine. This drug, although efficacious early in the course of the disease for alleviating rigidity but not tremor, wanes in its activity after about 5 to 10 years. When given chronically it produces complicating adverse effects (dyskinesia–involuntary rapid flowing movements of limbs, trunk or head). As a result, levodopa slow release preparations, dopamine agonists (bromocriptine, ropinirole, pramipexole, cabergoline, pergolide [an agonist that allows a 25% reduction in dose of levodopa]), amantadine, anticholingerics, and inhibitors of dopamine catabolism catecholamine-O-methyltransferase inhibitors (COMT inhibitors, monoamine oxidase B inhibitors) are used.[60]

Drug therapy generally is not initiated until lifestyle impairment such as slowness or imbalance occurs. Drug selection is based on the anticipated side effects and complications, and is initiated at the lowest effective dose. Adjunct medication such as controlled-release levodopa (Sinemet CR), dopamine agonists, or COMT inhibitors (entacapone) are introduced to diminish the motor fluctuations associated with levodopa. Dose adjustments are required when dyskinesias, immobility, psychosis, or other side effects develop. Amantadine, propranolol, mirtazapine, and benzodiazepines also have been used to improve dyskinesia control,[68] and clozapine is a reasonable alternative for treatment of tremor.[69] Physical therapy is important for showing patients safe methods for rising from a chair, walking around a room, traversing stairs and combating immobility and contractures.

If symptoms progress despite drug therapy, surgery involving replacement of dopamine neurons by grafting fetal nerve tissue[70] appears to be an encouraging alternative for those with advanced Parkinson's disease.[71] Newer modalities are focusing on halting neuronal loss by use of antioxidants, or the introduction (injection) of trophic factors using lentiviral delivery of a gene that encodes glial cell line-derived neurotrophic factor.[72] Deep brain stimulation of the Vim nucleus of the thalamus, thalamotomy or pallidotomy are reserved for advanced disease and severe disabling or intractable tremor.

DENTAL MANAGEMENT

MEDICAL CONSIDERATIONS

The dentist who manages adult patients plays an important role in recognizing the features of Parkinson's disease and making a referral to a physician for thorough evaluation of patients who exhibit features of the disease. Once the diagnosis has been made, concerns in dental management are twofold: (1) minimizing the adverse outcomes of muscle rigidity and tremor and (2) avoiding drug interactions.

Because the muscular defect and tremor can contribute to poor oral hygiene, the dentist should assess patients' ability to cleanse their dentition by demonstration. If a patient is unable to provide adequate home care, alternative solutions should be provided, such as the introduction of the Collis curve toothbrush, mechanical toothbrushes, assisted brushing, or chlorhexidine rinses.

Drug interactions of concern to dentistry are outlined in Table 22-2. Epinephrine vasoconstrictors should be used with caution and the dose limited in patients who take COMT inhibitors (tolcapone [Tasmar]; entacapone [Comtan]). Erythromycin should not be given to patients who take the dopamine agonist, pramipexole (Mirapex). The clinician should be aware that anti-Parkinsonian drugs can be CNS depressants, and a dentally prescribed sedative can have an additive effect.

Orthostatic hypotension and rigidity is common in patients who have Parkinson's disease. To reduce the likelihood of a fall from the dental chair, the patient should be assisted to and from the chair. At the end of the appointment the chair should be inclined slowly to allow for re-equilibration.

TREATMENT PLANNING MODIFICATIONS

The treatment plan for the patient with Parkinson's disease may require modification based on the patient's ability to cleanse the oral cavity. When communicating the treatment plan and other advice, the dentist should directly face the patient. This provides effective communication with a person who has the potential for cognitive impairment.

Patients should receive dental care at the time of day in which their medication has maximum effect (generally 2 to 3 hours after taking it). The presence of tremors or choreiform movements may dictate that the dentist use soft arm restraints or sedation procedures.

TABLE 22-2

Drugs Used in the Management of Parkinson's Disease

Class and Drug	Dose (mg)	Adverse Effects	Dental Consideration
Anticholinergic			
Trihexyphenidyl HCl (Artane)		Sedation, urinary retention, constipation	Dry mouth
Benztropine mesylate (Cogentin)			
Dopamine Precursor			
Levodopa			
Carbidopa/levodopa (Sinemet CR, Madopar CR)	25/100-25/250 bid	Dyskinesias, fatigue, headache, anxiety, confusion, insomnia, orthostatic hypotension	If choreiform movements, dyskinesias or tremors present may require sedation techniques to perform dentistry; caution when rising from dental chair
Dopamine Agonist			
Bromocriptine mesylate (Parlodel)*	5-10 tid	Dopaminergic effects: psychosis (hallucinations, delusions) orthostatic hypotension, dyskinesias, nausea.	Caution when rising from dental chair
Pergolide mesylate (Permax)†	0.1-1 tid		
	1-1.5 tid		
Pramipexole (Mirapex)	2-6 tid		Mirapex adversely interacts with erythromycin
Ropinirole HCl (Requip)			
Catechol-O-methyltransferase (COMT) Inhibitors			
Tolcapone (Tasmar)*	100-200 tid	Potentiate levodopa effects: dyskinesias, psychosis or orthostatic hypotension; nausea and diarrhea	Caution with use of vasoconstrictors. Monitor vital signs during and following administration of first carpule; limit dose to 2 carpules containing 1:100,000 epinephrine (36 μg) or less depending on vital signs and patient response; aspirate to avoid intravascular injection.
Entacapone (Comtan)	200 4 to 6 × d		
Monoamine Oxidase B Inhibitor			
Selegiline	5-20 once daily	Dizziness, orthostatic hypotension, nausea	Adrenergic agents (i.e., amphetamine, pseudoephedrine and tyramine) but not epinephrine or levonordefrin
Neurotransmitter Inhibitor			
Amantadine	100 b/tid	Sedation, urinary retention, peripheral edema, nausea, constipation, confusion	

*Can cause significant hepatic toxicity.
†Also has adverse vasoconstrictive properties.

ORAL COMPLICATIONS AND MANIFESTATIONS

Parkinson's disease is associated with staring, excess salivation and drooling from decreased frequency of blinking and swallowing. Muscle rigidity makes repetitive muscle movement and the maintenance of good oral hygiene difficult. In contrast, the drugs used to manage the disease (anticholinergics, dopaminergics, amantadine and L-dopa) often result in xerostomia, nausea and tardive dyskinesia. Dental recall visits should be more frequent for this population and specific measures (specialized toothbrushes—e.g., Collis curve toothbrush, mechanical brushes) should be devised to maintain adequate oral hygiene. If the patient is experiencing xerostomia, then dysphagia and poor denture retention is likely. Salivary substitutes are beneficial in alleviating symptoms. Topical fluoride should be considered for use in dentate patients with xerostomia to prevent root caries. Personal care providers should be educated in their role in assisting and maintaining the oral hygiene of these patients.

■ MULTIPLE SCLEROSIS ■

DEFINITION

Multiple sclerosis is the most common autoimmune disease of the nervous system. It is characterized by chronic and intermittent demyelination of the corticospinal tract neurons in the brain and periods of recovery. The demyelinated regions are limited to the white matter of the CNS and are randomly located and multiple (Fig. 22-10). The peripheral nervous system is not affected.

EPIDEMIOLOGY: INCIDENCE AND PREVALENCE

Approximately 300,000 persons suffer from multiple sclerosis (MS) in the United States, representing a prevalence of about 58 per 100,000 persons. The incidence is about 5 to 10 per 100,000 persons in the United States but has been increasing during the past century. The disease affects young adults between 20 and 40 years of age, and women twice as often as men. The prevalence is highest in the temperate regions of the world (i.e., northern and southern latitudes) and is infrequently seen along the equator.[73,74] Dentists who manages adult patients can expect to have at least one patient with this condition in their practice.

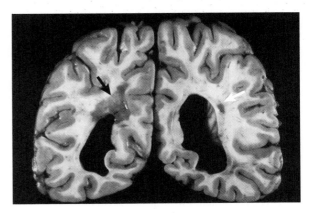

Fig. 22-10 Multiple sclerosis. Large periventricular "demyelinated plaque" (dark region above left ventricle, black arrow) and smaller "demyelinated plaque" (white arrow) lateral to right ventricle demonstrated in a coronal section of the brain of a patient who had multiple sclerosis. (Courtesy Daron G. Davis, Lexington, Ky.)

ETIOLOGY

Although the cause of MS remains unknown, it is widely held to be an autoimmune disease triggered by an infectious agent. Initial support for this arises from cluster studies of MS outbreaks in small regions.[75,76] During the past century several microbes (rabies, measles, herpes viruses, *Chlamydia pneumoniae*[77]) have been purported to be associated with MS. In recent years, human herpes virus type 6 has been identified in active demyelinated regions of the CNS in patients who have MS.[78,79] It is hypothesized that this neurotropic virus in combination with host genetic factors results in processes that cause immune-mediated demyelination. However, not all persons infected with human herpes virus type 6 develop MS, suggesting that genetic factors and other environmental factors are also important. Consistent with the role of genetic factor involvement, the concordance rate among monozygotic twins is 30%.[80,81] Risk is increased if human leukocyte antigen DR[2] is carried by a northern European.[82]

PATHOPHYSIOLOGY AND COMPLICATIONS

Demyelination of MS occurs in scattered white matter regions in the brain. Myelin loss ranges in size from 1 mm to several centimeters in diameter.[75] Affected regions show inflammatory demyelination with accumulation of macrophages, B and T lymphocytes and plasma cells. Inflammatory cytokines and

immunoglobulins accompany the acute MS lesion and influence macrophages to attack myelin, resulting in tissue destruction and swelling.[83] The demyelinated areas or "plaques" are impaired in axonal conduction producing the pathophysiologic defect. The most common demyelinated regions are the optic nerve, periventricular cerebral white matter and the cervical spinal cord.

A significant complication of MS is that 50% of patients will need help walking within 15 years of onset of the disease.[84] Continued muscle atrophy can cause restriction to a wheelchair or bed, thus increasing the chances for the development of pneumonia. The life expectancy for patients with MS is calculated to be 82.5% (approximately 58 years) of normal.[85]

CLINICAL PRESENTATION

SIGNS AND SYMPTOMS

The first clinical signs of MS often begin in young adulthood. Clinical signs are dependent upon the region of the CNS involved (motor or sensory region) and the degree of myelin sheath disruption. Disturbance in visual acuity (sometimes resulting in blindness) and abnormal eye movements (nystagmus and double vision) are the most common presenting symptoms. Common are motor disturbances affecting walking and use of the hands (incoordination, spasticity, difficulty in walking, loss of coordination or weakness, tremor or paralysis of a limb); bowel and bladder incontinence; spastic paresis of skeletal muscles (imprecise speech or tremor); and sensory disturbances, including loss of touch, pain, temperature, and proprioception (numbness, shock sensations, tingling). Fatigue is the major symptom, with worsening fatigue occurring in the afternoon. Symptoms are exacerbated by heat (hot baths, sun exposure) and dehydration, and generally appear over a few days then stabilize before improving a few weeks later. Recovery can be partial or complete.

A typical presentation is one of attacks and relapses that repeats for several years. The course is unpredictable and depends on the frequency of the attacks and extent of the recovery. Four categories have been used to describe the course of the disease. They are relapsing-remitting (occurs in 80% of patients), primary-progressive, secondary-progressive, or progressive-relapsing. Recovery in most cases is temporary because remyelination is not a feature of the disease. Repeated attacks can cause permanent physical damage, however intellectual function remains intact. Depression and emotional instability are common features accompanying the disease.

LABORATORY FINDINGS

The diagnosis of MS usually is made from the accumulation of information derived from the history, clinical examination, cerebral spinal fluid (CSF), sensory evoked potentials and imaging procedures. The CSF shows immune activation with immunoglobulin levels increased in 80% to 90% of patients. Oligoclonal bands can be detected by gel electrophoresis in 70% to 80% of patients. Myelin basic protein released by myelin destruction can be detected by radioimmunoassay in the CSF. Myelin destruction also causes a slowing of conduction velocity. The conduction response to visual stimuli (visual evoked potential) or somatosensory evoked stimuli is usually measured in a laboratory. Magnetic resonance scans are useful for delineating hypodense demyelinated regions in white matter usually near the ventricles, brainstem and cerebellum.[86]

MEDICAL MANAGEMENT

Patients having relapses of MS are given antiinflammatory medications: either intravenous corticosteroids (methylprednisolone), interferon beta-1a (Avonex), or beta-1b (Betaseron) injections.[86] The interferons reduce the proliferation of T cells and the production of tumor necrosis factor. Corticosteroids have many antiinflammatory functions, including the ability to block eicosanoid and cytokine release, and endothelial cell expression of intracellular and extracellular adhesion molecules (ICAM and ELAM, respectively) that attract neutrophils. Interferons and glatiramer acetate (Copaxone) are used during periods of remission to reduce the rate of clinical relapse.[86]

Complications of MS are managed with several drugs. Spasticity is managed with antispastic drugs such as baclofen (GABA agonist), benzodiazepines (GABA receptor activator), dantrolene (modifier of calcium release in muscle fibers), and tizanidine (Zanaflex; alpha2 adrenergic agonist). An implantable pump for intrathecal administration of baclofen sometimes is used. Poor bladder control is managed with anticholinergics such as oxybutynin (Ditropan) or tolterodine tartrate (Detrol). Fatigue is managed with afternoon naps, amantidine (Symmetrel), pemoline (Cylert), or methylphenidate HCL (Ritalin). Paroxysmal events respond to carbamazepine, phenytoin, gabapentin, and pergolide. Serotonin reuptake inhibitors (fluoxetine

[Prozac]) and tricyclic antidepressants are used to manage the accompanying depression.

DENTAL MANAGEMENT

MEDICAL CONSIDERATIONS

The dentist can play an important role in directing the undiagnosed patient who has MS to the appropriate health care provider for diagnosis. Complaints of abnormal facial pain (mimicking trigeminal neuralgia), numbness of an extremity, visual disturbances, or muscle weakness require the dentist to perform a neuromuscular examination and rule out MS. The disease should be suspected if the onset is progressive over several days, the patient is between 20 and 35 years old, and afternoon fatigue is present. Referral to a neurologist is the next step in confirming diagnosis for this patient.

Patients undergoing relapse are unfit for routine dental care. Emergency dental care can be provided but is impacted by the medications the patient takes. In particular, corticosteroids are immunosuppressive, and stressful surgical procedures could require an increase in dose (see Chapter 15, Adrenal Insufficiency). The physician should be consulted before the performance of emergency dental care in these patients.

The optimum time to treat patients with MS is during periods of remission. This care should be provided with the understanding that the medications these patients take can affect the practice of dentistry. In particular, the anticholinergics (oxybutynin [Ditropan], tolterodine tartrate [Detrol]), and tricyclic antidepressants can cause a dry or burning mouth that may require use of salivary substitutes to provide relief. If more relief is needed, the use of pilocarpine (see Appendix B) should be discussed with the physician.

TREATMENT PLANNING MODIFICATIONS

Treatment planning changes are dictated by the level of motor impairment and fatigue. Patients with stable disease and little motor spasticity or weakness can receive routine dental work. Patients with more advanced disease may require help transferring to and from the dental chair, have difficulty maintaining oral hygiene, and may be poor candidates for reconstructive and prosthetic procedures. Because fatigue is often worse in the afternoon, short morning appointments are advised.

ORAL COMPLICATIONS AND MANIFESTATIONS

The dentist should be aware of the oral manifestations of MS that have been reported to occur in 2% to 3% of those affected. The most common features include dysarthria, paresthesia, numbness of the orofacial structures or trigeminal neuralgia. The dysarthria produces slow, irregular speech with unusual separation of syllables of words, termed "scanning speech." During an attack, a patient's face may develop paresthesia and the muscles of facial expression (especially the periorbital) can undulate like waves. The term *myokymia* is used to describe the unusual muscle movement which resemble movement of a "bag of worms." Referral to a physician is advised if the condition has not been diagnosed. Relief of trigeminal neuralgic pain can be achieved through the use of carbamazepine, clonazepam, or amitryptiline.

Cerebrospinal Fluid Shunts

Within the spectrum of neurological disorders is the condition hydrocephalus – a disorder that has an increasing accumulating of CSF within the cerebral ventricles. This condition often requires shunting to reduce increased cerebrospinal fluid pressure. Several types of shunts are used to decrease fluid pressure. Ventriculoperitoneal, ventriculoatrial, and lumboperitoneal are the most common types of shunts.[87-89] In the United States, around 75,000 cerebrospinal fluid shunts are placed each year.[90]

With respect to dentistry, the most significant concern is the risk of CSF shunt infection. Overall, shunt infection rate ranges from about 5% to 15%, with most infections resulting from wound contamination.[91] Almost 70% of the infections are caused by skin flora staphylococcal organisms.[91] Cerebrospinal fluid shunt infections usually occur within 2 months after implantation.[92] The infection rate is higher for ventriculoperitoneal shunts than for ventriculoatrial shunts. However, other types of complications include thromboemboli, severe complications of infection, and shunt malfunctions that make ventriculoatrial shunts more risky.[87,89]

Ventriculoperitoneal and lumboperitoneal shunts do not appear to cause increased risk for infection from hematogenous seeding of bacteria.[87-90,93] However, ventriculoatrial shunts can become infected by transient bacteremias resulting from distant acute infection or invasive dental procedures, and patients with them usually are covered with antibiotics. The need for antibiotic prophylaxis should be established by medical consultation. When prophylaxis is selected, the standard regimen of the current American Heart Association's guidelines[94] should be used (see Chapter 2).

References

1. Pedley T: The Epilepsies. In Goldman L, Bennett JC, editors: *Cecil textbook of medicine*, ed 20, Philadelphia, 2000, WB Saunders.

2. Sutherland J, Eadie M: *The epilepsies: modern diagnosis and treatment*, ed 3, Edinburgh, 1980, Churchill Livingstone.

3. Commission on Classification and Terminology of the International League Against Epilepsy: Proposal for revised clinical and electroencephalographic classification of epileptic seizures, *Epilepsia* 489-501:489-501, 1981.

4. Dodson W et al: Management of seizure disorders: selected aspects, *J Pediatr* 89:527-540, 1976.

5. Sander J et al: National general practice study of epilepsy: newly diagnosed epileptic seizures in a general population, *Lancet* 336:1267-1271, 1990.

6. De la Courte A et al: Prevalence of epilepsy in the elderly: the Rotterdam study, *Epilepsia* 37:141-147, 1996.

7. Dalquist N, Mellinger J, Klass D: Hazard of video games in patients with light-sensitive epilepsy, *JAMA* 249:776-777, 1983.

8. Dichter M: The epilepsies and convulsive disorders. I: In Wilson JD, Braunwald E, Isselbacher KJ, editors: *Harrison's principles of internal medicine*, New York, 1991, McGraw-Hill.

9. Dichter M, Brodie M: New antiepileptic drugs, *N Engl J Med* 334:1583-1590, 1996.

10. Camfield P, Camfield C: Treatment of children with "ordinary" epilepsy, *Epileptic Disorders* (2)2245-2251, 2000.

11. Greenwood RS: Adverse effects of antiepileptic drugs. *Epilepsia* 41(Suppl 2):S42-S52, 2000.

12. George MS et al: Vagus nerve stimulation: a new tool for brain research and therapy, *Biol Psychiatry* 47:287-295, 2000.

13. *Drug information for the health care professional*, 19 ed, Rockville, Md, 1999, Pharmacopeial Convention.

14. Hassell TM et al: Valproic acid: a new antiepileptic drug with potential side effects of dental concern, *J Am Dent Assoc* 9:983-987, 1979.

15. Starreveld E, Starreveld A: Status epilepticus. Current concepts and management, *Can Fam Phys* 46:1817-1823, 2000.

16. Leppik IE et al: Double-blind study of lorazepam and diazepam in status epilepticus, *JAMA* 249:1452-1454, 1983.

17. Syrjanen S, Syrjanen K: Hyperplastic gingivitis in a child receiving sodium valproate treatment, *Proc Finn Dent Soc* 75: 95-98, 1979.

18. Anderson H, Rapley J, Williams D: Gingival overgrowth with valproic acid: a case report, *J Dent Child* 64:294-297, 1997.

19. Katz J, Givol N, Chaushu G, et al: Vigabatrin-induced gingival overgrowth, *J Clin Periodontol* 24:180-182, 1997.

20. Hassell T: Epilepsy and the oral manifestations of phenytoin therapy. In Myers H, editor: *Monographs in oral science*, Basel, 1981, S Karger.

21. Hall W: Dilantin hyperplasia: a preventable lesion? *Compendium* 14(suppl):5502-5505, 1990.

22. Handin R: Bleeding and thrombosis. In Wilson JD, Braunwald E, Isselbacher KJ, editors: *Harrison's principles of internal medicine*, New York, 1991, McGraw-Hill.

23. Philstrom B: Prevention and treatment of dilantin-associated gingival enlargement, *Compendium* 14(suppl):5506-5510, 1990.

24. Rzany B et al: Risk of Stevens-Johnson syndrome and toxic epidermal necrolysis during first weeks of antiepileptic therapy: a case-control study. Study Group of the International Case Control Study on Severe Cutaneous Adverse Reactions, *Lancet* 353:2190-2194, 1999.

25. Hoyert D, Kochanek K, Murphy S: Deaths: final data for 1997. In *National vital statistics reports*, US Department of Health and Human Services, CDC, National Center for Health Statistics: Hyattsville, 1999, Maryland.

26. American Heart Association: *2001 Heart and Stroke Statistical Update*, 2000, Dallas, American Heart Association. http://www.americanheart.org/statistics/pdf/HSSTATS2001_1.0.pdf.

27. Rosamond WD et al: Stroke incidence and survival among middle-aged adults: 9-year follow-up of the atherosclerosis risk in communities (ARIC) cohort, *Stroke* 30:736-743, 1999.

28. Centers for Disease Control and Prevention: Age-specific excess deaths associated with stroke among racial/ethnic minority populations—United States, 1997, *MMWR* 49(5):94-97, 2000.

29. Toole J: Vascular diseases. In Rowland L, editor: *Merritt's textbook of neurology*, Philadelphia, 1989, Lea & Febiger.

30. Gillman MW et al: Inverse association of dietary fat with development of ischemic stroke in men, *JAMA* 278:2145-2150, 1997.

31. Bostom AG et al: Nonfasting plasma total homocysteine levels and stroke incidence in elderly persons: the Framingham Study, *Ann Intern Med* 131:352-355, 1999.

32. Wu T et al: Periodontal disease and risk of cerebrovascular disease: the first national health and nutrition examination survey and its follow-up study, *Arch Intern Med* 160:2749-2755, 2000.

33. Kernan WN et al: Phenylpropanolamine and the risk of hemorrhagic stroke, *N Engl J Med* 343:1826-1832, 2000.

34. Abramowicz M, editor: *Phenylpropanolamine and other* OTC *alpha-adrenergic agonists*, Vol. 42. New Rochelle, NY, 2000, The Medical Letter, Inc.

35. Gillman MW et al: Protective effect of fruits and vegetables on development of stroke in men, *JAMA* 273:1113-1117, 1995.

36. Kiely D et al: Physical activity and stroke risk: the Framingham Study, *Am J Epidemiol* 140:608-620, 1994.

37. Markesbery W: The central nervous system. In Golden A et al, editors: *Pathology. Understanding human disease*, Baltimore, 1985, Williams & Wilkins.

38. Li Y et al: Temporal profile of in situ DNA fragmentation after transient middle cerebral artery occlusion in the rat, *J Cereb Blood Flow Metab* 15:389-397, 1995.

39. Ostuni E: Stroke and the dental patient, *J Am Dent Assoc* 125:721-727, 1994.

40. Wolf PA et al: Probability of stroke: a risk profile from the Framingham Study, *Stroke* 22:312-318, 1991.

41. Kase CS et al: Intellectual decline after stroke: the Framingham Study, *Stroke* 29:805-812, 1998.

42. Kistler J, Ropper A, Martin J: Cerebrovascular diseases. In Wilson JD, Braunwald, E, Isselbacher KJ, editors: *Harrison's principles of internal medicine*, New York, 1991, McGraw-Hill.

43. Furlan A et al: Intraarterial prourokinase for acute ischemic stroke. The PROACT II study: a randomized controlled trial. Prolyse in acute cerebral thromboembolism, *JAMA* 282:2003-2011, 1999.

44. The National Institute of Neurological Disorders and Stroke rt-PA Stroke Study Group: Tissue plasminogen activator for acute ischemic stroke. *N Engl J Med* 333:1581-1587, 1995.

45. Caplan L: Tissue plasminogen activator for acute ischemic stroke, *N Engl J Med* 341:1240-1241, 1999.

46. Albers GW et al: Intravenous tissue-type plasminogen activator for treatment of acute stroke: the Standard Treatment with Activase to Reverse Stroke (STARS) Study, *JAMA*, 283:1145-1150, 2000.

47. Fisher M, Schaebitz W: An overview of acute stroke therapy: past, present, and future, *Arch Int Med* 160:3196-3120, 2000.

48. Feigin VL et al: Calcium antagonists in patients with aneurysmal subarachnoid hemorrhage: a systematic review, *Neurology* 50:876-883, 1998.

49. Sacks FM et al: The effect of pravastatin on coronary events after myocardial infarction in patients with average cholesterol levels, *N Engl J Med* 335:1001-1009, 1996.

50. Stalenhoef A: Scandinavian Simvastatin Study (4S). *Lancet* 344:1766-1767, 1994.

51. Wahl M: Myths of dental surgery in patients receiving anticoagulant therapy, *J Am Dent Assoc* 131:77-81, 2000.

52. Niwa H, Satoh Y, Matsuura H: Cardiovascular responses to epinephrine-containing local anesthetics for dental use: a comparison of hemodynamic responses to infiltration anesthesia and ergometer-stress testing, *Oral Surg Oral Med Oral Pathol Oral Radiol Endod* 90:171-181, 2000.

53. Furlan AJ et al: PROACT II: recombinant prourokinase (r-ProUK) in acute cerebral thromboembolism initial trial result, *Stroke* 30:234, 1999.

54. Friedlander A, Maeder L: The prevalence of calcified carotid artery atheromas on the panoramic radiographs of patients with type 2 diabetes mellitus, *Oral Surg Oral Med Oral Pathol Oral Radiol Endod* 89:420-424, 2000.

55. Friedlander A, Baker J: Panoramic radiography: an aid in detecting patients at risk of cerebrovascular accident, *J Am Dent Assoc* 125:1598-1603, 1994.

56. Friedlander A, Friedlander I: Identification of stroke prone patients by panoramic radiography, *Aust Dent J* 43:51-54, 1998.

57. Carter LC et al: Use of panoramic radiography among an ambulatory dental population to detect patients at risk of stroke, *J Am Dent Assoc* 128:977-984, 1997.

58. Parkinson J: *An Essay on Shaking Palsy*, 1817, London: Sherwood Neely and Jones.

59. Jankovic J: Parkinsonism. In Goldman L, Bennett JC, editors: *Cecil textbook of medicine*, Philadelphia, 2000, WB Saunders.

60. Biziere K, Kurth M: *Living with Parkinson's disease*, New York, 1997, Demos Vermande.

61. Tanner C, Ben-Shlomo Y: Epidemiology of Parkinson's disease, *Adv Neurol* 30:153-159, 1999.

62. Polymeropoulos MH et al: Mutation in the alpha-synuclein gene identified in families with Parkinson's disease, *Science* (276)2045-2047, 1997.

63. Hughes A et al: Accuracy of clinical diagnosis of idiopathic Parkinson's disease: a clinico-pathological study of 100 cases, *J Neurol Neurosurg Psychiatry* 55:181-184, 1992.

64. Braak H, Braak E: Pathoanatomy of Parkinson's disease, *J Neurol* 247(Suppl 2):II3-110, 2000.

65. Alexi T et al: Neuroprotective strategies for basal ganglia degeneration: Parkinson's and Huntington's diseases, *Prog Neurobiol* 60:409-470, 1999.

66. Marsh L: Neuropsychiatric aspects of Parkinson's disease, *Psychosomatics* 41:15-23, 2000.

67. Wolters E: Dopaminomimetic psychosis in Parkinson's disease patients, *Neurology* 52(suppl 3):S10-S13, 1999.

68. Ahlskog J: Treatment of motor complications in advancing Parkinson's disease: which drugs and when? *Formulary* 35:654-668, 2000.

69. Trosch RM et al: Clozapine use in Parkinson's disease: a retrospective analysis, *Mov Disord* 13:377-382, 1998.

70. Perlow MJ et al: Brain grafts reduce motor abnormalities produced by destruction of nigrostriatal dopamine system, *Science* 204:643-647, 1979.

71. Hallett M, Litvan I: Evaluation of surgery for Parkinson's disease: a report of the Therapeutics and Technology Assessment Subcommittee of the American Academy of Neurology. The Task Force on Surgery for Parkinson's Disease, *Neurology* 53:1910-1921, 1999.

72. Kordower JH, Emborg ME, Bloch J, et al: Neurodegeneration prevented by lentiviral vector delivery of GDNF in primate models of Parkinson's disease, *Science* 290:767-773, 2000.

73. Ebers G, Sadovnick A: The geographic distribution of multiple sclerosis: a review, *Neuroepidemiol* 12:1-5, 1993.

74. Kurtzke J: Epidemiology of MS. In Hallpike JF, Adams CWM, Tourtellote WE, editors: *Multiple Sclerosis*, Baltimore, 1983, Williams & Wilkins.

75. Rudick R: Multiple sclerosis and related conditions. In Goldman L, editor: *Cecil Textbook of Medicine*, Philadelphia, 2000, WB Saunders.

76. Olek M: Multiple sclerosis–part I. Overview, pathophysiology, diagnostic evaluation, and clinical parameters, *J Am Osteopath Assoc* 99:574-588, 1999.

77. Sriram S et al: Chlamydia pneumoniae infection of the central nervous system in multiple sclerosis, *Ann Neurol* 46:6-14, 1999.

78. Carrigan D, Harrington D, Knox K: Subacute leukoencephalitis caused by CNS infection with human herpesvirus-6 manifesting as acute multiple sclerosis, *Neurology* 47:145-148, 1996.

79. Knox K et al: Human herpesvirus 6 and multiple sclerosis: systemic active infections in patients with early disease, *Clin Infect Dis* 31:894-903, 2000.

80. Ebers GC et al: A population based study of multiple sclerosis in twins, *N Engl J Med* (315)1638-1642, 1986.

81. Ebers GC, Sadovnick AD, Risch NJ: A genetic basis for familial aggregation in multiple sclerosis, *Nature* 377:150-151, 1995.

82. Altmann D, Sansom D, Marsh S: What is the basis for HLA-DQ associations with autoimmune disease? *Immunol Today* 12:267-270, 1991.

83. Steinman L: Multiple sclerosis: a coordinated immunological attack against myelin in the central nervous system, *Cell* 85:299-302, 1996.

84. Weinshenker BG et al: The natural history of multiple sclerosis: a geographically based study. I. Clinical course and disability, *Brain* 112:133-146, 1989.

85. National Center for Health Statistics: *Vital statistics of the U.S. 1992-Mortality*, Washington, DC, 1996, United States Department of Health and Human Services, US Government Printing Office.

86. Noseworthy JH et al: Multiple sclerosis, *N Engl J Med* 343:938-952, 2000.

87. Fan-Havard P, Nahata M: Treatment and prevention of infections of cerebrospinal fluid shunts, *Clin Pharm* 6:866- 880, 1987.

88. Fernell E et al: Ventriculoatrial or ventriculoperitoneal shunts in the treatment of hydrocephalus in children, *Z Kinderchir* 40:12-14, 1985.

89. Gardner P, Leipzig T, Sadigh M: Infections of mechanical cerebrospinal fluid shunts, *Curr Clin Top Infect Dis* 9:185-214, 1989.

90. Sugarman B, Young E: Infections associated with prosthetic devices: magnitude of the problem, *Infect Dis Clin North Am* 3:187-198, 1989.

91. Drucker MH et al: Thromboembolic complications of ventriculoatrial shunts, *Surg Neurol* 22:444-448, 1984.

92. Aoki N: Lumboperitoneal shunt: clinical applications, complications and comparison with ventriculoperitoneal shunt, *Neurosurgery* 26:998-1003, 1990.

93. Segreti J, Levin S: The role of prophylactic antibiotics in the prevention of prosthetic device infections, *Infect Dis Clin North Am* 3:357-371, 1989.

94. Dajani AS, Taubert KA, Wilson W: Prevention of bacterial endocarditis: recommendations by the American Heart Association, *Clin Infect Dis* 25:1448-1458, 1997.

Behavioral and Psychiatric Disorders

23
CHAPTER

$\mathcal{P}$roblems may be encountered in dental practice that stem from a patient's behavioral patterns rather than from physical conditions. A good dentist-patient relationship can reduce the number of behavioral problems encountered in practice and modify the intensity of emotional reactions. A positive dentist-patient relationship is based on mutual respect, trust, understanding, cooperation, and empathy. Role conflicts between the dentist and the patient should be avoided or identified and dealt with effectively. The anxious patient should be offered support that minimizes the damaging effects of anxiety, and the angry or uncooperative patient should be accepted and encouraged to share reasons for feelings and behavior, thus becoming a more peaceful and cooperative individual. Patients with emotional factors that contribute to oral or systemic diseases or symptoms and patients with more serious mental disorders can be managed in an understanding, safe, and empathetic manner.

The dentist may see patients with a variety of behavioral and mental disorders. The fourth edition of *Diagnostic and Statistical Manual of Mental Disorders*[1] (DSM-IV) and the fourth edition of *Diagnostic and Statistical Manual of Mental Disorders, Text Revision* (DSM-IV-TR) presents a classification system with which the dentist should be familiar to be better able to understand psychiatric diagnoses and associated symptoms. This system consists of five axes (axis I through axis V), or categories, used to describe mental disorders. Table 23-1 lists the five specific areas used to evaluate a patient's psychosocial health. Box 23-1 lists the clinical conditions encountered in axis I disorder.[1,2]

Mental disorders are common in today's society. Approximately one third of the population in the United States will have at least one psychiatric disorder during their lifetime, and 20% to 30% of adults in the United States will suffer from one or more psychiatric disorders during a 1-year period. About 10% of the adult population has a serious drug abuse or dependency problem; 6% to 10% of the population suffers from serious affective or mood disorders. Anxiety disorders are found in about 13%. Schizophrenic disorders are found in 1.1%, and severe cognitive disorders are found in about 3% of the population.[3-8]

Psychiatric problems impact the course and outcome of patients with various medical illnesses. Psychiatric problems increase length of treatment, decrease the functional level of the patient, and have a negative impact on overall prognosis and outcome. Disorders secondary to smoking, drinking, and drug use account for a significant portion of the health care dollar. The elderly population has a high prevalence of psychiatric complications associated with medical illnesses. About 15% to 20% suffer from depressive symptoms. Between 10% and 20% suffer from anxiety disorders, including phobias. Phobia is the most common psychiatric disorder in women over the age of 65 years. Approximately 20% of the elderly have a substance abuse disorder.[3]

The identification and management of patients with anxiety, depression, and mental illness outlined in Box 23-2 are considered. Then the drugs used to treat psychiatric disorders and their significant drug interactions and side effects are discussed as a separate heading. The *Dental Management* section includes short presentations on patients' attitude toward the dentist, psychological significance of the oral cavity, and behavioral reactions to illness.

■ ANXIETY DISORDERS ■

DEFINITION

Anxiety is a sense of psychological distress that may not have a focus. It is a state of apprehension that may involve an internal psychological conflict, an environmental

TABLE 23-1

System for Classification of Psychosocial Health

Type	Description
Axis I	Clinical disorders
	Other conditions that may be a focus of clinical attention
Axis II	Personality disorders
	Mental retardation
Axis III	General medical conditions
Axis IV	Psychosocial and environmental problems
Axis V	Global assessment of functioning

From American Psychiatric Association: *Diagnostic and statistical manual of mental disorders*, ed 4, Text Revision, Washington DC, 2000, American Psychiatric Association, p 27.

BOX 23-1

Axis I—Clinical Disorders, Other Conditions That May Be a Focus of Clinical Attention

Disorders usually first diagnosed in infancy, childhood, or adolescence
Delirium, dementia, and amnestic and other cognitive disorders
Mental disorders caused by a general medical condition
Substance-related disorders
Schizophrenia and other psychotic disorders
Mood disorders
Anxiety disorders
Somatoform disorders
Factitious disorders
Dissociative disorders
Sexual and gender identity disorders
Eating disorders
Sleep disorders
Psychological factors affecting medical conditions
Impulse-control disorders not elsewhere classified
Adjustment disorders
Other conditions that may be a focus of clinical attention

From American Psychiatric Association: *Diagnostic and statistical manual of mental disorders*, ed 4, Text Revision, Washington, DC, 2000, American Psychiatric Association, p 28.

stress, a physical disease state, a medicine or drug effect, or combinations of these. Anxiety can be purely a psychological experience with few somatic manifestations. In contrast it can present as purely a physical experience with tachycardia, palpitations, chest pain, indigestion, headaches, and so on, with no psychological distress other than concern about the physical symptoms. Why some individuals experience anxiety in a psychological way and others in a physical way is not clear.[6]

EPIDEMIOLOGY: INCIDENCE AND PREVALENCE

Anxiety disorders constitute the most frequently found psychiatric problem in the general population. Simple phobia is the most common of the anxiety disorders; however, panic disorder is the most common anxiety disorder in people seeking medical treatment. About 9% of persons experience at least one panic attack during their lives and about 3% have recurrent panic attacks.[6]

A *phobia* is defined as an irrational fear that interferes with normal behavior. Phobias are fears of specific objects, situations, or experiences. The feared object, situation, or experience has taken on a symbolic meaning for the patient. Both unconscious wishes and fears have been displaced from an original goal onto an external object.[6]

A *panic disorder* consists of the sudden, unexpected, overwhelming feeling of terror with symptoms of dyspnea, palpitations, dizziness, faintness, trembling, sweating, choking, flushes or chills, numbness or tingling sensations, and chest pains. The panic attack peaks in about 10 minutes and usually lasts for about 20 to 30 minutes.

Panic disorder, phobic disorders, and obsessive-compulsive disorders occur more frequently among first-degree relatives of people with these disorders than among the general population.[6,9] The prevalence of panic disorder in cardiac patients is about 9%. Generalized anxiety disorder has a community prevalence of 2.5% to 5%.[3]

ETIOLOGY

Anxiety represents a threatened emergence into consciousness of painful, unacceptable thoughts, impulses, or desires (anxiety may result from psychologic conflicts of the past and present). These psychologic conflicts or feelings stimulate physiologic changes that lead to clinical manifestations of anxiety.[6,10] Anxiety disorders may occur in persons under emotional stress, in those with certain systemic illnesses, or as a component of various psychiatric disorders. Panic disorders tend to be found in families. If one first-degree relative has a panic disor-

BOX 23-2

Classification of Behavioral and Psychiatric Disorders

Category	Specifics
Anxiety disorders	Panic disorders
	Agoraphobia
	Phobias
	Obsessive-compulsive disorder*
	Posttraumatic stress disorder
	Acute stress disorder
	Generalized anxiety disorder
	Anxiety disorder caused by a general medical condition
	Substance-induced anxiety disorder
Mood disorders	Depressive disorders
	Major depression
	Dysthymic disorder
	Depression not otherwise specified
	Bipoiar disorders
	Bipolar I–manic, mixed, depressed
	Bipolar II–hypomanic, depressed
	Cyclothymic disorder
	Bipolar not otherwise specified
Somatoform disorders	Body dysmorphic disorder*
	Conversion disorder
	Hypochondriasis
	Somatization disorder
	Pain disorder
Factitious disorders*	Predominantly psychological signs and symptoms
	Predominantly physical signs and symptoms
	Combined psychological and physical signs and symptoms
Psychologic factors affecting medical conditions*	Mental disorder affecting medical condition
	Stress-related physiological response affecting medical condition
Substance abuse disorders	Alcohol and other sedatives (barbiturates, benzodiazepines, and others)
	Opiates
	Stimulants (Amphetamine, cocaine)
	Cannabis
	Hallucinogens (LSD, PCP)
	Nicotine
	Others (steroids; inhalants such as paint, glue, gasoline)
Eating disorders	Anorexia nervosa, bulimia nervosa, eating disorders not otherwise specified

*Conditions not covered in this chapter.
From American Psychiatric Association: *Diagnostic and statistical manual of mental disorders,* ed 4, Text Revision, Washington DC, 2000, American Psychiatric Association; and Reus, VI: In Wilson JD et al, editors: *Harrison's principles of internal medicine,* ed 14, New York, 1998, McGraw-Hill, pp 2485-2502. *Continued*

BOX 23-2

Classification of Behavioral and Psychiatric Disorders——cont'd

Category	Specifics
Cognitive disorders	Delirium
	Dementia
	Primary (Alzheimer's type)
	Vascular
	HIV
	Parkinson's disease
	Amnestic disorder
Schizophrenia	Catatonic type
	Disorganized type
	Paranoid type
	Undifferentiated type
Delusional (paranoid) disorder*	Erotomania grandiosity, jealousy, persecution complex, somatic delusions

*Conditions not covered in this chapter.
From American Psychiatric Association: *Diagnostic and statistical manual of mental disorders*, ed 4, Text Revision, Washington DC, 2000, American Psychiatric Association; and Reus, VI: In Wilson JD et al, editors: *Harrison's principles of internal medicine*, ed 14, New York, 1998, McGraw-Hill, pp 2485-2502.

der, other relatives have about an 18% chance of developing a panic disorder.[6,10]

No single theory fully explains all anxiety disorders. No single biologic or psychologic cause of anxiety exists. Psychosocial and biological processes together may best explain anxiety. The locus coeruleus, a brain stem structure that contains the majority of noradrenergic neurons in the central nervous system (CNS) appears to be involved in panic attacks and anxiety. Panic and anxiety may be correlated with the dysregulated firing of the locus coeruleus caused by input from multiple sources, including peripheral autonomic afferents, medullary afferents, and serotonergic fibers.[6]

Other neurobiologic theories to explain panic attacks and anxiety involve lactate infusion, benzodiazepine receptors, the amygdala, and synaptic responses in the brain. Lactate infusion causes peripheral somatic sensations resembling those in natural panic attacks. Dysfunction of the benzodiazepine receptor may be responsible for some components of anxiety. The amygdala is a brain structure that influences fear, vigilance, and rage. Some think the amygdala plays a role in anxiety by interaction with various hypothalamic and brain stem structures.[6]

Another theory for anxiety states that stressors induce protein c-fos, a class of immediate early proteins that act early in the neural process, which through cascades may induce long-lasting biochemical and neurobiologic changes.[6]

Anxiety states also may be associated with organic diseases, other psychiatric disorders, use of certain drugs, hyperthyroidism and mitral valve prolapse. Anxiety also is associated with mood disorders, schizophrenia, or personality disorders.[3,6,8,10]

CLINICAL PRESENTATION AND MEDICAL MANAGEMENT

From a psychological aspect, anxiety can be defined as emotional pain or a feeling that all is not well—a feeling of impending disaster. The source of the problem usually is not apparent to the person with anxiety. The feeling is the same as that of patients with fear, but they are aware of what the problem is and why they are "fearful."

The physiologic reaction to anxiety and fear is the same and is mediated through the autonomic nervous system. Both sympathetic and parasympathetic components may be involved. Symptoms of anxiety caused by overactivation of the sympathetic nervous system include increased heart rate, sweating, dilated pupils, and muscle tension. Symptoms of anxiety resulting from stimulation of the parasympathetic system include urination and diarrhea.

Most individuals experience some anxiety. Anxiety can be a strong motivator; low levels of anxiety can increase attention and improve performance. Anxiety leads to dysfunction when it is constant or results in episodes of extreme vigilance, excessive motor tension, autonomic hyperactivity, and impaired concentration. Anxiety is part of the clinical picture in many patients with psychiatric disorders. Patients with mood disorders, dementia, psychosis, panic disorder, adjustment disorders, and toxic and withdrawal states often complain of anxiety.[6]

Phobias

Phobias consist of three major groups: agoraphobia, social, and simple. Agoraphobia is a fear of having distressful or embarrassing symptoms if one leaves home. It often accompanies panic disorder. Social phobias may be specific, such as fear of public speaking or as general as fear of being embarrassed when with people. Simple phobias include fear of snakes, heights, flying, darkness and needles. The two phobias that can affect medical or dental care are needle phobia and claustrophobia during magnetic resonance imaging (MRI) or radiation therapy.[3,6,10]

Panic Attack

About 15% of patients seen by cardiologists come to the doctor because of symptoms associated with a panic attack. The onset is usually between late adolescence and the mid 30s but may occur at any age. A key feature of panic is the adrenergic surge, which results in the fight or flight response. This response is an exaggerated sympathetic response. Panic attacks may be cued or uncued. An example of a cued attack would be the individual who is fearful of flying. Many patients report that they are unaware of any life stressors preceding the onset of panic disorder. These attacks would be classified as uncued. The major complication of repeated panic attacks is a restricted lifestyle adopted to avoid situations that might trigger an attack. Some patients develop agoraphobia, an irrational fear of being alone in public places, which can lead to being housebound for years. Sudden loss of social supports or disruption of important interpersonal relationships appears to predispose an individual to development of panic disorder.[6,9,10]

Generalized Anxiety Disorder

Some patients develop a persistent diffuse form of anxiety with symptoms of motor tension, autonomic hyperactivity, and apprehension. No familial or genetic basis for the disorder exists. It has a better outcome than panic disorder; however, it can lead to depression and substance abuse.[6,9,10]

Posttraumatic Stress Disorder

Posttraumatic stress disorder (PTSD) is a syndrome of psychophysiologic signs and symptoms that come after exposure to a traumatic event outside the usual range of human experience, such as combat exposure, a holocaust experience, rape, or a civilian disaster (e.g., a hurricane).[6] Most men with PTSD have been in combat and most women give a history of sexual or physical abuse. The three cardinal features of PTSD are hyperarousal; intrusive symptoms, or flashbacks of the initial trauma; and psychic numbing.[6] PTSD may appear after traumatic events that are anticipated or not anticipated, constant or repetitive, natural or malevolent. PTSD occurs when the onset of symptoms occurs at least 6 months after the trauma or the disorder has a duration longer than 3 months. The traumatic event is outside the range of usual human experience. It may be a serious threat to one's life or physical integrity; serious threat to one's children, spouse, or other loved ones; sudden destruction of one's home or community; or the result of having seen an accident or physical violence that seriously injures or kills another person(s).[9]

The diagnostic criteria for PTSD are a history of traumatic experience and the reexperience of the event by intrusive memories, disturbing dreams, "flashbacks," and psychologic or physical distress as result of the reminders of the event, in addition to the avoidance of things associated with the trauma. Symptoms include sleep problems, irritability, trouble concentrating, hypervigilance, startle responses, and psychic numbing consisting of detachment from others, reduced capacity for intimacy, and decreased interest in sex.[3,6,10]

Acute Stress Disorder

This is a new DSM-IV category of anxiety disorder. A patient with this disorder has been exposed to a traumatic event and has specific signs and symptoms resembling those of PTSD. In acute stress disorder the symptoms are of shorter duration and their onset occurs more rapidly after the trauma. The symptomatic reaction is limited to the time that the stressful event is occurring and its immediate aftermath.[6,9]

Treatment of Anxiety Disorders

Psychologic, behavioral and drug modalities are used to treat anxiety disorders. Psychologic treatment involves psychotherapy, which in general is used in the more severe cases. Behavioral treatment includes cognitive, biofeedback, hypnosis, relaxation imaging, desensitization and flooding. Drug treatment includes the use of tricyclic antidepressants, selective serotonin reuptake inhibitors, monoamine oxidase inhibitors, benzodiazepines, and beta-adrenoreceptor antagonists. The most commonly used drugs are the benzodiazepines (Table 23-2).[3,6,10]

TABLE 23-2

Commonly Used Benzodiazepines

	Range for Daily Oral Dose (mg)	Half-life (hr)
Anxiolytics		
Chlordiazepoxide (Librium)*	20 to 100	7 to 23
Diazepam (Valium)*	5 to 40	20 to 90
Lorazepam (Ativan)†	1 to 10	10 to 12
Oxazepam (Serax)†	30 to 120	3 to 20
Aiprazolam (Xanax)†	0.75 to 10.0	12 to 15
Sedative-hypnotics		
Flurazepam (Dalmane)‡	15 to 30	24 to 100
Temazepam (Restoril)‡	30	8 to 10
Trizolam (Halcion)‡	0.125 to 0.5	2 to 3

From Judd LL; In Wilson JD et al, editors: *Harrison's principles of internal medicine*, New York, 1991, McGraw-Hill, p 2139-2154.
*Prescribed in a daily or twice-daily regimen—diazepam, chlordiazepoxide.
†Prescribed in a three or four times daily regimen—lorazepam, oxazepam, aiprazolam (short acting).
‡Prescribed in a daily or bedtime regimen—flurazepam, temazepam, triazolam (long acting).

Systemic desensitization (patient is gradually exposed to the feared situation) and flooding (the patient is exposed directly to the anxiety provoking stimulus) are used in the treatment of phobias. Claustrophobia associated with MRI can be managed with a low dose of benzodiazepines and behavioral therapy. No drug has been shown to be widely effective in the treatment of PTSD. Phenelzine has been shown to be more effective for symptoms of nightmares and flashbacks. Early intervention in patients with PTSD can shorten the duration and severity of anxiety.[3,6,10]

■ MOOD DISORDERS ■

DEFINITION

Mood disorders represent a heterogeneous group of mental disorders characterized by extreme exaggeration and disturbance of mood and affect. These dis-orders have associated physiologic, cognitive, and psychomotor dysfunctions. Mood disorders tend to be cyclic. They include depression and bipolar disorder.[10-12]

EPIDEMIOLOGY: INCIDENCE AND PREVALENCE

About 5% of the adults in the United States have a significant mood disorder. Mood disorders are more common among women (Table 23-3). Major depression may begin at any age and is evenly distributed throughout adult life. Between 20% and 25% of adult women and 7% to 12% of adult men at some time experience a major depressive episode. About one third of these individuals require hospitalization, and 30% develop a chronic course with residual symptoms and social impairment.[4,13] The lifetime prevalence of dysthymia, a chronic, milder form of depression, is 2.2% in women and 4.1% in men.[4] Approximately 0.4% to 1.6% of adults in the United States have bipolar disorder.[4] In contrast to major depression, that is more than twice as common in females as in males, bipolar disorder occurs with equal frequency between both sexes.[8]

ETIOLOGY

Several theories have been presented to explain the etiology of mood disorders. Decreased brain concentrations of norepinephrine and serotonin, neurotransmitters, for some time have been thought to cause depression. Increased levels of these neurotransmitters have been related to the cause of mania. The etiology of depression and mania now appear to be more complex. Current research focuses on the interactions of norepinephrine and serotonin with a variety of other brain systems and on abnormalities in the function or quantity of receptors for the transmitters.[4] Thyrotropin release of thyroid-stimulating hormone and cortisol release by corticotropin-releasing factor and adrenocorticotropin over a chronic period of time may be involved with the development of depression. This model suggests that depression is the result of a stress reaction that has gone on too long.[4]

Genetic studies using epidemiologic samples have shown that recurrent affective disorders tend to cluster in families. Relatives of patients with affective disorders are two to three times more likely to be ill than persons in the general population. The genetic influence is greater with bipolar disorders than with unipolar depression. Studies of identical and fraternal twins show marked genetic links for mood disorders. Adoption studies also show a trend for mood disorders in adoptees to

TABLE **23-3**

Epidemiology of Mood Disorders

Variable	Depressive Disorders	Bipolar Disorders

Prevalence	Major depression point
	    Men: 2.3 % to 3.2%
	    Women: 4.5% to 9.3%
	Lifetime
	    Men: 7.0% to 12.0%
	    Women: 20% to 25%
	More common in divorced or separated individuals
	Dysthymia
	    Lifetime:
	        Men: 4. 1%
	        Women: 2.2%
		Bipolar I lifetime: 0.4 % to 1.6%
		
		Bipolar II lifetime: 0.5%
		
		More common in upper socio eco-
		    nomic classes
		Equal in sex and race
		High rates of divorce
		
		Cyclothymia lifetime: 0.4% to 1.0%

Age of onset	Late 20s or 30s Childhood possible May have much later onset Higher rate and earlier onset For individuals born after 1940 than those born before	Late teens or early 20s Childhood possible Cyclothymia may precede late onset of overt mania or depression

Family and genetic studies	Unipolar patients tend to have relatives with major depression
	    and dysthymic disorders and fewer with bipolar disorders
	Early onset, recurrent course, and psychotic depression
	    appear to be heritable
		Bipolar patients have many relatives
		    with bipolar disorder, cyclothymia,
		    unipolar depression, and schizoaf-
		    fective disorder

Twin studies	Concordance in monozygotic twins:
	    Recurrent depression 59%
	    Single episode only 33%
	Concordance rates for identical (monozygotic) twins is
	    4 times greater than found in fraternal (dizygotic) twins
		Concordance in monozygotic twins:
		    65% to 80%

From Kahn DA: Mood disorders. In *Saunders review series: Psychiatry*, Philadelphia, 1999, WB Saunders.

be related to their biologic parents rather than their adopted parents.[4,10]

Psychosocial theory focuses on loss as the cause of depression in vulnerable individuals. Mania receives much less attention because it is thought to be more of a biologically caused disorder. The psychoanalytical hypothesis suggests that unconscious mental conflicts and incomplete psychological development are important factors in the cause of some mental disorders, including depression. The interpersonal hypothesis states that social losses in a patient's current life contribute to depression and improved interpersonal relations may reduce or eliminate the depression. The cognitive hypothesis proposes that depression results from distorted thinking, which leads to unrealistically pessimistic and negative views of oneself and the world.[4]

CLINICAL PRESENTATION AND MEDICAL MANAGEMENT

Depressive Disorders

The DSM-IV lists three types of depressive disorders; major depression, dysthymic disorder, and depression not otherwise specified (NOS). Major depression (unipolar) is one of the main mood disorders. Patients with major depression are depressed most of the day, show a marked decrease in interest or pleasure in most activities, have a marked gain or loss in weight, and manifest insomnia or hypersomnia. These symptoms must be present for at least 2 weeks for a diagnosis of major depression. About 50% to 80% of individuals who have had a major depressive episode will have at least one more depressive episode; 20% of the individuals will have a

subsequent manic episode and should be reclassified as bipolar. A major depression usually will last about 8 to 9 months if the individual is not treated. Dysthymia represents a chronic, milder, form of depression with symptoms lasting at least 2 years. Depression NOS is a form of depression that falls short of the diagnostic criteria for major depression and has been to brief for dysthymic disorder.[4,10,14]

Bipolar Disorder

The DSM-IV lists four types of bipolar disorders: bipolar I, bipolar II, cyclothymic, and bipolar disorder NOS. Bipolar I disorder consists of recurrences of mania and major depression or mixed states that occur at different times in the patient or a mixture of symptoms occurring at the same time. The essential feature of a manic episode is a distinct period during which the person's mood is either elevated and expansive or irritable. Associated symptoms of the manic syndrome include inflated self-esteem, grandiosity, decreased need for sleep, excessive speech, flight of ideas, distractibility, psychomotor agitation, and excessive involvement in pleasurable activities. During a manic episode, the mood often is described as euphoric, cheerful, or "high." The expansive quality of the mood is characterized by unceasing and unselective enthusiasm for interacting with people. However, the predominant mood disturbance may be irritability and anger. The speech often is loud, rapid, and difficult to interpret. Behavior may be intrusive and demanding. The style of dress is often colorful and strange. Long periods without sleep are common. Poor judgment may lead to financial and legal problems. Drug and alcohol abuse often is seen.[4,10,14]

Bipolar II disorder consists of recurrences of major depression and hypomania (mild mania). Cyclothymic disorder consists of recurrent brief episodes of hypomania and mild depression. Bipolar disorder NOS is used to describe partial syndromes, such as recurrent hypomania without depression. Patients with bipolar disorders have at least 1 episode of mania or hypomania.[4,14]

The diagnosis of bipolar disorder is made as soon as a patient has one manic episode, even if that person has never had a depressive episode. Most patients who become manic will eventually experience depression. However, about 10% of patients diagnosed with bipolar disorder appear to have only manic episodes.[4]

Men tend to have more manic episodes and women more depressive episodes. Untreated individuals with bipolar disorder will have a mean of 9 affective episodes during their lifetime. Each cycle's length tends to decrease, although the number of cycles increases with age. Each affective episode lasts about 8 to 9 months. Bipolar patients have more episodes,

hospitalizations, divorces, and suicides than unipolar patients.[10]

Treatment of Mood Disorders

Table 23-4 shows the commonly used antidepressants. These agents are used to treat major depression, dysthymic disorder, and depression NOS and depression associated with bipolar disorder. Drug therapy is essential in bipolar disorder to achieve two goals: rapid control of symptoms in acute episodes of mania and depression, and prevention of future episodes or reduction of their severity and frequency. Mood disorders have a tendency

TABLE 23-4

Commonly Used Antidepressants

Drug	Daily Oral Dose (mg)
First-Generation Antidepressants	
Tricyclic derivatives	
Amitriptyline (Elavil)	150 to 300
Nortrptyline (Pamelor)	50 to 150
Imipramine (Tofranil)	150 to 300
Desipramine (Norpamin)	150 to 250
Doxepin (Sinequan)	150 to 300
Monoamine oxidase inhibitors	
Pheneizine (Mardil)	15 to 60
Tranylcypromine (Parnate)	20 to 30
Isocarboxazid (Marplan)	10 to 30
Second-Generation Antidepressants	
Heterocylic derivatives	
Clomipramine (Anaframil)	150 to 300
Ainoxapine (Asendin)	150 to 300
Maproliline (Ludiomil)	100 to 225
Selective serotonin reuptake inhibitors	
Fluoxetine (Prozac)	10 to 40
Paroxetine (Paxil)	10 to 40
Seitraline (Zoloft)	50 to 200
Serontonin and noradrenergic reuptake inhibitors	
Nefazodone (Serzimc)	300 to 600
Venlafaxine (Effexor)	75 to 375
Derivatives of other chemical classes	
Bupropion (Welibutrin)	200 to 300
Trazodone (Desyrel)	100 to 600

From Judd LL: In Wilson JD et al, editors: *Harrison's principles of internal medicine,* New York, 1994, McGraw-Hill, pp 2139-2154 and 2400-2419.

to recur. Affective episodes may occur spontaneously or be triggered by adverse events. Individuals with mood disorders and their families need to become aware of the early signs and symptoms of affective episodes so that treatment can be initiated. These individuals also must be aware of the need for medication compliance and be aware of the medication's side effects and possible complications.[10,11]

The mainstays of drug therapy are the mood-stabilizing drugs that generally act on both mania and depression. The three drugs used are lithium, valproate, and carbamazepine. The most widely used mood stabilizer is lithium carbonate. Lithium is most helpful in patients with euphoric mania. When lithium is ineffective or when medical problems prevent its use, the anticonvulsants valproate or carbamazepine are used. Electoconvulsive therapy is an effective antimanic treatment. It may be used in cases of manic violence, delirium, or exhaustion. It is also appropriate for use with patients who do not respond to medication taken for many weeks. When antidepressant drugs are given for bipolar depression, they can cause a switch to mania or a mixed state or may induce rapid cycling. The most common treatment for bipolar depression is an antidepressant combined with a mood stabilizer to prevent a manic switch or rapid cycling.[4]

Lithium takes about 7 to 10 days to reach full therapeutic effectiveness. Most of the antidepressant drugs have a delay (10 to 21 days) before full therapeutic benefits are achieved.[10,11]

Patients who have had two or three episodes of bipolar disorder, including depressive episodes, usually are treated indefinitely because of the near certainty of relapse. Prevention targets both manic and depressive episodes. Lithium is the treatment of choice. About one third of the patients will not have any further episodes and are considered cured. Another one third of the patients taking lithium will have less frequent or less severe episodes and function quite well. The remaining third of the patients will continue to have frequent and severe episodes with ongoing disability.[4]

An estimated 30,000 suicides occur each year in the United States. About 70% of these involve individuals with major depression. The physician must consider suicidal lethality in the management of patients with depression. In general, the risk for suicide is increased with the following: alcoholism, drug abuse, social isolation, being an elderly male, terminal illness, and undiagnosed/untreated mental disorders. Patients at greatest risk are those with a history of previous suicide attempts, drug or alcohol abuse, recent diagnosis of a serious condition, loss of a loved one, just retired,

living alone, or having poor social support. Patients with a plan and the means to carry out that plan are at highest risk of suicide. Once the patient with a mood disorder undergoes medical control, insight-oriented psychotherapy often is initiated as an adjunct to the patient's management.[10,14,15]

■ SOMATOFORM DISORDERS ■

DEFINITION

Individuals with somatoform disorders have physical complaints for which no general medical etiology is present. Associated unconscious psychological factors contribute to the onset, exacerbation, or maintenance of the physical symptoms. The following conditions are considered as somatoform disorders: somatization, conversion disorder, pain disorder, and hypochondriasis. Patients with somatization disorder experience multiple, unexplained somatic symptoms that may last for years.[16]

EPIDEMIOLOGY: INCIDENCE AND PREVALENCE

The lifetime prevalence for somatization disorder is less than 2%. Most of these occur in women. Patients with symptoms that do not meet the full criteria for somatization disorder are much more common. Conversion disorder, pain disorder, and hypochondriasis appear to be more common than somatization disorder.[3,16]

ETIOLOGY

In this group of disorders, physical symptoms suggest a physical disorder for which there is no demonstrable underlying physical basis. The symptoms are linked to psychologic factors. Somatization therefore is defined as the manifestation of psychologic stress in somatic symptoms.

A conversion reaction results when a psychologic conflict or need is expressed as an alteration or loss of physical function, suggesting a physical disorder. A person who views a traumatic event, for example, but has a conflict about acknowledging that event may develop a conversion disorder of blindness. In this case, the symptom of blindness has symbolic value and is a representation and partial solution to the underlying psychologic conflict. In contrast, patients with hypochondriasis or a factitious (self-inflicted) disorder are aware of the nature of their problem but may be unable to control it. Many patients with pain disorder give a history of a physical

injury that precedes the later onset of pain. The onset of pain is accompanied by environmental stress or emotional conflicts.[3,4,10,17]

Somatization Disorder

Somatization consists of multiple symptoms and usually begins before the age of 30 years. These patients experience multiple, unexplained somatic symptoms. The symptoms may be pain, diarrhea, bloating, vomiting, sexual dysfunction, blindness, deafness, weakness, paralysis, or coordination problems. This is a serious psychiatric illness. Many of these patients have concurrent anxiety, depression or personality disorders.[16]

Conversion Disorder

Conversion disorder is a monosymptomatic somatoform disorder that affects either the individual's voluntary motor system or sensory functions. The patient may experience blindness, deafness, paralysis, or inability to speak or to walk. The symptoms suggest a physical condition, but the etiology is psychological. The symptom is not intentionally produced. The symptom typically is a symbolic representation that relieves an underlying emotional conflict.[16]

Pain Disorder

Pain disorder causes the patient significant distress in important areas of functioning such as social, occupational and others. In patients with pain disorder, no organic pathology can be identified. Often a stressful event precedes the onset of pain. The pain often results in secondary gain; increased attention and sympathy from others.[16]

Hypochondriasis

Patients with hypochondriasis are preoccupied with the fear or belief that they have a serious disease. Their misinterpretations of normal bodily functions are generally to blame.[16]

Treatment

Treatment of patients with somatoform disorders often requires multiple therapeutic modalities, including psychotherapy for their interpersonal and psychological problems. Medication to treat underlying depressive disorder also may be needed. Group therapy is beneficial in some cases. Unneeded medical or surgical treatment must not be rendered and will not correct the

problem. It is costly and may lead to significant associated complications.[16]

■ SUBSTANCE-RELATED DISORDERS ■

DEFINITION

Substance-related disorders concerns symptoms and maladaptive behavioral changes associated with the regular use of psychoactive substances that affect the CNS. These disorders involve substance dependence, abuse, tolerance, and withdrawal symptoms.[3,7,10,18]

EPIDEMIOLOGY: INCIDENCE AND PREVALENCE

Alcohol dependence tends to cluster in families. Approximately 13% of the adult population has abused or been dependent on alcohol at some time in their lives.[3] Alcohol is involved in about 30% of suicides and 60% of homicides.[3] In addition, 1 in 5 male dental patients and 1 in 10 female dental patients are alcoholics. Most alcohol is consumed by a small percentage of people; 10% of alcohol drinkers consume 50% of the total amount. Most adults in the United States are light drinkers as 55% consume fewer than 3 alcoholic drinks a week. About 35% of adults abstain from alcohol. Drinking patterns vary by age and gender. For both genders, the prevalence of drinking is highest in the 21- to 34-year-old range. At all ages, 2 to 5 times more men than women are heavy drinkers.[7,18]

Cannabis is the most widely used illicit psychoactive substance in the United States. In 1995, 9.8 million persons in the United States were marijuana smokers and 1.5 million persons were cocaine users. Cocaine can be injected into a vein, snorted through the nose, smoked in a free-base form, or smoked as "crack" (cocaine base premade into solid pellet form).[7,19,20]

The annual high school senior survey in 1996 showed illicit drug use to be below the peak of 1980. Alcohol is the drug most often used by young people. Marijuana use continues to be a major problem among young people. Stimulants and inhalants also are commonly used illicit drugs among young people. Tobacco use is rising among youths.[7]

ETIOLOGY

A complex, unique set of variables influence the addictive behavior of individuals with alcohol or drug problems. Some evidence exists that genetic transmission is involved in alcoholism. Psychologic factors such as depression, self-medication (used to treat psychic distress), personality disorders, poor coping skills, and others ap-

TABLE **23-5**

Chronic Substance Use

Substance	Related Physical Complaints	Possible Physical Findings
Alcohol	Frequent injuries; abdominal pain, nausea, and vomiting (gastritis, pancreatitis); diarrhea; headaches; vague physical complaints; erectile dysfunction; convulsions; palpitations; insomnia	Hypertension; injuries (e.g., bruises, cigarette burns, unexplained burns); enlarged liver; cutaneous stigmas of liver disease (spider angioma, palmar erythema); ecchymoses on legs, arms, or chest; smell of alcohol on breath; myopathy; peripheral neuritis; congestive heart failure
Cocaine	Fatigue, sinusitis, sore throat, hoarseness, persistent fever, chest pain, sexual problems, bronchitis, weight loss, nausea and vomiting, headaches, muscle jerks and spasms, convulsions, arrhythmia	Cocaine: rhinitis, rash around nasal area, perforation of nasal septum, hypertension, tachycardia. Crack cocaine: hoarseness; parched lips, tongue, and throat; singed eyebrows or eyelashes; stigmas of IV use
Stimulants	Insomnia, weight loss	Worn-down teeth (from tooth grinding), scratches, skin ulcers, dyskinesia
Inhalants (hydrocarbons)	Weight loss, breathing difficulties, fatigue, nosebleeds, weakness, stomach upset, intellectual changes	Halitosis, rash around nose or mouth, mental status changes
Cannabis	Chronic dry cough, bronchitis, sinusitis, pharyngitis, laryngitis	Conjunctival suffusion; distinct odor of burnt leaves on breath and clothes; dilated, poorly reactive pupils
Opioids	False complaints of severe pain made to obtain drugs; infections (especially cellulitis, abscess, pneumonia, SBE	Needle track marks, skin lesions, constricted pupils, swollen nasal mucosa, thrombosis, lymphadenopathy
Other sedatives	Insomnia, restlessness, convulsions, pneumonia	Slurred speech; needle track marks if IV user (especially with barbiturates); pupillary constriction with glutethimide
Hallucinogens	Palpitations, chest pain (especially in older users); convulsions with PCP	Myopathy; renal failure with PCP

From Levin FR, Kleber HD: Alcohol and substance abuse disorders. In Cutler JL, Marcus ER, editors: *Saunders review series: Psychiatry,* 1999, Philadelphia, WB Saunders, p 140.

pear to be involved in addictive behavior. Social factors that may be involved include interpersonal, cultural, and societal influences.[16]

CLINICAL PRESENTATION AND MEDICAL MANAGEMENT

Substance dependence occurs when an individual takes a substance in larger amounts or over a longer period than was originally intended. A great deal of time may be spent in activities needed to get the substance, take it, or recover from its effects. The person gives up important social, occupational, and recreational activities because of substance use. A marked tolerance may develop to the substance (more than 50% increase); hence, larger amounts are needed to achieve intoxication or produce the desired effect. The person continues to take the substance despite having persistent or recurrent social, psychologic, and physical problems resulting from its use.[16]

Substance abuse denotes substance use that does not meet the criteria for dependence. This diagnosis most likely is to be applicable to people who have just started taking psychoactive substances. Examples of substance abuse may include the following: a middle-aged man who repeatedly drives his car while intoxicated (the man has no other symptoms) or a woman who keeps drinking although her physician has warned her it is responsible for exacerbating the symptoms of a duodenal ulcer (she has no other symptoms).[3,7,10,18] Table 23-5 lists the physical complaints

(symptoms) and possible physical findings (signs) that may be found in individuals with chronic substance use.

Withdrawal occurs when the person with substance dependence stops or reduces intake of the substance. Withdrawal symptoms vary based on the substance involved. Physiologic signs of withdrawal are common after prolonged use of alcohol, opioids, sedatives, hypnotics, and anxiolytics. Such signs are less obvious in withdrawal from cocaine, nicotine, amphetamines, and cannabis.[3,7,10,18]

Opioids Use

The main effects of the opioids (opiate-like drugs) are to decrease pain perception, cause modest levels of sedation, and result in euphoria. Drugs included in this category include heroin, morphine, codeine, and many nonsteroidal prescription analgesics. Semisynthetic drugs produced from the morphine or thebaine molecules include hydromorphone, heroin, and oxycodone. Synthetic opioids include meperidine, propoxyphene, diphenoxylate, fentanyl, buprenorphine, methadone, and pentazocine. Tolerance to any one opioid is likely to generalize to other drugs in the group.[21]

Opiates by direct effects in the CNS can result in nausea and vomiting, decreased pain perception, euphoria and sedation. Additives in street drugs can cause permanent damage to the nervous system including peripheral neuropathy and CNS dysfunction. Patients may experience constipation and anorexia. Respiratory depression occurs because of a decreased response of the brainstem to carbon dioxide tension. This effect is part of the toxic reaction to opiates described below, but also can be significant in patients with compromised lung activity. Cardiovascular effects of the opiates are mild with no direct effect on heart rhythm or myocardial contractility. Orthostatic hypotension can occur which is probably secondary to dilation of peripheral vessels. A major danger with the use of these drugs taken intravenous is using contaminated needles. This practice leads to increased risk for hepatitis B and C, bacterial endocarditis, and infection with HIV.[7,21]

Dependence on opiates can be seen in at least three groups of patients. A minority of patients with chronic pain syndromes misuse their prescribed drugs. The second group at high risk is physicians, dentists, nurses, and pharmacists. These individuals have easy access to drugs with abuse potential. Members of the third group buy their drugs on the street to get high. Once persistent opiate use is established the outcome is often very serious. More than 25% of such users are likely to die with 10 to 20 years of active use. Death results from suicide, homicide, accidents, and infectious diseases such as hepatitis or AIDS.[21]

Toxic reactions are seen with all opiates. They are more frequent and dangerous with the more potent drugs such as fentanyl, which is 80 to 100 times more powerful than morphine. IV overdose can lead immediately to slow, shallow respirations, bradycardia, drop in body temperature, and lack of responsiveness to external stimulation. Emergency treatment includes the support of vital signs using a respirator and a reversal agent such as naloxone injected IM or IV.[7,21]

In contrast to sedative withdrawal, the withdrawal from opiates is an unpleasant but not life threatening experience. Gastrointestinal upset, muscle cramps, rhinorrhea, and irritability are the prominent symptoms. Opiate users with memory impairment or cognitive dysfunction should be assessed for HIV infection by risk factors and blood screening of the patient after appropriate counseling.[7]

Cocaine Use

Cocaine is a stimulant and local anesthetic with potent vasoconstrictor properties. The drug produces physiologic and behavioral effects when administered orally, intranasally intravenously, or via inhalation by smoking. Cocaine has potent pharmacologic effects on dopamine, norepinephrine, and serotonin neurons in the central nervous system. Cocaine has a short plasma half-life of about one hour.[22]

Cocaine intoxication causes sense of well being, heightened awareness of sensory input, anorexia, decreased desire to sleep, restlessness, elation, grandiosity, agitation, and psychotic states (panic attack, paranoid ideation, delusions, as well as auditory and visual hallucinations). Physical findings of cocaine intoxication are tachycardia, cardiac arrhythmias, papillary dilation, and elevated blood pressure. Individuals in this condition may complain of headache and experience chills, nausea, and vomiting. Needle tracts ("skin popping") may be found on the arms of intravenous users of cocaine and heroin. Frequent or high-dose use of cocaine can produce psychiatric states similar to acute schizophrenic episodes. Pregnant women who are chronic uses of cocaine or heroin may give birth to infants who are "addicted."[7,19,22]

Cocaine overdoses can be life threatening. "Crack" cocaine, which is inhaled via "freebasing" or smoking, results in much higher blood levels of cocaine than "snorting" the drug. Myocardial infarctions, arrhythmias, strokes, and symptoms consistent with neuroleptic malignant syndrome have been related to cocaine use. Depression is common in cocaine addicts, particularly during periods of withdrawal, and under these conditions the drug may be taken in an attempt to commit suicide.[7]

Treatment of cocaine overdose is a medical emergency that involves resuscitation in an intensive care

unit. Intravenous diazepam has been shown to be effective for control of seizures. Ventricular arrhythmias can be managed by intravenous propranolol. Medication is not available that is both safe and effective for either cocaine detoxification or maintenance of abstinence.[22]

IV cocaine abusers are at increased risk for hepatitis B and exposure to the human immunodeficiency virus (HIV). Some IV cocaine abusers develop a pruritic rash on the chest (allergic reaction to a benzoic acid ester), and ester-type local anesthetics must be avoided in these patients.[7,19]

Amphetamine Use

Amphetamines and related drugs are CNS stimulants. Their psychoactive effects last longer than those of cocaine. Their peripheral sympathomimetic effects also may be more potent than those of cocaine. Many people develop dependence when first using amphetamines for their appetite suppressant effect in an attempt at weight control. Intravenous administration of amphetamine can lead to rapid development of dependence. Progressive tolerance is common in amphetamine dependence. Amphetamine use can result in the same symptoms and complications that are seen with cocaine abuse.[7,18]

Cannabis Use

Delta-9-tetrahydrocannabinol is the major psychoactive ingredient in substances causing cannabis dependence. Several different preparations of marijuana are available. These preparations, bhang, charas, ganja, or hashish, are known to vary in potency and quality. They usually are smoked but can be taken orally or are sometimes mixed with food. Current marijuana supplies are much more potent than those available in the 1960s. Most users describe an altered sense of time and distance perception. Acute intoxication may result in anxiety and paranoid ideation or frank delusions. Marijuana can destabilize patients whose schizophrenia is in remission. Social and occupational impairment occurs but is less than that seen with alcohol and cocaine use. Cannabis is the most widely used illicit psychoactive substance in the United States.[7,18]

Alcohol Dependence

The behavioral and physiologic effects of alcohol depend on the amount of intake, its rate of increase in plasma, the presence of other drugs or medical problems, and the past experience with alcohol. The effects of alcohol are more dramatic with rising blood levels of the agent. Ethanol alone or with other drugs such as benzodiazepines is probably responsible for more toxic overdose deaths than any other agent.[21]

The DSM-IV defines alcohol dependence as repeated alcohol-related difficulties in at least three of seven areas of functioning. These include any combination of tolerance, withdrawal, taking larger amounts of alcohol over longer periods than intended, an inability to control use, giving up important activities to drink, spending a great deal of time associated with alcohol use, and continued use of alcohol despite physical or psychological consequences. Thus the clinical diagnosis of alcohol dependence rests on the documentation of a pattern of difficulties associated with alcohol use and is not based on the quantity and frequency of alcohol consumption.[21]

In cases of abuse or dependence, three patterns of alcohol use are seen: regular daily intake of large amounts, regular heavy drinking limited to weekends, and long periods of sobriety interspersed with binges of daily heavy drinking. Chronic use of heavy alcohol intake can result in cognitive impairment even when the person is sober. Some individuals will develop an alcohol amnestic disorder and are unable to learn new material or to recall known material. An alcoholic blackout occurs in some individuals, which is an amnestic period for events occurring while intoxicated. A few individuals can develop an alcohol- induced dementia, which involves the loss of intellectual abilities, and the loss of abstract thinking, language, and judgment. Severe personality changes also may occur.[3,7,18] See Chapter 10 for a discussion concerning dental findings and dental management of chronic heavy alcohol abusers.

Treatment of alcoholics consists of three basic steps. The first and most important is a thorough physical examination for those individuals who are considering stopping drinking. It is needed to evaluate organ systems that could be impaired. This includes a search for evidence of liver failure, gastrointestinal bleeding, cardiac arrhythmia, and glucose or electrolyte imbalance (see Chapter 10). The second step in treating withdrawal is to give the patient adequate nutrition and rest. All patients should be given oral multiple B vitamins, including 50 to 100 mg of thiamine daily for at least a week or two. The third step is to recognize that the CNS symptoms were caused by the rapid removal of the brain-depressant effects of ethanol. Administering another CNS depressant and gradually decreasing the level of the drug over a 3- to 5-day period alleviate these symptoms. The agents most often used are benzodiazepines such as diazepam or chlordiazepoxide.[21]

Patients suffering from alcoholic withdrawal delirium (delirium tremens [DTs]) will have clouding of consciousness, disorientation, impaired attention and memory, incoherent speech, perceptual disturbances, illusions, and grand hallucinations. An episode of DTs is a serious medical event with a 5% mortality rate, and it requires immediate treatment in a medical intensive care unit. Other symptoms associated with alcohol withdrawal

include, hand tremors, malaise, weakness, anxiety, irritability, and depression. Physical findings include severe sweating, elevated blood pressure, and tachycardia.[7,23]

Once the treatment of withdrawal has been completed the alcoholic is educated about alcoholism. This includes teaching the family and friends to stop protecting the alcoholic from the problems caused by alcohol. Disulfiram has been used for some patients during alcohol rehabilitation. Disulfiram causes nausea, vomiting, and diarrhea when taken with ethanol. Naltrexone and acamprosate, may be used to decrease the amount of alcohol consumed or shorten the period during which alcohol is used in cases of relapse.[21]

Nicotine Addiction

Cigarette smoking is the main cause of preventable disease, disability, and premature death in the United States.[24] Yet more than a million children and teenagers start smoking each year, and established smokers have difficulty in quitting. Nicotine is addictive and accounts for most of this public health problem. To effectively deal with patients, tobacco use must be viewed as an addiction and nicotine as the addictive drug. Nicotine use produces a compelling urge to smoke, provides pleasurable alterations in mood, and motivates chronic tobacco using behavior. Smokers regulate their nicotine dose to obtain desired effects and to avoid withdrawal symptoms. The withdrawal syndrome consists of a craving for tobacco products, depressed mood, insomnia, irritability, anxiety, restlessness, difficulty concentrating, and an increased appetite.[24]

Large population studies have shown a strong association between cigarette smoking and several diseases. Atherosclerotic cardiovascular disease, cancer, and chronic obstructive pulmonary disease account for most of the excess mortality and morbidity due to smoking. Smoking during pregnancy has been shown to increase the risk for spontaneous abortion, fetal death, neonatal death, and sudden infant death syndrome. Gastric and duodenal ulcers are more prevalent in smokers than nonsmokers.[24]

Mortality rates of pipe and cigar smokers are substantially less than those of cigarette smokers. These differences are greatly reduced if the pipe and cigar smokers inhale. Death rates from cancer of the oral cavity, larynx and esophagus are elevated compared with those of nonsmokers and are similar among cigarette, pipe and cigar smokers. The use of chewing tobacco and snuff may produce plasma nicotine levels comparable to those of cigarette smokers and can lead to nicotine dependence or addiction. The use of chewing tobacco and snuff increases the risk for oral cancer, advanced periodontal changes, and halitosis.[21]

More than 90% of confirmed ex-smokers quit without formal assistance. Quitting "cold turkey" was the most common method used by these ex-smokers. Heavy smokers and those most addicted to nicotine may benefit from participation in an organized cessation program. These programs use a variety of approaches including self-help, physician advice and counseling, use of medication, group therapy, and behavioral training. The antidepressant, bupropion has been approved by the U.S. Food and Drug Administration as a smoking cessation agent. Medications now are available for nicotine dependence. The medications work by the principle of drug substitution. Nicotine gum, an intradermal nicotine patch, a nasal spray, and an oral nicotine inhaler are available.[7]

■ SCHIZOPHRENIA ■

DEFINITION

Disordered thinking, inappropriate emotional responses, hallucinations, delusions, and bizarre behavior characterize schizophrenia. The lifetime prevalence rate for schizophrenic disorders is about 1% (this includes all cultures and both genders). The age at onset is usually during adolescence or early adulthood. Studies have suggested an earlier onset in men than in women.[5]

ETIOLOGY

The etiology of schizophrenia is not known but appears to involve the interaction of genetic and environmental factors. Evidence for a genetic relationship comes from family, twin, and adoption studies. Family studies have shown a 13% risk for schizophrenia in children with one parent with schizophrenia. If both parents are schizophrenic the risk increases to 46%. The risk for developing schizophrenia for first-degree relatives is 5% to 10%, and for second-degree relatives it is 2% to 4%. Concordance in twins for schizophrenia is 46% for identical twins and 14% for nonidentical twins. However, 89% of the individuals with schizophrenia do not have a parent with the disease, and 81% do not have either a parent or a sibling with the disease. The identification of a specific gene that is causally linked to schizophrenia has been unsuccessful to date. A few studies have suggested that the defect in schizophrenia may involve chromosome 5 and possibly chromosome 10.[5,10,25]

The predominant biological hypothesis for a neurophysiologic defect in schizophrenia is the dopamine hypothesis. This hypothesis states that symptoms of schizophrenia are caused in part by a disturbance in the

dopamine-mediated neuronal pathways in the brain. This theory is supported by the blocking effect that most antipsychotics drugs have on the postsynaptic dopamine receptors. The disease is more common among persons in the lower socioeconomic classes. A separate risk factor is the chronic stress of poverty, which may have an adverse effect on the outcome of the illness.[5]

Schizophrenia appears to be triggered by certain environmental events operating in a genetically predisposed individual. Drugs, medical illnesses, stressful psychosocial events, viral infections, and family situations characterized by conflicting and self-contradictory forms of communication have been reported to precipitate schizophrenia in susceptible individuals.[5,10]

CLINICAL PRESENTATION AND MEDICAL MANAGEMENT

According to the DSM-IV definition, schizophrenia can be diagnosed in patients who have two or more of the following symptoms for at least one month: hallucinations, delusions, disorganized speech, grossly disorganized or catatonic behavior, or negative symptoms such as affective flattening, alogia, or avolition. In addition, the patient's social or occupational functioning must have deteriorated.

Patients with schizophrenia show psychotic symptoms consisting of delusions, hallucinations, incoherence, catatonic behavior, or flat or grossly inappropriate affect. Delusions and hallucinations are referred to as "positive" symptoms and withdrawal and reduction of affect as "negative" symptoms. The delusions usually are bizarre such as thought broadcasting or being controlled by a dead person. The hallucinations are prominent and occur throughout the day for several days or several times a week for several weeks. The four types of schizophrenic disorders are catatonic, disorganized, paranoid, and undifferentiated. Patients with schizophrenic disorders show deterioration in their level of functioning regarding work, social relations, and self care. They are often confused, depressed, withdrawn, anxious, and without emotion. Physically they may grimace and pace about or be rigid and catatonic. The vulnerability to a schizophrenic disorder is inherited, and life stresses appear to trigger the disorder.[3,5,10,25]

In schizophrenia two kinds of thought disturbances are seen: formal thought disorder and disorder of thought content. Formal thought disorders affect the relationships and associations among the words used to express thought. Thoughts may be strung together by incidental associations. Thoughts may be completely unrelated. Thought blocking is common with psychotic patients. Disorders of thought content involve the development of delusions. Delusions are fixed ideas based on incorrect perceptions of reality. Delusions are commonly paranoid or persecutory. Delusions also may be bizarre, somatic, grandiose, or referential (events the patient believes have special significance). Perceptual disturbances in schizophrenic patients include auditory, visual, tactile, olfactory and gustatory hallucinations. Auditory hallucinations consist of sounds being heard by the patient in the absence of any real auditory stimulus. Patients may hear sounds of bells, whistles, whispers, rustlings and other noises. The most common is to hear the sound of voices talking. Often visual, tactile, or olfactory hallucinations occur.[5]

The most common emotional change in schizophrenia is a general "blunting" or "flattening" of affective expression. The patient appears to be emotionally detached or distant. The patient may appear quite wooden and robotlike, and lack warmth or spontaneity. Paranoid patients may feel frightened or enraged in response to a perceived threat or a delusion of persecution. They can be very hostile and guarded to any perceived slight.[5]

The long-term course of illness is variable. About 25% of the patients will have a full remission of symptoms. Another 25% will have mild residual symptoms. The remaining 50% will have moderate to severe symptoms.[5]

Drug treatment has made the most dramatic impact on controlling the symptoms and improving the quality of life of patients with schizophrenia. Psychotherapy and other psychosocial treatments also are important because they provide patients with the human connection that helps them develop social skills, educates them about their illness and what to expect, and offers support throughout a long, difficult course of illness. Drug treatment of schizophrenic disorders consists of using antipsychotics medications that act selectively against specific target symptoms. These drugs are effective for "positive" symptoms such as hallucinations and psychotic agitation but are noneffective for "negative" symptoms such as social withdrawal or anhedonia (inability to get pleasure from or find interest in activities). The antipsychotics drugs are described later in this chapter.[3,5,8,26]

■ COGNITIVE DISORDERS ■

DEFINITION

The cognitive disorders include dementia and delirium. Dementia consists of the slow, progressive, chronic decline in intellectual abilities, including memory impairment, aphasia, decline in planning, organizing, sequencing, and abstracting. These cognitive defects can cause

significant impairment in social and occupational functioning. Patients suffering from delirium experience an acute change in mental status. The typical signs include confusion, periods of sleepiness, alternating with periods of agitation, deficits in attention and memory, failure to be able to perceive the outside world, and to use and understand language.

EPIDEMIOLOGY: INCIDENCE AND PREVALENCE

Dementia

The prevalence of dementia increases with age from 1% at age 60 to over 40% at age 85. Overall the course of dementia is chronic in 65% of the cases, partially treatable in 25% of the cases and reversible in only 10% of the cases. Most cases of dementia are nonreversible. These include Alzheimer's disease, vascular dementia, and dementia caused by Parkinson's disease. Approximately 6 million to 8 million people in the United States suffer from dementia, and more than half of these are the Alzheimer's type. More than $50 billion is spent annually in care for its victims. Women are at greater risk for developing the disease. Alzheimer's disease occurs predominantly in persons over the age of 65 years. About 11% of the individuals over age 65 have the disease. From the age of 70 the prevalence doubles every 5 years. By age 85 more than 40% of the individuals will have Alzheimer's disease. Vascular dementia accounts for about 12% to 20% of all cases.[3,27,28]

Delirium

Delirium is one of the most commonly encountered mental disorders found in medical practice. It will affect up to 30% of hospitalized and elderly medically ill patients. Delirium often is mistaken as depression, anxiety, dementia, personality disorder, or it may be overlooked completely.[28] Table 23-6 list the prevalence, age of onset, course and risk factors for dementia and delirium.

ETIOLOGY

Dementia

Various medical diseases can cause dementia. These include hepatic encephalopathy, acid-base disturbances, hypoglycemia, thyroid disease (low or high), uremia, primary or metastatic brain lesions, acquired immune deficiency syndrome (AIDS), trauma, syphilis, multiple sclerosis, and stroke. Drugs that can cause dementia include anticholinergics, benzodiazepines, digoxin, narcotics, phenytoin, and salicylates. Some of these conditions when treated will allow reversal of the symptoms of dementia.[3,27,28]

The etiology of Alzheimer's disease is unknown; however, several possibilities are under investigation includ-

ing genetics, nutrition, environment, and infectious agents. The cognitive deficits in Alzheimer's disease may be caused by dysfunction of cholinergic, mucarinic or nicotinic receptors. Neuritic plaques, neurofibrillary tangles, or cerebral atrophy are found in these areas in affected brains. These changes are not found in the motor, visual and somatosensory parts of the cerebral cortex. Genetic predisposition to Alzheimer's disease has a clear-cut pattern in some families. These are limited to less than 20% of all cases. In these cases the disease appears to be inherited via the apolipoprotein E4 allele located on chromosome 19. Three other chromosomes have been implicated to a lesser degree in the transmission of Alzheimer's disease, an amyloid precursor gene on chromosome 21, a presenilin-1 gene on chromosome 14, and a presenilin-2 gene on chromosome 1. Adults with trisomy 21 (Down syndrome) consistently develop the typical neuropathologic hallmarks of Alzheimer's disease if they survive beyond the age of 40 years. Numerous environmental factors such as aluminum, mercury, and viruses have been proposed as causes of Alzheimer's disease, but none have been proven to play a role.[27,28]

Vascular dementia is produced by occlusion of small vessels in the brain by damage from hypertension or arteriosclerosis. The occlusion leads to focal or lacunar infarctions. Often computed tomography (CT) scanning or MRI or both are needed to reveal these small infarcts.[28] Dementia occurs in 30% to 40% of patients with Parkinson's disease. This form of dementia is caused by an imbalance between dopaminergic inhibition and cholinergic stimulation in the basal ganglion, which may affect other neurotransmitters such as serotonin and norepinephrine. Dementia in patients with HIV infection can be caused by primary infection in the brain, effects of immunosuppressive secondary to the infection, or by the drugs used to treat the infection.[28]

Delirium

The impairment of attention and consciousness that are characteristic of delirium can develop over a short period of time and tend to fluctuate over the course of the day. The causes of delirium include systemic medical conditions (thyroid disease, hepatic failure, renal failure, primary brain tumors, metastatic lesions to the brain, lupus erythematosus, infections of the brain, and others), substance intoxication or withdrawal (alcohol or cocaine abuse), and multifactorial causes such as hyponatremia, hypoxia, anemia, and fever.[3,28,29]

Amnestic Disorder

Amnestic disorders may be caused by any illness that damages the deep brain structures that are associated with memory. These disorders are common in head trauma victims or patients with thiamine deficiency (seen in alcohol

TABLE 23-6

Epidemiology of Delirium and Dementia

Disorder	Prevalence	Age of Onset	Course	Risk Factors
Delirium	10-30% in hospitalized patients	Any age; most common after age 40 years	Variable, depending on etiology	Increases with age
Dementia	Age 60-69, 1.4-1000; age 70-79, 6.4/1000; age 80+, 20.5/1000	Most common after age 40 years	65% chronic, 25% partially treatable, 10% reversible	Increases with age and positive family history
Alzheimer's disease	Represents 50% of all dementias 1.5-2 million people in U.S. From age 70, prevalence doubles every 5 years; from age 90, almost 50%	Typically after 50s	Progressive downward deterioration	Increases with age; female gender; positive family history of first-degree relative with disorder; head trauma increases risk 3—4 times; Down syndrome; defects in apolipoprotein E4 allele
Vascular dementia	In 12-20% of patients with dementias	Earlier age than Alzheimer's	Stuttering course: deterioration and destabilization	Cardiovascular (hypertension, abnormal lipid profiles, smoking, history of arrhythmia); diabetes; more common in men; no family correlation known
Dementia because of HIV disease	33% of hospitalized HIV patients	Typically 20s or 30s	Chronic course: deterioration over time	Unknown for HIV dementia. Sexual contact, transfusions, sharing needles for HIV disease
Dementia because of Parkinson's disease	25% of Parkinson patients, usually in end stages	Usually begins between ages 50 and 65 years	Mild dementia for years; later, severe dementia possible in some cases	Males and females equally affected; in U.S. greater risk for African-Americans than whites, for northern inhabitants than southern, for rural areas than urban; family history

From Feinstein, RL, Cognitive and mental disorders due to general medical conditions. In Cutler JL, Marcus ER, editors: *Saunders review series: Psychiatry*, 1999, Philadelphia, WB Saunders, p 83.

abuse). Infections, neoplastic conditions, drugs (phencyclidine) and autoimmune disease such as vasculitis affecting the posterior cerebral artery can lead to amnestic disorders.

CLINICAL PRESENTATION AND MEDICAL MANAGEMENT

Dementia is a clinical condition characterized by a general decline in memory, intellect, and personality from a previously normal intellectual level occurring in the presence of an otherwise normal consciousness. Dementia has many causes (see Table 23-6). A relatively small percentage of cases are the result of potentially reversible causes and include such conditions as intoxication, infection, metabolic diseases, nutritional disorders, and intracranial lesions. The majority of cases, however, are the result of irreversible processes: Lewy body dementia, frontotemporal dementia, vascular dementia and Alzheimer's disease.[28,30]

Alzheimer's Disease
Alois Alzheimer first described this disease in 1907. It predominantly affects the elderly; however, the process

is seen in younger adults as well. The definitive diagnosis of Alzheimer's can be made only at autopsy. Gross examination of the brain reveals cortical atrophy and ventricular enlargement. Characteristic microscopic features include neurofibrillary tangles, neuritic plaques that contain A-beta amyloid, and accumulation of A-beta amyloid in the walls of cerebral vessels (amyloid angiopathy). These changes also are present but to a lesser degree in patients who do not have dementia. On a biochemical level, a deficiency of acetylcholine and its associated enzymes exists. This is significant because cholinergic neurons are intimately involved in cognition.[27,28] The only fully recognized risk factors for Alzheimer's disease are age, family history of dementia, and presence of the allele epsilon 4 of the apolipoprotein E gene.[31]

The onset of this disease usually is subtle and insidious, with the first sign being recent memory loss of or a change in personality or behavior. Slowly the cognitive problems start to interfere with daily activities such as keeping track of finances, following instructions on the job, driving, shopping, and housekeeping. Some patients remain unaware of these developing problems while others are aware of them and become frustrated and anxious. In the middle stages of the disease the patient is unable to work, is easily lost and confused, and requires daily supervision. Patients may become lost while taking walks or driving. Social graces, routine conversation, and superficial conversation may be maintained for varying periods of time. Language may be impaired, especially comprehension and naming of objects. Motor skills such as eating, dressing, or solving simple puzzles are lost. Patients are unable to do simple calculations or tell time. Loss of inhibitions and belligerence may occur. Nighttime wandering may become a problem with some patients. Anxiety and depression become more of a problem as the disease progresses. In end-stage of Alzheimer's disease patients often become rigid, mute, incontinent and bedridden often requiring a nursing facility. Generalized seizures may occur. Death usually results from malnutrition, secondary infections, or heart disease. The typical duration of Alzheimer's disease is 8 to 10 years. However, the course of the illness can range from 1 to 20 years. Some patients will have a steady down hill course while others may have prolonged plateaus without major deterioration.[27,28]

For the first time a better prognosis and improved quality of life appear to be available to patients in the early stages of Alzheimer's disease. Thus more emphasis is now being placed on the identification of predementia states.[31] The diagnosis of the disease is based solely on patient history and clinical findings. Criteria for making a

definitive diagnosis include the confirmation of dementia, at least two cognitive deficits, progressive worsening of memory, normal consciousness, onset between ages of 40 and 90 years, and the absence of any other condition that could account for the deficits. A clinical diagnosis of Alzheimer's disease established after careful evaluation is confirmed at autopsy about 85% to 95% of the time.[27]

No clinical laboratory tests exist that are diagnostic of Alzheimer's disease; however, conducting a battery of tests is useful in an attempt to identify correctable causes of dementia. These tests include a complete blood count, electrolyte panel, screening metabolic panel, thyroid function, vitamin B_{12} and folate levels, tests for syphilis and HIV antibodies, urinalysis, electrocardiogram, and chest radiograph. A CT scan or MRI of the brain, positron emission tomography, electroencephalogram, and lumbar puncture also are included when warranted. Of significant aid in diagnosis are neuropsychiatric tests, which are part of the necessary criteria for diagnosis.[27,28,32]

Once the dementia is determined to be Alzheimer's and not the result of a treatable condition, management is directed primarily toward symptomatic relief. At present many drugs are being developed for the treatment of dementia. Tacrine and donepezil (cholinesterase inhibitors), have been released for the treatment of Alzheimer's disease. These drugs appear to delay the progression of the disease by about six months. Tacrine and donepezil have limited effectiveness in reversing memory deficits. They both have a mild to moderate toxicity profile that somewhat limits their use.[27,28] A recent Canadian study showed that propentofylline, a neuroprotective agent, was effective for patients with mild to moderate Alzheimer's disease.[33] An older drug, velnacrine (a metabolite of tacrine), has been reported to produce modest but significant benefits in patients with Alzheimer's disease.[34]

Noncognitive symptoms respond to therapy. Although efforts are made to use nonpharmacologic approaches to manage symptoms such as anxiety, depression, irritability, and sleep disturbances, medications inevitably are required. Antidepressants, sedative-hypnotics, and antipsychiatrics are all used, with varying degrees of success. A small percentage of patients experience seizures and are treated with standard anticonvulsants.[27,28]

Delirium

Delirium is a transitory state primarily characterized by impaired attention and consciousness. Other cognitive changes may be present, such as memory impairment,

TABLE 23-7

Diagnosis and Epidemiology of Eating Disorders

Condition	Diagnosis	Epidemiology

Anorexia nervosa	1. Refusal to maintain body weight (less than 85% of expected)
	2. Fear of gaining weight
	3. Fear of becoming fat
	4. Disturbance in body image
	5. Amenorrhea
		1. Prevalence—0.5% to 1.0%
		2. Mean age at onset—17 yrs
		3. Rare after 40 years of age
		4. Mortality—10%
		   a. Starvation
		   b. Suicide
		   c. Electrolyte imbalance
		5. Females 90% to 95% of cases

Bulimia nervosa	1. Recurrent episodes of binge eating:
	   a. Large amounts of food
	   b. Discrete period of time
	   c. Lack control over eating
	2. Binge eating—at least 2 times per week over at least a 3-month period
	3. Inappropriate behavior to prevent weight gain:
	   a. Self-induced vomiting
	   b. Laxatives
	   c. Diuretics
	   d. Enemas
	   e. Ipecac (induce vomiting)
	   f. Fasting
	   g. Excessive exercise
	4. Self-evaluation is unduly influenced by body shape and weight
		1. Prevalence—1% to 3%
		2. Over 30% abuse alcohol and stimulants
		3. 50% have personality disorders
		4. Long-term outcome not known
		5. Females 90% to 95% of cases

Eating disorders not otherwise specified	Fall short of the criteria for either anorexia nervosa or bulimia nervosa. (For example individual uses laxatives or induces vomiting but is not a binge eater.)	Difficult to establish the prevalence of this group of eating disorders

disorientation, language disturbance, and perceptual disturbance. Symptoms last hours to days and tend to change during the day. Recognizing delirium is important because it often leads to the diagnosis of the underlying medical disease or drug use. Treatment of the medical disorder will in most cases correct the delirium. Patients with delirium may appear withdrawn, agitated, or psychotic.

Agitated behaviors associated with delirium are managed with neuroleptics, benzodiazepines, or a combination of the two. Partial or complete restraints may be needed for some patients to prevent injury. Delirious patients should not drive or walk in areas with traffic.[3,29]

■ **EATING DISORDERS** ■

DEFINITION

The two major eating disorders are anorexia nervosa and bulimia nervosa (Table 23-7). Anorexia nervosa is characterized by severe restriction of food intake, leading to weight loss and the medical sequelae of starvation. Bulimia nervosa is characterized by attempts to restrict food intake, but with a different form than found in anorexia nervosa. In bulimia the attempts at restriction are interspersed with binge eating followed by various methods of trying to rid the body of the

food. These include induced vomiting (finger in the throat, syrup of ipecac), laxatives and diuretics.

EPIDEMIOLOGY: INCIDENCE AND PREVALENCE

These disorders cause psychological and physical morbidity in women (90% to 95%) and to a much lesser extent, men (5% to 10%).[35] Anorexia nervosa affects an estimated 1% of women between 12 and 25 years of age.[36] The overall incidence is 0.24 to 7.3 cases per 100,000 per year.[35] Bulimia nervosa is more common than anorexia nervosa. Its prevalence is estimated at 1% to 5% for most populations with some as high as 15%.[35,36]

ETIOLOGY

The cause of the eating disorders is unknown. Genetic, cultural, and psychiatric factors appear to play a role in the etiology of these disorders. In addition, primary dysfunction of the hypothalamus has been suggested to play a role in the etiology of eating disorders. However, the recognized hypothalamic abnormalities revert to normal with weight gain and thus appear to be secondary in nature.[35-37]

Family and twin studies suggest a weak genetic component for the etiology of both anorexia nervosa and bulimia nervosa. In anorexia nervosa a 50% concordance exists in monozygotic twins and 7% in dizygotic twins.[35] In bulimia nervosa a 23% concordance exists in monozygotic twins and 9% in dizygotic twins.[35] For both disorders, first-degree relatives of probands are at increased risk for eating disorders, affective disorders, and substance abuse. A genetic predisposition indicates increased risk if the right cultural and psychological stresses are present.[35]

Cultural issues are important in the etiology of eating disorders. The quest for health and slimness is a powerful force in modern society and may reinforce the fear of fatness in patients with an eating disorder or tip the borderline case into overt disease. Certain hobbies and occupations (modeling, skating, gymnastics, wrestling, track, and ballet dancing) that emphasize body shape, weight, and appearance may play a role in eating disorders.[36,37]

Some evidence indicates that dysfunction in serotonin-mediated neurotransmission may play a role in the development of eating disorders. The peptide leptin (a product of the ob gene) is released into blood from adipose tissue and inhibits formation or release in the hypothalamus of a neuropeptide Y, a powerful feeding signal. Serotonin may function as a neurotransmitter linking leptin and neuropeptide Y inhibition.[37]

CLINICAL PRESENTATION AND MEDICAL MANAGEMENT

Anorexia nervosa and bulimia nervosa are eating disorders usually found in young, previously healthy women who develop a paralyzing fear of becoming fat. The population at risk consists largely of white women from middle-class backgrounds. The disorders rarely occur in black or oriental women, in the poor, or in men. The driving force is the pursuit of thinness, all other aspects of life being secondary. In anorexia nervosa this aim is achieved primarily by radical restriction of food intake, the end result being emaciation. In bulimia induced vomiting and excessive use of laxatives follow massive binge eating. Weight loss in bulimic subjects is not great despite the obsession with food. Some authors consider the two disorders to be distinct illnesses while others classify bulimia as a variant of anorexia nervosa. Overlap syndromes exist since emaciated patients fulfilling the criteria of true anorexia nervosa may exhibit bulimic behavior and subjects with bulimia often pass through a phase of anorexia.[37]

The diagnosis of the eating disorders is made on clinical grounds (see Table 23-7). In anorexia nervosa amenorrhea is a consistent feature. The weight criterion for diagnosis is 85% or less than expected ideal weight. An expressed intense fear of gaining weight or becoming fat, even when underweight, and a disturbance of body image completes the diagnostic triad[37] The diagnosis of bulimia is made if a history of binge eating without major weight gain, evidence of purging (induced vomiting or regular use of laxatives or diuretics), obsessive/compulsive behavior, and antisocial activity or self-mutilation exist.[37]

Anorexia nervosa usually begins around puberty but may appear later, usually by the middle 20s age range. Despite severe weight loss patients deny hunger, thinness or fatigue. They are often physically active and participate in ritualized exercise. Constipation and cold intolerance are common. Amenorrhea usually accompanies or comes after weight loss. In advanced cases bradycardia, hypothermia, and hypotension are found. Little or no body fat is evident and bones protrude through the skin. Parotid glands may be enlarged. The skin may be dry and scaly and is often yellow because of carotenemia. Patients with eating disorders may show other dermatologic manifestations; alopecia, xerosis, hypertrichosis, and nail fragility that are secondary to starvation.[37,38]

Patients with bulimia ("ox-hunger") nervosa experience episodic, compulsive ingestion of large amounts of food. They are aware that the eating is abnormal and have a fear that they cannot stop the eating and have feelings of depression at the completion of the eating. Bulimic patients have a morbid fear of becoming fat.

Secrecy about the eating-vomiting sequence is common. The episodes of binge eating are followed by induced vomiting using a finger, an object or a drug such as ipecac, with or without the subsequent ingestion of laxatives. Bloating, constipation, abdominal pain, and nausea are common. Binge eating generally occurs daily; large amounts of food are consumed, usually high-carbohydrate foods such as ice cream, bread, candy, and doughnuts. Dental caries becomes a problem because of the high carbohydrate content of the diet.[37]

The serum amylase has been reported to be elevated in 45% of bulimic patients.[39] In the same study the serum amylase was found to be elevated in pregnant women with hyperemesis but not in nonvomiting pregnant women. The authors of the study[39] concluded that vomiting rather than the binge eating increases the serum amylase in bulimic patients. They speculated that the increased amylase came from the salivary gland. Another study[40] found that parotid gland size was enlarged in 36% of bulimic patients and correlated with frequency of bulimic symptoms and with serum amylase concentrations.

Patients with anorexia nervosa are vulnerable to sudden death from ventricular tachyarrhythmias. The risk of death becomes high when weight declines below 35% of ideal weight. Complications of bulimia are aspiration of vomitus, esophageal or gastric rupture, hypokalemia with cardiac arrhythmias, pancreatitis and ipecac-induced myopathy and cardiomypathy.[37]

The prognosis is better for anorexia nervosa than bulimia nervosa. About 49% of patients with anorexia nervosa achieve normal weight, 20% improve but remain underweight, 20% continue anorexic, and 5% become obese and 6% or more die. Death is caused by cardiac arrhythmias associated with starvation or suicide. Bulimia patients have a poorer outcome because of more severe psychiatric disturbances leading to a higher suicide rate and the medial complications of gorging. About 40% of treated patients remain bulimic after 18 months of treatment. Relapse occurs in about two thirds the patients within a year of recovery.[37]

The treatment of anorexia nervosa cannot proceed in a meaningful way in the absence of weight gain. The patient's nutritional status and medical stability are first evaluated. Patients with electrolyte disturbances or with ECG abnormalities may require hospitalization. Once the patient is medical stable psychiatric treatment can begin. Behavior modification techniques are used to assist the patient in weight gain. The efficacy of psychotherapy has not been established. Drug therapy (antipsychotics, cyproheptadine, antidepressants) has not significantly improved the outcome of patients with anorexia nervosa. The antidepressant fluoxetine has been shown to be useful in preventing relapse in patients who have gained back their weight.[35,37]

Antidepressant medication, cognitive-behavior therapy, and interpersonal therapy are all effective in bulimia nervosa. Most patients are treated on an outpatient basis. Those patients with medical complications such as extreme electrolyte imbalance or severe bulimic symptoms may require hospitalization.[35] Supportive care by an understanding physician also can be helpful for the bulimic patient. Attempts should be made to stop the gorging-regurgitation cycle or at least limit the load of food ingested to minimize the chance of aspiration or gastric rupture. Potassium supplementation may be needed in vomiters or laxative users.[37]

DRUGS USED TO TREAT PSYCHIATRIC DISORDERS

ANTIDEPRESSANT MEDICATIONS

Tricyclics
The major group of drugs used to treat depression is tricyclics. The first tricyclic used to treat depression was imipramine. Tricyclics inhibit neural reuptake of norepinephrine and 5-hydroxytryptamine (5-HT), resulting in down- regulation of their respective receptors. The tricyclics are all equally effective in the management of depression, but they differ in their associated side effects. Amitriptyline and doxepin are the most sedating, and this side effect is taken advantage of by using these drugs just before bedtime. Two combinations of drugs are available for treating depression and other psychotic symptoms. Triavil (Amitriptyline and perphenazine) is used to treat patients with depression and agitation or psychotic behavior. Limbitrol (Amitriptyline and chlordiazepoxide) is used to treat patients with depression and anxiety.[3,41,42] Table 23-4 shows the drugs used to treat depression.

The adverse side effects associated with tricyclics include dry mouth, constipation, blurred vision, cardiac dysrhythmias such as tachycardia, hypotension, blurred vision, allergic reactions, and important drug interactions (Table 23-8). Tricyclic drugs should be used with caution in patients with cardiac conditions because a risk exists for atrial fibrillation, atrial ventricular block, or ventricular tachycardia. Tricyclics can lower the seizure threshold and must be used with care in patients with a history of seizures. They can increase intraocular pressure in patients with glaucoma. Urinary retention can be increased if they are used in patients with prostate hypertrophy. Erectile or ejaculatory disturbances occur in up to 30% to 40% of the patients. If used in certain patients with bipolar disorder, tricyclics can reduce the time between episodes, induce manic episodes, and cause rapid cycling of episodes.

TABLE **23-8**

Side Effects and Drug Interactions of Antidepressant Drugs

Complications	Heterocyclics	MAO Inhibitors	SSRIs	SNRIs
Side Effects	Dry mouth	Dry mouth	Dry mouth	Dry mouth
	Nausea and vomiting	Nausea and vomiting	Nausea and vomiting	Nausea and vomiting
	Constipation	Constipation	Diarrhea	Constipation
	Urinary retention	Urinary retention	Anorexia	Somnolence
	Postural hypotension	Drowsiness	Weight loss	Weight loss/gain
	Nervousness	Confusion	Blurred vision	Blurred vision
	Insomnia	Anorexia	Insomnia	Dizziness
	Drowsiness	Weight gain	Nervousness	Anorexia
	Sleepiness	Tremor	Sexual dysfunction	Impotence
	Reflux	Fatigue	Sweating	Loss of libido
	Anorgasmia (women)	Insomnia	Sedation (paroxetine)	
	Erectile problems (men)	Anorgasmia (women)	Akathisia	
	Loss of libido	Erectile problems (men)		
	Gynecomastia (men)			
Serious Side Effects	Mania	Mania	Mania	Mania
	Seizures	Hypertensive crisis	Seizures	Hypertensive (venlafaxine)
	Obstructive jaundice	Orthostatic Hypotension	Orthostatic Hypotension	
	Leukopenia	Peripheral edema	Anemia	
	Tachycardia	Anemia	Bleeding (platelet effect)	
	Arrhythmias	Leukopenia	Hypothyroidism	
	Myocardial infarction	Thrombocytopenia		
	Stroke	Agranulocytosis		
Drug Interactions				
Barbiturates	CNS depression	CNS depression		
Benzodiazepines	CNS depression	CNS depression	CNS depression	
SSRIs	Dangerous—don't use	Dangerous—don't use		Serotonin syndrome Seizures
SNRIs	Dangerous—don't use	Dangerous—don't use		
MAO Inhibitors	Anticholinergic toxicity	Don't use two or more agents	Dangerous—don't use	Dangerous—don't use
Heterocyclics	Dangerous—don't use	Dangerous—don't use	Dangerous—don't use	Dangerous—don't use
Anticonvulsants	Interfers with action of anticonvulsants	Interfers with action of anticonvulsants		
Antihistamines	CNS depression	CNS depression		
Beta blockers	Anticholinergic toxicity	Sinus bradycardia	Bradycardia	

From Feinstein, RL, Cognitive and mental disorders due to general medical conditions. In Cutler JL, Marcus ER, editors: *Saunders review series: Psychiatry*, 1999, Philadelphia, WB Saunders, p 83.

TABLE **23-8**

Side Effects and Drug Interactions of Antidepressant Drugs—cont'd

Complications	Heterocyclics	MAO Inhibitors	SSRIs	SNRIs
Warfarin	Warfarin metabolism inhibited—can lead to increased INR values		Warfarin metabolism inhibited—can lead to increase INR values	
Cimetidine	Inhibits clearance—can lead to toxicity		Inhibits clearance—can lead to toxicity	
Erythromycin	Interferes with action of the antibioitic			
Opioid analgesics	Increased sedative effect			
Vasoconstrictors	Actions are enhanced; use with caution			
Epinephrine		Actions enhanced		
Levonordefrin		Use with caution		
Phenylephrine		Best to avoid		
		Avoid		
Foods/beverages				
Tyramine	Avoid	Hypertension/Arrhythmias—must avoid these agents		
Caffeine	Avoid			
Ethanol	CNS depression	CNS depression		

From Feinstein, RL, Cognitive and mental disorders due to general medical conditions. In Cutler JL, Marcus ER, editors: *Saunders review series:* Psychiatry, 1999, Philadelphia, WB Saunders, p 83.

Drug interactions reported with the use of tricyclics include the following: (1) tricyclics potentiate the effects of other CNS depressants such as ethanol and benzodiazepines; (2) they also potentiate the actions of anticholinergic drugs such as antihistamines; (3) they are reduced in levels by oral contraceptives, alcohol, barbiturates, and Dilantin; and (4) they produce other drug interactions, including potentiation of the pressor effects of sympathomimetic agents such as epinephrine and levonordefrin, blockage of the antihypertensive effect of guanethidine, and induction of a hypertensive crisis if taken with or soon after a monoamine oxidase inhibitor (see Table 23-8). Overdosage with a tricyclic can cause death from cardiac arrhythmias or respiratory failure.[3,41,42]

Monoamine Oxidase Inhibitors

The traditional monoamine oxidase (MAO) inhibitors, which are both non-selective and irreversible, were the first effective drugs used in the treatment of depression. There are now only three drugs on the market that are from that group of MAO inhibitors: phenelzine (Nardil), tranylcypromine (Parnate), and isocarboxazid (Marplan). These drugs act by inhibiting the two forms of MAO, type A and type B. Inhibition of type A MAO results in the antidepressant effect seen with MAO inhibitors. More than 80% of type A MAO must be bound to serum proteins before the drug effects can be seen clinically. Resynthesis of new enzyme takes 10 to 14 days. If a patient is changing from an MAO inhibitor drug to a tricyclic drug, 2 weeks or more must elapse after stopping the MAO inhibitor before starting the tricyclic. Significant drug interactions occur between MAO inhibitors and opioids and sympathomimetic amines. MAO inhibitors potentiate the depressant activity of the opioids. They can produce a hypertensive crisis if combined with certain sympathomimetic amines (see Table 23-8).[3,4,43,44]

Phenyletholamine and phenylephrine must not be given to patients taking MAO inhibitors. MAO metabolizes these agents, and their use with an MAO inhibitor could lead to significant potentiation of their pressor effects (see Chapter 4). These adverse effects are not seen with epinephrine and levonordefrin. Many over-the-counter cold remedies contain phenylephrine and should not be prescribed for patients taking MAO inhibitors (see Table 23-8).

Tyramine is a naturally occurring amine that releases norepinephrine from sympathetic nerve endings. Dietary tyramine is deaminated by gastrointestinal MAO-A. In the presence of MAO inhibitors, dietary tyramine is rapidly absorbed into the circulation, and a hypertensive crisis can result. Foods that contain high concentrations of tyramine must be avoided by these patients. Food with high tyramine levels include aged foods such as cheeses, red wines, pickled fish, bananas, and chocolate.[3,4,43,44]

Second Generation Antidepressant Drugs

Selective Serotonin Reuptake Inhibitors. The group of drugs known as selective serotonin reuptake inhibitors (SSRIs) includes fluoxetine (Prozac), sertraline (Zoloft), paroxetine (Paxil) and citalopram. As a group these drugs are just as effective as the tricyclics but are not any more effective. These drugs are better tolerated than the tricyclics. The tricyclics are generally more lethal in overdose than the newer antidepressants. The SSRIs are considerably more expensive than the traditional tricyclic agents. Nausea, in up to 25% of patients using these drugs, is the most frequent problem associated with their use. Higher doses of the SSRIs drugs more often are associated with nervousness and insomnia (see Table 23-8). Many physicians consider a serotonin reuptake inhibitor as the first-line drug for the treatment of depression.[3,44,45]

Other Antidepressants. Amoxapine (Asendin), bupropion (Wellbutrin), trazodone (Desyrel), maprotiline (Ludiomil), nefazodone (Serzone), mianserin, and venlafaxine (Effexor) are other nontricyclics used as antidepressants. Bupropion has a greater tendency to produce seizures than the other antidepressants. Nefazodone does not cause sexual side effects. Mianserin was one of the first antidepressants to have a significantly improved toxicity profile after overdose. However, blood dyscrasias have been reported with its use. Venlafaxine is a drug from the new class of antidepressants, the serotonin-noradrenaline reuptake inhibitors (see Tables 23-4 and 23-8). Venlafaxine has a similar side-effect profile to the SSRIs. It also has been reported to increase blood pressure in higher doses.[3,43,44,46] Table 23-4 shows the dosage of some of the second-generation antidepressant drugs.

MOOD-STABILIZING DRUGS

Lithium

Lithium has some antidepressant effects, but its main role is in the treatment of bipolar disorders. Its mode of action is unclear. Lithium is used to treat acute manic episodes and to prevent manic episodes in a patient with bipolar disorder. It is effective when used alone in 60% to 80% of classic bipolar patients. Lithium should not be used if renal disease is present. Lower doses also must be used in older patients. The dose ranges from 600 to 3000 mg/day. It takes 7 to 10 days to reach full therapeutic effect. The patient on maintenance therapy should be evaluated every 3 to 6 months for serum levels of lithium, sodium, potassium, creatinine, T_4, thyroid-stimulating hormone, and free T_4 index. Medical complications associated with chronic lithium use include nontoxic goiters and hypothyroidism, arrhythmias, T wave depression, and a vasopressin-resistant nephrogenic diabetes insipidus. All these complications are related to the effect of lithium on adenylate cyclase activity.[3,4,43,44]

Drug interactions with lithium include erythromycin and nonsteroidal antiinflammatory drugs (NSAIDs) increasing the serum lithium levels that could lead to toxicity.

Carbamazepine

Carbamazepine, an anticonvulsant drug, has been successful in the treatment of manic episodes in bipolar patients who do not respond to lithium or cannot take lithium because of its complications. The dose is 600 to 1600 mg/day. Side effects include nausea, blurred vision, ataxia, leukopenia, and aplastic anemia.[3,4,43,44]

ANTIANXIETY (ANXIOLYTIC) DRUGS

The benzodiazepines are used to treat the various anxiety states (see Table 23-2). These drugs selectively but indirectly enhance gamma-aminobutyric acid neurotransmission. This may occur by the drugs' increasing neuronal receptor sensitivity to gamma-aminobutyric acid. The benzodiazepines are very effective for short-lived reactive states of tension and anxiety. They are the drugs of choice for generalized anxiety disorders. Tricyclics and MAO inhibitors are the drugs of choice for panic disorders. Benzodiazepines are used for the treatment of anticipatory anxiety associated with panic disorders. They also are used in the treatment of other forms of anxiety associated with panic disorders and for anxiety symptoms found in patients with phobic disorders.[3,6,10,47]

Diazepam is the standard for antianxiety therapy. No other anxiolytic drug has shown better antianxiety efficacy. Treatment with anxiolytic drugs should continue

only for a period of 4 weeks or less. To avoid the development of drug tolerance, these drugs often are given for 7 to 10 days, with a 2- to 3-day period after that without the drug. An early sign of drug tolerance occurs when increased dosage is required. Symptoms of drug withdrawal include muscle aches, agitation, restlessness, insomnia, confusion, delirium, and, on rare occasions, grand mal seizures. Some patients may experience rebound anxiety after the drug has been stopped.[3,6,10,47,48]

Drug side effects of the benzodiazepines include daytime sedation, mild cognitive impairment, and aggressive and impulsive behavior responses. The benzodiazepines can potentiate the CNS effects of opioids, barbiturates, and alcohol. Benzodiazepines are hazardous or contraindicated in the following cases: driving or operating machinery; patients with depressive mood disorders or psychosis; and in moderate-to-heavy drinkers, pregnant women, and the elderly. Tolerance and habitual and physical dependence can occur with therapeutic doses. Actions of the benzodiazepines are additive and usually synergistic with psychotropic agents. Drug interactions have been reported with cimetidine and erythromycin.[3,6,10,47,48]

Buspirone has mixed agonist/antagonist actions at serotonergic receptors that are thought to be involved in anxiety. It appears to have anxiolytic effects comparable with those of benzodiazepines without sedative, anticonvulsant or muscle relaxant effects. The anxiolytic effects are delayed in onset, taking up to 3 weeks before becoming clinical clinically obvious. The drug is recommended for short-term use only. At this time buspirone is not a first-line drug for the treatment of anxiety.[5,10,47]

A number of tricyclic and other antidepressants have additional sedative or anxiolytic effects. They appear to be as effective as benzodiazepines in generalized anxiety and superior in panic disorder and agoraphobia. Selective serotonin reuptake inhibitors and monoamine oxidase inhibitors also are effective in phobic states and panic disorders. The disadvantages of these drugs are their slow rate of onset; they may initially exacerbate anxiety symptoms, and some are toxic in overdose and have many adverse side effects.[47]

ANTIPSYCHOTIC (NEUROLEPTIC) DRUGS

The introduction of chlorpromazine in the 1950s revolutionized the practice of psychiatry. Other agents have been introduced since chlorpromazine, but none represent any real improvement beyond this prototypic agent. The popularity of these drugs is shown by the fact that two thirds of all prescriptions for antidepressant and antipsychotic (neuroleptic) drugs are written by physicians other than psychiatrists. The antipsychotic drugs appear to work by antagonizing the effects of dopamine in the basal ganglia and limbic portions of the forebrain. The antipsychotic drugs should be used only when they are clearly the drugs of choice because of significant adverse reactions associated with their use.[5,8,10,49,50]

The antipsychotic drugs sedate, tranquilize, blunt emotional expression, attenuate aggressive and impulsive behavior, and cause disinterest in the environment. They leave higher intellectual functions intact but ameliorate the bizarre behavior and thinking of psychotic patients. They all have significant anticholinergic side effects and produce dystonias and extrapyramidal symptoms.[5,8,10,49,50] The commonly used antipsychotic drugs are shown in Table 23-9.

Side effects of the antipsychotic drugs are numerous and often significant (Box 23-3). Patients become sedated, lethargic, and drowsy when first placed on these drugs; however, after several days they develop a tolerance to these effects. The anticholinergic actions produced by these drugs include dry mouth, postural hypotension, constipation, and urinary retention. Other side effects observed are obstructive jaundice, retinal pigmentations, lenticular opacities, skin pigmentation, and male impotence.[5,8,10,49,50]

The extrapyramidal side effects (motor or movement disorders) include acute and chronic conditions. During the first 5 days of treatment with an antipsychotic agent, acute muscular dystonic reactions or a Parkinsonlike syndrome may occur. Akathisia, or extreme motor restlessness, also may develop early in treatment. Symptoms consist of involuntary repetitive movements of the lips (lip smacking), the tongue (tongue thrusting), the extremities, and the trunk. The risk increases for patients over age 60 years and those with preexisting CNS pathology (70% risk). Many of the acute extrapyramidal side effects are reversible if the drug is stopped or anticholinergic agents are given.[5,10,50]

Tardive dyskinesia is the most common late extrapyramidal side effect associated with the use of antipsychotic drugs. It usually presents after antipsychotic medication has been used for several years. The chief sign is involuntary movements of the lips, tongue, mouth, jaw, upper and lower extremities, or trunk. The classic tardive dyskinesia affects the buccal, lingual, and masticatory muscles, leading to "flycatcher's tongue," "bonbon sign," grimaces, or chewing movements. Flycatcher's tongue refers to the tongue's darting in and out of the mouth. Bonbon sign is the pushing of the tongue against the cheek wall so that it looks as though a piece of candy is pressed against the cheek. An early sign of tardive dyskinesia is wormlike movements of the tongue while it is at rest in the mouth. Tardive dyskinesia develops in about 20% of schizophrenic patients who are treated for years. Patients treated with antipsychotics

TABLE **23-9**

Commonly Used Antipsychotic Medications

	Range of Oral Dosage (mg)	Potency Ratio Compared to 100 mg of Chlorpromazine
1. Phenothiazines		
a. Aliphatics		
Chlorpromazine (Thorazine)	400 to 800	1:1
b. Piperazines		
(1) Fluphenazine (Prolixin)	4 to 20	1:50
(2) Perphenazine (Trilafon)	8 to 32	1:10
(3) Trifluoperazine (Stelazine)	6 to 20	1:20
c. Piperidines		
Thioridazine (Mellaril)	200 to 600	1:1
2. Butyrophenones		
Haloperidol (Haldol)	8 to 32	1:50
3. Thioxanthenes		
a. Clorprothixene (Taractan)	400 to 800	1:1
b. Thiothixene (Navane)	15 to 30	1:25
4. Oxoidoles		
Molindone (Moran, Lidone)	40 to 200	1:10
5. Dibenzoxazepines		
Loxapine (Loxitane, Dazolin)	60 to 100	1:10

From Judd LL: In Wilson JD et al, editors: *Harrison's principles of internal medicine*, 1994, New York, McGraw-Hill; pp 2400-2419.

who are followed longitudinally, will develop tardive dyskinesia at the rate of about 4% per year. Elderly patients appear to have a much higher risk of developing tardive dyskinesia early in their treatment.[5,10,42,50]

Additional side effects of the anticholinergic antipsychotics drugs include hormonal effects, postural hypotension, and photosensitivity. The hormonal effects are primarily influenced by the effect of these drugs on prolactin. This may result in galactorrhoea, missed menstrual periods and loss of libido. Orthostatic hypotension is a potentially serious side effect, which is most common with the low-potency agents. Dehydrated patients are at greatest risk for this complication.[5,50]

Several atypical antipsychotic drugs are available for the treatment of schizophrenia, including clozapine (Clozaril), risperidone (Risperdal), olanzapine (Zyprexa), and quetiapine. Clozapine does not cause extrapyramidal side effects or risk of tardive dyskinesia. It also can be effective for improving the negative symptoms of schizophrenia. Unfortunately, a 1% to 2% incidence of agranulocytosis exists. Patients treated with Clozapine must be monitored weekly with complete blood cell counts. Clozapine is effective in some schizophrenic patients who

do not respond to standard antipsychotics drugs. Risperidone is a combined serotonin-dopamine antagonist. In contrast to the standard neuroleptics, which have little or no effect on the "negative" symptoms, risperidone is effective for both "negative" and "positive" symptoms of schizophrenia. All the atypical antipsychotics have a lower affinity for binding to D2 receptors and a lower risk for extrapyramidal side effects.[3,5]

Antacids can diminish the absorption of neuroleptic drugs from the gut. Neuroleptic drugs can decrease the blood levels of warfarin sodium. Neuroleptics and tricyclic antidepressants reduce the metabolism of each other, allowing for increased plasma concentrations of both drugs. Thioridazine can prevent the metabolism of phenytoin, allowing toxic blood levels to occur. Smoking can decrease the blood levels of antipsychotic agents. When neuroleptic drugs are used with tricyclic antidepressants or antiparkinsonian drugs, a powerful anticholinergic effect can result.[5,8,50,51]

Malignant neuroleptic syndrome represents a rare but very serious side effect of antipsychotics drugs. This syndrome combines autonomic dysfunction, extrapyramidal dysfunction, and hyperthermia. The patient develops tachycardia, labile blood pressure, dyspnea, masked fa-

**Side Effects and Drug Interactions
of Antipsychotic Drugs**

1. **Significant Side Effects**
   a. Agranulocytosis
   b. Visual impairment
   c. Cholestatic jaundice
   d. Excessive or abnormal involuntary movements
      Dystonia, akathisia
   e. Parkinson-like symptoms
      Dyskinesia, tardive dyskinesia
   f. Xerostomia
   g. Hypotension—orthostatic hypotension
   h. Tachycardia
   i. Seizures
   j. Neuroleptic malignant syndrome

2. **Significant Drug Interactions**
   a. Prolong and intensify effects of following drugs, which can lead to severe respiratory depression
      (1) Sedatives
      (2) Hypnotics
      (3) Opioids
      (4) Antihistamines
   b. Produce hypotensive crisis—Epinephrine
      (1) No more than two cartridges of 2% lidocaine with 1:100,000 epinephrine
      (2) Avoid more concentrated forms of epinephrine

cies, tremors, muscle rigidity, catatonic behavior, dystonia, and marked elevation in temperature (106° F). The syndrome was first reported in 1960, and since that time more than 200 cases have been described. It occurs after the use of neuroleptic drugs given in therapeutic doses. Malignant neuroleptic syndrome is most common in young male adults with mood disorders. The symptoms continue 5 to 10 days after the drug has been stopped. Mortality rate is 10% to 20%. Treatment consists of stopping all neuroleptic medication, body cooling, rehydration, and treatment with bromocriptine (a dopamine agonist).[5,8,10,49,50]

DENTAL MANAGEMENT

PATIENTS' ATTITUDE TOWARD THE DENTIST

Childhood experiences and learned social roles of the patient are important factors in the development of the patient's feelings and attitudes toward the dentist. Children learn role expectations through the teaching of physicians, dentists, parents, and peers. The patient may come to believe that the physician and dentist are powerful and dangerous and thus may feel awe, envy, and wonder in their presence. Other emotions, attitudes and actions associated with the patients' relationship with their parents also may be transferred to the dentist. Those of respect and politeness can be helpful. However, those for a need of unending love, a demand for unceasing attention, feelings of resentment and hate can be destructive. The more that dentists reveal of themselves to the patient from the first contact, the less likely are these attitudes and feelings to be encouraged. Unrealistic expectations and inappropriate behavior should be open for discussion between the dentist and patient if a solid relationship is to be developed and maintained.[52-55]

PSYCHOLOGIC SIGNIFICANCE OF THE ORAL CAVITY

The soft tissues of the mouth are an important and highly emotional part of the body. The mouth is the area of the body that early in life is involved with feelings of pleasure and satisfaction during feeding or with frustration and anger if the feeding is late or difficult. The mouth is an area of the body that may be involved with sexual sensations and is used to show the expression of an emotion that a person is feeling. The mouth is important for speech, appearance, and aesthetics. It is involved in our society with the images of health, sex, and youth. Dental treatment and manipulation in the mouth may allow the patient to become aware of many of these feelings.[52]

Teeth also have important psychologic significance. They may be symbolic of the expression of aggression because they were the first weapons of the child. A patient's body image may be reflected in that patient's attitude toward teeth. To some people, the loss of teeth means body destruction. Individuals who have a tendency toward self-destructive feelings may view the need to lose teeth as a means of gaining some degree of satisfaction for having these feelings. A person may view the loss of teeth as an indication of premature aging; or it may be seen as a loss of sexual potency and youthful optimism.

The dentist may not be aware of the source of a patient's strong feelings expressed in the dental setting, but the dentist should appreciate the fact that these feelings may have origins having nothing to do with the procedure being performed.

BEHAVIORAL REACTIONS TO ILLNESS

The DSM-IV calls attention to the interplay of psychologic and behavioral factors with medical illness under the diagnostic category psychologic factors affecting medical

conditions. All patients with medical illness experience psychologic reactions to being ill. The reactions a patient has will vary based on the nature of the illness and the nature of the patient. Significant aspects of the illness include severity, chronicity, and the site and nature of the symptoms. Important patient characteristics include age, level of maturity, character style, previous experience with illness, and social supports.[2,56]

Regression, denial, anxiety, depression, and anger are general responses to illness that are common to all human beings. These responses originate in the various meanings that people attribute to physical illness, the fears typically raised by being ill, and the means used to cope with the illness.[1,56]

Depressive thoughts and feelings are common psychological reactions to medical illness. Being ill usually is experienced as a loss. The loss may be experienced as a loss of physical abilities, loss of bodily integrity, to the loss of organs or limbs. Feelings of loss of control are very common among hospitalized patients. These patients may feel that they cannot do some of the things they have always done that are important part of their identities. These include being unable to fulfill family roles, taking care of professional responsibilities and participating in recreational and social activities. All medical patients suffer the loss of their sense of being healthy. Transient depressed thoughts and feelings are common in medically ill patients. Major depression in medically ill patients is not normal and must be aggressively identified and treated.[56]

Patients commonly experience anger about being ill. However, some patients become enraged; in an effort to feel less helpless, guilty, or afraid they lash out at the people around them. These patients can become hostile, suspicious, and accusatory toward family members and health care providers. The most common causes of anger, irritability, and suspiciousness in medically ill patients are medications and substances of abuse. Certain groups of patients are at high risk for paranoid reactions. These include elderly patients, those with depression or cognitive impairment, and those with prior history of psychotic illness.[56]

Severe and chronic illnesses foster a certain dependency by the patient on others. Severely disabled patients will have a greater need to relay on others. Some individuals cannot accept this dependency and become anxious and try to deny their need for help. Feelings of resentment, anger, and hostility can develop toward persons in contact with such a patient. Once again, an understanding of this process will allow individuals caring for such a patient to be empathetic and supportive.

Sick people tend to view the world around them as being small and develop a preoccupation with their sickness, needs, and fears. They may retreat to highly personal or magical notions about the cause of their illness.

For example, cancer patients may believe that their illness is a punishment for swearing at their mother or for some "evil" thoughts they may have had.

PATIENT MANAGEMENT

Anxiety

Generalized Anxiety. The dentist may detect anxiety in persons by their physical appearance, speech, dress, and the presence of certain signs and symptoms.

The anxious person looks overalert, displaying it in such ways as sitting forward in a chair; moving fingers, arms, or legs; getting up and moving; pacing around the room; checking certain parts of clothing; straightening ties or scarves, and so on. On the other hand, sloppy dress habits and other signs, just the opposite of a concern with perfection, may be seen. Anxious persons may show signs of being watchful of possessions, always trying to keep them in sight.

The anxious person may speak mechanically and rapidly and at times may seem to block out or not connect thoughts together. The anxious person may respond to questions quickly, often not allowing the dentist to finish a question.

Signs of sweating, tension in muscles, increased breathing, and rapid heart rate may be seen. The patient may complain of an inability to sleep, may wake at an early hour, and may not be able to go back to sleep. Attacks of diarrhea and increased frequency of urination may occur. In general, anxious persons are overalert and tense, feel apprehensive, and have a sense of impending disaster that has no apparent cause. Insomnia, tension, and apprehension lead to fatigue, which makes it even more difficult for the individual to deal with anxiety.

The dentist should talk with the patient and show personal interest. Verbal and nonverbal communication must be consistent. The dentist should confront the patient with the observation that the patient appears anxious then ask if the individual would like to talk about feelings, which may include the person's attitude toward the dentist. During these discussions, tension-free pauses should be allowed to develop between ideas, allowing a temporary state of regression to occur that will help the patient to restore a more anxiety-free state. Some patients may respond well to this approach without ever indicating why they were anxious.

If the patient remains anxious in the dental situation, the dentist may plan to use hypnosis, oral or parenteral sedation agents or nitrous oxide, and oxygen to better manage the dental treatment (Box 23-4).

PTSD. Veterans with PTSD may view the dentist as an authority figure who misled them and sent them to war. They may associate dental treatment with loss of control; hence, the dentist must attempt to establish communication and trust with these patients. Those pa-

BOX 23-4

Dental Management of the Anxious Patient

1. Preoperative
   a. Behavioral
      (1) Establish effective communication with the patient
      (2) Be open and honest, let the patient see who you are
      (3) Ensure consistent verbal and nonverbal communication
      (4) Explain procedures and answer any questions
      (5) If there may be discomfort with a procedure, explain this
      (6) Explain what you will do to make procedures "pain free"
      (7) May confront patient about appearing anxious, using such statements as "You seem tense today" "Would you like to talk about it?"
   b. Pharmacologic: Oral sedation—Benzodiazepines
      (1) Night before appointment—aid in getting a good night's sleep
      (2) Day of appointment—reduce anxiety prior to appointment
      (3) Select a fast acting drug and as low a dosage as to be effective
2. Operative
   a. Behavioral
      (1) Allow patient to ask questions about what is happening
      (2) Let patient know if any discomfort is about to be felt
      (3) Reassure patient that procedure is going well
   b. Pharmacologic
      (1) Effective local anesthesia
      (2) Oral sedation—benzodiazepines
      (3) Inhalation sedation—nitrous oxide
      (4) Intramuscular sedation—midazolam, promethazine, meperdine
      (5) Intravenous sedation—diazepam, midazolam, fentanyl
3. Postoperative
   a. Behavioral
      (1) Explain what usually occurs after the procedure
      (2) Explain what the patient needs to do
      (3) Explain what the patient needs to avoid
      (4) Describe complications that can occur such as:
         (a) Pain
         (b) Bleeding
         (c) Infection
         (d) Allergic reaction to medication
      (5) Tell patient to inform you if any complications develop
   b. Pharmacologic
      (1) Effective postoperative pain control is essential
      (2) Select the most appropriate medication for pain control
         (a) Analgesics—NSAIDs, salicylates, acetaminophen, codeine, oxycodone, fentanyl, morphine, and others
         (b) Adjunctive medications—antidepressants, muscle relaxants, steroids, anticonvulsants, and antibiotics

tients with IV drug habits may be carriers of the hepatitis B virus (HBsAg positive) and HIV. Those who are heavy drinkers may have liver and bone marrow involvement and be at an increased risk for infection, excessive bleeding, delayed healing, and altered drug metabolism. During the depressive stage of PTSD, patients often show a total disregard for oral hygiene procedures and are at an increased risk for dental caries, periodontal disease, and pericoronitis. They may complain of glossodynia, temporomandibular joint (TMJ) disorder, and bruxism.

Depression

During the depth of a depressive episode, a significant impairment of all personal hygiene may occur, including a total lack of oral hygiene. Salivary flow may be reduced, and patients may complain of dry mouth, increased rate of dental caries, and periodontal disease. In addition, complaints of glossodynia and various facial pain syndromes are common.[57]

Signs of low-grade chronic depression include tiredness even after enough sleep; difficulty getting up in the morning; restlessness; loss of interest in family, work, and sex; inability to make decisions; anger and resentment; chronic complaining; self-criticism; feelings of inferiority; and excessive daydreaming. Signs of more severe depression in a patient include excessive crying, change in sleeping habits, thoughts of food making one sick, weight loss without dieting, strong feelings of guilt, nightmares, thoughts about suicide, feeling unreal or in a "fog," and an inability to concentrate.

BOX 23-5

Dental Management of the Patient with Depression or Bipolar Disorder

1. Preoperative
   a. Consult with patient's physician
      (1) Determine patient's current status
      (2) Confirm drugs patient is taking
      (3) Determine drugs to be avoided or used in reduced dosage
   b. Refer severely depressed patients
      (1) Risk of suicide is increased
      (2) Suicidal thoughts should be inquired about
      (3) Spouse or relatives may need to share in concerns
   c. Examine for signs of the following:
      (1) Abrasion of teeth—excessive brushing seen in some manic patients
      (2) Gingival injury—excessive flossing
      (3) Xerostomia—drug side effect
      (4) Thrombocytopenia—drug side effect
      (5) Leukopenia—drug side effect

2. Operative
   a. Patients taking antidepressants or neuroleptic drugs
      (1) Epinephrine:
         (a) Can use 1:100,000 epinephrine in local anesthetic
         (b) Limit to two cartridges
         (c) Aspirate, and inject slowly
         (d) Avoid more concentrated forms of epinephrine retraction cord, control of bleeding
         (e) Avoid or use in reduced dosages (Sedative agents, hypnotic agents narcotics for pain control)

3. Postoperative
   a. Avoid or use in reduced dosage
      (1) Sedative agents
      (2) Narcotics for pain control
      (3) Hypnotic agents
   b. Manage xerostomia if present

Depressed patients often have poor oral hygiene because of lack of interest in caring for themselves. The effects of the poor oral hygiene may be compounded by xerostomia, which is a side effect of medications the patient may be taking. Only small amounts of epinephrine should be used in local anesthesia. Sedative medication may have to be given in reduced dosage to avoid over depression of the CNS. No medical contraindication exists for dental treatment during a depressive episode. However, most depressed patients may be best managed by dealing with their immediate dental needs only during the depression. Once the patient has responded to medical treatment, more complex dental procedures can be performed (Box 23-5).

Patients with severe depression must be referred for medical evaluation and treatment. If the patient is not responsive to this recommendation, the problem should be shared with a family member and every attempt made to get the individual in for medical attention. During severe depression, suicide is an ever-possible outcome; however, medical treatment currently is able to reduce this possibility.

Bipolar Disorder

From a dental standpoint, lithium, used to manage bipolar disorders, can cause xerostomia and stomatitis. However, no adverse drug interactions exist between lithium and other agents used in dentistry other than NSAIDs and erythromycin that can cause lithium toxicity.[3,57,58]

Patients who do not respond to lithium or those who can no longer take lithium usually are treated with a phenothiazine type of drug. Phenothiazines can cause bone marrow suppression and fluctuations in blood pressure. The dentist must be aware of these side effects and examine the patient for signs of thrombocytopenia and leukopenia (see Chapters 19 and 20) because serious problems with infection and/or excessive bleeding can occur. Phenothiazine drugs potentiate the sedative action of sedative medications, and serious respiratory depression could occur when using these agents in their normal dosage. Therefore, if these agents must be used, the dosage needs to be reduced. The dentist should consult with the patient's physician regarding this point. Epinephrine used in normal amounts usually will produce no adverse effects when used in patients taking phenothiazine-type drugs (see Box 23-5). The primary effect of epinephrine/phenothiazine interaction is hypotension and should be monitored.[3,59]

Somatoform Disorder

The characteristics of a somatoform disorder include the following: no identifiable lesion or pathologic condition can be found, the disorder or reaction has an emotional cause, it is not dangerous to the patient, and it is a defense for the patient in terms of reducing the level of anxiety. The reduction of anxiety by converting it into a symptom is called the *primary gain*. These patients also

may have secondary gains resulting from their condition; for example, because of their symptom they may not be able to work or they may receive increased attention from their family.

The following are examples of oral symptoms that can be produced by somatoform disorders: burning tongue, painful tongue, numbness of soft tissue, tingling sensations of oral tissues, and pain in the facial region. The diagnosis of a somatoform disorder should be made only under the following circumstances: (1) a thorough search from a clinical standpoint has failed to provide any evidence of a disease process that could explain the symptoms; (2) the symptoms have been present long enough that if they were related to a disease process, a lesion would have developed; (3) the symptoms have not followed known anatomic distribution of nerves; or (4) the underlying systemic conditions that could produce the symptoms have been ruled out by laboratory tests or by a referral to a physician. Systemic conditions that must be ruled out include anemia, diabetes, cancer, and a nutritional deficiency (vitamin B complex).[3,17]

The process of establishing the diagnosis of somatoform disorders is slow and time consuming. Dental treatment should not be performed on the basis of the patient's symptoms unless a dental cause can be found. Many patients have had needless extractions, root canals, and other procedures performed in an attempt to correct somatoform symptoms. Complex dental care should not be attempted until the somatoform problem has been managed. The diagnosis of a somatoform disorder should not be reached until a thorough search has been made over a period of time that fails to uncover pathologic findings that could explain the symptoms.

After a diagnosis of an oral somatoform disorder has been established, the patient can be managed as follows. First, the findings should be discussed with the patient in the presence of a close relative, husband, or wife. During this discussion, the dentist should point out that no organic source for the patient's problem could be found, that the patient does not have oral cancer, and that the pain or symptom is real to the patient. Next, the possibility that feelings of "unhappiness" are the source of the symptoms should be pointed out, which will be difficult for the patient to understand and accept, but it is important to establish this "groundwork." Complex or unnecessary dental procedures should not be performed, even it the patient demands them in the belief that this will cause the symptoms to disappear.

Dentists should pay close attention to their feelings toward the patient. The symptoms may be viewed only as a device to gain attention and sympathy, and this may cause feelings of hostility and anger on the part of the dentist, which will not help in proper management of the patient. The dentist should try to feel empathy toward the patient and understand the cause of the problem, and react in a positive manner.

An attempt should be made by the dentist to manage the patient with a mild somatoform disorder (mild in the sense that the patient is able to function at a reasonable level even with the symptom, the patient's emotional status appears to be "stable," and the patient has shown or expressed no suicidal tendencies). Such patients should be assured that they do not have a life-threatening disease such as cancer. A series of regular short appointments should be scheduled to reexamine the patient for possible signs of disease, to discuss symptoms, and to reassure the individual that no tissue changes are present. The patient should be charged for this time and told what the fee will be before the appointments are set up.

Patients with a severe somatoform disorder should be referred to a psychiatrist; however, once a patient has been referred, the dentist still should be willing to be involved. The patient may need to be reexamined and the psychiatrist consulted concerning the findings. If patients feel that the dentist only wants to get rid of them, the suggestion of referral will not be helpful or effective.

Stress-Related Disorders

Oral diseases that are thought to have a significant psychological component involved in their clinical presentation (the older term was psychophysiologic disorders) include acute necrotizing ulcerative gingivitis, aphthous ulcers, lichen planus, TMJ dysfunction, myofascial pain, and geographic tongue.[60-62] Examples of some of these lesions are shown in Figs. 23-1 and 23-2.

In these disorders, an identifiable lesion with an emotional component to the clinical presentation exists. The pathologic process is potentially dangerous to the patient. The disorder does not reduce the level of anxiety or depression but rather increases it, and the increased anxiety or depression can aggravate the condition. These disorders can be treated using the indicated regimen in Appendix B. The anxious patient can be sedated using one of the agents shown in Table 23-4. Patients with TMJ dysfunction or myofascial pain are often treated with an antidepressant medication.

Substance Abuse

The dentist should be on the alert for the signs and symptoms that may indicate substance abuse (see Table 23-5). Telltale cutaneous lesions often indicate parenteral abuse of drugs. These include subcutaneous abscesses, cellulitis, thrombophlebitis, skin "tracks" (chronic inflammation from multiple injections), and infected lesions. Skin tracks usually appear as linear or bifurcated erythematosus lesions, which become indurated and

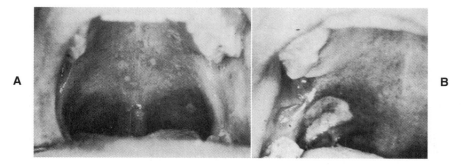

Fig. 23-1 Emotional factors appear to play a role **A,** in some cases of aphthous stomatitis, and **B,** in some cases of major aphthous.

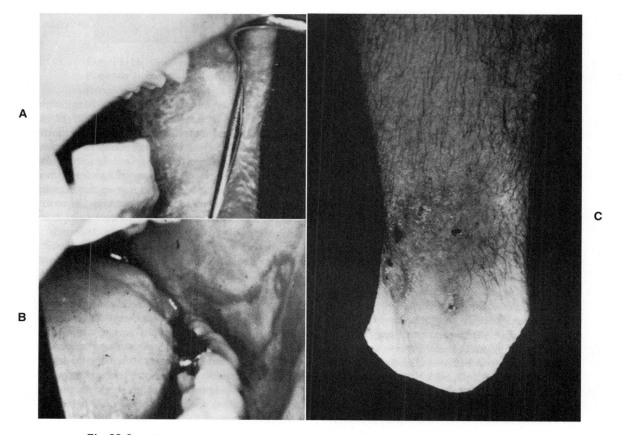

Fig. 23-2 A, Lichen planus involving the gingival and buccal mucosac. **B,** Erosive lichen planus involving the buccal mucosa. **C,** Skin lesions of lichen planus. Many patients with this disorder have a history of emotional crisis occurring just before the onset of oral or skin lesions.

hyperpigmented. An ill-defined febrile illness also can indicate a possible problem with parenteral drug abuse.[63]

Drug abusers may try to obtain drugs from dentists. This may occur by their demanding pain medication for a dental problem they refuse to have treated. The opioid abuser may claim to be allergic to codeine in an attempt to obtain a stronger drug such as morphine or hydrocodone. The dentist should not let patients know where drugs are kept, leave prescription pads out where they can be taken, and not use prewritten prescription forms.[63]

Drug abuse occurs more often in dentists than in the general population because of the ready availability of opioid analgesics and sedative-hypnotic drugs. The inhalation of nitrous oxide is one form of drug abuse common among dentists.[63]

Cocaine. Patients who are "high" on cocaine should not receive any dental treatment for at least 6 hours after the last administration of cocaine.[19] Peak blood levels occur within 30 minutes and usually are gone by 2 hours. The danger of significant myocardial ischemia and cardiac arrhythmias is the main concern in patients who are high on the drug. Local anesthetics with epinephrine or levonordefrin must not be used during the 6-hour waiting period after cocaine administration because cocaine potentiates the response of sympathetically innervated organs to sympathomimetic amines, which could result in a hypertensive crisis, cerebral vascular accident, or a myocardial infarction.[19]

Before treating a patient who is in a cocaine treatment program, the dentist should consult the patient's physician concerning medications the patient may be taking and how to manage the patient in pain. Patients with substance abuse should not be prescribed addictive substances.

Alcohol. The dental management of the patient at risk or with alcohol abuse problems is presented in Chapter 10.

Pain Control. Drug abusers often take their favorite drug to counteract dental fears and anxiety before dental appointments. If determined that this has occurred the dental appointment should be rescheduled and the patient counseled to not use drugs before the next appointment. Tolerance to sedative drugs and local anesthetics may occur, particularly in parenteral drug abusers. The need for larger doses of these agents carries the risk of increased incidence of adverse effects. Treatment of pain and anxiety in the recovering or reformed substance abuser presents a problem to the dentist. Before beginning dental treatment for these patients, the dentist needs to establish the patient's attitude towards drug treatment. Many patients will refuse mood-altering drugs. In addition, the dentist should never administer a drug, or another of its class, that has been abused by the patient in the past. For control of anxiety in these patients oral propranolol can be considered. NSAIDs can usually manage postoperative pain.[63]

Nicotine. The dentist is in the unique position of being able to observe the oral effects of tobacco use and to use this information as motivation for patients to stop the habit. Tobacco use counseling and cessation programs are important preventive services that dentists should provide to their patients. Cessation programs are incorporated easily into the dental practice. Patients must be informed of the medical problems associated with tobacco use (cardiovascular disease, chronic obstructive pulmonary disease, chronic bronchitis, gastric ulcers, low birth weight babies, spontaneous abortions, and cancer of the larynx, esophagus, pancreas, bladder, colon, oral cavity, and lung).

The dental office should be identified as a smoke-free area. The dentist's visible commitment to a smoke-free office sends a strong health message to patients. All ashtrays should be removed. The smoke-free signs can be rotated periodically to maintain the attention of patients and staff. Tobacco cessation materials should be provided in the reception area. Only magazines that do not carry tobacco advertising should be placed in the reception area.[64]

The dentist can help patients quit their tobacco use by applying the four A's: ask, advise, assist, and arrange.[65] The counseling process starts by asking tobacco use-related questions in the medical and dental history. These questions cover such topics as whether the patient smokes cigarettes; if so, for how long a time and how many per day; whether the patient ever has attempted to quit smoking and what happened. The history should inquire whether the patient smokes a pipe or a cigar; if so, for how long and whether the patient inhales the smoke. Patients should be asked if they use smokeless tobacco; if so, for how long, what types, and where they place it. The history also may ask whether the patient who uses tobacco is interested in stopping the habit. The dental record should clearly show whether the patient is a tobacco user and, if so, the type and pattern of use.

During the initial oral examination signs of tobacco-related oral conditions should be identified and shown to the patient. These would include periodontal diseases,[66] tooth loss,[67] necrotizing ulcerative gingivitis, halitosis, tooth staining, delayed healing, leukoplakia, erythroplakia, non-healing ulcers, and other lesions that may represent oral or pharyngeal cancer (see Chapter 21). Findings from the medical and dental history and from the clinical examination that may be tobacco related should be discussed with the patient and used to motivate the patient to seek further information about tobacco use cessation.

All patients who are tobacco users should be advised to stop the habit. Patients with medical or dental conditions known to be associated with tobacco use should strongly be advised to quit. The effect of tobacco on the patient's conditions should be made clear. The addictive effect of nicotine should be discussed.

TABLE 23-10

Pharmaceutical Agents Approved by the Federal Drug Administration for Smoking Cessation

Type	Nicotine Dosage	How Available	Maximum Dosage
Nicotine Patch			
Habitrol	21, 14, and 7 mg	Prescription	
Nicoderm CQ	21, 14, and 7 mg	Over the counter	
Nicotrol	15 mg	Over the counter	
Prostep	22 and 11 mg	Over the counter	
Nicotine Gum	2 and 4 mg	Over the counter	
Other Nicotine Replacement Products			
Nicotrol nasal spray	1 mg/dose (0.5 mg/spray)	Prescription	5 doses/hour or 40 doses per day
Nicotrol inhaler	2 mg absorbed	Prescription	6 to 16 cartridges per day
Non-Nicotine Medications			
Zyban SR (bupropion hydrochloride sustained-release tablet)	150 mg (1 tablet QAM for 3 days, then 1 tablet BID for 7 to 12 weeks)	Prescription	

From: Indiana Tobacco Control Center, http://iumeded.med.iupui.edu/tobacco/nrtinfo.htm

The dentist can assist by recommending the use of nicotine transdermal patches (Nicoderm CQ, Nicotrol, or Prostep) or nicotine gum (Nicorette Gum) to aid during the withdrawal period.[68] In some cases the antidepressant bupropion (hydrochloride sustained-release [Zyban SR]) can be prescribed.[69,70] Table 23-10 shows the dosage for the various agents used for smoking cessation.[71] The combination of bupropion and a nicotine patch or nicotine gum has been effective for some patients.[72] Psychosocial self-help materials can be provided to the patient. Some patients may want access to support groups dealing with cessation of tobacco use; others may want to be referred for behavioral modification therapy. Highly motivated patients may chose to quit "cold turkey." In all cases the dentist should work with the patient to establish a quit date within the upcoming 4 weeks. The degree of motivation the patient has expressed to quit should be recorded in the patient's dental record as low, moderate, or high.

The dentist should arrange for a follow-up appointment 1 or 2 weeks after the quit date. Patients should be asked about their tobacco-use status. Relapse is common; if it happens the patient should be encouraged to try again immediately. A second follow-up appointment should be made in 1 to 2 months. The dentist should discuss with patients who have relapsed the circumstances of the relapse and be supportive of their attempt to quit

the habit. This process should be continued at all recall appointments.

Schizophrenia

Routine dental treatment of the schizophrenic patient should not be attempted unless the patient is under medical management. Even then, these patients may be difficult to deal with. An attendant or family member should accompany the patient to maximize comfort and familiarity. Patients should be scheduled for morning appointments. Confrontation and an authoritative attitude on the part of the dentist should be avoided.[13,73] If such an approach does not allow for proper dental management, the dentist should consider sedation or tranquilization, which should be done in consultation with the patient's physician. Chlorpromazine (Thorazine), chloral hydrate, diazepam (Valium), or oxazepam can be considered.[13]

Alzheimer's Dementia

Alzheimer's patients are managed best by an understanding and empathetic approach. A patient's attention should be kept, and the dentist should explain what is going to happen before doing it. The dentist should communicate using short words and sentences and should repeat instructions and explanations. Nonverbal communication can be very helpful. Facial motion and body posture of the dentist should show support, cues

that the patient is understood and that the dentist cares for the patient. Positive nonverbal communication includes direct eye contact, smiling, touching the patient on the arm, and so on. Patients with Alzheimer's disease should be placed on an aggressive preventive dentistry program including 3-month recall, oral examination, prophylaxis, fluoride gel application, oral hygiene education, and adjustment of prosthesis.[74] Patients with advanced dementia may require sedation and short appointments. The choice of the sedative medication should be made in consultation with the patient's physician. Chloral hydrate and benzodiazepines have been used with some success.[61,75]

Eating Disorders

The major role of the dentist in the management of patients with bulimia nervosa is to deal with the results of their diet (dental caries), and the effects of chronic vomiting on the teeth (erosion). One study[76] found the average pH of vomitus was 3.8, which with chronic exposure can lead to severe erosion of teeth. The dentist's role as a case finder is important to the patient. The dentist may be the first person to become aware of the eating disorder by finding a pattern of erosion of the teeth consistent with regurgitation of stomach contents. This can lead to referral and medical diagnosis and treatment. However, patients often deny this is a problem. The erosive pattern involves the lingual surfaces of the teeth, primarily the maxillary teeth as the tongue protects the mandibular teeth. This particular type of erosion is known as *perimylolysis*. In some cases the erosion also can affect the occlusal surfaces of molar and premolar teeth where the process can be accelerated by attrition.[76-78] The serious medial complications of bulimia nervosa must be pointed out to the patient (gastric rupture, esophageal tears, cardiac arrhythmia, and death) and that these can be avoided with proper medial and psychological therapy.[35,37]

The diet of some bulimic patients is rich in carbohydrates and carbonated liquids and can lead to extensive dental caries and additional erosion of the teeth. The increase in dental caries most often occurs in patients with poor oral hygiene. For these patients the dentist's goal is to improve the patient's oral hygiene. This will include tooth brushing instructions, use of dental floss, and topical fluoride application. The patient is instructed to use a baking soda mouth rinse and to brush the teeth following induced vomiting.[76] Tooth sensitivity can be managed using desensitizing toothpastes, fluoride applications and other means.

Patients with anorexia nervosa may be more difficult to identify and deal with in a dental practice. About 40% to 50% of the patients with anorexia nervosa are also bulimic and may show the dental signs of bulimia.[35,79]

Young patients who appear to be anorexic should be confronted concerning the weight loss. If no symptoms or history of serious medial diseases such as cancer or diabetes mellitus are noted the possibility of self-starvation should be discussed with the patient. The serious medical complications, including death (mortality rate is as high as 15% to 18%), of anorexia nervosa need to be discussed in a straightforward manner. Again when young patients are involved their parents need to be informed. Every attempt should be made to refer these patients to a physician for evaluation and treatment.

Suicidal Patient

Suicide is one of the leading causes of death for individuals under the age of 45 years. It also is far too common in the elderly. Since 1980 a dramatic increase has occurred in the rate of suicide in persons 5 to 19 years of age and persons 65 years or older. Men are three times more successful in their suicide attempts than are women. However, women are 10 times more likely to attempt suicide. Patients with suicidal symptoms often say that they feel frustrated, helpless, or hopeless. They frequently are angry, self-punishing, and harshly self-critical. Suicide is a hazard for individuals who suffer from any of the following conditions: chronic physical illness, alcoholism, drug abuse, and depression. Suicide statistics show that men, adolescents, and the elderly are at greatest risk. A history of a previous suicide attempt greatly increases the risk. A history of recent psychiatric hospitalization increases the risk. A recent diagnosis of a serious condition such as cancer or AIDS also increases the risk for suicide. The recent loss of a loved one or recent retirement may increase the risk for suicide. If any of the above occur in the individual who lives alone or has little or no social support, the risk for suicide increases. Patients who are at highest risk are those who are perturbed, state a plan for suicide, and have the means to carry it out.[80]

The dentist should ask if the very depressed patient has had any thoughts about suicide. Studies have shown that questions about suicide do not prompt the act in these patients. Patients who state they have had these thoughts must be referred for immediate medical care. If possible, members of the family need to be involved.[3,15]

DRUG INTERACTIONS AND SIDE EFFECTS

Tricyclic Antidepressants

Many of the heterocyclic antidepressants can cause hypotension, orthostatic hypotension, tachycardia, and cardiac arrhythmias. When sedatives, hypnotics, barbiturates, and narcotics are used with the heterocyclic antidepressants, severe respiratory depression can result. If these agents must be used, the dosage needs to be reduced.

Atropine should be used with care in these patients because increased intraocular pressure can result. Small amounts of epinephrine (1:100,000) can be used in patients taking heterocyclic antidepressants if the dentist aspirates before injecting and injects the anesthetic slowly. No more than two cartridges should be injected at any appointment (see Box 23-5). Other, more concentrated, forms of epinephrine must be avoided. Levonordefrin is contraindicated in patients taking tricyclics due to the possibility of an exaggerated hypertensive response.[41,42]

Monoamine Oxidase Inhibitors

Patients taking MAO inhibitors can receive small amounts of epinephrine in local anesthetics as described previously. Other forms of epinephrine (retraction cord, topical for control of bleeding) must be avoided. Phenylephrine must not be used in patients taking MAO inhibitors. MAO inhibitors may interact with sedatives, narcotics, nonnarcotic analgesics, antihistamines, and atropine to prolong and intensify their effect on the CNS[41,42] (see Table 23-8).

Antianxiety Drugs

Important drug interactions can occur between benzodiazepines and barbiturates, opioids, psychotropic agents, cimetidine, and erythromycin. In general, these agents will potentiate the CNS depressant effects of benzodiazepines. Regarding the use of these agents, two situations of concern to the dentist exist: (1) barbiturates and opioids used for dental sedation or pain control must be administered with caution in decreased dosages in patients taking a benzodiazepine for an anxiety disorder; (2) on the other hand, the dentist may prescribe a benzodiazepine for sedation to control dental-related anxiety, but care must be taken in dealing with the individual being treated with psychotropic agents for a psychiatric disorder. Usually the dosage of the medication can be reduced to avoid over depression of the CNS. The dentist should consult with the patient's physician before using these drug combinations. During treatment the patient can be monitored using a Pulseoximeter.[48,49,81,82]

Antipsychotic Drugs

Several important drug interactions can occur in patients taking neuroleptic drugs. Extreme care must be taken if sedatives, hypnotics, antihistamines, and opioids are used in patients taking neuroleptic agents because neuroleptic drugs increase the respiratory depressant effect of these agents. This can be dangerous, particularly in patients with compromised respiratory function. If these types of drugs must be used, the dosage needs to be reduced. The dentist must consult with the patient's physician before using these agents.[41,42]

Epinephrine must be used with great care in patients receiving a neuroleptic drug because a severe hypotensive episode can result. Small amounts of epinephrine (1:100,000) can be used in patients taking neuroleptic drugs if the dentist aspirates before injecting, injects the anesthetic solution slowly, and uses no more than two cartridges. Epinephrine in retraction cords or for topical application for control of bleeding is contraindicated (see Box 23-3).

Older patients taking antipsychotic drugs present several important problems concerning drug usage. These patients usually have decreased levels of serum albumin; hence, many of them have a higher percentage of the drug in an unbound state. This increases the risk for toxic reaction. In addition, many of these patients have marginal liver function; hence, drugs metabolized by the liver may remain in circulation for longer periods and in increased concentrations.

TREATMENT PLANNING CONSIDERATIONS

The goals of treatment planning for patients with psychiatric disorders are to maintain oral health, comfort, and function, and to prevent and control oral diseases. Without an aggressive approach to prevention, many of these patients will be susceptible to dental caries and periodontal disease. Susceptibility to such diseases increases because of the side effect of xerostomia associated with most of the medications and the fact that some of the psychiatric conditions for which these patients are being treated reduce interest in or the ability to perform oral hygiene procedures. Also, many of these patients' diets contain foods or drinks that increase the risk for dental disease.[81,83]

The dental treatment plan should contain the following elements. The daily oral hygiene procedures must be identified. The treatment plan must be realistic for the patient's psychiatric disorder and physical status. The plan must be dynamic to take into account changes in the status of the psychiatric disorder and the patient's physical status. For example, a patient with Alzheimer's disease has progression to more severe symptoms that will make dental care most difficult in the later stages of the disorder. The patient with advanced dementia is often anxious, hostile, and uncooperative in the dental office. Complex dental procedures should be done, if at all, in such a patient before the disease has reached the advanced stage. Prosthetic appliances are misplaced, lost, or improperly worn. In advanced cases, removable prosthetic devices may need to be taken from the patient because of the danger of self-injury. Another example of the need for a flexible, dynamic treatment plan is for patients with major depression or bipolar disorder. During affective episodes, the emphasis should be on maintenance and prevention. Complex dental procedures should be performed only when the patient is in a stable condition

regarding the mood disorder. The treatment plan should minimize any stress of the dental visit. This can best be accomplished by effective patient management efforts and the use of nonverbal communication.[83]

The dental team should communicate to the patient and the family members a positive, hopeful attitude toward maintenance of the patient's oral health. The dental team should determine if the patient is legally able to make rational decisions. This should be discussed with the patient and a loved one. Treatment planning often will involve input and permission from a loved one so that decisions can be made.

The last aspect of the treatment plan deals with the selection of medications to be used in the dental treatment of the patient. Certain agents may need to be avoided, while others will require a reduction in their usual dosage. Medical consultation is suggested to establish the patient's current status, confirm the medications the patient is taking, identify any complications that may be present, and confirm dental medications and doses that will minimize possible drug interactions.[83]

Treatment planning for the patient with Alzheimer's disease demonstrates some of these principles. In a patient with mild dementia, good oral health should be quickly restored because of the progressive nature of the disease. Subsequent care should concentrate on preventing dental disease as the dementia progresses. A patient with moderate dementia may not be as amenable to dental treatment as the patient in earlier stages of the disease. For such patients, treatment consists of maintaining the dental status and minimizing any deterioration.[83] A patient with advanced dementia often is very difficult to treat and most likely will require sedation, short appointments, and noncomplex procedures.[83]

Bulimic patients should not be treatment planned for complex restorative procedures until the gorging and vomiting cycle has been broken. In a few cases, full coverage may be required in an attempt to save teeth. Once the patient is stable and wants to have the teeth with severe erosion restored this can be done. The dentist and patient need to be aware that relapse is common and complex restorations may fail with recurrence of chronic vomiting.

ORAL COMPLICATIONS AND MANIFESTATIONS

Antipsychotic drugs can cause agranulocytosis, leukopenia, or thrombocytopenia. Oral lesions associated with this reaction may occur. If the dentist notes oral lesions, fever, or sore throat in patients taking antipsychotic drugs, the patient must be evaluated for possible agranulocytosis.

Patients who are taking antipsychotic agents may develop muscular problems (dystonia, dyskinesia, or tardive dyskinesia) in the oral and facial regions. If the dentist first observes symptoms of dysfunction, the patient should be referred to the patient's physician for evaluation and management.[81]

Patients with psychiatric disorders may engage in painful self-destructive acts. Acts of orofacial mutilation such as eye gouging, pushing sharp objects into the ear canal, lip biting, cheek biting, tongue biting, burning of oral tissues with the tip of a cigarette, or mucosal injury with a sharp or blunt object have been reported.[60-62]

Patients with severe psychiatric disorders may not have the interest or the ability to care for themselves. Hence oral hygiene is poor and increased dental problems develop. Most of the medications used to treat psychiatric disorders contribute to increased dental problems in such patients because xerostomia is one of their main side effects. This may lead to an increased incidence of smooth surface caries and candidiasis. Stiefel et al[84] reported on the oral health of persons with and without chronic mental illness in community settings. Patients with chronic mental illness were found to have a significantly higher incidence of dry mouth, mucosal lesions, coronal smooth surface caries, and severity of plaque, and calculus buildup.

Patients with dementia often have oral injuries from falls and ulcerations of the tongue, cheeks, and alveolar mucosa from accidents with forks, spoons, or mastication.[74] They also may have poor oral hygiene with an increased incidence of periodontal disease, root and crown caries, missing teeth, attrition and abrasion of teeth, and migration of teeth. Edentulous patients misplace or lose their dentures and at times even attempt to wear the upper denture on the lower arch and vice versa.[73]

Patients with bulimia may develop severe erosion of the lingual and occlusal surfaces of their teeth. Severe erosion can cause increased tooth sensitivity to touch and cold temperature. Dental caries may be more prevalent in these patients. The amount of saliva produced may be decreased. Patients often complain of dry mouth. Patients with poor oral hygiene have increased periodontal disease. The parotid gland may be enlarged. Patients with anorexia nervosa may have decreased salivary flow, dry mouth, atrophic mucosa, and enlarged parotid gland.[76,79,85-87]

References

1. *Diagnostic and statistical manual of mental disorders* (DSM-IV) ed 4 Washington DC, 1994, American Psychiatric Association.

2. Association AP. DSM-IV Classification. In *Diagnostic and statistical manual of mental disorders—text revision* (DSM-IV-TR), 4 ed. Washington DC, 2000, American Psychiatric Association.

3. Goldberg RJ: *Practical guide to the care of the psychiatric patient,* St Louis, 1995, Mosby.

4. Kahn DA: Mood disorders. In Cutler JL, Marcus ER, editors: *Saunders text and review series: Psychiatry*, Philadelphia, 1999, WB Saunders.

5. Horwath E, Courinos F: Schizophrenia and other psychotic disorders. In Cutler JL, Marcus ER, editors: *Saunders text and review series: Psychiatry*. Philadelphia, 1999, WB Saunders.

6. Vogel LR, Muskin PR: Anxiety disorders. In Cutler JL, Marcus ER, editors: *Saunders text and review series: Psychiatry*. Philadelphia, 1999, WB Saunders.

7. Levin FR, Kleber HD: Alcohol and substance abuse disorders. In Cutler JL, Marcus ER, editors: *Saunders text and review series: Psychiatry*. Philadelphia, 1999, WB Saunders.

8. Reus VI: Psychiatric disorders. In Fauci AS et al, editors: *Harrison's principles of internal medicine*, ed 14, New York, 1998, McGraw-Hill.

9. Anxiety Disorders. In *Diagnostic and statistical manual of mental disorder–text revision* (DSM-IV-TR), ed 4, Washington DC, 2000, American Psychiatric Association.

10. Judd LL, Britton KT, Braff DL: Mental disorders. In Isselbacher KJ, Brauwald E et al, editors: *Harrison's principles of internal medicine*, ed 13, New York, 1994, McGraw-Hill.

11. Judd LL et al: Psychiatric disorders. In Wilson JD et al, editors: *Harrison's principles of internal medicine*, ed 12, New York, 1991, McGraw-Hill.

12. *Diagnostic and statistical manual of mental disorders*, ed 3, Washington DC, 1987, American Psychiatric Association.

13. Friedlander AH, Brill NQ: Dental management of patients with schizophrenia, *Spec Care Dent* 6(5):217-219, 1986.

14. Mood Disorders. In *Diagnostic and statistical manual of mental disorders–text revision* (DSM-IV-TR), ed 4, Washington DC, 2000, American Psychiatric Association.

15. Adelman SA, Scott ME: Depression. In Greene H et al, editors: *Clinical medicine*, ed 2, St Louis, 1996, Mosby.

16. Hyler SE: Somatoform and factitious disorders. In Cutler JL, Marcus ER, editors: *Saunders text and review series: Psychiatry*, Philadelphia, 1999, WB Saunders.

17. Somatoform Disorders. In *Diagnostic and statistical manual of mental disorders–text revision* (DSM-IV-TR), ed 4, Washington DC, 2000, American Psychiatric Association.

18. Substance-Related Disorders. In *Diagnostic and statistical manual of mental disorders–text revision* (DSM-IV-TR), ed 4, Washington DC, 2000, American Psychiatric Association.

19. Friedlander AH, Gorelick DA: Dental management of the cocaine addict, *Oral Surg* 65:45-48, 1988.

20. Balster RL: Drug and substance abuse. In Brody TM LJ, Minneman KP, Neu HC, editors: *Human pharmacology–molecular to clinical*, ed 2, St Louis, 1995, Mosby.

21. Schuckit MA: Alcoholism and drug dependency. In Fauci AS et al, editors: *Harrison's principles of internal medicine*, ed 14, New York, 1998, McGraw-Hill.

22. Mendelson JH, Mello NK: Cocaine and other commonly abused drugs. In Fauci AS et al, editors: *Harrison's principles of internal medicine*, ed 14, New York, 1998, McGraw-Hill.

23. Friedlander AH, Soloman DH: Dental management of the geriatric alcoholic patient, *Gerodontics* 4(1):23-27, 1988.

24. Holbrook JH: Nicotine Addiction. In Fauci AS et al, editors: *Harrison's principles of internal medicine*, ed 14, New York, 1998, McGraw-Hill.

25. Schizophrenia and other psychotic disorders. In *Diagnostic and statistical manual of mental disorders* ed 4, Washington DC, 2000, American Psychiatric Association.

26. Bennett JPJ: Antipsychotic agents. In Brody TM LJ, Minneman KP, Neu HC, editors: *Human pharmacology–molecular to clinical*, ed 2, St Louis, 1995, Mosby.

27. Bird TD: Alzheimer's disease and other primary dementias. In Fauci AS et al, editors: *Harrison's principles of internal medicine*, ed 14, New York, 1998, McGraw-Hill.

28. Feinstein RE: Cognitive and mental disorders due to general medical conditions. In Cutler JL, Marcus ER, editors: *Saunders text and review series: Psychiatry*, Philadelphia, 1999, WB Saunders.

29. Brown MM, Hachinski VC: Acute confusional states, amnesia, and dementia. In Isselbacher KJ et al, editors: *Harrison's principles of internal medicine*, ed 13, New York, 1994, McGraw-Hill.

30. Bolla LR, Filley CM, Palmer RM: Dementia DDx. Office diagnosis of the four major types of dementia, *Geriatrics* 55(1): 34-46, 2000.

31. Bazin N, Fremont P: Alzheimer type dementia: is early diagnosis significant?, *Presse Med* 29(15):871-875, 2000.

32. McKhann G et al: Clinical diagnosis of Alzheimer's disease: report of the NINCDS-ADRDA Work Group, *Neurology* 34:939-944, 1984.

33. Bachynsky J et al: Propentofylline treatment for Alzheimer disease and vascular dementia: an economic evaluation based on functional abilities, *Alzheimer Dis Assoc Disord* 14(2):102-111, 2000.

34. Antunono PG: Effectiveness and safety of velnacrine for the treatment of Alzheimer's disease: a double-blind placebo-controlled study, *Arch Intern Med* 155(Sep 11):1766-1773, 1995.

35. Devlin MJ. Eating Disorders. In: Cutler JL, Marcus ER, editors. *Saunders text and review series: Psychiatry*. Philadelphia, 1999, WB Saunders.

36. McSherry J. Eating Disorders; 1997, written personal communication.

37. Foster DW: Anorexia nervosa and bulimia nervosa. In Fauci AS et al, editors: *Harrison's principles of internal medicine*, ed 14, New York, 1998, McGraw-Hill.

38. Glorio R et al: Prevalence of cutaneous manifestations in 200 patients with eating disorders, *Int J Dermatol* 39(5):348-353, 2000.

39. Robertson C, Millar H: Hyperamylasemia in bulimia nervosa and hyperemesis gravidarum, *Int J Eat Disord* 26(2):223-227, 1999.

40. Metzger ED: Salivary gland enlargement and elevated serum amylase in bulimia nervosa, *Biol Psychiatry* 45(11):1520-1522, 1999.

41. Felpel LP: Psychopharmacology: antipsychotics and antidepressants. In Yagiela JA, Neidle EA, Dowd FJ, editors: *Pharmacology and therapeutics for dentistry*, ed 4, St Louis, 1998, Mosby.

42. Russakoff LM: Psychopharmacology. In Cutler JL, Marcus ER, editors: *Saunders text and review series: Psychiatry*. Philadelphia, 1999, WB Saunders.

43. Bennett JP: Drugs for affective (mood) disorders. In Brody TM LJ, Minneman KP, Neu HC, editors: *Human pharmacology–molecular to clinical*, ed 2 St. Louis, 1995, Mosby.

44. Pratt JP: Affective disorders. In Walker R, Edwards C, editors: *Clinical pharmacy and therapeutics*, ed 2, London, 1999, Churchill Livingston.

45. Parker NG, Brown CS: Citalopram in the treatment of depression, *Ann Pharmacother* 34(6):761-771, 2000.

46. Zanardi R et al: Venlafaxine versus fluvoxamine in the treatment of delusional depression: a pilot double-blind controlled study, *J Clin Psychiatry* 61(1):26-29, 2000.

47. Ashton CH: Insomnia and anxiety. In Walker R, Edwards C, editors: *Clinical pharmacy and therapeutics*, ed 2, London, 1999, Churchill Livingston.

48. Smith CM: Antianxiety drugs. In Smith CM, Reynard AM, editors: *Textbook of pharmacology*, Philadelphia, 1992, WB Saunders.

49. Winter JC: Antipsychotic drugs (antipsychotics). In Smith CM, Reynard AM, editors: *Textbook of pharmacology*, Philadelphia, 1992, WB Saunders.

50. Branford D: Schizophrenia. In Walker R, Edwards C, editors: *Clinical pharmacy and therapeutics*, ed 2, London, 1999, Churchill Livingston.

51. Black JL: Antipsychotic agents: a clinical update, *Mayo Clin Proc* 60:777-789, 1985.

52. Bloom SW: *The doctor and his patient: a sociological interpretation*, New York, 1963, Russell Sage.

53. Blum LH: Psychological aspects and the dentist-patient relationship, *NY State Dent J* 39:8-10, 1969.

54. Blum LH: Psychological aspects and the dentist-patient relationship, II, *NY State Dent J* 39:51-55, 1969.

55. Adelson H. The psychodynamics of the doctor-patient relationship. *NY State Dent J* 1970;36:95-103.

56. Caligor E: Psychological factors affecting medical conditions. In Cutler JL, Marcus ER, editors: *Saunders text and review series: Psychiatry*, Philadelphia, 1999, WB Saunders.

57. Friedlander AH, West LJ: Dental management of the patient with major depression, *Oral Surg Oral Med Oral Pathol* 71(5):573-578, 1991.

58. Roth JA: Drugs used in the treatment of mood disorders. In Smith CM, Reynard AM, editors: *Textbook of pharmacology*, Philadelphia, 1992, WB Saunders.

59. Friedlander AH et al: Dental management of the geriatric patient with major depression, *Special Care Dent* 13(6):249-253, 1993.

60. Brightman VJ: Oral symptoms without apparent physical abnormality. In Lynch MA, editor, *Burket's oral medicine, diagnosis and treatment*, ed 7, Philadelphia, 1977, JB Lippincott.

61. Mitchell RJ: Burket's oral medicine, diagnosis and treatment. Etiology of temporomandibular disorders, *Curr Opin Dent* 1:471-475, 1991.

62. Michels R, Schoenberg BB: Psychogenic disturbances. In: Zegarelli EV, editor: *Diagnosis of diseases of the mouth and jaws*, ed 2, Philadelphia,1978,Lea & Febiger.

63. Abel PW, Bockman CS: Drugs of Abuse. In Yagiela JA, Neidle EA, Dowd FJ, editors: *Pharmacology and therapeutics for dentistry*, ed 4, St Louis, 1998, Mosby.

64. Medical Educational Resources Program/Division of Continuing Education: *Guide to smoking cessation: for physicians and office staff in assisting patients*, 2000, Indiana Tobacco Control Center. http://iumeded.med.iupui.edu/tobacco/phys4a.htm

65. Glynn TJ, Manley MW: *How to help your patients stop smoking: a National Cancer Institute manual for physicians*, 1997, US Department of Health and Human Services, National Institutes of Health.

66. Haber J: Cigarette smoking: a major risk factor for periodontitis, *Compend Contin Educ Dent* 8:1002, 1994.

67. Holm G: Smoking as an additional risk for tooth loss, *J Periodontal* 65:996, 1994.

68. Cooper TM, Clayton RR: Stop smoking program using nicotine reduction therapy and behavior modification for heavy smokers, *J Am Dent Assoc* 118(1):47-51, 1989.

69. Hughes JR, Stead LF, Lancaster T: Antidepressants for smoking cessation (Cochrane Review). *Cochrane Database Syst Rev* 2000;4 Accession Numbers 11034670 Issue 4, pages CD000031.

70. West R, McNeill A, Raw M: Smoking cessation guidelines for health professionals: an update, *Thorax* 55(12):987-999, 2000.

71. Medical Educational Resources Program/Division of Continuing Education: *Characteristics of FDA approved smoking cessation pharmaceutical agents*, Indiana Tobacco Control Center; 2000. http://iumeded.med.iupui.edu/tobacco/natinfo.htm

72. Prochazka AV: New developments in smoking cessation, *Chest* 117(4 Suppl 1):169S-175S, 2000.

73. Steinberg BJ, Brown S: Dental treatment of the health compromised elderly: medical and psychological considerations, *Alpha Omegan* 79:34-41,1986

74. Friedlander AH, Jarvik LF: The dental management of the patient with dementia, *Oral Surg* 64:549-553, 1987.

75. Magarian GJ, Middaugh DA, Linz DH: Hyperventilation syndrome: a diagnosis begging for recognition, *JAMA* 155:732-740, 1983.

76. Milosevic A, Brodie DA, Slade PD: Dental erosion, oral hygiene, and nutrition in eating disorders, *Int J Eat Disord* 21(2):195-199, 1997.

77. Milosevic A: Eating disorders and the dentist, *Br Dent J* 186 (3):109-113, 1999.

78. Scheutzel P: Etiology of dental erosion–intrinsic factors, *Eur J Oral Sci* 104(2|Pt 2|):178-90,1996.

79. Roberts MW, Li SH: Oral findings in anorexia nervosa and bulimia nervosa: a study of 47 cases, *J Am Dent Assoc* 115(3):407-410, 1987.

80. Feinstein RE: Suicide and violence. In Cutler JL, Marcus ER, editors: *Saunders text and review series: Psychiatry*, Philadelphia, 1999, WB Saunders.

81. Judd L: The therapeutic use of psychotropic medications. In Wilson JD et al, editors: *Harrison's principles of internal medicine*, ed 12, New York, 1991, McGraw-Hill.

82. VanDer Bijl P: Benzodiazepines in dentistry: a review, *Compendium* 13(1):46-49, 1992.

83. Niessen L, Jones JA: Professional dental care for patients with dementia, *Gerodontology* 6(2):67-71,1987.

84. Stiefel DJ et al: A comparison of oral health of persons with and without chronic mental illness in community settings, *Spec Care Dent* 10(1):6-12, 1990.

85. Ohrn R, Enzell K, Angmar-Mansson B: Oral status of 81 subjects with eating disorders, *Eur J Oral Sci* 107(3):157-163, 1999.

86. Rytomaa I et al: Bulimia and tooth erosion, *Acta Odontol Scand* 56(1):36-40, 1998.

87. Robb ND, Smith BG, Geidrys-Leeper E: The distribution of erosion in the dentitions of patients with eating disorders, *Br Dent J* 178(5):171-5, 1995.

Arthritic Diseases

24

CHAPTER

*A*rthritis is a nonspecific term that means inflammation of the joints. Arthritic disease encompasses a group of disorders of the rheumatic diseases that affect bones, joints, and muscles. The term *arthritis* often is used interchangeably by laypersons with the term *rheumatism*, denoting aches, pains, and stiffness in the joints and muscles. More than 100 arthritic (or rheumatic) diseases affect different parts of the body. Some of the more common types include rheumatoid arthritis, osteoarthritis, systemic lupus erythematosus, juvenile arthritis, scleroderma, Sjögren's syndrome, gout, ankylosing spondylitis, Lyme disease, fibromyalgia, and psoriatic arthritis.

Arthritic diseases have significant personal and economic impact. According to the Arthritis Foundation,[1] more than 37 million Americans suffer from the various forms of arthritis, and more than 7 million of these are disabled. In terms of its overall economic impact, arthritis costs the American economy more than $14 billion annually, with a loss of 26.6 million workdays per year.

Although arthritis is a large group of important diseases, this chapter is limited to a discussion of rheumatoid arthritis, osteoarthritis, systemic lupus erythematosus, Lyme disease and Sjögren's syndrome, which are among the most common forms encountered and can serve as models for the other forms.

■ RHEUMATOID ARTHRITIS ■

DEFINITION

INCIDENCE AND PREVALENCE

Rheumatoid arthritis (RA) is an autoimmune disease of unknown etiology characterized by symmetric inflammation of joints, especially the hands, feet, and knees. The

severity of the disease varies widely from patient to patient and from time to time in the same patient. Determination of prevalence is somewhat difficult because of lack of well-defined markers of the disease; however, estimates of prevalence range from 1% to 2% of the population.[1,2] The disease onset is usually between ages 35 and 50 years and is more prevalent in women than men by a 3:1 ratio. This gender differentiation implies involvement of sex hormones in the susceptibility and sensitivity of the disease. Other factors, such as socioeconomic status, education, and psychosocial stress, have been suggested to play predisposing roles.[3]

ETIOLOGY

The cause of RA is unknown; however, evidence seems to implicate an interrelationship of infectious agents, genetics, and autoimmunity. A theory suggests that a viral agent alters the immune system in a genetically predisposed individual and leads to destruction of synovial tissues.[1,2] Many persons who develop RA have a genetic predisposition in the form of a tissue marker called HLA-DR4; however, not everyone with this tissue type develops the disease. Some questions have been raised as to whether vitamins or foods are implicated in RA. Currently, circumstantial evidence exists that food could have a role in the etiology and therapy of RA; however, present studies are of limited value and further research is warranted.[4]

PATHOPHYSIOLOGY AND COMPLICATIONS

With RA, the fundamental abnormality is microvascular endothelial cell activation and injury.[2] Primary changes occur in the synovium, which is the inner lining of the joint capsule. Edema of the synovium occurs, followed by thickening and folding. This excessive tissue, com-

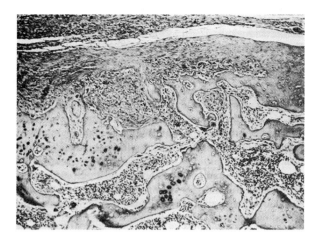

Fig. 24-1 The joint surface *(top)* has lost its cartilage and consists of granulation tissue with scar tissue. Subchondral bone shows degenerative changes and areas of necrosis. (Courtesy A. Golden, Lexington, Ky.)

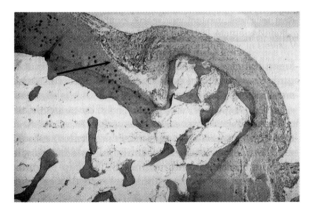

Fig. 24-2 A micrograph of a pannus resulting from severe synovitis in rheumatoid arthritis. The pannus is eroding articular cartilage and bone *(arrow)*. (Courtesy Richard Estensen, Minneapolis, Minn.)

posed of proliferative and invasive granulation tissue, is referred to as *pannus* (Fig. 24-1). In addition, a marked infiltration of lymphocytes and plasma cells into the capsule occurs. Eventually, granulation tissue covers the articular surfaces and destroys the cartilage and subchondral bone through enzymatic activity (Fig. 24-2). This process also extends to the capsule and ligaments, causing distention and rupture. New bone or fibrous tissue then is deposited, resulting in fusion or loss of mobility.[5]

A likely sequence of events begins with a synovitis that stimulates immunoglobulin G (IgG) antibodies. These antibodies form antigenic aggregates in the joint space and lead to the production of rheumatoid factor (autoantibodies). Rheumatoid factor then complexes with IgG complement and produces an inflammatory reaction that injures the joint space.[5]

An associated finding in 20% of patients with RA is the presence of subcutaneous nodules, commonly found around the elbow and finger joints.[6] These nodules are thought to arise from the same antigen-antibody complex that is found in the joint. Vasculitis confined to small- and medium-sized vessels also may occur and is probably caused by the same complexing.[7]

The course and severity of RA are unpredictable but characterized by remissions and exacerbations. The most progressive period of the disease occurs during the earlier years and thereafter slows. Approximately 10% of patients will undergo permanent remission within the first 2 years.[8,9] Another 10% will experience relentless crippling, leading to nearly complete disability.[31] For the majority of patients, however, the disease is a sustained, lifelong problem that can be controlled or modified to allow a normal or nearly normal life.

The life expectancy of persons with severe RA is shortened by 10 to 15 years. This increased mortality rate usually is attributed to infection, pulmonary and renal disease, and gastrointestinal bleeding.[10]

Many complications may accompany RA. Included among these are digital gangrene, skin ulcers, muscle atrophy, keratoconjunctivitis sicca (Sjögren's syndrome), temporomandibular joint (TMJ) involvement, pulmonary interstitial fibrosis, pericarditis, amyloidosis, anemia, thrombocytopenia, neutropenia, and splenomegaly (Felty's syndrome).[11]

CLINICAL PRESENTATION

SIGNS AND SYMPTOMS

The usual onset of RA is gradual and subtle (Table 24-1), and is commonly preceded by a prodromal phase of general fatigue and weakness with joint and muscle aches. Characteristically, these symptoms come and go over varying periods. Then painful joint swelling, especially of the hands and feet, occurs in several joints and progresses to other joints in a symmetric fashion. Joint involvement persists and gradually progresses to immobility, contractures, subluxation, deviation, and other deformities. Characteristic features include pain in the affected joints aggravated by

movement, generalized joint stiffness after inactivity, and morning stiffness of greater than 1 hour's duration.[11] The joints most commonly affected are fingers, wrists, feet, ankles, knees, and elbows. Multiple joint changes in the hands are seen and include a symmetric spindle-shaped swelling of the proximal interphalangeal (PIP) joints, with dorsal swelling and characteristic volar subluxation of the metacarpophalangeal (MCP) joint[12] (Fig. 24-3). The TMJ is reported to be involved in up to 75% of patients.[13]

Extraarticular manifestations include rheumatoid nodules, vasculitis, skin ulcers, Sjögren's syndrome, interstitial lung disease, pericarditis, C-spine instability, entrapment neuropathies, and ischemic neuropathies.[12] The American Rheumatism Association[14] has developed revised criteria for the diagnosis and classification of RA to be used in clinical trials and epidemiologic studies (Box 24-1). These criteria have high specificity (89%) and sensitivity (91% to 94%) compared with controls when used to classify patients with RA. For the diagnosis of RA to be made, 4 of 7 criteria must be present.

LABORATORY FINDINGS

No laboratory tests exist that are pathognomonic or diagnostic of RA, although they are used in conjunction with clinical findings to confirm the diagnosis. Laboratory findings most commonly seen in RA include an increased erythrocyte sedimentation rate, the presence of C-reactive protein, positive rheumatoid factor in 85% of affected patients, and a hypochromic-microcytic anemia. In patients with Felty's syndrome (RA with splenomegaly) a marked neutropenia may be present.[11,12]

TABLE **24-1**

Comparison of Rheumatoid Arthritis and Osteoarthritis

Rheumatoid Arthritis	Osteoarthritis
Multiple symmetric joint involvement	Usually one or two joints (or groups) involved
Significant joint inflammation	Joint pain usually without inflammation
Morning joint stiffness longer than 1 hour	Morning joint stiffness of less than 15 minutes
Symmetric spindle-shaped swelling of proximal interphalangeal joints and volar subluxation of metacarpophalangeal joints and Bouchard's nodes of proximal interphalangeal joints	Heberden's nodes of distal interphalangeal joints
Systemic manifestations (fatigue, weakness, malaise)	No systemic involvement

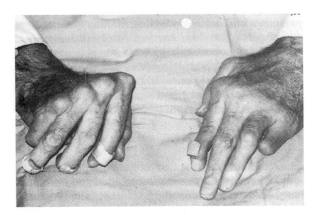

Fig. 24-3 Hands of a patient with severe rheumatoid arthritis. Note effects of digital gangrene.

BOX **24-1**

Criteria for the Diagnosis of Rheumatoid Arthritis*

Morning stiffness
Arthritis of three or more joint areas
Arthritis of hand joints
Symmetric arthritis
Rheumatoid nodules
Serum rheumatoid factor
Radiographic changes

*At least four must be present to make a diagnosis of RA. From Arnett FC, Edworthy SM, Bloch DA, et al: *Arthitis Rheum* 31:315-324, 1988.

MEDICAL MANAGEMENT

The treatment of RA is, by necessity, palliative because no cure as yet exists for the disease. Treatment goals are to reduce joint inflammation and swelling, relieve pain and stiffness, and facilitate and encourage normal function. These goals are accomplished by a basic treatment program consisting of patient education, rest, exercise, physical therapy, and aspirin or other nonsteroidal antiinflammatory drugs (NSAIDs).[15] The NSAIDs, especially aspirin, constitute the cornerstone of treatment. Aspirin may be prescribed in large doses on an individual basis. A common approach is to start a patient on three 5-grain tablets four times a day then adjust the dosage based on patient response.[16] The most common sign of aspirin toxicity is tinnitus. Should this occur, dosage is decreased. In addition to aspirin, many NSAIDs are available for use. Some of the more common of these include the new COX-2 inhibitors: rofecoxib (Vioxx) and celecoxib (Celebrex), ibuprofen (Motrin, Advil, Rufen, Nuprin), naproxen (Naprosyn, Aleve), sulindac (Clinoril), tolmetin (Tolectin), fenoprofen (Nalfon), piroxicam (Feldene), diclofenac (Voltaren), flurbiprofen (Ansaid), diflunisal (Dolobid), etodolac (Lodine), and nabumetone (Relafen). All the NSAIDs can cause a qualitative

platelet defect that may result in prolonged bleeding, especially in high doses. Aspirin's effects are irreversible for the life of the platelet (10 to 12 days), and thus this effect remains until new platelets have replaced the old. The effect of the other NSAIDs on platelets is reversible and lasts only as long as the drug is present in the plasma (see Chapter 19).

In addition to NSAIDs, a variety of other drugs are used to treat RA (Table 24-2). Many of these drugs can cause blood dyscrasias that can lead to increased infections, delayed healing, and prolonged bleeding.

Disease-modifying antirheumatic drugs (DMARDs) are commonly employed in the treatment of RA. There are several groups of these which each have multiple drugs (i.e., antimalarials, penicillamine, gold compounds, etc.) (see Table 24-2).

Gold compounds may be effective in decreasing inflammation and retarding the progress of the disease, but the incidence of toxicity is high, and dermatitis with mucosal ulceration, proteinuria, neutropenia, and thrombocytopenia may result.[7] Antimalarial drugs (chloroquine, hydroxychloroquine) are also used to treat RA, usually in combination with aspirin or corticosteroids. Side effects include severe eye damage and blue-black intraoral pigmentation.[15] Penicillamine also

TABLE **24-2**

Drugs Used in the Management of Rheumatoid Arthritis and Systemic Lupus Erythematosus

Generic Name (Trade Name)	Dental and Oral Considerations
Salicylates Aspirin, Ascriptin, Bufferin, Anacin, Ectotrin, Empirin	Prolonged bleeding but not usually clinically significant
Nonsteroidal Antiinflammatory Drugs Ibuprofen, Fenoprofen, Indomethacin, Naproxen Meclofenamate, Piroxicam, Sulindac, Tolmetin Diclofenac, Flurbiprofen, Diflunisal, Etodolac Nabumetone, Motrin, Nalfon, Indocin, Feldene Naprosyn, Meclomen, Clinoril, Tolectin Voltaren, Ansaid, Dolobid, Lodine, Relafen, Oxaprozin, Ketoralac	Prolonged bleeding, but not usually clinically significant; oral ulceration, stomatitis
COX-2 Inhibitors Celecoxib Rofecoxib	None
TNF-Alpha Inhibitors Etanercept Infliximab	None

Continued

TABLE 24-2

Drugs Used in the Management of Rheumatoid Arthritis and Systemic Lupus Erythematosus—cont'd

Generic Name (Trade Name)	Dental and Oral Considerations
Injectible Glucocorticoids	
Triamcinolone hexacetonide	Adrenal suppression, masking of oral infection, impaired healing
Triamcinolone acetonide	
Prednisolone tebutate	
Methylprednisolone acetate	
Dexamethasone acetate	
Hydrocortisone acetate	
Triamcinolone diacetate	
Betamethasone sodium phosphate and acetate	
Dexamethasone sodium phosphate	
Prednisolone sodium phosphate	
Systemic Glucocorticoids	
Hydrocortisone, Cortisone, Prednisone	Adrenal suppression, masking of oral infection, impaired healing
Prednisolone, Dexamethasone	
Methylprednisolone	
(Deltasone, Meticorten, Orasone, Articulose-50, Delta-Cortef, Medrol)	
Disease-Modifying Antirheumatic Drugs	
Anti-malarial agents	
Hydroxychloroquine, Quinine	
Chloroquine (Plaquenil)	
Penicillamine	Increased infections, delayed healing, prolonged bleeding, oral
(Cuprimine, Depen)	ulcerations
Gold compounds	Increased infections, delayed healing, prolonged bleeding,
Gold sodium thiomalate	glossitis, stomatitis
(Auranofin, Aurothioglucose, Myochrysine Ridaura, Solganal)	
Aralen	Increased infections, delayed healing, prolonged bleeding, intraoral pigementation
Sulfasalazine	Increased infections, delayed healing, prolonged bleeding
Azulfidine	
Immunosuppressives	
Azathioprine, Cyclophosphamide	
Methotrexate, Cyclosporine, Chloambucil	Increased infections, delayed healing, prolonged bleeding,
(Imuran, Cytoxan, Rheumatrex)	stomatitis

is used in the treatment of RA. Both the antimalarials and penicillamine, however, are associated with significant toxicity, which limits their use. Corticosteroids (prednisone, prednisolone) frequently are useful in controlling acute symptoms; however, because of multiple side effects, long-term usage is avoided if possible. One of the more potentially significant side effects is adrenal suppression (see Chapter 15).

In cases of refractory disease, immunosuppressive therapy has been used successfully and may include methotrexate, cyclophosphamide, or azathioprine. These drugs are associated with significant side effects including severe oral ulcerations. Methotrexate also can result in hepatic toxicity. More recently the COX-2 inhibitors and TNF-alpha inhibitors have proven to also be effective in relieving the symptoms of RA (see Table 24-2).

The COX-2 inhibitors (celecoxib [Celebrex] and rofe-coxib [Vioxx]) recently have shown considerable efficacy in inflammatory pain relief in rheumatoid arthritis. Standard NSAIDs inhibit both cyclooxygenases (COX-1 and COX-2): the enzymes involved in the production of prostaglandins. Whereas COX-2 is active on demand, COX-1 is critical for normal cellular function. A complication from the use of NSAIDs for arthritis (and other conditions) is the side effect of gastrointestinal distress. Since COX-2 inhibitors are selective for that enzyme, they produce less adverse side effects on the gastrointestinal system.

In two recent studies reported in the *New England Journal of Medicine*,[17,18] the biological agents etanercept and infliximab, both TNF-alpha inhibitors, were shown to be very effective for treating early rheumatoid arthritis when compared with the gold standard, methotrexate. Although costly and difficult to administer (intravenous route), etanercept (Enbrel, Immunex, etc.) was shown to reduce significantly RA symptoms and slow joint damage compared with methotrexate.[17] Infliximab (costly and somewhat difficult to administer by subcutaneous injection) likewise when used with methotrexate significantly reduced RA symptoms and slowed joint damage compared with methotrexate therapy alone.[18] Although these biological agents are novel and show great promise, their widespread use for RA therapy presently is limited.

Surgical management of severely deformed or dysfunctional joints often is necessary and may involve a variety of procedures, including arthroplasty, reconstruction, synovectomy, and total joint replacement.

DENTAL MANAGEMENT

MEDICAL CONSIDERATIONS

Because patients may have multiple joint involvement with varying degrees of pain and immobility, dental appointments should be kept as short as possible, and the patient should be allowed to make frequent position changes as needed (Box 24-2). The patient also may be more comfortable in a sitting or semisupine position as opposed to a supine one. Physical supports, such as a pillow or rolled towel, may be needed to provide support for deformed limbs, joints, or neck.

The most significant complications associated with RA are drug related (see Table 24-2). Aspirin and other NSAIDs can interfere with platelet function and cause prolonged bleeding; however, this generally is not found to be a significant clinical problem.[19,20] A patient who is taking both aspirin and a corticosteroid may be more of a concern, and a pretreatment bleeding time may be ad-

---

BOX 24-2

Dental Management of the Patient with Rheumatoid Arthritis

1. Short appointments
2. Ensure physical comfort
   a. Frequent position changes
   b. Comfortable chair position
   c. Physical supports as needed (pillows, towels, etc.)
3. Drug considerations
   a. Aspirin and NSAIDs—bleeding may be increased but usually is not clinically significant
   b. Gold salts, penicillamine, antimalarials, immunosuppressives—get complete blood cell count with differential; bleeding time; treat stomatitis symptomatically
   c. Corticosteroids—adrenal suppression possible
4. Joint prosthesis—prophylactic antibiotics are suggested by some authors (cephalosporin or clindamycin)
5. Technical treatment modification dictated by patient's disabilities
6. Temporomandibular joint pain/dysfunction—sudden occlusal changes possible
   a. Decrease jaw function
   b. Soft, nonchallenging diet
   c. Moist heat or ice to face/jaw
   d. Medication as directed by physician
   e. Occlusal appliance to decrease joint loading
   f. Consideration of surgery for persistent pain or dysfunction

---

visable. Even if the bleeding time is moderately prolonged (up to 20 minutes), the risk is not great, and patients usually can be treated, as long as curettage or surgery is performed conservatively in small segments with attention to good techniques.[20] Bleeding times greater than 20 minutes should be discussed with the physician (see Chapter 19).

Patients taking gold salts, penicillamine, sulfasalazine, or immunosuppressives are susceptible to bone marrow suppression that can result in anemia, agranulocytosis, and thrombocytopenia. As a rule, these patients should be followed closely by their physician to detect this problem. If a patient has not had recent laboratory tests, ordering a complete blood cell count with a differential white blood cell count and bleeding time is advised. Abnormal results should be discussed with the

physician. If corticosteroids are used for prolonged periods, the potential for adrenal suppression exists. Management of this problem is discussed in Chapter 15. Corticosteriods also may induce a number of side effects. These are presented in Table 24-2.

Prosthetic Joints

A potential long-term complication of chronic rheumatoid arthritis is the ultimate destruction of the particular joint structures to the degree that the joint must be replaced with synthetic materials. Patients with prosthetic joints often are encountered in dental practice, and when that occurs, the question arises concerning the need for antibiotic prophylaxis to prevent infection of the prosthesis. This is a legitimate concern; however, the issue is whether bacteremias from dental procedures can cause prosthetic joint infections (PJI). This issue has been debated for many years with little scientific data upon which to base decisions. Recommendations to place dental patients on prophylactic antibiotics have been made empirically by orthopedic surgeons, in spite of a lack of evidence that dentally induced bacteremias cause PJI.

While reports in the literature weakly associate PJI with dentally induced bacteremias, authors have questioned the validity of these reports.[21] Examining the microbiology of PJI is instructive. Pallasch and Slots[22] reviewed the cumulative data from 281 isolates from 6 clinical studies of PJI caused by hematogenous bacterial spread. They found that two thirds of the PJI were the result of staphylococci, only 4.9% caused by *viridans streptococci* of possible oral origin, and 2.1% caused by Peptostreptococcus species. This suggests either wound contamination or skin infections as the source of the vast majority of the infections. Even the few cases of PJI caused by presumably oral bacteria more likely were the result of physiologically occurring bacteremias or bacteremias resulting from acute or chronic infection rather than from being related to invasive dental procedures.[21]

A study often cited as evidence of hematogenous PJI involves an animal model demonstrating that PJI can occur as a result of blood-borne bacteria. To produce PJI, large inocula of staphylococci were injected into a group of rabbits, creating such an overwhelming septicemia that it resulted in the almost immediate death of one third of the animals. It also caused death within a few days of another one third and with subsequently 10 animals surviving developing PJI. This model is not applicable to usual clinical situations and thus does not provide support for any conclusion relating normal bacteremias with PJI. Unfortunately, however, many orthopedic surgeons have persisted in requesting that their patients receive antibiotic prophylaxis for dental procedures.[21]

BOX 24-3

High-Risk Patients with Prosthetic Joints

Immunocompromised/Immunosuppressed Patients

Inflammatory arthropathies: rheumatoid arthritis, systemic lupus erythematosis disease-, drug- or radiation-induced immunosuppression

Other Patients

Insulin-dependent (Type 1) diabetes
First 2 years following joint replacement
Previous prosthetic joint infections
Malnourishment
Hemophilia

In an effort to clarify the issue, an advisory statement made in 1997 jointly by the American Dental Association and the American Academy of Orthopedic Surgeons was published. This advisory statement is presented and debated in an article by Little.[21] This advisory statement concluded that scientific evidence does not support the need for antibiotic prophylaxis for dental procedures to prevent PJI. It further stated that antibiotic prophylaxis is not indicated for dental patients with pins, plates, and screws, nor is it routinely indicated for most patients with total joint replacement. The statement did indicate, however, that antibiotic prophylaxis should be considered for some "high risk" patients who are at increased risk for infection and undergoing dental procedures likely to cause significant bleeding (Box 24-3). No evidence exists that even these "higher risk" patients are at increased risk from dentally induced bacteremias, and in fact the microbiology of PJI in them is the same as for other patients with PJI.[21] A more appropriate interpretation is that these patients are at increased risk for PJI from the usual sources such as wound contamination and acute infection from distant sites. The advisory statement also is clear that the final decision on whether or not to provide antibiotic prophylaxis lies with the dentist who must weigh perceived potential benefits against the risks. The advisory statement provides suggested antibiotic regimens should the practitioner elect to provide antibiotic prophylaxis (Box 24-4). The opinion of the authors of this is book is that no patient with a prosthetic joint requires antibiotic prophylaxis to prevent PJI secondary to a dentally induced bacteremia.[22,23] However, if by informed consent the patient selects to be prophylaxed, then one of the regimens shown in Box 24-4 can be utilized.

BOX 24-4

BOX 24-4

Suggested Antibiotic Prophylaxis Regimens

Patients Not Allergic to Penicillin: Cephalexin, Cephadine or Amoxicillin
2 grams orally 1 hour before dental procedure

Patients Not Allergic to Penicillin and Unable to Take Oral Medications: Cephazolin or Ampicillin
Cefazolin 1 gram or ampicillin 2 grams intramuscularly or intravenously 1 hour before dental procedure

Patients Allergic to Penicillin: Clindamycin
600 mg orally 1 hour before the dental procedure

Patients Allergic to Penicillin and Unable to Take Oral Medications: Clindamycin
600 mg IV 1 hour before dental procedures

TREATMENT PLANNING MODIFICATIONS

Treatment planning modifications are dictated by the patient's physical disabilities. An individual with marked systemic disability or limited or painful jaw function due to TMJ involvement should not be subjected to prolonged or extensive treatment, such as complicated crown and bridge procedures. If replacement of missing teeth is desired, consideration should be given to a removable prosthesis because of the decreased chair time needed for mouth preparation and the ease of cleansability of the appliance. If a fixed prosthesis is desired, ease of cleansability must be a significant factor in design. Unpredictable, progressive, or abrupt occlusion changes are possible because of erosion of the condylar head. Therefore, the dentist and patient should take these potential occlusal changes into consideration when considering significant reconstructive treatment.

Disabled patients may have significant difficulty cleaning their teeth. Cleaning aids such as floss holders, toothpicks, irrigating devices, and mechanical toothbrushes may be recommended. Manual toothbrushes can be modified by placing acrylic or a rubber ball on the handle to improve the grip.

RA is a progressive disease that ultimately may lead to severe disability and crippling in some patients, which can make providing dental care difficult. Therefore, the dentist should be aggressive in providing ongoing preventive care and should attempt to identify and treat or eliminate potential problems before the disease progresses.

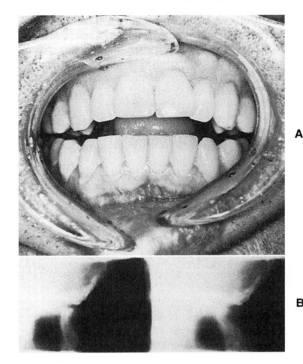

Fig. 24-4 **A,** Anterior open bite deformity in a patient with rheumatoid arthritis of the temporomandibular joints. Contact is present only on the second molars. **B,** Radiograph of the temporomandibular joints of this patient demonstrates extreme destruction and deformity of the condylar heads.

ORAL COMPLICATIONS AND MANIFESTATIONS

The most significant complication of the oral and maxillofacial complex in RA is TMJ involvement found in up to 45% to 75% of patients with RA.[13,24] This may present as bilateral preauricular pain, tenderness, swelling, stiffness, and decreased mobility of the TMJs, or it may be asymptomatic. periods of remission and exacerbation may occur as with other joint involvement. Fibrosis or bony ankylosis can occur. Clinically, patients may present with tenderness over the lateral pole of the condyle, crepitus, limited opening, and radiographic evidence of structural change. Radiographic changes initially may show increased joint space. Later these changes are primarily erosive and can involve both the condyles and fossa.

A particularly disturbing event is the development of an anterior open bite caused by the destruction of the condylar heads and the loss of condylar height (Fig. 24-4). This sudden retrognathia and anterior open bite can be

severe and has been reported to cause obstructive sleep apnea.[25,26] Although palliative treatment such as interocclusal splints, physical therapy, and medication may prove to be helpful, surgical intervention often becomes necessary to decrease pain, improve appearance, or restore function.

An additional complication that may be seen in patients with RA is a severe stomatitis occurring after the administration of drugs such as gold compounds, penicillamine, or immunosuppressives. This may be an indication of drug toxicity and should be reported to the physician. Palliative treatment for this problem may include bland mouth rinses, diphenhydramine elixir, or a topical emollient such as Orabase (see Appendix B).

■ OSTEOARTHRITIS ■

DEFINITION

INCIDENCE AND PREVALENCE

Osteoarthritis (OA, degenerative joint disease) is another of the rheumatic diseases and is the most common form of arthritis.[1,27] Almost everyone past the age of 60 years will have OA to some degree. Most people will be minimally symptomatic; however, approximately 17 million people in the United States have OA to the extent that it results in pain. OA is the leading cause of disability among the elderly.[1,27]

OA is considered a regional disease and usually affects often-used joints such as hips, knees, feet, spine, and hands. The TMJ also is affected. Women are afflicted twice as often as men; however, men are afflicted at an earlier age. It is generally a disease of middle to older age, first appearing after the age of 40. Racial differences exist for both prevalence of OA and the pattern of joint involvement.[28]

ETIOLOGY

The exact cause of OA is not known and has been thought to be the end result of normal wear and tear on joints over a long period. However, other factors are now thought to be of significance. Preexisting structural joint abnormalities, intrinsic aging, metabolic factors, genetic predisposition, obesity leading to overloaded joints, and macrotrauma or microtrauma are considered causative or contributory factors in the origin of the disease.

PATHOPHYSIOLOGY AND COMPLICATIONS

In the early stages of the disease, the articular cartilage actually becomes thicker than normal, with an in-

crease in water content and the synthesis of proteoglycans.[29] This reflects a repair effort by the condrocytes and may last for several years. Ultimately, however, the joint surface thins, proteoglycan concentration decreases, leading to a softening of the cartilage.[28] Progressive splitting and abrasion of cartilage down to the subchondral bone occurs. The exposed bone becomes polished and sclerotic, resembling ivory (eburnation). Some resurfacing with cartilage may occur if the disorder is arrested or stabilized. New bone forms at the margin of articular cartilage, in the nonweightbearing part of the joint, creating osteophytes (or spurs), often covered by cartilage, that augment the degree of deformity.[5]

In contrast to RA, OA has a more favorable prognosis and less serious complications, depending on the joint or joints involved. The two most important complications with osteoarthritis are pain and disability. Although RA is a more serious disease, OA has a thirtyfold greater economic impact, resulting in 68 million lost work days per year compared with 2 million for RA.[30] Conservative treatment often can retard the progress of the disease; however, surgery may be required to restore function and decrease pain.

CLINICAL PRESENTATION

SIGNS AND SYMPTOMS

The primary symptom of OA is pain localized to one or two joints (see Table 24-1). The pain is described as a dull ache accompanied by stiffness typically that is worse in the morning or after a period of inactivity. The pain and stiffness usually last 15 minutes or less.[33] Joint noises or grinding sounds (crepitus) may be detected with movement. Redness and swelling usually are not associated with OA.

The most common sign of OA is a painless bony growth on the medial and lateral aspects of the distal interphalangeal joints called Heberden's nodes. When these enlargements occur on the distal interphalangeal joints, they are called Bouchard's nodes (Fig. 24-5). On occasion, some pain may be associated with these nodes.

Depending on which joint or group of joints is involved, patients may experience varying degrees of incapacitation. Hip and knee joints are particularly troublesome and are a common source of disability.

A form of OA called primary generalized osteoarthritis is characterized by involvement of three or more joints or groups of joints. It appears most often in women, and affects hands, knees, hips, and spine.[31]

Radiographic signs of OA include narrowing of the joint space, articular surface irregularities and remodelings, and

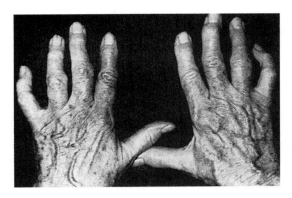

Fig. 24-5 Heberden's nodes and Bouchard's nodes in osteoarthritis.

osteophytes or spurs. In addition, subchondral sclerosis (eburnation) and ankylosis may be seen.[31] Symptoms often are not well correlated with radiographic signs.

LABORATORY FINDINGS

Laboratory findings in OA are essentially unremarkable. The erythrocyte sedimentation rate usually is normal, except for a mild elevation in primary generalized cases.

MEDICAL MANAGEMENT

The management of OA is palliative. Drug therapy basically is limited to analgesics. Acetaminophen frequently is effective in the management of OA and is recommended as a first-line drug.[16] Aspirin or NSAIDs also are commonly employed when acetaminophen is not effective. Narcotic analgesics are generally only used for acute flares for short periods. Intraarticular steroid injections may be used for acute flares for short periods. Intraarticular steroid injections may be used intermittently to reduce acute pain and inflammation. Patient education, physical therapy, mild exercise, weight reduction, and joint protection are all important aspects of management. Surgery may be required to improve function or for the relief of pain.

DENTAL MANAGEMENT

MEDICAL CONSIDERATIONS

Depending on which joints are involved, patients may not be comfortable in a supine position in the dental chair. Consideration should be given to providing a more

---

BOX 24-5

Dental Management of the Patient with Osteoarthritis

1. Short appointments
2. Physical comfort of patient
   a. Frequent position change
   b. Comfortable chair position
   c. Physical supports as needed (pillow, towel, etc.)
   d. Drug considerations
3. Aspirin and NSAIDs—bleeding may be increased but usually is not clinically significant
4. Joint prosthesis-generally prophylactic antibiotics are not required unless diabetes mellitus or immunosuppressed; if so, use cephalosporin or clindamycin
5. Technical treatment modifications dictated
6. TMJ pain/dysfunction usually self-limiting
   a. Painless jaw function encouraged
   b. Soft, nonchallenging diet
   c. Moist heat or ice to face/jaw
   d. Acetaminophen, aspirin, or NSAIDs for analgesia
   e. Occlusal appliance to decrease joint loading
   f. Surgery consideration for persistent pain or dysfunction

---

upright chair position, using neck, back, and leg supports, and the scheduling of short appointments (Box 24-5). Decreased platelet function because of large doses of aspirin or other NSAIDs can lead to prolonged bleeding, but this is generally not a clinically significant problem.[19,20] A pretreatment platelet function test or bleeding time can be obtained if desired, however. Elevated results of 15 to 20 minutes do not pose a significant risk as long as procedures that result in bleeding are kept to a minimum and other bleeding problems are not present[20] (see Chapter 19). Grossly abnormal bleeding times (more than 20 minutes) should be discussed with the physician.

Adrenal suppression generally is not a concern with occasional intra-articular injections of steroids. Patients with OA who have a joint prosthesis usually will not require antibiotic prophylaxis for dental treatment unless a concomitant condition exists such as diabetes mellitus, or the patient is otherwise immune suppressed.[37] If that is the case, consideration of antimicrobial prophylaxis with cephalosporin or clindamycin as the drugs of choice is recommended.

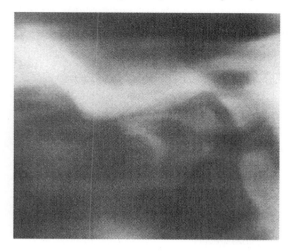

Fig. 24-6 Osteoarthritic changes in the temporomandibular joint.

TREATMENT PLANNING MODIFICATIONS

As with RA, the technical modifications of dental treatment for OA are dictated by a patient's disabilities. For instance, severe disabilities of hip, knee, or other joint, or TMJ involvement may prevent lengthy appointments; therefore, extensive treatment such as reconstruction or a long surgical procedure may not be appropriate. Patients with hand disabilities may have difficulty cleaning their teeth, and aids such as floss holders or electric toothbrushes may be helpful. Modified toothbrush handles also are recommended to facilitate cleaning.

ORAL COMPLICATIONS AND MANIFESTATIONS

The TMJ may be affected with OA and may constitute a problem for the patient. As would be expected, most people over age 40 years show some degree of histologic and radiographic changes in their TMJs, but most have no symptoms. Occasional TMJ pain caused by OA occurs. The usual finding in patients with OA of the TMJ is an insidious onset of unilateral preauricular aching and pain with stiffness after a period of inactivity that decreases with mild activity. Severe pain may be elicited on wide opening, and pain occurs with normal function and worsens during the day. Adjacent muscle splinting and spasm may occur. Crepitus is a common finding in the affected joint. In most cases, osteoarthritic pain in the TMJ will resolve within 8 months of onset.[33] Radiographic changes include decreased joint space, sclerosis, remodeling, and osteophytes (Fig. 24-6). No correlation exists between TMJ symptoms and radiographic or histologic signs of OA.

In the past, uncertainty has existed over the relationship between disk displacement and OA. Reports[34,35] of a 30-year longitudinal study now provide evidence that, for patients with a reducing anterior disk displacement, about a 50% chance exists that no progression of the disorder will occur, nor will any significant radiographic changes happen in the TMJ hard or soft tissue structures. For the remaining 50%, a likelihood exists of progression to a nonreducing disk displacement or dislocation (closed lock). These patients can experience a period of variable pain and dysfunction, but it appears to be self-limiting in most patients. Also, 86% of patients with nonreducing disks demonstrate significant radiographic changes in the condyle and fossa on plain films, and disk changes on magnetic resonance imaging. These changes occur rapidly during the first 3 years, then a stable, persistent, quiescent period is attained. Thus most patients with disk displacement, whether reducing or nonreducing, can be managed successfully by conservative, reversible therapies.

Treatment of OA of the TMJ consists of acetaminophen, aspirin or NSAIDs, muscle relaxants, limiting jaw function, physical therapy (heat, ice, ultrasound, controlled exercise), and occlusal splints to decrease joint loading. Conservative therapy is successful in controlling symptoms in most cases; however, should pain or dysfunction be severe and persistent, TMJ surgery may be necessary.

■ SYSTEMIC LUPUS ERYTHEMATOSUS ■

DEFINITION

Lupus erythematosus has two forms: one predominantly affecting the skin (discoid, DLE) and a more generalized one affecting multiple organ systems (systemic, SLE).[27,34] DLE is characterized by chronic, erythematous, scaly plaques on the face, scalp, or ears. Most patients with DLE do not have systemic manifestations and the course tends to be more benign.[36] SLE involves the skin and many other organ systems and is the more serious form. This section will focus on SLE.

INCIDENCE AND PREVALENCE

SLE is a prototypical autoimmune disease that predominantly affects women of childbearing age, with a female-male ratio of 5:1, and is more common and severe in blacks and Hispanics than in whites.[36,37] A defining feature of SLE is the almost invariable presence in the blood of antibodies directed against one or more components

of cell nuclei; certain manifestations of the disease are associated with the presence of one or more of these different antinuclear antibodies.[36]

ETIOLOGY

The etiology of SLE is unknown, although it is clearly an autoimmune disease. A strong familial aggregation exists, with a much higher frequency among first-degree relatives of patients. Studies of patients with SLE suggest that the disease is caused by genetically determined immune abnormalities that can be triggered by both exogenous and endogenous factors. Among these triggering factors are infectious agents, stress, diet, toxins, drugs, and sunlight.[37]

PATHOPHYSIOLOGY AND COMPLICATIONS

The production of pathogenic antibodies and immune complexes, and their deposition with resultant inflammation and vasculopathy, is the basic abnormality underlying SLE. Antibodies are formed in response to some antigenic stimulus, and the reaction between antigen and circulating antibodies forms antigen-antibody complexes, which are deposited in a wide variety of tissues and organs including the kidney, skin, blood vessels, muscle and joints, heart, lung, brain, gastrointestinal tract, lymphatics, and eye.[37,38] The clinical expression of the disease reflects the organs or tissues involved and the extent of that involvement.

Despite advances in diagnosis and management, complications attributable to SLE or its treatment continue to cause substantial morbidity.[39] Of hospitalizations for SLE, one third were for neurologic or psychiatric involvement, whereas infections, coronary artery disease, and osteonecrosis also were major reasons.[40]

Several studies have documented substantial improvement in the survival of patients with SLE, with 5-year survival rates of 90% or greater, and 10-year survival rates of greater than 80%.[41-43] The leading causes of death in patients with SLE are infectious complications and clinical manifestations related to lupus itself including acute vascular neurologic events, renal failure, and cardiovascular or pulmonary involvement.[38]

CLINICAL PRESENTATION

SIGNS AND SYMPTOMS

Because of the widespread systemic involvement of SLE, multiple manifestations are found through many tissues and organs. Although malaise, overwhelming fatigue,

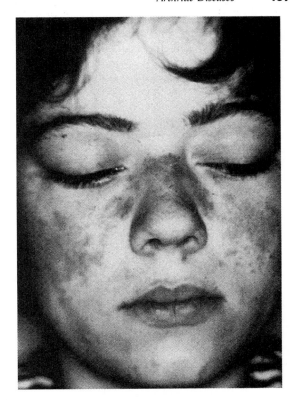

Fig. 24-7 Female patient with butterfly-shaped rash of systemic lupus erythematosus. (From Langlais RP, Miller, CS: *Color atlas of common oral diseases*, Philadelphia, 1992, Lea & Febiger.)

fever, and weight loss are nonspecific manifestations that effect most patients at some time in their disease, the classic picture of SLE is that of a young woman with polyarthritis and a butterfly-shaped rash across the nose and cheeks (Fig. 24-7). The presentation of SLE, however, varies widely from mild to severe and depends largely on the extent and selection of organ involvement.

Arthritis is the most common manifestation of SLE and is seen in as many as 76% of patients.[44] It affects the small joints, is migratory, and the pain typically is out of proportion to the signs. The classic butterfly rash of the nose and cheeks is found in only about one third of patients with SLE; however, a rash on the upper trunk or areas of exposed skin is more common.[45] Recurrent noninfectious pharyngitis and oral ulcerations also are common.[46]

Serious renal abnormalities occur in less than one third of patients with SLE, although most patients will demonstrate some abnormality on renal biopsy.[41] Renal failure is one of the most serious problems and is the best clinical indicator of a poor prognosis.[47]

Neuropsychiatric symptoms are common and include organic brain syndrome, psychosis, seizures, stroke, movement disorders and peripheral neuropathy.[38] Thromboembolism associated with antiphospholipid antibody is an important cause of abnormalities in the central nervous system.

Pulmonary manifestations include pleuritis, infection, pulmonary edema, pneumonitis, and pulmonary hypertension. Cardiac involvement is common and consists of pericarditis, myocarditis, endocarditis, and coronary artery disease. Valvular abnormalities can be identified by echocardiography in 25% of patients but rarely result in serious valvular dysfunction.[48] However, Libman-Sacks endocarditis (nonbacterial verrucous endocarditis) is found in 50% of patients with SLE at autopsy.[49] Unfortunately, this is not always demonstrated by echocardiography or by clinical examination. This condition is thought to predispose patients to infective endocarditis.[50-51] A retrospective study of 313 patients with SLE suggested that the risk for bacterial endocarditis was similar to that in patients with rheumatic heart disease and prosthetic heart valves.[51] A clinically detectable heart murmur was found in 18.5 % of the patients that required further investigation to determine its significance. Approximately 4% of the patients had cardiac valve abnormalities that placed them in the moderate risk group for endocarditis. However, none of the cases demonstrated a relationship between endocarditis and SLE. Based upon current American Heart Association guidelines, the 4% of those SLE patients with cardiac valve abnormalities that placed them in the moderate risk group for endocarditis, should receive the standard regimen for antibiotic prophylaxis for the designated bacteremia-producing dental procedures. The dentist should consult with the patient's physician to properly identify those patients and decide upon prophylaxis.

A study by Rhodus[52] indicated that patients with SLE may have a higher potential for arrhythmias and electrocardiographic abnormalities. The diagnosis of SLE is based on criteria suggested by the American Rheumatism Association.[27,50] Although these criteria were primarily intended for research purposes, they are nevertheless clinically useful, requiring at least 4 of 11 criteria to make a diagnosis.

LABORATORY FINDINGS

The antinuclear antibody test is the best screening test for SLE, as it is positive in 95% of patients. It also occurs in patients with other rheumatic diseases, however. Anti-DNA assays, double helix and single helix, also are elevated in 65% to 80% of patients with active untreated SLE.[27,53-55]

Hematologic abnormalities include hemolytic anemia, leukopenia, lymphopenia, and thrombocytopenia.[53,55] The leukopenia in SLE usually is not associated with recurrent infections.[55] Autoimmune thrombocytopenia occurs in as many as 25% of patients with SLE and may be severe in 5% of these.[38] Patients with severe thrombocytopenia are at risk for bleeding either spontaneously or after trauma. This is rare, however, if the platelet count is greater than 50,000/mm.[12,56]

A variety of clotting abnormalities may be seen, the most common being the lupus anticoagulant, which is associated with an elevation of the partial thromboplastin time (PTT). This can result in thromboembolic events rather than increased bleeding, and invasive surgery can be performed without correction of this laboratory abnormality.[55] The erythrocyte sedimentation rate often is elevated but does not reflect disease activity. With active nephritis, proteinuria will be present as will hematuria and cellular or granular casts. Other abnormalities include false-positive serologic tests for syphilis.[55]

MEDICAL MANAGEMENT

A cure for SLE does not exist; thus all treatment is of a symptomatic or palliative nature. Patients with SLE are advised to avoid sun exposure as this may trigger onset or exacerbate the disease.[45] Many of the drugs used to treat rheumatoid arthritis also are used in the management of SLE (see Table 24-2). These include aspirin and NSAIDs for mild disease, antimalarials for dermatologic disease, glucocorticoids for more severe symptoms, and cytotoxic agents for symptoms unresponsive to other therapies or as adjuncts in severe disease. Several experimental approaches to therapy are under investigation, including plasmapheresis, lymph node irradiation, cyclosporine injections, sex hormone therapy, cyclosporin, and immune gamma globulin.[27]

DENTAL MANAGEMENT

MEDICAL CONSIDERATIONS

Because SLE is such a varied disease with so many potential problems caused by the disease or its treatment, pretreatment consultation with the patient's physician is advised (Box 24-6). As in rheumatoid arthritis, drug considerations and side effects in SLE are of major importance. Table 24-2 lists the dental and oral considerations with the use of these drugs. The leukopenia common in SLE usually is not associated with a significant increase in infection; however, when combined with corticosteroids

BOX 24-6

Dental Management of Patient with Systemic Lupus Erythematosus

1. Consultation with physician
   a. Patient status and stability
   b. Extent of systemic manifestations (i.e., kidney, heart)
   c. Hematologic profile (complete blood cell count - CBC; with differential; prothrombin time—PT; partial thromboplastin time—PTT, bleeding time-BT)
   d. Drug profile
2. Drug considerations
   a. Aspirin and NSAIDs—bleeding may be increased but is not usually clinically significant; if patient is concurrently taking corticosteroids, bleeding more likely—suggest obtaining pretreatment bleeding time (<20 minutes)
   b. Gold salts, antimalarials, penicillamine, and cytotoxic drugs can cause leukopenia and thrombocytopenia; also severe stomatitis—treat symptomatically
   c. Corticosteroids can cause adrenal suppression
3. Hematologic considerations
   a. Leukopenia with corticosteroids or cytotoxic drugs can predispose patient to infection; use of postoperative antibiotics with surgical procedures can be considered
   b. Platelet count <50,000/mm^3 may result in severe bleeding—consultation with physician
   c. Elevated PTT associated with lupus anticoagulant usually does not cause increased bleeding surgery can be performed
4. Infective endocarditis is a potential problem—antibiotic prophylaxis using American Heart Association recommendations should be prescribed for dental procedures likely to cause bleeding

or cytotoxic drugs, the likelihood of infection is increased. Therefore in patients taking corticosteroids or cytotoxins who also have leukopenia, the use of prophylactic antibiotics for periodontal and oral surgical procedures can be considered. Patients taking corticosteroids also may develop significant adrenal suppression and could require supplementation, especially for surgical procedures or in cases of extreme anxiety (see Chapter 15).

Abnormal bleeding is a potential problem in some patients with SLE because of thrombocytopenia. A coagulation profile should be obtained, especially noting the platelet count, bleeding time, and PTT. Bleeding times less than 20 minutes, and a platelet count greater than 50,000/mm^3 are indications of adequate platelet activity. Otherwise, abnormalities should be discussed with the physician. As previously mentioned, an elevated PTT associated with the lupus anticoagulant is not a risk factor for increased bleeding.

Because cardiac valvular abnormalities are found in 25% to 50% of patients with SLE and often are not clinically detectable, the potential for bacterial endocarditis resulting from dentally induced bacteremias exists. Therefore, prudence suggests that patients with SLE are candidates for antibiotic prophylaxis for dental treatment likely to result in gingival bleeding (see Chapter 3). The current American Heart Association regimen for endocarditis prophylaxis is suggested (see Chapter 2). Finally, patients with SLE-associated renal failure have the potential for altered drug metabolism, hematologic disorders, and infection (see Chapter 19 for management recommendations).

TREATMENT PLANNING CONSIDERATIONS

No specific treatment planning modifications are required. Consideration, however, should be given to physical disabilities secondary to arthritis and myalgias. Additionally, systemic complications such as renal impairment, cardiac problems such as arrhythmias and valvular defects may exist. For patients with SLE, the establishment and maintenance of optimum oral health are of paramount importance.

ORAL COMPLICATIONS AND MANIFESTATIONS

Oral lesions of the lips and mucous membranes have been reported to occur in up to 5% to 25% of patients with SLE.[56,57] The lesions are rather nonspecific and may be erythematous with white spots or radiating peripheral lines and also can demonstrate painful ulcerations (Fig. 24-8). They frequently resemble lichen planus or leukoplakia. When lesions occur on the lip, a silvery, scaly margin, similar to that seen on the skin may develop. Skin and lip lesions frequently occur following exposure to the sun. Treatment of these lesions is symptomatic, with avoidance of future sun exposure (see Appendix B). Other oral manifestations of SLE may include xerostomia and hyposalivation, dysgeusia, and glossodynia.[57,59] The dentist should always remain alert to oral eruptions and lesions secondary to any of a variety of the medications used to treat SLE, for they may be a sign of toxicity. Similarly, some medications (hydralazine) have been associated with causing lupus-like eruptions.

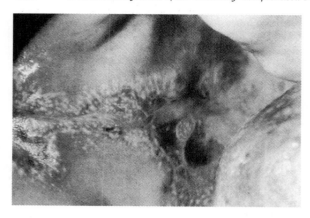

Fig. 24-8 Systemic lupus erythematosus lesions of the buccal mucosa. (From Neville BW et al: *Color atlas of clinical oral pathology,* Philadelphia, 1991, Lea & Febiger.)

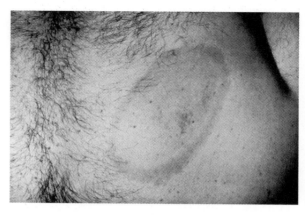

Fig. 24-9 Classic *Erythema migrans* lesion for Lyme disease. (Courtesy Richard Estensen, Minneapolis, Minn.)

■ LYME DISEASE ■

DEFINITION

Lyme disease is a multisystemic inflammatory disease caused by the tick-borne spirochete *Borrelia burgdorferi.* The disease was first identified in the United States in 1975 from an outbreak around Lyme, Connecticut, of an inflammatory condition presumed to be juvenile rheumatoid arthritis. The classical pattern of Lyme disease is a characteristic macular skin rash (*erythema migrans*), which appears within a month after the tick (*Ixodes dammini*) bite. Then several different manifestations may occur, including neurologic, articular and cardiac manifestations.[27]

INCIDENCE AND PREVALENCE

Lyme disease has been reported in North America, Europe, and Asia. In the United States more than 90% of all cases of Lyme disease have been reported in only 8 states (New York, Connecticut, Pennsylvania, Massachusetts, Rhode Island, New Jersey, Wisconsin, and Minnesota). Differences in the organism and in the immunogenetics of the affected population may explain the differences in the clinical presentation of Lyme disease.

PATHOPHYSIOLOGY AND COMPLICATIONS

Precisely how *B. burgdorferi* causes Lyme disease is not clear. The organism does not make toxins or cause tissue damage. It may activate proteolytic enzymes and induce spirochetemia. Local inflammation results from host response mechanisms. Vasculitis has been implicated in some cases of perripheral neuropathy and a vascular lesion resembling endarteritis obliterans has been identified in meninges and synovium of Lyme disease patients.[61]

The clinical manifestations of Lyme disease can be divided into three phases: early localized, early disseminated, and late disease. Patients with a diagnosis of Lyme disease may not be identified until the later stages of the disease.[61] Early localized disease includes *erythema migrans* and associated findings. E. *migrans* occurs in 50% to 80% of infected patients within on month of the tick bite. Only about 30% of patients will recall an associated tick bite. The E. *migrans* presents as a "target" or "bull's eye" lesion typically appears in or near the axilla or beltline because the ticks like the warm, moist areas of the human body (Fig. 24-9). Most often the lesion is asymptomatic although it may itch, burn or hurt. The lesion typically expands and enlarges over the course of a few days. Some sources have reported that 50% of patients will have multiple E. *migrans* lesions because of spirochetemia. Patients also may have an acute viremialike syndome with fever, malaise, nausea, myalgia, fatigue, headache, and athralgias.

The next phase of clinical presentation is early disseminated disease, which may occur in a few days to a few months after the tick bite and may occur without the preceeding erythema migrans.[61] The primary clinical manifestations of this phase are cardiac and neurologic problems. In the absence of treatment, about 8% of patients infected with Lyme disease will manifest some cardiac problems, including heart block and myopericarditis. In the majority of cases, the carditis begins to resolve even without antibiotic therapy. Neurologic damage occurs in approximately 10% of untreated patients with

Lyme disease. Primary manifestations include lymphocytic meningitis, cranial nerve pallsies (especially the facial nerve), and radiculoneuritis.[61] In the late disease stage, which may occur months to years after the infection and may not be preceded by the earlier manifestations, musculoskelatal problems are the main manifestation. Intermittent, migratory episodes of polyarthritis occur in approximately 50% of patients, which mimics the "juvenile arthritis" originally described in cases of Lyme disease. Chronic arthritis of the knee is common with erosion of bone and cartilage. Chronic inflammatory joint disease may last for 5 to 8 years.[61]

Late neurologic manifestations of Lyme disease called *tertiary neuroborreliosis* include encephalopathy, neurocognitive dysfunction, and peripheral neuropathy. The symptoms may be subtle, causing headache and fatigue in addition to cognitive, mood, and sleep disturbances. Neuropsychologic testing may be useful in the diagnosis. Patients also may manifest distal neuropathies. Fibromyalgia is common in patients with Lyme disease.[63]

LABORATORY FINDINGS

While the diagnosis of Lyme disease is found primarily upon clinical grounds, serologic testing may prove useful. Current practice is to confirm all enzyme-linked immunosorbant assay (ELISA) results with Western blot analysis. Many other conditions may mimic Lyme disease (Epstein-Barr virus-infections [EBV], SLE, infective endocarditis), therefore laboratory testing should be done to arrive more precisely at a definitive diagnosis. Serologic testing has not been standardized between various laboratories, which may be problematic. Antibody responses may be undetectable in infections of less than 6 weeks and early antibiotic therapy based on symptoms may render the infected patient seronegative. Most patients with late disease manifestations are strongly seropositive.

MEDICAL MANAGEMENT

Antibiotic therapy of B. *burgdorferi* infections is effective. Prompt antibiotic therapy when early symptoms exist usually prevents progression to later stages of Lyme disease. Oral therapy with 100 mg bid of doxycycline for 3 to 4 weeks is the first-line of treatment for early infections. Alternatively, tetracycline of amoxicillin (250-500 mg qid) for the same time period may be used. In the late disseminated stages of Lyme disease, intravenous antibiotics may be necessary. The third generation cephalosporins (ceftriaxone: 2g qid or cef-

taxmime: 3g bid), penicillin G (20 million units in 6 divided doses), or chloramphenicol (50 mg/kg/day in 4 divided doses) may be used. Some physicians treat all pregnant women only with the IV route. Some patients with arthritis are refractory to antibiotic therapy. These patients may benefit from intraarticular corticosteroid injections or hydroxychloroquine. Adequate therapy for neurologic damage is elusive and recovery may be very slow.[61-62]

DENTAL MANAGEMENT

MEDICAL CONSIDERATIONS

The major dental consideration of Lyme disease is the identification of unusual symptoms in the absence of a clear medical condition. Symptoms of fatigue, malaise, arthralgia, neuritis or neuralgia including facial palsy may indicate the possibility of Lyme disease and referral for proper medical diagnosis. Numerous reports exist of facial nerve palsy closely resembling Bell's palsy resulting from Lyme disease.[63] The presentation of this facial palsy may be combined with other neurologic deficits or may stand alone. The involvement of the parotid glands (acute parotitis) has been reported.[64] Cases also have been identified during pregnancy.[65] With facial nerve palsy, facial and dental neuralgia, and temporomandibular joint symptoms also have been reported with Lyme disease.[66]

■ SJÖGREN'S SYNDROME ■

DEFINITION

Sjögren's syndrome (SS) is an autoimmune disease complex classified among the many rheumatic diseases, which causes exocrinopathy and affects the salivary and lacrimal glands. SS is characterized by a triad of clinical conditions: keratoconjunctivitis sicca, xerostomia and a connective tissue disease (usually rheumatoid arthritis). SS presents in two different forms: primary SS and secondary SS. Primary SS (SS-1) clinically manifests with the primary ocular complication of keratoconjunctivitis sicca and in the oral cavity presents as various levels of salivary gland dysfunction (xerostomia). Secondary SS (SS-2) manifests as the presence of either keratoconjunctivitis sicca or xerostomia, in the presence of a diagnosed systemic connective tissue disease. The connective tissue disorder for which SS is secondary most commonly is rheumatoid arthritis, with systemic lupus erythematosus, primary biliary cirrhosis, fibromyalgia, mixed connective tissue disease, polymyositis, Raynaud's

syndrome and several others among the associated inflammatory conditions.[67-69]

INCIDENCE AND PREVALENCE

According to the World Health Organization, the prevalence of SS is unknown.[69] A recent epidemiological study in Sweden estimated the prevalence in the adult population to be 2.7%.[70] Today the prevalence of SS in the United States is estimated at more than 1 million.[71] Originally named for an ophthalmologist from Sweden, SS has been reported in nearly every major country, and the geographic distribution of cases, although accurate data is lacking, appears to be relatively uniform. SS is primarily a disease of women as more than 90% of all SS patients are female.[67-71]

SS typically presents during the fourth or fifth decade of life, although the condition usually progresses insidiously over several years, going unrecognized. Therefore some individuals actually may begin developing SS at a much earlier age than when actually diagnosed. Isolated cases of SS have been reported in children.[70]

ETIOLOGY

The precise etiology of Sjögren's syndrome, as with many of the autoimmune rheumatic disorders, is unknown, although several contributing factors have been identified. A theory is that the pathology results from complications from a viral infection with EBV.[71] Exposure to or reactivation of EBV elicits expression of the HLA (human lymphocyte antigen) complex, and this is recognized by the T-cell 1 (CD-4+) lymphocytes, resulting in the release of cytokines (TNF, IL-2, IFN-g, and others). Chronic inflammation, infiltration of lymphocytes and ultimate destruction of exocrine gland tissue follows.[67-71]

PATHOPHYSIOLOGY AND COMPLICATIONS

SS is a chronic, progressive autoimmune disorder characterized by exocrinopathy and generalized lymphoproliferation primarily affecting the salivary and lacrimal glands. A genetic marker, HLA-DR4, has been identified specific for SS.[71]

Labial salivary gland histopathology almost universally has been accepted as the *prima facia* diagnostic indicator for definitive diagnosis of SS. The classic histopathology of the minor salivary glands in SS is a lymphocytic infiltration that includes benign lymphosialadenopathy (focal lymphocytic sialadenitis or benign lymphoepithelial lesion in the major salivary glands). The benign lymphosialadenopathy may manifest as parotid hypertrophy, particularly in patients with primary SS. Small clusters of intralobular ducts enlarge to replace the acinar epithelial

TABLE 24-3

Clinical Manifestations (with approximate frequency) for Sjögren's Syndrome Subjects*

Clinical Manifestation	Prevalence (% of SS patients)
Orcheilosis/angular cheilitis	75
Glossitis	60
Mucositis	30
Glossodynia	45
Dysgeusia	75
Dysphagia	45
Candidiasis	75
Dental caries	100
Periodontitis	60-100

*From 62 consecutive SS patients presenting to the University of Minnesota Xerostomia Clinic data published in part in Rhodus, NL: Xerostomia and glossodynia in patients with autoimmune disorders, *Ear Nose Throat J* 68:791-794, 1989 and Rhodus NL et al: Quantitative assessment of dysphagia in patients with primary and secondary Sjögren's syndrome. *Oral Surg Oral Med Oral Pathol Oral Rad Endod* 79:305-310, 1995.

parenchyma. The lesion comprises primarily CD-4+ T-cell lymphocytes along with late acquisition of polyclonal B-cells and plasma cells. In the lymphocytic foci approximately 75% are T-cells with 5-10% B cells.[69,71] As the inflammatory process progresses, fibrosis and atrophy of the salivary glands occur and hyposalivation progresses. Progression to lymphoma is a possibility in SS and will be discussed in the *Patient Management* section.[69,71]

CLINICAL PRESENTATION

SIGNS AND SYMPTOMS

The oral clinical manifestations of SS typically include hyposalivation, glossitis, mucositis, parotid gland hypertrophy, angular cheilosis, dysgeusia (taste dysfunction), secondary infections, and a significantly increased caries rate[69-71] (Table 24-3).

SALIVARY GLAND DYSFUNCTION AND HYPOSALIVATION

Saliva in normal quantity and composition is rich in constituents that have potent antimicrobial, antacid, lubricative, and homeostatic properties. Saliva contains ap-

proximately 60 important, protective constituents, including immunoglobulins, electrolytes, buffers, antimicrobial enzymes, digestive enzymes, and many others, all of which make saliva an essential contributor to the health and homeostasis of the oral cavity. Obviously, when saliva is diminished in quantity or altered in composition, as in SS, deterioration of oral soft and mineralized tissues can occur.[69-72]

Patients with SS also demonstrate increased levels of dysphagia as compared with controls. Studies have shown that patients with SS have difficulty tasting, tolerating and swallowing certain foods. These SS patients have demonstrated resulting nutritional intake inadequacies.[69-73]

Among its many beneficial constituents, saliva has been shown to be rich in proteins that have potent antifungal properties, thus it plays an important role in host defense and protection from yeasts such as *Candida* species. Therefore with the reduction in salivary flow in SS, *Candida* infections become very common.[69,74]

The results of a recently published study indicated that the presence and density of *Candida albicans* in the SS subjects at baseline was extremely high and was evidenced by clinical signs in most subjects (especially those with the highest counts). The study also found that the prevailing clinical manifestation of infection with C. *albicans* (before *and* after pilocarpine HCl administration) was the erythematous form (63% and 25%, respectively).[69,74] A few recent studies also have indicated that patients with SS exhibit more periodontal disease, especially clinical attachment loss.[69,75]

DIAGNOSIS

The precise diagnostic criteria for SS remain controversial although most certainly specific laboratory tests are available for the major diagnostic categories of salivary and tear production, histopathologic changes, and serological inflammatory markers. Sets of published criteria total 5 for the diagnosis of SS with several common characteristics with some variations and modifications[69] (see Box 24-7).

LABORATORY FINDINGS

Serologically, hypergammaglobulinemia is the most frequent laboratory finding (80%) of patients with SS. Hyperactivity of B-lymphocytes results in increased rheumatoid factor antibodies, antinuclear antibodies (ANA) and antibodies against organ-specific antigens, such as salivary duct epithelia or thyroid tissue.[69,71] The ANA are the SS-A (Ro), which is present in approximately 70% of patients with SS-1 and 15% to 90% with SS-1 and SS-B (La) antibodies, which are present in approximately 50% of patients with SS-1 and 5% to 30% with SS-2. These ANA also

---

BOX 24-7

Diagnostic Criteria (European Criteria) for Sjögren's Syndrome* Used at the University of Minnesota

Ocular Symptoms (1:3)	**Ocular Signs (1:2)**
Daily dry eyes > 3 mos.	+ Shirmer's test
Sand or gravel sensitivity	(<5mm/5min.)
Use of tear substitutes	Rose bengal score
(> tid)	(>4.vBs)
Oral Symptoms (1:3)	**Salivary Function (1:3)**
Daily dry mouth > 3 mos.	+ scintigraphy
Swollen salivary glands	+ sialography
Need fluids to swallow	WUSF<1.5 ml/ 15 min.
food	(0.1 ml/min.)
Labial SG Histology	**Autoantibodies (1:2)**
focus score >1/4 mm	anti- SS- Ro
>50 mononuclear cells	anti- SS- La

*Subjects must meet 4:6 criteria; must include either labial biopsy or serology.

---

may be found in other autoimmune disorders.[27,32] Elevated erythrocyte sedimentation rate (ESR) mild anemia (approximately 25%) and leukopenia (approximately 10%) also are found in patients with SS. The laboratory tests used to diagnose SS are summarized in Box 24-7.

Sialometry
Sialometry is useful both as an initial screening tool for hyposalivation associated with SS and to assess the level of severity of SS. Salivary flow collection must be performed precisely according to the type of gland and over a period of at least 5 minutes (often up to 15 minutes) to be valuable as a diagnostic technique.

Imaging
Radiographic findings may appear in advanced stages of fibrosis of the salivary glands. Sialograms are performed by injecting a radiocontrast dye into the salivary ductal system before conventional radiography. Sialograms may reveal punctate radioopaque calcifications or, if more advanced, larger, lobular calcifications. Sialectasis in portions of the ductal system may occur or appear dilated or may appear with areas of absent acinar parenchyma. MRI sialography has been shown to be much more accurate in demonstrating the level of salivary gland destruction in SS.[69] Salivary scintigraphy with 99m technetium pertechnetate (sodium pertechnetate, a radioisotope of technetium) can be performed to

TABLE 24-4

Management of Salivary Dysfunction*

Moisture and Lubrication (Continuous, as Needed)

General	*Specific**
Drink (sip water, liquids)	Oral Balance (especially at night)
Use sugarless candy or gum	Pilocarpine hydrochloride, 2% (Salagen, 5 mg, 3 times daily)
Avoid ethanol	Mouthkote (artificial saliva)
Avoid tobacco	Optimoist (artificial saliva)
Avoid coffee, tea, and other caffeinated beverages	Salivart (artificial saliva)
	Sodium carboxymethylcellulose, 05% sin

Soft Tissue Lesions and Soreness (Treatment and Maintenance)

General	*Specific**
Oral Balance	Benadryl + Maalox + nystatin elixir†
	(Carafate, optional)
	(Lidocaine, 2%, optional, for acute lesions)
	Decadron 0.5 mg/5 mL elixir‡ (for acute lesions)
Biotene mouthwash	Triamcinolone, 0.1% (in Orabase) (for acute lesions)
	Orabase-HCA (for acute lesions)
	Mycelex 60-mg troches (for candidiasis)
	Mycolog II ointment (lips and tongue)

Prevention of Caries and Periodontal Disease (Continuous)

General	*Specific**
Meticulous perioral hygiene	Biotene toothpaste (neutral sodium fluoride, 1.0%, trays)
Avoid acids	
Regular hygiene and prophylaxis recalls	Prevident, 5000 pm§
Sodium bicarbonate rinses (optional)	(Optional) Peridex (chlorhexidine gluconate)
Halitosis (Retardex)	Waterpik

*Specific treatments are dependent on the diagnosis.
†Benadryl, 25 mg/10 mL + Maalox, 64 mL + nystatin, 100,000 IU/mL = 16 mL.
‡Decadron elixir, 0.5%/5 mL. Dispense 100 mL. To be swished and expectorated, 5 mL 3 times daily.
§Prevident neutral sodium fluoride, 1.0%, to be applied in trays 2 times daily.
Manufacturers: Oral Balance, Laclede Pharmaceuticals; Salagen, MGI Pharmaceuticals; Mouthkote, Parnell Pharmaceuticals; Optimoist, Colgate-Hoyt; Salivart, Gebauer; Biotene, Laclede Pharmaceuticals; Benadryl, Parke-Davis; Maalox, Novartis Pharmaceuticals; Carafate, Hoechst, Marion, Roussel Pharmaceuticals; Decadron, Merck & Co. Pharmaceuticals; Orabase, Colgate-Palmolive; Mycelex, ALZA Prevident, Colgate-Hoyte; Peridex, Procter & Gamble; Waterpik, Teledyne.
Published in part by Rhodus et al.

assess the function of the salivary glands by measuring the rate and density of technetium uptake.

DENTAL MANAGEMENT

MEDICAL CONSIDERATIONS

No known cure exists for SS. Patient management for SS traditionally has been palliative and preventive. Relief of the primary symptoms of dryness (oral and ocular) and the secondary burning and discomfort is the main goal. Restoration and maintenance of a normal homeostatic oral environment is a secondary goal.[69]

Therapy for the oral component of SS may be classified into three major categories: (1) provision of moisture and lubrication by either stimulation or simulation, (2) treatment of secondary mucosal conditions (such as mucositis or candidiasis) and (3) prevention of oral disease, maintenance, and general support (such as nutrition).[69] These therapeutic strategies are outlined in Table 24-4.

MOISTURE AND LUBRICATION

Patients with SS will be quite thirsty but should be counseled to drink plenty of water (8 to 10 glasses per day) and to avoid diuretics such as caffeine, tobacco, and alcoholic beverages. Obviously certain medications (more than 400) may contribute to and compound the xerostomia, so some may need to be modified or avoided if possible.[69] Any changes in the patient's medication must be coordinated with the patient's physician. While salivary substitutes, oral moisturizers and artificial salivas may provide some relief for the xerostomia experienced by patients with SS, by and large they are inadequate. Most are compounds of carboxymethylcellulose or hydroxymethylcellulose and are either too viscous or not viscous enough for most patients. The retentivity or longevity of their effect is very short-lived, providing little more relief than water. To date, these simulated salivas appear to be of little benefit to the patient with SS. Some artificial salivas from Europe (including Saliva Orthana) seem to be effective. On the other hand, pharmacological stimulation of the salivary glands can be quite successful. Recently the Food and Drug Administration has approved the use of pilocarpine HCl (Salagen) and cevimiline HCL (Evoxac) for the treatment of signs and symptoms of hyposalivation in patients with SS.[69,72]

Systemic administration of pilocarpine or cevimiline effectively stimulates only the salivary acinar tissue which remains functional. Therefore SS patients who have lost most salivary acinar tissue capable of fluid production will benefit little from this drug. Conversely, those patients with functional tissue remaining will experience an increase in salivary secretion after the administration of pilocarpine relative to the ability of the tissue to become stimulated. The dosage of pilocarpine ranges from 2.5 to 15 mg administrated from 2 to 6 times daily. The dosage of cevimiline is 30 mg, 2 to 4 times daily.

Other pharmacological sialogogues have been shown to stimulate salivary flow, such as bethanechol chloride, bromhexine and anethole trithione, but none has withstood extensive clinical evaluation in the United States for safety and efficacy, and none has been approved by the Food and Drug Administration as of this writing. Very recently clinical trials have been undertaken on the safety and efficacy of human IFN-alpha for the treatment of SS. This NSAID appears to have significant promise as a new therapy for SS.[69,72]

ORAL COMPLICATIONS AND MANIFESTATIONS

Among the most common oral symptoms associated with SS aside from xerostomia is glossodynia (burning tongue). The tongue often becomes depapillated, and fis-

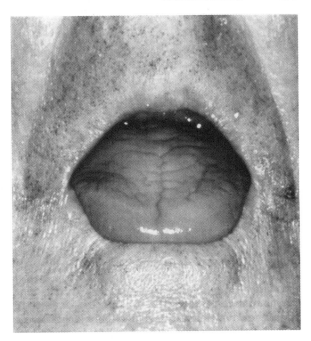

Fig. 24-10 Dry, atrophic oral mucosa, cheilosis, and glossitis in a patient with salivary hypofunction with Sjögren's syndrome.

sured (with a scrotal appearance), the dorsal epithelium often is atrophic or eroded, erythematous and potentially secondarily infected (Fig. 24-10). Pain and burning may be spontaneous or elicited with acidic or spicy food such as those containing ascorbic or acetic acid.[69,73] The tongue is commonly infected (as high as 83% of SS patients) with C. *albicans* in patients with SS. Not only must the acute Candidal infection be treated, but also some type of maintenance therapy to prevent recurrence of the fungal infection must be instituted. As long as the oral environment is adversely affected by hyposalivation, susceptibility to recurrence of the oral infection and continued deterioration will exist.[69,74] Atrophy of the epithelium in the dry environment may render the tissue susceptible to painful excoriation and ulceration. Therefore clinical follow-up and some phased maintenance therapy will be necessary. Generally these oral mucosal conditions are treated as if occurring independently (i.e., antifungal agents, topical antiinflammatory agents including corticosteriods, analgesics, or anesthetics as indicated[69,74] (see Table 24-4).

PREVENTION AND MAINTENANCE

The patient with SS may have less than 5% of the normal quantity of saliva to protect the oral cavity. The

risk for caries as well as enamel erosion then is extremely high. Of particular risk is the cervical, cementoenamel junction portion of the tooth. Meticulous oral hygiene with minimally abrasive fluoridated dentifrices and irrigation devices is paramount. In the xerostomic environment, abrasion of the tooth surface should be minimized as much as possible. Frequent professional hygiene recall intervals is also extremely important.

The frequent application of concentrated fluorides delivered either as a direct brush-on or by custom-made trays is imperative to prevent the rapid progression of caries. Over the counter fluoride rinses are inadequate; 5000 ppm sodium fluoride is preferred because of the unpleasant metallic taste of stannous fluoride, which also may cause some burning symptoms in the xerostomic patient and staining of the enamel. Special dentifrices have been found to be well accepted by patients with SS[69] (see Table 24-4).

Lymphoma

Most lymphomas occur in SS-1. The prevalence is approximately 5%.[76] Kassan et al in 1983 predicted the relative risk in SS patients to be 44 times normal; even higher (67 times) in those SS-1 patients with chronic parotid enlargement and whether patients had other cancers or irradiation therapy or chemotherapy (then the relative risk may be as high as 100 times).[76] Progression to lymphoma in patients with SS is thought to be related to chronic inflammatory challenge as the case of *Helicobacter pylori* in gastric Ca. In the presence of continued and chronic inflammation (mediated first by type-1 cytokines: TNF-a, IL-2, IFN-g, then later with type-2 cytokines, IL-4, IL-6 and IL-10) the B-cells undergo oligoclonality and sometimes eventually monoclonality. These SS patients may then manifest non-Hodgkin's lymphoma. B-cell monoclonality seems to be predictive of lymphomas arising outside the salivary glands.[69,71,76]

Associated clinical findings with lymphoma include anemia, cryoglobulinemia, lymphopenia, cutaneous vasculitis, and peripheral neuropathy. Lymphadenopathy is common with enlarged cervical and axillary nodes (86%). Evidence exists that the initial transformation to lymphoma occurs in the salivary glands and that the presence of B-cell monoclonality in LMSG tissue is associated with progression to malignancy.[77]

The most common type of lymphoma in SS is the mucosa-associated lymphoid tissue; 70% are low-grade, non-aggressive lymphomas with 15% high grade lymphoblastic. IL-6 and TNF-a are associated with lesions that go on to transform to lymphoma.[76,77]

References

1. Arthritis Foundation: *Basic facts*, Atlanta, 2000, Arthritis Foundation.
2. Wilder RL: Rheumatoid arthritis. A. Epidemiology, pathology and pathogenesis. In Schumacher HR Jr, editor: *Primer on the rheumatic diseases*, ed 10, Atlanta, 1993, Arthritis Foundation.
3. Goemaere S et al: Onset of symptoms of rheumatoid arthritis in relation to age, sex, and menopausal transition, J Rheumatol 17:1620-1622, 1990.
4. Wordsworth P, Pile K: Rheumatoid arthritis. Etiology. In Klippel JH, Dieppe PA; editors: *Rheumatology*, St Louis, 1994, Mosby-Year Book.
5. Golden A, Powell DE, Jennings CD: *Pathology: understanding human disease*, ed 2, Baltimore, 1985, Williams & Wilkins.
6. Matteson EL, Cohen MD, Conn DL: Rheumatoid arthritis. Clinical features-systemic involvement. In Klippel JH, Dieppe PA; editors: *Rheumatology*, St Louis, 1994, Mosby.
7. Lightfoot RW: Treatment of rheumatoid arthritis. In McCarty DJ, editor: *Arthritis and allied conditions*, ed 10, Philadelphia, 1985, Lea & Febiger.
8. Ragan C, Farrington E: The clinical features of rheumatoid arthritis. Prognostic indices, J Am Med Assoc 2:16, 1959.
9. Short CL, Bauer W, Reynolds E: *Rheumatoid arthritis*, Boston, 1957, Harvard University Press.
10. Pisetsky DS: Systemic lupus erythematosus. A. Epidemiology, pathology, and pathogenesis. In Schumacher HR Jr, editor: *Primer on rheumatic diseases*, ed 10, Atlanta, 1993, Arthritis Foundation.
11. Lipsky, PE: Rheumatoid arthritis. In Wilson JD et al, editors: *Harrison's principles of internal medicine*, ed 12, New York, 1991, McGraw-Hill.
12. Anderson RJ: Rheumatoid arthritis. B. Clinical features and laboratory. In Schumacher HR Jr, editor: *Primer on rheumatic diseases*, ed 10, Atlanta, 1993, Arthritis Foundation.
13. Kent JN, Carlton DM, Zide MF: Rheumatoid disease and related arthropathies. II. Surgical rehabilitation of the temporomandibular joint, Oral Surg 61:423-439, 1986.
14. Arnett FC, et al: The American Rheumatism Association 1987 revised criteria for the classification of rheumatoid arthritis, Arthritis Rheum 31:315- 324, 1988.
15. Williams HJ: Rheumatoid arthritis. C. Treatment. In Schumacher HR, editor: *Primer on rheumatic diseases*, ed 10, Atlanta, 1993, Arthritis Foundation.
16. Bradley JD et al: Comparison of an antiinflammatory dose of ibuprofen, an analgesic dose of ibuprofen, and acetaminophen in the treatment of patients with osteoarthritis of the knee, N Engl J Med 325:87-91, 1991.
17. Baton J et al: A comparison of etanercept and methotrexate in patients with early rheumatoid arthritis, N Engl J Med 343:1586-1593, 2000.
18. Lipsky P et al: Infliximab and methotrexate in the treatment of patients with early rheumatoid arthritis, N Eng J Med 343:1594-1602, 2000.
19. Amrein PC, Ellman L, Harris WH: Aspirin-induced prolongation of bleeding time and perioperative blood loss, J Am Med Assoc 245:1825-1828, 1981.

20. Ferraris VA, Swanson E: Aspirin usage and perioperative blood loss in patients undergoing unexpected operations, *Surg Gynecol Obstet* 156:439-442, 1983.

21. Little JW: Patients with prosthetic joints: Are they at risk when receiving invasive dental procedures? *Spec Care Dent* 17(5):153-160, 1997.

22. Pallasch T, Slots J: Antibiotic prophylaxis and the medically compromised patient, *Periodontology* 10:107-138, 1996.

23. Little JW: Managing dental patients with joint prostheses, *J Am Dent Assoc* 215:1374-1378, 1994.

24. Celiker R, Gokce-Kutsal Y, Eryilmaz M: Temporomandibular joint involvement in rheumatoid arthritis. Relationship with disease activity, *Scand J Rheumatol* 24:22-25, 1995.

25. Pepin JL et al: Sleep apnea syndrome secondary to rheumatoid arthritis, *Thorax* 50:692-694, 1995.

26. Sugahara T et al: Obstructive sleep apnea associated with temporomandibular joint destruction by rheumatoid arthritis: report of case, *J Oral Maxillofac Surg* 52:876-880, 1994.

27. A primer on the Rheumatic Diseases, 210-217, Arthritis Foundation, 2000. Wilder RL: Rheumatoid arthritis. A. Epidemiology, pathology and pathogenesis. In Schumacher HR Jr, editor: *Primer on the rheumatic diseases*, ed 10, Atlanta, Arthritis Foundation.

28. Brandt KD, Slemenda CW: Osteoarthritis. Epidemiology, pathology, and pathogenesis. In Schumacher HR Jr, editor: *Primer on rheumatic diseases*, ed 10, Atlanta, 1993, Arthritis Foundation.

29. Adams ME, Brandt KD: Hypertrophic repair of canine articular cartilage in osteoarthritis after anterior cruciate ligament transection, *J Rheumatol* 18:428-435, 1991.

30. Kramer JS, Yelin EH, Epstein WY: Social and economic impacts of four musculoskeletal conditions: a study using national community-based data, *J Rheumatol* 26:901-907, 1983.

31. Moskowitz RW, Goldberg VM: Osteoarthritis. B. Clinical features and treatment. In Schumacher HR Jr, editor: *Primer on rheumatic diseases*, ed 10, Atlanta, 1993, Arthritis Foundation.

32. Kreutziger KL, Mahan PE: Temporomandibular degenerative joint disease. I. Anatomy, pathophysiology and clinical description, *Oral Surg* 40:165-182, 1995.

33. deLeeuw R et al: Radiographic signs of temporomandibular joint osteoarthrosis and internal derangement 30 years after nonsurgical treatment, *Oral Surg Oral Med Oral Pathol Oral Radiol Endod* 79:382-392, 1995.

34. Prystowsky SD, Herndon JH Jr, Gilliam JN: Chronic cutaneous lupus erythematosus (DLE)-clinical and laboratory investigation of 80 patients, *Medicine (Baltimore)* 55:183-191, 1976.

35. Pincus T, Callahan LF: Early mortality in RA predicted by poor clinical status, *Bull Rheum Dis* 41:14, 1992.

36. Boumpas DT et al: Systemic lupus erythmatosus: emergency concepts. Part 2: Dermatologic and joint disease, the antiphospholipid antibody syndrome, pregnancy and hormone therapy, morbidity and mortality, and pathogenesis, *Ann Intern Med* 123:42-53, 1995.

37. Klippel JH: Systemic lupus erythematosus. Treatment-related complications superimposed on chronic disease, *JAMA* 263:1812-1815, 1990.

38. Petri M, Genovese M: Incidence of and risk factors for hospitalizations in systemic lupus erythematosus: a prospective study of the Hopkins lupus cohort, *J Rheumatol* 19:1559-1565, 1992.

39. Pistiner M et al: Lupus erythematosus in the 1980s: a survey of 570 patients, *Semin Arthritis Rheum* 21:55-64, 1991.

40. Seleznick MJ, Fries JF: Variables associated with decreased survival in systemic lupus erythematosus, *Semin Arthritis Rheum* 21:73-80, 1991.

41. Swaak AJ et al: Systemic lupus erythematosus: I. Outcome and survival: Dutch experience with 110 patients studied prospectively, *Ann Rheum Dis* 48:447-454, 1989.

42. Cronin ME: Musculoskeletal manifestations of systemic lupus erythematosus, *Rheum Dis Clin North Am* 14:99-116, 1988.

44. Callen JP: Mucocutaneous changes in patients with lupus erythematosus: the relationship of these lesions to systemic disease, *Rheum Dis Clin North Am* 14:79-97, 1988.

44. Burge SM et al: Mucosal involvement in systemic and chronic cutaneous lupus erythematosus, *Br J Dermatol* 121:727-741, 1989.

45. McLaughlin J et al: Kidney biopsy in systemic lupus erythematosus. II. Survival analyses according to biopsy results, *Arthritis Rheum* 34:1268-1293, 1991.

46. Sturfelt G et al: Cardiovascular disease in systemic lupus erythematosus: a study of 75 patients from a defined population, *Medicine (Baltimore)* 71:216-223, 1992.

47. Bulkley BH, Roberts WC: The heart in systemic lupus erythematosus and the changes induced in it by corticosteroid therapy, *Am J Med* 58:243-264, 1975.

48. Lehman TA et al: Bacterial endocarditis complicating systemic lupus erythematosus, *J Rheumatol* 10:655-658, 1983.

49. Luce EB, Montgomery MT, Redding SW: The prevalence of cardiac valvular pathosis in patients with systemic lupus erythematous, *Oral Surg Oral Med Oral Pathol* 70:590-592, 1990.

50. Mills JA: Systemic lupus erythematosus, *N Engl J Med* 330:1871-1879, 1994.

51. Hiser DG et al: Risk of infective endocarditis in patients with systemic lupus erythematosus, *Oral Surg Oral Med Oral Pathol* 80:423, 1995.

52. Rhodus NL, Johnson DA: Electrocardiographic abnormalities in dental patients with systemic lupus erythematosus, *Spec Care Dent* 4(6):46-51, 1990.

53. Zweiman B, Lisak RP: Autoantibodies: autoimmunity and immune complexes. In Henry JB, editor: *Clinical diagnosis and management by laboratory methods*, ed 18, Philadelphia, 1991, WB Saunders.

54. Gladman DD, Urowitz MB: Systemic lupus erythematosus. B. Clinical features. In Schumacher HR Jr, editor: *Primer on rheumatic diseases*, ed 10, Atlanta, 1993, Arthritis Foundation.

55. Kimberly RP: Systemic lupus erythematosus. In Paget SA, Fields TR, editors: *Rheumatic disorders*, Boston, 1992, Anover Medical Publishers.

56. Neville BW et al: *Oral and maxillofacial pathology*, Philadelphia, 1995, WB Saunders.

57. Rhodus NL, Johnson DK: The prevalence of oral manifestations of systemic lupus erythematosus, *Quint Int* 21:231-239, 1990.

58. Rhodus NL: Glossodynia and xerostomia associated with autoimmune diseases, *Ear Nose and Throat J* 68:791-796, 1989.

59. Rhodus NL et al: Dysphagia in patients with salivary gland dysfunction of three different etiologies, *Ear Nose Throat J* 74(1):39-46, 1995.

60. Sigal LH: Summary of the first 100 cases seen at a Lyme disease referral center, *Am J Med* 88:587-591, 1990.

61. Steere AC, Schoen RT, Taylor E: The clinical evolution of Lyme arthritis, *Ann Int Med* 107:725-727, 1987.

62. Dotevall L, Hageberg L: Successful oral doxycycyline treatment of Lyme disease and associated facial palsy and meningitis, *Clin Inf Dis* 28:569-573, 2000.

63. Lotgric-Furan S et al: Lyme borreliosis and facial palsy, *Wien Klin Wochenschr* 111:970-975, 2000.

64. Kawagishi N et al: A case of Lyme disease with parotitis, *Dermatology* 197:386-387, 1999.

65. Grandsaerd MJ, Meulenbroeks AA: Lyme borreliosis as a cause of facial palsy during pregnancy, *Eur J Obstet Gynecol Reprod Biol* 91(1):99-10, 2000.

66. Heir GM, Fein LA: Lyme disease: considerations for dentistry, *J Orofac Pain* 10(1):74-86, 1996.

67. Daniels TE, Fox PC: Salivary and oral components of Sjögren's syndrome, *Rheum Dis Clin N Amer* 18(3)571-589, 1992.

68. Rhodus NL: Diagnosis and management of the patient with Sjögren's syndrome, *Comp Cont Dent Ed* 8(8):578-593, 1987.

69. Rhodus NL: Sjögren's syndrome, *Quint Int* 29:231-23,1999.

70. Ostuni PA: Juvenile onset of primary Sjögren's syndrome: report of ten cases, *Clin Exper Rheumatol* 14(6):689-693, 1996.

71. Fox RI: Clinical features, pathogenesis, and treatment of Sjögren's syndrome, *Curr Opin Rheum* 8(5): 438-445, 1996.

72. Rhodus NL, Schuh MJ: The effects of Pilocarpine on salivary flow in Sjögren's syndrome patients, *Oral Surg Oral Med Oral Path Oral Radiol Endod* 72(11):545-549,1991.

73. Rhodus NL et al: Quantitative assessment of dysphagia in patients with primary and secondary Sjögren's syndrome, *Oral Surg Oral Med Oral Pathol Oral Radiol Endod* 79:305-310, 1995.

74. Rhodus NL: Candida albicans levels in patients with Sjögren's syndrome before and after long-term use of pilocarpine hydrochloride, *Quint Int* 29:705-710, 1998.

75. Rhodus NL et al: Salivary s-IgA and cytokine levels in Sjögren's patients before and after pilocarpine HCl administration, *J Clin Invest* 2:1-5, 1999.

76. Kassan S, Thomas T, Moutsopoulos HM: The increased risk of lymphoma in sicca syndrome, *Ann Int Med* 89:888-892, 1978.

77. Jordan RCK, Speight PM: Lymphoma in Sjögren's syndrome from histopathology to molecular pathology, *Oral Surg Oral Med Oral Pathol Oral Radiol Endod* 81(3):808-820, 1996.

Organ Transplantation

25

CHAPTER

Nobel laureate, Dr. Joseph E. Murray, performed the first successful human organ transplant in 1954, using a kidney donated by the patient's identical twin brother.[1] Then Murray performed the first successful kidney allograft transplant in 1959, applying total-body irradiation as immunosuppression, and the first successful human kidney cadaver transplant in 1962, introducing Imuran (azathioprine), an immunosuppressive drug.[1,2] Before these early transplants, patients with renal failure, hypertension, and azotemia were undergoing renal dialysis, which was not nearly as successful.[3] Since those early days more than 473,000 kidney transplants have been performed in the United States.[4] Since 1984, renal transplants have averaged nearly 10,000 per year nationwide.[5] At the University of Minnesota Hospital, more than 300 renal transplants are performed each year. This statistic is true for about 12 other transplant centers around the United States.[1] A total of 581 centers perform kidney transplants in the United States.[4] Improvements in preparation of the patient before the transplant, with better immunosuppressive techniques, have increased the success of the procedure and extended the longevity of the transplant recipient. The 1-year survival rate of the renal transplant patient is greater than 90%, and the 5-year survival rate is greater than 80%.[5]

The first human heart transplantation was performed in 1967. During 1968, 102 heart transplants were performed, with a 1-year survival rate of only 22%.[6,7] Presently, more than 53,000 heart transplants have been performed at the rate of approximately 3,400 per year at more than 250 U.S. hospitals. The 1-year survival rate is greater than 80%, with the 5-year survival rate nearly 70%[6] (Table 25-1).

The first orthotopic liver transplantation was performed in 1963. However, the first transplant resulting in an extended survival of 13 months was not achieved until 1967.[8] By 1980, only 300 liver transplants had been performed, with a 1-year survival rate of 28%. Since then more than 8300 liver transplants have been performed each year, with about the same number on the waiting list for a liver transplant. More than 80,000 liver transplants have been performed in the United States.[4] The 1-year survival rate is more than 85% with a 5-year survival rate of greater than 70%.[9,10]

The first pancreas transplant was performed in 1966, by Kelly and Lillehei at the University of Minnesota, along with a duodenum and a kidney, for a patient with diabetic nephropathy.[11,12] More than 300 pancreas transplants are performed each year with a total of more than 3000. The 5-year survival rate is greater than 75%. Recently, pancreatic islet-cell transplants also have shown considerable success.

In 1990 only 5 lung transplants had been performed: Since that time, more than 10,000 lungs have been transplanted at 119 centers, most within the last 5 years. The first heart-lung combination transplant was performed in 1981. Since that time, more than 800 have been performed, with a 1-year survival rate of 60%.[13-15]

To date, only a few small bowel transplants performed (some combined with liver transplants) at only a few transplant centers (Cambridge, England; London, Ontario; Pittsburgh, and Omaha). However, much progress is being made in this area for the treatment of end-stage intestinal failure, with the current 1-year survival rate at 70%.[16]

The modern era of bone marrow transplantation (BMT) was ushered in by the seminal experiments of Jacobsen (1950) and Lorenz (1951) and their colleagues, who demonstrated that mice could be protected from the lethal radiation that was used to treat severe aplastic anemia or leukemia by shielding the spleen or intravenous infusion of bone marrow.[17-19] By 1956, several laboratories had demonstrated that the protective effects

TABLE 25-1

Numbers of Transplants with Survival Rates

Organ	CUMULATIVE NUMBERS				SURVIVAL RATES (%)	
	1989	1991	1994	1999	(1 yr)	(5 yr)
Heart	13,119	19,445	29,990	53,880	83	70
Lung	146	653	2,478	6,745	62	49
Liver	12,824	21,324	34,225	80,221	85	67
Renal	201,680	241,048	285,900	473,597	87	76
Pancreas	524	1,066	2,144	3,070	85	75
Heart-lung	316	418	590	841	60	—
Small bowel	—	—	<50	267	70	—
Bone marrow	32,028	41,766	48,000	88,909	50-90	30-70*

*Survival rate varies depending on underlying pathology indication for BMT.
Compiled from data in Kahan B: *Surg Clin North Am* 74:1055-1075, 1994, and Cecka JM, Terasaki PI: *Clinical transplants*, UCLA Immunogenetics Center, 1999.

against otherwise lethal doses of total-body irradiation were caused by the colonization of the recipient bone marrow by the infused donor cells.[17,19]

In 1957, E. Donnell Thomas[20] described the clinical technique of large quantities of marrow infused intravenously into patients with leukemia with safety and efficacy and demonstrated a transient bone marrow transplant in humans.[18,20,21] In 1958, BMT was performed in 6 victims of a radiation accident.[19]

Most early BMTs were performed in only terminally ill patients, and the grafts could not be evaluated because the patient did not live long enough. The few successful allogeneic grafts were followed by lethal immunologic reaction of graft–versus–host disease (GVHD).[17,18,22-24] Many years of research in rodents, then dogs and monkeys, paved the way for the ultimate success of BMT in humans.[18,23,25] Recent advances in the knowledge of histocompatability typing, in the prevention of GVHD, as well as more supportive measures for the patient, have resulted in greater success and more frequent BMTs.[14,19,26]

The first attempts at transplantation in the 1950s and 1960s were all followed by increased activity in transplantation that resulted in very poor survival rates. A period followed during which few transplants were attempted. Increased research activity in the 1960s led to techniques that dealt with the major limiting factor in organ transplantation rejection of the organ by the host immune system.

With the development of effective immunosuppressive agents, improved surgical techniques (including percutaneous biopsy of solid transplanted organs to monitor

rejection), and the acceptance of the concept of "brain death" as a definition for determining the death of potential donors, major advances in organ transplantation have occurred.[8,9,19,27]

Transplantation of the heart, liver, and kidney is no longer considered an experimental procedure and is available as a treatment option for selected patients with end-organ disease. Transplantation of the pancreas also is considered a major treatment option for uremic diabetic patients who are receiving a kidney transplant.[3] BMT is an indicated treatment for patients with myelogenous leukemia and for other blood dyscrasias[19] (see Table 25-1).

DEFINITION

Organ transplants are common today and may be performed in several organ systems, depending on the mix of recipients and donors. Heart, liver, kidney, pancreas, heart-lung, bone marrow, and other transplants may be available for the appropriate recipient. The ideal combination involves the transplantation of an organ from an identical twin to the other twin (syngeneic). The next best match for organ survival is transplantation of an organ from one living relative to another (allogeneic). This is followed by transplantation of an organ between living nonrelated individuals (xenograft). Each of these combinations, however, is limited by the fact that unless two organs are present, the donor could not survive. Thus these types of matches are basically limited to kidney and

bone marrow donors. Nevertheless, recent studies have shown success with transplantation of a portion of a liver or pancreas from living donors. The largest organ pool for transplantation is cadaver organs, but the match also is poorest.

INCIDENCE AND PREVALENCE

Since 1987, all organ transplant procedures performed in the United States have been reported to the United Network for Organ Sharing (UNOS). In 1980, the Registry of the International Society for Heart Transplantation was established. Similar international registries have been established for other organ transplants.[14,17,23,25,28] By the end of 1991, a total of 1,342 pancreas transplants had been performed in the United States. This represented more than half of the 2,144 transplants that were reported worldwide to the International Registry. More than half of all the pancreas transplants reported to the UNOS Registry (United States) were performed in 1990.[29,30] By the end of 2000, the figure for the United States had grown to more than 3,000[12,31] (see Table 25-1). As of October 1, 1990, data from more than 14,500 heart transplant patients were collected by the Registry of the International Society for Heart Transplantation.[14] Before 1980, fewer than 100 heart transplantations were performed annually. In 1988, about 2,450 heart transplants were reported worldwide. Within a year, this figure had doubled. More than 85% of all heart transplantations performed worldwide have been done since 1985. In the United States, more than 200 centers perform heart transplantations. Presently, nearly 54,000 heart transplants have been performed worldwide.[4,31-33] Further in the annual number of heart transplant procedures is now limited by the supply growth of donor organs.[14]

Approximately 800 combination heart-lung transplants have been performed. This procedure has only recently become more available. The 1-year survival rate for these transplants is approximately 60%.[15]

During 1988 and 1989, some 3,343 patients received their first orthotopic liver transplantation as reported to UNOS. Most patients received a single liver graft; however, some patients received multiple liver grafts. From 1988 to 1989, a 25% increase occurred in the number of liver transplantations performed. At present, more than 30,000 liver transplants have been performed. Survival for patients receiving transplants in 1988 was 75.5% at 1 year and 68.6% at 2 years following the operation. The 1-year survival rate for patients receiving transplants in 1989 was 73.45%. The difference in 1-year survival between 1988 and 1989 was not statistically significant.[27,31] Presently, the survival rates

have increased slightly to approximately 80% for 1 year and 70% for 5 years.[9,33]

The International Bone Marrow Transplant Registry reported that more than 20,000 patients had received allogenic bone marrow transplants between 1955 and 1987. More than 50% of these were performed during the 3 years between 1985 and 1987. By 1991, that figure had doubled, and through 1999 nearly 90,000 BMTs had been performed. Bone marrow transplants are the treatment of choice for patients with aplastic anemia and chronic myelogenous leukemia, those who fail conventional therapy for acute leukemia, and patients with a variety of immune deficiency disorders.[16,34,35] Table 25-1 shows the numbers of all types of transplants reported through the end of 1999.

The Cincinnati Transplant Tumor Registry since 1968 has collected and analyzed data from transplant centers throughout the world. As of November 1990, 5435 posttransplant malignancies were reported, occurring in 5103 recipients. The incidence of cancer in patients with transplanted organs ranged from 1% to 18%, with a mean of 6%.[35]

ETIOLOGY

The most common indications for heart transplantation are cardiomyopathy and severe coronary artery disease. The most common diseases in adults for which liver transplantation is indicated are primary biliary cirrhosis, chronic hepatitis, sclerosing cholangitis, fulminant hepatic failure, and metabolic disorders. In children, most liver transplants are performed for extrahepatic biliary atresia or metabolic disorders. Common indications for kidney transplantation are bilateral chronic disease or end-stage renal disease. Glomerulonephritis, pyelonephritis, diabetic nephropathy, and congenital renal disorders are the most frequent conditions leading to end-stage renal disease. The most common indication for pancreas transplantation is severe diabetes leading to end-stage renal disease. Diabetic patients who are going to receive a kidney transplant also are good candidates for pancreas transplantation. The most common indications for bone marrow transplantation are acute and chronic myelogenous leukemia, acute lymphoblastic leukemia, aplastic anemia, and immune deficiency syndromes.[4]

PATHOPHYSIOLOGY AND COMPLICATIONS

All candidates for heart, liver, and bone marrow transplantation have severe end-stage organ disease and would die without transplantation. Patients with end-stage renal disease can be kept alive by hemodialysis.

However, the quality of their lives can be greatly improved by renal transplantation. Patients with severe diabetes also can be kept alive with daily insulin injections, but their lives also may be greatly improved by pancreas transplantation.[5,29,30,36,37]

CLINICAL PRESENTATION

SIGNS AND SYMPTOMS

Signs and symptoms for the diseases necessitating transplantation are discussed in the chapters indicated:
- Advanced cardiac disease, Chapters 4, 5, and 6
- End-stage renal disease, Chapter 9
- Advanced liver disease, Chapter 10
- Advanced diabetes mellitus, Chapter 14
- Bone marrow transplantation, Chapters 20 and 21

LABORATORY FINDINGS

Laboratory findings of particular importance to the dentist who may be involved with patients before transplantation include bleeding time, differential white blood cell count, prothrombin time, hematocrit, partial thromboplastin time, blood urea nitrogen, aspartate aminotransaminase, serum creatinine, specific gravity of urine, platelet count, white blood cell (WBC) count, serum bilirubin, alkaline phosphatase, and testing urine for proteins. Elevation of aspartate aminotransaminase, alkaline phosphatase, prothrombin time, and serum bilirubin would suggest advanced liver disease. Increased bleeding time, low platelet count, decreased WBC count, and decreased hematocrit are associated with many of the blood dyscrasias. Elevation of serum creatinine and blood urea nitrogen and increased specific gravity of urine and proteinuria are associated with advanced renal disease. In addition, a low hematocrit, prolonged partial thromboplastin time, and decreased WBC count can be found in patients with advanced renal disease. These patients may be potential bleeders, prone to infection, and build up toxic levels of drugs that are metabolized by the liver or kidney, depending on the organ involved (Table 25-2).

MEDICAL AND SURGICAL MANAGEMENT

IMMUNOSUPPRESSION

The immunosuppressive agents now used for most heart, liver, kidney, and pancreas transplantations are cyclosporine, azathioprine, prednisone, and an antilymphocyte agent. Since the 1980s cyclosporine has been the standard immunosuppressive drug used to prevent organ graft rejection. Antilymphocyte agents include the Minnesota antilymphocyte globulin, equine antithymocyte globulin, rabbit antithymocyte globulin, or Orthoclone monoclonal antibody. The best clinical results are obtained with triple-drug immunosuppressive therapy, cyclosporine, prednisone and azathioprine, or mycophenolate mofetil (MMF). Antilymphocyte agents are used at the time of induction of immunosuppression and for acute rejection episodes. A newer immunosuppressive agent, Tacrolimus (FK 506), is being used with organ transplants. Tacrolimus is a xenobiotic immunosuppressive drug that was discovered in Japan in 1984 and has been proven effective in the prevention of graft rejection. It is now used in organ transplantation recipients as a primary immunosuppressive drug or as a rescue-drug in cases of therapy-resistant acute rejection. It seems to produce less adverse side effects than other forms of immunosuppressive therapy. The immunosuppression regimens vary from center to center in terms of dosage, timing, and duration of use of the various agents. After transplantation, doses of the immunosuppression agents are reduced as much as possible to prevent rejection of the graft.[29,34,37,38]

The year 1999 was the first of the extended clinical use of the new anti-interleukin–2 antibodies (IL-2 R-alpha), daclizumab (humanized anti-IL-2 R-alpha) and basiliximab (chimeric-anti-IL-2 R-alpha). These agents have proven quite successful in furthering the immunosupression.[4] Another important new drug is sirolimus, which is a macrocyclic lactone and blocks IL-2 receptors. Organ rejection and the need for antilymphocyte globulin have been reduced by sirolimus.

Total-body irradiation (1000 cGy) has been the most effective means of conditioning a bone marrow graft recipient. Cyclophosphamide usually is used in the immunosuppressive phase before (4 to 5 days) transplantation. Busulfan also has been used for conditioning the graft recipient. Cyclosporine, prednisone, and methotrexate are used after marrow transplantation to prevent or ameliorate GVHD.[3,4,9,34,39]

SURGICAL PROCEDURE

Heart Transplantation

Heart transplantation involves the surgical removal of the heart from the donor by one surgical team and the removal of the recipient's diseased heart and the attachment of the donor's heart to the major vessels of the recipient's heart by a second surgical team (Fig. 25-1). In addition to the immunosuppressive agents given to the recipient, other medications are given at the time of transplantation. These include agents such as dipyridamole (for platelet suppres-

TABLE **25-2**

Screening Laboratory Tests Used to Evaluate Status of Kidney, Liver, Pancreas, and Bone Marrow Function*

Test	Normal Range	Abnormal Result	Organ
Alanine aminotransferase (ALT)	0 to 45 U/L	Elevated	Liver
Alkaline phosphatase	1 to 4 Bodansky units		
	3 to 13 King-Armstrong units	Elevated	Liver
Aspartate aminotransferase (AST)	8 to 50 U/L	Elevated	Liver
Bleeding time (BT)	1 to 6 seconds (Ivy)	Prolonged	Kidney
Differential WBC			
Neutrophils	43% to 47%	Decreased	Bone marrow
Lymphocytes	17% to 47%		
Monocytes	0% to 9%		
Platelet count	140,000 to 400,000/mm^3	<80,000/mm^3	Bone marrow, kidney, liver
Prothrombin time (PT)	11 to 15 seconds	Prolonged	Liver
Activated partial thromboplastin time (APTT)	21 to 30 seconds	Prolonged	Liver, Kidney
Serum albumin	3.3 to 5 mg/dl	Elevated	Kidney
Serum amylase	60 to 180 U/L	Decreased	Pancreas
Serum bilirubin	0.2 to 0.1.5 mg/dl	Elevated	Liver
Serum chloride	95 to 103 mmol/L	Elevated	Kidney
Serum glucose	70 to 100 mg/dl (fasting),	>126 mg/dl	Pancreas
Serum creatinine	0.6 to 1.2 mg	Elevated	Kidney
Serum potassium	3.8 to 5 mmol/L	Elevated	Kidney
Serum sodium	136 to 142 mmol/L	Elevated	Kidney
Thrombin time (TT)	9 to 13 seconds	Prolonged	Liver
Urinalysis			
Specific gravity	1.003 to 1.03	Elevated	Kidney
pH	4.8 to 7.5	Decreased	Kidney
Protein	2 to 8 mg/dl	Elevated	Kidney
Glucose	<180 mg%	Elevated	Pancreas
BUN	8 to 18 mg	Elevated	Kidney
Amylase	35 to 260 Somogyi units	Decreased	Pancreas
White blood cell count (WBC)	4,000 to 10,000/mm^3	Decreased	Bone marrow

*Normal values may vary depending on techniques used.

sion), sulfa-methoxazole-trimethoprim (to prevent infection), and nystatin (Mycostatin) (*Candida* prophylaxis). Surveillance right-ventricular endomyocardial biopsies are obtained after transplantation to check for signs of acute or chronic rejection. Starting 1 year after transplantation, coronary angiography often is performed to look for evidence of coronary artery disease.[6,32]

Heart-Lung Transplantation
In addition to the surgical protocol for the cardiac transplant, the lungs are generally combined in patients with primary pulmonary hypertension, pulmonary fibrosis, cystic fibrosis, certain congenital heart conditions, and primary cardiac disease accompanied by secondary pulmonary hypertension.[15,40] Heart-lung transplantation also involves the surgical removal of the heart and lungs from the donor by one surgical team and the removal of the recipient's diseased heart and lungs and the attachment of the donor's heart and lungs with anastomotic sites at the trachea, the right atrium, and the aorta by the second surgical team (Fig. 25-2). The typical immunosuppressive agents are used as in heart transplants.[15]

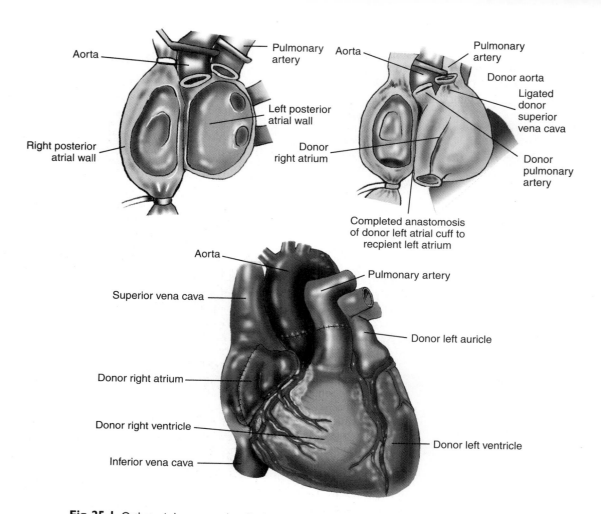

Fig. 25-1 Orthotopic heart transplant. By this procedure, a patient's atria and ventricles are completely replaced. (Dedrawn from Herman M: *Am J Nurs* 80(10):1786, 1980.)

Fig. 25-2 Anastomotic sites in a completed combination heart-lung transplant: *1*, aorta; *2*, right atrium; *3*, trachea.

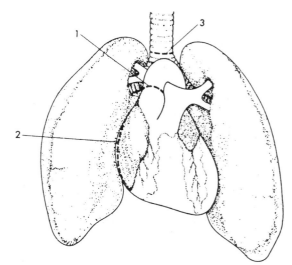

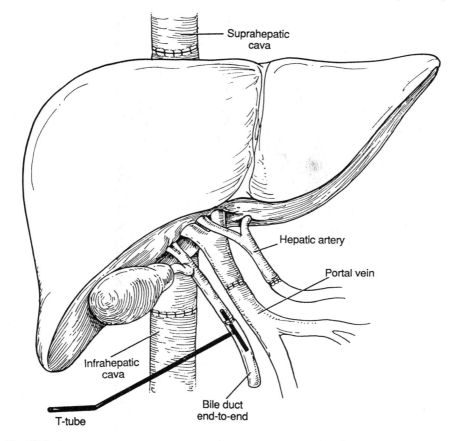

Fig. 25-3 Completed liver transplant. Vascular anastomoses include the suprahepatic vena cava, infrahepatic vena cava, portal vein, and hepatic artery. A choledochocholedochostomy biliary reconstruction is depicted. (From Howard TK et al: In Kaplowitz N, editor: *Liver and biliary diseases*, Baltimore, 1992, Williams & Wilkins.)

An additional complication, however, that may be seen in heart-lung combination transplants is the implantation response. The incidence of this particular complication most commonly occurs between 4 to 21 days after transplantation. It is a reversible condition characterized by fever, tachypnea, diffuse pulmonary infiltrates on the chest radiograph, decreased arterial oxygen pressure (pO_2) and increased arterial carbon dioxide pressure (pCO_2). The cause is lymphatic interruption, ischemia, denervation, and surgical trauma. The patient may need short-term mechanical ventilation. Acute rejection of the transplanted organs is also a major complication and the most common cause of death within the first year.[15]

Liver Transplantation

Liver transplantation involves the excision of the diseased recipient's liver with reconstruction of the vena cava, portal vein, and biliary tree (Figs. 25-3 and 25-4).

The transplant procedure is commonly divided into three phases: (1) dissection, during which the recipient's liver is dissected free of surrounding structures; (2) anhepatic, when blood flow through the vena cava, portal vein, and hepatic artery is interrupted (during this time, the recipient's liver is resected and the donor liver revascularized); and (3) reperfusion, in which the implanted donor's liver is filled with blood. The final step is biliary anastomosis.[30,34]

Liver transplants have been performed in patients with hemophilia, and their factor VIII deficiency has been corrected. Therefore factor VIII is produced by the liver and not endothelial cells.[10,38]

Small Bowel Transplantation

Few small bowel transplantations (SBTs) have been performed.[16] Because of its quasi-experimental nature, SBT currently is restricted to patients with end-stage

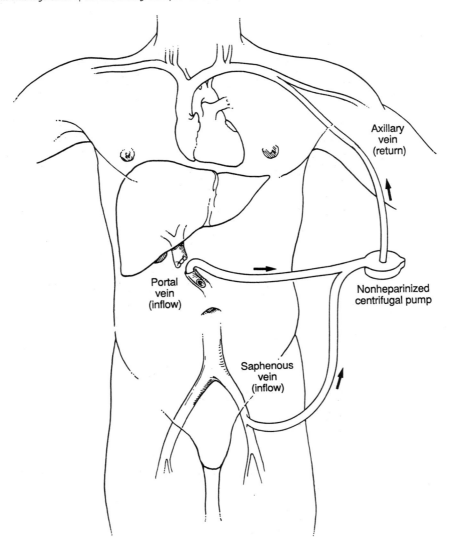

Fig. 25-4 Venovenous bypass. The portal vein is divided, and devascularization of the liver is completed. Then the portal vein is cannulated and a second cannula is placed in the iliac vein via the saphenous vein. The blood is pumped by a centrifugal pump through a nonheparinized system and returned to the patient via a cannula placed in the axillary vein. Flows of 2 to 5 L/min are commonly attained. Flow must be maintained above 700 to 1000 ml/min to prevent thrombosis. (From Howard TK et al: In Kaplowitz N, editor: *Liver and biliary diseases*, Baltimore, 1992, Williams & Wilkins.)

intestinal failure who have failed conventional treatments. Intestinal failure is characterized by the inability to maintain nutrition and intestinal fluid and electrolyte balance. Several causes of this condition exist, the most common being massive small bowel resection and the "short gut syndrome," which results in rapid intestinal transit without proper absorption of nutrients. Nearly

2 million patients per year in the United States have this condition. SBT is commonly performed in conjunction with liver transplantation.[16] The small bowel is unique among solid-organ transplant grafts because of the large amount of lymphoid tissue contained in the mesenteric lymph nodes, Peyer's patches, and lamina propria, and the heavy colonization with microorgan-

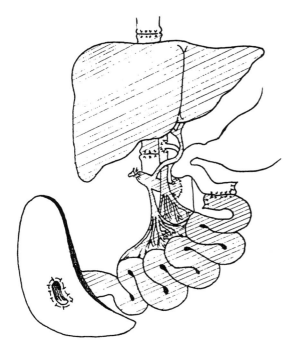

Fig. 25-5 Small bowel transplantation. Anastomoses are at the superior end of the small intestine at the jejunum, and the terminus is exteriorized in a stoma. Here the liver also has been transplanted. (From Asfar S, Zhong R, Grant D: *Surg Clin North Am* 74(5):1197-1207, 1994.)

isms and large quantities of antigens on the surface of the intestinal epithelium. These factors contribute to a high rate of GVHD, graft rejection, and sepsis.

The surgical technique for SBT is shown in Figure 25-5. The transplanted small bowel has anastomotic sites at the superior end of the native gastrointestinal tract at the jejunum, and at its distal end a stoma is created exteriorly. The superior mesenteric artery is attached to the native aorta below the renal arteries.[16]

Kidney Transplantation

Patients who have a living related donor available for kidney transplantation usually are admitted to the hospital 2 days before transplantation. When a kidney recipient is to receive a cadaver kidney, the patient is admitted to the hospital on an urgent basis. Current preservation techniques allow kidney storage for up to 72 hours.[5,41]

The indications for renal transplantation generally includes chronic renal disease or end-stage renal disease (ESRD). ESRD is a progressive, bilateral deterioration of kidney nephrons that results in uremia and, ultimately, death. ESRD is associated with glomerulonephritis,

nephrosclerosis, pyelonephritis, diabetic nephropathy, congenital renal disorders, drug-induced nephropathy, obstructive uropathy, and hypertension.[1,5]

Accompanying hypertension, diabetes, congestive heart failure, infections, volume depletion, urinary tract obstruction, hypercalcemia, and hyperuricemia must be constantly managed. After conservative care (i.e., drug therapy, dietary restrictions, management of underlying disease), to control waste products, fluid balance, and electrolyte levels becomes inadequate, renal dialysis is the next step. As renal disease progresses, and more nephrons are destroyed, azotemia cannot be controlled, and the patient must have the blood artificially filtered. Therefore the therapy of peritoneal dialysis or hemodialysis begins.[1,5]

More than 80,000 patients are currently being maintained on hemodialysis in the United States.[1,5,18] Hemodialysis treatment must be performed every 2 to 3 days and requires 4 to 5 hours each treatment. The cost in terms of time, money, patient inconvenience, and so on is enormous and extremely confining (see Chapter 9). An alternative to dialysis is transplantation of a kidney from either a living donor or from a cadaver. The transplant frees the patient from not only the burden of dialysis but also most all of the chronic consequences of ESRD. Renal transplantation has become a standard surgical procedure in most major hospitals today.[1,5]

The recipients of a kidney transplant require immunosuppressive preparation so that they will not reject the graft. As with all major transplant procedures, the major problem in renal transplantation is rejection of the graft. The type of preparation depends on the nature of the underlying renal disease. Intensive chemotherapy is commonly used. Chemotherapy with cytotoxic agents (azathioprine) or steroids (prednisone) and administration of antilymphocytic globulin (ALG) are effective. However, greater success has been attained with cyclosporine instead of prednisone or azathioprine.[1,5]

With the immunosuppression, the patient is rendered susceptible to infection and poor wound healing. Sepsis is a major complication in renal transplant patients. Adrenal function may be suppressed and likewise endogenous cortisol production[1,5,18] (Box 25-1).

In addition to being given immunosuppressive medications, the patient receives a bladder injection of antibiotic solution by means of a Foley catheter and a second-generation cephalosporin. The donor renal artery usually is anastomosed to the aorta and the renal vein to the vena cava in children. In adults, the renal artery is anastomosed to either the internal or the external iliac artery. After the kidneys are reperfused, urethral implantation is done. The antibiotics that were started just before surgery are stopped 3 days after surgery, and the

BOX 25-1

**Signs of Overimmunosuppression
in Posttransplantation Patients**

Viral infections (HSV, CMV, HBV, HIV)
Bacterial infections (respiratory, wound, etc.)
Fungal infections (candidiasis, pulmonary, etc.)
Delayed healing
Excessive bleeding
Hypertension
Cushingoid reaction (edema, ascites, etc.)
Addison's reaction (adverse reaction to stress, etc.)
Diabetes mellitus
Anemia
Osteoporosis
Tumors

HSV, Herpes simplex virus, CMV, cytomegalovirus; HBV, hepatitis B virus; HIV, human immunodeficiency virus.

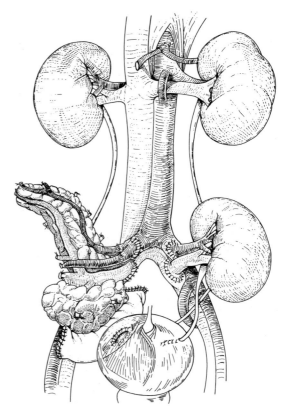

Fig. 25-6 Pancreaticoduodenocystostomy. Combined kidney and pancreas transplants. (From Groshek M, Smith VL: In Norris MK, House MA, editors: *Organ and tissue transplantation*, Philadelphia, 1991, FA Davis, p 159.)

patient is given trimethoprim/sulfamethoxazole (Bactrim) daily for as long as the graft is functioning. Acyclovir and nystatin usually are given for the first 3 months to prevent herpes simplex virus (HSV), cytomegalovirus (CMV), and *Candida* infections.[1,5,18]

Pancreas Transplantation

Pancreas transplantation can be done (1) simultaneously with kidney transplantation (Fig. 25-6), (2) after kidney transplantation, or (3) as a separate procedure (Figs. 25-7 and 25-8). Living related donor grafts usually are used for recipients of pancreas transplants alone or a pancreas transplant after a previous kidney. However, cadaver grafts can be transplanted to all recipient categories. Cadaver donor pancreas grafts can be preserved by cold storage in a silica gel-filtered plasma solution for about 10 to 24 hours. In most grafts, the pancreatic duct is drained into the bladder. Urine amylase levels (25% reduction) are used in bladder-drained patients to monitor for rejection. Decreased urinary amylase activity precedes hyperglycemia as a manifestation of rejection. In patients who have simultaneous kidney and pancreas transplants, an increase in serum creatinine indicates the possible onset of rejection before changes in urinary amylase are detected.[23,29,37]

A relatively new, revolutionary technique that may have far-reaching implications for the management of diabetes is transplantation of islet cells from a donor's pancreas into the liver of the recipient.[27] The response to the transplanted beta cells has helped in many cases of diabetes. One impediment to the success of this technique has been to avoid immune attacks from the recipient on the transplanted donor cells. However, this technique certainly holds much promise for the future.[27]

Bone Marrow Transplantation

Patients who are going to receive a BMT are prepared using different preoperative regimens, depending on the patient's disease. The greatest chance of success from BMT is in patients with chronic myelogenous leukemia. Commonly, patients with aplastic anemia, lymphoma, Hodgkin's disease, neuroblastoma, or genetic diseases (i.e., immunodeficiency, Hurler's syndrome) undergo BMT as well. Chronic myelogenous leukemia is 100% fatal without BMT but with BMT is approximately 60% to 70% successful.[35] Acute myelogenous leukemia is 40% to 60% curable, and acute lymphoblastic leukemia has a 20% to

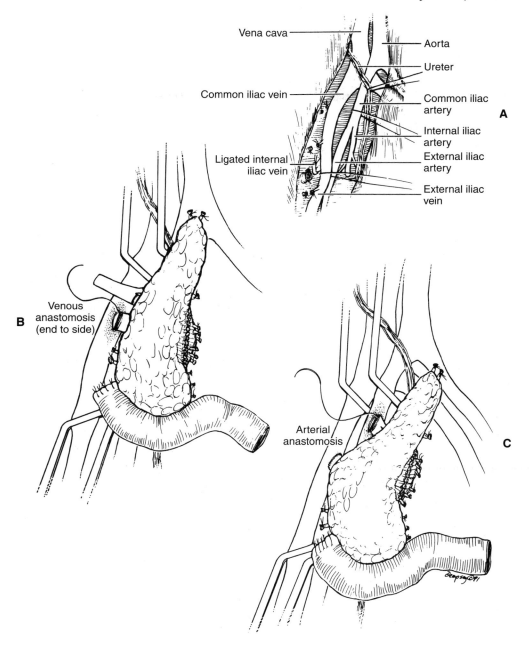

Fig. 25-7 Transplantation of the pancreaticoduodenal allografts. **A,** Preparation of the recipient vessels. Note that all deep branches of the common and external iliac veins are ligated and divided. The vein is brought lateral to the artery. The ureter is mobilized and brought medial to the artery. **B,** The venous anastomosis is performed end-to-side, with the portal vein of the pancreas graft anastomosed to the proximal external or distal common iliac vein. **C,** The arterial anastomosis is performed after the venous anastomosis and placed superior to the venous anastomosis. The common iliac artery of the recipient is used as the site for the arterial anastomosis. (From Brayman KL et al: In Cameron JL, editor: *Current surgical therapy,* ed 4, St Louis, 1992, Mosby, p 466.)

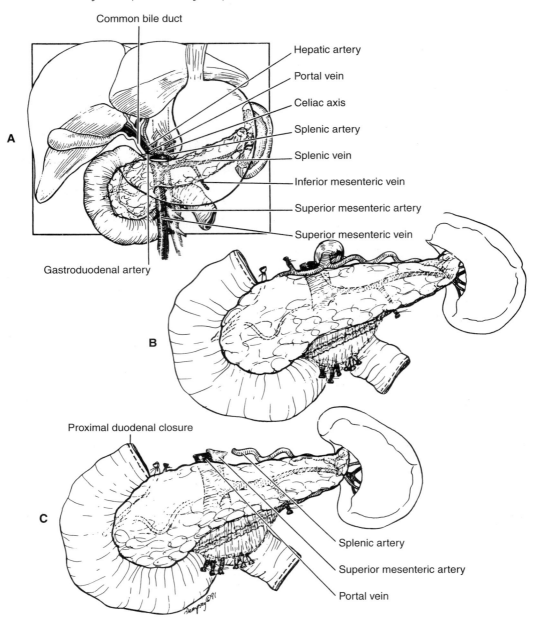

Fig. 25-8 Procurement of the pancreaticoduodenal allograft. **A,** Vascular anatomy of the liver and pancreas. Note the gastroduodenal artery, which is divided during simultaneous procurement of the liver and the pancreas but not during procurement of the pancreas alone. **B,** Pancreaticoduodenal allograft following procurement (nonliver donor). Note that the proximal duodenum has been divided with the GIA stapler. The mesentery of the small intestine inferior to the pancreas also has been ligated and divided following placement of two parallel rows of TA 90 staples. **C,** Pancreaticoduodenal allograft following procurement from a donor whose liver also was procured. Note the splenic and superior mesenteric arteries, which require ex vivo reconstruction. (From Brayman KL et al: In Cameron JL, editor: *Current surgical therapy,* ed 4, St Louis, 1992, Mosby, p 461.)

25% cure rate. Cyclophosphamide and total-body irradiation or busulfan may be used for patients with leukemia. Patients with a lymphoma may be given cyclophosphamide and total-body irradiation, busulfan and cyclophosphamide, or busulfan alone. Patients with aplastic anemia may be given cyclophosphamide alone. The preoperative regimens start 7 to 10 days before transplantation. At transplantation, the donor's marrow is infused into the recipient. The recipient of a syngeneic marrow graft (from an identical twin) requires no immunosuppressive preparation. Similarly, the patient with severe immunologic deficiency requires no immunosuppressive preparation because of the very nature of the disease. However, all other recipients of BMT must undergo some form of immunosuppressive therapy so that they will not reject the graft. The type of preparation depends on the nature of the underlying disease. BMT is not the cure for the cancer. The intensive chemotherapy or total-body irradiation kills the cancer. However, these treatments also may kill the patient, so BMT is a method to "rescue" the patient from the lethal effects of the chemoradiation therapy. The marrow is harvested from the donor's iliac bones by numerous needle aspirations under spinal anesthesia in an operating room environment. The typical quantity of marrow obtained per needle aspiration is 1 to 3 ml (from 400 to 800 ml is required). Generally, the procedure is well tolerated and involves few complications.[8,9,17,19,20]

In nonmalignant conditions (i.e., aplastic anemia), the preparation of the recipient can be directed solely toward the problem of immunosuppression without worrying about destroying cancerous cells. In malignant disorders, however, specifically acute myelogenous leukemia, the preparation of the recipient must not only accomplish immunosuppression, but likewise kill all or nearly all of the malignant leukemic cells. Total-body irradiation (1000 cGy) has been the most effective means of conditioning a bone marrow graft recipient. Cyclophosphamide (50 mg/kg) is used in the immunosuppressive phase prior (4 to 5 days) to the transplantation.[8,9,17,19,20]

Histocompatibility. Matching of blood type and human lymphocyte antigens (HLA) with tissue compatibility tests usually results in longer graft and patient survival. The best matching occurs in identical twins; however, with appropriate screening tests, acceptable matches can be found for other potential organ recipients and living or cadaver donors.[8,9,17,19,20]

Syngeneic or isogeneic human marrow transplantation involves donors and recipients carrying the same tissue antigens, as in identical twins. Consequently, no immunologic barrier exists to transplantation. An autologous marrow graft refers to the transplantation of the patient's own marrow, which was harvested from the same patient and set aside before the intense chemotherapy or total radiation therapy and until used in the transplantation. An allogeneic marrow graft involves a donor and a recipient of different genetic origin within the same species (usually 50% to 70% of transplants). Siblings are the best and partially match (haploidentical), or parents may donate the marrow (providing usually 30% to 50% of BMTs). Allogeneic grafts also may involve unrelated donors (usually 10% to 15%). These transplants involve moderate to severe histoincompatibility and present a bidirectional immunologic barrier to transplantation. The recipient may react adversely to the donated marrow and reject it, or secondly, the infused marrow cells from the donor transplant, containing immunologically competent cells, react against the host to produce GVHD.[8,9,17,19,20]

In humans, the major histocompatibility complex (H-2) involves two closely associated serologically detected loci, the first, or "LA" locus and the second, or "4" locus. (HLA-A4). Marrow grafts between unrelated humans carry a high probability of major histocompatibility problems because of the complex polymorphism of the histocompatibility complex. Members of the same family, however, simplify the situation considerably, because only 4 haplotypes can be involved. HLA typing of the family can therefore identify the most ideal donor.[8,9,17,19,20]

Before the grafting procedure begins, almost all marrow recipients undergo a period of no marrow function because of their underlying disease and immunosuppressive preparation. After the transplant, 10 to 20 days elapse before the transplanted marrow begins to function. Naturally, this is a critical period for the patient's recovery and success of the BMT. The posttransplant period consists of three phases of recovery: the pancytopenic phase (absolute neutrophil count greater than 500 for 4 to 6 weeks), the immune recovery phase (3 to 12 months), and the long-term immunocompetent phase (1 to 3 years). Most patients are given cyclosporine, methotrexate, or steroids following transplantation. Patients testing positive for HSV are given prophylactic IV acyclovir. Patients usually are given an antifungal medication such as IV miconazole to prevent *Candida* infection. These medications are continued after bone marrow transplantation throughout the critical period needed for the transplanted marrow to begin functioning. This critical period may last up to 20 days or more. Once the transplanted marrow starts to function, the risk of infection decreases. However, long-term therapy using broad-spectrum antibiotics such as Bactrim is needed to reduce the risk of infection.

TABLE **25-3**

Major Medical Complications Associated with Transplantation

Excessive immunosuppression
  Infection
  Tumors
  Delayed healing
Rejection of allograft
Graft failure—heart, kidney, liver, pancreas
Increased risk for excessive bleeding-liver, kidney, bone marrow
Overdosage—if drugs metabolized or excreted by kidney or liver are administered in normal amounts
Death or retransplantation—heart, liver, bone marrow
Insulin, hemodialysis or retransplantation—kidney, pancreas
Side effects caused by immunosuppressent agents
  Hypertension
  Diabetes mellitus
  Infection
  Excessive bleeding
  Anemia
  Osteoporosis
  Adrenal crisis (significant stress from surgery, trauma)
Special organ complications:

Heart transplants	Accelerated coronary artery atherosclerosis
Bone marrow transplants	Graft-versus-host disease

Patients who develop evidence of GVHD are treated with methotrexate.[8,9,17,19,20]

COMPLICATIONS

Complications associated with organ transplantation generally consist of technical problems involving the surgical procedure, problems related to immunosuppression, and special problems specific to the organ transplanted. A discussion of the surgical complications is beyond the scope of this text and would seldom apply to the dentist's management of such patients (Table 25-3).

IMMUNOSUPPRESSION

Excessive immunosuppression increases the risk for infection and must be avoided. Invasive (biopsy) and non-invasive techniques are used to evaluate patients for signs of excessive immunosuppression. Clinical evidence of such immunosuppression are opportunistic infections and tumors known to be related to these agents. When evidence of excessive immunosuppression is found, the dosage of the immunosuppressant drugs must be reduced.[9,14,36,40]

Of course, signs of overimmunosuppression can exist in all of the types of transplant patients. These signs include infections, delayed healing, hypertension, diabetes, Addison's reactions, Cushingoid reactions (e.g., edema, ascites, buffalo-hump, moon facies), increased susceptibility to infection, weakness, fatigue (see Box 25-1).

REJECTION

Rejection of the transplanted organ is evidenced when signs and symptoms of organ failure begin to occur. Organ biopsies are used to confirm the rejection reaction (Fig. 25-9). When evidence of acute rejection is found, the dosage of the immunosuppressive agents usually is increased.

Chronic rejection occurs insidiously and is progressive. It cannot be reversed with intensified therapy. Chronic rejection of the organ graft is associated with signs and symptoms of organ failure. Classic evidence of chronic rejection is found by biopsy.[9,11,14,29]

DRUG SIDE EFFECTS

The agents used for immunosuppression have several important side effects. A major side effect of azathioprine is bone marrow suppression with resulting leukopenia, thrombocytopenia, and anemia. These changes place the patient at greater risk for infection and excessive bleeding. Cyclosporine has replaced azathioprine as the key agent for immunosuppression in transplant patients because it does not suppress the bone marrow. However, cyclosporine does have important side effects. It may cause severe kidney and liver changes, which can lead to hypertension, bleeding problems, and anemia; and it may potentiate renal injury caused by other agents. Cyclosporine also is related to an increased incidence of gingival hyperplasia, hirsutism, gynecomastia, and cancer of the skin and cervix. Antithymocyte globulin (ATG) and ALG both act as lymphocyte-selective immunosuppressants. Important side effects associated with these agents include fever, hemolysis, leukopenia, thrombocytopenia, tumor development, and increased risk for infection.[9,18,19,38,42,43]

Prednisone has important side effects including hypertension, diabetes mellitus, osteoporosis, impaired healing, mental depression, psychoses, and increased risk for

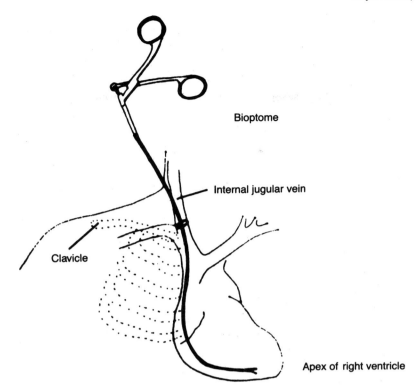

Fig. 25-9 Endomyocardial biopsy technique showing the bioptome in place in the right ventricle. (From Copeland JG, Stinson EB: *Curr Probl Cardiol* 4(8):1-5, 1979.)

infection (see Chapter 24 for side effects of corticosteroids). In addition to these side effects, prednisone therapy may cause adrenal gland suppression. If adrenal suppression occurs, the patient is unable to produce and release increased amounts of steroids needed to deal with the stress of infection, trauma, surgery, or extreme anxiety.[3,9]

Immunosuppressed patients have an increased incidence of certain cancers. Overall, approximately 6% of these patients develop various forms of cancer. Cancers commonly seen in the general population (carcinomas of lung, breast, prostate, and colon) show no change in occurrence in immunosuppressed patients. However, two types of cancer found commonly in the general population are found with increased frequency in immunosuppressed patients: squamous cell carcinoma of the skin and in situ carcinomas of the uterine cervix.[35,43] Cancers that are uncommon in the general population but that occur with increased frequency in immunosuppressed patients are lymphomas, lip carcinomas, Kaposi's sarcoma, carcinomas of the kidney, and carcinomas of the vulva and perineum (Table 25-4). Cancer is a complication of

TABLE 25-4

Cancer Development in the General Population and in Transplant Patients

Tumor	General Population (%)	Transplant Patients (%)
Lymphomas	<5.3	20
Lip carcinomas	<0.3	28
Kaposi's sarcoma	<0.1	26
Carcinoma of kidney	2.1	25
Carcinoma of vulva and perineum	<0.6	2

From Najarian JS, Sutherland DER: *Transplant Proc* 24(4):1293-1926, 1992.

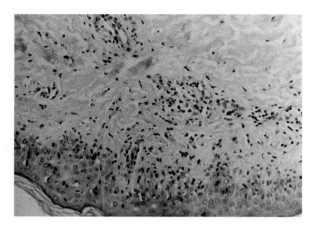

Fig. 25-10 Photomicrograph of GVHD in a post-BMT patient.

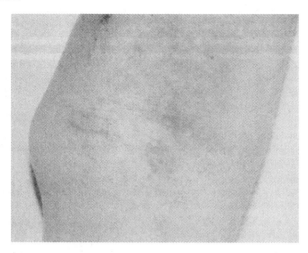

Fig. 25-11 GVHD in bone marrow transplant patient. Note areas of necrosis. (Courtesy Norma Ramsay, University of Minnesota Hospital.)

intense immunosuppression per se, rather than being related to the use of any particular agent. However, certain agents may play a more direct role. Cyclosporine is one of these agents, as well as monoclonal antibodies. Both these agents are associated with a higher incidence of lymphoma. Such lymphomas tend to occur earlier and show more nodal involvement.[35]

SPECIAL ORGAN COMPLICATIONS

The major specific organ complications of immunosuppression involve the heart and bone marrow. Recent improvements in immunosuppressant agents have not altered the development of graft coronary artery disease.[6,9,32] In one study, the incidence of coronary artery disease in transplanted patients was 10% at 1 year, 25% at 3 years, and 36% at 5 years. Coronary artery disease was responsible for 60% of late deaths.[32] A study showed a possible association between CMV infection and coronary atherosclerosis in transplanted hearts.[44]

GVHD is an important and often lethal complication of allogenic bone marrow transplantation. Acute GVHD occurs within the first 2 months after transplantation and is characterized by skin, liver, and gastrointestinal tract involvement (see Figures 25-10, 25-11, and 25-12). Chronic GVHD occurs later and is characterized by skin changes similar to scleroderma, sicca syndrome, malabsorption, and features of autoimmunity. Cyclosporine appears to be more effective than methotrexate in preventing GVHD in HLA-identical siblings who have received a bone marrow transplant for severe aplastic anemia. Methotrexate appears to be more effective for acute leukemia.[17,19,34]

DENTAL MANAGEMENT

PRETRANSPLANT MEDICAL CONSIDERATIONS

A number of significant medical problems must be considered during the dental management of patients being prepared for transplantation. The problems associated with advanced coronary artery disease, significant cardiac arrhythmias, and congestive heart failure are discussed in Chapters 5, 6, and 7. The medical considerations that affect the dental treatment of patients with renal failure and end-stage liver are discussed in Chapters 9 and 10. The medical considerations impacting on dental treatment for severe diabetic patients being considered for pancreas and kidney transplantation are covered in Chapters 9 and 14.

The patient who is a candidate for a bone marrow transplant is generally very ill and prone to infection, bleeding, and delayed healing because of thrombocytopenia and leukopenia (see Chapters 20 and 21).

POSTTRANSPLANT MEDICAL CONSIDERATIONS

Medical considerations of importance to the dentist in the management of the transplanted patient fall into three stages: (1) immediate posttransplant period, (2) stable transplant period, and (3) chronic rejection period.[19,24,34,35]

During the immediate posttransplant period, which is generally for the first 3 months after the transplant, the patient will be started on immunosuppressive therapy to

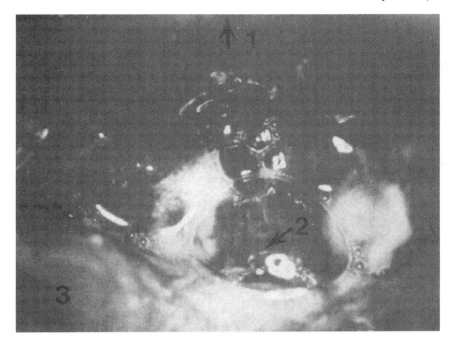

Fig. 25-12 Oral mucositis/candidiasis in BMT: *1*, soft palate; *2*, oropharynx; *3*, tongue. (Courtesy Norma Ramsay, University of Minnesota Hospital.)

prevent cytotoxic T-cells from destroying the graft. This is the time that the patient is at the greatest risk for technical complications, acute rejection, and infection. The length of this period will vary depending on a number of factors. Cyclosporine, prednisone and other immunosuppresive agents (azothioprine, antilymphocyte globulin, etc.) have great benefit in increasing the survival and prevent rejection in posttransplant patients. However, these agents also have significant major side effects and place the patient at substantial risk for infection. Also, many drugs exist that may adversely interact with cyclosporine and other immunosuppresive agents, including several dentists may use (i.e., erythromycin, ketoconazole, carbamazepine, phenytoin, and others).[4] The dentist needs to consult with the patient's physician to confirm the patient's status, the level and severity of immunosuppression and to determine whether the patient has progressed beyond this critical stage.

Medical complications are relatively common during the immediate posttransplant period. The patient may have acute respiratory distress syndrome, viral, bacterial and fungal infections of varying types and severity, bleeding problems, hypertension, acute renal and or hepatic failure, acute pancreatitis, and other problems. For these reasons, during the first 3 months after an organ trans-

plant the patient should have only emergency dental treatment and elective procedures should be postponed. Even the emergency dental treatment must be provided in close association with the patient's physician(s). Antibiotic prophylaxis should be used during this time because of the immunosuppression and increased risk of infections.[45] The type of agents and regimen for this antibiotic prophylaxis is special for transplant patients and is presented in Table 25-5.

The next stage is the period when the graft is stable and functional. In most cases, this is approximately 3 months posttransplantation. The patient has undergone graft healing and the new organ should be functioning nearly normally. In most cases, the coagulation factors and susceptibility to bleeding, the blood chemistry profiles etc., will have returned to normal limits, although this should be confirmed by the patient's physician. The medical considerations during this stage relate to the effects of immunosuppressive agents. The patient will still be susceptible to infections, but now the major concern is overimmunosuppression, which increases the risk for infection, and underimmunosuppression, which increases the risk for acute rejection. If rejection of the graft occurs, the organ begins to fail, and the problems associated with end-stage heart, liver, kidney, and pancreas

TABLE 25-5

Recommended Standard Prophylactic Regimen for Dental–Oral Procedures in the Post-transplant Patient*

Medication	Regimen
Amoxicillin	2 g orally 1 hour before procedure.
plus Metronidizole,	500 mg orally 1 hour before procedure.
Amoxicillin-penicillin allergy*	
Vancomycin: 1 gm IV	Infused slowly over one-hour preoperatively.
or	
Imipenum 1 gm IV	Infused slowly over one-hour preoperatively.
Unable to take oral medication	
Ampicillin	2 g intravenously 1 hour before procedure.
plus Metronidazole,	500 mg intravenously 1 hour before procedure.

*For the prevention of spontaneous bacterial peritonitis
Note: Clindamycin: should not be used in most organ transplant patients because of acute liver toxicity.

failure will have to be considered and managed when present.

The side effects of the immunosuppressive agents may present significant medical problems during any of the stages following transplantation. However, those occurring during the stable graft stage are of greatest concern to the dentist. These side effects may increase the risk for infection; excessive bleeding; bone fractures; circulatory collapse following significant emotional, physical, or surgical stress; hypertension; diabetes mellitus; and anemia.[1,3,4,19,32,45,46]

Posttransplant patients are also particularly susceptible to fungal infections, especially with *Candida albicans*. Therefore prevention and aggressive management with antifungal agents should be a consideration. Special organ complications found in heart and bone marrow transplantation recipients must be considered during the stable graft period. Symptomatic coronary artery disease develops in many of the heart transplantation patients. However, one important clinical feature of coronary insufficiency or myocardial infarction is missing in these patients. The transplanted heart has no nerve supply; thus pain is not associated with angina or infarction.

Bone marrow transplantation patients may develop GVHD following transplantation. Acute GVHD occurs dur-

ing the immediate posttransplant period, whereas the chronic form of the disease may appear in the stable period. The patient is particularly susceptible to community-based infections such as influenza and pneumonia so precautions such as vaccination should be taken to prevent those.

The chronic rejection period begins with signs and symptoms usually associated with organ failure along with histologic findings on biopsy indicating chronic rejection of the graft. This reaction is not reversible and will lead to retransplantation or death in heart and liver recipients. Kidney patients will require dialysis or retransplantation. Pancreas patients will require insulin or retransplantation.[1,3,4,19,32,45,46]

TREATMENT PLANNING CONSIDERATIONS

PRETRANSPLANT PATIENTS

Patients being prepared for transplantation should be referred for an evaluation of their dental status. Whenever possible, patients found to have active dental disease should receive indicated dental care before the transplant operation. Patients with advanced periodontal disease may best be advised to have their teeth extracted and dentures constructed. The same consideration would be involved for patients who have extensive caries and have demonstrated little interest or ability to improve their level of oral hygiene or to modify their diet.

Patients who have a very good level of dental health should be encouraged to keep their teeth, but they must be advised of the risks and problems involved if significant dental disease were to develop following transplantation. The need for effective preventive dental procedures and more frequent recall visits to the dentist following transplantation must be pointed out to the patient.[1,3,4,19,32,45,46]

Recommendations concerning retention of teeth for patients who have a dental status that falls between the extremes of poor and very good are more difficult to make. The risks involved regarding infection, the steps needed to prevent these complications, and the costs involved must be discussed with the patient and transplant surgeon. Patients with poor oral hygiene who have failed to become motivated to improve their level of home care should be encouraged to consider the extraction of teeth and the construction of dentures.[1,3,4,19,32,45,46]

Before transplantation, all nonrestorable teeth and teeth with advanced periodontal disease should be extracted in those patients deciding to retain their dentition. Nonvital teeth should be endodontically treated or

extracted, and all active carious lesions should be restored in these patients. Preventive dentistry techniques including toothbrushing and flossing, diet modification, and the use of topical fluorides should be initiated, reviewed, and implemented. The importance of using effective hygiene procedures, including antiseptic mouth rinses such as chlorohexidine or Listerine, and the need for maintenance of good oral hygiene must be emphasized.[1,3,4,19,32,45,46]

Before invasive dental procedures are performed on the patient, before transplantation, the dentist must consult with the patient's physician to establish the degree of organ dysfunction, need for prophylactic antibiotics to prevent local or distant infection, the ability of the patient to tolerate dental treatment, and the need to obtain other management suggestions. In most cases, the earlier that most dental treatment should be performed before the transplant, the better.[1,3,4,19,32,45,46]

No data exist to show that prophylactic antibiotics are indicated in the dental management of patients with advanced heart, liver, kidney, and pancreatic disease unless patients are subject to endocarditis or endarteritis (heart or kidney patients on hemodialysis). In patients with a depressed WBC count, a case can be made for using prophylactic antibiotics. The presence of infection in the operative field might be used as an additional indication for the use of antibiotics. Patients being prepared for bone marrow transplantation may require antibiotic prophylaxis. The need for prophylactic antibiotic treatment for invasive dental procedures in patients with advanced heart, liver, kidney, or bone marrow disease should be discussed with the patient's physician before treatment.[9,45] The possibility exists of spontaneous bacterial periotonitis after transplantation, and therefore antibiotic prophylaxis may be indicated.[45] If the decision is made to use prophylactic antibiotics for certain patients, no general agreed-on antibiotic, dosage, or duration of administration exists. The current American Heart Association's standard regimen used for prevention of endocarditis appears to be adequate for this need (see Table 25-5). Patients facing bone marrow transplantation may require a more aggressive prophylactic regimen than do those with advanced heart, liver, and kidney disease.[1,3,4,19,32,45,46]

Results of selective screening tests shown in Table 25-3 should be reviewed. If they are not available through medical consultation, they should be ordered before any invasive dental procedure is performed. If the screening tests reveal significant alterations in bleeding time and/or coagulation status (prothrombin time, thrombin time, and activated partial thromboplastin time), the dentist should consider using antifibrinolytic agents, fresh frozen plasma, vitamin K, and platelet replacement. The approach selected should be based on consultation with the patient's physician. The physician also should be consulted regarding drug selection and dosage modification.[1,3,4,19,32,45,46]

In patients with end-stage liver or kidney disease, the dentist should not use drugs that are metabolized by these organs or reduce the dosage to prevent increased or unexpected effects (Table 25-6). Patients with severe diabetes mellitus must be managed as described in Chapter 14. If infection is present, an increase in insulin dosage may be required. Again, the dentist should consult with the patient's physician to confirm the patient's current status and specific management needs (Box 25-2).

POSTTRANSPLANT PATIENTS

The dental management of the patient after transplantation can be divided in three phases: (1) immediate posttransplant period, (2) stable graft period, (3) chronic rejection period (Box 25-3), or, in bone marrow transplants, the onset of significant graft-versus-host disease.

Immediate Posttransplant Period
During this phase, when operative complications and acute rejection of the graft are the major medical concerns, no routine dentistry is indicated. Only emergency dental care should be provided, following medical consultation, and it should be as noninvasive as possible.[1,3,4,19,32,45,46]

Stable Posttransplant Period
Once the graft has healed and the acute rejection reaction has been controlled, the patient is considered to be in the stable phase. This period should be confirmed by medical consultation with the transplant surgeon. Usually any indicated dental treatment can be performed during this period if the procedures shown in Box 25-3 are adhered to completely. Many of the dental management problems with stable graft patients are similar regardless of the organ that was transplanted. However, some problems are unique to patients with specific transplanted organs.[1,3,4,19,32,45,46]

Risk of Infection. Many posttransplantation infections may occur (Table 25-7). The healthcare professional must be aware of the clinical appearance, signs, and symptoms of these various infections. In some cases, specific prophylaxis may be indicated.[41]

The increased risk for infection in the immunosuppressed transplant patient makes the case for use of prophylactic antibiotics stronger. Many transplant centers recommend prophylactic coverage for all dental procedures that can produce transient bacteremias in

TABLE 25-6

Common Dental Drugs Metabolized Primarily by the Liver and Kidney and Therefore Should Be Avoided or Adjusted Before Dental Treatment

Drug	OK to Use Normal Dosage	Dose Adjustment
Lidocaine (Xylocaine)	Yes	n/a
Aspirin	No	Increase interval between doses (avoid if possible)
Acetaminophen (Tylenol)	No	Increase interval between doses (avoid if possible)
Ibuprofen (Motrin)	Yes	n/a
Propoxyphene (Darvon)	Yes	n/a
Codeine	Yes	n/a
Meperidine (Demerol)	Yes	n/a
Penicillin V	No	Increase interval between doses
Erythromycin	Yes	n/a
Cephalexin (Keflex)	No	Increase interval between doses
Tetracycline (Doxycycline)	No	Increase interval between doses (avoid if possible)
Diazepam (Valium)	Yes	n/a

Modified from Bennet WM et al: *Am J Kidney Dis* 3:155-176, 1983.

BOX 25-2

Dental Management of the Patient Being Prepared for Transplantation

Complete dental evaluation
1. Poor dental status—consider extractions and dentures
2. Good dental status—maintain dentition
3. Other—decide on individual patient basis

Patients maintaining their dentition
1. Extract all nonrestorable teeth
2. Extract all teeth with advanced periodontal disease
3. Perform endodontic treatment or extraction of nonvital teeth
4. Initiate an active, effective, oral hygiene program
   a. Toothbrushing, flossing
   b. Diet modification if indicated
   c. Topical fluorides
   d. Plaque control, calculus removal
   e. Chlorhexidine or Listerine mouthwash

Patients receiving dental treatment including dental prophylaxis:
1. Medical consultation
   a. Degree of organ failure
   b. Current status of patient
   c. Need for antibiotic prophylaxis (WBC count depressed)
   d. Need to modify drug selection or dosage (kidney or liver failure)
   e. Need to take special precautions to avoid excessive bleeding
   f. Other special management procedures that may be required
2. Laboratory tests (surgical procedures planned)
   a. Access to current PT, APTT, BT, platelet count
   b. Access to WBC count and differential

BOX 25-3

Dental Management of the Patient with Transplanted Organs

Immediate Post-Transplant Period (6 months)
1. Avoid routine dental treatment
2. Continue oral hygiene procedures
3. Provide emergency dental care as needed
   a. Medical consultation
   b. Conservative selection of treatment

Stable Graft Period
1. Maintain effective oral hygiene procedures
2. Initiate active *recall* program every 3 to 6 months
3. Schedule *medical consultation* regarding patient status and management
4. Treat all new *dental disease*
5. Use *universal precautions* in controlling infection
6. Have staff *vaccinated* against HBV infection
7. Avoid *infection*
   a. Medical consultation-need for antibiotic prophylaxis
   b. Screening tests-WBC count, differential, CD4 and CD8 counts
   c. American Heart Association (AHA) standard regimen as option

8. Avoid excessive *bleeding*
   a. Screening tests-BT, PT, APTT, platelet count
   b. Special precautions
9. Alter *drug-selection* or reduced dosage
   a. Liver or kidney failure
   b. Avoid drugs toxic to liver or kidney
10. Establish need for *steroid supplementation* and be able to identify and deal with acute adrenal crisis if it should occur
11. Examine for oral signs and symptoms of *overimmunosuppression* or *graft rejection*
12. Monitor blood pressure for patients taking cyclosporine or prednisone; if blood pressure increases above baseline established, refer for medical evaluation

Chronic Rejection Period
1. Render immediate or emergency dental treatment
2. Follow recommendations for patients with stable grafts if dental treatment is needed

TABLE 25-7

Potential Post-Transplantation Infections

	Time of Onset After Surgery	Susceptibility Period
Viral infections		
Hepatitis B	Immediate	4 to 5 weeks
Hepatitis C	3 to 4 weeks	Continuous
HIV	3 to 4 weeks	Continuous
HSV	3 to 4 weeks	8 to 10 weeks
CMV	4 to 5 weeks	Continuous
Bacterial infections		
Staphylococcal wound	Immediate	4 to 5 weeks
Staphylococcal pneumonia	Immediate	4 to 5 weeks*
Urinary tract infection (bacteremia/ pyelonephritis)	Immediate	4 to 5 weeks
Tuberculosis *Pneumocystis carinii* pneumonia, toxoplasmosis	4 to 5 weeks	25 to 30 weeks
Fungal infections	4 to 5 weeks	Continuous

*Community-acquired pneumonia may occur/recur after approximately 6 months. Adapted from Rubin RH, et al: Am J Med 70:405-411, 1981.

these patients. The rationale for this practice is based on the increased risk for local and systemic infection resulting from suppression of the immune system. Again, no data indicate if this practice is effective or necessary for all immunosuppressed transplant patients. To further complicate the situation, the oral flora in these patients is altered by the immunosuppressive therapy, making the selection of the best antibiotics for prophylaxis difficult. In addition, repeated antibiotic prophylaxis itself may alter the oral flora. Patients who have shown evidence of rejection and are receiving an increased dose of immunosuppressive agents are considered to be at greater risk for infection. A stronger case for the use of prophylactic antibiotics could be made for these patients.[45,46]

Based on the lack of scientific information indicating any benefit from antibiotic prophylaxis in the prevention of local or systemic infection in organ transplant patients receiving invasive dental procedures, antibiotic use should be determined on an individual patient basis. Thus the decision to use antibiotic prophylaxis and the regimen to follow should be made in consultation with the patient's transplant physician. Patients in excellent-to-good dental health, whose grafts are stable, and who are not undergoing extensive dental procedures may not require prophylaxis. By contrast, patients needing increased dosage of immunosuppressants, or those with active dental infection (chronic periodontitis), may best be managed using antibiotic prophylaxis for invasive dental procedures (see Table 25-5).

The recommendations for antibiotic prophylaxis in posttransplant patients are somewhat different from those for prevention of infective endocarditis. Part of the rationale for this is the susceptibility of posttransplant patients to subacute bacterial peritonitis.[45] The basic prophylactic regimen is with amoxicillin 2 gm 1 hour before the dental procedure plus Metronidiazole 500 mg 1 hour before the dental procedure. In patients allergic to amoxicillin, Vancomycin, or imipenem 1 gm infused slowly over 1 hour before the dental procedure should be used. Clindamycin may be toxic to the liver and kidneys and therefore should not be used in most posttransplant patients. In patients who cannot take a drug by the oral route, intravenous Ampicillin 1 gm with Metronidazole 500 mg 1 hour before the dental procedure should be used.[45,46] (see Table 25-5).

The immunosuppressive agents used in the transplant patient may mask the early signs and symptoms of oral infection, making the diagnosis of the problem more difficult. When acute infection does occur, it often is more advanced and severe than that found in normal patients. The dentist should examine carefully for any evidence of acute infection in all transplant patients. The overimmunosuppressed patient can be more prone to oral infection as can be the patient with bone marrow suppression caused by the side effects of azathioprine, ALG, or ATG.[45,46]

Viral Infections. Posttransplant patients may be especially susceptible to viral infections. The agents include: herpes simple viruses (HSV), Epstein-Barr virus (EBV), cytomegalovirus (CMV), hepatitis B and hepatitis C virus (HBV, HCV) and human immunodeficiency virus (HIV). The most common infection in these patients is CMV.[47,48] Effective infection control procedures must be used when transplant patients receive dental treatment. Patients who receive a transplant because of chronic hepatitis complications may still be infected with HBV or HCV. In addition, during transplant surgery, additional blood is used, increasing the risk of infection with HBV or HCV. A few transplant patients also become HIV infected[49] (see Table 25-7). Excessively immunosuppressed patients may be infected with HSV, CMV, EBV, or other microorganisms that could be transmitted to dental staff or other patients.[49] Patients also are at increased risk for infection transmitted to them in the dental operatory. The use of barrier techniques and the practice of universal precautions (recommended for all patients being treated in the dental office) are considered adequate to manage transplantation patients with stable grafts. In addition, hepatitis B vaccine should be administered to all dental staff to protect against infection from HBV.

Excessive Bleeding. Liver transplant patients may be taking anticoagulants to prevent recurrence of hepatic vein thrombosis. Heart transplant patients may be taking anticoagulants to prevent thrombosis of the coronary vessels. Transplant patients taking anticoagulants may need to have the dosage reduced by their physician before any dental surgical procedures. If the level of anticoagulation is greater than 2.5 times the normal prothrombin time (PT) (greater than 3.5 international normalized ratio), the dosage of the medication may need to be reduced by the patient's physician (see Chapter 19). At least 3 to 4 days are required for the effect of the reduced dosage to lower the PT. When the patient's prothrombin time ratio (or international normalized ratio) has been appropriately reduced, the surgery can be performed. If the PT still is above 2.5 times normal or the international normalized ratio is greater than 3.5, the surgery may need to be delayed. Following surgery, the dentist must be prepared to deal with excessive bleeding, if it should occur, by use of splints, thrombin, antifibrinolytic agents, and so on.

Liver, kidney, and bone marrow transplant patients who are not taking anticoagulants still could be potential bleeders if rejection of the graft or GVHD and significant organ dysfunction occurs. Therefore before any dental surgical procedure, the patient's physician should be consulted to determine the patient's current status. If necessary, selected screening tests should be ordered (a PTT, PT, bleeding time, etc.).[1,3,4,19,32,45,46]

Adverse Reaction to Stress. Transplant patients who are receiving steroids may not be able to adjust to the stress of various dental surgical procedures because of adrenal suppression and may require additional steroids before and after these surgical procedures to protect against an acute adrenal crisis (see Chapter 15). The need for supplemental steroids should be established by medical consultation. If steroid supplementation is recommended, the dosage and timing in relation to the dental procedure should be confirmed with the patient's physician. Dental treatment such as surgery or extensive appointments may require supplementation. If postoperative pain or complications are anticipated, the need for supplementation is increased. Patients taking a very large daily dose of prednisone usually will not require supplementation (see Chapter 19). Also, many routine dental procedures, such as examinations, orthodontics, prophylaxis, simple restorations, and even minor oral surgery, may not need supplementation.

Even though precautions are taken and patients are managed with increased steroid levels, the dentist should remain alert to the possibility of an acute adrenal crisis. Signs and symptoms of acute adrenal insufficiency include hypotension, weakness, nausea, vomiting, headache, and, frequently, fever. Immediate treatment of this complication is required and consists of 100 mg of hydrocortisone (SoluCortef), intravenously or intramuscularly, and emergency transportation to a medical facility (see Chapter 15).[1,3,4,19,32,45,46]

Hypertension. An important side effect of cyclosporine is renal damage and associated hypertension. Prednisone also can cause hypertension. The dentist must determine, by medical consultation once the graft is stable, what the "baseline" blood pressure is for each patient treated with cyclosporine or prednisone. As a part of each visit to the dentist, the patient's blood pressure should be measured and, if it becomes elevated above the patient's baseline level, the patient's physician should be consulted immediately.[1,3,4,19,32,45,46]

Chronic Rejection Period

The third posttransplant period begins when significant signs and symptoms appear of chronic rejection of the graft or GVHD. This phase should be established by medical consultation. In general, only emergency or immediate dental needs should be treated during this period.

ORAL COMPLICATIONS AND MANIFESTATIONS

Oral complications associated with advanced heart, liver, and kidney diseases are discussed in Chapters 5, 6, 7, 9, and 10. Oral complications found in patients with blood dyscrasias are covered in Chapter 20. Oral complications found in patients with organ transplants usually are caused by (1) rejection, (2) overimmunosuppression, (3) side effects of the immunosuppressive agents, and (4) in bone marrow transplants, GVHD.

Oral findings associated with graft rejection are the same as those found in patients with organ failure before transplantation. If lesions are found by the dentist that could be associated with organ failure, the patient immediately should be referred to the transplant physician for evaluation of possible organ rejection (Figs. 25-11 and 25-12). Management of ulcerative or infectious lesions is described in Appendix B.

Oral findings that may indicate overimmunosuppression include mucositis, herpes simplex infections, herpes zoster, CMV, candidiasis, large and slow-to-heal aphthous ulcers and other ulcerations, unusual alveolar bone loss, and, on occasion, lymphoma, Kaposi's sarcoma, squamous cell carcinoma of the lip, and hairy leukoplakia.[14,16,19,23,24,32,33,49]

In addition, the potential is present for progressive gingival and periodontal disease. The presence of any of these lesions may indicate the transplant patient is overimmunosuppressed.[49]

Oral complications associated with the side effects of the immunosuppressive agents include infection, bleeding, poor healing, and tumor formation. Azathioprine may cause bone marrow suppression, and, when it occurs, patients may develop oral ulceration, petechiae, and bleeding. ATG and ALG may cause bone marrow suppression, thus increasing the risk for bleeding and infection. Cyclosporine may cause poor healing, increase the risk for infection, and produce gingival hyperplasia.[7] The increased incidence of lymphoma in transplant patients is related to immunosuppression in general but also is related to the side effects of cyclosporine and antilymphocyte monoclonal antibodies.[1,3,4,19,32,45-47] Oral ulcerations following liver transplantation were found to decrease once the dosage of the immunosuppressive agent (tacrolimus) was decreased.[38] After proper investigation, the transplant physician may need to reduce the dosage of the immunosuppressant agents. The dental management of these lesions is covered in Chapter 15 and Appendix B.

References

1. Rhodus NL, Little JW: Dental management of the renal transplantation patient, *Comp Cont Educ Dent* 14(4):518-532, 1993.

2. Friskopp J, Klintmalm G: Gingival enlargement: a comparison between cyclosporine and azathioprine-treated renal allograft recipients, *Swed Dent J* 10(3):85-92, 1986.

3. Little JW, Rhodus NL: Dental management of the liver transplant patient, *Oral Surg* 73:419-426, 1992.

4. Cecka JM, Terasaki PI: Clinical transplants. UCLA Immunogenetics Center. 1999.

5. Browne BJ, Kahan BD: Renal transplants in horizons in organ transplantation, *Surg Clin North Am* 74(5):1097-1111, 1994.

6. Frazier OH, Macris M: Heart transplants in horizons in organ transplantation, *Surg Clin North Am* 74(5):1169-1181, 1994.

7. Lansman SL, Ergin MA, Grieff RB: History of cardiac transplantation. In Wallwork J, editor: *Heart and heart-lung transplantation*, Philadelphia, 1989, WB Saunders.

8. Starzl TE et al: Evolution of liver transplantation, *Hepatology* 2:614-636, 1982.

9. Kahan BA, Ghobrial R: Immunosuppressive drugs in horizons in organ transplantation, *Surg Clin North Am* 74(5):1015-1027, 1994.

10. Ozaki CF et al: Liver transplants in horizons in organ transplantation, *Surg Clin North Am* 74(5):1197-1207, 1994.

11. Matas AJ, Najarian JS: Therapeutic approaches to renal transplantation. In *Current therapy in allergy, immunology, and rheumatology*, ed 4, St Louis, 1992, Mosby.

12. Sollinger HW, Geffnew SR: Pancreas transplants in horizons in organ transplantation, *Surg Clin North Am* 74(5): 1183-1193, 1994.

13. Cheng DCH, Demajo W, Sandler AN: Lung transplants. Organ transplantation, *Anesth Clin North Am* 12:635-641, 1994.

14. Kriett JM, Tarazi RY, Kaye MP: The registry of the international society for heart transplantation. In Terasaki P, editor: *Clinical transplants*, Los Angeles, 1990, UCLA Tissue Typing Laboratory.

15. Jhaveri R, Tardiff B, Stanley TE: Anesthesia in heart-lung transplantation. Organ transplantation, *Anesth Clin North Am* 12(4):729-747, 1994.

16. Asfar S, Zhong R, Grant D: Small bowel transplants in horizons in organ transplantation, *Surg Clin North Am* 74(5):1197-1207, 1994.

17. Heimdahl A et al: The oral cavity as a port of entry for early infections in patients treated with bone marrow transplantation, *Oral Surg* 68:711-716, 1989.

18. Henderson RG: Complications of immunosuppression. In Hunter AR et al, editors: *Transplant surgery: anesthesia and perioperative care*, New York, 1988, Elsevier Science Publishing.

19. Rhodus NL, Little JW: Dental management of the bone marrow transplantation (BMT) patient, *Comp Cont Educ Dent* 13(11):1040-1052, 1992.

20. Thomas ED et al: Intravenous infusion of bone marrow in patients receiving radiation and chemotherapy, *N Engl J Med* 257:491-496, 1957.

21. White DG: Immunosuppression for cardiac transplantation. In Wallwork J, editor: *Heart and heart-lung transplantation*, Philadelphia, 1989, WB Saunders.

22. Belle SH et al: Liver transplantation in the United States: 1988 to 1989. In Terasaki P, editor: *Clinical transplants*, Los Angeles, 1990, UCLA Tissue Typing Laboratory.

23. Heck CF, Shumway SJ, Kaye MP: The registry of the International Society for Heart Transplantation: sixth official report-1989, *J Heart Transplant* 8(4):271-276, 1989.

24. Itin P: Oral hairy leukoplakia in a HIV-negative renal transplant patient: a marker for immunosuppression? *Dermatologica* 177:127-128, 1988.

25. Starzl TE, Demetris AJ, Van Thiel D: Liver transplantation: I, *N Engl J Med* 321:1014-1021, 1989.

26. First MR: Annual review of transplantation. In Terasaki P, editor: *Clinical transplants*, Los Angeles, 1990, UCLA Tissue Typing Laboratory.

27. Lacy PE: Treating diabetes with transplanted islet cells, *Sci Am* (7):50-55, 1995.

28. Worldwide transplantation: Reports of various registries. In Terasaki P, editor: *Clinical transplants*, Los Angeles, 1991, UCLA Tissue Typing Laboratory.

29. Najarian JS, Sutherland DER: Pancreas transplantation-1991, *Transplant Proc* 24(4):1293-1296, 1992.

30. Sutherland DER, Moudry-Munns KC: International Pancreas Transplantation Registry analysis, *Transplant Proc* 22(2):571-574, 1990.

31. Van Buren CT, Barakat O: Organ donation trends in horizons in organ transplantation, *Surg Clin North Am* 74(5):1055-1075, 1994.

32. Olivari MT et al: Five-year experience with triple-drug immunosuppressive therapy in cardiac transplantation, *Circulation* 82(suppl 5):276-280, 1990.

33. Robinette MA: Organ donation resources in organ transplantation, *Anesth Clin North Am* 12(4):635-641, 1994.

34. Horowitz MM, Bortin MM: Current status of allogenic bone marrow transplantation. In Terasaki P, editor: *Clinical transplants*, UCLA Tissue Typing Laboratory, 1990, Los Angeles.

35. Penn I: Occurrence of cancers in immunosuppressed organ transplant recipients. In Terasaki P, editor: *Clinical transplants*, Los Angeles, 1990, UCLA Tissue Typing Laboratory.

36. Nicholson V, Johnson PC: ProHorizons in organ transplantation, *Surg Clin North Am* 74(5):1219-1238, 1994.

37. Sutherland DER et al: A 10-year experience with 290 pancreas transplants at a single institution, *Ann Surg* 210:274-288, 1989.

38. Hernandez G et al: Resolution of oral ulcerations after decreasing the dosage of tacrolimus in a liver transplant recipient, *Oral Surg Oral Med Oral Pathol Oral Radiol Endod* 92:26-31, 2001.

39. Svirsky JA, Saravia ME: Dental management of patients after liver transplantation, *Oral Surg* 67:541-546, 1989.

40. Muirhead AS: Heart-lung transplants in organ transplantation, *Anesth Clin North Am* 12(4):90-111, 1994.

41. Rubin RH et al: Infections in the renal transplant patient, *Am J Med* 70:405-411, 1981.

42. Seymour RA, Smith DG, Rogers SR: The comparative effects of azathioprine and cyclosporin on some gingival health parameters of renal transplant patients: a longitudinal study, J Clin Periodontol 14(10):610-613, 1987.

43. King GN et al: Increased prevalence of dysplastic and malignant lip lesions in renal transplant patients, N Engl J Med 332:1052-1057, 1995.

44. Harms KA, Bronny AT: Cardiac transplantation: dental considerations, J Am Dent Assoc 112(5):677-781, 1986.

45. Douglas LR et al: Oral management of the patient with end-stage liver disease and the liver transplant patient. Oral Surg Oral Med Oral Path Oral Radiol Endod 86:55-64, 1998.

46. Little JW, Rhodus NL: Dental management of the heart transplant patient, Gen Dent 40(2):127-131, 1992.

47. Barkholt LM et al: Cytomegalovirus infections inpost liver transplant patients, Transplant Proc 22:235-237, 1990.

48. Grattan MT et al: Cytomegalovirus infection is associated with cardiac allograft rejection and atherosclerosis, JAMA 261:3561-3566, 1989.

49. Seymour RA, Thomason JM, Nolan A: Oral lesions in organ transplant patients, J Oral Pathol Med 26:297-304, 1997.

Dental Management of Older Adults

26

*A*fter reaching the age of 40 years, people experience a progressive decline in homeostatic control and the ability to respond to stress and change. The World Health Organization defines the population between 65 and 75 years as "elderly." The term "old" is used for individuals between 76 and 90 years and "very old" for those over age 90. Elderly and old individuals are often very different with respect to their physiologic function, burden of illness, and any associated disability.[1] This chapter uses the term *older adults* for individuals 65 years or older.

DEFINITION

EPIDEMIOLOGY: INCIDENCE AND PREVALENCE

Older adults by the year 2040 are expected to account for approximately 21% of the population of the United States, a significant increase from the 4% in 1900 and 12% in 1990. The 85 and older age group is the most rapidly growing segment of the U.S. population.[2] Nearly 90% of all older adults have a chronic illness.[3] At present 30% of the individuals over age 65 have 3 or more chronic illnesses and account for more than 33% of the costs for health care in the United States.[2] The most common illnesses found in older American adults are arthritis, hypertension, impaired hearing, heart disease, and impaired vision, in that order.[1-3] The 3 leading causes of mortality in older adults are cardiovascular disease, cancer, and cerebrovascular disease, and they account for approximately 75% of all deaths.[1,2]

Cardiovascular disease remains the leading cause of death in older adults but has experienced a significant reduction since 1940. Since then a marked reduction in cardiovascular deaths for all age groups has occurred.

The 85 years and older group has had the least reduction, which was 20%.[4]

Cancer (lung, breast, prostate and colon) is the second-most-common cause of death in older adults. Since 1940 a 20% increase has occurred in cancer deaths for persons 55 years of age or older. Statistics show that 37% of men and 22% of women ages 60 to 79 years will develop invasive cancer. The risk for invasive cancer from birth to death is 50% in men and 30% in women. The most marked increase has been in cancer of the lung in both men and women.[5]

The third-leading cause of death in older adults is cerebrovascular disease. The incidence has been decreasing since 1960.[1,2] Approximately 10 stroke patients exist per 1000 population in the United States.[6] Prevalence rises in men from 14.6 per 1000 adults at 45 to 64 years to 77.5 for men ages 75 and older, and from 15.9 to 79.6 in the respective age groups in women.[6]

Based on the above information, a dramatic increase is expected in the number of older adults in this country and the proportion with significant chronic illnesses. These older adults will need dental care at an increasing level in the years to come. Dentists must be aware of the special management needed to treat this group of patients. For example, drug dosages and duration of treatment may have to be modified, certain drugs may have to be avoided, antibiotic prophylaxis may have to be administered, and special precautions may have to be made before surgery to avoid excessive bleeding.[2]

ETIOLOGY

Normal aging can be subdivided into successful and usual aging. Successful aging describes individuals who demonstrate minimal physiologic decline from aging alone. Healthful strategies such as exercise, modification

TABLE 26-1

Older Adults' Life Expectancy and Number of Years Free of Dependency in Activities of Daily Living

Age	LIFE EXPECTANCY, AVERAGE		DISABILITY-FREE YEARS REMAINING	
	Men	Women	Men	Women
65-69	13	20	9	11
70-74	12	16	8	8
75-79	10	13	7	7
80-84	7	10	5	5
85 and older	7	8	3	3

From Resnick NM: Geriatric Medicine. In Fauci AS et al, editors: *Harrison's principles of internal medicine*, McGraw-Hill, New York, 1998, page 37.

of diet, social and intellectual stimulation, and cessation of smoking enhance a person's quality of life and promote successful aging. Usual aging refers to the more common mode of aging. It is associated, for example, with the observed decline in renal, immune, visual, musculoskeletal and hearing function.[1] Table 26-1 shows the estimated life expectancy and number of years free of dependency in activities of daily living for different age groups.

Theories of Aging

Of 5 theories, 2 main ones have been put forward to explain the aging process. The 2 theories are not exclusive and may interact in the aging process. The first states that aging is a genetically programmed process. Studies of identical twins have supported this theory. Also, diseases that cause early aging, progeria, and Werner's syndrome support the theory. This theory suggests destructive genes are expressed later in life. An expression of genes may occur in older adults that has an opposite effect on fitness characteristics.[2] Telomeres are regions of DNA that cap the ends of linear chromosomes. In somatic cells the telomers shorten progressively with every cell division, reducing the number of tandem repeat sequences. Eventually the chromosomes become unstable and the cell is no longer able to replicate. This acts like an inherent biological clock, limiting the number of divisions the cells can accomplish. In contrast, germ cells do not undergo telomeric shortening and have relatively unlimited capacities for cell division.[7]

The second theory is that aging is the result of accumulation of damage to critical cellular and tissue constituents. This theory has several variations: metabolic rate, free radical effect, toxic effect of glucose, and somatic mutation. An inverse relationship between metabolic rate and life span has been observed in many animal species. Thus the faster the metabolic rate the shorter the life span. However, exceptions exist to this relationship, as seen in birds. Free radicals resulting from oxidative metabolism have been suggested to cause aging. The free radicals suggested to be involved are supraoxide, hydroxyl, and hydrogen peroxide. Protective enzymes against these free radicals, such as catalase, may be genetically encoded to decline with age. Examples of free radical damage with aging are lipid peroxidation, protein oxidation, and DNA oxidation.[2]

The toxic effect of glucose, the result of advanced glycosylation products, may cause aging by cross-linking or otherwise modifying biologic molecules. Somatic mutation may lead to the accumulation of DNA damage in cells that will accelerate the aging process. Animal studies have shown that food restriction retards DNA alterations. Also, the mutation frequency in cells from patients with Werner's syndrome suggests that these patients age prematurely because of accelerated accumulation of DNA or mutations.[2]

The immune system may play a role in aging. With increasing age the immune system loses some of its effectiveness and the ability to recognize one's own cells. Thus aging results from active self-destruction mediated by the immune system.[1]

In summary, 5 hypotheses have been advanced in an attempt to explain the aging process: (1) free radical, (2) error and somatic mutation, (3) wear and tear, (4) pacemaker, and (5) immunologic.[1,2] Each likely contributes in some degree to the aging process.

PATHOPHYSIOLOGY AND COMPLICATIONS

Human aging after age 40 years is accompanied by physiologic deterioration. However, this decline is highly variable among older persons and within organ systems of any given individual.[2] Recent studies suggest that by maintaining good nutrition, exercise, and social activities, older adults can maintain better health.[2,8] For example, this approach has been reported to delay the onset of type 2 diabetes in older adults genetically programmed for this disease.

Certain homeostatic regulators appear to be affected by aging (Table 26-2). Muscle mass decreases, body fat increases, and total body water decreases with aging. The increase in body fat and decrease in body water has an important impact on drug usage in older adults. The

TABLE **26-2**

Selected Age-Related Changes and Their Consequences

Organ/System	Age-Related Physiologic Changes	Consequences of Age-Related Change	Consequences of Disease, Not Age
General	Increased fat	Increase volume for fat soluble drugs	Obesity
	Decreased body water	Decrease volume for water soluble drugs	Anorexia
Endocrine	Impaired glucose	Increase glucose in response to illness	Diabetes mellitus
	Decreased thyroxine clearance and production	Decrease T_4 dose in hypothyroidism	Thyroid dysfunction
	Increased ADH, decreased renin, and decreased aldosterone		Decrease Na^+, Increase K^+
	Decrease testosterone		Impotence
	Decrease vitamin D absorption and activation	Osteopenia	Osteomalacia, fracture
Respiratory	Decrease lung elasticity and increase chest wall stiffness	Ventilation/perfusion mismatch and decrease PO_2	Dyspnea, hypoxia
Cardiovascular	Decrease arterial compliance	Hypotensive response to increase heart rate, volume depletion	Syncope
	Increase systolic pressure		
	Decrease β-Adrenergic response	Decrease cardiac output and HR response to stress	Heart failure
	Decrease baroreceptor sensitivity and decrease SA node automaticity	Impaired BP response to standing, volume depletion	Heart block
Gastrointestinal	Decrease hepatic function	Delayed metabolism of some drugs	Cirrhosis
	Decrease gastric acidity	Decreased Ca^+ absorption	Osteoporosis, B_{12} def.
	Decrease colonic motility	Constipation	Fecal impaction
	Decrease anorectal function		Fecal incontinence
Renal	Decrease GFR	Impaired excretion of some drugs	Increase serum creatinine
	Decrease urine concentration/dilution	Delayed response to salt or fluid restriction/overload; nocturia	Increase decrease Na^+
Musculoskeletal	Decrease lean body mass, muscle		Functional impairment
	Decrease bone density	Osteopenia	Hip fracture
Nervous system	Brain atrophy	Benign forgetfulness	Dementia, delirium
	Decrease catechol synthesis		Depression
	Decreased dopaninergic synthesis	Stiffer gait	Parkinson's disease
	Decrease righting reflexes	Increased body sway	Falls

Changes generally observed in healthy elderly subjects free of symptoms and detectable disease in the organ system studies. The changes are usually important only when the system is stressed or other factors are added such as drugs, disease, or environmental challenge. Abbreviations: T_4, thyroxine: BP, blood pressure; HR, heart rate; ADH, antidiuretic hormone; and GFR, glomerular filtration rate. Resnick, NM: Geriatric medicine. In *Harrison's principles of internal medicine*, Fauci AS et al, editors: New York, McGraw-Hill, 1998, p 37.

increase in fat volume affects the actions of lipophilic drugs, such as diazepam, by decreasing their initial effect and prolonging their action. The decrease in total body water has the opposite effect on water-soluble drugs, such as acetaminophen, by producing an exaggerated initial effect. These drugs often must be given in reduced dosage to older adults.[2,9,10]

The baroreflex sensitivity is impaired with aging. This leads to increased orthostatic hypotension and decreased thermoregulation. Increased orthostatic hypotension increases the risk of falls and serious injury. Also, the hypotensive effect of antidepressants, nitrates, and antihypertensives can be compounded by decreased baroreflex sensitivity. The impaired thermoregulation results in absence of shivering, failure of the metabolic rate to rise, poor vasoconstriction, and insensitivity to low body heat. These effects increase the risk for hypothermia and heat stroke in older adults. Certain drugs such as chlorpromazine and alcohol should be used with caution in these individuals as they may cause hypothermia.[2,9]

The activity of aortic and carotid chemoreceptors has been reported to decrease in older adults. The use of normal adult dosage of morphine can lead to severe respiratory depression in these individuals. Neurologic control of bowel and bladder function can be altered in older adults. Anticholinergic drugs—such as antidepressants, antihistamines, antipsychotics, and many cold preparations—must be used with care in these patients.[2,9]

Organ Systems Effected by Aging

Cardiovascular. In older adults the heart may become less compliant or stiffer because of the increase of connective tissue and ventricular hypertrophy (see Table 26-2). Early left ventricular diastolic filling is decreased and increased reliance develops on atrial contraction to maintain adequate left ventricular filling. These events can lead to symptoms of pulmonary congestion. This diastolic dysfunction in older adults is important because medical management differs from traditional heart failure. Digoxin serves no purpose in the management of congestive heart failure caused by fibrosis in the older adult and can be harmful. Instead the treatment is to use gentle diuresis and aggressive control of coexistent hypertension.[2,9]

The heart of a 65-year-old person beating at an average of 70 times per minute has opened and closed the heart valves 2,391,500,000 times. Not surprisingly, the valves show evidence of degenerative change, which is the most common cause of valve disease in these patients. The aortic and mitral valves are most often affected. Aortic stenosis, in persons 50 to 59 years of age, is most often caused by degeneration of a congenitally abnormal aortic valve. When occurring for the first time in a 60-year-old or older individual aortic stenosis usually is caused by degeneration of a normal aortic valve. Older adults with valvular heart disease are more prone to atrial fibrillation than younger adults with similar lesions.[11]

Atrial fibrillation (AF) in community-dwelling individuals 75 years of age or older is about 11% or 110 cases per 1000. The prevalence of atrial fibrillation increases with age. Atrial fibrillation is an important precipitating cause of congestive heart failure (CHF) and increases the risk for stroke. It increases the risk of stroke fivefold in the absence of rheumatic heart disease and twentyfold in the presence of rheumatic heart disease.[12] The incidence of all ventricular arrhythmias in older adults ranges from 69% to 96%. Ventricular tachycardia occurs in 2% to 13% of older adults. The higher frequency, 13%, is found in patients with known heart disease.[12]

Arrhythmias in older adults often require the use of pacemakers (see Chapter 6). In addition, many older adults are treated with coumadin to prevent thrombosis and embolism (see Chapter 19).

Endocarditis is a rare, far less than 1 case per 1000, disease that has become more common in older adults. More than 50% of the patients having the first episode of endocarditis are 60 years of age or older. The clinical presentation of endocarditis in older adults is often atypical. The patient may be asymptomatic, or complain of vague nonspecific symptoms such as anorexia, nausea and vomiting. Only 50% to 70% of the older adults will have fever. Neurologic symptoms, such as confusion, occur in about 33% of the older adults. The diagnosis of endocarditis must be considered in any older adult with heart murmur, malaise and fever[11] (see Chapters 2 and 3).

The prevalence of CHF increases dramatically with age. The average annual incidence of CHF increases from 9 per 1000 in 65- to 74-year-old men to 31 per 1000 in 85 to 94 year old men.[6] Older adults with CHF have a poor prognosis; 30% have a first-year mortality and 50% have a third-year mortality. CHF is the most frequently recorded hospital discharge diagnosis for older adults[12] (Fig. 26-1).

Arteriosclerotic heart disease (ASHD) is the most common category of heart disease found in older adults, with a prevalence of 168.9 per 1000.[6] ASHD is the leading cause of death for all ethnic groups of older adults in the United States. The incidence of ASHD increases in men and women until age 75. By age 80, the incidence of ASHD is 20% in both men and women.[12]

Pulmonary. A decrease in lung elasticity may occur with aging, particularly in inactive individuals. Arterial oxygen tension will decrease as a result of ventilation-perfusion imbalance caused by airway collapse. Thus, pulmonary function often decreases with aging. The ventilatory response to hypoxia and hypercapnia also will be

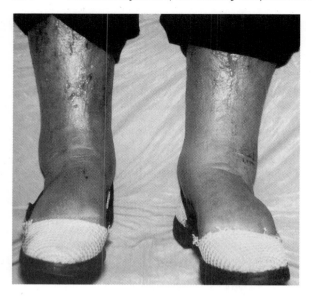

Fig. 26-1 Ankle edema in an older adult with congestive heart failure. (Courtesy Robert Henry, Lexington, Ky.)

decreased in these patients.[2] In addition, the risk for infection of the lungs is increased.[1] Oral organisms may contribute to pulmonary infection in older adults.

Gastrointestinal. Several significant functional changes occur as the result of aging. A decreased parietal cell function develops. The gastric pH increases with aging. Gastric emptying rate is slowed and the splanchnic blood flow is reduced. Overall gastrointestinal motility is slowed and a reduction of absorptive surface develops. The net effect of these changes is decreased absorption of most drugs given orally.[9] The following are the more common medical problems found in older adults involving the gastrointestinal tract: gastroesophageal reflux, esophagitis, gastritis, peptic ulcer, enteritis, intestinal obstruction, diverticulitis, hemorrhoids, and colorectal carcinoma.[13]

Renal. As the adult ages a decrease develops in renal mass, particularly of the renal cortex. A decrease occurs in the number of glomeruli. The remaining glomeruli show an increased amount of glomerulosclerosis. Although variable, the glomerular filtration rate tends to decrease. A decrease in sodium conservation—getting sodium from urine—occurs, which in part is caused by age-related decline in renin and aldosterone levels. These changes lead to impaired urinary concentrating ability after water deprivation. Also, thirst and drinking responses to water deprivation are decreased in older adults. The urinary concentrating defect and reduced thirst in these individuals

increases the risk of dehydration during illness. The renal changes also can impair the clearance of drugs that are primarily cleared by the kidney.[2,9]

Hepatic. After a person reaches 40 years of age, liver mass decreases by about 1% per year. The older adult may have decreased liver function because of it. In addition, the blood flow to the liver decreases by 40% to 45% with age. The result of these and other changes is to lower the plasma albumin level, decrease microsomal enzyme activity in the liver and slow hepatic blood flow. Significant decreases in plasma albumin (seen in hospitalized or poorly nourished older adults) can result in greater amounts of free or unbound drug, which may cause greater drug affect.[9] However, the rate of hepatic metabolism of a drug is not predictable based on the above alterations in hepatic function.[1,2,9]

Endocrine. Glucose tolerance decreases independent of obesity and physical inactivity. The primary cause of this decrease is insulin resistance in peripheral tissues, primarily skeletal muscle, at the post-receptor level. Pituitary secretion of growth hormone decreases in older adults. The anabolic effects of growth hormone are mediated by insulin-like growth factor-1 (IGF-1). IGF-1 is produced in liver and other tissues in response to growth hormone. Thus, as growth hormone secretion is reduced with aging, IGF-1 levels also decrease. The decrease in lean body composition seen in aging is in part caused by these decreases in hormone levels. Support for this relationship has been shown when growth hormone is given to healthy older adult men with low IGF-1 levels. Their lean body mass increases and fat mass decreases.[1,2]

Other age-related changes in the endocrine system result in increased levels of norepinephrine, insulin, and parathormone and increased vasopressin secretion. They also result in decreased plasma rennin activity, aldosterone concentration, conversion of thyroxine to triiodothyronine, metabolism of thyroxine, and secretion of estrogens and androgens. These and other changes result in impaired extracellular volume regulation, sodium homeostasis, glucose tolerance, and response to catecholamine stimulation.[1]

Immune System. T-cell proliferation decreases with aging. Several factors including defective transduction of mitogenic signals, decreased interleukin-2 synthesis and receptor expression, and thymic involution with loss of thymic hormones appear to be responsible for the decrease in T-cell production. A decrease in humoral immunity (B-cell) also exists in older adults. A decreased antibody response to foreign antigens and increase production of autoantibodies occurs. The effect of the decreased immune response is to increase the risk for infection and cancer in older adults.[1,2]

Hematopoietic System. Increased marrow fat is found with aging that results in decreased amount of active bone marrow. Once menstrual bleeding stops in a woman (i.e., post-menopausal) the red blood cell mass increases. In general no significant age-related changes occur in laboratory tests values, such as white blood cell count, hematocrit, hemoglobin, or platelet count.[1] However, the gender difference in hematocrit and hemoglobin levels decreases in aging, with women's levels increasing and men's decreasing slightly.[14]

Nervous System. About a 5% to 7% decrease in brain weight occurs in old and very old adults. Also, a significant decrease occurs in blood flow to the brain in these individuals. Decreased baroreflex sensitivity often is found in the older adult. An increased rigidity of the iris and decreased elasticity of lens often occur. A loss of cochlear neurons is found in many older adults. These and other changes increase the risk of cognitive loss, syncope, glaucoma, impaired vision in darkness and glare, cataracts and hearing loss for pure tones, particularly higher frequencies.[1]

Musculoskeletal System. Aging in older adults often leads to decreased bone mass, muscle mass, lean body mass, osteoblastic cell activity, number of muscle fibers, and intervertebral disk space. Women have increased susceptibility to osteoporosis with aging, with the major impact occurring after menopause. Microfractures of bone take longer to repair due to decreased osteoblastic cell activity. Also occuring is flattening of the arch of the feet. These and other changes lead to osteoporosis, decreased muscle strength, loss of height, curvature of the spine, and gait impairment.[1]

Oral and Dental. Age does not appear to play a major role in the decline of oral health. Oral cancer can lead to death by local extension or metastasis. Radiation therapy for head and neck cancer can lead to oral disorders such as mucositis, dental caries, xerostomia, or osteoradionecrosis. Cancer elsewhere in the body can metastasize to the oral cavity (represents about 1% of cancers found in the oral cavity) and in some cases (about 20%) be the first sign of the presence of a distant primary cancer.[15]

Older adults underutilize dental services. Less than one third of older adults have annual dental visits, and almost one half have not seen a dentist in 5 years.[16] Dentistry should be involved with an aggressive educational program to get older adults to be seen and evaluated by a dentist. Other health professionals need to provide their older adult patients with an oral screening assessment and refer to dentistry those with oral disease.[16]

Many adults 40 years ago thought that tooth loss was part of "aging." In 1957 only 40% of older adults had all or some of their natural teeth. This increased to more than 66% in 1994.[16] Tooth loss in young patients is usually due to caries or trauma. Tooth loss in adults (30 to 64 years of age) most often is caused by periodontal disease. Tooth loss in older adults is caused by periodontal disease and dental caries. Recurrent caries (involving margins of restorations) and root surface caries account for the vast majority of lesions found in older adults. Older adults are predisposed to caries and tooth loss related to certain aging changes. These include diminished tooth sensation, root exposure, gingival recession, compromised oral hygiene, changes in the composition of saliva, and decreased salivary flow.[16,17]

The most common age-related changes in teeth are occlusal attrition, pulpal recession, fibrosis, and decreased cellularity. Severe attrition can lead to loss of vertical dimension of occlusion. Secondary and reparative dentin leads to acellular and dehydrated dentin and a decrease in the number of nerve fibers in the pulp of teeth occurs with aging. With aging the teeth undergo staining, chipping, and cracking, and become more susceptible to fracture.[17]

Older adults often feel no pain with advancing carious lesions. Acute, throbbing pain is not a common symptom of caries in the older adult as it is in younger individuals. Older adults most often seek treatment because of food impacting in the carious lesion, or fracture of the tooth, which is unsightly or lacerates oral soft tissues.[16]

Older adults show evidence of gingival recession and loss of periodontal attachment and bony support. Changes in the periodontium because of aging alone are not sufficient to cause tooth loss.[16] However, the additional effect of poor oral hygiene, systemic diseases, and medication affects leads to increased periodontal disease and dental caries resulting in tooth loss. Gingival recession makes the teeth more susceptible to caries by increasing the total tooth surface that the patient must maintain and by exposing tooth surfaces not covered by enamel (e.g., cementum).[16]

Physical and cognitive impairment in older adults can interfere with the patient's ability to perform oral hygiene procedures. In many cases caregivers have to take over these procedures. In cases where no caregivers are able to aid with oral hygiene procedures, dental problems such as dental caries, tooth abscess, tooth fractures, gingival and periodontal disease can be expected.[16]

In healthy older adults no general diminution exists in the volume of saliva produced.[16] Many older adults complain of a dry mouth and some of these have diminished salivary output. Systemic diseases such as diabetes mellitus can cause dry mouth. Radiation therapy for head and neck cancer can decrease salivary flow. Medications taken by older adults also can cause this problem. More

than 400 drugs exist that have been reported to cause dry mouth.[16] The following groups of drugs are most noted to cause xerostomia: tricyclic antidepressants, sedatives and tranquilizers, antihistamines, antihypertensives, cytotoxic agents, and anti-Parkinsonian drugs.[17]

Prolonged salivary dysfunction leads to numerous oral and pharyngeal problems in older adults. These problems include dry and friable oral mucosa, fissured tongue, decreased antimicrobial activity, diminished lubrication, caries, periodontal disease, fungal infection, burning, pain, and difficulty with mastication, and swallowing.[17] Early diagnosis and treatment can prevent the problems associated with prolonged dry mouth. Diagnostic procedures may include review of the patient's history and physical findings, sialometry, sialograms, labial gland biopsies, and T[99] pertechnetate scintiscans.[17] (The management of xerostomia is covered in Chapter 21.)

Changes in mastication, swallowing and oral muscular posture occur with aging. These changes may not have any adverse effects on healthy older adults. However, when compounded with systemic diseases (e.g., strokes, Parkinson's disease) and drug regimens (e.g., tardive dyskinesia associated with antipsychotic drugs) serious complications can occur with chewing and swallowing, such as choking or aspiration.[17]

Older adults may complain of reduced food recognition and enjoyment and altered smell and taste function. Taste function undergoes few age-related changes. However, smell is dramatically diminished across the human life span.[17] Decreased smell capacity combined with changes in oral motor, salivary, and other sensory functions appear to account for the loss of flavor perception and interest in food in older adults.[17] These patients require nutritional counseling to prevent malnutrition and dehydration.[17]

Most oral cancers, squamous cell carcinomas are found in persons older than 50 years of age. Hodgkin's disease is found in two peaks: early adulthood and around the fifth decade of life. Non-Hodgkin's lymphoma is found in all age groups. Both benign and malignant salivary gland neoplasms are more common in older adults.

Other Considerations

Cognitive. Dementia is the loss of established intellectual ability that interferes with occupational and social function. It includes impairment of memory, language, perception, calculation, abstract thinking, judgment, and executive function. More than 50% of the cases of dementia are caused by Alzheimer's disease, which is irreversible. The next most-common cause of dementia is small multiple infarcts of the brain, which also is irreversible. Between 10% and 20% of the cases of dementia are classified as reversible.[2] The reversible dementias may be associated with the following medical diseases: hepatic encephalopathy, acid-base disturbances, hypoglycemia, thyroid disease, uremia, AIDS, trauma, syphilis, multiple sclerosis, and stroke.

Dementias are more fully discussed in Chapter 23. Alzheimer's disease is discussed here briefly as it is the most common type of dementia. Global cognitive impairment exists in Alzheimer's disease. Approximately 10% of older adults over age 65 years and 45% over age 85 have Alzheimer's disease. A new drug, tacrine (Cognex) has shown short-term gain in the treatment of Alzheimer's disease but with no evidence of long-term benefit. Tacrine has a high rate of drug toxicity.[2,9] Another new drug, donepezil (Aricept), has shown about the same level of benefit as tacrine but without the high rate of toxicity. Tacrine and donepezil are cholinesterase inhibitors.[18] Velnacrine, a metabolite of tacrine, also has been used to treat Alzheimer's disease with limited results.[19] In Europe and Canada a neuroprotective agent, propentofylline, has been shown to be effective for patients with mild to moderate Alzheimer's disease.[20]

Depression. Although depression is common in older adults, age itself is not a significant risk factor. Illness and loss of a spouse or loved one are the most striking risk factors for depression. In treatment settings the prevalence of depression in older adults is (1) 9% to 15% in primary care practices; (2) 15% to 25% in geriatric clinics; (3) 33% to 45% in hospitals and nursing homes. Medical or psychotherapy both offer about the same treatment benefit, which is significant. Treatment should be offered to all older adults with depression.[2]

Falls. Accidental falls usually exclude those resulting from syncope, stroke, or seizure. Approximately 33% of community-dwelling older adults fall each year. In nursing homes more than 50% fall at least once per year. Across all settings 1 of every 6 falls results in injury, usually to soft tissue; 1 in 20 results in fracture of hip, rib, or wrist; and 1 of every 100 results in hospitalization. Injury is the sixth-leading cause of death in older adults (Table 26-3). Intrinsic risk factors for falls in older adults are decrease in physical function (strength, balance, gait); neurologic disorders (stroke, dementia, Parkinsonism, arthritis); sensory deficits (vision, hearing); and postural hypotension. Extrinsic risk factors for falls include poor fitting shoes, long loose garments, slick floors, loose rugs, obstacles, poor lighting, lack of hand rails, and the number and type of medications being taken. Multiple drugs, regardless of the type, increase the risk for falls in older adults.[2] Certain drugs, however, pose greater risk (i.e., those that affect central nervous system function and balance, such as benzodiazepines).

TABLE **26-3**

Intrinsic Risk Factors for Falling and Possible Intervention

Risk Factor	Medical	Rehabilitative or Environmental
Reduced visual acuity, dark adaptation and perception	Refraction: cataract extraction	Home safety assessment
Reduced hearing	Removal of cerumen: audiologic evaluation	Hearing aid if appropriate: reduction in background noise
Vestibular dysfunction	Avoidance of drugs affecting the vestibular system: neurologic or ear evaluation if indicated	Habituation exercises
Proprioceptive dysfunction, cervical degenerative disorders, and peripheral neuropathy	Screen for vitamin B_{12} deficiency and cervical spondylosis	Balance exercises, walking aid; correct sized footwear, home safety assessment
Dementia	Detection of reversible causes; avoid sedative or centrally acting drugs	Supervised exercise and ambulation; home safety assessment
Musculoskeletal	Appropriate diagnostic evaluation	Balance and gait training; muscle-strengthening exercises; walking aid; home safety assessment
Foot disorders (calluses, bunions, deformities, edema)	Shaving of calluses; bunionectomy; treatment of edema	Trimming of nails; appropriate footwear
Postural hypotension	Assessment of medications; rehydration; possible alteration in situational factors such as meals, change of position	Dorsiflexion exercises; pressure-graded stockings; elevation of head of bed; use of a tilt table if condition is severe
Use of medications sedative: benzodiazepines, phenothiazines, antidepressants; antihypertensives; others: anti-arrhythmics anticonvulsants, diuretics, alcohol	Steps to be taken: 1. Attempt to reduce number of medications being taken 2. Assessment of risks and benefits of each drug 3. Select medication with least affect and shortest acting 4. Prescription of lowest effective dose 5. Frequent reassessment of risks and benefits	

Resnick, NM: Geriatric medicine. In Fauci AS et al, editors: *Harrison's principles of internal medicine*, New York, 1998, McGraw-Hill.

Infectious Disease. From 1981 to 1996, more than 10% of all AIDS cases were reported in adults 50 years of age or older. When comparing the number of AIDS cases in the 50-year and older age group reported in 1991 with those reported in 1996 a 20% increase was noticed.[21] In 1996 severe immunosuppression was found to be the AIDS-defining condition in more than 52% of individuals 50 years or older.[21] The vast majority of these cases oc-curred in homosexual men, blood transfusion recipients, injecting-drug use, heterosexual contact, and men who have sex with men who are injecting-drug users.[21,22]

The prognosis for HIV infection in individuals over age 50 years is much worse than for younger adults. HIV infection in older adults leads more quickly to subclinical immunodeficiency. Survival time after the diagnosis of AIDS is inversely related to age. Leading causes of death

in older adults is the same as for younger adults—opportunistic infections and bacterial infection.[22]

Older adults are prone to develop complications when infected with the influenza virus. The aging process decreases the ability to clear secretions and to protect the airway. Older adults with chronic illness are especially at risk for the complications of influenza. Older adults account for 80% to 90% of all influenza-related deaths.[23]

Pneumonia is a very serious disease in older adults often resulting in death. The increased risk is due to the age-related deterioration of the immune system, underlying chronic illnesses, weakened cough reflex, decreased mobility, and oral bacteria. Older adults often do not display the classic symptoms of pneumonia (fever, chills, anorexia, and general malaise) seen in younger adults. The older adult with pneumonia often will have symptoms of dehydration, confusion, and increased respiratory rate. *Streptococcus pneumoniae* is the leading cause of community-acquired pneumonia in older adults, accounting for approximately 25% of the cases. Nosocomial pneumonia in older adults is most often caused by *Staphylococcus aureus*.[23]

Diabetes. Type-2 diabetes represents 90% to 95% of the diagnosed cases, and most of these individuals are 40 years of age or older. Approximately 50% of individuals with diabetes are 65 years of age or older.[24] The prevalence of type-2 diabetes increases from 0.08 per 1000 at age 15 years to 1.63 per 1000 at age 65. The disease occurs about equally in men and women.[24] For every known person with type-2 diabetes is one undiagnosed person with diabetes. A 1989 survey found that 43% of persons with diabetes were treated with insulin and 49% with oral anti-diabetic drugs. Since that time even more persons with diabetes are being treated with insulin to better control blood glucose variation, which has been shown to slow the onset of the complications of diabetes. Type-2 diabetics over age 65 years have the highest rate of comorbidity—coronary artery disease, hypertension and osteoarthritis.[2]

Hypertension. More than 45% to 50% (450 to 500 per 1000) of older adults are estimated have high blood pressure.[25] Several years ago the benefit of treating mild elevation of diastolic (90 to 99 mm of Hg) blood pressure was established. Little or no attention was paid to elevation of the systolic pressure. Isolated systolic hypertension (ISH) in older adults was thought to be a normal part of aging. Recent reports have shown that even mild ISH results in significant complications in older adults.[26-28] Current guidelines recommend the treatment of persistent systolic hypertension in older adults.[26-28]

A National Health Survey in 1990 showed the prevalence of hypertension to be 60% in older whites, 71% in older African-Americans, and 61% in older Hispanics. In a screen for systolic blood pressure in 5566 persons 75 years of age or older, 75% were found to have systolic hypertension.[29] In England, a study of ISH reported that 12.6% of persons age 70 years and 23.6% at age 80 had systolic blood pressures of 160 mm Hg or higher.[30]

Unlike younger persons with hypertension, older adults with hypertension often have a decrease in cardiac output, increased systemic vascular resistance, arteriolar narrowing, and central arterial stiffening. Ischemic (some areas are not supplied with enough blood) and high-pressure (effects of the elevated blood pressure) threats coexist in the older adult with hypertension. Thus treatment goals are to protect organs from damage caused by high pressure and ischemic injury, and to maintain blood flow to key organs. In older adults with ISH of 180 mm Hg or higher, the initial goal is to lower it to less than 160 mm Hg. In older patients with ISH in the range of 160 to 179 mm Hg, the initial treatment goal is to lower the pressure by 20 mm Hg. If the diastolic pressure also is elevated, the goal is to lower it to below 90 mm Hg.[29]

LABORATORY FINDINGS

The laboratory tests used to evaluate the older adult patient are covered in the chapter dealing with the specific illness being considered. Little variation is found in the complete blood count, calcium, blood urea nitrogen, and cortisol or growth hormone with increased age. Age-related decrease in levels of aldosterone, androgens, angiotensin II, and parathyroid hormone are found in older adults. In addition, age-related increase in levels of thyroid stimulating hormone, triiodothyronine, and vasopressin occur in these individuals.[1]

DENTAL MANAGEMENT

Table 26-4 lists some of the problems the dentist will face in treating older adults. A health questionnaire may be impossible for an older adult with vision loss to fill out. The history of the patient should be obtained whenever possible; this can be done by oral means. In cases of severe dysfunction that does not allow the patient to participate effectively, relatives or care providers will have to be involved with the medical history of the patient.

Of particular importance are the medications older adults may be taking. Each medication the patient is taking needs to be identified, including prescription and over-the-counter drugs. Many older adults are taking multiple drugs; thus the medication history is even more important in this group of patients. Within a one-year time frame, each older adult is estimated to receive an average of 17 to 20 prescription drugs.[10]

TABLE 26-4

Selected Problems Older Adults May Have Regarding Dental Care

Condition	Problem	Possible Solutions
Dementia, physical disability, advanced illness	Difficult to follow directions, sit still during appointment, render effective home care	May need to apply sedation; make short appointments; request spouse or relatives render home care
Poor eyesight	Difficult to fill out health and dental questionnaire	Have spouse or relative fill out questionnaire or dentist take an oral history from the patient
Patient taking multiple medications	Possible drug overdose, drug interactions, and potential problems with medications dentist may need to use	Refer patient with obvious toxic drug effects or interactions; confirm with physician that medications are current; use the lowest possible effective dose of drugs needed for dental care and avoid drug interactions
Noncompliant patient; hypertensive patient not taking medication	Elevated blood pressure, possible risk of stroke, angina, myocardial infarction.	Refer patient for reevaluation by the physician; select a drug without the side effects the patient may be concerned about
Patient with signs and symptoms of systemic disease, such as leukemia, diabetes, hypertension, renal disease, liver disease	Patient may be at great risk of infection, bleeding or a cardiovascular complication	Refer to physician for diagnosis and treatment as indicated
Patients under medical treatment of cardiovascular disease	Sudden increase or decrease in blood pressure may indicate onset of complication	Monitor patient's blood pressure and pulse during dental treatment; leave blood pressure cuff on during treatment and take the blood pressure every 10 to 15 minutes (Pulseoximeter can be used to monitor the heart rate)
Patient taking an anticoagulant	Surgical procedures could cause excessive bleeding	Consult with patient's physician; (surgery can be preformed if INR is 3.5 or less or the PTR is 2.5 or less; higher values of INR or PTR usually require reduction in the anticoagulant dosage before surgery requires 3 to 5 days after dosage reduction for the INR or PTR to fall)
Patient with prosthetic heart valve, history of endocarditis, congenital heart disease, recent open heart surgery to correct cardiovascular problem or acquired valvular heart disease	Dental bacteremias could cause bacteria endocarditis: extractions, oral surgery, periodontal surgery, tooth cleaning, placement of dental implants and cleaning of dental implants are dental procedures that are recommended for prophylaxis (see chapter 2)	Use the appropriate American Heart Association (1997) prophylactic regimen for the prevention of endocarditis (single dose regimens given one hour before the dental procedure [see chapter 2])
Patient taking antihypertensive, antidepressant, antipsychotic, or other medications that cause xerostomia	Increases the risk for dental caries, periodontal disease, fungal infection and mucositis	Ask if physician can change medication; use topical fluoride, good home care including brushing and flossing, saliva substitutes, saliva stimulants (see Appendix B)

The dentist needs to know what drugs the patient is taking to prevent drug interactions with agents the dentist needs to prescribe. When problems with the patient's medications are identified, such as signs and symptoms of overdose or drug interaction, the dentist should communicate those findings to the patient's physician. Also, the older adult who is taking multiple medications and who has not seen a physician within the last year should be directed to make an appointment so the doctor can review the current appropriateness of the patient's medications.

The clinical examination may be more difficult in some older adults. For example patients with arthritis of the temporomandibular joint; head and neck cancer treated by surgery or radiation, neurologic disease, disorders of the musculoskeletal system, or with side effects of antipsychotic drugs such as Parkinson-like symptoms or tardive dyskinesia. These patients may have difficulty in opening their mouths, being able to hold still, and cooperating with the dentist's instructions for mouth or head positioning. The dentist may need to spend additional time and use sedative agents to complete the clinical exam. The dentist will need to speak louder, face the patient, and use shorter statements when giving directions or asking question of patients with hearing loss or dementia. By gentle hand or finger pressure the patient can be directed to move the head or jaws to facilitate the examination. In some patients complex examination procedures will not be able to be performed.

The clinical examination should include inspection of the exposed skin of the arms, legs, neck, face, and intra-oral soft tissues for signs of benign and malignant lesions. Basal cell carcinoma and squamous cell carcinoma of the skin are common lesions found in older adults. Also, squamous cell carcinoma of the oral cavity is more common in older adults (see Chapter 21). Psoriasis is a dermatologic disorder common in older adults (and in adolescence) (Fig. 26-2). Another common skin lesion found in older adults is seborrheic keratosis (Fig. 26-3).

Blood pressure should be taken on all new dental patients including those already identified as being hypertensive and at all recall appointments (see Chapter 4). Medically compromised patients may be best managed by taking their blood pressure at the start of every dental appointment and at key times during prolonged, complex dental procedures. The current upper limit for normal blood pressure is 140 mm Hg for systolic and 90 mm Hg for diastolic.[26] The blood pressure should be taken early during the first dental appointment then again later in the appointment. The average of the two recordings should be used to evaluate the patient's blood pressure (see Chapter 4).

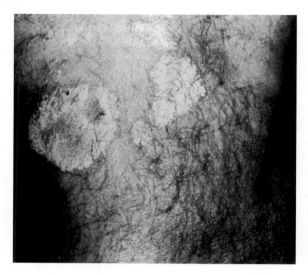

Fig. 26-2 Psoriasis on the leg of an older adult male. (Courtesy Richard Estensen, Minneapolis, Minn.)

Any patient with a mean initial diastolic pressure of 110 mm Hg or greater should be referred at once for medical evaluation and diagnosis. Patients with initial diastolic pressures between 90 and 109 mm Hg should have their blood pressure taken again at the next dental visit. If the mean repeat diastolic pressure is greater than 90 mm Hg, the patient should be referred for medical evaluation.

Any patient with an initial mean normal diastolic pressure and a mean systolic pressure of 180 mm Hg or higher should be referred at once for medial evaluation and diagnosis. Patients with an initial normal diastolic pressure and an initial systolic pressure between 140 to 179 mm Hg should have their blood pressure taken again at the next dental visit. If the mean repeat systolic pressure is greater than 140 mm Hg, the patient should be referred for medical evaluation. A Pulseoximeter (Oxycount(r) Mini Pulseoximeter, Weinmann, e-mail, b.bataryk@weinmann.de) can be used to monitor the pulse for patients with AF or pacemakers.

Lesions of senile purpura (Fig. 26-4) seen on the face, legs, and arms of many older adults, don't indicate an underlying bleeding problem. These lesions result from decreased fat content in the subcutaneous tissue and age changes in the connective tissue that allow for increased mobility. The increased mobility of the skin produces shearing forces that rupture small blood vessels. The blood lost by this bleeding takes about 1 to 3 weeks to be cleared from the skin. Senile purpura is more common in older women. The platelet count and

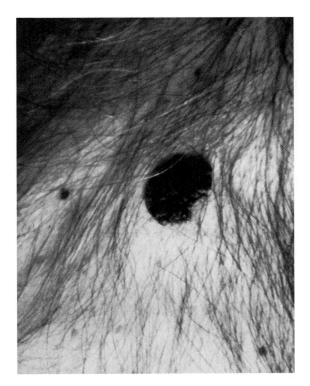

Fig. 26-3 Seborrheic keratosis of the scalp. (Courtesy Richard Estensen, Minneapolis, Minn.)

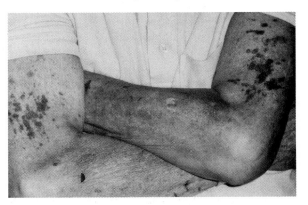

Fig. 26-4 Multiple lesions of senile purpura on the skin of the arms of an older adult male. (Courtesy Robert Henry, Lexington, Ky.)

platelet function are normal in these patients.[31] However, bruising can be a sign of thrombocytopenia or a bleeding tendency (Fig. 26-5).

Oral lesions may be found in patients with pemphigus vulgaris, cicatricial pemphigoid, lichen planus, lupus erythematosus, erythema multiforme, leukemia, neutropenia, anemia, salivary gland tumors, cancer and a host of other conditions. History, clinical findings, laboratory tests, cytology, and biopsy are used to establish the diagnosis of oral lesions (see Appendix B). If the dentist is unable to establish the diagnosis for a particular lesion he or she should refer the patient to an oral medicine specialist, oral maxillofacial surgeon, or an oral maxillofacial pathologist.

WHEN TO REFER/CONSULT

Older adults with advanced organ disease such as liver, kidney, lung, or heart disease may be at increased risk for invasive or prolonged dental treatment. The dentist should consult with the patient's physician to establish the patient's current status and confirm all drugs the patient is taking before the performance of any dental treatment. Special management procedures being planned for the patient should be reviewed with the patient's physician for input and modification when indicated.

Older adults found to be hypertensive need to be referred to a physician for diagnosis and treatment. Patients with signs or features of oral cancer should be referred for further diagnosis and treatment. Patients with signs and symptoms suggesting untreated systemic disease, such as diabetes, or AIDS, should be referred for diagnosis and treatment.

When surgery is planned for older adults taking anticoagulants (Coumadin), the dentist should consult with the patient's physician to determine the prothrombin time (PT) ratio and international normalized ratio (INR). Most dental surgery can be performed for patients being maintained in the low- to mid-therapeutic ranges of anticoagulation (PT ratio 1.5 to 2.5 or INR of 1.5 to 3.5) without any adjustment of dosage. Patients with a PT ratio greater than 2.5 or an INR greater than 3.5 should have their dosage of Coumadin reduced by their physician 3 to 5 days before dental surgery.

A dentist prescribing drugs for older adults should use the following guidelines: (1) the patient's medical problems should be known, (2) all drugs, including over-the-counter preparations being taken by the patient, must be identified, (3) the dentist must know the pharmacology of the drugs, (4) a new drug should be started using a small dose and additional doses titrated based on response, (5) dosage regimens should be kept as simple as possible, and (6) visual, motor or cognitive impairment can lead to errors or noncompliance, and relatives or caregivers may have to be involved in drug administration.

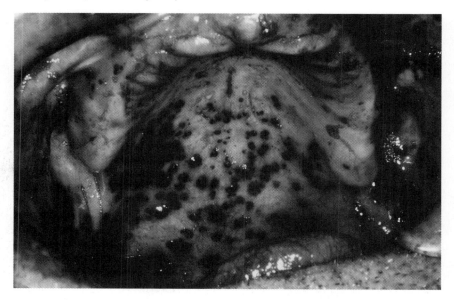

Fig. 26-5 Lesions of thrombocytopenic purpura on the mucosa of the oral cavity. (Courtesy Robert Henry, Lexington, Ky.)

The patient's physician should review the drugs being taken on a regular basis. If it has been longer than one year since the older adult dental patient has seen the physician, the patient should be referred for this review. The dentist and physician must consider that new symptoms or problems could be drug induced.[9] Multiple drug use must be avoided whenever possible.

Individuals complaining of dry mouth who are taking medications that have been reported to cause xerostomia (the dentist should measure salivary flow to determine if it is reduced) can best be served by the dentist's consulting with their physician to see if another drug without this side effect could be used to control the patients systemic condition.

General anesthetics should not be used on older adults in the general dentist's office and must not be used on medically compromised older adults. The amide local anesthetics must be used with care or not at all in patients with advanced liver disease. As a general guideline, no more than 2 cartridges of 2% lidocaine with 1:100,000 epinephrine should be used during any dental appointment for older adults with cardiovascular disease. Older adults with refractory arrhythmias, recent myocardial infarction, unstable angina, uncontrolled hyperthyroidism, recent coronary artery bypass graft, uncontrolled congestive heart failure, and uncontrolled hypertension should not be given any vasoconstrictor with a local anesthetic (see Chapters 4, 5, and 6).

Sedatives and hypnotics must be used with extra care in the older adult as they may precipitate cognitive impairment. These medications should be started at the lowest dose possible. The dose can then be increased gradually to the minimum effective one.[32] The use of short acting agents such as triazolam (Halcion) is suggested. Nitrous oxide analgesia can be used but care must be taken to make sure adequate amounts of oxygen are being supplied. These patients will require an escort to get home.

Older adults are often more easily stressed by dental treatment. In general mid-morning or early afternoon appointments (1:00 PM to 2:00 PM) are best for this group of patients. Medical complications are more common in these patients in the early morning as their blood pressure is rising. By the late afternoon these patients may be stressed by the days activities. Medically compromised older adults should be seen by the dentist early in the week so that if postoperative complications develop the patients can be seen promptly. Medically compromised older adults should have their blood pressure and pulse monitored at the start of the dental appointment and several times during it (every 15 to 30 minutes; Pulseoximeters are useful for this assessment). Long appointments should not be scheduled for these patients. Stress reduction can be obtained using oral, inhalation (nitrous oxide), intramuscular, or intravenous sedation. Care must be taken to avoid over-dosing with these agents.

The most common bleeding problems in older adults are caused by anticoagulation drugs (heparin, Coumarin, aspirin, and nonsteroidal antiinflammatory drugs [NSAIDs]), liver disease, renal disease, and cancer and the agents used to treat it. These causes of bleeding are not related to aging itself. For example, the platelet count does not change with increasing age. Although liver mass decreases with age, it has little or no effect on production of adequate amounts of coagulation factors for control of bleeding. Age related renal changes, if severe, might lead to bleeding problems by effecting platelet function.[33] Usually only persons with mild forms of inherited bleeding disorders will survive to old age. The dental management of the patient who may be a bleeder is covered in Chapter 19.

The side effects associated with antihypertensive drugs are covered in Chapter 4, with the most common being dry mouth, orthostatic hypotension, depression, sexual dysfunction, weakness, flushing, and altered taste. Drug interactions with antihypertensive drugs and agents used by the dentist also are presented in Chapter 4. In general, only small amounts of epinephrine, maximum of 0.036 mg, should be used with these agents. NSAIDs may reduce the effectiveness of some of the antihypertensive drugs.

Patients with congestive heart failure or chronic obstructive pulmonary disease may have difficulty breathing in a supine position for dental work. These patients will do much better if put in an upright or semi-supine position. Care should be taken when changing the chair position for older adults. The incidence of orthostatic hypotension increases with age and is a side effect of many drugs these patients may be taking. A sudden change from the semi-supine to the upright position may cause this type of hypotension. Of particular concern is when the older adult first gets out of the dental chair. Orthostatic hypotension at this time may lead to syncope (fainting) and a fall that could cause serious injury. Patients should be put to an upright position slowly, allowed to sit for a minute then supported by the dentist or dental assistant when getting out of the dental chair.

Selection of a postoperative oral analgesic requires knowledge of systemic health and medicines taken by the older adult patient. The most common adverse reaction of aspirin and the NSAIDs is gastrointestinal upset. These agents should not be used in older adults with gastrointestinal disorders such as ulcers, gastritis or hiatal hernia. In other older adults these agents can be used, but care should be taken to avoid gastrointestinal irritation. This can be done by giving them with food, milk, water (a full glass), or by having the patient take a liquid antacid with the aspirin or NSAIDs.

NSAIDs, aspirin, and acetaminophen in high doses should not be used with patients taking Coumadin or other anticoagulants. Aspirin and NSAIDs must not be used in patients with bleeding disorders such as thrombocytopenia, hemophilia, and advanced liver disease.[10] Tylenol (acetaminophen) should not be used or should be done so with care in patients with liver disease or kidney disease. The combination of acetaminophen and aspirin or a NSAID for chronic use must be avoided as they increase the risk for nephropathy. (See Chapters 9, 10, and 19 for a more detailed discussion of the use of analgesics in patients with renal disease, liver failure and bleeding disorders.)

Patients who had their dosage of Coumadin reduced before surgery (PT ratio greater than 2.5 or INR greater than 3.5 or other patients whose physician recommended a dose reduction before surgery) should be contacted within 24-72 hours to determine whether postoperative bleeding is occurring. The patient should then be seen at least 72 hours after surgery. If healing is progressing normally, their physician should be called and the patient returned to the normal Coumadin dosage.

Older adults who have been given antibiotic prophylaxis to prevent endocarditis should be told to return to the dentist or contact the physician if symptoms of anorexia, nausea and vomiting, fever, confusion, or anemia develop. These are the symptoms associated with endocarditis in older adults.

In the past antibiotic prophylaxis had been recommended for surgical procedures performed in patients with controlled diabetes mellitus and hemophilia, and in patients taking anticoagulants. The adverse reactions associated with antibiotics (super infection, bacterial resistance, severe allergic reactions, pseudomembranous colitis) no longer support this use. If postoperative infection develops in these older adults, the infection can be dealt with at that time using local and systemic treatments.

References

1. Ferri FF, Fretwell MD, Wachtel TJ: *Practical guide to the care of the geriatric patient*, ed 2, St Louis, 1997, Mosby.
2. Katz MS, Gerety MB: Gerontology and geriatric medicine. In Stein JH, editor: *Internal medicine*, 1998, St Louis, Mosby.
3. Eliopoulos C: *Manual of gerontologic nursing*, ed 2, 1999, St Louis, Mosby.
4. Fein Leib M, Zarate AD: Reconsidering age adjustment procedures: workshop proceedings, National Center for Health Statistics, *Vital Health Stat* 4(29):5-17, 1992.
5. Landis SH et al: Cancer statistics, 1998, CA *Cancer J Clin*, 48:6-29, 1998.
6. Kannel WB, Thom TJ: Incidence, prevalence, and mortality of cardiovascular diseases. In Hurst JW, editor: *The heart, arteries, and veins*, New York, 1990, McGraw-Hill.

7. Mera SL, The role of telomeres in aging and cancer, Br J Biomed Sci, 55(3):221-225, 1998.
8. American Diabetes Association 57th Annual Meeting and Scientific Sessions, June 21-24, Boston, Mass., Clinical Reviews 7(8):162-165, 1997.
9. Thornburg JE, Gerontological pharmacology. In Brody TM, Larner J, Minneman KP, editors: Human pharmacology: molecular to clinical, 1994, St Louis, Mosby.
10. Rho JP, Wong FS: Principles of prescribing medications. In Yoshikawa TT, Cobbs EL, Brummel-Smith K: editors: Practical ambulatory geriatrics, 1998, St Louis, Mosby.
11. Channer KS: Valvular heart disease in old age. In Tallis R, Fillit H, Brocklehurst JC, editors: Geriatric medicine and gerontology, 1998, New York, Churchill Livingstone.
12. Trumble TJ, Taffet GE: Cardiac problems. In Yoshikawa TT, Cobbs EL, Brumel-Smith K, editors: Practical ambulatory geriatrics, 1998, St Louis, Mosby.
13. Dudley-Brown S, Gastrointestinal function. In Lueckenotte AG, editor: Gerontologic nursing, 1996, St Louis, Mosby.
14. Tripp TR: Laboratory and diagnostic tests. In Lueckenotte AG, editor: Gerontologic nursing, 1996, St Louis, Mosby.
15. Zacharides N: Neoplasms metastatic to the mouth, J Craniomaxillofac Surg 17(6):283-290, 1989.
16. Lloyd PM: Oral and dental problems. In Yoshikawa TT, Cobbs EL, Brummel-Smith K, editors: Practical ambulatory geriatrics, 1998, St Louis, Mosby.
17. Ship JA, Mohammad AR, editors: Clinician's guide to oral health in geriatric patients, 1999, Baltimore, American Academy of Oral Medicine.
18. Scharre DW, Cummings JL, Dementia. In Yoshikawa TT, Cobbs EL, Brummel-Smith K, editors: Practical ambulatory geriatrics, 1998, St Louis, Mosby.
19. Antunono PG: Effectiveness and safety of velnacrine for the treatment of Alzheimer's disease: A double-blind placebo-controlled study, Arch Intern Med, 155(Sep 11):1766-1773, 1995.
20. Bachynsky J et al: Propentofylline treatment for Alzheimer disease and vascular dementia: an economic evaluation based on functional abilities, Alzheimer Dis Assoc Disord 14(2):102-111, 2000.
21. Control CFD, AIDS Among Persons Aged >= 50 Years—United States, 1991-1996, MMWR, 47(2):21-27, 1998.
22. Williams GD, Jogerst GJ: HIV infection in older persons. In Reichel W, editor: Care of the elderly; clinical aspects of aging, 1995, Baltimore, Williams & Wilkins.
23. Weltitz PB: Respiratory function. In Lueckenotte AG, editor: Gerontologic nursing, 1996, St Louis, Mosby.
24. Stilliman RA, Diabetes mellitus in the elderly patient. In Reichel W, editor: Care of the elderly: clinical aspects of aging, 1995, Baltimore, Williams & Wilkins.
25. Steven D, Kirk-Gardner R: Cardiovascular function. In Lueckenotte AG, editor: Gerontologic nursing, 1996, St Louis, Mosby.
26. Joint National Committee on Prevention, Evaluation, and Treatment of High Blood Pressure: The Sixth Report of the Joint National Committee on Prevention, Detection, Evaluation, and Treatment of High Blood Pressure, 1997, Washington DC, National Institutes of Health, National Heart, Lung, and Blood Institute.
27. Ofili EO et al: Effect of treatment of isolated systolic hypertension on left ventricular mass, JAMA, 279(10):778-780, 1998.
28. Staessen JA et al: Subgroup and par-protocol analysis of the randomized European trial on isolated systolic hypertension in the elderly, Arch Intern Med, 158(15):1681-1691, 1998.
29. Mahnensmith RL: Hypertension in the elderly. In Reichel W, editor: Care of the elderly: clinical aspects of aging, 1995, Baltimore, Williams & Wilkins.
30. Scott AK: Hypertension. In Tallis R, Fillit H, Brocklehurst JC, editors: Geriatric medicine and gerontology, 1998, New York, Churchill Livingstone.
31. Freedman ML, Sutin DG: Blood disorders and their management in old age. In Tallis R, Fillit H, Brocklehurst JC, editors: Geriatric medicine and gerontology, 1998, New York, Churchill Livingstone.
32. Fretwell MD: Optimal pharmacotherapy. In Ferri FF, Fretwell MD, Wachtel TJ, editors: Practical guide to the care of the geriatric patient, 1997, St Louis, Mosby.
33. Erban JK: Hematologic problems of the elderly. In Reichel W, editor: Care of the elderly: clinical aspects of aging, 1995, Baltimore, Williams & Wilkins.

Infection Control

APPENDIX A

*T*he American Dental Association (ADA) and the Centers for Disease Control have recommended that all dental patients be considered as potentially infectious and that universal precautions be used. These guidelines have been available since 1985 and were updated in 1993.[1] The basis for these recommendations is that dental patients and dental healthcare workers (DHCWs) may be exposed to a variety of microorganisms via blood, oral or respiratory secretions, and aerosolization.

The federal government, through the Occupational Safety and Health Administration (OSHA), has expanded these guidelines to include how to prevent blood-borne pathogen transmission in the workplace and how to protect the healthcare worker. The standards, which apply to dental offices with at least one employee, went into effect on March 6, 1992, with all provisions being enforced after July 6, 1992. OSHA requires a written exposure control plan for the dental office and information and training programs on infection control offered to all employees. Other aspects of the regulations pertain to personal protection equipment, housekeeping, engineering and work controls, hepatitis vaccination, postexposure follow-up, medical records on all employees, and the posting of the OSHA poster in the dental office.[2,3,4]

Dentists should check with the OSHA office in the state in which they practice to obtain a copy of the regulations. A state plan for the program may differ slightly from the federal program. By law the state plan must be as effective as the federal program. Through their state's health department, dentists need to gain access to the state regulations as well as those of OSHA.[5] The ADA published a question-answer paper on the new OSHA standards and on Infection Control Recommendations.[6] These documents are available on request from the ADA.[3]

By law, OSHA cannot give advanced notice of an inspection. Most dental office inspections OSHA has conducted, during the time temporary regulations were being enforced, were based on employee complaints. However, random spot check inspections have been conducted. In all 75% of the inspections conducted resulted in citations. Violations fell into the following categories: (1) willful, (2) repeated, (3) serious, (4) other than serious, and (5) no display of the OSHA poster.[5,7] Fines for willful or repeated violations can be as high as $70,000. The fine for not displaying the OSHA poster was $1,000. The dentist has 15 days to pay the fine and correct the problem, call the regional office for a conference, or contest the citation. Most (66%) of the citations issued in the early 1990s were related to serious violations that carried a fine of up to $7,000.[5,7] The fine for serious violations has been raised to a maximum of $10,000. From October 1999 to September 2000 OSHA issued 82 citations with the average penalty being $134.*

PROCEDURES

The following steps for sterilization, disinfection, barrier protection, universal precautions, and office management meet OSHA standards.

VACCINATION

OSHA requires that healthcare employers make hepatitis B vaccinations available without cost to their employees who may be exposed to blood or other infectious materials.

---

*http://www.osha.gov/cgi_bim/std/stdseri, accessed 12/20/01

PROTECTIVE ATTIRE

Gloves

Disposable medical gloves (latex or vinyl) always must be worn by DHCWs when the potential exists for contacting blood, blood-contaminated saliva, or mucous membranes.[1] One pair is required in the treatment of each patient, unless tears occur that would require new gloves immediately. Hand washing should be done before and after treatment of each patient (after gloves have been removed) with antimicrobial soaps that have residual action. Gloves should not be washed.

Face Shielding

Chin-length plastic face shields or a disposable surgical mask and protective eye ware should be worn for all procedures that may induce splashing, spattering, or aerosolization. Side shields should be used with corrective glasses.[2,4] Masks should be changed when soiled; the shield should be cleaned when soiled.

Protective Clothing

A clinic gown should be worn and changed, at least once per day, or anytime it becomes soiled. Impervious gowns are not required by OSHA. Long sleeves are recommended. Work clothes (such as gowns) should not be worn away from the workplace and must not be laundered at home.[3,8]

Disposable Barriers for Contact Surfaces

Disposable barriers should be used, whenever possible, to reduce the need for surface disinfection. Aluminum foil, plastic wrap, plastic bags, or plastic-lined paper can be used as disposable barriers for equipment and surfaces.[3,8] Between the treatment of patients, the coverings should be discarded and replaced. DHCWs should limit contact with inanimate objects during treatment.

Infectious Conditions

DHCWs who have exudative lesions or weeping dermatitis, particularly on the hands, should refrain from all direct patient care and from handling equipment associated with dental healthcare.

Adjunctive Devices

A rubber dam and high-speed air evacuation should be used to minimize transmission of droplets, spatter, and aerosols.

Sharps Disposal

A sharps disposal system is needed. The sharps container must be rigid, puncture proof, leak resistant, sterilizable or burnable, and labeled. Needles, sutures, scalpel blades, burrs, glass, pointed instruments, anesthetic capsules, and orthodontic wire should be discarded in it. Used needles should never be recapped or bent. A one-handed scoop technique or a specific resheathing device should be used to resheath needles.[8,3]

STERILIZATION

Sterilization is required for all critical instruments that penetrate soft tissue or bone. Sterilization is recommended for all semicritical instruments that contact oral tissues but do not penetrate soft tissue or bone. Noncritical instruments that come into contact only with intact skin may be reprocessed between patients with disinfection.

Instruments should be cleaned before sterilization. Ultrasonic cleaning is an effective method for removing debris. Cleaned instruments are rinsed and, if still visibly dirty, they are hand scrubbed. If ultrasonic cleaning is not used, all instruments should be hand scrubbed. If ultrasonic cleaning is used, the ultrasonic machine needs to be tested on a regular basis to ensure that energy is being delivered throughout the tank and power is not being lost. These procedures should be performed while dental personnel are wearing nitrile utility gloves to reduce the possibility of puncture wounds. Clean instruments are placed into heat sterilization bags that meet ADA acceptance standards. Packaging of instruments protects them from being contaminated after sterilization.[9] Studies have demonstrated that these sterile packs can be stored up to 12 months without loss of sterile integrity.[10]

Steam under pressure, prolonged dry heat, and unsaturated chemical vapor sterilization are the preferred methods for sterilization (Table A-1). The efficiency of office sterilization procedures should be monitored by the dentist. Chemically treated indicator tapes and biologic monitors are used to check for proper functioning of an office sterilizer. Indicator tapes should be used inside the instrument pack for every cycle; a color change in the tape indicates sterilizing conditions occurred. Calibrated biologic monitors guarantee sterilization. Proof of spore destruction by culturing after exposure to the sterilization cycle indicates that all microorganisms exposed to the same conditions have been destroyed. Weekly use of biologic monitors is adequate for most dental practices (Table A-2). A record of all test results must be kept for at least 3 years.[2]

A number of products are on the market for immersion sterilization and surface disinfection. Those for im-

TABLE A-1

Suitable Methods for Sterilizing Common Dental Instruments and Items*

Materials	Steam Autoclave†	Dry Heat Oven	Chemical Vapor	Ethylene Oxide
General hand instruments				
Stainless steel	1	1	1	1
Carbon steel	3	1	1	2
Mirrors	2	1	1	2
Burrs‡				
Steel	2	1	1	1
Carbon steel	3	1	1	1
Tungsten-carbide	2	1	2	2
Stones				
Diamond	2	1	1	2
Polishing	1	2	1	1
Sharpening	1	1	1	2
Polishing wheels and disks				
Rubber	2	3	3	1
Garnet and cuttle	4	3	3	1
Rag	1	3	2	1
Rubber dam equipment				
Carbon or carbide steel clamps	13	1	1	1
Stainless steel clamps	1	—	1	1
Punches	3	1	1	1
Plastic frames	3	3	3	1
Metal frames	1	1	1	1
Impression trays				
Aluminum metal, chrome plated	1	1	1	1
Custom acrylic resin	4	4	4	1
Plastic (discarding is preferred)	4	4	4	2
Fluoride gel trays				
Heat-resistant plastic	1	4	3	1
Non–heat-resistant plastic	4	4	3	1
Orthodontic pliers				
High-quality stainless	1	1	1	1
Low-quality stainless	4	1	1	1
With plastic parts	4	4	4	1

*1, Indicates preferred method with minimum risk of damage; 2, indicates that materials should withstand treatment with minimum risk of damage; 3, indicates that treatment usually is not suitable and may damage materials, manufacturer should be consulted; 4, indicates that materials are likely to be damaged or process may be ineffective.

†Chemical protection of certain nonstainless instruments may permit steam autoclaving. A rust-preventive dip (1% sodium nitrate) is recommended before sterilization.

‡Steel burrs may be sterilized in hot endodontic sterilizer for 15 to 20 seconds at 475° F (256° C), but the process may not be suitable for carbide burrs.

TABLE **A-1**

Suitable Methods for Sterilizing Common Dental Instruments and Items—cont'd

Materials	Steam Autoclave†	Dry Heat Oven	Chemical Vapor	Ethylene Oxide
Endodontic instruments				
Reamers and files, broaches, stainless metal handles	1	1	1	1
Nonstainless metal handles	4	1	1	1
Stainless with plastic handles	1	1	3	1
Pluggers and condensers	1	1	1	2
Glass slabs	1	2	1	2
Dappen dishes	1	2	1	2
Handpieces§				
High speed	1	3	2	1
Low-speed straight	2	3	2	2
Prophy angles	2	2	2	2
Contra-angles	1	3	1	1
Radiographic equipment				
Plastic film holders, columating devices	1	4	2	1
Stainless steel surgical instruments	1	1	1	2
Ultrasonic scaling tips	2	4	4	1
Electrosurgical tips and handles	4	2	4	2
Needles				
Disposable (do not reuse)	4	4	4	4
Nitrous oxide				
Hose/nose piece	1	4	1	1

§Some common latch-type contra-angles cannot withstand repeated heat sterilization; short, heat-sterilizable contra-angle handpieces are now available. Confirm with manufacturer.

TABLE A-2

Sterilization Method, Biologic Indicator Spore Type, and Incubation Temperature

Sterilization Method	Spore Type*	Incubation Temperature (C)
Autoclave	Bacillus stearothermophilus	56°
Chemical vapor		
Dry heat	Bacillus subtilis	37°
Ethylene oxide		

*For most dental practices, weekly verification should be adequate. Contact Council on Dental Materials, Instruments, and Equipment of the ADA for information regarding monitoring services.
Based on Merchant VA: *Dent Teamwork* 1990, pp 13-15.

mersion sterilization use glutaraldehyde as the active ingredient. However, the use of liquid chemical germicides to gain "cold sterilization" is generally discouraged. For heat-sensitive instruments, this procedure may take 6 to 10 hours and may be ineffective if the solution is not prepared properly.[6,8,3]*

---

*For more than 9 years Clinical Research Associates has been evaluating the effectiveness of the various products for use in infection control in the dental office. The company is involved with continuous evaluations and issues monthly updates concerning its findings. When selecting a glutaraldehyde-based disinfectant, the dentist should consider that the agencies approving the use of these agents do not actually test disinfectants to confirm efficacy. These agencies (Environmental Protection Agency, Food and Drug Administration, Center for Disease Control, and ADA) use reports submitted by the companies to establish efficacy, and these reports may not always be accurate. For example, testing of 12 brand names of glutaraldehyde-based disinfectants by Clinical Research Associates found that (1) disinfectants with similar active ingredients had equivalent performance despite diverse label claims, (2) contact time needed to be increased beyond the conventional 10 minutes, (3) contact time increased as the active agent(s) were diluted, and (4) all solutions tested were effective if the clinician was willing to tolerate the increased contact time needed for products with diluted active agents.

DISINFECTION

Environmental surfaces should be cleaned before they are disinfected. Diluted iodophors, chlorines, or synthetic phenolics are good cleaners in addition to being effective disinfectants (Table A-3). Products with high alcohol content are generally poorer cleaners. Alcohol will precipitate proteins in saliva and blood, making it more difficult to clean the surface. A recommended method for surface cleaning and disinfection is the "spray-wipe-spray" technique. The first spray and wipe is for cleaning; the second spray is for disinfection. If the product is a good cleaner, it can be used for both steps. A disinfectant that is registered by Environmental Protection Agency as a "hospital disinfectant" (and accepted by the ADA) and labeled "tuberculocidal" should provide adequate antimicrobial and virucidal activity. Utility gloves should be worn when using chemical disinfectants or cleaning the operatory.[2,4]

Handpieces
Handpieces should be sterilized after each use. The equipment manufacturer's directions should be consulted to ensure compatibility.

Air and Water Syringes
Air and water syringes should be cleaned and sterilized in accordance with the manufacturer's directions.

Dental Unit Water Lines
Antiretraction valves should be installed and routinely maintained (in accordance with manufacturer's directions) to prevent water and saliva from being drawn into the fluid line. Water and air should be discharged from high-speed handpieces for a minimum of 20 to 30 seconds after each patient. Overnight or weekend microbial accumulation in water lines can be reduced substantially by removing the handpiece and allowing water lines to run and to discharge water for several minutes at the beginning of each day. Water lines to all instruments should be flushed thoroughly after treatment of each patient and at the start of each clinic day.

Impressions
Dental impressions should be rinsed with water then disinfected. Diluted sodium hypochlorite is effective for all impression materials except zinc oxide eugenol (ZOE) impression paste. Glutaraldehydes are suggested for zinc oxide eugenol. The manufacturer's directions for disinfection should be followed. The impression can be immersed in the disinfectant for no more than

Office Sterilization and Asepsis Procedures Research Foundation (OSAP) Guide to Chemical Agents for Disinfection and Sterilization

Products	EPA Reg. No.	TB Directions (Test Timer Temp)*	ADA Accepted	Sterilization	Sterilant Reuse (Days)
Immersion only					
Multicide Plus	1043-36	1:32, 20 min, 20°C† (AOAC)	No	No	None
CoeSteril, ColdSpor	55195-2	1:20, 10 min, 20°C (AOAC)	Yes	1:5, 6 hr, 20°C 1:20, 12 hr, 20°C	30
Sporicidin	8383-5	1:16, 10 min, 20°C (AOAC)	Yes	FS*, 6 ¾ hr, 20°C	1 to 14 (1:8, 8 hr); 15 to 30 (1:8, 10 hr)
Glutarex	7182-4	FS, 10 min, 20°C (AOAC)	Yes	FS, 10 hr, 20°C	Not established
Banicide Sterall	15136-1	1:4 or FS* 30 min (AOAC)	Yes	FS, 10 hr, 21°C	30
Wavicide 01	"	"			
Cidex Plus (3.2%)	7078-14	FS, 20 min, 25°C† (Quant)	Yes	FS, 10 hr, 20°C	28
Cidex 7	7078-1	FS, 90 min, 20°C (AOAC)	Yes	FS, 10 hr, 25°C	28
Germ-X	10352-29	FS, 10 min, 20°C (AOAC)	Yes	FS, 10 hr, 20°C	Not established
Baxter/Omnicide	46851-2	FS, 45 min, 20°C (AOAC)	Yes	FS, 10 hr, 20°C	28
Glutall	"	"			
K-Cide	"	"			
Omnicide	"	"			
Procide	"	"			
CoeCide XL	46781-2	FS, 20 min, 20°C (AOAC)	Yes	FS, 6 hr, 20°C	30
Maxicide	"				
Metricide	"	FS, 20 min, 25°C† (AOAC)			
Protect-Top	"	"			
Vitacide	"	"			
Surface only					
Alcide LD	45631-15	10:1 : 1, 3 min, 20°C	Yes	No	None
Exspor	45631-03	4:1 : 1, 3 min, 20°C	No	4 : 1 : 1, 6 hr, 20°C	None
Bleach (5.25%)	—	1:10, 10 min, 20°C	Yes	No	None
Sporicidin Spray	8383-3	10 min, 20°C (AOAC)	Yes	No	None
Lysol Spray	777-53	10 min, 20°C (AOAC)	Yes	No	None
Coe Spray—The Pump	334-417	10 min, 20°C (AOAC)	Yes	No	None
Procide Spray	46851-5	10 min, 20°C (AOAC)	Yes	No	None

*Test used for TB label claim: FS, full strength; AOAC, Association of Official Analytical Chemists: *Quant*, Quantitative TB Test.
†210°C = 25°C = 77°F

From Cottone JA, Molinari JA: J *Am Dent Assoc* 122(9):33-41, 1991.

Management of Biopsy Specimens

Place usual specimen container with fixative into rigid container for transport.

Require laboratory personnel to wear gloves and mask when processing specimen.

Remind laboratory personnel to be extremely careful to avoid accidental injury.

30 minutes. An optional method of disinfection is to spray the disinfectant onto the impression then place it in a plastic bag. Stone models can be sprayed with an iodophor solution. The impression should be rinsed with water before and after disinfection. A suggested disinfectant for dental prostheses being sent to a dental laboratory is an iodophor. Prostheses, following disinfection, should be rinsed with water before being placed into the patient's mouth.[4,9,12] Table A-3 and Box A-1 summarize the precautions that the dental laboratory and clinical laboratory personnel should take in dealing with impressions, dental prostheses, and biopsy specimens.

References

1. Centers for Disease Control: Recommended infection-control practices for dentistry, 1993, MMWR 42(RR-8):1-12, 1993.
2. Council on Dental Materials, Instruments, and Equipment; Council on Dental Practice; and Council on Dental Therapeutics: Infection control recommendations for the dental office and dental laboratory, J Am Dent Assoc 116:341-343, 1988.
3. Council on Scientific Affairs, American Dental Association: OSHA's bloodborne pathogens standard: questions and answers, J Am Dent Assoc 123(suppl):1, 1992.
4. Schaefer ME: Infection control in dental laboratory procedures, Can Dent Assoc J 13(10):81-84, 1985.
5. Conners, ME: Be ready for inspections: OSHA official stresses planning. An ADA official stresses planning, ADA News, 23(2), January 1992.
6. American Dental Association: Infection control recommendations, 1992.
7. OSHA issues regulations: ADA foresees unnecessary costs, ADA News, 23(2), January 1992.
8. Cottone JA, Molinari JA: State-of-the-art infection control in dentistry, J Am Dent Assoc 122(9):33-41, 1991.
9. Merchant VA: Infection control and prosthodontics, J Calif Dent Assoc 17(2):49-53, 1989.
10. Butt WE et al: Evaluation of the shelf life of sterile instrument packs, Oral Surg 72:650-654, 1991.
11. Mitchell EW: Chemical disinfecting/sterilizing agents, Can Dent Assoc J 13(10):64-67, 1985.
12. Miller CH: Barrier techniques for infection control, Can Dent Assoc J 13(10):54-59, 1985.

Therapeutic Management of Common Oral Lesions

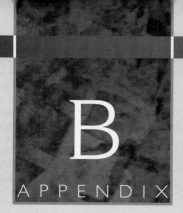

APPENDIX B

This is a quick reference to the etiologic factors, clinical description, currently accepted therapeutic management, and patient education of the more common oral conditions. Some of the recommended treatments have been more thoroughly investigated than others, but all have been reported to be of clinical value.

No cure exists for many oral conditions described here, but treatment modalities are available that can relieve discomfort, shorten the clinical duration and frequency, and minimize recurrences.

Clinicians are reminded that an accurate diagnosis is imperative for clinical success. Every effort should be made to determine the diagnosis before initiating treatment. Infection and malignancy must be ruled out. Where signs, symptoms, microscopic and other laboratory evidence do not support a definitive diagnosis, empirical treatment may be initiated and evaluated as a therapeutic trial basis.

Patient management should be governed by the natural history of the oral condition and that either a palliative, supportive, or curative treatment exists. Referral of patients should be made when the patient's problems are beyond the scope of the clinician trial. Further treatment can be determined by the patient's response. However, when healing of a lesion or when an expected response to treatment is not achieved within an expected period of time, a biopsy is recommended.

Note: The treatment protocols included herein were adapted with permission from Siegel MA, Silverman S, Sollecato TP, editors: *Clinician's guide to treatment of common oral conditions*, ed 5, Baltimore, 2001, American Academy of Oral Medicine. Certain portions of that text are reprinted here with permission of the American Academy of Oral Medicine. For further information or to purchase a copy of the Clinician's Guide to Treatment of Common Oral Conditions, contact: American Academy of Oral Medicine, 2910 Lightfoot Drive, Baltimore, MD 21209.

All drugs require a prescription unless identified as over-the-counter (OTC) drugs. Please note that the Food and Drug Administration (FDA) has been active in recent years with allowing OTC status for drugs formerly available by prescription only. Be sure to check on the dosages of the newly released OTC drugs, as they are usually of a different strength than those available by prescription.

SUPPORTIVE CARE

Management of oral mucosal conditions may require topical and systemic interventions. Therapy should address patient nutrition and hydration, oral discomfort, oral hygiene, management of secondary infection, and local control of the disease process. Depending on the extent, severity, and location of oral lesions, consideration should be given to obtaining a consultation from a dentist who specializes in oral medicine, oral pathology or oral surgery. When a question arises involving a medical condition, a physician should be consulted.

Symptomatic relief of painful conditions can be provided with topical preparations such as 2% viscous lidocaine hydrochloride, or 0.5% dyclonine hydrochloride. Topical anesthetics can be used as a rinse in adults but should be applied with a cotton swab in a child so that the child does not swallow the medication. Swallowing these anesthetics is contraindicated, in part, because they may interfere with the patient's gag-reflex. Symptomatic relief also can be obtained by mixing equal parts of diphenhydramine hydrochloride elixir and magnesium hydroxide/aluminum hydroxide. Children's formula diphenhydramine hydrochloride elixir does not contain alcohol. Sucralfate suspension also may be used before meals. The diphenhydramine mixture and the sucralfate coat the ulcerated lesions and may allow the patient to eat more comfortably.

Meticulous oral hygiene is absolutely mandatory for these patients. Mucosal lesions contacting bacterial plaque present on the dentition are more likely to become secondarily infected. Patients should be seen by the dentist or hygienist for scaling and root planing, under local anesthesia when necessary, in all cases where oral hygiene is sub-optimal. Patients must be encouraged to brush and floss their teeth after meals in a gentle yet efficient manner. This may be enhanced by placing a soft toothbrush under hot water to further soften the bristles. Tartar control toothpastes containing calcium pyrophosphate should be avoided because of their caustic nature and reported involvement in circumoral dermatitis.

HERPES SIMPLEX

Infection with the herpes simplex virus produces a disease that has a primary, or acute, phase and a secondary, or recurrent, phase.

 PRIMARY HERPETIC GINGIVOSTOMATITIS

Etiology: A transmissible infection with herpes simplex virus, usually type I or, less commonly, type II.

Clinical description: Clear, then yellowish, vesicles develop intraorally and extraorally. These rupture within hours and form shallow, painful ulcers. The gingivae often are red, enlarged, and painful. The patient may have systemic signs and symptoms, including regional lymphadenitis, fever, and malaise. Usually it is self-limiting, with healing in 7 to 10 days.

Rationale for treatment: Relieve symptoms, prevent secondary infection, and support general health. Supportive therapy includes forced fluids, protein, vitamin and mineral food supplements, and rest. Systemic acyclovir is effective in treating herpes in immunocompromised patients. Topical steroids should be avoided as they tend to permit spread of the viral infection on mucous membranes, particularly ocular. Patients should be cautioned to avoid touching the herpetic lesions and then touching the eyes, genital, or other body areas because of the possibility of self-inoculation.

TOPICAL ANESTHETICS AND COATING AGENTS

Rx
Diphenhydramine (Benadryl) elixir 12.5 mg/5 ml (Note: elixir is Rx and syrup [Benylin] is OTC) 4 oz mixed with Kaopectate OTC 4 oz (to make a 50% mixture by volume).

Disp: 8 oz
Sig: Rinse with 1 teaspoonful every 2 hours and spit out. Maalox OTC can be used in place of Kaopectate. Dyclonine (Dyclone) HCl 0.5% 1 oz may be added to the above for greater anesthetic efficacy.

Rx
Diphenhydramine (Benadryl) elixir 12.5 mg/5 ml (Note: elixir is Rx and syrup [Benylin] is OTC)
Disp: 4-oz bottle
Sig: Rinse with 1 teaspoonful for 2 minutes every 2 hours and before each meal and spit out.

Rx
Dyclonine HCl (Dyclone) 0.5% or 1%
Disp: 1-oz bottle
Sig: Rinse with 1 teaspoonful for 2 minutes before each meal and spit out.

SYSTEMIC ANTIVIRAL THERAPY

Acyclovir oral capsules may relieve and decrease the duration of symptoms.

Rx
Acyclovir (Zovirax) capsules 200 mg
Disp: 50 (or 60) capsules
Sig: Take 1 capsule 5 times a day for 10 days (or 2 capsules 3 times a day for 10 days).
(Current FDA recommendation is that systemic acyclovir be used to treat oral herpes only for immunocompromised patients.)

SYSTEMIC ANTIBIOTICS

(For secondary bacterial infection in susceptible individuals. Do not use routinely.)

Rx
Penicillin V tablets 500 mg
Disp: 40 tablets
Sig: Take 1 tablet qid.
For patients allergic to penicillin:

Rx
Erythromycin tablets 250 mg
Disp: 40 tablets
Sig: Take 1 tablet qid.
If nausea or stomach cramps occur, prescribe enteric-coated preparations (E-Mycin, ERYC, PCE, etc.) or a second-generation erythromycin, e.g., clarithromycin (Biaxin).

NUTRITIONAL SUPPLEMENTS

Rx
Meritene (protein-vitamin-mineral food supplement) OTC
Disp: 1-lb can (plain vanilla, chocolate, and eggnog flavors)

Sig: Take 3 servings daily. Prepare as indicated on the label. Serve cold.

Rx

Ensure Plus (protein-vitamin-mineral food supplement) OTC

Disp: 20 cans

Sig: Drink 3 to 5 cans in divided doses throughout the day as tolerated. Serve cold.

ANALGESIC

Rx

Acetaminophen tablets 325 mg OTC

Sig: Take 2 tablets q4h prn for pain and fever. Limit 4 g per 24 hours.

For moderate to severe pain:

Acetaminophen 300 mg with codeine 30 mg (Tylenol #3)

Sig: Take 1 or 2 tablets q4h for pain (requires Drug Enforcement Agency; DEA; number).

■ RECURRENT (OROFACIAL) ■ HERPES SIMPLEX

Etiology: Reactivation of the latent virus that resides in the sensory ganglion of the trigeminal nerve. Precipitating factors include fever, stress, exposure to sunlight, trauma, and hormonal alterations.

Clinical description: *Intraoral*–single or small clusters of vesicles that quickly rupture, forming painful ulcers. The lesions usually occur on the keratinized tissue of the hard palate and gingiva.

Labialis–clusters of vesicles on the lips that rupture within hours and then crust.

Rationale for treatment: Should be initiated as early as possible in the prodromal stage, with the objective of reducing the duration and symptoms of the lesion. Oral acyclovir, prophylactically and therapeutically, may be considered where frequent recurrent herpetic episodes interfere with daily function and nutrition. (Current FDA recommendation is that systemic acyclovir be used to treat oral herpes only for immunocompromised patients.)

PREVENTION

Rx

PreSun 15 sunscreen lotion (OTC)

Disp: 4 fl oz

Sig: Apply to susceptible area 1 hour before sun exposure and every hour thereafter.

Rx

PreSun 15 lip gel (OTC)

Disp: 15 oz

Sig: Apply to lips 1 hour before sun exposure and every hour thereafter.

If a recurrence on the lips usually is precipitated by exposure to sunlight, the lesion may be prevented by the application to the area of a sunscreen with a high skin protection factor (SPF 15 or higher).

TOPICAL ANTIVIRAL AGENTS

Antiviral creams and ointments are of minimal efficacy for recurrent herpes simplex. Their value may be attributable to the coating of the lesion by the petrolatum vehicle, which reduces the possibility of self-inoculation. Constant or intermittent application of ice to the area for 90 minutes during the prodromal phase may result in aborting the lesion. Cocoa butter ointment, lanolin-based lip preparations, or petrolatum (Vaseline) as an emollient may be palliative.

Rx

Penciclovir (Denavir) topical ointment 5%

Disp: 15-g tube

Sig: Apply to area q2h during waking hours, beginning when symptoms first occur.

Rx

Docosanol (Abreva) cream (OTC)

Disp: 2 gm tube

Sig: Dab on lesion 5 times per day during waking hours for 4 days, beginning when symptoms first occur.

VARICELLA ZOSTER (SHINGLES)

Etiology: Reactivation of latent herpes-varicella virus present since an original varicella infection through chickenpox. Precipitating factors include thermal, inflammatory, radiologic, or mechanical trauma.

Clinical description: Usually painful segmental eruption of small vesicles that later rupture to form punctate or confluent ulcers. Acute zoster follows a portion of the trigeminal nerve distribution in approximately 20% of cases. It is rare in the young, more common in the elderly.

Rationale for treatment: Promptly initiate antiviral therapy to reduce duration and symptoms of the lesions. Patients older than 60 years of age are particularly prone to postherpetic neuralgia. In the absence of specific contraindications, consideration should be given to prescribing short-term, high-dose corticosteroid prophylaxis for postherpetic neuralgia, in conjunction with oral acyclovir.

Rx

Acyclovir (Zovirax) capsules 200 mg

Disp: 200 capsules

Sig: Take 4 capsules 5 times daily for 10 days.

Rx
Valacyclovir (Valtrex) HCl caplets 500 mg
Disp: 42 capsules
Sig: Take 2 capsules 3 times daily for 7 days.
Use with caution in immunocompromised patients.
Rx
Prednisone tablets 10 mg
Disp: 50 tablets
Sig: Take 6 tablets in the morning, then reduce the number by 1 each successive day.

RECURRENT APHTHOUS STOMATITIS

Etiology: An altered local immune response is the predisposing factor. Patients with frequent recurrences should be screened for disease such as anemia, diabetes mellitus, vitamin deficiency, inflammatory bowel disease, and immunosuppression.

Precipitating factors include stress, trauma, allergies, endocrine alterations, and dietary components such as acidic foods and juices, and foods that contain gluten. Inspect the oral cavity closely for sources of trauma.

Clinical description: Minor aphthae (canker sore), less than 0.6 cm, small, shallow, painful ulceration covered by a gray membrane and surrounded by a narrow erythematous halo. They usually occur on nonkeratinized (moveable) oral mucosa.

Major aphthae, greater than 0.6 cm, large painful ulcers. A more severe form of aphthae that may last weeks or months. They may mimic other diseases such as granulomatous or malignant lesions.

Herpetiform ulcers, crops of small, shallow, painful ulcers. They may occur anywhere on nonkeratinized oral mucosa and resemble recurrent intraoral herpes simplex clinically but are of unknown etiology.

Rationale for treatment: Effective treatment involves barriers, amlexanox, topical or systemic corticosteroids, and immunosuppressants or combination therapy, when indicated. Treatment should be initiated as early in the course of the lesions as possible. Identification and elimination of precipitating factors may serve to minimize recurrent episodes. Medications such as mycophenolate mofetil, pentoxifylline, and thalidomide are used to treat patients with severe, persistent recurrent aphthous ulcers but should not be routinely used.

Nonsteroidal:
Rx
Amlexanox oral paste 5 %
Disp: 5 gm tube
Sig: Dab on affected area qid until healed.
Rx
Orabase Soothe-N-Seal Protective Barrier (OTC)

Disp: 1 package
Sig: Apply as per the package directions every six hours when necessary.

Therapies with steroids and immunomodulating drugs are presented to inform the clinician that such modalities are available. Because of the potential for side effects, close collaboration with the patient's physician is recommended if these medications are prescribed. These modalities may be beyond the scope of clinical experience of general dentists, and referral to a specialist in oral medicine or to an appropriate physician may be necessary.

Topical Steroids:
Prolonged use of topical steroids (greater than two weeks continuous use) may result in mucosal atrophy, secondary candidiasis, and may increase the potential of systemic absorption. It may be necessary to prescribe antifungal therapy with steroids.
Rx
Triamcinolone acetonide (Kenalog) in Orabase 0.1%
Disp: 5 gm tube
Sig: Coat the lesion with a thin film after each meal and at bedtime.
Other topical steroid preparations (cream, gel rinse, ointment) include:
Ultra-Potent:
Clobetasol propionate (Temovate) 0.05%
Halobetasol propionate (Ultravate) 0.05%
Potent:
Dexamethasone (Decadron) 0.5 mg/5ml
Intermediate:
Betamethasone valerate (Valisone) 0.1%
Triamcinolone acetonide (Kenalog) 0.1%
Low:
Hydrocortisone 1%
(Mixing ointments with equal parts of Orabase B paste promotes adhesion.)
Rx
Dexamethasone (Decaderon) elixir 0.5 mg/5 ml
Disp: 100 ml
Sig: Rinse with 1 teaspoon for 2 minutes qid and expectorate. Discontinue when lesions become asymptomatic.

Oral candidiasis may result from topical steroid therapy. The oral cavity should be monitored for emergence of fungal infection on patients who are placed on therapy. Prophylactic antifungal therapy should be initiated in patients with a history of fungal infections with previous steroid administration (see Candidiasis/Candidosis).

SYSTEM STEROIDS AND IMMUNOSUPPRESSANTS

For severe cases:
Rx
Dexamethasone (Decadron) elixir 0.5 mg/5ml
Disp: 320 ml

Sig:

1. For 3 days, rinse with 1 tablespoon (15 ml) qid and swallow. Then
2. For 3 days, rinse with 1 teaspoonful (5 ml) qid and swallow. Then
3. For 3 days, rinse with 1 teaspoonful (5 ml) qid and swallow every other time. Then
4. Rinse with 1 teaspoonful (5 ml) qid and spit out. Discontinue medication when mouth becomes comfortable.

If mouth discomfort recurs, restart treatment at step 3. Rinsing should be done after meals and at bedtime. Refill one time.

Rx

Prednisone tablets 5 mg

Disp: 40 tablets

Sig: Take 5 tablets in the morning for 5 days, then 5 tablets in the morning every other day until gone.

For very severe cases:

Rx

Prednisone tablets 10 mg

Disp: 26 tablets

Sig: Take 4 tablets in the morning for 5 days, then decrease by 1 tablet on each successive day.

Therapy with medications such as systemic steroids, immunosuppressants, and immunomodulators are presented to inform the clinician that such modalities have been reported effective for patients suffering from severe, persistent, recurrent aphthous stomatitis. Medications such as azathioprine, pentoxifylline, levamisole, colchicine, dapsone, and thalidomide are used to treat patients with severe, persistent recurrent aphthous stomatitis but should not be routinely used because of the potential for side effects. Close collaboration with the patient's physician is recommended when these medications are prescribed.

CANDIDIASIS

Etiology: *Candida albicans*, a yeastlike fungus. *Candida* is an opportunistic organism that tends to proliferate with the use of broad-spectrum antibiotics, corticosteroids, medicines that reduce salivary output, and cytotoxic agents. Conditions that contribute to candidiasis include xerostomia, diabetes mellitus, poor oral hygiene, prosthetic appliances, and suppression of the immune system (i.e., AIDS or the side effects of some medications). It is important to determine the predisposing factors.

Clinical description: The disease is characterized by soft, white, slightly elevated plaques that usually can be wiped away, leaving an erythematous area (pseudomembranous type). Candidiasis also may appear as generalized erythematous, sensitive areas (atrophic or erythematous type) or as confluent white areas (hypertrophic form). When the clinical diagnosis is questionable, it is advisable to culture for *Candida albicans* concurrent with starting medication.

Rationale for treatment: To reestablish a normal balance of oral flora and improve oral hygiene. Medication should be continued for 48 hours after disappearance of clinical signs to prevent immediate recurrence.

TOPICAL ANTIFUNGAL AGENTS

Rx

Nystatin (Mycostatin, Nilstat) oral suspension 100,000 units/ml

Disp: 60 ml

Sig: Take 2-5 ml qid. Rinse for 2 minutes and swallow. Nystatin suspension has a high sugar content; therefore good oral hygiene should be reinforced. A few drops of nystatin oral suspension can be added to the water used for soaking acrylic prostheses.

Rx

Nystatin ointment

Disp: 15-g tube

Sig: Apply a thin coat to inner surface of denture and to the affected area after each meal.

Rx

Nystatin topical powder

Disp: 15 g

Sig: Apply a thin layer under the prosthesis after each meal.

Rx (Mycostatin)

Nystatin pastilles 200,000 u

Disp: 50 pastilles

Sig: Let 1 pastille dissolve in mouth 5 times a day.

Rx

Nystatin vaginal suppositories 100,000 u

Disp: 40

Sig: Let suppositor dissolve in mouth qid. Do not rinse for 30 minutes.

Rx

Clotrimazole (Mycelex) troches 10 mg

Disp: 70 troches

Sig: Let 1 troche dissolve in mouth 5 times a day. If concern exists about sugar content of the nystatin and clotrimazole troches, vaginal tablets can be substituted.

Rx

Ketoconazole (Nizoral) cream 2%

Disp: 15 gm tube

Sig: Apply thin coat to inner surface of denture and affected areas after meal.

Rx

Clotrimazole (Gyne-Lotrimin, Mycelex-G) vaginal cream 1% (OTC)

Disp: 1 tube

Sig: Apply small dab to tissue side of denture or to the infected oral mucosa four times a day.

Rx

Miconazole (Monistat 7) vaginal cream 2% (OTC)

Disp: 1 tube

Sig: Apply small dab to tissue side of denture or to the infected oral mucosa 4 times a day

SYSTEMIC ANTIFUNGAL AGENTS

Note: In many cases, combinations of these antifungal preparations (liquids, troches and ointments) may be employed depending upon clinical considerations and response to therapy.

When topical therapy is not practical or is ineffective, ketoconazole (Nizoral) and fluconazole (Diflucan) are effective, well tolerated, systemic drugs for mucocutaneous candidiasis. They should be used with caution in patients with impaired liver function (i.e., with history of alcoholism or hepatitis). Liver function tests should be performed initially and conducted monthly when ketoconazole is prescribed for an extended period. Several drug interactions have been reported with ketoconazole.

Rx

Ketoconazole (Nizoral) tablets 200 mg

Disp: 20 tablets

Sig: Take 1 tablet daily with a meal or orange juice.

Rx

Fluconazole (Diflucan) tablets 100 mg

Disp: 20 tablets

Sig: Take 2 tablets stat, then 1 tablet daily.

Rx

Itraconazole (Sporanox) tablets 100 mg

Disp: 28 tablets

Sig: Take 1 tablet bid or 2 tablets daily with meal or orange juice

Rx

Amphotericin B (Fungizone) oral suspension 100 mg/ml

Disp: 48 ml

Sig: 1 ml qid. Swish in mouth 3-4 minutes then swallow.

CHEILITIS AND CHEILOSIS

■ ANGULAR CHEILITIS ■ AND CHEILOSIS

Etiology: Fissured lesions in the corners of the mouth are caused by a mixed infection of the microorganisms *Candida albicans*, staphylococci, and streptococci. Predisposing factors include local habits, drooling, a decrease in intermaxillary space, anemia, immunosuppression, and an extension of oral infections.

Clinical description: The commissures may appear wrinkled, red, fissured, cracked, or crusted.

Rationale for treatment: Identification and correction of predisposing factors and elimination of the secondary infection and inflammation.

Rx

Nystatin plus triamcinolone acetonide (Mycolog II) ointment

Disp: 15 gm tube

Sig: Apply to affected area after each meal and at bedtime. Concomitant intraoral antifungal treatment may be indicated.

Rx

Ketoconazole (Nizoral) cream 2%

Disp: 15 gm tube

Sig: Apply a small dab to corners of mouth daily at bedtime

Rx

Clotrimazole (Gyne-Lotrimin, Mycelex-G) vaginal cream 1% (OTC)

Disp: 1 tube

Sig: Apply small dab to corner of mouth qid.

Rx

Miconazole (Monistat 7) nitrate vaginal cream 2% (OTC)

Disp: 1 tube

Sig: Apply small dab to corner of mouth qid.

■ ACTINIC CHEILITIS ■ AND SOLAR CHEILOSIS

Etiology: Prolonged exposure to sunlight results in irreversible degenerative changes in the vermilion of the lips, especially the everted lower lip.

Clinical description: The normal red translucent vermilion with regular vertical fissuring of a smooth surface is replaced by a white flat surface that may exhibit periodic ulceration.

Rationale for treatment: If exposure to the ultraviolet light in the sun's rays is allowed to continue, the degenerative changes may progress to a malignancy. Sunscreens with a high skin protection factor (SPF greater than 15) should be used constantly.

Rx

Several over-the-counter sunscreen preparations are available (e.g., PreSun 15 lotion and lip gel). For those patients allergic to paraaminobenzoic acid, nonparaaminobenzoic acid sunscreens should be prescribed.

GEOGRAPHIC TONGUE (BENIGN MIGRATORY GLOSSITIS; ERYTHEMA MIGRANS)

Etiology: The etiology is unknown. Since its histologic appearance is similar to psoriasis, some have associated it with psoriasis. This may be purely coincidental. Oral

lesions should not be associated with psoriasis if no cutaneous signs exist of this disorder. It also has been associated with Reiter's syndrome and atopy.

Clinical description: A benign inflammatory condition caused by desquamation of superficial keratin and filiform papillae. It is characterized by both red denuded irregularly shaped patches of the tongue dorsum and lateral borders surrounded by a raised white-yellow border.

Rationale for treatment: Generally no treatment is necessary as most patients are asymptomatic. When symptoms are present, they may be associated with secondary infection with *Candida albicans* (see Supportive Care). Topical steroids, especially in combination with topical antifungal agents, are the treatment modality of choice. Patients must be told that this condition does not suggest a more serious disease and is not contagious. In most cases, biopsy is not indicated because of the pathognomonic clinical appearance.

Rx
Nystatin-triamcinolone acetonide (Mycolog II, Mytrex) ointment
Disp: 15 gm tube
Sig: Apply to affected areas after meals and at bedtime.

Rx
Clotrimazole-betamethasone dipropionate (Lotrisone) cream
Disp: 15 gm tube
Sig: Apply to affected area after each meal and at bedtime.

Rx
Betamethasone Valerate ointment, 0.1%
Disp: 15 gm tube
Sig: Apply to affected areas after meals and at bedtime.

Rx
Nystatin ointment
Disp: 15 gm tube
Sig: Apply to affected areas after meals and at bedtime.

XEROSTOMIA

Etiology: Acute or chronic reduced salivary flow may result from drug therapy, mechanical blockage, dehydration, emotional stress, infection of the salivary glands, local surgery, avitaminosis, diabetes, anemia, connective tissue diseases, Sjögren's syndrome, radiation therapy, and congenital factors (e.g., ectodermal dysplasia) (see Box 21-9).

Clinical description: The tissues may be dry, pale, or red and atrophic. The tongue may be devoid of papillae, atrophic, fissured, and inflamed. Multiple carious lesions may be present, especially at the gingival margin and on exposed root surfaces.

Rationale for treatment: Salivary stimulation or replacement therapy to keep mouth moist, prevention of caries and candidal infection, and palliative relief.

SALIVA SUBSTITUTES

Rx
Sodium carboxymethyl cellulose 0.5% aqueous solution (OTC)
Disp: 8 fl oz
Sig: Use as a rinse as frequently as needed.
Saliva substitutes (OTC) Optimoist, MouthKote, Sage Moist Plus, Xero-Lube, Salivart, Moi-Stir, Orex
Commercial oral moisturizing gels (OTC) Sage Mouth Moisturizer, Oral Balance
Relief from oral dryness and accompanying discomfort can be achieved conservatively by sipping water frequently all day long, letting ice melt in the mouth, restricting caffeine intake, not using mouth rinses that contain alcohol, humidifying sleeping area, coating lips with Blistex or Vaseline

SALIVA STIMULANTS

Chewing sugarless gum and sucking sugarless mints are conservative methods to temporarily stimulate salivary flow in patients with medication xerostomia or with salivary gland dysfunction. Patients should be cautioned against using products that contain sugar.

Rx
Pilocarpine HCl solution 1 mg/ml
Disp: 100 ml
Sig: Take 1 teaspoonful qid. (The dosage should be adjusted to increase saliva while minimizing the adverse side effects [sweating, stomach upset].)

Rx
Pilocarpine HCl 5 mg tablets (Salagen)
Disp: 100 tablets
Sig: Take 1 tablet tid. An *extra tablet* (10 mg) may be taken at bedtime.

Rx
Cevimiline HCl (Evoxac) 30 mg tablets
Disp: 100 tablets
Sig: Take 1 tablet po tid or qid

Rx
Bethanechol (Urecholine) 25 mg
Disp: 21 tablets
Sig: Take 1 tablet tid.

CARIES PREVENTION

Rx
Stannous fluoride gel 0.4%

Disp: 4.3 oz

Sig: Apply to teeth daily for 5 minutes; 5-10 drops in a custom tray. Do not swallow the gel.

SnF_2 gels available include IDP Gel-Oh, Stan-Gard, Perfect Choice, Flo Gel, True Gel, Nova Gel, Omni-Gel, Control, Gel-Pro, Perfect Choice, Basic Gel, Gel-Tin, IDP Gel-Oh, Gel-Kam, Stan-Gard, Easy-Gel, Thera-Flur

When the taste of acidulated SnF_2 gels is poorly tolerated, or where there is etching of ceramic restorations, neutral pH sodium fluoride gel 1% (Thera-Flur-N) should be considered.

Rx

Neutral NaF gel (Thera-Flur-N) 1.0% or PreviDent (Colgate) 1.1% neutral NaF

Disp: 24 ml

Sig: Place 1 drop per tooth in custom tray; apply for 5 minutes daily. Avoid rinsing or eating for 30 minutes following treatment.

FDA regulations have limited the size of bottles of fluoride due to toxicity if ingested by infants. Since most preparations do not come in childproof bottles, the sizes of topical fluoride preparations vary; 24 ml is approximately a 2-week supply for application to a full dentition in custom carriers. Xerostomia provides an excellent environment for the overgrowth of *Candida albicans*. The patient is likely to require treatment for candidiasis along with the treatment for dry mouth. In a dry oral environment, plaque control becomes more difficult. Scrupulous oral hygiene is essential.

LICHEN PLANUS

Etiology: Postulated to be a chronic mucocutaneous autoimmune disorder with a genetic predisposition that is initiated by a variety of factors, including emotional stress, hypersensitivity to drugs, dental products or foods.

Clinical description: Lichen planus varies in clinical appearance. Oral forms of this disorder include lacy white lines representing Wickham's striae (reticular), an erythematous form (atrophic), and an ulcerating form that is often accompanied by striae peripheral to the ulceration (ulcerative).

The lesions are commonly found on the buccal mucosa, gingiva, and tongue, but can be found on the lips and palate. Lichen planus lesions are chronic and also may affect the skin.

Any refractory lesion should be considered for a biopsy to establish a diagnosis and to rule out a malignancy.

Rationale for treatment: To provide oral comfort if the lesions are symptomatic. No known cure exists.

Systemic and local relief with antiinflammatory and immunosuppressant agents is indicated. Identification of any dietary, component, dental product, or medication (lichenoid drug reaction) should be undertaken to ensure against a hypersensitivity reaction. Treatment or prevention of a secondary fungal infection with a systemic antifungal agent also should be considered.

Therapies with steroids and immunomodulating drugs are presented to inform the clinician that such modalities are available. Because of the potential for side effects, close collaboration with the patient's physician is recommended when these medications are prescribed. These modalities may be beyond the scope of clinical experience of general dentists, and referral to a specialist in oral medicine or to an appropriate physician may be necessary.

Topical steroids:

Prolonged use of topical steroids (for a period of greater than two weeks continuous use) may result in mucosal atrophy and secondary candidiasis, and may increase the potential of systemic absorption. The prescribing of antifungal therapy with steroids may be necessary. Therapy with topical steroids, once the lichen planus is under control, should be tapered to alternate day therapy or less depending on control of the disease and the tendency to recur.

Rx

Fluocinide (Lidex) gel 0.05%

Disp: 30 gm tube

Sig: Coat the lesion wit a thin film after each meal and at bedtime.

Rx

Dexamethasone (Decadron) elixir 0.5 mg/5 ml

Disp: 100 ml

Sig: Rinse with 1 teaspoonful for 2 minutes qid and spit out. Discontinue when lesions become asymptomatic.

Other topical steroid preparations (cream, gel ointment) include:

Ultra-potent:

Clobetasol propionate (Temovate) 0.05%

Halobetasol propionate (Ultravate) 0.05%

Potent:

Dexamethasone (Decadron) 0.5 mg/5 ml

Fluocinonide (Lidex) 0.05%

Intermediate:

Betamethasone valerate (Valisone) 0.1%

Triamcinolone acetonide (Kenalog) 0.1%

Low:

Hydrocortisone 1%

Oral candidiasis may result from topical steroid therapy. The oral cavity should be monitored for emergence of fungal infection on patients who are placed on therapy. Prophylactic antifungal therapy should be initiated in patients with a history of fungal infection with prior steroid administration (see Candidiasis/Candidosis).

SYSTEMIC STEROIDS
AND IMMUNOSUPRESSANTS

For severe cases:
Rx
Dexamethasone (Decadron) elixir 0.5 mg/5 ml
Disp: 320 ml
Sig:

1. For 3 days, rinse with 1 tablespoonful (15 ml) qid and swallow. Then
2. For 3 days rinse with 1 teaspoonful (5 ml) qid and swallow. Then
3. For 3 days, rinse with 1 teaspoonful (5 ml) qid and swallow every other time. Then
4. Rinse with 1 teaspoonful (5 ml) qid and expectorate.

Rx
Prednisone tablets 10 mg
Disp: 26 tablets
Sig: Take 4 tablets in the morning for 5 days, then decrease by 1 tablet on each successive day.

Rx
Prednisone tablets 5 mg
Disp: 40 tablets
Sig: Take 5 tablets in the morning for 5 days, then 5 tablets in the morning every other day until gone.

If oral discomfort recurs, the patient should return to the clinician for reevaluation.

Many studies suggest that oral lichen planus has an intrinsic property predisposing to malignant transformation. However, the etiology is complex, with interaction between genetic, infectious agents environmental, and lifestyle factors. Prospective studies have demonstrated that lichen planus patients have a slightly increased risk to develop oral squamous cell carinoma. All patients exhibiting lichen planus intraorally, particularly those who have had the ulcerative form, should receive periodic follow-up.

Therapy with medications such as systemic steroids, immunosuppressants, and immunomodulators is presented to inform the clinician that such modalities have been reported effective for patients suffering from ulcerative lichen planus. Medications such as azathioprine, mycophenolate mofetil, tacrolimus hydro-xychloroquinesulfate, acitretin, and cyclosporine-A are used to treat patients with severe persistent ulcerative lichen planus but should not be routinely used because of the potential for side effects. Close collaboration with the patient's physician is recommended when these medications are prescribed.

PEMPHIGUS AND MUCOUS MEMBRANE PEMPHIGOID

Pemphigus and mucous membrane pemphigoid are relatively uncommon lesions. They should be suspected when chronic, multiple oral ulcerations and a history of oral and skin blisters exist. Often they may occur only in the mouth. Diagnosis is based on history, histologic, and immunofluorescent characteristics of a biopsy of the primary lesion.

Etiology: Both are autoimmune diseases with autoantibodies against antigens appearing in different portions of the epithelium (mucosa). In pemphigus the antigens are within the epithelium (desmosomes) while in pemphigoid the antigens are located at the base of the epithelium in the hemidesmosomes.

Clinical characteristics: In pemphigus the lesion may stay in one location for a long period of time with small placid bullae. The bullae may rupture, leaving an ulcer. Approximately 80% to 90% of the patients have oral lesions. In approximately two thirds of the patients the oral manifestations are first sign of the disease. All parts of the mouth may be involved. The bullae rupture almost immediately in the mouth but may stay intact for some time on the skin. One of the classic signs, the Nikolsky's sign (blister formation induced with gentle rubbing of an affected mucosal site) is positive in pemphigus but is not pathognomic because it also has been found positive in other disorders. Because the vesicle or bullae are intraepithelial, they are often filled with clear fluid. Histologically a cleavage (Tzank cells, acantholytic cells) exist within the spinous layer of the epithelium.

In pemphigoid the cleavage or split is beneath the epithelium, resulting in bullae that are usually blood filled. Mucous membrane pemphigoid is often limited to the oral cavity, but some patients have ocular lesions (symblepharon, ankyloblepharon) that need to be evaluated by an ophthalmologist. Gingiva is the most common oral site involved. Pemphigoid may appear clinically as a red, nonulcerated gingival lesion.

Rationale for treatment: Since both pemphigus and pemphigoid are autoimmune disorders, the primary treatment is topical or systemic steroids or other immunomodulating drugs. Custom trays may be utilized to localize topical steroid medications on the gingival tissues (occlusive therapy). Because they can resemble other ulcerative bullous diseases, a biopsy is necessary for a definitive diagnosis. Specimens should be submitted for light microscopic, immunofluorescent and immunologic testing. Because of the potential serious nature, referral to specialist in oral medicine, dermatology, and ophthalmology must be considered. When eye lesions are present an ophthalmologist must be consulted immediately to prevent blindness.

Therapy with medications such as systemic steroids, immunosuppressants, and immunomodulators are presented to inform the clinician that such modalities have been reported effective for patients suffering from vesiculo-bullous disorders such as pemphigus vulgaris and mucous membrane pemphigoid. Therapies such as dapsone,

methotrexate, mycophenolate mofetil, cyclosporine-A, niacinamide with tetracycline, and plasmaphoresis are used to treat patients with vesiculo-bullous disorders such as pemphigus vulgaris and mucous membrane pemphigoid but should not be routinely used because of the potential for side effects. Close collaboration with the patient's physician is recommended when these medications are prescribed.

INJECTABLE STEROIDS

Dexamethasone phosphate injectable, 1 ampule (4 mg/ml), may be used in the following manner. After anesthetizing the area with lidocaine, inject 0.5 to 1 ml around margins of ulcer with a 25-gauge needle twice a week until ulcer heals. Therapy with systemic or injectable steroids should be coordinated with the patient's physician due to side effects and potential systemic complications.

ORAL ERYTHEMA MULTIFORME

Etiology: Oral erythema multiforme is believed to be an autoimmune condition. It may occur at any age. Drug reactions to medications such as penicillin and sulfonamides may play a role in some cases. It has been observed in a few patients who develop oral erythema multiforme that a herpetic infection occurred immediately before the onset of clinical signs.

Clinical description: Signs of oral erythema multiforme include "blood crusted" lips, "targetoid" or "bull's eye" skin lesions, and a nonspecific mucosal slough. The name multiforme is used because its appearance may take multiple different forms.

A severe form of erythema multiforme is called Stevens'-Johnson syndrome, or Erythema multiforme Major. Erythema multiforme as a skin disease occurs most frequently because of an allergic reaction.

Rationale for treatment: Treatment is primarily antiinflammatory in nature. Steroids are initiated then tapered. Because of the possible relationship or oral erythema multiforme with herpes simplex virus, suppressive antiviral therapy may be necessary before initiation of steroid therapy. Patients should be questioned carefully about a previous history of recurrent herpetic infections and prodromal symptoms that might have preceded the onset of the erythema multiforme.

Dosing must be titrated to specific situations.
Steroid therapy:
Rx
Prednisone tablets 10 mg
Disp: 100 tablets
Sig: Take 6 tablets in the morning until lesions recede, then decrease by 1 tablet on each successive day.

Suppressive antiviral therapy:
Renew as needed to following:
Rx
Acyclovir (Zovirax), 400 mg capsules
Disp: 90 capsules
Sig: Take 1 tablet 3 times daily.
Rx
Valacyclovir (Valtrex), 500 mg capsules
Disp: 30 capsules
Sig: Take 1 tablet daily.

DENTURE SORE MOUTH

Etiology: Discomfort under oral prosthetic appliances may result from combinations of candidal infections, poor denture hygiene, an occlusive syndrome, overextension, or excessive movement of the appliance. This condition may be erroneously attributed to an allergy to dentrue material, which is a rare occurrence. The retention and fit of the denture should be idealized and mechanical irritation should be ruled out.

Clinical description: The tissue covered by the appliance, especially one made of acrylic, is erythematous and smooth or granular and it may be asymptomatic or associated with burning.

Rationale for treatment: Therapy is directed toward controlling all possible etiologies and improving oral comfort. If therapy is ineffective, consider underlying systemic conditions such as diabetes mellitus and poor nutrition.

Treatment:
1. Institute appropriate antifungal medication (see Candidiasis/Candidosis).
2. Improve oral and appliance hygiene. The patient may have to leave the appliance out for extended periods of time and should be instructed to leave the denture out overnight. The appliance should be soaked in a commercially available denture cleanser or soaked in a 1% sodium hypochlorite solution (1 teaspoon of sodium hypochlorite in a denture cup of water) for 15 minutes and thoroughly rinsed for at least 2 minutes under running water.
3. Reline, rebase, or construct a new appliance.
4. Apply an artificial saliva or oral lubricant gel, such as LaClede Oral Balance or Sage gel, to the tissue contact surface of the denture to reduce frictional trauma.

If all the above fail to control symptoms, a biopsy or short trial of topical steroid therapy may be used to rule out contact mucositis (an allergic reaction to denture materials). If a therapeutic trial fails to resolve the condition, a biopsy should be performed to establish the diagnosis.

BURNING MOUTH SYNDROME

Etiology: Multiple conditions have been implicated in the causation of Burning Mouth syndrome. Current literature favors neurogenic, vascular, and psychogenic etiologies. However, other conditions such as xerostomia, candidiasis, referred pain from the tongue musculature, chronic infections, reflux of gastric acid, medications, blood dyscrasias, nutritional deficiencies, hormonal imbalances, allergic and inflammatory disorders need to be considered.

Clinical description: Burning Mouth syndrome is characterized by the absence of clinical signs.

Rationale for treatment: To reduce discomfort by addressing possible etiologic factors.

Treatment: On the basis of history, physical evaluation, and specific laboratory studies, rule out all possible organic etiologies. Minimal blood studies should include CBC and differential fasting, glucose, iron, ferritin, folic acid, and B-12, and a thyroid profile (TSH, T3, T4).

Rx
Diphenhydramine (Children's Benadryl) elixir 12.5 mg/5 ml (OTC)
Disp: 1 bottle
Sig: Rinse with 1 teaspoon for 2 minutes before each meal and swallow.
Children's Benadryl is alcohol free.

When the burning mouth is considered psychogenic or idiopathic, a tricyclic or benzodiazepine in low doses exhibit the properties of analgesia and sedation, and are frequently successful in reducing or eliminating the symptoms after several weeks or months. The dosage is adjusted according to patient reaction and clinical symptomatology.

Rx
Clonazepam (Klonopin) tablets 0.5 mg
Disp: 100 tablets
Sig: Take 1 tablet tid, then adjust dose after 3-day intervals. This therapy is probably best managed by an appropriate specialist or the patient's physician at this time.

Rx
Amitriptyline (Elavil) tabs 25 mg
Disp: 50 tablets
Sig: Take 1 tablet at bedtime for 1 week, then 2 tablets hs. Increase to 3 tablets hs after 2 weeks and maintain at that dosage or titrate as appropriate.

Rx
Chlordiazepoxide (Librium) tablets 5 mg
Disp: 50 tablets
Sig: Take 1 or 2 tablets tid.

Rx
Alprazolam (Xanax) tablets 0.25 mg
Disp: 50 tablets
Sig: Take 1 tablet tid.

Rx
Diazepam (Valium) tablets 2 mg
Disp: 50 tablets
Sig: Take 1 or 2 tablets

The dosage should be adjusted according to the patient's response. Anticipated side effects are dry mouth and morning drowsiness. The rationale for the use of tricyclic antidepressant medications and other psychotropic drugs should be thoroughly explained to the patient, and the patient's physician should be made aware of the therapy. Those medications have a potential for addiction and dependence.

Rx
Tabasco sauce (Capsaicin) (OTC)
Disp: 1 bottle
Sig: Place 1 part tabasco sauce in 2-4 parts of water. Rinse for 1 minute qid and expectorate.

Rx
Capsaicin (Zostrix) cream 0.025% (OTC)
Disp: 1 tube
Sig: Apply sparingly to affected site(s) qid
Wash hands after each application and do not use near the eyes.
Topical capsaicin may serve to improve the burning sensation in some individuals. As with topical capsaicin, an increase in discomfort for a 2-3 week period should be anticipated.

CHAPPED OR CRACKED LIPS

Etiology: Alternate wetting and drying, resulting in inflammation and possible secondary infection.

Clinical description: The surface of the vermilion is rough, peeling, and may be ulcerated with crusting. The normal vertical fissuring may be lost.

Rationale for treatment: An interrupted and chronically inflamed surface invites secondary infection. An antiinflammatory agent in a petrolatum or adhesive base will interrupt the irritating factors and allow healing.

Rx
Betamethasone valerate (Valisone) ointment 0.1%
Disp: 15-g tube
Sig: Apply to lips after each meal and at bedtime.
Prolonged use of corticosteroids can result in thinning of the tissue. Their use should be closely monitored.
For maintenance, the frequent application of lip care products (e.g., Blistex, Chapstick, Vaseline, or cocoa butter) should be suggested.
If the lesions do not resolve with treatment, consider biopsy to rule out dysplasia or malignancy.

GINGIVAL ENLARGEMENT

Etiology: Phenytoin sodium (Dilantin), calcium channel blocking agents (nifedipine and others), and cyclosporine therapy are drugs known to predispose some patients to gingival enlargement. Blood dyscrasias and hereditary fibromatosis should be ruled out by history and indicated laboratory tests.

Clinical description: The gingival tissues, especially in the anterior region, are dense, resilient, insensitive, and enlarged but essentially of normal color.

Rationale for treatment: Local factors, such as plaque and calculus accumulation, contribute to secondary inflammation and the hyperplastic process. This further interferes with plaque control. Specific drugs tend to deplete serum folic acid levels, which results in compromised tissue integrity. Folic acid and drug serum levels should be determined every 6 months. This should be coordinated with the patient's physician.

Treatment: Treatment consists of (1) meticulous plaque control, (2) gingivoplasty when indicated, and (3) folic acid oral rinse.

Rx
Folic acid oral rinse 1 mg/ml
Disp: 16 oz
Sig: Rinse with 1 teaspoonful for 2 minutes bid and spit out.
Rx
Chlorhexidine gluconate (Peridex) 0.12%
Disp: 16 oz
Sig: Rinse with 1/2 oz bid for 30 seconds and spit out.

TASTE DISORDERS

Etiology: Taste acuity may be affected by neurologic and physiologic changes and drugs. Diagnostic procedures should first rule out a neurologic deficiency, an olfactory deficit, and systemic influences such as malnutrition, metabolic disturbances, drugs, chemical and physical trauma, and radiation sequelae. Blood tests for trace elements should be conducted to identify any deficiencies.

Rationale for treatment: A reduction in salivary flow may concentrate the electrolytes in the saliva, resulting in a salty or metallic taste. (See treatment for xerostomia.) A deficiency of zinc has been associated with a loss of taste (and smell) sensation.

FOR ZINC REPLACEMENT (in patients with proven zinc deficiency)

Rx
Orazinc capsules 220 mg (OTC)
Disp: 100 capsules
Sig: Take 1 capsule with milk 3 times a day for at least 1 month.
Rx
Z-Bec tablets (OTC)
Disp: 60 tablets
Sig: Take 1 tablet daily with food or after meals.

MANAGEMENT OF PATIENTS RECEIVING ANTINEOPLASTIC AGENTS AND RADIATION THERAPY

Etiology: Cancer chemotherapy and radiation to the head and neck tend to reduce the volume and alter the character of the saliva. The balance of the oral flora is disrupted, allowing overgrowth of opportunistic organisms (e.g., *Candida albicans*). Also, anticancer therapy damages fast-growing tissues, especially the oral mucosa.

Clinical description: The oral mucosa becomes red and inflamed. The saliva is viscous or absent.

Rationale for treatment: The treatment of these patients is symptomatic and supportive. Patient education, frequent monitoring, and close cooperation with the patient's physician are important. The oral discomfort may be relieved with topical anesthetics, such as diphenhydramine elixir (Benadryl), and dyclonine (Dyclone). Artificial salivas (i.e., Sage Moist Plus, Moi-Stir, Salivart, Xero-Lube) will reduce oral dryness. Mouth moisturizing gels (i.e., Sage Mouth Moisturizer or OralBalance gel) also may be helpful. Nystatin and clotrimazole preparations will control fungal overgrowth. Chlorhexidine rinses help control plaque and candidiasis. Fluorides are applied for caries control. A patient information sheet that follows this topic can be reproduced and given to the patient.

MOUTH RINSES

Rx
Alkaline saline (salt/bicarbonate) mouth rinse. (Mix 1/2 teaspoonful each of salt and baking soda in a glass of water.)
Sig: Rinse with copious amounts qid.
Commercially available as Sage Salt and Soda Rinse.

GINGIVITIS CONTROL

Rx
Chlorhexidine gluconate mouthwash (Peridex) 0.12%
Disp: 32 oz
Sig: Rinse with 1/2 oz bid for 30 seconds and spit out. Avoid rinsing or eating for 30 minutes following treatment. (Rinse after breakfast and at bedtime.)

In xerostomic patients, chlorhexidine (Peridex) should be used concurrently with an artificial saliva to provide the needed protein binding agent for efficacy and substantivity.

CARIES CONTROL

(See Xerostomia.)

Rx

Neutral NaF gel (Thera-Flur-N) 1.0%

Disp: 24 ml

Sig: Place 1 drop per tooth in the custom tray; apply for 5 minutes daily. Avoid rinsing or eating for 30 minutes after treatment.

TOPICAL ANESTHETICS

Rx

Diphenhydramine (Benadryl) elixir 12.5 mg/5 ml. (Note: elixir is Rx and syrup (Benylin) is OTC 4 oz, mixed with Kaopectate (OTC) 4 oz (to make a 50% mixture by volume).

Disp: 8 oz

Sig: Rinse with 1 teaspoonful every 2 hours and spit out.

Maalox (OTC) can be used in place of Kaopectate. Dyclonine (Dyclone) HCl 0.5% 1 oz may be added to the above for greater anesthetic efficacy.

Rx

Diphenhydramine (Benadryl) elixir 12.5 mg/5 ml. (Note: elixir is Rx and syrup [Benylin] is OTC.)

Disp: 4-oz bottle

Sig: Rinse with 1 teaspoonful for 2 minutes before each meal and spit out.

Rx

Dyclonine HCl (Dyclone) 0.5% or 1%

Disp: 1-oz bottle

Sig: Rinse with 1 teaspoonful for 2 minutes before each meal and spit out.

5. Antifungals

(See Candidiasis.)

Rx

Clotrimazole (Mycelex) troches 10 mg

Disp: 70 troches

Sig: Let 1 troche dissolve in the mouth 5 times a day.

Rx

Nystatin pastilles 200,000 u

Disp: 50 pastilles

Sig: Let 1 pastille dissolve in the mouth 5 times a day. (see Candidiasis for additional antifungal therapy.)

KEY POINTS TO REMEMBER

- When topical anesthetics are used, patients should be warned about a reduced gag reflex and the need for caution while eating and drinking to avoid possible airway compromise. Allergies are rare, but may occur.
- In immunocompromised patients, herpes simplex virus lesions can occur on any mucosal surface and may have atypical appearances. They can resemble major aphthae and allergic responses.
- Mixing ointments with equal parts of Orabase promotes adhesion.
- The therapy with systemic steroids and immunosuppressants is presented to inform the clinician that such modalities are available. Because of the potential for side effects, close collaboration with the patient's physician is recommended when these medications are prescribed.
- Although some consultants disagree with the use of vaginal creams intraorally, the efficacy of the creams has been observed clinically in selected cases where other topical antifungal agents have failed.
- Generic carboxymethyl cellulose solutions may be prepared by a pharmacist. These cholinergics should be prescribed in consultation with a physician because of significant side effects.
- The rationale for the use of tricyclic antidepressant medications and other psychotropic drugs should be thoroughly explained to patients, and their physician also should be made aware of the therapy. These medications have a potential for addiction and dependency.
- When testing for serum folate level, it is judicious to also check for the vitamin B_{12} level because a B_{12} deficiency can be masked by the patient's use of folic acid supplement. The phenytoin level also should be assessed for future reference.

PATIENT INFORMATION SHEET

The oral regimen for patients receiving chemotherapy and radiotherapy is outlined earlier in this chapter. The following are general guidelines to be individualized by your doctor. Follow your doctor's advice or discuss any questions with your doctor if these guidelines differ from what you've been told or have heard.

A. Rinses
　　1. Rinse with warm, dilute solution of sodium bicarbonate (baking soda) or salt and bicarbonate every 2 hours to bathe the tissues and control oral acidity. Take 2 teaspoonfuls of bicarbonate (or 1 teaspoonful of table salt plus 1 teaspoonful of bicarbonate) per quart of water.
　　2. If you are experiencing pain, rinse with 1 teaspoonful of elixir of Benadryl before each meal. Be careful when eating while your mouth is numb to avoid choking.
　　3. If your mouth is dry, sip cool water frequently (every 10 minutes) all day long. Allowing ice chips to melt in the mouth is comforting. Artificial salivas (e.g., Moi-Stir, Salivart, Xero-Lube, Orex) can be used as frequently as needed to make the mouth moist and "slick." Keep the lips lubricated with petrolatum or a lanolin-containing lip preparation. Commercial mouthrinses with alcohol or coffee, tea, and colas should be avoided as they tend to dry the mouth.
　　4. If an oral yeast infection develops, antifungal medications can be prescribed.
　　　　a. Nystatin pastille,* let one dissolve in mouth 5 times a day or
　　　　b. Let a 10-mg clotrimazole (Mycelex)* troche dissolve in the mouth 5 times a day.
B. Care of teeth and gums
　　1. Floss your teeth after each meal. Be careful not to cut the gums.
　　2. Brush your teeth after each meal. Use a soft even-bristle brush and a bland toothpaste containing fluoride (e.g., Aim, Crest, Colgate). Brushing with a sodium bicarbonate-water paste is also helpful. Arm & Hammer Dental Care toothpaste and tooth powder are bicarbonate based. If a toothbrush is too irritating, cotton-tip swabs (Q-Tips) or foam sticks (Toothettes) can provide some mechanical cleaning.
　　3. A pulsating water device (e.g., Water-Pik) will remove loose debris. Use warm water with a half teaspoonful of salt and baking soda and low pressure to prevent damage to tissue.
　　4. Have custom, flexible vinyl trays made by your dentist to self-apply fluoride gel to the teeth for 5 minutes once a day after brushing.
　　5. Rinse with an antiplaque solution (Peridex) (if prescribed by your dentist) 2 or 3 times a day when you cannot follow other oral hygiene procedures.
　　6. Follow any alternative oral hygiene instructions prescribed by your dentist.
C. Nutrition
　　Adequate nutrition and fluid intake are very important for oral and general health. Use diet supplements (e.g., Carnation Instant Breakfast, Meritene, Ensure). If your mouth is sore, a blender may be used to soften food.
D. Maintenance
　　Have your oral health status reevaluated at regularly scheduled intervals by your dentist.
E. Supportive
　　A humidifier in the sleeping area will alleviate or reduce nighttime oral dryness.

---

*Drugs that must be prescribed by your dentist or physician.
The above regimen is also applicable to patients with AIDS.

Suggested Readings

1. Boger J, Araujo O, Flowers F: Sunscreens: efficacy, use and misuse, *South Med J* 77:1421-1427, 1984.
2. Brooke RI, Sapp JP: Herpetiform ulceration, *Oral Surg Oral Med Oral Pathol* 42:182-188, 1976.
3. Brown RS, Bottomley WK: Combination immunosuppressant and topical steroid therapy for treatment of recurrent major aphthae, *Oral Surg Oral Med Oral Pathol* 69:42-44, 1990.
4. Browning S et al: The association between burning mouth syndrome and psychosocial disorders, *Oral Surg Oral Med Oral Pathol* 64:171-174, 1987.
5. Burns RA, Davis WJ: Recurrent aphthous stomatitis, *Am Fam Physician* 32:99-104, 1988.
6. Bystryn JC: Adjuvant therapy of pemphigus, *Arch Dermatol* 120:941-951, 1984.
7. Dilley D, Blozis G: Common oral lesions and oral manifestations of systemic illnesses and therapies, *Pediatr Clin North Am* 29:585-611, 1982.
8. Drew H et al: Effect of folate on phenytoin hyperplasia, *J Clin Periodontol* 14:350-356, 1987.
9. Duxbury AJ et al: Clinical trial of a mucin-containing artificial saliva, *IRCS Med Sci* 13:1197-1198, 1985.
10. Fardal O, Turnbull RS: A review of the literature on use of chlorhexidine in dentistry, *J Am Dent Assoc* 112:863-869, 1986.
11. Feinmann C: Pain relief by antidepressants: possible modes of action, *Pain* 23:1-8, 1985.
12. Fenske NA, Greenberg SS: Solar-induced skin changes, *Am Fam Physician* 25:109-117, 1982.
13. Fharav V et al: The analgesic effect of amitriptyline on chronic facial pain, *Pain* 31:199-207, 1987.
14. Fox PC et al: Systemic therapy of salivary gland hypofunction, *J Dent Res* 66:689-692, 1987 (special issue).
15. Gabriel SA et al: Lichen planus: possible mechanisms of pathogenesis, *J Oral Med* 40:56-59, 1985.
16. Gorsku M, Silverman S, Chinn H: Clinical characteristics and management outcome in the burning mouth syndrome, *Oral Surg Oral Med Oral Pathol* 72:192-195, 1991.
17. Gorsline J, Bradlow HL, Sherman MR: Triamcinolone acetonide 21-oic acid methyl ester: a potent local anti-inflammatory steroid without detectable systemic effects, *Endocrinology* 116:263-273, 1985.
18. Greenberg MS: Oral herpes simplex infections in immunosuppressed patients, *Compendium* 9(suppl):289-291, 1988.
19. Grushka M: Clinical features of burning mouth syndrome, *Oral Surg Oral Med Oral Pathol* 63:30-36, 1987.
20. Hay KD, Reade PC: The use of an elimination diet in the treatment of recurrent aphthous ulceration of the oral cavity, *Oral Surg Oral Med Oral Pathol* 57:504-507, 1984.
21. Holst E: Natamycin and nystatin for treatment of oral candidiasis during and after radiotherapy, *J Prosthet Dent* 51:226-231, 1984.
22. Huff JC et al: Therapy of herpes zoster with oral acyclovir, *Am J Med* 85:85-89, 1988.
23. Hughes WT et al: Ketoconazole and candidiasis: a controlled study, *J Infect Dis* 147:1060-1063, 1983.
24. Katz S: The use of fluoride and chlorhexidine for the prevention of radiation caries, *J Am Dent Assoc* 104:164-169, 1982.
25. Lamey PJ et al: Vitamin status of patients with burning mouth syndrome and the response to replacement therapy, *Br Dent J* 160:81-84, 1986.
26. Lang NP, Brecx MC: Chlorhexidine digluconate—an agent for chemical plaque control and prevention of gingival inflammation, *J Periodont Res* 43(suppl):74-89, 1986.
27. Lever WF, Schaumburg-Lever G: Treatment of pemphigus vulgaris: results obtained in 84 patients between 1961 and 1982, *Arch Dermatol* 120:44-47, 1984.
28. Lozada F, Silverman S Jr, Migliorati C: Adverse side effects associated with prednisone in the treatment of patients with oral inflammatory ulcerative diseases, *J Am Dent Assoc* 109:269-270, 1984.
29. Lucatorto FM et al: Treatment of refractory oral candidiasis with fluconazole: A case report, *Oral Surg Oral Med Oral Pathol* 71:42-44, 1991.
30. Lundeen RC, Langlais RP, Terezhalmy GT: Sunscreen protection for lip mucosa: a review and update, *J Am Dent Assoc* 111:617-621, 1985.
31. O'Neil T, Figures K: The effects of chlorhexidine and mechanical methods of plaque control on the recurrence of gingival hyperplasia in young patients taking phenytoin, *Br Dent J* 152:130-133, 1982.
32. Owens NJ et al: Prophylaxis of oral candidiasis with clotrimazole troches, *Arch Intern Med* 144:290-293, 1984.
33. Poland JM: The spectrum of HSV-1 infections in nonimmunosuppressed patients, *Compendium* 9(suppl):310-312, 1988.
34. Porter SR, Sculy C, Flint S: Hematologic status in recurrent aphthous stomatitis compared with other oral disease, *Oral Surg Oral Med Oral Pathol* 66:41-44, 1988.
35. Raborn GW et al: Oral acyclovir and herpes labialis: a randomized, double-blind, placebo-controlled study, *J Am Dent Assoc* 11:38-42, 1987.
36. Rhodus NL et al: Candia albicans levels in patients with Sjögren's syndrome before and after long-term use of pilocarpine hydrochloride, *Quintessence International* 29:705-710, 1998.
37. Rhodus, NL, Schuh, MJ: The effects of pilocarpine on salivary flow in patients with Sjögren's syndrome, *Oral Surg Oral Med Oral Path;* 72:545-549.36, 1991
38. Rowe NJ: Diagnosis and treatment of herpes simplex virus disease, *Compendium* 9(suppl):292-295, 1988.
39. Schiffman SS: Taste and smell in disease (pts a and b), *N Engl J Med* 308:1275-1279, 1337-1343, 1983.
40. Scully C, Mason DK: Therapeutic measures in oral medicine. In Jones JH, Mason DK, editors: *Oral manifestations of systemic disease*, London, 1980, WB Saunders.
41. Silverman S Jr et al: Oral mucous membrane pemphigoid, *Oral Surg Oral Med Oral Pathol* 61:233-237, 1986.
42. Silverman S et al: A prospective of findings and management in 214 patients with oral lichen planus, *Oral Surg Oral Med Oral Pathol* 72:665-670, 1991.
43. Sonis ST, Sonis AL, Lieberman A: Oral complications in patients receiving treatment for malignancies other than of the head and neck, *JAMA* 97:468-471, 1978.
44. Straus SE, moderator: Herpes simplex virus infection: biology, treatment, and prevention, *Ann Intern Med* 103:404-419, 1985.

45. Thompson PJ et al: Assessment of oral candidiasis in patients with respiratory disease and efficacy of a new nystatin formulation, *Br Med J* 292:699-700, 1986.
46. Vincent SD et al: Oral lichen planus: the clinical, historical and therapeutic features of 100 cases, *Oral Surg Oral Med Oral Pathol* 70:165-171, 1990.
47. Wood MJ et al: Efficacy of oral acyclovir treatment of acute herpes zoster, *Am J Med* 85:79-83, 1988.
48. Wright WE et al: An oral disease prevention program for patients receiving radiation and chemotherapy, *J Am Dent Assoc* 110:43-47, 1985.

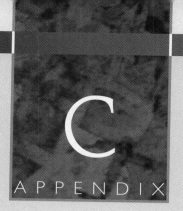

Drug Interactions of Significance to Dentistry

APPENDIX C

TABLE C-1

Dental Drug	Interacting Drug	Medical Condition/ Situation	Effect
Antibiotics			
Antibiotics	Oral contraceptives (BCP)	Contraception	Decreased effectiveness of oral contraceptives has been suggested for several antibiotic classes because of elimination of gut bacteria responsible for second round cleavage and activation of contraceptive. However, most well-designed studies do not show any reduction in estrogen serum levels in patients taking antibiotics (except rifampin). **RECOMMENDATION: Okay to use dental antibiotics.**
Beta Lactams (penicillins, cephalosporins)	Allopurinol (Lopurin, Zyloprim)	Gout	Incidence of minor allergic reactions to ampicillin is increased. Other penicillins have not been implicated. **RECOMMENDATION: Avoid ampicillin.**
	Beta-blockers (e.g., Tenormin, Lopressor, Inderal, Corgard)	Hypertension	Serum levels of altenolol are reduced after prolonged use of ampicillin. Anaphylactic reactions to penicillins or other drugs may be more severe in patients taking beta-blockers because of increased mediator release from mast cells. **RECOMMENDATION: Use ampicillin cautiously, advise patient of potential reaction.**
	Tetracyclines and other bacteriostatic antibiotics	Infection, acne or periodontal disease	Effectiveness of penicillins and cephalosporins may be reduced by bacteriostatic agents. **RECOMMENDATION: Avoid interaction.**

TABLE C-1

Dental Drug	Interacting Drug	Medical Condition/ Situation	Effect
Antibiotics—cont'd			
Tetracyclines	Antacids	Dyspepsia, gastroesophageal reflux, peptic ulcer	Antacids, dairy products, and other agents containing divalent and trivalent cations will chelate tetracyclines and limit their absorption in the gut. Doxycycline is least influenced by this interaction. **RECOMMENDATION: Avoid interaction.**
	Insulin	Diabetes mellitus	Doxycycline and oxytetracycline have been documented as enhancing the hypoglycemic effects of exogenously administered insulin. **RECOMMENDATION: Select different antibiotic, or increase carbohydrate intake.**
Metronidazole	Ethanol	Alcohol use or abuse	Severe disulfiram-like reactions are well documented. **RECOMMENDATION: Avoid interaction.**
	Lithium	Manic depression	Inhibits renal excretion of lithium leading to elevated/toxic levels of lithium. Lithium toxicity produces confusion, ataxia and kidney damage. **RECOMMENDATION: Avoid interaction.**
Antibiotics/Anti-fungals metabo-lized by CYP3A4 and CYP1A2 (e.g., erythromycin, clarithromycin, ketaconazole (Nizoral)—cont'd	Benzodiazepines	Anxiety	Delayed metabolism of benzodiazepine, increasing the pharmacologic effects can result in excessive sedation and irrational behavior. **RECOMMENDATION: Reduce dose of benzodiazepine.**
	Carbamazepine (Tegretol)	Seizure disorder	Increased blood levels of carbamazepine leading to toxicity, symptoms include drowsiness, dizziness, nausea, headache, and blurred vision. Hospitalization has been required. **RECOMMENDATION: Avoid interaction.**
	Cyclosporine	Organ transplant	Enhanced immunosuppression and nephrotoxicity. **RECOMMENDATION: Avoid interaction/monitor patient.**
	H_1 Histamine blocker astemizole (Hismanal)	Allergy	Block metabolism of parent molecule resulting in accumulation of antihistamine and ventricular arrhythmia (torsade de pointes) potentially life-threatening. **RECOMMENDATION: Avoid interaction.**
	Lovastatin, pravastatin, simastatin, and other statins	Hyperlipidemia	Muscle (eosinophilia) myalgia and rhabdomyolysis. **RECOMMENDATION: Avoid interaction.**

Continued

TABLE **C-1**

Dental Drug	Interacting Drug	Medical Condition/ Situation	Effect
Antibiotics—cont'd			
Antibiotics/Antifungals metabolized by CYP3A4 and CYP1A2 (e.g., erythromycin, clarithromycin, ketaconazole (Nizoral)—cont'd	Prednisone, methylprednisolone	Autoimmune disorders, organ transplant	Increased risk of Gushing's syndrome and immunosuppression. **RECOMMENDATION: Monitor patient, shorten duration of antibiotic administration if possible.**
	Theophylline (Theodur)	Asthma	Erythromycins inhibit the metabolism of theophylline leading to toxic serum levels toxicity (symptoms of toxicity: headache, nausea, vomiting, confusion, thirst, cardiac arrhythmias, and convulsions). Conversely, theophylline reduces serum levels of erythromycin. **RECOMMENDATION: Avoid prescribing erythromycin.**
Antibiotics (especially Erythromycin and Tetracycline)	Digoxin (Lanoxin)	Congestive heart failure	Alters GI flora and retards metabolism of digoxin in roughly 10% of patients, resulting in dangerously high digoxin serum levels that may persist for several weeks after discontinuation of antibiotic. Strongest documentation has been for erythromycin and tetracycline. Patients should be cautioned to report any signs of digitalis toxicity (salivation, visual disturbances and arrhythmias) during antibiotic therapy. **RECOMMENDATION: Safe in 90%, should have digoxin levels monitored during antimicrobial therapy.**
Antibiotics cephalosporins, erythromycin, clarithromycin metronidazole	Warfarin (Coumadin)	Atrial fibrillation, myocardial infarction, post-major surgery, stroke prevention	Anticoagulant effect of warfarin may be increased by several antibiotic classes. Reduced synthesis of vitamin K by gut flora is a putative mechanism, but several antibiotics have antiplatelet and anti-coagulant activity. Cephalosporins, macrolide antibiotics and metronidazole have the most convincing documentation. **RECOMMENDATION: Penicillins, tetracyclines and clindamycin would be preferred choices, but must be used cautiously.**
Analgesics Acetaminophen	Alcohol	Alcohol use and abuse	Increased risk of liver toxicity, especially during fasting state or $\geq$ 4 gram of acetaminophen per day. **RECOMMENDATION: Use lower dose, encourage discontinuation of alcohol use.**

TABLE **C-1**

Dental Drug	Interacting Drug	Medical Condition/ Situation	Effect
Analgesics—cont'd			
Aspirin	Oral hypoglycemics, e.g., (sulfo-nylureas: Glyburide, Chlorpropamide, Acetohexamide)	Diabetes type 2	Increased hypoglycemic effects. **RECOMMENDATION: Avoid interaction.**
Aspirin NSAIDs	Anticoagulants (coumarins)	Atrial fibrillation, myocardial infarction, post-surgery	Increased risk of gastrointestinal bleeding. **RECOMMENDATION: Avoid interaction.**
Aspirin NSAIDs	Alcohol	Alcohol use and abuse	Increases risk of gastrointestinal bleeding. **RECOMMENDATION: Lower dose, encourage discontinuation of alcohol use.**
NSAIDs	Beta-blocker ACE inhibitor	Hypertension, post-myocardial infarction	Decreased anti-hypertensive effect. **RECOMMENDATION: Limit duration of NSAID dosage to about 4 days.**
NSAIDs	Lithium	Manic depression	Produces symptoms of lithium toxicity including nausea, vomiting slurred speech and mental confusion. **RECOMMENDATION: NSAIDs should not be prescribed to patients with manic depression who take lithium. It can result in toxic levels of lithium.**
NSAIDs	Methotrexate (MTX)	Connective tissue disease, cancer therapy	Toxic level of methotrexate may accumulate. **RECOMMENDATION: Avoid interaction if on high dose MTX for cancer therapy. Low dose MTX for arthritis is not a concern.**
Anesthetics			
Lidocaine	Bupivacaine		Additive effect of these two local anesthetics increasing the risk **RECOMMENDATION: Limit dose of each.**
Mepivacaine	Meperidine (Demerol)		Sedation with opioids may increase risk of local anesthetic toxicity; especially in children. **RECOMMENDATION: Reduce anesthetic dose.**
Sedatives			
Barbiturates	Digoxin, theophylline, corticosteroids, oral anticoagulants	Congestive heart failure, asthma, autoimmune disease, atrial fibrillation	Barbiturates bind p450 cytochrome system in liver, enhance metabolism of many drugs. **RECOMMENDATION: Limit dose, observe for adverse effects.**

Continued

TABLE **C-1**

Dental Drug	Interacting Drug	Medical Condition/ Situation	Effect
Sedatives—cont'd			
Barbiturates— cont'd	Benzodiazepines, alcohol, antihistamines	Anxiety, alcohol use and abuse, seasonal allergies	Additive effects for sedation and respiratory depression. **RECOMMENDATION: Reduce dose, administer combination of sedatives with extreme caution.**
Benzodiazepines (BZDP) (e.g., alprazolam, chlordiazepoxide, diazepam)	Cimetidine, oral contraceptives, fluoxetine, isoniazid (INH), alcohol,	Peptic ulcer disease, depression, tuberculosis, alcohol use and abuse	Delayed metabolism of BZDP, increasing the pharmacologic effects can result in excessive sedation and irrational behavior. **RECOMMENDATION: Reduce dose of benzodiazepine.**
	Digoxin (Lanoxin), phenytoin, theophylline (Theodur)	Congestive heart failure, epilepsy, asthma	Serum concentrations of digoxin, phenytoin may be increased, resulting in toxicity. Antagonize sedative effects of .benzodiazepine **RECOMMENDATION: Avoid interaction.**
	Protease inhibitors (Indinavir, Nelfinavir)	HIV and AIDS	Increased bioavailability and effects of benzodiazepines especially triazolam and oral midazolam. **RECOMMENDATION: Avoid interaction.**
Vasoconstrictor Epinephrine and Levonordephrine (Neocobefrin)	Nonselective β blockers: Propranolol (Inderal), nadolol (Corgard), penbutolol (Levatol), pindolol (Visken), sotalol (Betapace), timolol (Blocadren)	Angina pectoris, hypertension, glaucoma, migraine, headache, hyperthyroidism, panic syndromes	Unopposed α effects—increased blood pressure with secondary bradycardia. **RECOMMENDATION: Initial dose is ½ carpule containing 1:100,000 epinephrine, aspirate to avoid intravascular injection, inject slowly. Monitor vital signs, if no adverse cardiovascular change, up to two cartridges containing a vasoconstrictor can be administered at 5-minute intervals with continual monitoring. Avoid epinephrine-containing retraction cord and higher concentrations of epinephrine in the dental anesthetic.**

TABLE C-1

Dental Drug	Interacting Drug	Medical Condition/ Situation	Effect
Vasoconstrictor—cont'd			
	Cocaine	Illicit use, topical anesthetic for mucous membrane procedures	Blocks reuptake of norepinephrine and intensifies postsynaptic response to epinephrine-like drugs. This potentiates the α adrenergic effects on the heart with the potential for a heart attack. **RECOMMENDATION: Recognize signs and symptoms of cocaine abuse; avoid use of vasoconstrictors in these patients until cocaine has been withheld for at least 24 hours.**
	Halothane	General anesthetic for surgical procedures	Stimulation of α_1 and β receptors resulting in arrhythmia at doses that exceed 2 µg/kg. **RECOMMENDATION: Limit dose to remain below 2 µg/kg threshold, aspirate to avoid intravascular injection. Monitor vital signs. Avoid epinephrine-containing retraction cord and concentrations of epinephrine higher than 1:100,000.**
	Tricyclic antidepressants (amitriptyline [Elavil], doxepin [Sinequan], imipramine [Tofranil])	Depression, severe anxiety, neuropathic pain, attention deficit disorder	Blocks reuptake of norepinephrine resulting in unopposed α effects—increased blood pressure, increased heart rate—potential cardiac arrhythmias; effect is greater with levonordefrin. **RECOMMENDATION: Avoid levonordefrin; limit dose to 2 carpules containing 1:100,000 epinephrine (36 µg), aspirate to avoid intravascular injection. Monitor vital signs. Avoid epinephrine-containing retraction cord and higher concentrations of epinephrine in the dental anesthetic.**

Continued

TABLE **C-1**

Dental Drug	Interacting Drug	Medical Condition/ Situation	Effect
Vasoconstrictor—cont'd			
Epinephrine and Levonordephrine (Neocobefrin)—cont'd	Peripheral adrenergic antagonists (reserpine [Serpasil], guanethidine [Ismelin], guanadrel [Hylorel])	Hypertension	Potential for increased sensitivity of adrenergic receptors to epinephrine and levonordefrin. **RECOMMENDATION: Administer cautiously. Monitor vital signs during and following administration of first carpule. Limit dose to 2 carpules containing 1:100,000 epinephrine (36 μg) or less depending on vital signs and patient response. Aspirate to avoid intravascular injection. Avoid epinephrine-containing retraction cord and higher concentrations of epinephrine in the dental anesthetic.**
	Catechol O-methyl-transferase inhibitors (tolcapone [Tasmar], entacapone [Comtan])	Parkinson's disease	Potential for increased sensitivity of adrenergic receptors to epinephrine and levonordefrin resulting in increased heart rate, blood pressure and arrhythmias. **RECOMMENDATION: Administer cautiously. Monitor vital signs during and after administration of first carpule. Limit dose to 2 carpules containing 1:100,000 epinephrine (36 μg) or less depending on vital signs and patient response. Aspirate to avoid intravascular injection. Avoid epinephrine-containing retraction cord and higher concentrations of epinephrine in the dental anesthetic.**

Index

Page numbers followed by *f* indicate figure; *t*, table; *b*, box.

Nucleoside analogs, 231*b*
Nutrition
  in alcoholic liver disease, 175*t*, 183
  in hyposalivation, 408-409
  supplements in herpes simplex virus and, 549-550
NVE. *See* Native valve endocarditis.
Nydrazid. *See* Isoniazid.
NYHA. *See* New York Heart Association.
Nystatin
  for angular cheilitis and cheilosis, 553
  for geographic tongue, 554
  for oral candidiasis, 552
    HIV/AIDS-associated, 242
    radiation and chemotherapy-associated, 406

O

OA. *See* Osteoarthritis.
Obesity in type 2 diabetes, 251
Occupation Safety and Health Administration
  infection control guidelines form, 541-547
  on tuberculosis exposure, 143-144
Occupational transmission of hepatitis, 166-167
Oclassen. *See* Podofilox.
Ofloxacin
  for gonorrhea, 206
  for tuberculosis, 140*b*, 143*t*
Older adult, DM72-75, 526-540
  bacterial endocarditis in, 22
  dental management of, 534-539, 535*t*, 536*f*, 537*f*, 538*f*
  etiology of, 526-527, 527*t*
  incidence and prevalence of, 526
  pathophysiology and complications in, 527-534, 528*t*
Omeprazole, 192*t*
Ophthalmopathy in Graves' disease, 290*f*, 290-291, 291*f*
Opioid abuse, 449*t*, 450
Opioid analgesics, 461*t*
Opportunistic infection
  chemotherapy and radiotherapy-related, 390, 405-407, 406*f*
  in HIV/AIDS, 231*t*, 231-233
  in leukemias, 383-384
Optimoist, 409
Oral Balance, 409
Oral cancer, 398*b*, 398-401, 399*f*, 400*f*, 401*t*
  alcoholic liver disease and, 184
  TNM staging of, 390*b*
Oral candidiasis
  associated with HIV/AIDS, 232, 236*f*, 237*f*, 240*t*, 241*t*, 241-242, 242*t*, 244*t*
  associated with renal disease, 150
  in bone marrow transplantation, 517*f*
  in diabetes mellitus, 268
  management of, 552-553
  in peptic ulcer disease, 194
  secondary to radiation and chemotherapy, 405-406, 406*f*
  Sjögren's syndrome and, 494
Oral care during cancer treatment, 403

Oral cavity
  effects of aging on, 531
  psychologic significance of, 465
Oral complications and manifestations
  in alcoholic liver disease, 183-184
  in allergy, 327*b*, 327*f*, 327-330, 328*f*, 329*b*
  in anemia, 381*f*, 381-382, 382*f*
  in asthma, 136
  in behavioral and psychiatric disorders, 475
  in bleeding disorders, 362
  in cardiac arrhythmias, 112, 112*t*
  in chronic obstructive pulmonary disease, 130
  in chronic renal failure, 157
  in congestive heart failure, 123
  in diabetes mellitus, 266-268, 267*f*, 268*f*
  in dialysis treatment, 159
  in epilepsy, 422-423, 423*f*
  in hepatitis, 174-175
  in HIV/AIDS, 236*f*, 236-245, 237*f*, 238*f*, 239*b*, 239*t*, 240*t*, 241*t*, 242*t*, 243*f*, 244*t*
  in hypertension, 76-77, 77*f*
  in hypothyroidism, 301
  in inflammatory bowel disease, 198-199, 199*f*
  in ischemic heart disease, 91-92
  in multiple sclerosis, 435
  in osteoarthritis, 488*f*, 488-489
  in Parkinson's disease, 433
  in peptic ulcer disease, 194*f*, 194-195
  during pregnancy and breast-feeding, 311*f*, 311-312
  in rheumatoid arthritis, 485-486, 486*f*
  in sexually transmitted diseases, 217-218, 218*f*
  in Sjögren's syndrome, 497, 497*f*
  in stroke, 428, 428*f*
  in systemic lupus erythematosus, 492, 492*f*
  in thyrotoxicosis, 300-301
  in transplantation, 523
  in tuberculosis, 142-143, 144*f*
  in white blood cell disorders, 382*f*, 382-385, 383*f*, 384*f*, 385*f*
Oral contraceptives, 564*t*, 568*t*
Oral erythema multiforme, 557
Oral glucose tolerance test, 257
Oral gonorrhea, 205*f*, 205-206
Oral hygiene
  aging and, 531
  in seizure disorders, 422, 423
  in white blood cell disorders, 380, 382-383, 383*f*
Oral hypoglycemic agents, 258, 259, 260, 260*t*, 328, 567*t*
Oral lesions, management of, 548-563
  burning mouth syndrome, 558
  candidiasis, 552-553
  chapped or cracked lips, 558-559
  cheilitis and cheilosis, 553
  denture sore mouth, 557-558
  geographic tongue, 553-554
  gingival enlargement, 559
  herpes simplex virus, 549-550
  herpes zoster, 550-551